LIA Handbook of Laser Materials Processing

Editor in Chief
John F. Ready

Associate Editor
Dave F. Farson

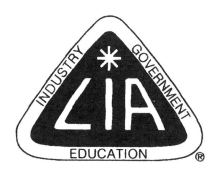 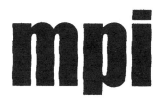

Laser Institute of America
Magnolia Publishing, Inc.

LIA HANDBOOK OF LASER MATERIALS PROCESSING

Editor in Chief : John F. Ready
Associate Editor: Dave F. Farson
Editor for Rapid Prototyping: Terry Feeley

Editorial Board:

Conrad M. Banas
Prem Batra
David A. Belforte
Sidney S. Charschan
Terry Feeley
Steven Llewellyn
Stan Ream
E. Swenson
Vivian Merchant

International Advisory Board:

H. W. Bergmann, Erlangen, Germany
Eckhard Beyer, Dresden, Germany
Milan Brandt, Lindfield, Australia
Friedrich Dausinger, Stuttgart, Germany
Volodymyr S. Kovalenko, Kiev, Ukraine
Claes Magnusson, Lulea, Sweden
William M. Steen, Liverpool, United Kingdom

Library of Congress Control Number (LCCN) 2001088071

LIA handbook of laser materials processing / editor in chief,
　John F. Ready ; associate editor, Dave F. Farson.
　– 1st ed.
　p. cm.
　Includes bibliographical references and index.
　ISBN: 0-912035-15-3 (Laser Inst.)
　ISBN: 0-941463-02-8 (Magnolia Pub.)

　1. Lasers–Industrial applications–Handbooks, manuals, etc.
　2. Manufacturing processes. I. Ready, John F., 1932- II
　Farson, Dave F. III. Laser Institute of America.

　TA1677.L53 2001　　　　　621.36'6
　　　　　　　　　　　　　　QBI01-200117

Copyright © 2001 by Laser Institute of America
All rights reserved.

This copyright applies to both *form and content*.

This Handbook in whole or in part may not be reproduced, copied, transmitted or be entered into an information storage or retrieval system without the written permission of the copyright owner. These restriction apply no matter the technology or means of reproducing, copying, etc., and include optical, mechanical, electronic, magnetic, acoustical technologies or combinations of these technologies, as well as manual entry.

Requests for permission should be mailed to Rights and Permission, Laser Institute of America,
13501 Ingenuity Drive, Suite 128, Orlando, FL 32826; lia@laserinstitute.org.

———

Printed in the United States of America

9 8 7 6 5 4 3 2

Table of Contents

Contributing Authors		XV
Acknowledgements		XXI
Foreword		XXIII
Preface		XXV

Chapter 1   Overview of Laser Materials Processing   1

- 1.0 Introduction   1
- 1.1 Laser Parameters – Paul Kelley   1
  - 1.1.1 Laser Beam Parameters   1
  - 1.1.2 Polarization   3
- 1.2 Absorption of Laser Energy – John F. Ready   4
  - 1.2.1 Reflection   4
  - 1.2.2 Absorption   5
  - 1.2.3 Focusing of Laser Light   5
  - 1.2.4 Laser Damage   7
- 1.3 Laser Configurations – John J. Zayhowski   9
  - 1.3.1 Modal Characteristics – John J. Zayhowski   9
  - 1.3.2 Temporal Behavior – John J. Zayhowski   11
  - 1.3.3 Survey of Active Media – John J. Zayhowski   13
  - 1.3.4 Commercial Lasers for Materials Processing – M. J. Weber   16
- 1.4 Laser Systems   17
  - 1.4.0 Introduction – David A. Belforte   17
  - 1.4.1 Subsystems – David A. Belforte   17
  - 1.4.2 Illustrations of Complete Materials Processing Systems – David A. Belforte   19
  - 1.4.3 Illustrations of Time- and Energy-Sharing Systems – Richard J. Coyle and Ronald M. Gagosz   23

Chapter 2   Lasers for Materials Processing   27

- 2.0 Introduction – John F. Ready
- 2.1 Carbon Dioxide Lasers   27
  - 2.1.1 Basic Principles – Jack Davis   27
  - 2.1.2 Laser Configurations – Jack Davis   28
  - 2.1.3 Optics – Jack Davis   32
  - 2.1.4 Power Sources, Accessories and Controls – Jack Davis   34
  - 2.1.5 Lifetime, Care and Maintenance – Jack Davis   34
  - 2.1.6 Laser Gases for CO_2 Laser Resonators – Joachim Berkmanns   35
- 2.2 Nd:YAG Lasers – Thomas R. Kugler   37
  - 2.2.1 Basic Principles   37
  - 2.2.2 Laser Configurations   38
  - 2.2.3 Pump Sources   41
  - 2.2.4 Power Control   42
  - 2.2.5 Lifetime, Care and Maintenance   42
  - 2.2.6 Output Beam Quality   42
- 2.3 Other Solid State Lasers – Stephen A. Payne   44
- 2.4 Excimer Lasers – James Higgins   47
  - 2.4.1 Basic Principles – James Higgins   47
  - 2.4.2 Wavelengths – James Higgins   48
  - 2.4.3 Resonator Configurations – James Higgins   48
  - 2.4.4 Optical Configurations – James Higgins   49
  - 2.4 5 Power Sources – James Higgins   49
  - 2.4.6 Lifetime, Care and Maintenance – James Higgins   49
  - 2.4.7 Gas for Excimer Lasers – Joachim Berkmanns   50
- 2.5 Other Lasers   52
  - 2.5.0 Introduction – John F. Ready   52
  - 2.5.1 CO Lasers – Tomoo Fujioka   52
  - 2.5.2 Metal Vapor Lasers – Richard Slagle   53
  - 2.5.3 Ion Lasers – Kurt G. Klavuhn   55
  - 2.5.4 Diode Lasers   60
    - Introduction to Diode Lasers – Bodo Ehlers   60
    - High-Power Diode Lasers for Materials Processing – Richard W. Solarz   64
  - 2.5.5 Iodine Lasers   66
    - The Chemical Oxygen Iodine Laser (COIL) – William P. Latham and Aravinda Kar   66
    - Photolytic Iodine Lasers – Philip R. Cunningham and L. A. (Vern) Schlie   67
  - 2.5.6 Nonlinear Optical Effects in Crystals – Ratan S. Adhav   69
  - 2.5.7 Free-Electron Lasers – John F. Ready   78
  - 2.5.8 X-Ray Lasers – Pierre Jaegle   78
  - 2.5.9 Ultrafast Lasers for Materials Processing – M. D. Perry, B. C. Stuart, P. S. Banks, M. D. Feit and J. A. Sefcik   82
- 2.6 Water Chiller Considerations for Laser-Cooling Applications – Terry L. Armbruster   83
  - 2.6.0 Introduction   83
  - 2.6.1 Capacity of Cooling System   83
  - 2.6.2 Power Requirements   83
  - 2.6.3 Chiller System Components   84
  - 2.6.4 Water Issues   89

Chapter 3   Optics and Optical Systems   91

- 3.0 Introduction   91
- 3.1 Properties of Laser Beams
  - 3.1.1 Monochromaticity – William P. Latham and Aravinda Kar   91
  - 3.1.2 Directionality – William P. Latham and Aravinda Kar   91
  - 3.1.3 Coherence – William P. Latham

		and Aravinda Kar	93
	3.1.4	Brightness – William P. Latham and Aravinda Kar	94
	3.1.5	Stable Resonator Modes – James T. Luxon	95
	3.1.6	Polarization – James T. Luxon	96
3.2	Beam Delivery Before Focusing		96
	3.2.0	Introduction	96
	3.2.1	Conventional Beam Delivery – Daniel A. Bakken	96
	3.2.2	Fiber Optic Beam Delivery: Diode Lasers – Chandrasekhar Roychoudhuri	98
	3.2.3	Fiber Optic Beam Delivery: Nd:YAG Lasers – Daniel A. Bakken	101
	3.2.4	Robotic Applications – Daniel A. Bakken	102
3.3	Focusing and Depth of Focus		104
	3.3.1	Focusing – John F. Ready	104
	3.3.2	Depth of Focus – William P. Latham and Aravinda Kar	105
3.4	Mode Quality – William P. Latham and Aravinda Kar		106

Chapter 4		Components for Laser Materials Processing Systems	109
4.0	Introduction		109
4.1	Components for Beam Delivery Systems – Marius Jurca		109
	4.1.1	General Remarks on Beam Delivery Systems and Design Criteria	109
	4.1.2	Components for Beam Delivery	110
	4.1.3	Adjustment/Alignment of Beam Delivery Systems	114
4.2	Focusing optics		116
	4.2.0	Introduction	116
	4.2.1	Lenses – Daniel L. Sherman	116
	4.2.2	Mirrors – Daniel L. Sherman	122
	4.2.3	Diffractive Optics – Daniel L. Sherman	125
	4.2.4	Focusing Head and Integrated Actuators – Marius Jurca	125
4.3	Other Optical Components – Walter J. Spawr		128
	4.3.1	Beam Shaping Optics	128
	4.3.2	Scanners	130
	4.3.3	Beam Splitters	132
	4.3.4	Polarizers	133
	4.3.5	Isolators	133
	4.3.6	IR and UV Transmitting Materials	134
4.4	Photodetectors		139
	4.4.1	Basics of Photodetectors – John F. Ready	139
	4.4.2	Commonly Used Detectors – Marius Jurca	144
4.5	Beam Monitoring and Measurement		144
	4.5.1	Beam Samplers – Francis Audet	144
	4.5.2	Energy Meters – Francis Audet	146
	4.5.3	Power Meters – Francis Audet	147
	4.5.4	Optimizing Meters – Francis Audet	148
	4.5.5	Positioning of Power Monitors – Marius Jurca	149
	4.5.6	Beam Profilers – John F. Ready, Karthnik Nagarathnam and Jyoti Mazumder	149
4.6	Components for Motion Systems – John F. Ready		151
	4.6.1	Basic Considerations	151
	4.6.2	Guiding Methods	151
	4.6.3	Drive Units	152
4.7	Controllers – David B. Veverka		153
	4.7.1	Laser and Motion Control	153
	4.7.2	Laser System Control	153
	4.7.3	Programming	154
	4.7.4	CAD/CAM and Off-Line Programming	154
4.8	Process Gas Nozzles		155
	4.8.0	Introduction	155
	4.8.1	Nozzle Configurations – Gary S. Settles	155
	4.8.2	Nozzle Selection – D. W. Moon	156
	4.8.3	Process Gas Nozzles for Cutting – Jim Fieret	157
4.9	Process Monitoring Systems		159
	4.9.1	Optical Penetration Sensing – W. W. Duley	159
	4.9.2	Optical Plasma Intensity Monitoring – W. W. Duley	160
	4.9.3	Acoustic Sensing – W. W. Duley	161
	4.9.4	Neural Networks – W. W. Duley	161
	4.9.5	Seam Tracking Basic Considerations – W. W. Duley Evaluation of Seam Tracking Methods – Marius Jurca	162 162
	4.9.6	Measurement of Keyhole Depth – Marius Jurca	165
	4.9.7	Infrared Monitoring – John F. Ready	166

Chapter 5		Laser–Material Interactions	167
5.0	Introduction		167
5.1	Materials Characteristics – Rolf E. Hummel		167
	5.1.1	Optical Properties	167
	5.1.2	Thermal Properties	171
5.2	Laser Characteristics		173
	5.2.1	Important Laser Properties – E. A. Metzbower	173
	5.2.2	Pulsed versus CW Characteristics – E. A. Metzbower	174
	5.2.3	Focusing Characteristics – E. A. Metzbower	174
	5.2.4	Irradiance – E. A. Metzbower	174
	5.2.5	Important Lasers for Materials Processing Applications – John F. Ready	174

Table of Contents

5.3 Reflectivity and Absorptivity of Opaque Surfaces
– Michael F. Modest ... 175
    5.3.1 Definitions ... 175
    5.3.2 Predictions from Electromagnetic Wave Theory ... 176
    5.3.3 Reflectivities of Metals ... 176
    5.3.4 Reflectivities in Nonconductors ... 178
    5.3.5 Polarization Effects ... 180
    5.3.6 Effects of Surface Conditions ... 180
    5.3.7 Summary ... 181
5.4 Absorption of Laser Radiation ... 182
    5.4.1 Absorption Coefficients – Michael F. Modest ... 182
    5.4.2 Semitransparent Sheets – Michael F. Modest ... 183
    5.4.3 Variation During Irradiation – John F. Ready ... 183
5.5 Energy Transport in Laser-Irradiated Materials
– P. S. Mohanty and Jyoti Mazumder ... 184
    5.5.0 Introduction ... 184
    5.5.1 Parameters ... 189
    5.5.2 Heat Balance ... 189
    5.5.3 Conduction ... 190
    5.5.4 Convection ... 194
    5.5.5 Vaporization ... 195
    5.5.6 Mass Diffusion ... 197
    5.5.7 Specific Examples ... 198
5.6 Phase Changes – Vladimir Semak ... 200
5.7 Plasma Shielding – J. Thomas Schriempf ... 202
    5.7.0 Introduction ... 202
    5.7.1 Atmospheric Breakdown ... 202
    5.7.2 Laser-Supported Absorption Waves ... 202
    5.7.3 Consequences of Plasma Shielding ... 203
5.8 Regimes of Irradiance and Interaction Time
– John F. Ready ... 204

Chapter 6 Hazards and Safety Considerations ... 205
6.0 Introduction ... 205
6.1 Health Hazards and Personnel Safety – Terry L. Lyon, Rodney L. Wood and David H. Sliney ... 205
    6.1.1 Specific Biological Effects ... 205
    6.1.2 Hazard Classification: Classes of Lasers ... 206
    6.1.3 Safety Measures ... 207
6.2 Safety with Industrial Lasers – Terry L. Lyon, Rodney L. Wood, and David H. Sliney ... 208
    6.2.1 Industrial Laser Systems ... 208
    6.2.2 Workplace Surveillance ... 208
6.3 Specific Systems and Applications ... 211
    6.3.1 Portable Laser Welders – An Example – Terry L. Lyon, Rodney L. Wood and David H. Sliney ... 211
    6.3.2 Beam Alignment Hazards – Marius Jurca ... 212
6.4 Nonbeam Hazards – LIA Nonbeam Hazard Subcommittee with Additions by C. Eugene Moss ... 214
    6.4.1 Types of Nonbeam Hazards ... 214
    6.4.2 Laser-Generated Chemical Hazards ... 214
    6.4.3 Physical Hazards ... 216
    6.4.4 Personnel Protective Equipment ... 217
    6.4.5 Biological/Medical Hazards ... 218
6.5 Laser Safety Standards – Robert Weiner ... 218
    6.5.1 Terms and Abbreviations ... 218
    6.5.2 United States Standards ... 219
    6.5.3 International Standards ... 219
    6.5.4 European and Other Nations' Standards and Directives ... 220
    6.5.5 Sources ... 220

Chapter 7 Surface Treatment: Heat Treatment ... 223
7.0 Introduction ... 223
7.1 Principles of Transformation Hardening – Charles E. Albright ... 223
7.2 Laser and Optics For Heat Treating ... 224
    7.2.1 Lasers – Wolfgang Bloehs ... 224
    7.2.2 Optics – Wolfgang Bloehs ... 227
    7.2.3 Optics For Uniform Beam Profiles – Charles E. Albright ... 231
7.3 Results of Laser Heat Treatment ... 232
    7.3.0 Introduction – Karthik Nagarathnam and Jyoti Mazumder ... 232
    7.3.1 Irradiance versus Interaction Time – Karthik Nagarathnam and Jyoti Mazumder ... 232
    7.3.2 Summary of Laser Heat Treatment Data – Karthik Nagarathnam and Jyoti Mazumder ... 233
    7.3.3 Effect of Process Variables – Karthik Nagarathnam and Jyoti Mazumder ... 233
    7.3.4 Residual Stresses in Laser Heat Treatment – Karthik Nagarathnam and Jyoti Mazumder ... 238
    7.3.5 Laser Heat Treatment Hardness Data – Karthik Nagarathnam and Jyoti Mazumder ... 239
    7.3.6 Surface Hardening with Diode Lasers – Bodo Ehlers ... 241
7.4 Materials and Testing – Klaus Müller and Hans Wilhelm Bergmann ... 243
    7.4.1 Alloy Effects ... 243
    7.4.2 Surface Condition ... 249
7.5 Surface Properties ... 249
    7.5.0 Introduction – Leonid F. Golovko ... 249
    7.5.1 Chemical Composition – Leonid F. Golovko ... 249
    7.5.2 Hardness and Its Distribution Along the Surface – Leonid F. Golovko ... 251
    7.5.3 Residual Stresses – Leonid F. Golovko ... 252

7.5.4	Residual Deformation – Leonid F. Golovko	255	
7.5.5	Mechanical Characteristics – Leonid F. Golovko	256	
7.5.6	Heat Resistance – Leonid F. Golovko	257	
7.5.7	Corrosion Resistance – Leonid F. Golovko	257	
7.5.8	Wear Resistance – Vivian E. Merchant	258	

7.6 Applications of Heat Treating 258
    7.6.1 Steering Gear Assemblies – David A. Belforte 258
    7.6.2 Diesel Engine Cylinder Liners – David A. Belforte 259
    7.6.3 Turbine Blade Hardening – John F. Ready 260
7.7 Comparison with Other Technologies – Vivian E. Merchant 260
    7.7.1 Advantages/Disadvantages 260
    7.7.2 Economic Considerations 261

Chapter 8 Surface Treatment: Glazing, Remelting, Alloying, Cladding, and Cleaning 263

8.0 Introduction – John F. Ready 263
8.1 Rapid Melting 263
    8.1.1 Melting Kinetics – John F. Ready 263
    8.1.2 Absorption Mechanism – Menachem Bamberger 264
    8.1.3 Effects of Convection – Menachem Bamberger 264
    8.1.4 Temperature Distribution in the Melt – Menachem Bamberger 266
8.2 Rapid Solidification and Microstructure – Menachem Bamberger 268
    8.2.1 Solidification 268
    8.2.2 Temperature Distribution During Cooling 269
    8.2.3 Dendrite Spacing 269
8.3 Appropriate Lasers and Optics – Walter J. Spawr 271
    8.3.1 Nd:YAG Lasers 271
    8.3.2 CO_2 Lasers 271
8.4 Laser Glazing 271
    8.4.1 The Glazing Process – Vivian E. Merchant 271
    8.4.2 Rapid Cooling – John F. Ready 272
8.5 Surface Remelting 273
    8.5.1 Surface Remelting of Bearings – Dennis W. Hetzner 273
    8.5.2 Melting Cast-Iron Surfaces – Menachem Bamberger 276
8.6 Surface Alloying 279
    8.6.1 Basics of Laser Alloying – John F. Ready 279
    8.6.2 Materials Deposition Techniques – Volodymyr S. Kovalenko 279
    8.6.3 Mixing Characteristics – Volodymyr S. Kovalenko 281
    8.6.4 Enhanced Surface Properties – Volodymyr S. Kovalenko 283

8.7 Surface Cladding – Thomas Aaboe Jensen 284
    8.7.0 Introduction 284
    8.7.1 Cladding Techniques 284
    8.7.2 Feeding Principles 285
    8.7.3 Process Characteristics 285
    8.7.4 Cladding Characteristics 286
    8.7.5 Cladding Materials 286
    8.7.6 Process Benefits 286
    8.7.7 Process Drawbacks 287
    8.7.8 Applications 287
    8.7.9 Special Applications 287
8.8 Cleaning 287
    8.8.0 Introduction – Martin C. Edelson 287
    8.8.1 Surface Cleanings – Martin C. Edelson 287
    8.8.2 Contaminant Removal – Mary Helen McCay 289
    8.8.3 Removal of Paint, Dielectric and Other Coatings – Alan E. Hill 293
8.9 Disk Texturing – Ronald D. Schaeffer 297

Chapter 9 Brazing/Soldering 299

9.1 Process Definition – E. Schubert, I. Zerner and G. Sepold 299
9.2 Appropriate Lasers – E. Schubert, I. Zerner and G. Sepold 299
9.3 Beam Manipulation Techniques – E. Schubert, I. Zerner and G. Sepold 300
9.4 Applications and Results – E. Schubert, I. Zerner and G. Sepold 301
    9.4.1 Brazing of Steel – E. Schubert, I. Zerner and G. Sepold 301
    9.4.2 Brazing of Titanium – E. Schubert, I. Zerner and G. Sepold 302
    9.4.3 Joining Of Dissimilar Materials – E. Schubert, I. Zerner and G. Sepold 302
    9.4.4 Soldering Applications with Diode Lasers – Bodo Ehlers 303

Chapter 10 Conduction Welding 307

10.0 Introduction – John F. Ready 307
10.1 Basic Description of Laser Welding 307
    10.1.1 Use of Laser Welding – George Chryssolouris and Stefanos Karagiannis 307
    10.1.2 Metal Reflectivity – Thomas R. Kugler 308
    10.1.3 Thermal Properties of Metals – Thomas R. Kugler 309
    10.1.4 Fusion Front Penetration – Thomas R. Kugler 310
    10.1.5 Thermal Conduction Limitations – Thomas R. Kugler 313
10.2 Welding Procedures 314
    10.2.1 Laser Characteristics – Thomas R. Kugler 314
    10.2.2 Optics – Thomas R. Kugler 316
    10.2.3 Focus Position – Thomas R. Kugler 317
    10.2.4 Surface Conditions – Thomas R. Kugler 318

Table of Contents

	10.2.5	Joint Design: Configurations and Tolerances – Dave F. Farson	318
	10.2.6	Joint Design: Choice – Thomas R. Kugler	320
	10.2.7	Elements of Quality – Thomas R. Kugler	320
	10.2.8	Processing Gases – Joachim Berkmanns	322
	10.2.9	Guidelines – Dave F. Farson	325
10.3	Laser Welding Results		325
	10.3.1	Nd:YAG Laser Welding – George Chryssolouris and Stefanos Karagiannis	325
	10.3.2	Nd:YAG Laser Welding Guidelines – David Havrilla	334
	10.3.3	Nd:YAG Laser CW Seam Welding of Common Materials – Dale U. Chang	338
	10.3.4	Nd:YAG Pulsed-Seam Welding – Thomas R. Kugler	339
	10.3.5	Spot Welding with Pulsed Nd:YAG Lasers – Hansjoerg Rohde	342
	10.3.6	Microjoining with Nd:YAG Lasers – Joseph J. Kwiatkowski	344
	10.3.7	Conduction Welding with CO_2 Lasers – John F. Ready	347
	10.3.8	Welding with Low Power CO_2 Lasers – John F. Ready	348
	10.3.9	Welding with Diode Lasers – Bodo Ehlers	348
	10.3.10	Welding with Photolytic Iodine Lasers (PILS) – Philip R. Cunningham and L. A. (Vern) Schlie	351
10.4	Materials Issues		352
	10.4.1	Tabulation of Materials and Weldability – R. F. Duhamel	352
	10.4.2	Welding of Dissimilar Materials – Kevin J. Ely	354
10.5	Comparison of Laser Welding with Other Technologies		357
	10.5.1	Advantages/Limitations – Vivian E. Merchant	357
	10.5.2	Economic Considerations – Vivian E. Merchant	358
	10.5.3	Comparison of Welding Results – George Chryssolouris and Stefanos Karagiannis	359

Chapter 11 Penetration Welding 361

11.0	Introduction – John F. Ready	361
11.1	Description of Penetration Welding	361
	11.1.1 The Deep Penetration Process – Dan Gnanamuthu	361
	11.1.2 Motion of the Keyhole – John F. Ready	363
	11.1.3 Penetration – John F. Ready	363
	11.1.4 Lasers for Penetration Welding – John F. Ready	364
	11.1.5 Melting Efficiency – John F. Ready	364
11.2	Welding Procedures - Conrad M. Banas	365
	11.2.1 Laser Choice	365
	11.2.2 Optics	366
	11.2.3 Focus Position	367
	11.2.4 Surface Conditions	368
	11.2.5 Joint Design	368
	11.2.6 Edge Preparation	369
	11.2.7 Fixturing	369
	11.2.8 Shielding and Plasma Control	370
	11.2.9 Preheating	372
	11.2.10 Spatter Control	372
	11.2.11 Process Monitoring Systems	373
	11.2.12 Post Treatment	373
	11.2.13 Filler Material Considerations	374
11.3	Welding Data Summary	375
	11.3.1 High-Power Laser Welding of Common Materials – Keng H. Leong and Paul G. Sanders	375
	11.3.2 CO_2 Laser CW Seam Welding of Common Materials; Conditions for Penetration Welding – Robert J. Steele	379
	11.3.3 CW CO_2 Laser Welding of Common Materials – E. A. Metzbower	381
	11.3.4 Pulsed CO_2 Laser Welding of Common Metals – Chris Rickert	383
	11.3.5 Nd:YAG CW Welding of Common Materials – C. L. M. Ireland	383
	11.3.6 Nd:YAG Laser-Pulsed Welding of Common Materials – David C. Weckman and Hugh W. Kerr	387
	11.3.7 Comparison of Penetration Welding with Nd:YAG and CO_2 Lasers – David Havrilla	399
	11.3.8 Laser Welding with Filler Wire – Andreas Gebhardt	400
	11.3.9 Welding with Other Lasers – Sunichi Sato	404
	11.3.10 Operating Costs for Penetration Welding – David Havrilla	407
11.4	Industrial Applications of High-Power Laser Welding	409
	11.4.1 Introduction – Geoff J. Shannon	409
	11.4.2 Key Aspects – Geoff J. Shannon	409
	11.4.3 Welding Thin Sheet Material (< 0.5 mm) – Geoff J. Shannon	411
	11.4.4 Sheet Material (1–3 mm) – Geoff J. Shannon	411
	11.4.5 Welding Plate Material (4–12 mm) – Geoff J. Shannon	412
	11.4.6 Weld Tolerances – Geoff J. Shannon	412
	11.4.7 Hybrid Welding – Geoff J. Shannon	413
	11.4.8 Weld Testing – Geoff J. Shannon	413
	11.4.9 Plastic Welding – Geoff J. Shannon	413
	11.4.10 Material Welding Summary – Geoff J. Shannon	414

11.4.11	Laser-Welded Tailored Blanks – Dave F. Farson	414
11.4.12	Automotive Applications – Andreas Gebhardt	417

11.5 Comparison of Laser Welding to Other Welding Technologies   418

11.5.1	Alternate Welding Technologies – Geoff J. Shannon	418
11.5.2	Key Aspects of Comparison – Geoff J. Shannon	421
11.5.3	Laser Welding Comparisons – Dan Gnanamuthu	423
11.5.4	Comparison of Welding Technology Results – David Havrilla	423

Chapter 12 Laser Cutting   425

12.1 Basic Description of Laser Cutting   425

12.1.1	Cutting Processes – Dirk Petring	425
12.1.2	Power Balance – Dirk Petring	428
12.1.3	Appropriate Lasers – Dirk Petring	431
12.1.4	Gas Assist Techniques – Dirk Petring	431
12.1.5	Cutting of Complex Shapes – Dirk Petring	432
12.1.6	Post-Cutting Operations – Dirk Petring	433
12.1.7	Polarization Effects in Laser Cutting: Basics – Flemming O. Olsen	433
12.1.8	Control of Beam Polarization Effects in Cutting – John Powell	436

12.2 Laser Cutting of Metals   437

12.2.1	The Metal Cutting Process – Leonard Migliore	437
12.2.2	Characteristics of Laser-Cut Edges – Leonard Migliore	438
12.2.3	Laser Cutting of Specific Metals – Leonard Migliore	439
12.2.4	CO_2 Laser Cutting of Metals – John Powell	439
12.2.5	Nd:YAG Laser Cutting – John Powell Thickness Versus Cutting Speed – David Havrilla	446
12.2.6	Microcutting of Metals with Pulsed Nd:YAG Lasers – Hansjoerg Rohde	448
12.2.7	Cutting of Metals with Other Lasers Cutting with a CO Laser – Tomoo Fujioka	450 450
	Cutting with a Chemical Oxygen-Iodine Laser – William P. Latham and Aravinda Kar	453
	Cutting with Photolytic Iodine Lasers – Philip R. Cunningham and L. A. (Vern) Schlie	453

12.3 Laser Cutting of Nonmetals   456

12.3.1	Cutting Mechanisms and Cut Quality – John Powell	456
12.3.2	CO_2 Laser Cutting – Volodymyr S. Kovalenko	456
12.3.3	Cutting of Nonmetals with Nd:YAG Lasers – John Powell	459
	Nd:YAG Laser Cutting Data – Volodymyr S. Kovalenko	460
12.3.4	Cutting Jewelry Materials – David M. Marusa	462

12.4 Costs of Laser Cutting   463

12.4.1	Conventional CO_2 Laser Cutting System – David Havrilla	463
12.4.2	Conventional Nd:YAG Laser Cutting System – David Havrilla	463

12.5 Comparison of Laser Cutting with Other Technologies   464

12.5.1	Advantages and Drawbacks of Laser Cutting – David Havrilla	464
12.5.2	Comparison of CO_2 Laser Cutting with Other Profiling Techniques – John Powell	464
12.5.3	Advantages and Limitation of Laser Cutting of Nonmetals – Volodymyr S. Kovalenko	470

Chapter 13 Hole Drilling   471

13.1 Basic Description of Laser Drilling   471

13.1.1	Surface Reflectivity – Xiangli Chen	471
13.1.2	Thermal Properties – Xiangli Chen	472
13.1.3	Physical Processes: Melting, Vaporization, Flushing, Percussion – Xiangli Chen	473
13.1.4	Appropriate Lasers: Power/Irradiance, Pulse Duration – Xiangli Chen	473
13.1.5	Percussion Drilling and Trepanning – Dana Elza and Steven R. Maynard	474

13.2 Drilling of Metals   474

13.2.0	Introduction	474
13.2.1	Nd:YAG Laser Drilling – Hansjoerg Rohde	475
13.2.2	CO_2 Lasers for Metal Drilling – Marshall G. Jones	479
13.2.3	CO_2 Laser Drilling – Hansoerg Rohde	479
13.2.4	Drilling with Copper Vapor Lasers – Roland Mayerhofer and Hans Wilhelm Bergmann	479
13.2.5	Applications of Copper Vapor Laser Drilling – Richard Slagle	483

13.3 Drilling of Nonmetals   484

13.3.1	General Considerations – Dana Elza and Steven R. Maynard	484
13.3.2	Nd:YAG Laser Drilling – Suwas Nikumb	484
13.3.3	CO_2 Laser Drilling – Dana Elza and Steven R. Maynard	490
13.3.4	Excimer Laser Drilling – Heinrich Endert and Dirk Basting	491
13.3.5	Copper Vapor Laser Drilling – Roland Mayerhofer and Hans Wilhelm Bergmann	494

Table of Contents

13.4 Aerospace Applications – Robert T. Brown 496
    13.4.1 Hole Requirements 496
    13.4.2 Laser Type 496
    13.4.3 Typical Focus-Head Arrangement 497
    13.4.4 Percussion Drilling 497
    13.4.5 Trepan Drilling 498
13.5 Ultrashort-Pulse Laser Machining – M. D. Perry, B. C. Stuart, P. S. Banks, M. D. Feit, and J. A. Sefcik 499
    13.5.0 Introduction 499
    13.5.1 Dielectrics 499
    13.5.2 Metals 503
13.6 Comparison With Other Technologies – Todd J. Rockstroh 508
    13.6.1 Consideration of Quantity of Holes Drilled 508
    13.6.2 Large Diameter Holes > 0.025 mm (0.001 in.) 509
    13.6.3 Small Diameter Holes < 0.025 mm (0.001 in.) 510
    13.6.4 Laser Costs and Other Factors 511
    13.6.5 Summary 512

Chapter 14 Balancing 513
14.1 Basics of Balancing – Hatto Schneider 513
    14.1.0 Introduction 513
    14.1.1 Conditions for Balancing 513
    14.1.2 Balancing Procedures 514
    14.1.3 Balancing Process 514
    14.1.4 Example: A Typical Balancing Task 515
14.2 Laser Balancing Procedures – Michael Martin 515
    14.2.0 Introduction 515
    14.2.1 Advantages/Limitations of Laser Balancing 516
    14.2.2 Balancing Systems 516
14.3 Some Applications of Laser Balancing – Hatto Schneider 518
    14.3.1 Timing Wheel Balancing 518
    14.3.2 Clutch Disk Balancing 519
    14.3.3 Frequency Spindle Balancing 519
    14.3.4 Other Applications 520

Chapter 15 Marking 521
15.1 Basic Principles – Terry McKee 521
15.2 Materials – Terry McKee 522
15.3 Appropriate Lasers 525
    15.3.1 CO_2 Lasers – Robert K. Brimacombe 525
    15.3.2 NdYAG Lasers – Martin Matthews 527
    15.3.3 Excimer Lasers for Marking – Heinrich Endert and Dirk Basting 528
15.4 Dot Matrix Marking – Andrew John Chambers 529
    15.4.1 Techniques 529
    15.4.2 Results 530
15.5 Engraving – Peter Becher, Phil DeBoer and Arlene Zdrazil 530
    15.5.1 Techniques 530
    15.5.2 Lasers 531
    15.5.3 Surface Effects 532
    15.5.4 Beam Motion Systems 532
    15.5.5 Masking 532
    15.5.6 Engraving Recommendations 533
15.6 Image Micromachining – Brian Norris 534
    15.6.1 Techniques 534
    15.6.2 Results 534
15.7 Applications – Terry McKee 535
    15.7.1 CO_2 Lasers – Terry McKee 535
    15.7.2 Nd:YAG Lasers – Terry McKee 535
    15.7.3 Excimer Lasers – Heinrich Endert and Dirk Basting 536
15.8 Comparison with Other Techniques – Terry McKee 537

Chapter 16 Rapid Prototyping 541
16.0 Introduction and Glossary – Terry Feeley and Paul F. Jacobs 541
16.1 Basics of Laser-Based Rapid Prototyping – Allan Lightman 542
    16.1.1 Rapid Prototyping: An Overview 542
    16.1.2 Lasers Parameters for RP 542
    16.1.3 Scanning Exposure Factors 543
    16.1.4 Small Spot Systems 544
16.2 Stereolithography 545
    16.2.1 The Stereolithography Process – Paul F. Jacobs 545
    16.2.2 Materials for Stereolithography – Stephen D. Hanna 548
    16.2.3 Lasers for Stereolithography – Kenneth G. Ibbs 550
    16.2.4 Stereolithography in Product Development – Thomas J. Mueller 552
16.3 Selective Laser Sintering 554
    16.3.1 The Selective Laser Sintering Process – Brent Stucker 554
    16.3.2 Materials for SLS – Sundar V. Atre and Randall M. German 556
    16.3.3 Lasers for Selective Laser Sintering – Damien F. Gray 557
    16.3.4 Directed Light Fabrication – Gary K. Lewis 559
    16.3.5 The Laser Engineered Net Shaping Process – David M. Keicher 561
    16.3.6 Results – Kevin P. McAlea 563
16.4 Laminated Object Manufacturing 564
    16.4.1 The LOM Process – Sung S. Pak 564
    16.4.2 Applications – Sung S. Pak 565
    16.4.3 Laser Cutting-Based Rapid Prototyping Options for Metal and Ceramic Components – Curtis W. Griffin and Alair Griffin 566
16.5 CAM-LEM Processing of Ceramic and Metal Parts – James D. Cawley 567
    16.5.0 Introduction 567

	16.5.1	Material Properties	568
	16.5.2	Machine Variables	570

16.6 Coating of Rapid Tools by Pulsed Laser Deposition
– Larry R. Dosser 572

16.7 Adaptation of RP Technology to the Manufacture
of Die Casting Tools – Peter J. Hardro 573

16.8 Table: Comparison of Rapid Prototyping Systems
– Peter J. Hardro 577

Chapter 17 Trimming 583

17.0 Introduction 583
17.1 Basics of Laser Trimming – Rodger Dwight 583
    17.1.1 Physical Processes – Rodger Dwight 583
    17.1.2 Overview of a Laser Trimming System
        – Rodger Dwight 585
    17.1.3 Types of Laser Trims – Rodger Dwight 585
    17.1.4 Appropriate Lasers – Rodger Dwight 585
17.2 Trimming Techniques – Philip DeLuca 586
    17.2.1 Thick-Film Trimming – Philip DeLuca 586
    17.2.2 Thin Film on Ceramic Laser Trimming
        – Philip DeLuca 587
    17.2.3 Chip Resistor Laser Trimming
        – Philip DeLuca 587
    17.2.4 Thin Film on Silicon Resistor Trimming
        – Philip DeLuca 587
    17.2.5 Interference Effects – Yunlong Sun 587

Chapter 18 Laser Marking/Branding 589

18.0 Introduction 589
18.1 Package Marking and Branding – Donald V. Smart
and Jose Downes 589
    18.1.1 Laser Marking in Production 589
    18.1.2 The Marking Process 589
    18.1.3 Mark Quality Criteria 590
18.2 Wafer Serialization – Jim Scaroni, Jerry Becker
and Terry McKee 590
    18.2.1 Techniques 590
    18.2.2 Results 591
18.3 Marking of Electronic Components
– Terry McKee 592

Chapter 19 Link Cutting/Making 595

19.1 Basics of Link Processing with Lasers 595
    19.1.0 Introduction – Donald V. Smart 595
    19.1.1 Basics of Link Cutting – John F. Ready 595
    19.1.2 Memory Repair Goals – Donald V. Smart 595
    19.1.3 Processing Concerns – Donald V. Smart 596
    19.1.4 Lasers for Link Cuttig – Donald V. Smart 597
    19.1.5 Positioning Systems – Donald V. Smart 598
    19.1.6 Optics – Donald V. Smart 598
    19.1.7 Pulse Control – Donald V. Smart 599
    19.1.8 Energy Coupling – Donald V. Smart 599
    19.1.9 Link Materials – Donald V. Smart 600
    19.1.10 Link Design – Donald V. Smart 600
    19.1.11 Link Groups – Donald V. Smart 601
    19.1.12 Accuracy – Donald V. Smart 602
    19.1.13 Alignment Strategy – Donald V. Smart 604
19.2 Redundancy for Memory Yield Enhancement 604
    19.2.0 Introduction 604
    19.2.1 Development of Redundancy
        – Edward J. Swenson 604
    19.2.2 Laser Choice – Edward J. Swenson 605
    19.2.3 Hardware Description
        – Edward J. Swenson 606
    19.2.4 Absorptivity Considerations
        – Edward J. Swenson 606
    19.2.5 Spot Size Consideration
        – James A. Dumestre 607
19.3 Link Making – Joseph B. Bernstein
and Wei Zhang 608
    19.3.0 Introduction 608
    19.3.1 Earlier Work 609
    19.3.2 Principles 609
    19.3.3 Reliability 611
    19.3.4 Implementation 612
    19.3.5 Laser Energy 613
    19.3.6 Summary 613
19.4 Personalization – Meir Janai 614
    19.4.1 Definitions and Basic Terms 614
    19.4.2 Personalization by Link Cutting
        – Choice of Laser 614
    19.4.3 The Personalization Process 614

Chapter 20 Repair 617

20.1 Repair Needs – Thomas A. Wassick 617
20.2 Substrate Repair – Thomas A. Wassick 617
    20.2.1 Repair of Shorts 617
    20.2.2 Repair of Opens 618
20.3 Laser-Based Photomask Repair – John F. Ready 621

Chapter 21 Applications in Photolithography 623

21.1 Overview – J. J. Dubowski 623
21.2 Laser Sources for Microlithography Exposure Tools
– Toshihiko Ishihara 623
    21.2.1 Excimer Lasers – Toshihiko Ishihara 625
    21.2.2 Diode Pumped Harmonic Nd:YAG Lasers
        – Roy D. Mead 626
21.3 Advantages of Laser Microlithography Compared to
Other Sources – John J. Shamaly 628
21.4 Laser-Based Photolithography System Issues
– John J. Shamaly 629

Table of Contents

21.5 Deep Ultraviolet Laser Photolithography
 – Timothy A. Brunner 629
   21.5.1 Overview 629
   21.5.2 High Resolution Lithography 630
   21.5.3 Deep Ultraviolet Lithography Issues 632

Chapter 22 Flat Panel Display 635
22.0 Introduction 635
22.1 Repair – Floyd R. Pothoven 635
   22.1.1 Short Removal 635
   22.1.2 Open Repair 636
22.2 Marking – Floyd R. Pothoven 638
22.3 Laser Patterning Indium Tin Oxide Coated Flat Panel Displays – Rodney Waters and Terry Pothoven 637
   22.3.1 Nature of Indium Tin Oxide 637
   22.3.2 Maskless Pattern Generation 637
   22.3.3 Laser Choices 637
   22.3.4 Laser Cutting 638
22.4 Annealing of Thin-Film Transistors – Heinrich Endert and Dirk Basting 638

Chapter 23 High-Temperature Superconductors 641
23.0 Introduction 641
23.1 Procedures – S. P. Pai, R. D. Vispute and T. Venkatesan 641
   23.1.1 Targets and Ablation 641
   23.1.2 Appropriate Lasers and Systems 642
   23.1.3 Film Growth 642
23.2 Results of HTSC Deposition – Quanxi Jia 644
   23.2.1 Characterization 644
   23.2.2 Comparison with Other Techniques 646
23.3 Laser Treatment of HTSC Films – Emil N. Sobol 647
   23.3.1 Modification 648
   23.3.2 Polishing of Thin HTSC Films 650

Chapter 24 Laser Produced Microstructures 651
24.1 Basic Laser Microstructuring Procedures – J. J. Dubowski 651
   24.1.0 Introduction 651
   24.1.1 Microstructuring by Laser Direct Ablation 651
   24.1.2 Microstructuring by Laser Etching 652
24.2 Other Methods of Laser Microstructuring – J. J. Dubowski 655
   24.2.1 Laser-LIGA Processing 655
   24.2.2 Laser Microstructuring of Glass 655
   24.2.3 Laser Microstructuring of Semiconductors 657

Chapter 25 Electronic Packaging: Electrical Interconnects 661
25.0 Introduction 661
25.1 Via Drilling – Mark D. Owen 661
   25.1.1 Lasers for Via Drilling 661
   25.1.2 Optical Configurations 662
   25.1.3 Applications and Results 663
25.2 Bonding/Soldering 665
   25.2.1 Laser Tape Automated Bonding (TAB) – James Hayward 665
   25.2.2 Laser Reflow Soldering – Gary M. Freedman 667
25.3 Wirestripping 672
   25.3.0 Introduction 672
   25.3.1 Important Parameters in Laser Wirestripping – James H. Brannon and Andrew C. Tam 672
   25.3.2 Lasers for Wirestripping – James H. Brannon and Andrew C. Tam 673
   25.3.3 Wirestripping Procedures – Ronald D. Schaeffer 675

Chapter 26 Electronic Packaging: Package Sealing and Ceramic Processing 677
26.0 Introduction 677
26.1 Package Welding – Phillip W. Fuerschbach 677
   26.1.1 General Considerations 677
   26.1.2 Weld Schedule Development 679
   26.1.3 Process Monitoring 682
26.2 Cutting and Scribing of Substrates – William H. Shiner and Steven R. Maynard 684
   26.2.0 Introduction 684
   26.2.1 Laser Selection 684
   26.2.2 Process Parameters 684
   26.2.3 Pulse Parameters 685
   26.2.4 Optical Considerations 686
   26.2.5 Assist Gas and Nozzle Configuration 686
   26.2.6 Hardware Considerations 687
   26.2.7 Comparison of Scribing and Cutting 687
   26.2.8 Laser Scribing Results – John F. Ready 687
26.3 Hole Drilling in Ceramics 688
   26.3.0 Introduction 688
   26.3.1 Advantages and Laser Choice – Ronald D. Schaeffer 688
   26.3.2 Procedures and Results – William H. Shiner and Steven R. Maynard 689

Chapter 27 Film Deposition and Doping 691
27.1 Thin Film Deposition – Ying Tsui 691
   27.1.1 Laser Chemical Vapor Deposition 691
   27.1.2 Coatings made by LCVD 693
   27.1.3 Direct Write Processing using LCVD 694
   27.1.4 Pulsed Laser Deposition 695
27.2 Deposition of Thick Films of Electronic Ceramics – D. B. Chrisey, J. S. Horwitz, P. C. Dorsey and L. A. Knauss 697

27.3 Gas Immersion Laser Doping (GILD)
– Michael O. Thompson, T. W. Sigmon
and Patrick M. Smith   700
   27.3.1   Theory of Operation   700
   27.3.2   GILD Equipment and Sample Preparation   701
   27.3.3   Laser Sources   701
   27.3.4   Gas Sources   702
   27.3.5   Process Monitoring and Calibration   702
   27.3.6   Doping Profiles   703
   27.3.7   Wafer Throughput   704

INDEX   705

Contributing Authors:
*Current address at end of list

Ratan S. Adhav
Quantum Technology Inc.
108 Commerce Street
Lake Mary, FL 32746-6313

Charles E. Albright
Ohio State University
Welding Engineering
1248 Arthur Adams Drive
Columbus, OH 43210

Terry L. Armbruster
Koolant Koolers
2625 Emerald Drive
Kalamazoo, MI 49001

Sundar V. Atre
Pennsylvania State University
P/M Lab
118 Research West
University Park, PA 16802

Frank Audet
Gentec, Inc.
2625 Dalton Street
Ste-Foy, Quebec
Canada GIP 3S9

Daniel A. Bakken
F-22 Program Manager
Laser Applications Inc.
7645 Baker Street
Minneapolis, MN 55432

Menachem Bamberger
Department of Materials and Engineering
Technion
32000 Haifa
Israel

Conrad M. Banas
56 Volpi Road
Bolton, CT 06043

Paul S. Banks*
Lawrence Livermore National Laboratory
PO Box 808
Mail Code L - 477
Livermore, CA 94550

Dirk Basting
Lambda Physik, Inc.
3201 West Commercial Boulevard
Fort Lauderdale, FL 33309

Peter Becher
Laser Machining, Inc.
500 Laser Drive
Somerset, WI 54025

Jerry Becker
GSI Lumonics
130 Lombard Street
Oxnard, CA 93030

David A. Belforte
Belforte Associates
P. O. Box 245
Sturbridge, MA 01566

Hans Wilhelm Bergmann
University of Bayreuth
Institut fur Materialforschung
Lehrstuhl Metallische Werkstoffe
Ludwig-Thoma-Strasse 36b
D-95440 Bayreuth
Germany

Joachim Berkmanns
AGA Gas Inc.
989 James L. Hart Parkway
Ypsilanti, MI 48197

Joseph B. Bernstein
Department of Materials and Nuclear
    Engineering
2100 Marie Mount Hall
University of Maryland
College Park, MD 20742-7531

Wolfgang Bloehs
AUDI AG
I/PG-63
Technologie-Entwicklung Fertigungstechnik
85045 Ingolstadt
Germany

James H. Brannon
IBM Storage Systems Division
5600 Cottle Road
E25/50-1
San Jose, CA 95193

Robert K. Brimacombe*
GSI Lumonics, Inc.
105 Schneider Road
Kanata, Ontario
Canada 2K 1Y3

Robert Brown
P. O. Stop 129 - 48
United Technologies Research Center
411 Silver Lane
East Hartford, CN 06108

Timothy A. Brunner
IBM-SDRC
Zip AP1
1580 Route 52
Hopewell Junction, NY 12533

James D. Cawley
Case Western Reserve University
Department of Materials Science and
    Engineering
Room 500   White Building
10900 Euclid Avenue
Cleveland, OH 44106 - 7204

Andrew John Chambers
Rofin-Sinar UK Ltd.
Yorkway
Willerby, Hull
HU10 6HD
United Kingdom

Dale U. Chang
Laser Applications
6371 North Orange Blossom Trail
Orlando, FL 32810

Xiangli Chen
KWC285
Research and Development Center
General Electric Company
P. O. Box 8
Schenectady, NY 12301

D. B. Chrisey
Code 6372
Naval Research Laboratory
Washington, DC 20375

George Chryssolouris
Laboratory for Manufacturing Systems
Department of Mechanical Engineering and
    Aeronautics
University of Patras
GR -26110 Rion Patras
Greece

Richard J. Coyle
Lucent Technologies
Bell Laboratories
P. O. Box 900
Princeton, NJ 08540-0900

Philip Cunningham
AOESC/POB 339
Edgewood, NM 87015-0339

Jack Davis (Deceased)

Phil deBeor
Laser Machining, Inc.
500 Laser Drive
Somerset, WI 54025

Philip G. DeLuca
Electro Scientific Industries, Inc
13900 NW Science Park Drive
Portland, OR 97229-5497

Handbook of Laser Materials Processing

P. C. Dorsey
Code 6372
Naval Research Laboratory
Washington, DC 20375

Larry R. Dosser
Mound Laser and Photonics Center
P.O. Box 223
Miamisburg, OH 45343

Jose Downes*
GSI Lumonics
Laser Systems Division
60 Fordham Road
Wilmington, MA 01887

J. J. Dubowski
Institute for Microstructural Sciences
National Research Council Canada
Building M-50
Montreal Road Campus
Ottawa, Ontario K1A OR6
Canada

Raymond F. Duhamel
Director of Applications
Convergent Energy
300 Pleasant Valley Road
South Windsor, CT 06074

W. W. Duley
Faculty of Science
Department of Physics
University of Waterloo
Waterloo, Ontario
Canada N2L 3G1

James A. Dumestre
Electro Scientific Industries, Inc
13900 NW Science Park Drive
Portland, OR 97229

Rodger Dwight
Electro Scientific Industries, Inc
13900 NW Science Park Drive
Portland, OR 97229-5497

Martin C. Edelson
Ames Laboratory
130 Spedding Hall
Ames, Iowa 50011

Bodo Ehlers
Fraunhofer USA
Center for Laser Technology
46025 Port Street
Plymouth, MI 48170

Kevin J. Ely
Edison Welding Institute
1210 Arthur E. Adams Drive
Columbus, OH 43221

Dana Elza
Convergent Energy
1 Picker Road
Sturbridge, MA 01566

Heinrich Endert
IMRA America, Inc.
1044 Woodridge Avenue
Ann Arbor, MI 48105

Dave F. Farson
Ohio State University
Welding Engineering
1248 Arthur Adams Drive
Columbus, OH 43210

Terry Feeley
Laser Fare, Inc.
70 Dean Knauss Drive
Narrangansett, RI 02882

M. D. Feit
Lawrence Livermore National Laboratory
Mail Code L - 439
P. O. Box 808
Livermore, CA 94550

Jim Fieret
Exitech Ltd.
Hanborough Park,
Long Handborough
Oxford OX8 8LH
United Kingdom

Gary M. Freedman
Compaq Computer Corp.
200 Forest Street
Marlboro, MA 01752

Philip W. Fuerschbach
Sandia National Laboratory
MS 0367
P. O. Box 5800
Albuquerque. NM 87185 - 0367

Tomoo Fujioka
Tokai University
Vice Chairman, Institute of
 Laser Technology
2-5-5-1 Tomioka, Koto-ku
Tokyo, 135
Japan

Ronald M. Gagosz
GBG Technical Services
P. O. Box 122
Farmington, CT 06032-0122

Andreas Gebhardt
Eginhardstrasse 28
D-52070 Aachen
Germany

Randall M. German
Pennsylvania State University
P/M Laboratory
118 Research West
University Park, PA 16802-6809

D. Gnanamuthu
1556 Aldercreek Place
Westlake Village, CA 91362-4211

Leonid F. Golovko
Laser Technology and Materials Science
 Department
National Technical University of Ukraine
(Kiev Polytechnic Institute)
Prospect Peremohy 37
252056, Kiev, Ukraine

Damien F. Gray*
1611 Headway Circle
Bldg Z
Austin, TX 78754

Alair Griffin
Javelin
Lone Peak Engineering, Inc.
470 West Lawndale
Suite G
South Salt Lake, Utah 84115

Curtis W. Griffin
Javelin
Lone Peak Engineering, Inc.
470 West Lawndale
Suite G
South Salt Lake, Utah 84115

Stephen D. Hanna
3D Systems, Inc.
26081 Avenue Hall
Valencia, CA 91355

Peter Hardro*
Department of Industrial and
 Manufacturing Engineering
Gilbreth Hall
University of Rhode Island
Kingston, RI 02881

David Havrilla
Rofin-Sinar
45701 Mast Street
Plymouth, MI 48170-6008

James Hayward
Advanced Micro-Devices Inc.
MS 58, P. O. Box 3453
Sunnyvale, CA 94088 - 3453

Dennis W. Hetzner
Timken Research
Box 6930
RES-04
Canton, OH 44706-0930

James Higgins
GSI Lumonics, Inc.
105 Schneider Road
Kanata, Ontario K2K 1Y3
Canada

Alan E. Hill
17 El Arco Road
Albuquerque, NM 87123

J. S. Horwitz
Code 6372
Naval Research Laboratory
Washington, DC 20375

Rolf E. Hummel
Department of Materials Science
 and Engineering
216 Rhines Hall
University of Florida
Gainesville, FL 32611-6400

Kenneth G. Ibbs
Marketing and Sales
LICONIX
3281 Scott Boulevard
Santa Clara, CA 95054

C.L.M. Ireland
88 Hillmorton Road
Rugby, Warwickshire CV22AH
England

Toshihiko Ishihara*
Amterra
4475 Mission Blvd. #203
San Diego, CA 92109

Paul F. Jacobs
Laser Fare, Inc.
70 Dean Knauss Drive
Narragansett, RI 02882

Pierre Jaegle
Laboratoire de Spectroscopie Atomique et
 Ionique
University of Paris-Sud, bat 350
91405 Orsay
France

Meir Janai
Chip Express
2323 Owen Street
Santa Clara, CA 95059

Thomas Aaboe Jensen
FORCE Institute
Welding and Production Technology
Park Allø 345
DK-2605 Broendby
Copenhagen, Denmark

Quanxi Jia
Mail Stop K763
Los Alamos National Laboratory
Los Alamos, NM 87545

Marshall G. Jones
G. E. Corporate Research
 and Development Center
MS KWC - 289
1 Research Center
Schenectady, NY 12301

Marius Jurca
My Optical Systems GmbH
Industriestr, 9
D-63796 Kahl am Main
Germany

Aravinda Kar
CREOL
P. O. Box 162700
University of Central Florida
Orlando, FL 32816-2700

Stefanos Karagiannis
Laboratory for Manufacturing Systems
Department of Mechanical Engineering and
 Aeronautics
University of Patras
GR -26110 Rion Patras
Greece

David M. Keicher
Optomec Design Company
2701-D Pan American Freeway NE
Albuquerque, NM 87107

Paul Kelley
Department of Electrical Engineering and
 Computer Sciences
Tufts University
Medford, MA 01801

Hugh W. Kerr
Department of Mechanical Engineering
University of Waterloo
Waterloo, Ontario
Canada N2L 3G1

Kurt G. Klavuhn*
Spectra-Physics Headquarters
1344 Terra Bella Ave
Mountain View, CA 94039

L. A. Knauss
Code 6372
Naval Research Laboratory
Washington, DC 20375

Volodymyr S. Kovalenko
Head, Laser Technology and Materials
 Science Department
National Technical University of Ukraine
(Kiev Polytechnic Institute)

Prospect Peremohy 37
252056, Kiev, Ukraine

Thomas R. Kugler
GSI Lumonics
19776 Haggerty Road
Livonia, MI 48152

Joseph J. Kwiatkowski
Precision Joining Technologies, Inc.
P. O. Box 531
Miamisburg, OH 45343 - 0531

William P. Latham
AFRL/DE BLDG. 499
Room 115a
3550 Aberdeen Avenue, S. E.
Kitkland Air Force Base
Albuquerque, NM 87117-5776

Keng H. Leong *
Argonne National Laboratory
9700 South Cass Avenue
Argonne, IL 60439

Gary K. Lewis
MS G - 770
Los Alamos National Laboratory
Los Alamos, NM 87545

Allan Lightman
ARDAL Electronics, Inc.
1165 Sessions Dr.
Dayton, OH 45459-8710

James Luxon
GMI Engineering and Management Institute
1700 West 3rd Avenue
Flint, MI 48502-2276

Terry L. Lyon
Laser/Optical Radiation Program
US Army CHPPM
Aberdeen Proving Grounds, MD 21010-5422

Michael Martin
Advanced Products Group
Mechanical Technology, Inc.
967 Albany-Shaker Road
Latham, NY 12110

David M. Marusa
P. O. Box 647
Ashland, OH 44805-0647

Martin Matthews
GSI Lumonics
105 Schneider Road
Kanata, Ontario
Canada K2K 1Y3

Roland Mayerhofer
University of Bayreuth

Handbook of Laser Materials Processing

Institut fur Materialforschung
Ludwig-Thoma-Strasse 36b
D-95440 Bayreuth
Germany

Steven R. Maynard
Convergent Energy
1 Picker Road
Sturbridge, MA 01566

Jyoti Mazumder
Center for Laser Aided Intelligent Manufacturing
University of Michigan
2141 GG Brown Building
2350 Hayward Drive
Ann Arbor, MI 48109-2125

Kevin McAlea
DTM Corporation
1611 Headway Circle
Bldg 2
Austin, TX 78754

Mary Helen McCay
The University of Tennessee
 Space Institute
B. H. Goethert Parkway
Tullahoma, TN 37388-8897

Terry McKee*
GSI Lumonics
105 Schneider Road
Kanata, Ontario
Canada K2K 1Y3

Roy Mead
Aculight Corporation
11805 North Creek Parkway S
Suite 113
Bothell, WA 98011

Vivian E. Merchant
Wilson Greatbatch Ltd.
10,000 Wehrle Drive
Clarence, N.Y. 14031

Edward A. Metzbower
Naval Research Laboratory
Code 6320
Washington, DC 20375-5343

Leonard Migliore
Laser Kinetics, Inc.
406 West Dana Street
Mountain View, CA 94041

Michael F. Modest
Pennsylvania State University
Department of Mechanical Engineering
301C Reber Building
University Park, PA 16802

P. S. Mohanty
Center for Laser Aided Intelligent
 Manufacturing.
University of Michigan
2141 GG Brown Building
2350 Hayward Drive
Ann Arbor, MI 48109-2125

D. W. Moon
Naval Research Laboratory
Code 6320
Washington, DC 20375-5343

C. Eugene Moss
PAAEB-NIOSH
MS R13
Robert E. Taft Laboratories
4676 Columbia Parkway
Cincinnatti, OH 45226-1998

Thomas J. Mueller
Mueller and Flynn
2314 Magnolia Court East
Buffalo Grove, IL 60089

Klaus Müller
University of Bayreuth
Institut fur Materialforschung
Lehrstuhl Metallische Werkstoffe
Ludwig-Thoma-Strasse 36b
D-95440 Bayreuth
Germany

Karthik Nagarathnam
Research Faculty
Applied Research Center
Old Dominion University
12050 Jefferson Avenue, Suite 717
Newport News, VA 23606

Suwas K. Nikumb
National Research Council
Integrated Manufacturing Technologies
 Institute
800 Collip Circle
London, Ontario N6G 4X8
Canada

Brian Norris
GSI Lumonics
105 Schneider Road
Kanata, Ontario M2K 143
Canada

Flemming O. Olsen
Institut For Procesteknik
Danmarks Tekniske Universitet
Bygning 425
DK-2800 Lyngby
Denmark

Mark D. Owen
MV Technology

16075 NW Telshire Drive
Beaverton, OR 97006

S. P. Pai
Center for Superconducting Research
Department of Physics
University of Maryland
College Park, MD 20742

Sung S. Pak
Helisys, Inc.
24015 Garnier Street
Torrance, CA 90505

Stephen A. Payne
Lawrence Livermore National Laboratory
P. O. Box 808, L-441
Livermore, CA 94551

Michael D. Perry*
Lawrence Livermore National Laboratory
Mail Code L - 439
P. O. Box 808
Livermore, CA 94550

Dirk Petring
Fraunhofer Institute for Laser Technology
 (ILT)
Steinbachstrasse 15
D-52074 Aachen
Germany

Floyd R. Pothoven
International Technology Works
10134 Artesian Place
Bellflower CA 90706

Terry Pothoven
Laserod Inc.
1846-A West 169th Street
Gardena, CA 90247

John Powell
Technical Director, Laser Expertise Ltd.
Unit H, Acorn Park Industrial Estate
Harrimans Lane, Dunkirk, Nottingham
NG7 2TR United Kingdom

John F. Ready
4401 Gilford Drive
Edina, MN 55435

Chris Rickert
TWB
1600 Nadeau
Monroe, Michigan 48162

Todd J. Rockstroh
MD D-83
General Electric Company
Laser Applications Center
1 Neumann Way
Cincinnati, OH 45215

Hansjoerg Rohde*
LASAG AG Industrial Lasers
Mittlere Strasse 52
CH-3600 Thun
Switzerland

Chandrasekhar Roychoudhuri
Photonics Research Center
University of Connecticut
54 Ahern Lane, U - 192
Storrs, CN 06269-5192

Paul G. Sanders*
Argonne National Laboratory
Building 207
Laser Applications Laboratory
9700 South Cass Avenue
Argonne, IL 60439

Shunichi Sato
Institute of Research and Innovation
Laser Laboratory
1201 Takada
Kashiwa-Shi Chiba-Ken
277 Japan

Jim Scaroni
GSI Lumonics
105 Schneider Road
Kanata, Ontario K2K 1Y3
Canada

Ronald D. Schaeffer
Photomachining, Inc.
29 Batch Elder Road
Mason, NH 03048

L. A. (Vern) Schlie
Air Force Research Laboratory
AFRL/DELO, Bldg 244
Kirtland AFB, New Mexico 87185

Hatto Schneider
SHENCK RoTec GmbH
64293 Darmstaadt
Germany

J. Thomas Schriempf
Applied Research Laboratory
Pennsylvania State University
Electro-Optics Center
West Hills Industrial Park
77 Glade Drive
Kittanning, PA 16201

E. Schubert
BIAS
Klangenfurter Strasse 2
28359 Bremen
Germany

Joseph A. Sefcik
Lawrence Livermore National Laboratory

P. O. Box 808, L-359
Livermore, CA 94551

Vladimir Semak
Department of Physics
Box 3001
New Mexico State University
Las Cruces, NM 88003

G. Sepold
BIAS
Klangenfurter Strasse 2
28359 Bremen
Germany

Gary Settles
Department of Mechanical Engineering
Pennsylvania State University
301D Reeber
University Park, PA 16802

John J. Shamaly
Silicon Valley Group
77 Danbury Road
Wilton, CT 06897-0877

Geoff J. Shannon
Synrad Inc.
6500 Harbor Heights Parkway
Mukilteo, WA 98275

Daniel L. Sherman
Laser Power Optics
12777 High Bluff Drive
San Diego, CA 92130-2094

William H. Shiner
Convergent Energy
1 Picker Road
Sturbridge, MA 01566

T. W. Sigmon*
Information Science and Technology
Lawrence Livermore National Laboratory
L-395
700 East Avenue
Livermore, CA 94551

Richard Slagle
Oxford Lasers Inc.
29 King Street
Littleton, MA 01460-1528

David H. Sliney
Laser/Optical Radiation Program
US Army CHPPM
Aberdeen Proving Grounds, MD 21010-5422

Donald V. Smart
GSI Lumonics.
Laser Systems Division
60 Fordham Road
Wilmington, MA 01887

Patrick M. Smith
Lawrence Livermore National Laboratory
Livermore, CA 94551

Emil N. Sobol
Institute of Laser and Information Technologies
2, Pionerskaya str.
Troitsk, 142092
Russia

Richard W. Solarz
Lawrence Livermore National Laboratory
P. O. Box 808
L - 590
Livermore, CA 94550

Walter J. Spawr
Spawr Industries, Inc.
Optics Division
P. O. Box 2490
Lake Havasu, AZ 86405

Robert J. Steele
Naval Air Warfare Center
Code 475 - 1000
Mail Stop 216 D
China Lake, CA 93555-6001

Brent C. Stuart
Lawrence Livermore National Laboratory
P. O. Box 808, L-477
Livermore, CA 94550

Brent Stucker
University of Rhode Island
Department of Industrial and Manufacturing Engineering
Gilbreth Hall
2 East Alumni Ave.
Kingston, RI 02881

Yunlong Sun
Electro Scientific Industries, Inc.
13900 NW Science Park Drive
Portland, OR 97229-5497

E. Swenson
Electro Scientific Industries, Inc.
13900 NW Science Park Drive
Portland, OR 97229-5497

Andrew C. Tam
IBM Almaden Research Center
K63/52K63/E-3
650 Harry Road
San Jose, CA 95120-6099

Michael O. Thompson
Deptartment of Materials Science
Bard Hall 329
Cornell University
Ithaca, NY 14853

Handbook of Laser Materials Processing

Ying Tsui
Department of Electrical
  and Computer Engineering
University of Alberta
Edmonton, Alberta
Canada T6G 2G7

Dr. T. Venkatesan
Center for Superconducting Research
Department of Physics
University of Maryland
College Park, MD 20742

David B. Veverka
Fanuc Robotics
3900 West Hamlin Boulevard
Rochester Hills, MI 48309

R. D. Vispute
Center for Superconducting Research
Department of Physics
University of Maryland
College Park, MD 20742

Thomas A. Wassick
IBM Microelectronics Division
1580 Route 52, MS/20A
Hopewell Junction, NY 12533

Rodney Waters
Laserod Inc.
1846-A West 169th Street
Gardena, CA 90247

M. J. Weber
Mail Stop 55-121
Lawrence Berkeley National Laboratory
1 Cyclotron Road
Berkeley, CA 94720

David C. Weckman
Department of Mechanical Engineering
University of Waterloo
Waterloo, Ontario
Canada N2L 3G1

Robert Weiner
Weiner Associates
544 23rd Street
Manhattan Beach, CA 90266

Rodney L. Wood
Laser/Optical Radiation Program
US Army CHPPM
Aberdeen Proving Grounds, MD 21010-5422

John Zayhowski, Gr. 82
MIT Lincoln Laboratory
244 Wood Street
Lexington, MA 02420-9108

Arlene Zdrazil
Laser Machining, Inc.
500 Laser Drive
Somerset, WI 54025

I. Zerner
BIAS
Klangenfurter Strasse 2
28359 Bremen
GERMANY

Wei Zhang
Department of Materials and Nuclear
  Engineering
2100 Marie Mount Hall
University of Maryland
College Park, MD 20742-7531

*Currently at:

Paul Banks
GA Photonics
P. O. Box 85608
Mail Stop 13-266
San Diego, CA 92186-9784

Robert K. Brimacombe
Nortel Networks
1341 Baseline Road
Ottawa, Ontario
Canada K2C 0A7

Jose Downes
Nortel Networks
299 Ballardvale Street
Wilmington, MA 01887

Dr. Damien F. Gray
National Instruments
11500 North Mopac Expressway
Austin, Texas, 78759-3504

Peter J. Hardro
Naval Undersea Warfare
Center Division Newport
1176 Howell Street
Newport, RI 02841

Toshihiko Ishihara
Cymer Laser Technologies
16750 via del Campo
San Diego, CA 92127

Dr. Kurt G. Klavuhn
Staff Development Engineer
Coherent Star
1249 Quarry Lane
Suite 100
Pleasanton, CA 94566

Keng H. Leong
Applied Research Laboratory
Pennsylvania State University
Electro-Optics Center
West Hills Industrial Park
77 Glade Drive
Kittanning, PA 16201

Terry McKee
K2H 8C3
JDS Uniphase
570 West Hunt Club Road
Nepean, Canada K2G 5W8

Michael D. Perry
GA Photonics
3550 General Atomics Court
Mail Stop 13-265
San Diego, CA 92186-9784

Hansjoerg Rohde
Baasel Lasertechnik GmbH
Petersbrunner Strasse 1b
D-82319 Starberg
Switzerland

Paul G. Sanders
Safety Research and Development
Ford Research Laboratory
P. O. Box 2053, MD 2115
Dearborn, MI 48121-2053

T. W. Sigmon
Dept of Electrical Engineering and
  Microelectronics
Center for High Technology Materials
The University of New Mexico
1313 Goddard, S. E.
Albuquerque, NM 87106

Acknowledgements

Section 2.1: The editors wish to acknowledge and express their thanks to Tommy Walling of Convergent Prima for preparing the figures for this section.

Section 2.5.6: Table 8 was adapted with permission from the table that appeared in the chapter by Peter F. Bordui and Martin M. Fejer in Annual Review of Materials Science, Volume 23, © 1993, published by Annual Reviews (http://www.AnnualReviews.org).

Section 2.6: This section is a revised and expanded version of a Koolant Koolers, Inc. information paper written several years ago by Robert R. Corrion.

Section 3.2.2: The author (Chandrasekhar Roychoudhuri) acknowledges the support of Ken Chen and Doug Bradway of the Photonics Research Center, in preparing this manuscript and Robert Brown of the United Technologies Research Center for many useful discussions. Support for related research work was provided by Connecticut Innovations of the State of Connecticut.

Sections 3.6.4 and 3.6.5: The author (Walter J. Spawr) wishes to express his thanks to John Q. Adams, Consultant, for his assistance in preparing these sections and to Laser Power Optics, Lincoln Laser and Janos Technology, Inc. for permission to publish their product descriptions, illustrations, photographs, data, tables and graphs.

We wish to thank Professor Dr. H. Huegel for kindly letting us use in 4.1.2 illustrations that appeared in H. Huegel, Optiken für die Materialbearbeitung mit Hochleistungslasern-Anforderungen und Qualifizierung, Proceedings of the 2nd LAF'90 (LaserAndwenderForum), Nov. 1990 Bremen, Germany, pages 151-158 and H. Huegel, F. Dausinger, Innovative Ansätze zur laserbasierten Füge-und Oberflächentechnik, Proceedings of the 3rd LAF'97 (LaserAndwenderForum), Sept. 1997, Bremen, Germany, Band 5, Pages 103-111.

Section 4.5: The author (Francis Audet) wishes to thank his colleague, Olivier Plomteux, for providing him with information that he had used for an article on optimizing laser meter performance that appeared in Laser Focus World in 1996.

Section 6.4: The editors thank the LIA Non-Beam Hazard Sub-Committee for providing the material on which this section was based and to C. Eugene Moss for preparing an outline of topics that, along with his further notes, was incorporated into the section. This section was put into final form by the editorial staff of MPI.

Sections 9.1 – 9.4.3: The authors (E. Schubert, I. Zerner and G. Sepold) wish to acknowledge the thesis work at the University of Bremen of C. Radscheidt and at the University of Erlangen of H. Hanebuth, each of whose work provided information of value in the preparation of these sections.

Section 10.2.8: The author (Joachim Berkmanns) would like to thank Gert Broden, AGA AB, Mark Faerber, AGA Gas GmbH and Ed Warzyniec, AGA Gas Inc. for their support.

Section 11.3.1: This section was prepared when the authors (Keng H. Leong and Paul G. Sanders) were at Argonne National Laboratory. The authors wish to thank the Laboratory for its support of their work on this section and for providing the release for its publication in this Handbook.

Section 11.3.1 has been authorized for publication in this Handbook by a contractor of the U.S. Government under contract No. W-031-109-ENG-38.

Section 11.3.6: Kapton is a tradmark of E. I. du Pont Demours and Co., Inc., Wilmington, Delaware.

Section 11.3.7: The authors (D.C. Weckman and H.W. Kerr) gratefully acknowledge the contributions of their former students and research associates, M. Biela, H. N. Bransch, M. P. Graham, D. M. Hirak, J. T. Liu, E. Michaud, T. Nguyen and Z. Y. Wang, who, they said, "led us and pushed us towards our better understanding of the science and technology of pulsed Nd:YAG laser welding".

Section 13.2.1: All photographs in this section are courtesy of LASAG AG Industrial Lasers.

Sections 13.5.0 - 13.5.2: The authors (M. D. Perry, B. C. Stuart, P.S. Banks, M. D. Feit, and J. A. Sefcik) would like to acknowledge the pioneering work in the field of Ultrashort-Pulse Laser Machining by P. Callen, E. Glenzer, W. Kautek, C. Momma, G. Mourou, and S. Nolte and thank them for many helpful discussions, and also thank P. Armstrong, N. Frank, B. Pyke, D. Shipley and others involved in the design and construction of the femtosecond machining system. This work was performed under the auspices of the U.S. Department of Energy by Lawrence Livermore National Laboratory under contract No. W-7405-ENG-48.

Section 15.5.3: NovaLine 100, NovaLine LITHO, and Nova Tube are registered trademarks of Lambda Physik, Inc.

Chapter 16: The following registered trademarks are among those cited in this chapter: SLS®, DTM™ DTM Corporation, Austin, TX), QuickCast (3D Systems, Inc. Valencia, CA), 3D Keltool (3D Systems, Inc. Valencia, CA), ExpressTool (Infinite Group, Warwick, RI), Nickel Ceramic Composite (CEMCOM, Corp. Baltimore, MD), ACES (3D Systems, Inc. Valencia, CA), Laminated Object Manufacturing (LOM) ™ (Helisys, Inc., Torrance, CA).

Section 16.4.2: Lone Peak Engineering would like to thank Dr. William Coblenz, DARPA, for support of the work described in this section under contracts DAAH01-93-C-R350 and DAAH01-94-CO-R324 and the Small Business Innovative Research (SBIR) program.

Section 16.6: The author (Larry R. Dosser) wishes to acknowledge a private communication from Dr. P. T. Murray that was useful in the preparation of this section.

Section 22.3: The authors (Rodney Waters and Terry Pothoven) have incorporated information received in private communications from Saleem Shaik (Thin Film Devices, Anaheim, CA) and Peter Barbee (Fluke Corp., Everett, WA).

Handbook of Laser Materials Processing

Foreword

The Laser Institute of America (LIA), a professional society, was founded in 1968. Its mission is to *foster lasers, laser applications and laser safety worldwide*. LIA publishes the *Journal of Laser Applications®*, sponsors international conferences, offers short courses, especially on laser safety, publishes the ANSI laser safety standards and many other publications.

LIA's International Congress on Applications of Lasers & Electro-Optics (ICALEO®) is recognized as the premier congress on laser materials processing, giving us access to the premier worldwide researchers in the field. So publishing this definitive and comprehensive handbook on laser materials processing is a natural consequence of this connection. Most of the editorial board and a large percentage of the contributors are LIA members. A work of this scope required that we draw on the expertise of specialists in all parts of the world, so the Handbook is a truly international collaboration.

LIA turned to Magnolia Publishing, Inc., a company whose personnel over the past thirty years created a number of significant technical works for major American scientific and technical publishers. We are pleased that Magnolia Publishing joined us as full partners in this venture, working closely with editors and LIA members, John F. Ready and Dave F. Farson, on this project.

We decided to go against traditional wisdom and the advice of a number of composition houses; we were cautioned that a stalemate might result in trying to convert standard word processing files from 200 different domestic and foreign sources into a platform suitable for presswork. We had hoped that our instructions to authors would carry the day, and for the most part they did; we had very little rekeyboarding to do. However, a small percentage of art came to us overly compressed (some contributors saved their figures at screen resolution) or in software that did not communicate as well we would have liked with the final program that went to the printer. Some of the figures - fortunately not many - show the result of the compromises we had to make.

It is important to note the following:

The information in this handbook is intended for individuals knowledgeable in the proper and safe use of lasers and the practice of laser processing. Inherent in the use of lasers and in doing laser processing are a range of safety and health concerns. Laser radiation, direct and reflected, can cause permanent eye damage and skin burns. It can ignite materials and react violently with certain gases. In processing materials it can produce hazardous gasses and plumes. Chapter 6 on laser safety is not a manual on the subject. Its purpose is to make one aware of the safety and health implications of working with and near lasers and how to go about obtaining information on setting up a safe facility. Additional information can be obtained from the Laser Institute of America.

Updated information and comments about the Handbook, our other products and services and membership information can be found on the LIA website, www.laserinstitute.org. Messages can be sent to us at lia@laserinstitute.org.

Peter M. Baker
Executive Director

To Claire,

With my thanks for your support and understanding
during the years it took to bring this Handbook to fruition.

Jack

Preface

This Handbook is for engineers, materials scientists, optical scientists and physicists. It is designed to help solve problems in laser processing of metals, ceramics and other materials. The Handbook contains a great deal of basic as well as advanced information and covers a broad range of pertinent topics: materials, instruments, procedures, industrial and laboratory equipment, monitoring, processes, processing systems, processing results and prototyping. A full range of applications are covered as they apply to many industries including aerospace, automotive, computer and electronic.

The Handbook features well established laser applications such as cutting and welding, but also covers developing applications such as diode laser processing. In addition, important reference material on available lasers, basic optics, accessory instrumentation and safety are to be found in its pages.

The Handbook is structured as a ready reference source. Thus, complete information on a given topic is contained within the section devoted to the topic. A corollary of this approach is redundancy. For example, the chapter on cutting has information that also appears in the chapter on welding, although not presented in the same way. Limiting redundancy while achieving chapters that would be able to stand on their own was one of the challenges in editing this work.

Tabulated numerical values are given for a variety of processes and for laser parameters. These allow the user to determine the potential of a given laser for use in a particular process. In many instances laser technologies are compared with non-laser technologies or the capabilities and limitations of the processes are outlined.

The Handbook does not treat the underlying theory of laser operations for the most part. Rather than dwell on theoretical considerations, we have chosen to stress the results of theory as they apply to processing operations.

Similarly, the Handbook is not highly mathematical. However, where pertinent, equations important for estimating the results of processing operations are provided, *sans* derivations.

Tabulated and graphed data must be interpreted as indicating a range of results. The exact results obtained for an operation depend on a wide variety of parameters which may vary from one laser installation to another. These parameters are often not specified well enough to allow the exact duplication of the conditions for a particular operation. The user must optimize the parameters for a particular processing operation experimentally in order to obtain the best results. An example would be the penetration depth and processing rate for a particular operation.

The Handbook excludes a major subject: biomaterials. Adding the necessary pages for biomaterials would have increased the size of the handbook and diluted its focus.

The number of references in each section has been held to a minimum, consistent with the nature of a handbook contribution as, say, opposed to a review paper. Those sections containing a fair number of references have been permitted to retain them because they may help the user determine the exact conditions for a particular processing operation. Reference to the *Handbook of Chemistry and Physics* is made by a number of contributing authors who, typically, cite the editions in their personal libraries. Since each edition of HBC&P deletes some material to make room for new data, there was a possibility that the referenced material might not be in the most current edition. We used our judgement as to when to update a citation to a recent edition and when to let the referenced edition stand.

A number of illustrations borrowed from non-English language publications required that they be used as camera copy. Several of these figures have foreign language legends as part of the art. However, the meaning in each case is quite obvious.

A word should be said about units. A significant number of contributions employ English units which, indeed, are widely used in industry. The editors have found that individuals who use other systems of units are generally quite conversant with the English system, whereas those who work in the English system are often uncomfortable with other systems. Hence, as a practical matter, we decided to retain the units used by each author. Irradiance is commonly given in "mixed units", watts per square centimeter (W/cm^2), and therefore appears throughout the Handbook in this form.

We wish to express our deep appreciation to the many people who worked with us in developing this Handbook. We thank the advisory boards who aided in the original formulation of the outline and who provided suggestions for authors. We especially thank the many contributing authors for their diligence in preparing the individual contributions to this work and for sharing their expertise.

For the specialized field of rapid prototyping, the editors turned to Terry Feeley and asked him to organize and edit the chapter on that subject. We thank him for his excellent work.

Many thanks are due to Heather Allan for her invaluable and dedicated work on the electronic files and to Melanie Lee whose sharp eye and sharp pencil are an invisible presence throughout these pages.

John F. Ready, Editor in Chief
Dave F. Farson, Associate Editor
February, 2001

Chapter 1

Overview of Laser Materials Processing

1.0 Introduction

This chapter presents introductory concepts fundamental to laser-based materials processing.

Section 1.1 defines the laser parameters that affect the results of a materials processing operation. Section 1.2 covers concepts relevant to the absorption of laser energy and its role in influencing the deposition of energy in a workpiece. Section 1.3 presents the spatial and temporal characteristics of laser light and introduces important types of lasers. Section 1.4 describes how numerous components of which the laser is one, may be assembled to form a complete laser processing system.

The level of the chapter is fairly elementary; it provides an introduction to the subject matter that underlies the technology of laser materials processing.

1.1 Laser Parameters

Lasers can be characterized by physical parameters such as the spatial and temporal properties of the output light, the active element producing the light, the pumping method, and the resonator design. Also important are considerations such as size, weight, power required, efficiency, stability, and reliability.

The behavior of the light is determined by properties such as spatial and temporal coherence, operation in a continuous or pulsed mode, spectral content, and state of polarization. Coherent laser light has important attributes that light from incoherent sources does not have. In the laser amplification process, the electromagnetic field grows in amplitude while maintaining its phase characteristics in space and time.

This section introduces some of the important optical and system parameters for lasers. These parameters will be discussed more fully in the descriptions of specific lasers.

1.1.1 Laser Beam Parameters

Laser beam parameters describe the physical state of the light coming from a laser. These parameters include the output power and pulse energy, spatial beam parameters such as shape and extent, temporal parameters such as pulse duration, and spatial and temporal coherence. Of these, one of the most important characteristics for material processing is spatial coherence.

Spatial Properties

In materials processing, spatial properties of the laser light, such as the ability to focus the light to a small spot, are very important. Coherent laser light has very different spatial behavior in comparison to other artificial light sources or the sun. A spatially coherent light field has a smooth, well-behaved wavefront in space, while spatially incoherent light field has a random, rapidly varying wavefront. This difference in spatial character is the reason that laser light can be focused to a very small spot size while focal spot sizes for incoherent light are typically much larger.

To get some idea of the difference between the coherent source and an incoherent source, we compare a focused laser beam with focused sunlight (1). The expressions given in this section will also allow the user to estimate accurately the delivery of power by focused laser beams.

A diffraction-limited (2) Gaussian profile laser beam with a diameter (3) D, defined to contain 99% of the power, has a diffraction-limited full angle, $\theta_{diff} \approx 2\lambda/D$. The diffraction-limited angle describes both how a coherent beam will spread in the far field (4) and how well it can be focused. For $D = 30$ mm and visible light, $\theta_{diff} \approx 3 \times 10^{-5}$ rad. In contrast, the angular subtense of the sun at the earth is $\theta_{sun} \approx 0.6° \approx 0.01$ rad. Again, this angle describes how a beam of sunlight will spread and focus after passing through an aperture or lens. In both cases, the focal spot diameter is given by $d_{focus} = \theta f$, where f is the focal length of the lens. For a lens with $f = 100$ mm and visible light, the laser focal spot diameter is 3 μm, while the diameter of the spot of focused sunlight is 1 mm.

The intensity of sunlight at the surface of the earth is $I_{sc} \approx 1.4$ kW/m², where the sc subscript stands for the solar constant. Assuming a focal length of 100 mm, the intensity at the focus, after passing through a 30-mm-diameter lens, is $I_{focus} = I_{sc} D^2/(\theta_{sun} f)^2 = 1000 I_{sc} = 1400$ kW/m². To achieve the same peak focused intensity with a diffraction-limited laser beam requires a peak laser intensity at the lens of $I_{laser} \approx I_{focus}(\pi\lambda f)^2/D^4 = I_{sc}(\pi\theta_{diff}/2\theta_{sun})^2 = 0.04$ W/m². To put it another way, the power of the laser required to give a focal spot intensity equal to the sun is $P_{laser} \approx (\pi/2)I_{sc}(\lambda/\theta_{sun})^2$. For a visible laser, $P_{laser} \approx 5$ μW.

The foregoing analysis demonstrates an important advantage of a spatially coherent source compared to a spatially incoherent source. However, there are other important considerations that

---

[1] This analysis is for an untruncated Guassian beam of laser radiation. The Gaussian distribution is defined in Section 1.3. Lenses truncate laser beams and will change the values given by a small amount. A full description of untruncated Gaussian beam propagation is given in A.E. Siegman, *Lasers* (University Science Books, Palo Alto, 1986).

[2] The term *diffraction-limited* refers to the beam divergence angle defined by the fundamental physical phenomenon of diffraction. It is the minimum possible beam divergence angle for a given geometry.

[3] This definition of diameter is related to the $1/e^2$ power radius, w, by $D = \pi w$.

[4] The near-field and far-field regions of Gaussian beams are important concepts. The near-field region occurs when the phase of the beam wavefront is flat; the far-field occurs when the phase of the beam wavefront is spherical. As a beam that is initially near-field propogates, it is transformed by diffraction into a far-field beam. The distance required is several times a characteristic distance $z_R = D^2/\pi\lambda$, which is known as the Rayleigh range.

ISBN 0-912035-15-3

bear mention here. Lasers whose output is not diffraction-limited cannot deliver the small spot sizes or high intensities that are possible at the same output power from a diffraction-limited laser. Typically, laser beam quality ranges from close to the diffraction limit to tens of times diffraction limited, where "times diffraction limited" or XDL is defined as $XDL = \theta_{actual}/\theta_{diff}$. While small laser focal spot sizes allow the very precise delivery of energy to localized regions, there are applications that do not require such great spatial precision. Thermal and mechanical transport can limit the amount of energy delivered per unit volume. The smaller the area irradiated, the shorter the transport-limited time becomes. In this case, it is often important to use lasers designed to deliver energy in short pulses.

When laser beams vary from the ideal diffraction-limited output, they often do not produce uniform intensity spots when focused. The nonuniform delivery of energy caused by "hot spots" in the beam can have undesirable consequences in materials processing. Beams with hot spots can be homogenized by adding random phase variations across the wavefront before the beam is focused. These parameters describing focused laser beams and the relevant defining equations are summarized in Table 1.

Table 1. Parameters Describing Focused Laser Beams

Parameters	Symbol-defining equation
Beam power	P
Width of the portion of the unfocused beam containing 99% of the power	D
Wavelength	λ
Full-width diffraction angle	$\theta_{diff} = 2\lambda/D$
Focal spot diameter	$d_{focus} = \theta_{diff} f = 2\lambda f/D$
Peak intensity at focus	$I_{focus} = 2P/d_{focus}^2$
Times diffraction limited	$XDL = \theta_{actual}/\theta_{diff}$

The collimation of laser radiation is limited by diffraction. An initially parallel (flat phase front) diffraction-limited Gaussian profile beam will remain nearly parallel up to a distance, called the Rayleigh range or near-field distance, given by $z_R = D^2/\pi\lambda$. After several times this distance, the beam is in the far-field region and will spread at an angular rate equal to the diffraction angle given in Table 1. Radiation that is not diffraction-limited will spread at a higher angular rate determined by the XDL factor given in the table.

Laser Cavity Modes

Cavity modes derive from the requirement that the cavity waves must repeat on one round trip in the cavity. Modes determine both the operating frequencies and the spatial characteristics of the laser output. Temporal and spatial coherence occurs when the phases of the modes have a fixed, nonrandom relationship. There are two types of modes in the open resonators that are used as cavities for lasers, longitudinal and transverse modes. The number of transverse modes produced by the laser determines the spatial characteristics of the laser output. If only the lowest-order transverse mode is excited, the beam will diffract at the minimum diffraction-limited rate. If several transverse modes are excited with random phases, the beam will diffract at a much higher rate. Operation in one or more longitudinal modes, but only the lowest-order transverse mode, will not affect the diffraction-limited character of the radiation. The spatial patterns characteristic of different transverse modes are presented in Section 1.3.1.

Operation in one or more longitudinal modes can have significant effect on the temporal character of the of the laser output. If all the longitudinal modes are locked in phase, the laser can produce a periodic train of short pulses. If the phases of the longitudinal modes are random, random power spikes will occur. In material processing, the time response characteristics of the medium will determine whether the periodic pulses or random spiking have an effect on the processing or whether the material responds only to the average power.

The modes described above are appropriate for empty resonators. In many lasers, the spatial characteristics of the beam are also determined the material medium inside the laser cavity; this medium can be very inhomogeneous, as is often the case with very high power solid-state lasers. The diffraction limit, however, provides a benchmark for comparison.

Temporal Properties

Lasers can be operated in a variety of temporal modes, either continuously (CW) or in pulses ranging from milliseconds to a few femtoseconds. In most material processing applications either CW or Q-switched operation is used. In Q-switched operation, pulses are produced by keeping laser cavity losses higher than the gain until the laser upper levels have maximum occupation; the cavity loss is then decreased quickly so that gain greatly exceeds loss. The stored energy is extracted in the short time, typically several nanoseconds, required to convert the material excitation into laser radiation. If substantially shorter pulses are required, the laser can be modelocked to produce pulses with duration in the picosecond regime. Further discussion of the methods of achieving different types of temporal operation will be discussed in Section 1.3.2.

Spectral Properties

The wavelengths of operation of lasers are determined predominantly by the spectral characteristics of the laser material's gain profile. Gas lasers typically have one or more operating wavelengths, each having narrow lines in the range of tens of MHz to a few GHz. Solid-state and liquid lasers typically have much broader ranges of operation, ranging from a few wavenumbers (one wavenumber = 30 GHz) for rare-earth-doped solid-state lasers to more than one thousand wavenumbers for dye lasers and Ti:Sapphire lasers.

Chapter 1: Overview of Laser Materials Processing

Polarization

Polarization relates to the orientation of the electric field vector with respect to the coordinate axes normal to the direction of propagation of the light. Normally laser radiation has a specific direction of polarization. In materials processing, the coupling of radiation into a material is affected by the state of polarization of the field when the radiation is incident on the surface in directions away from the surface normal (see Chapter 5).

1.1.2 System Parameters

In evaluating the use of lasers in practical areas such as materials processing, issues such as size, weight, power requirements, reliability, and serviceability must be taken into consideration. In what follows, we will give definitions and examples of important system parameters.

Optical

The optical components of a laser include a cavity containing the active laser material and various elements to control the temporal and spatial properties of the emitted radiation. In the case of optical pumping, other optical elements are used to condition and efficiently deliver the pump radiation to the active medium.

Pumping

The production of the population inversion required for a laser is called *pumping*. Pumping can be achieved either through optical excitation, direct electrical excitation, or excitation provided by a chemical reaction. Examples of optically pumped lasers include rare-earth- and transition-metal-doped, solid-state lasers. Semiconductor diode lasers are electrically pumped by reverse biasing a *p-n* junction. Gas lasers such as the CO_2 laser, the Ar-ion laser, and the KrF and ArF excimer lasers are examples of electrically excited gas discharge lasers. Chemical reaction pumped lasers include the HF and DF lasers and the oxygen-iodine laser.

Electrical

Most material processing lasers use electrical power either directly or indirectly. The type of laser including its efficiency has an important bearing on electrical power requirements. Semiconductor lasers can have a 50% electrical-to-optical efficiency. When they are used in arrays for pumping solid-state lasers, very high current supplies are required because of the low bias voltages. Argon lasers, which have very low efficiency, require high electrical powers even for modest optical power output. If the laser power source is not well controlled, fluctuations in laser power can occur, particularly if the laser is operated near an unstable point.

Mechanical

As with other optical systems, mechanical design is important for lasers. Because of the short wavelength of light, tolerances of fractions of a micrometer must be maintained for the best operational stability. If the laser is not properly designed, the fluctuations in laser power, beam quality, and direction of propagation can occur.

Efficiency

Laser efficiency is a very important characteristic. It strongly impacts the power and cooling requirements for the laser. For example, the argon-ion laser, which has an efficiency $< 10^{-3}$, has significant power and cooling system requirements. The CO_2 laser, another important gas laser used in material processing, has an efficiency of the order of 10%. Semiconductor lasers, with an electrical-to-optical efficiency of up to 50%, are the most efficient lasers. Diode pumped rare-earth-doped, solid-state lasers can have efficiencies in the 5–10% range, while lamp-pumped lasers are in the 1–2% range.

Size and Weight

Laser heads, the portion of the laser containing the laser material, the cavity resonator, and other ancillary optical elements required for laser operation, together with the equipment for applying the excitation and cooling to the laser material, typically are tens of cubic centimeters up to one or two cubic meters. The size depends primarily on the efficiency, average power, and type of medium, and to a lesser extent on the pumping method and the method used to control the spatial and temporal output. Weights vary from hundreds of grams to several hundred kilograms. Ancillary equipment such as power supplies, cooling systems, and control devices can have size and weight that are comparable to or exceed the size of the laser head.

Thermal Effects and Cooling

Optical distortion, loss of efficiency, and material failure due to thermal stress are all important problems in laser operation. Most often the temperature of the laser material must be controlled; however, heating of optical windows, cavity mirrors, and intracavity elements can cause loss of optical quality and damage. To avoid deleterious thermal effects, cooling must often be used. In the case of the Ar-ion laser, which has very low efficiency, extensive cooling must be used.

Environmental

Dust and smoke, vibration, and extreme temperatures can adversely affect laser operation. A careful assessment of the operating environment must be made. Suitably designed lasers should be used, and steps need to be taken to isolate sensitive lasers from unfavorable conditions.

Reliability and Servicing

Operational and shelf life are important considerations in evaluating laser systems. Life cycle cost must be considered, including the cost of laser maintenance. Lasers that have frequent component failures and require frequent servicing are of dubious utility. In a production environment, excessive downtime can be very costly. Redundant laser systems may be needed to reduce downtimes in critical production lines.

Safety

Lasers can be hazardous electrically, optically, and chemically. Laser power supplies can be lethal, and several deaths have occurred from careless laser operation.

ISBN 0-912035-15-3

The most important source of optical damage to humans is damage to the retina of the eye. The danger is significant because of the focusing effect of the eye and the invisibility of some of the laser wavelengths that can penetrate to the retina. Several cases of permanent retinal damage have been reported. Temporary corneal burns from ultraviolet laser light have also occurred.

Chemical hazards can also be significant, particularly for dye lasers and gas lasers such as chemical and excimer lasers. Several important laser dyes are known to be carcinogenic.

Laser systems must be designed with interlocks and other safety features. Installations should also include additional safety systems recommended by manufacturers and experts in laser safety. Workers must be equipped with appropriate personal safety equipment and properly trained in laser safety. This includes not only the operators of the lasers but also workers who face potential laser hazards. A more extensive discussion of laser safety is presented in Chapter 6.

PAUL KELLEY

1.2 Absorption of Laser Energy

The most important feature of lasers for materials processing is their ability to deliver very high values of irradiance to a selected spot on a workpiece, such as cannot be matched by any other optical source. This can produce rapid heating in a very small region. The localized nature of the heating leads to many of the applications of lasers in materials processing.

In this section we shall consider the absorption of laser energy by target materials, including the losses of energy that result from reflection, the depth within which the energy is absorbed, the focusing of laser energy to a small spot, and the usually undesirable damage that occurs when high-power laser energy is absorbed in normally transparent materials.

1.2.1 Reflection

A parameter that affects laser processing is the reflectivity of the workpiece surface. Reflectivity is a dimensionless number between zero and unity. It is defined as the ratio of the radiant power reflected from the surface to the radiant power incident on the surface. The light that is reflected is lost and is not available to produce heating within the target. This discussion summarizes briefly how the reflectivity affects absorption of laser light by the workpiece; more information on reflectivity is presented in Section 5.1.

We first consider metals. The reflectivity of metals is often high, near unity, so that much of the incident light is lost. Values of the reflectivity as a function of wavelength from the ultraviolet to the far infrared are presented in Table 1 for several metals. The values given in the table are for normal incidence of the light and for commercially pure samples of the metals with smooth, unoxidized surfaces. The exact value of the reflectivity is a function of variable conditions, including composition, surface finish, and state of oxidation.

The table shows several important features. The reflectivity of all metals becomes high at long infrared wavelengths. For infrared wavelengths, reflectivity is strongly dependent on electrical conductivity. Metals with high electrical conductivity have higher values of infrared reflectivity. The reflectivity of silver is higher than that of copper, which in turn is higher than that of steel and tungsten.

Table 1. Reflectivity of Metals

Wavelength (μm)	Metal					
	Copper	Nickel	Steel	Tungsten	Chromium	Silver
			(99% Fe, 1% C)			
0.251	0.259	0.378	0.38	0.15	0.32	0.341
0.305	0.253	0.442	0.44	0.25	0.37	0.091
0.357	0.273	0.488	0.50	0.28	0.41	0.745
0.500	0.437	0.608	0.560	0.493	0.55	0.927
0.700	0.834	0.688	0.580	–	0.56	0.946
1.0	0.901	0.720	0.63	0.623	0.57	0.964
2.0	0.955	0.835	0.77	0.846	0.63	–
3.0	0.971	0.887	0.83	0.905	0.70	0.981
5.0	0.979	0.944	–	0.940	0.81	0.981
9.0	0.984	0.956	0.93	0.905	0.92	–

Source: Adapted from G. G. Gubareff, J. E. Janssen, and R. H. Torborg, *Thermal Radiation Properties Survey,* 2nd ed., Minneapolis Honeywell Regulator Co., Minneapolis, MN, 1960.

The amount of light absorbed by a metallic surface is proportional to $1-R$, where R is the reflectivity. At the CO_2 laser wavelength of 10.6 μm, R is near unity, and $1-R$ is small. This means that much of the incident laser light is lost and that only a relatively small fraction of the energy is absorbed and available for heating the workpiece.

The difference in the value of R is especially important at long infrared wavelengths. For copper or silver at 10.6 μm, $1-R$ is about 0.02, whereas for steel it is about 0.05. Steel then absorbs about 2.5 times as much of the incident energy as more conductive metals. This means that steels are easier to weld with a CO_2 laser than are conductive metals.

The wavelength variation of R may affect the choice of laser for a particular operation. At shorter wavelengths, the factor $1-R$ is much larger than at long infrared wavelengths. This means that more light is absorbed from a shorter-wavelength laser for equal irradiance incident on the surface. In some cases it will be preferable to use a Nd:YAG laser rather than a CO_2 laser, especially for conductive metals. We note also that the reflectivity may be even lower in the ultraviolet. This fact may favor the use of excimer lasers for some operations.

It is possible for the initially high reflectivity to decrease during the laser interaction. This allows the laser energy to be absorbed more effectively by the material, because the average reflectivity during the irradiation may be lower than the initial value of the reflectivity. This variation of reflectivity during irradiation is discussed further in Section 5.4.3. Because of this decrease of reflectivity, CO_2 lasers can be effective for welding of metals that are not highly conductive, like steel. For high-conductivity metals, like copper, the use of a shorter-wavelength laser may be desirable.

For nonmetals, the wavelength variation of reflectivity is more complicated than for metals and the values may be lower. Table 2 presents values of reflectivity for some materials. There is no systematic increase of reflectivity with wavelength, as there is with metals, and in some cases, reflectivity is low and the light can be effectively absorbed. For a specific application, the laser should be chosen so that the workpiece has high absorption at the laser wavelength. For many nonmetallic materials, the value of reflectivity is low at the CO_2 laser wavelength, so that CO_2 lasers are used for many applications involving processing of these materials. As an example, for processing alumina ceramic, CO_2 laser light is absorbed well, but Nd:YAG laser light is reflected.

1.2.2 Absorption

When light strikes an opaque surface, it is absorbed within a thin layer located near the surface. The light is absorbed according to the equation

$$I(x) = I_0 \exp(-ax) \quad (1)$$

where I_0 is the incident intensity, $I(x)$ is the intensity reaching depth x from the surface, and a is the absorption coefficient, with units of reciprocal centimeters. The light (at least 63% of it) is absorbed within a depth of $1/a$ from the surface. Then it can be transported to greater depth by thermal conduction. See Section 5.4 for more details.

The absorption coefficients for metals are typically large. Table 3 shows values of absorption coefficient for a number of metals at various wavelengths in the ultraviolet and visible spectra. The values are relatively large, of the order of 10^5 or more; this means the light will be absorbed within a depth less than 10^{-5} cm from the surface. The variation of the absorption coefficient with wavelength in this region is typically rather slow.

For nonmetals, the absorption coefficient can vary significantly with wavelength. For transparent materials, it is near zero. For semiconductors, it will be large at shorter wavelengths and then drop rapidly as the wavelength increases past the band edge of the semiconductor. Thus, for scribing silicon, the Nd:YAG laser wavelength is well absorbed but the CO_2 laser wavelength is absorbed poorly.

Conversely, almost all organic materials have high absorption near 10 μm, but many are transparent or weakly absorbing near 1 μm. Hence, CO_2 lasers are often a good choice for processing organic materials.

1.2.3 Focusing of Laser Light

The localization of laser heating effects is also strongly influenced by the fact that laser light can be focused to a very small spot. This leads to high values of irradiance, even if the power is not extremely high. Of course one cannot focus the beam to an infinitesimal point. There is a minimum spot size that is determined ultimately by diffraction. In any optical system, there is a limit, termed the *diffraction limit*, which determines the minimum focal area and hence the maximum irradiance that can be attained.

Table 2. Reflectivity of Some Nonmetals

Wavelength (μm)	0.60	4.4	8.8
Asphalt	0.148	-	-
Indiana limestone	0.429	0.203	0.050
Quartz powder	0.810	0.079	0.090
Slate	0.067	0.134	0.200
White marble, unpolished	0.535	0.064	0.051
Black velvet	0.0187	0.037	0.027
MgO white pigment	0.86	0.16	0.03

Source: Adapted from G. G. Gubareff, J. E. Janssen, and R. H. Torborg, *Thermal Radiation Properties Survey*, 2nd ed., Minneapolis Honeywell Regulator Co., Minneapolis, MN, 1960.

Table 3. Absorption Coefficients (in cm^{-1}) for Metals

Wavelength (μm)	Metal					
	Aluminum	Gold	Silver	Copper	Nickel	Iron
0.231	-	-	6.04 X 10^5	5.71 X 10^5	-	-
0.257	-	-	-	-	6.94 X 10^5	4.27 X 10^5
0.298	-	-	-	4.43 X 10^5	-	-
0.398	-	-	-	-	5.37 X 10^5	3.50 X 10^5
0.400	-	3.55 X 10^5	-	-	-	-
0.431	8.31 X 10^5	-	-	-	-	-
0.450	-	-	6.67 X 10^5	5.31 X 10^5	-	-
0.460	-	3.28 X 10^5	-	-	-	-
0.486	8.14 X 10^5	-	-	-	-	-
0.500	-	4.70 X 10^5	7.39 X 10^5	5.10 X 10^5	-	-
0.508	-	-	-	-	5.10 X 10^5	3.17 X 10^5
0.527	8.08 X 10^5	-	-	-	-	-
0.540	-	10.05 X 10^5	-	-	-	-
0.550	-	-	7.56 X 10^5	-	-	-
0.589	7.81 X 10^5	-	7.76 X 10^5	-	4.57 X 10^5	2.26 X 10^5
0.600	-	-	-	11.54 X 10^5	-	-
0.657	7.50 X 10^5	-	-	-	-	-
0.660	-	21.32 X 10^5	-	10.99 X 10^5	-	-
0.668	-	-	-	-	4.10 X 10^5	2.03 X 10^5
0.700	-	24.41 X 10^5	-	-	-	-

Source: Adapted from G. G. Gubareff, J. E. Janssen, and R. H. Torborg, *Thermal Radiation Properties Survey,* 2nd ed., Minneapolis Honeywell Regulator Co., Minneapolis, MN, 1960.

Focusing of laser beams will be considered in detail in Section 3.3. For this section, we point out that the equation

$$d = f\theta \quad (2)$$

where f is the focal length of the lens used for focusing and θ is the beam divergence angle, is commonly used to estimate the minimum diameter d of the focal spot. Table 4 presents some values for d determined by use of this equation for a beam divergence angle of 0.001 rad, a value that is typical of many lasers. Also the values of focal area and the irradiance for a power of 1000 W are presented. The parameters assumed for this calculation are modest, but the very high values of irradiance are striking. The use of short-focal-length lenses is required to produce small focal spots. But it is easy to produce very high values of irradiance with simple optics.

Lens aberrations must also be considered; aberrations will degrade the performance of the focusing optics and increase the size of the focal area. For a monochromatic, collimated laser beam incident along the axis of the lens, many of the aberrations considered in elementary optics are unimportant. The most significant lens aberration is spherical aberration, which causes the light rays from a point source that enter the lens at different

Table 4. Calculated Focal Diameter, Focal Area, and Irradiance for a Focused Laser Beam

Lens focal length (cm)	Focal diameter (μm)	Focal area (cm^2)	Irradiance (W/cm^2)
10	100	7.8 x 10^{-5}	1.27 X 10^7
5	50	1.96 X 10^{-5}	5.29 X 10^7
2	20	3.14 x 10^{-6}	3.18 x 10^8
1	10	0.78 x 10^{-6}	1.27 x 10^9

Beam divergence 0.001 rad, power 1000 W.

ISBN 0-912035-15-3

distances from its axis to be focused to a blurred circle, rather than a single point. Spherical aberration becomes more serious as the focal length of the lens decreases. This fact sets a practical lower limit on the focal length that can be used.

Spherical aberration can be reduced by the use of best-shape lenses, compound (multielement) lenses, or aspheric lenses with specially ground shapes. In this section we consider only single spherical lenses. For use in the visible or near-infrared portions of the spectrum, a planoconvex lens, with the convex side toward the laser, gives spherical aberration near the minimum. In the far-infrared spectrum, near 10 μm, the optimum lens shape is a meniscus (concave-convex) lens, again with the convex side toward the laser. Under favorable conditions, one can focus a laser beam to a spot of single-wavelength dimension.

To summarize methods for focusing the beam to a small spot, first one should use a laser with a Gaussian beam profile. This minimizes the beam divergence angle. Then one should choose a lens with as short a focal length as possible, consistent with the desired depth of focus and the lens aberrations. The shape of the lens should be chosen to give minimum spherical aberration, that is, planoconvex in the visible and near infrared and meniscus (concave-convex) in the far infrared.

1.2.4 Laser Damage

High-power laser pulses can cause sudden, catastrophic damage to the laser material itself and also to mirrors, lenses, and other optical components in the beam. The damage phenomena are most often observed with Q-switched and mode-locked lasers, with short pulse duration. Lasers with longer pulse durations are less susceptible to damage. Common lower-power gas lasers, like helium-neon and argon, are not vulnerable to dramatic catastrophic damage of the type discussed here.

Crystals, mirrors, and other optical components exposed to laser light with high values of irradiance all show degradation, more or less rapidly. This fact is of practical economic interest to users of lasers. Many of the components in high-power lasers and components used for beam delivery are expensive. so that frequent replacement can be an economic hardship.

High-power laser light can produce damage in materials that are transparent to the light at low intensity. Optical damage or optical breakdown begins at some threshold value of laser irradiance. Below the threshold, the light is transmitted through the material, apparently without harmful effect to the material. But if the irradiance increases above the threshold value, catastrophic breakdown occurs and produces damage in the material. The breakdown is usually accompanied by a flash of light and by a sharp sound. The resulting damage takes many different forms, including pitting, cracking, formation of internal voids, and vaporization of material. The optical component, whether laser rod, window, or lens, has its performance much degraded. The damage grows worse as additional laser pulses are incident on the component.

The value of the breakdown threshold depends in a complicated way on many factors, including the nature of the material, the previous history of laser irradiation, the wavelength of the laser light, the duration of the exposure, the presence of impurities and imperfections in the material, and the surface condition. Even for nominally identical conditions, the breakdown threshold may exhibit statistical fluctuations. In many cases, the statistical fluctuations may be small enough that one can define the breakdown threshold reasonably well.

Voluminous literature exists describing laser-induced damage, the value of the damage threshold, and the physical mechanisms that produce it. An annual conference, the so-called "Laser Damage Conference" (more exactly Laser-Induced Damage in Optical Materials) is held in Boulder, CO, and a volume of each conference's proceedings is published. It is not the intent of this section to provide a complete review of the phenomena involved, but we shall summarize some pertinent conclusions.

It is now generally believed that optical breakdown of transparent materials is similar to dielectric breakdown caused by a high electric field. Dielectric breakdown of an insulating material involves so-called avalanche ionization. This process starts with a very small number of free electrons in the material. The electrons are accelerated by the electric field of the light wave, collide with bound electrons, and free them from their parent atoms, producing more free electrons in the material. These electrons also gain energy from the light wave and produce still more free electrons. This avalanche process yields an absorbing plasma that can absorb a large fraction of the laser energy, producing damage in the material.

Multiphoton absorption of laser energy is also involved in breakdown of nominally transparent optical materials. When the photon energy becomes greater than half the band gap energy of the transparent material, two-photon absorption becomes possible. Models that include both avalanche ionization and excitation of electrons across the band gap of an insulating material by simultaneous absorption of several quanta give better agreement with experiment than models that include only one of these mechanisms.

The threshold for damage usually is lower at the surface of a material than in the bulk. This results from the presence of small imperfections, such as scratches, pits, and voids, near the surface. Suitable polished surfaces free of defects have shown breakdown thresholds comparable to those of bulk material.

Some rough rules of thumb have been formulated for laser damage. These rules are commonly quoted for determining how the damage threshold scales with important parameters. One should note that many experiments have supported these approximate rules, but there have been other experiments whose results have deviated from them.

1. Wavelength scaling. The laser damage threshold often scales as the inverse fourth power of the laser wavelength. Thus ultraviolet lasers are especially susceptible to laser damage.

TABLE 5. Damage Thresholds (J/cm²) for Thin Film Optical Coatings

Material	Thickness[a]	Wavelength (mm)							
		1.06		0.53		0.353		0.26	
		Pulse duration (ns)							
		5	15	5	15	5	15	5	15
MgF_2	1	9.2	13.1	3.6	7.9	3.6	4.2	2.9	2.4
	1/2	-	15.8	6.9	12.1	-	-	-	2.0
	1/4	11.5	16.9	7.2	14.4	2.7	4.7	1.9	2.9
	1/8	27.4	37.0	8.9	13.9	2.3	5.4	1.3	3.0
Al_2O_3	1	11.4	15.1	-	13.2	3.2	6.6	1.5	2.3
	1/2	-	16.3	6.5	11.7	-	-	-	-
	1/4	13.5	20.1	7.3	13.2	2.7	6.0	2.2	2.0
	1/8	20.0	21.5	8.5	14.0	2.9	5.9	1.7	2.3
MgO	1	10.2	9.8	-	11.4	-	-	-	-
	1/2	14.9	15.0	6.1	10.6	-	-	-	-
	1/4	-	-	6.8	16.2	2.8	3.9	1.3	2.3
	1/8	12.2	12.8	10.6	14.2	2.8	4.3	1.6	2.6
TiO_2	1	8.8	-	4.3	-	0.1	-	-	-
	1/2	11.4	-	4.8	-	-	-	-	-
	1/4	14.9	13.8	6.5	11.8	0.1	-	-	-
	1/8	10.0	9.8	6.4	10.8	0.6	-	-	-
SiO_2	1	-	-	-	-	-	-	-	-
	1/2	-	7.8	-	-	-	-	-	-
	1/4	22.4	45.0	9.4	19.6	5.6	10.7	0.9	1.6
	1/8	41.4	47.3	21.1	48.4	-	13.5	2.2	2.5

Source: T. W. Walker, A. H. Guenther, and P. E. Nielsen, *IEEE J. Quantum Electron.* QE-17, 2041 (1981).
[a] In units of 1.06 μm.

2. Surface roughness scaling. The damage threshold for a surface increases as the inverse square root of the root mean square of the surface roughness.

3. Pulse duration scaling. The damage threshold scales with the square root of the duration of the irradiation. The damage threshold in terms of the laser energy per unit area increases proportionately to the square root of the duration. The threshold in terms of the irradiance decreases proportionately to the square root of the duration. Thus, if a certain total energy per unit area is to be delivered, one should make the pulse duration as long as possible to avoid damage. If a certain peak power per unit area is needed, one should make the pulse duration as short as possible.

In order to show specific examples of the type of data available and the values of damage threshold that have been measured, Tables 5 to 7 present values of laser damage thresholds. Table 5

Table 6. Damage Threshold as a Function of Pulse Duration for a Common Nd-Doped Laser Glass, at a Wavelength of 1.06 μm

Pulse duration (ns)	Damage threshold (GW/cm²)
0.02	750
0.12	183
2	17
40	1.32

Source: Based on data from Owens-Illinois, Inc.

Table 7. Damage Thresholds of Optical Materials for 1-ns-Duration Pulses

Material	Wavelength (μm)	Threshold (GW/cm²)
NaCl	10.6	20
SiO_2	1.06	360
SiO_2	0.53	200
LiF	0.26	2

is relevant to thin film optical coatings for the indicated laser wavelengths and pulse durations. Table 6 presents data for a common type of Nd-doped laser glass for a wavelength of 1.06 μm. Table 7 presents typical values for damage thresholds for optical materials for a 1-ns duration laser pulse for several wavelengths. Each material is transparent in the indicated wavelength at low laser intensity.

This discussion is a very brief introduction to the complex subject of catastrophic breakdown of nominally transparent materials produced by high laser power. It has economic importance because lenses, windows, and other components placed in the path of a laser beam will be damaged if the irradiance becomes too high. The components then will have to be replaced. The user should determine the damage threshold for the particular materials and keep the laser irradiance below the threshold for damage.

References
H. E. Bennett et al. (Eds.), "Laser-Induced Damage in Optical Materials: 1991," SPIE Proceedings, Vol. 1624, SPIE, Bellingham, WA (1992). This is the proceedings of a conference (the so-called "Laser Damage Conference") held annually in Boulder, CO, and is one of an extensive series of proceedings of this conference.
R. M. Wood, "Laser Damage in Optical Materials," Adam Hilger, Bristol and Boston (1986).

JOHN F. READY

1.3 Laser Configurations

A laser generally consists of three components: (1) an active gain medium with energy levels that can be selectively populated, (2) a pump to produce population inversion between some of these energy levels, and (usually) (3) a resonant electromagnetic cavity (resonator) that contains the active medium and provides feedback to maintain the coherence of the electromagnetic field. This section starts by looking at the effect of the cavity on the properties of the output radiation. It then reviews the temporal behavior of lasers, and concludes with a brief survey of several different types of gain media.

1.3.1 Modal Characteristics

The electromagnetic field in a resonator has well-defined modes that have patterns both transverse to and along the cavity axis. The transverse modes determine the spatial profile of the output beam; the axial modes give rise to the spectral performance.

Spatial Profile

Some lasers employ waveguides to confine the radiation to the amplifying medium and to force the laser to operate in a single transverse mode. Notable examples are semiconductor and fiber lasers. More frequently, laser resonators are open in the sense that the transverse structure is defined only by axial mirrors or lenses. Open resonators formed with convergent optics (optics that confine light near the cavity axis) are "stable," and generally have the lowest diffraction losses. Resonators formed with divergent optics are "unstable." Stable and unstable resonators are illustrated schematically in Figure 1.

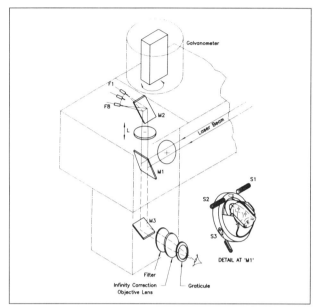

Figure 1. Schematic illustration of stable and unstable resonators.

A stable laser cavity confines the oscillating fields near the axis of the cavity, typically in well-defined modes with a Gaussian (lowest-order, TEM_{00} mode), Hermite-Gaussian (higher-order, rectangular symmetry), or Laguerre-Gaussian (higher-order, cylindrical symmetry) profile. Some of the low-order modes for a stable resonator with square and circular symmetry are shown in Figure 2. The TEM_{mn} indicates that the modes have nearly transverse electric and magnetic fields with, for the Hermite-Gaussian modes, m nodes vertically and n nodes horizontally. For the Laguerre-Gaussian modes, it indicates n nodes radially and $2m$ nodal lines running radially outward from the mode axis. A linear superposition of two like higher-order circularly symmetric modes, one rotated by 90° about the axis relative to the other, is designated by an asterisk. For example, the TEM_{01*} mode is made up of two TEM_{01} modes, and has a "donut" profile. This mode is often used in material processing.

The intensity profile of the lowest-order (TEM_{00}), Gaussian mode is given by

$$I = I_0 \exp(-2r/\omega_0)$$

where I_0 is the intensity at the center of the beam, r is the radial coordinate, and ω_0 is the Gaussian beam waist. Typically, this mode has the largest net gain and is the first transverse mode to oscillate. Single-transverse-mode lasers operating in the TEM_{00} mode have optimal "spatial brightness." The divergence (half-

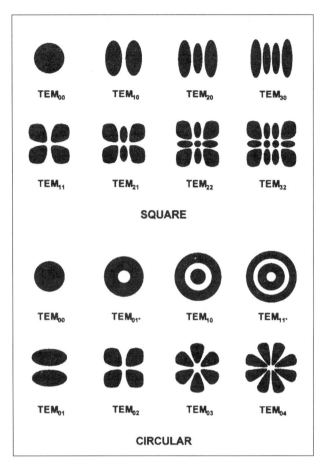

Figure 2. Low-order transverse modes for a stable resonator with square and circular symmetry.

Many unstable resonators use hard-edged mirrors, as illustrated in Figure 1. The disadvantages of these cavities are:

1. The output beam is in the form of a ring with a dark hole in the middle;

2. The amplitude profile is not as smooth as for a stable cavity; and

3. The cavity is often more sensitive to perturbations than a stable cavity.

These disadvantages can be overcome with a variable-reflectivity output coupler for the unstable cavity.

Spectral Performance

Cavity modes have a frequency spacing that is determined primarily by the cavity length. The spacing between longitudinal (axial) modes (free spectral range) is the inverse of the round-trip transit time for light in the cavity. For a standing-wave gas laser, the spacing is $c/2L_c$, where c is the velocity of light. Laser operation tends to occur at the longitudinal-mode frequency (or frequencies) closest to the gain peak. For most lasers, the frequency spacing between adjacent longitudinal modes is much less than the gain bandwidth. Consequently, lasers tend to oscillate at several frequencies simultaneously.

There are many techniques for obtaining single-frequency operation from a laser. Several of these involve introducing an element into the cavity such that the cavity sees a frequency-dependent loss, thereby decreasing the net gain bandwidth and selecting an individual longitudinal cavity mode. Examples of such elements are a prism, a grating, a Fabry-Perot etalon, and the combination of a birefringent filter and a polarizing element (Lyot filter). In some cases, a cavity may require more than one device in order to obtain enough frequency selectivity to ensure single-frequency operation.

Single-frequency operation has also been obtained by reducing the length of the cavity so that the longitudinal mode spacing is comparable to, or less than, the gain bandwidth. This is most easily done with gas lasers, which have a narrow gain bandwidth, but has also been achieved in very short solid-state lasers, sometimes referred to as microchip lasers.

Alternatively, single-mode operation can be achieved in a laser with a homogeneously broadened gain medium by reducing or eliminating the effects of spatial hole burning. A unidirectional ring cavity has a uniform optical intensity within the cavity, rather than the sinusoidal intensity distribution of a standing-wave cavity. Spatial hole burning is therefore eliminated, and such a laser may operate at a single frequency well above threshold.

Lasers can have very narrow linewidths and, therefore, very high "spectral brightness" (power per unit spectral interval). Linewidths as narrow as a fraction of a hertz have been obtained (one hertz stability corresponds to a fractional stability of about 2×10^{-15} for visible lasers).

angle) θ_d of the output beam is near the minimum value for the spot size of the laser on the output mirror, and is given by

$$\theta_d = \left(\frac{\lambda}{\pi \omega_0}\right)$$

where λ is the oscillating wavelength. Such a beam is said to be diffraction limited.

For a stable cavity, the beam radius for fundamental-transverse-mode operation is of the order

$$\omega_0 \approx \left(\frac{L_c \lambda}{2\pi}\right)^{1/2}$$

where L_c is the cavity length. For a 1-m-long cavity oscillating at 1 μm, the beam radius is ~0.5 mm. For multimode operation, the beam radius will be slightly larger.

The small beam size of a stable cavity limits the amount of power (or energy) that can be obtained from the laser. Unstable cavities can have much larger beam diameters and, therefore, produce much higher output powers (or energies). Consequently, they are often used when high output power (or energy) is required.

ISBN 0-912035-15-3

The first step in achieving narrow-line operation is to design the laser to operate in a single longitudinal and transverse mode. Once single-mode operation has been obtained, the linewidth of the output is determined by technical and fundamental noise. Technical noise arises from sources that can be controlled, such as power-supply fluctuations, variations in the thermal environment, environmental vibrations, etc. Fundamental noise arises from sources that cannot be eliminated, such as spontaneous emission and fundamental thermal fluctuations. The random effect of noise causes the laser frequency to drift. The influence of noise can often be reduced by adjusting controllable parameters such as cavity lifetime. In addition, the frequency drift can be reduced by measuring the frequency of the laser and providing feedback to adjust the cavity mode frequency to compensate for the drift.

Frequency tuning of a laser can occur in one of two ways. If the mode spacing of the laser cavity is much less than the gain bandwidth, the cavity is capable of supporting several longitudinal modes, each at a different frequency. A single frequency is then selected by inserting an element into the cavity such that the cavity sees a frequency-dependent loss. In most of the examples listed above, a small repositioning of the frequency-selective element results in a new longitudinal mode (and hence a new operating frequency) being selected. The frequency-selective element is used to select one of the several cavity modes, and discrete tuning is obtained. Fast tuning can be obtained using electro-optic frequency-dependent components.

The other way a laser can be tuned is to change the frequency of a given cavity mode by changing the optical length of the cavity. Since the cavity length can be changed continuously, this leads to continuous tuning. This type of tuning is usually limited by the free spectral range of the cavity. Once the cavity modes are shifted by a full free spectral range, an adjacent cavity mode is positioned at the frequency where the initial mode started. For the same reasons that the initial mode was originally favored, the adjacent mode is now favored, and the laser will have a tendency to mode hop back to the original frequency.

Single-frequency operation and accurate wavelength control are desirable for many applications, including holography and spectroscopy. They usually result in reduced output power, however, and are typically not required for material processing.

Polarization

For each spatial mode of a resonator, there are two orthogonal polarization modes. Typically, these modes are linearly polarized. It is often desirable for a laser to oscillate in a single linear polarization. In some solid-state lasers, the polarization is fixed by the gain medium. For lasers with isotropic gain media, an intracavity polarizing element, such as a Brewster plate, is often used to fix the polarization. In single-frequency devices, the presence of any tilted optical element may be sufficient to polarize a laser because the reflectivity of surfaces is often different for *s*- and *p*-polarized light; only a small amount of discrimination is needed to select one of two frequency-degenerate polarizations.

1.3.2 Temporal Behavior

It is often desirable to control the amplitude of the output of a laser either in a continuous way or by pulsing it. Short pulses of laser radiation can be made in a variety of ways including gain switching, Q-switching, cavity dumping, and mode locking.

Relaxation Oscillations

Relaxation oscillations occur whenever the population inversion of a laser is disturbed from its equilibrium value. They are a result of the coupling between the population inversion and the photon density within the laser cavity. For a single-mode laser, a small disturbance in the inversion density results in damped oscillations with an oscillation frequency

$$\omega = \left(\frac{P/P_{thresh}-1}{\tau_c \tau}\right)^{1/2}$$

and a damping constant

$$\tau_0 = 2\tau \, \frac{P_{thresh}}{P}$$

where P is the pump power, P_{thresh} is the pump power required to reach threshold, τ_c is the cold-cavity lifetime, and τ is the lifetime of the upper laser level. Note that if $1/\tau_0 > \omega$, the oscillations are overdamped and spiking will not occur. Although this condition is not satisfied in solid-state lasers, it is common in gas lasers.

Amplitude Modulation

The output power of a laser can be controlled by changing the pump power, the output coupling, or the intracavity loss. This type of amplitude modulation is usually limited to frequencies below the frequency of the relaxation oscillations. Near the relaxation frequency there is resonant enhancement of the modulation response; above the relaxation frequency the response rolls off.

Methods used for direct amplitude modulation of a laser may have the side effect of introducing frequency modulation as well. For example, changing the pump power affects the thermal load on the gain medium, and therefore the temperature. This, in turn, affects the refractive index, changing the optical length of the cavity and the oscillating frequency. For applications where frequency stability is critical, it is often better to modulate the laser power external to the cavity.

Long-Pulse Operation

Long-pulse, or quasi-CW, operation refers to a pulsed laser with a pulse duration long enough for all relevant parameters within the system to come to their steady-state value. Although the behavior of the system is CW-like at the end of the pulse, it can be quite different at the beginning of the pulse.

When a single-mode laser is rapidly turned on, there is often regular spiking at the beginning of the pulse. The process is damped, however, and with time, the intensity of the spikes decreases. Spiking eventually gives way to damped relaxation oscillations and finally CW-like behavior. This behavior is illustrated in Figure 3. In a multimode laser, the interaction between modes often leads to mode hopping, mode beating, and very irregular spiking that may never damp out.

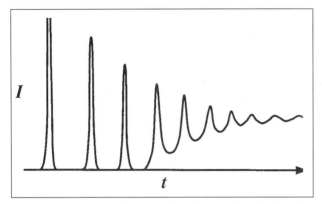

Figure 3. Illustration of the intensity spikes and oscillations that typically occur when a single-mode laser is rapidly turned on. *I*, intensity; *t*, time.

Gain-Switched Operation

The initial spike that occurs when a laser is rapidly turned on often reaches an intensity well in excess of the CW intensity of the laser. This relatively short output pulse contains most of the energy that was deposited by the pump during the pulse buildup time. The pump can then be turned off before depositing energy for a second output pulse. The technique of obtaining short pulses from a laser by pulsing the pump source is known as *gain switching*.

Q-Switched Operation

A common technique used to obtain short, high-peak-power pulses from a laser is Q switching. With this technique, a large population inversion is obtained in a relatively lossy cavity. The cavity losses are then quickly decreased so that the inversion density is well in excess of its new threshold value. The large inversion density allows an intracavity optical field to develop rapidly. This field then depletes the population inversion and turns itself off. The cavity loss is subsequently increased to prevent the development of a second pulse. This technique is known as Q switching since the quality factor, or Q, of the optical cavity is changed.

Q switching relies on the fact that the lifetime of the population inversion is much longer than the output pulse. The gain medium is therefore able to store energy, which can be quickly released in a short pulse of light.

The minimum pulse width (full width at half-maximum) that can be obtained from a Q-switched laser is

$$t_w = \frac{8.1 t_{rt}}{\ln(G_{rt})}$$

where t_{rt} is the round-trip transit time of light in the resonator and G_{rt} is the round-trip small-signal gain. (The same minimum pulse width applies to gain-switched lasers if G_{rt} is interpreted as the round-trip gain just before the output pulse forms.) Typically, the buildup time of the pulse is an order of magnitude longer than the pulse, and the output pulse may contain up to 95% of the available energy in the gain medium. The duration of Q-switched pulses is typically in the nanosecond range.

Methods for Q switching a laser include the use of electro-optic shutters, mechanical devices, and acousto-optic Q switches. Passive Q switching can be obtained with an intracavity saturable absorber. To obtain optimal performance from a Q-switched laser, it must be possible to change the cavity Q in a time that is comparable to, or shorter than, the pulse buildup time. Q-switched pulses are frequently used in materials-processing applications, like resistor trimming.

Cavity-Dumped Operation

Cavity dumping allows the optical energy in a laser cavity to be output in a time comparable to the round-trip transit time of light in the cavity. The concept is to rapidly (within a cavity round-trip time) introduce a large output coupling (nearly 100%) into a cavity that previously had no output coupling. Methods for cavity dumping include the use of an electro-optic Pockels cell and polarizing beam splitter, and acousto-optic devices.

Mode-Locked Operation

Mode locking refers to the situation when the phases of several cavity modes are fixed (or locked) with respect to each other such that the electric fields add coherently and constructively for a short period of time. This allows the generation of a train of high-peak-power, ultrashort pulses, with durations typically in the femtosecond to picosecond range. When the phases of all of the modes are locked so that the output pulse has its minimum possible width, the pulse is referred to as a transform-limited pulse, since its temporal profile is the Fourier transform of its spectral profile. This need not be the case — it is possible to obtain longer pulses, but not shorter pulses.

The spacing between the output pulses of a mode-locked laser is equal to the round-trip transit time of light within the cavity. (Harmonic mode locking can be used to produce two or more equally spaced pulses per cavity round-trip time.) Therefore, the maximum pulse energy that can be obtained from a CW mode-locked laser is equal to the energy deposited during the round-trip time. Mode locking can be combined with Q switching or cavity dumping to increase the pulse energy, and peak power, that can be obtained. It is worth noting that, unlike the other pulsed schemes described in this section, a mode-locked laser is a CW device and there is phase coherence between pulses.

Mode locking can be obtained actively or passively. Active mode locking can be broken into two categories, AM mode locking and FM mode locking. In AM mode locking, the loss of some element in the laser cavity is modulated at the round-trip cavity frequency. Light circulating in the cavity will see less loss, and therefore more net gain, when it is incident at the loss element during the time of minimum loss. This encourages short-pulsed operation and mode locking can be induced. The same result occurs if the gain of the cavity is modulated. Gain modulation through modulation of the pump source is known as *synchronous pumping*.

In FM mode locking, the optical length of the laser cavity (length or refractive index) is modulated at the round-trip cavity frequency. For simplicity, consider the case where one of the mirrors is moved sinusoidally along the direction of the cavity axis. Light incident on the mirror during its motion will be Doppler shifted. Consequently, it will not reproduce itself after one round trip, and will not produce a coherent oscillating mode. Light incident on the mirror at its turning points (maximum or minimum cavity length) sees a stationary mirror and will not experience a Doppler shift. The net result is that mode-locked pulses will tend to form. Modulation of the refractive index at some point in the cavity has the same effect. The output of an FM mode-locked laser tends to have a frequency chirp, and not be transform limited.

Passive mode locking can occur when a laser cavity contains a nonlinear optical element, such as a saturable absorber. In this case, the more intense the light incident on the saturable absorber, the less the total absorption. The total loss of the cavity is therefore minimized by putting all the energy into short pulses. This is essentially self-induced AM mode locking. A similar effect is obtained by putting a Kerr lens and an aperture within the cavity. Other techniques include the use of interferometric elements containing nonlinear media.

Passive mode locking must be initiated by the presence of a pulse within the cavity. If the optical intensity within the cavity is uniform in time, there is no loss or gain element that is modulated at the round-trip cavity frequency to induce mode locking. Noise, however, is capable of introducing a small amplitude modulation on the optical field. In some lasers, this small modulation is sufficient to start the mode-locking process. Such lasers are referred to as *self starting*. In other systems, a pulse (or AM modulation) must be intentionally introduced into the cavity to start the mode-locking process. Once started, however, mode locking can persist for long times.

The introduction of an appropriate nonlinear optical element into a laser cavity is not sufficient to guarantee mode locking. For passive mode locking to work, the relative phases of all the longitudinal modes must remain constant after completing a round trip in the laser cavity. One effect that can destroy the phase relationship, and therefore prevent mode locking, is dispersion. Passively mode-locked lasers must be dispersion free if mode locking is to occur. To accomplish this, prisms are often introduced into the laser cavity to compensate the dispersion of other intracavity elements, such as the gain medium. In a properly compensated cavity, non-mode-locked operation can be unstable.

Another effect that can destroy the phase relationship between the spectral components in a mode-locked pulse train is spontaneous emission, or noise. The phase of the noise is unrelated to the phase of the oscillating mode. The net phase is shifted when the two are combined.

The duration of mode-locked pulses, typically between several femtoseconds and several hundred picoseconds, is too short for most materials-processing applications; such lasers are not frequently encountered in materials processing.

Pulse Compression

External pulse-compression techniques can be used to reduce the pulse width of a laser system. The optical Kerr effect (change in refractive index proportional to optical intensity) can cause short pulses, typically 0.1–10 ps in duration from a mode-locked laser, to acquire a frequency chirp (i.e., change in frequency during the pulse). By sending the chirped pulses through a frequency-dispersive delay line, such as a grating or prism pair, pulses as short as 5 fs can be obtained. Pulses of similar duration have been obtained directly from mode-locked lasers — external pulse compression can be used to obtain extremely short pulses from a laser system with a gain bandwidth that is too narrow to support the direct generation of the pulse. Again, such short pulses have not often been used in materials processing.

1.3.3 Survey of Active Media

A rich variety of physical systems has been exploited to produce laser radiation over a five-decade range of wavelengths. This section briefly describes some of the most significant of these. Several of these laser systems, the ones most important for materials processing, are discussed in detail in Chapter 2.

Gas Lasers

Several methods have been used to produce population inversion and lasing in gaseous media. Inversion can exist between energy levels of the constituents in an electrical discharge. The most efficient and powerful of the molecular gas-discharge lasers is the CO_2 laser. One version of this laser makes use of a dilute mixture of CO_2 in N_2. The N_2 molecules are excited to their first excited vibrational state by collisions with electrons. This excitation is resonantly transferred by molecular collisions to preferentially excite CO_2 molecules to a particular vibrational state. These molecules, in turn, undergo radiative transitions to lower vibrational levels. The vibrational transitions couple to rotational transitions to give rise to clusters of potential lasing lines with wavelengths near 10.6 and 9.6 μm. The gas-discharge CO_2 laser has better than 10% electrical-to-optical conversion efficiency and is capable of producing CW output powers of many kilowatts. CO_2 lasers are discussed in detail in Section 2.1. Other important molecular gas-discharge lasers make use of vibration-rotational or pure rotational transitions of H_2O, CO (see Section 2.5.1), and HCN, and produce emission at (78 μm, 119 μm), 5.3 μm, and (337 μm, 311 μm), respectively.

Lasers operating at shorter wavelengths make use of transitions between electronic states. One subclass of these makes use of neutral atoms in gaseous or vapor form. The neutral-noble-gas lasers oscillate in the infrared (1–10 μm), with the notable exception of the He-Ne laser. In the He-Ne laser, a gas discharge excites He atoms to their first excited level. This excitation is resonantly transferred to the Ne. The Ne decays radiatively to a lower electronic state, giving rise to CW laser emission in the red at 632.8 nm with an output power up to tens of milliwatts. Other Ne transitions produce emission at 543 nm, 1.15 μm, and 3.39 μm.

Neutral-metal-vapor lasers provide intense sources of pulsed radiation in the visible. Copper-vapor lasers produce average output powers of tens of watts in high-repetition-rate (up to ~20 kHz) pulsed operation (~50-ns pulse duration) at 510 and 578 nm. Gold-vapor lasers operate in the red at 628 nm. Metal-vapor lasers are discussed in Section 2.5.2.

Ion lasers tend to operate at shorter wavelengths than neutral-gas lasers. The argon-ion laser produces tens of watts of CW blue-green output in clusters of lines near 488 and 514 nm. The He-Cd laser produces 50–100 mW of CW output at 325 and 416 nm. Ion lasers are discussed in Section 2.5.3. Gas-discharge lasers have also been made to operate further into the UV, but special problems arise in this frequency range; these are discussed below.

So far, all the lasers discussed are pumped through a gas discharge. A number of other methods of generating laser radiation in gases have also been devised. UV photodecomposition of CH_3I (methyl iodide) has produced powerful pulses of laser radiation at 1.3 μm. Photolytic iodine lasers are discussed in Section 2.5.5. In the gas-dynamic laser, a nonthermal distribution of molecular vibrational energy levels is produced by the rapid expansion of a hot gas through a nozzle. This method has produced tens of kilowatts of CW output at 10.6 μm from CO_2 gas. In chemical lasers, two molecular species react to produce a product that is left in an excited vibration-rotation state. The product returns to the ground state radiatively. One example is the HF (DF) laser, which oscillates in the 2.5- to 3.5-μm region when H_2 (D_2) and F_2 gases react.

Other types of gas lasers include TEA (transversely excited atmospheric-pressure) lasers, electron-beam-excited lasers, UV-preionized electric-discharge lasers, and optically pumped lasers. CO_2 laser radiation has been used to pump other gases, such as NH_3 (output at 291 μm) and CH_3OH (output at 164 and 205.3 μm), yielding far-infrared emission.

Solid-State Lasers

The term solid-state laser, as it is used here, excludes semiconductor lasers. While semiconductors are solids, they are differentiated from laser media involving optically active ions in ionic hosts because of their markedly different physical and technological characteristics. Semiconductor lasers are discussed in a separate subsection below.

Most solid-state lasers are derived from optically pumped transitions among electronic levels of ions in a crystal or other solid-state host. One important subclass of solid-state gain media includes crystals and glasses doped with rare-earth ions. The most extensively developed of the rare-earth lasers are the Nd:YAG (Nd^{3+} in $Y_3Al_5O_{12}$) laser and the Nd-glass (Nd^{3+} in glass) laser, oscillating in the vicinity of 1.06 μm. Nd:YAG lasers have produced CW outputs in excess of 1 kW, several joules in low-repetition-rate (10 Hz) pulsed operation, and tens of millijoules in high-repetition-rate (1 kHz) pulsed operation. Typically, Q-switched pulses from a Nd:YAG laser are of the order of 10 ns in duration, although pulses as short as 100 ps have been obtained from microchip Nd:YAG lasers. Nd:YAG lasers are discussed in detail in Section 2.2. Large Nd-glass lasers have produced tens of joules at repetition rates of several hertz, and several kilojoules at very low repetition rates (~1 per hour). These lasers are discussed in Section 2.3. Nd^{3+} has additional transitions that produce emission near 1.32 and 0.95 μm.

Other rare-earth lasers are based on Er^{3+} (operating near 3.0 or 1.5 μm), Ho^{3+} (operating near 2.1 μm), Tm^{3+} (operating near 2.0 μm), and Yb^{3+} (operating near 1 μm). Er:YAG and Ho:YAG lasers are also discussed in Section 2.3. The optical transitions of interest in all the rare-earth ions correspond to transitions among an incomplete set of $4f$ electrons that are generally well shielded from the host crystal field by a complete xenon shell. The transition energies vary little from host to host and are characterized by relatively narrow linewidths (~10^{11}–10^{12} Hz for crystals, somewhat broader for glasses) and long lifetimes (~0.1–10 ms). The long lifetimes are particularly useful for pump-energy storage and the generation of high peak power via Q switching of the laser cavity (see Section 1.3.2).

Rare-earth-doped glass fiber lasers are of utility in optical communications. Er^{3+} fiber lasers produce output powers of the order of 100 mW and are in use as amplifiers in long-distance fiber transmission. More recently, fiber lasers have emerged as high-power devices, producing several tens of watts of TEM_{00} output.

A second major subclass of dopant materials for solid-state lasers includes the transition-metal ions. Primary among these are Cr^{3+}, Cr^{4+}, Ti^{3+}, Ni^{2+}, and Co^{2+}. These are especially interesting in cases where the ion–host interaction results in a broadly tunable system.

Cr^{3+} is the active ion in the ruby laser ($Cr:Al_2O_3$), the first laser system to be demonstrated. This three-level laser is typically pumped by a xenon flashlamp and produces narrow-band pulsed emission at 694 nm, with pulse energies of about 1 J.

The optical transitions in Cr^{3+} are extremely sensitive to the host and can be the basis of a broadly tunable, four-level laser. Such is the case for alexandrite ($Cr:BeAl_2O_4$), in which the laser transition can terminate on a variety of final vibrational states. Consequently, this laser is tunable from 700 to 818 nm, and has pulsed output energies similar to the ruby laser. The $Ti:Al_2O_3$ laser has even broader tunability, covering a range from 660 nm to beyond 1.1 μm. Pumped by an argon-ion laser, it has operated CW at power levels up to 17 W; when pumped by a frequency-doubled Nd:YAG laser, $Ti:Al_2O_3$ lasers produce pulses with energies of hundreds of millijoules. Because of their broad emission spectra, $Ti:Al_2O_3$ lasers can be mode locked to produce pulses as short as 7 fs (see Section 1.3.2).

Lasers based on color centers in alkali-halide crystals provide wavelength coverage over a range from 0.82 to 3.3 μm, with CW output powers ranging from tens of milliwatts to over a watt. Stability of the color centers can be a problem, and low-temperature storage is required for many of these crystals.

Dye Lasers

When illuminated with visible or ultraviolet radiation, many organic dyes exhibit strong, broadband fluorescence at longer wavelengths. One problem with dyes is the existence of long-lived nonradiative traps, which interfere with laser action. This can be largely circumvented by circulating the dye solution through the laser cavity. Dye lasers can be flashlamp pumped or pumped with other lasers. With a single dye, they can be tuned over as much as 40 nm. A battery of dyes placed in an optical cavity can give tunable output over a range from roughly 1 μm to 400 nm.

The broad bandwidth of dye fluorescence has a tendency to produce broad laser emission lines. The laser lines can be greatly narrowed using a diffraction grating in place of one of the cavity mirrors. Even narrower linewidths are obtained using intracavity etalons, and single-longitudinal-mode operation can be achieved. Alternatively, the large gain bandwidths of dyes are well suited for mode-locked operation. CW mode-locked dye lasers have produced pulses of less than 10-fs duration.

Semiconductor Lasers

A periodic crystal has bands of allowed energy levels separated by forbidden energy gaps. The optical transitions in semiconductor lasers occur across the band gaps. Using modern crystal growth techniques, one can engineer the band gaps to allow lasing at any wavelength from the ultraviolet to far infrared.

The most technologically important type of semiconductor laser is the semiconductor diode laser. These devices are fabricated in the form of a carefully engineered *p-n* junction diode. When a voltage is applied in the forward direction, electrons are injected from the *n* region into the depletion region of the junction (a region of the junction about 1 μm thick). At the same time, holes are injected from the *p* region. As the electrons and holes recombine, they emit radiation at a frequency near the energy gap. When the injection current density is sufficiently high, population inversion and lasing are induced. Semiconductor diode lasers are discussed in detail in Section 2.5.4.

AlGaAs and InGaAs diode lasers have been operated CW in the wavelength range of 0.8–1.0 μm at room temperature with output powers in the range of several watts. Single-mode diodes produce outputs up to several hundred milliwatts. Linear arrays of diodes, in the form of multiple stripes in a 1-cm bar, have given a total output of over 50 W. In addition, electrical-to-optical power conversion efficiencies of greater than 50% have been obtained. CW room-temperature operation has also been obtained in the quaternary alloy system InGaAsP, in the wavelength range of 1.3–1.8 μm. In the visible region, using the quaternary alloy AlGaInP, CW room-temperature operation has been obtained at wavelengths as short as 640 nm, and pulsed operation has been obtained down to 603 nm. Recently, operation in the visible to violet region has been demonstrated in InGaN devices.

Lead-salt lasers (PbSnTe, PbSSe) operate at cryogenic temperatures. These alloy systems are particularly interesting since, in these small-gap semiconductors, the band gap is a sensitive function of temperature, giving rise to temperature-tunable laser output. These tunable sources have been used extensively for high-resolution infrared spectroscopy in the 5- to 20-μm region.

In addition to being very useful laser sources unto themselves, semiconductor diode lasers are nearly ideal pump sources for many ionic solid-state lasers, and for other semiconductor systems where electrical junctions are difficult to fabricate. Semiconductor systems have also been pumped with electron beams.

Ultraviolet and X-Ray Lasers

Stimulated emission in the ultraviolet and x-ray spectral regions presents special problems. The spontaneous radiative lifetime of excited electrical states typically varies with the transition wavelength as λ^3. As a result, the nitrogen gas-discharge laser, which radiates in the near ultraviolet (337 nm), can operate only in a pulsed mode, and must be pumped by a powerful intermittent source. Another problem is the difficulty of devising resonant structures, since the reflectivity of materials becomes very small in the vacuum-ultraviolet and x-ray regions. Consequently, directionally amplified spontaneous emission (superradiance) must frequently be used in these spectral regions, where the directional amplification is achieved by the geometry of the pumped region.

The nitrogen and hydrogen discharge lasers make use of radiative transitions between two bound electronic levels. On the other hand, excimer lasers use radiative transitions between a bound excited state and a free or very weakly bound ground state. For example, Xe and Kr form the excited molecular states Xe_2^* and Kr_2^*; these diatomic molecules are unstable in their ground states. Pumped by powerful electron-beam sources, these gases emit superradiantly at 172 and 145.7 nm, respectively. At somewhat longer wavelengths, rare-gas–halide excimers, such as ArF^* at 248 nm, KrF^* at 193 nm, $XeCl^*$ at 308 nm, and XeF^* at 351 nm, have been operated both by electron-beam pumping and by transversely excited discharge. These lasers can produce multijoule pulses at 100-Hz repetition rates. Excimer lasers are discussed in Section 2.4.

X-ray lasers present an even more difficult challenge. A high-power visible laser can create inversion in a laser-generated plasma. This approach has been used to achieve operation near 21 nm in Se XXV. Alternatively, the x-rays from a laser plasma can be used to pump a separate x-ray laser medium. X-ray lasers are discussed in Section 2.5.8.

Free-Electron Lasers

Relativistic electrons traveling in a periodically alternating transverse magnetic field (wiggler) can be stimulated to give up radiation to a co-propagating electromagnetic field of wavelength

$$\lambda = \frac{\lambda_w}{2\gamma^2}$$

where λ_w is the wiggler period and γ is the ratio of the electron energy to its rest mass energy. Free-electron lasers do not have the wavelength restrictions imposed on other lasers. However, the requirements on the electron beam and wiggler are demanding, and become more demanding as the wavelength decreases. Furthermore, these systems have the large sizes associated with relativistic electron-beam sources.

Frequency Conversion

Nonlinear optical techniques can be used to extend the frequency coverage of lasers, converting the output of practical lasers to regions where primary laser sources may not exist or may not be very practical. The most commonly used frequency-conversion techniques are second-harmonic and sum-frequency generation. Typically, the output of infrared lasers in the 1-μm region, such as Nd:YAG, is frequency doubled into the green. Conversion efficiencies as high as 75% have been reported, and average powers of greater than 50 W have been obtained. Shorter wavelengths can be obtained by summing the green radiation with the infrared, or frequency doubling the green.

Difference-frequency generation and optical parametric oscillators (OPOs) provide tunable sources in the infrared. CW difference-frequency generation is typically inefficient and produces low average-power output. OPOs, on the other hand, are highly efficient. Stimulated Raman scattering has been used to generate large pulse energies with nearly unity quantum efficiency at a variety of wavelengths. Nonlinear frequency conversion is discussed in more detail in Section 2.5.6.

JOHN J. ZAYHOWSKI

1.3.4 Commercial Lasers for Materials Processing

Commercial lasers are now available with an astonishingly large range of properties—wavelengths from the ultraviolet through the infrared, pulse lengths from femtoseconds to microseconds to continuous wave, operating with predicted lifetimes in some cases of greater than 10^6 hours, highly monochromatic or tunable, and with peak powers of hundreds of joules and CW powers of tens of kilowatts.

Of the over 15,000 lasing transitions that have been reported (1) and the many types of lasers that have been demonstrated, only a comparatively few lasers are available commercially, and the number used for materials processing applications is even smaller. These include (1) gas lasers: atomic (He-Cd), ionic (Ar, Kr), excimer (F_2, KrF, ArF, XeF, XeCl), molecular (CO_2 and CO), and metal vapor (principally Cu), (2) solid-state lasers: lanthanide and iron group ions in crystals and glasses, and (3) single-element and multielement semiconductor lasers.

Tables 1 and 2 present listings of continuous-wave and pulsed lasers that have been employed in materials processing. These tables list the laser wavelength, type of laser, and output levels available; for pulsed lasers, typical pulse durations are also given (these may vary with repetition rate). These data are compiled from recent (1997–1999) laser buyers guides (1) and manufacturers' literature and are representative rather than exhaustive; thus they may not be the only lasers available commercially nor may the lasers still be manufactured. Performance figures may also be expected to change because of advances in technology.

A more complete listing of commercial lasers and wavelengths available is given in Section 6 of the *Handbook of Laser Wavelengths* (2). For descriptions of the properties and operating characteristics of various lasers, see *The Laser Guidebook* (3).

Table 1. Commercial Continuous-Wave Lasers

Wavelength (μm)	Laser	Output
Gas lasers		
0.325	He-Cd	0.01–0.1 W_{00}
[0.351–0.676]	Kr ion	1–5 W
0.4416	He-Cd	0.01–0.2 W
0.4416	He-Cd	0.10 W_{00}
[0.455–0.515]	Ar ion	0.3–50 W
[0.458–0.676]	Ar-Kr ion	1–3 W
0.510/0.578	Cu vapor	10–100 W
0.628	Au vapor	2 W
[5–7]	CO	1–35 W
[9.2–11.4]	CO_2	0.2–45 kW
10.6	CO_2	1–400 W_{00}
Solid-state lasers		
0.266 (FH)	Nd:YAG	0.02–0.6 W_{00}
0.355 (TH)	Nd:YAG	0.05–4 W_{00}
0.370 (SH)	alexandrite	0.01 W_{00}
0.523 (SH)	Nd:YLF	1 W_{00}
0.527 (SH)	Nd:YLF	25–30 W
0.527 (SH)	Nd:YLF	1–5 W_{00}
0.532 (SH)	Nd:YAG	15–60 W
0.532 (SH)	Nd:YAG	0.1–8 W_{00}
0.6943	ruby	7 W
0.7–0.8	alexandrite	0.1–2 W_{00}
0.700–1000	Ti:Sapphire	0.2–5 W_{00}
1.047	Nd:YLF	0.5–4 W_{00}
1.047	Nd:YLF	2–85 W
1.053	Nd:YLF	2–45 W_{00}
1.064	Nd:YAG	1–50 W_{00}
1.064	Nd:YAG	1–2500 W
[2.01–2.02]	Ho:YAG	0.05–1 W_{00}
[2.02–2.03]	Ho:YLF	0.05–1 W_{00}
Semiconductor lasers		
[0.75–0.85]	GaAlAs	0.001–0.2 W_{00}
[0.75–0.85]	GaAlAs array	1–40 W_{00}

Wavelengths enclosed in brackets denote the extremes of a group of discrete laser lines or chemical compositions/structures.

Abbreviations: SH, second harmonic; TH, third harmonic; FH, fourth harmonic; J_{00}, W_{00}, TEM_{00} mode; YAG, $Y_3Al_5O_{12}$; YLF, $LiYF_4$; alexandrite, $BeAl_2O_4$:Cr; ruby, Al_2O_3:Cr.

ISBN 0-912035-15-3

Table 2. Commercial Pulsed Lasers

Wavelength (μm)	Laser	Output	Pulse duration
Gas lasers			
0.157	F_2 excimer	0.01–0.06 J	~20 ns
0.193	ArF excimer	0.01–0.6 J	~20 ns
0.248	KrF excimer	0.1–1.2 J	~20 ns
0.308	XeCl excimer	0.1–0.6 J	~20 ns
0.3371	nitrogen (N_2)	0.1–3 J	≤10 ns
0.351	XeF excimer	0.1–0.5 J	~20 ns
[0.48–0.54]	Xe ion	0.6 J	0.1–0.4 μs
0.510/0.578	Cu vapor	1–20 J	~20 ns
0.628	Au vapor	0.2–0.6 mJ	~0.1 μs
[9.2–11.4]	CO_2	1–20 J	~1 μs
[9.2–11.4]	CO_2	1–500 J	1 ms
Solid-state lasers			
0.263 (FH)	Nd:YLF	0.2–2 mJ_{00}	~10 ns
0.266 (FH)	Nd:YAG	2–150 J	~10 ns
0.266 (FH)	Nd:YAG	10–100 mJ_{00}	5 ns
0.347 (SH)	ruby	0.1–0.3 J	25 ns
0.351 (TH)	Nd:glass^a	0.1–8 J	20 ns
0.355 (TH)	Nd:glass^b	0.3–2 J	10 ns
0.355 (TH)	Nd:YAG	10–500 J	~5 ns
0.355 (TH)	Nd:YAG	10–500 mJ_{00}	5 ns
0.380 (SH)	alexandrite	0.1 J	0.1 μs
0.523 (SH)	Nd:YLF	1–15 mJ_{00}	~10 ns
0.527 (SH)	Nd:glass^a	1–5 J	—
0.53 (SH)	Nd:glass^b	0.2–22 J	20 ns
0.532 (SH)	Nd:YAG	0.01–1 kJ	4–8 ns
0.532 (SH)	Nd:YAG	0.01–1 J	6–8 ns
0.6943	ruby	1–100 J	—
0.6943	ruby	1–25 J_{00}	25 ns
0.7–1.1	Ti:Sapphire	0.01–3 J	~10 ns
0.72–0.82	alexandrite	0.1–3 J	—
1.047	Nd:YLF	0.5 J	~20 ns
1.053	Nd:YLF	0.1–10 J	~20 ns
1.054	Nd:glass^a	1–80 J	20 ns
1.061	Nd:glass^b	1–20 J	10 ns
1.064	Nd:YAG	20–2000 J	5–10 ns
1.064	Nd:YAG	0.1–2.5 J_{00}	5–10 ns
[2.09–2.10]	Ho:YAG	0.1–0.25 J_{00}	—
[2.09–2.10]	Ho:YAG	1–5 J	—
Semiconductor lasers			
[0.75–0.85]	GaAlAs	10–20 mJ	~200 μs
[0.78–0.91]	GaAlAs array	20–120 mJ	~200 μs

a Phosphate glass.
b Silicate glass.

References

1. See, for example, *Laser Focus World Buyers Guide*, Pennwalt Publishing Company, Tulsa, OK.
2. Weber, M. J., 1998: *Handbook of Laser Wavelengths*, CRC Press, Boca Raton, FL.
3. Hecht, J., 1992: *The Laser Guidebook* (second edition), McGraw-Hill, New York.

M. J. WEBER

1.4 Laser Systems

1.4.0 Introduction

A laser beam with a large amount of energy is appropriate for processing a wide range of industrial materials. However, this energy, unless focused to a usable spot size, may not be sufficient, when absorbed by a material and converted to heat, to produce a significant physical change in the material.

Assuming a means to focus this energy is present, the processing procedure may require the movement of this energy over the surface of the material. This motion may be simply point-to-point or along a continuous path.

Finally, the laser energy may be required to synchronize with the material contours or, perhaps, be delivered intermittently, on demand, to produce a certain response on or in the material.

In short, a laser processing system closely resembles a generic machine tool where energy is transferred to a material, under some form of control, in a process that enhances the use of this material in a manufacturing operation. While this concept of a machine tool removes some of the glamour from laser processing, it is appropriate because, in fact, the laser is, in most applications, a controlled source of heat that, when applied properly, produces changes in materials with minimal residual effect on that material.

It is not by accident that industrial laser systems resemble conventional machine tools. When lasers were first utilized in industrial applications, system designers chose conventional machine tools to integrate the laser into the process. The first successful laser systems were modified machine tools, the ubiquitous Bridgeport milling machine, for example. It so happened that replacing the cutting tool on the quill with a laser beam focus head provided a stable base for laser processing. And the speeds and travel of the worktable were consistent with the work capacity of those early laser beams.

As lasers evolved in terms of output power and reliability, system suppliers entered the marketplace, adapting their conventional systems to laser processing. Thus it is not unusual to see a laser sheet metal cutter bearing a strong resemblance to a conventional turret punch press. And the familiar arc welding robot has had its end effector adapted for laser processing, while retaining its rugged assembly-line characteristics.

1.4.1 Subsystems

An industrial laser system is composed of specific subsections: the laser and its associated ancillary equipment, a beam delivery system, a work fixture with motion system and associated controller, and a feedback system to close the process control loop. An important option may be a means to monitor and adapt the process to procedural changes. A brief summary of these subsystems follows.

Laser

The two most popular industrial lasers are the pulsed or continuous carbon dioxide (CO_2) laser, a gaseous unit with output power up to 45 kW, and the pulsed or continuous Nd:YAG laser, a solid-state unit with average output power to 4 kW and peak pulsed power in the tens of kilowatts range. A less widely used unit, the excimer laser, is a pulsed gas laser with extremely short pulse widths (nanoseconds) and very high peak power (megawatts).

For industrial applications these lasers should have stable output beam characteristics and be capable of operation in an industrial environment. The qualities of the laser beam, coherence, monochromaticity, low divergence, and high brightness, are factors that affect the amount and quality of energy directed to the workpiece material. Typically, high-quality beams are applicable in cutting, drilling, welding, and marking applications. Beams with less quality are useful in certain welding and surface treatment applications.

Generally, as power increases, so do the laser's physical characteristics, dimensions, weight, and size. A 10-W sealed-off CO_2 laser with an integral power supply can be the size of a loaf of bread, while a continuous 45-kW unit resembles a panel van.

Solid-state lasers (Nd:YAG) tend to be physically smaller than equivalent-power CO_2 lasers, but they are limited in average output power. CO_2 lasers in the popular 1.5–3 kW power range are relatively compact and highly integratable with motion systems. Flowing gas CO_2 lasers require a source of laser gas that must be delivered to a gas distribution panel in the laser control system. Most lasers require a closed-cycle cooling system to optimize output performance. These cooling systems are an ancillary subsystem and, depending on laser cooling requirements, may be large and require additional electrical power.

Lasers may be located on a motion system (the Bridgeport concept) or remote from the workstation, at rather long distances (100 m is typical in certain electronics plants). So some form of beam delivery system is necessary. This can be as simple as a single focusing lens or as complex as a beam expander and multimirror integrator.

Beam Delivery

Laser beams travel in a straight line; so any necessary change in direction is accomplished by mirrors or prisms of appropriate size and material. Other optical elements can shape the beam or split it into multiple beams as required. Most of today's solid-state lasers use a fiber optic delivery system, even for simple fixed optic applications, because these provide a safe beam delivery path to the workpiece.

If beam motion is required, the selection of the beam delivery subsystem is more complex. Essentially, there are three choices for beam motion: move the laser, move the beam, or a combination of beam and workpiece motion. This summary on beam delivery will discuss only beam motion. The other options will be addressed in the motion section.

As stated, whenever the beam is required to change direction, some optical components are used. In a multiaxis, three-dimensional CO_2 laser processing system, up to a dozen mirrors may be required to direct the beam from a fixed laser through jointed tubes to a point on the workpiece. Beam alignment can be a serious task. With Nd:YAG lasers, which are fiber optic compatible, only simple beam insertion and focus optics are necessary. Currently, fibers compatible with high-power CO_2 laser beams are unavailable; so fiber-delivered, high-power Nd:YAG lasers are finding greater acceptance in online processing applications. Single and multiple beams from one laser can be either time or energy shared for flexible processing requirements.

Some CO_2 lasers can produce multiple beams, and all lasers can have their output beam divided into multiple beams through the use of mirrored beam splitters. This allows multiple processing operations as an option for a cost-effective processing solution. Each division of the output beam reduces the delivered energy by the number of divisions. Nd:YAG lasers with beam splitters and fiber delivery are common. Low-power systems, < 75 W units, typically employ two to four fibers on a time-share or energy-share basis. Time sharing the beam is exemplified by a system that utilizes 28 fibers from one laser in a multispot-welding application.

Motion

Once the beam is delivered to the workstation there are several options for processing. The simplest system, a fixed focus with a fixed workpiece, represents a large number of laser applications. In this system, part loading and workpiece fixturing are the design considerations. Simple, single spot welding is an example.

If processing is to occur at several locations of the workpiece, then part manipulation or beam manipulation is required. Because optics are light weight, many designers favor beam motion over conventional part manipulation. The availability of multiple fiber optic systems enhances applications such as multispot welding.

Work motion systems can be simple *X/Y* tables, higher-volume dial feed tables, or the more exotic robot manipulator. In any of these options the laser beam is generally focused at a predetermined point in space and the workpiece is indexed into the focused beam. The design of the part motion is a system engineer's function and most designs generally use accepted machine tool practices. Because the noncontact beam does not impose pressure on the workpiece, fixture and motion system design is simplified. Since part load/unload cycles can be longer than the laser process time, multistation processing has become popular, using a split beam (with fiber optic delivery) or time-shared beams.

A time-shared beam is a rapid switching operation that directs the beam to the appropriate workstation for only the time required to perform the process.

When continuous operations, such as seam welding or part cutting, are involved, the worktable motion must be synchronized to the laser output. Because laser processing is fast, rapid, and accurate, motion is a necessity. Work motion systems capable of moving sheet metal 1.5 m by 3 m at slew speeds of 60 m/min are now common.

An option called hybrid motion defines a combination of workpiece and beam motion, properly synchronized, that reduces the average motion dimensions, saving floorspace. In these systems moving hard optics or fiber optics are used to shift the beam at processing speeds, while work is moved in opposition. The number of axes of motion of each is the designer's choice. Today hybrid systems for sheet metal cutting produce cuts at rates of 30 m/min.

Full beam motion offers attractive possibilities for multiaxis applications. In sheet metal cutting, for example, full beam motion provides the smallest system footprint. These were mentioned earlier in the beam delivery section. Accuracy and repeatability are factors involved in the design of these modern systems.

A final option, less used today, except with low-power CO_2 lasers, is full laser motion. Moving a laser in multiple directions is an interesting processing solution and, when implemented, reduces the number of optics and shortens the beam path to work distances. In reality, a moving laser is the perfect solution for beam movement, but it is hampered by high-power laser size and the necessary connections to the power supply and ancillaries. The rapid acceptance of compact sealed-off CO_2 lasers has led to growth in moving laser applications.

When anthropomorphic robots are used to manipulate the beam, an infinite variety of beam motions is made available, but accuracy and repeatability suffer somewhat, leading to creative end effector treatments, such as the trepanning head mounted on the robot end effector, used to produce accurate holes. Fiber-delivered energy, robot manipulated, is an excellent solution to online, multiaxis laser processing.

Feedback Control

Most systems used to control material processing also control the laser output characteristics. The commonly used CNC controls found on conventional machine tools, supplied by leading international suppliers, are typically used.

Today's laser systems are increasingly controlled by personal computers. The power of low-cost PCs has enabled system designers to install software that allows a semiskilled operator to select the proper operating conditions, laser and motion, for the required procedure. An example can be found in flat-sheet cutters sold today that provide material/process data in a database that leads to accurate, repeatable high-quality parts.

High-speed, 32-bit CNC controls supplied with the laser are compatible with motion systems such that functions like rapid quality cutting of shallow angles in sheet metal is now a straightforward task. The advent of high-speed computing capability now enables cutting of profiled shapes in sheet metal at rates up to 30 m/min.

Adaptive Process Control

Currently in the initial stages of introduction are a variety of devices that provide real-time process control. Sensors monitor the beam/material interaction zone to detect changes in process intensity, by visual and audio techniques. Collected data are compared to stored data to determine the efficiency of the process. Deviations detected can be corrected in real time, leading to higher productivity.

Devices are already available on the market to monitor cut and weld quality, the latter important in applications such as tailored blank welding for warranty traceability requirements.

The next step will be the ability to detect material changes, prior to laser processing, for automatic parameter adjustment. Also in development are new techniques to maximize the efficiency of the laser process to enhance productivity.

Safety

Laser systems present potential hazards to exposed operating personnel. Federal and State regulations and other voluntary safety standards control the use of lasers. Manufacturers assemble systems to comply with the safety standards.

Potential users should be aware of the standards and have an understanding of the safety requirements, from both laser and process standpoints. Information on laser safety standards is readily available from the Laser Insitute of America. Laser safety is discussed more fully in Chapter 6.

1.4.2 Illustrations of Complete Materials Processing Systems

The subsystems that make up a typical industrial laser materials processing system were described above. In this section specific examples of commercially available processing systems are presented.

The systems selected for this overview represent a variety of laser, beam delivery, processing motion, and floor space arrangement configurations. The selection includes systems that are sold to a significant portion of the manufacturing market. Each of the systems shown in this section is produced by one of several suppliers and, therefore, is representative of a generic solution to a common processing application.

Handbook space precludes the inclusion of other systems such as markers, circuit trimmers, microvia drillers, rapid prototyping systems, as well as special systems that are not sold to a large sector of the industry.

Fixed Beam Systems

Most of the early systems installed in manufacturing applications were simple in concept. A fixed beam delivery system produced a spot of laser energy on a workpiece that was held stationary, was held in proper relationship to the focused spot, or utilized conventional X/Y or rotary motion of the workpiece to accomplish the process. Examples are systems for turbine blade drilling, pacemaker welding, and hermetic sealing of integrated circuits.

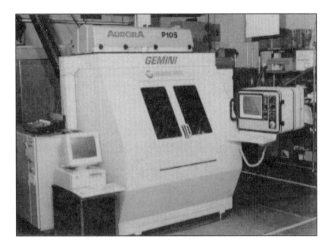

Figure 1. Typical laser machining center with a pulsed Nd:YAG laser. (Convergent Energy).

These early systems, grouped under the generic title of "laser machining centers" were offered as flexible processing systems. Current workstation units are exemplified by the system shown in Figure 1. The unit shown integrates a Nd:YAG laser mounted on top of the workstation with either fixed optic or fiber optic beam delivery to a point above an X/Y table that can carry work fixtures or rotary motion drives.

Motion system accuracy of ±12 μm and repeatability of 6 μm are typical for high-precision systems. Table motion with less accuracy and repeatability are available at a lower selling price. Table travel is typically 30 x 30 or 60 x 60 cm.

This system's PC-based CNC uses a dedicated processor that controls laser and operating parameter functions. Control can be located at the workstation, as shown, or remotely. The PC offers operator friendliness and ease of programming. Also, its lower cost greatly reduces system selling price.

Safety is provided by enclosing the beam so that it does not emerge from the enclosure. A full-view, eye-safe window allows observation of the process. Other systems employ a CCTV system to monitor and display the procedure. With the doors closed, this system meets factory floor safety requirements.

Systems can employ CO_2, Nd:YAG, or excimer lasers. Chillers sized for the laser's output are typically built into the workstation cabinet.

Variations of this system can include automatic part feeding or pay/off and takeup reels for roll material processing.

Flat Sheet Cutters with Work Motion

A conventional flat sheet system, shown in Figure 2, is the least complex of all the laser cutters. A laser, in most cases a fast-axial-flow, kilowatt-level CO_2 unit, is located adjacent to the workstation with the beam brought, through beam ducts, to a fixed focus head immediately above the workpiece. Any necessary changes in beam direction are accomplished with mirrors, and the beam enclosure is flooded with clean dry air.

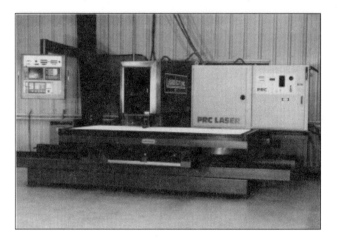

Figure 2. This sheet metal cutting system employs two axes of worktable motion (Lasercut, Inc.).

At the focus head a sensor, tactile or noncontact, measures the spacing between the focus lens and the work, automatically adjusting the Z dimension to maintain focus. In the system shown, the Z motion is 90 mm.

The X/Y motion table can travel up to 2 by 4 m at cutting rates up to 13 m/min and rapid traverse rates up to 25 m/min. Positioning accuracy is ±0.2 mm/254 mm and repeatability is ±12 μm. Load capacity is 1000 kg. Tables are servo-motor-driven by a heavy-duty rotating nut ball screw on tool steel ways.

System control uses a high-speed, 32-bit microprocessor with part program storage. Conventional machine tool CNCs, with software adapted for laser cutting, are employed.

Work support systems, in this example spike pins, and a dross tray for scrap removed, are standard. Clamping to hold the sheet during high acceleration traversing are included.

This flat sheet cutter requires up to 6.4 by 4.4 m of floor space, including the laser and chiller.

Laser power ranges up to 3 kW, which enables high-speed cutting of sheet and plate up to 17 mm thick.

Systems installed in metal fabricating plants are not usually safety enclosed. Instead, safety for this type of system relies on the measures described in Chapter 6.

Hybrid Motion Cutters

With the trend to high cutting speeds, system manufacturers have responded with a combination beam/workpiece motion unit that provides cutting speeds up to 30 m/min (with linear motion drive). The system shown in Figure 3 employs X-axis laser beam movement to allow sheets of 1.5 by 2.8 m to be cut.

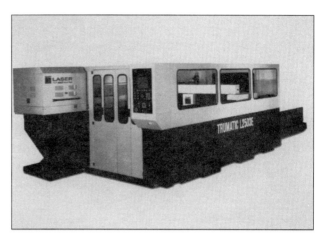

Figure 4. Moving optics add to this system's processing flexibility (Trumpf, Inc.).

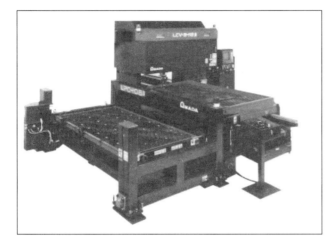

Figure 3. A combination of beam and workpiece motion offers accuracy in high-speed metal cutting (Amada America, Inc.).

The system, shown with an automatic pallet changer, has accuracy and repeatability figures comparable to those of moving table cutters. Table capacity is up to 350 kg, with sheets being clamped to hold position during high-speed traversing.

Systems are powered by high-beam-quality, fast-axial-flow DC or RF excited CO_2 lasers, usually rated at 2.6 kW, to produce cuts.

A work chute allows easy retrieval of cut parts and scrap to maintain high system throughput capability.

The system shown in Figure 3 occupies a 5.6 by 2.8 m floor space, not including the shuttle table.

Flying Optics Systems

The design of gantry-style, flying optics systems provides users with flexible laser processing of large workpieces in a minimum amount of floor space. The unit shown in Figure 4 is a typical shuttle-table-fed, gantry-style sheet or plate cutter.

The focusing optics are mounted on a Y-axis travel mechanism that is suspended from a portal-type gantry that moves the cutting head, under synchronous control, along the length of X-axis rails, racks, or tracks. With this design, sheets and plates of metal up to 1.5 by 3 m can be cut accurately.

The portal design allows shuttle tables to enter the cutting area with uncut metal and to exit after cutting with finished parts and scrap. Shuttle tables contain sheet supporters and trays to capture slag. Fume removal is automatic.

Standard with all cutters is a Z-motion capability to adapt the focused laser beam to changes in the distance to the workpiece.

The system shown can cut sheet metal and plate up to 17 mm thick using the power produced by the RF excited compact CO_2 laser located to the left side of the protective enclosure.

Like most of the metal cutters available today, a 32-bit CNC control provides the computing power necessary to cut at high speeds.

Flying optic systems offer a small floor space footprint. The system shown occupies a space 3 by 6 m, not including the shuttle table.

Moving Laser Systems

Although the system shown in Figure 4 has a small footprint, an even smaller one can be obtained if the laser is moved as part of the process motion capability. Moving lasers require units that are compact, lightweight, and rugged, with a reduction in the size and number of umbilical connections. Sealed-off CO_2 lasers meet these criteria, and units ranging in power up to 500 W are incorporated in several types of moving laser applications.

On the higher end of the power scale, a diffusion-cooled, semisealed 2-kW CO_2 meets most of the moving laser criteria. Shown in Figure 5 is a laser plate cutter that mounts two of these 2-kW units on either side of a portal gantry system used in plate cutting applications.

End track mounting of these lasers requires only a connection to their power supply, control console, and cooling system. The number of mirrors required to deliver the beam to the cutting area is reduced as the beam is brought to either one or two cutting heads that move along the gantry Y axis. The motion of the

ISBN 0-912035-15-3

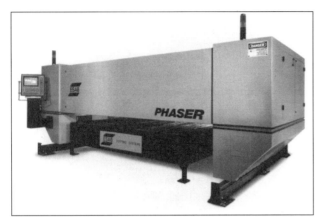

Figure 5. Thick-plate cutter with gantry end carriage mounted diffusion-cooled CO_2 laser (ESAB L-Tec Cutting Systems).

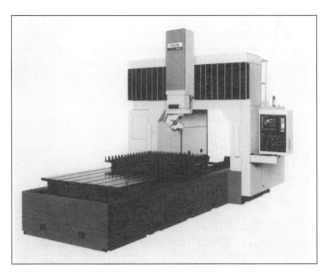

Figure 6. Five-axis combination laser/workpiece motion processing system (Mazak Nissho Iwai Corp.).

gantry along rails in the X direction provides cutting areas up to 6.4 m wide by almost unlimited length.

Other versions of these moving-beam plate cutters employ conventional fast-axial-flow CO_2 lasers up to 6 kW that move on massive bridge-type gantry systems up to 50 m in length.

Depending on laser power and beam quality, cut thicknesses up to 40 mm have been made with square edges, and bevel cuts to 19 mm have been accomplished.

Machine accuracy of the unit shown is 0.1 µm over a 1016 by 1016 mm area with repeatability of 0.05 mm over the same area. High-speed turnover is 19 m/min.

Multiaxis Systems

Processing three-dimensional parts is accomplished in multiaxis systems that are available with up to 10 axes of beam and workpiece motion. Most of these systems employ the portal-type design with beam motion provided by flying optic designs.

Figure 6 is a combination system with four axes of beam motion Y, Z, A, and B and one table motion, X. This arrangement is a favorite of companies processing large, heavy, or bulky parts. The combination motion system provides tight tolerance processing, ±0.005 mm, for the X, Y, and Z axes, with ±0.01° for the A and B axes.

The system shown has the capacity to handle workpieces of 1.5 by 3.05 m, with a rapid traverse speed up to 24 m/min.

Laser power is typically 1.5 to 2 kW, which produces processing rates consistent with the system travel speeds.

Figure 7 is another variation of a gantry-style, multiaxis system. This version, which has been installed with up to 10 axes of combined beam and workpiece motion, has sophisticated control software that offers automatic focus control, feature finders, fixture I.D., in-fixture gauging, and auto-normal. The latter capability maintains beam focus perpendicular to the workpiece at all times.

This moving beam system offers X travel of 2.4 m, Y travel of 1.8 m, and Z travel of 0.9 m. Rotary motion is ±450° and tilt is ±135°.

Feed rates in the X and Y axes are up to 20 m/min, with linear travel accuracy of ±0.013 mm per 305 mm. Repeatability in the X, Y, and Z axes is 0.038 mm and in the rotary motion is 15 arc second.

This unit can be supplied with either a CO_2 or Nd:YAG laser.

CO_2 Laser/Robots

CO_2 lasers can be coupled, through a telescoping articulated arm, to the end effector of an anthropomorphic (human-like) robot. The unit shown in Figure 8 is a conventional heavy-duty robot with an end-of-arm capacity of 200 kg. Travel accuracy and repeatability are on the order of ±0.3 mm. Consequently, without some adaptation such as a trepanning head, these units lack the accuracy of gantry-style, multiaxis units.

Power from a remotely located multikilowatt CO_2 laser is delivered to the focus head through telescoping tubes. The beam direction may be changed by reflection from copper mirrors. In the installation shown, three mirrors direct the beam to the focusing lens. In many applications the laser is located above the work area to limit floor space requirements.

Special part fixturing and clamping devices ensure fit-up for welding applications. In the figure, a rolling wheel is used to close a wide gap in the weld joint.

Chapter 1: Overview of Laser Materials Processing

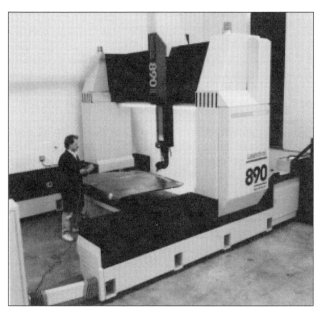

Figure 7. Five-axis portal mounted flying optic laser processing system (Lumonics-Laserdyne).

Advocates of CO_2 laser robots point to very high output power, good beam quality, and low investment cost as benefits of this system.

Nd:YAG Laser/Robots

The obvious disadvantage of articulated CO_2 beam delivery is eliminated by the use of high-power, continuous Nd:YAG lasers with fiber optic beam delivery. Fiber delivery allows

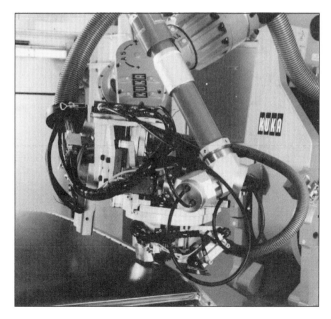

Figure 8. Free-arm robot with CO_2 laser beam delivery for auto roof welding (Kuka Roboter GmbH).

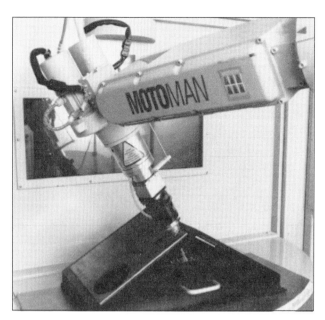

Figure 9. Six-axis robot with a fiber-delivered Nd:YAG laser beam for auto body cutting (Motoman, Inc.).

the Nd:YAG laser to be located remotely from the workstation, up to 100 m.

With available laser power to 4 kW, systems are installed in on-line welding applications in the auto industry. One disadvantage, eye safety, associated with the Nd:YAG laser, is overcome by housing the laser/robot in a cabin that also offers operator protection from robot motion.

Figure 9 is a typical Nd:YAG laser/robot installation with the fiber connected to a remote 2-kW Nd:YAG laser. At the focus head a rotating trepanning optic allows precise hole cutting in auto components.

This six-axis robot has a repetitive positioning accuracy of ±0.3 mm and an extended reach of 2 m, affording processing on large parts.

In the configuration shown this unit can cut round holes up to 6.7 m/min with a diameter of 4 to 30 mm. A 32-bit, RISC architecture computer allows high performance in a factory environment.

DAVID A. BELFORTE

1.4.3 Illustrations of Time- and Energy-Sharing Systems

Foundations for Beam Sharing

While the practice of using lasers for materials processing encompasses a wide variety of applications (see Parts II and III), the vast majority of these are dedicated systems. As described in Section 1.4.2, dedicated systems employ a single laser, single

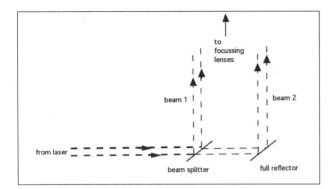

Figure 10. Schematic representation of a basic multiple beam generation system.

workstation, and a single controller. In many of these situations, the selection of laser processing is based upon its ability to provide a unique processing capability under CNC control, for example, localized heat treating and cladding, complex shape cutting, deep penetration welding, and drilling. Often, significant cost savings are achieved with laser processing compared to conventional processing methods.

Although significant cost savings can be achieved with these single-ended systems, further improvements in productivity and manufacturing cost reductions can be achieved for a broader class of applications by sharing the laser output using a variety of beam-sharing configurations (1). Because the laser generally is the most expensive component in the system, significant savings in capital investment costs can result from sharing its output. Those configurations employing a single laser generally fall into two classes: time sharing and energy sharing. In either of these configurations the application is generally limited to a single processing type (for example welding, cutting, or drilling). A third class uses more than one laser and can, therefore, employ both energy-sharing and time-sharing principles, thereby eliminating the single process limitation and maximizing the flexibility and productivity of the system (2). Systems with multiple lasers and flexible work cells may require complex or sophisticated computer control (3).

One of the most important parameters in laser processing is the beam brightness, M^2, which is a function of the beam diameter and beam divergence (see Section 3.4). M^2 is a measure of the mode quality of the laser beam and of its performance relative to the diffraction limit. Just as it is important to maintain stable laser beam mode quality in a conventional single-beam system, it is perhaps more important to determine and maintain the beam quality when considering the conversion of a single system to a sharing system or the new design of a shared system.

As mentioned above, beam sharing is generally accomplished in two ways, either by splitting the beam into several components and using each component in a separate workstation (energy sharing) or directing the beam at different times to a separate workstation (time sharing).

Beam-Sharing Principles — Energy Sharing

The simplest method for energy sharing is achieved by coupling the laser energy simultaneously from both ends of the laser cavity. Similarly, multiple discharge tube gas lasers have been modified to deliver an output beam from each discharge tube, thereby providing the desired multiple beams. If only a single output beam is available, or one wishes to split a multiple output system further, the output beam energy can be divided with beam splitters or partially reflecting mirrors as shown in Figure 10. The divided beams can then be directed simultaneously to a number of work locations. These locations can be on the same, or separate, workstations depending upon workpiece requirements. In general, the accommodation of multiple beam processing is easiest when the individually split beam energies are comparable and when processing tolerances permit slight variations in energy without affecting the finished quality. In high-average-power lasers systems it may be more advantageous spatially to divide the laser beam (by inserting a 100% reflector partially into the beam and skimming, or scraping off portions of the beam) to avoid any thermal distortions from the absorption of energy within the beam splitter.

Beam-Sharing Principles — Time Sharing

Time sharing the laser output beam is advantageous when the workpiece handling time is significantly greater than the workpiece processing time. The simplest form of time sharing is, therefore, to direct the beam to a second workstation during this handling, or loading, interval. This can be done by replacing the beam splitter in Figure 10 with a full reflector. For industrial applications this is best accomplished with a switchable rotary or translational mirror. More rotary mirrors may be arranged sequentially to add additional workstation capability if the interval time permits.

In pulsed systems, the mirrors can be operated continuously to direct successive pulses to a number of beam locations, on the same workstation or onto separate workstations as needed. This method is applicable for low-repetition-rate lasers and is therefore more suited for solid-state laser systems.

System Application Principles

As indicated above, the adaptation of multiple beams to laser processing is driven by the need economically to justify the implementation into manufacturing. The success of that adaptation will depend upon several factors, not the least of which is the maintenance of M^2, the mode quality of the laser beam. It is imperative that the multiple beam generating apparatus does not introduce any beam distortion into the system that could alter the processing characteristics from that characteristic of a single system. Similarly, the multiple beam apparatus should provide consistent beam quality between the individual beams. That is, each individual beam of the multiple should duplicate the original single-beam characteristics, within allowable tolerances, and maintain that condition with time.

For example, consider a cutting operation with a pulsed solid-state laser that may require 100 W of average power to provide

Chapter 1: Overview of Laser Materials Processing

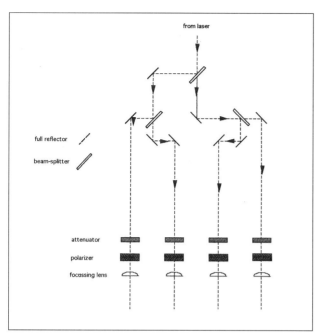

Figure 11. Schematic representation of a conceptual four-beam design.

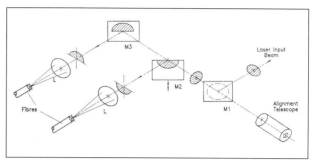

Figure 12. Illustration of a commercial application of a dual-beam fiber optic delivery system (courtesy of GSI Lumonics Inc., Livonia, MI).

optimum cut quality. The beam quality, M^2, is inversely dependent on average power and degrades at elevated power levels, thereby adversely affecting the focusability of the beam and its ability to do work. Therefore, simply generating four beams and raising the operating power to 400 W does not produce the desired improvement in productivity unless other changes are made. In this example, a shorter-focal-length lens can be used to compensate for the M^2 change and to produce the expected results. A shorter-focal-length lens, however, shortens the working distance to the workpiece and may reduce lens life expectancy as well as affect cut quality.

Figure 11 illustrates conceptually a typical multiple beam arrangement that may be employed for an energy-sharing system and the components required for beam-to-beam consistency. The same illustration could be used to depict a time-sharing system if switchable mirrors are used instead of the beam splitters. With Nd:YAG solid-state lasers, flexible fibers can be employed instead of the plane mirrors to direct the split beams to the focusing lenses (4). Fibers offer the additional advantages of flexibility of beam location and separation, as well as reducing any spatial inhomogeneity introduced by the multiple-beam apparatus (5).

Regardless of the splitting system or beam delivery system employed, Figure 11 illustrates several characteristics that should be present to develop a useful working system. In this figure, the total path length from laser to focusing lens should be the same for each beam. This ensures the replication of spot size for each beam at the workpiece. Attenuators, located in each beam, provide the means to adjust individual beam energy into balance with the others and ensure comparable energy densities

and working efficiencies at the workpiece. Finally, circular polarizers may be required to compensate for any polarizations shifts introduced by the beam splitters and turning mirrors. This ensures uniform coupling of each beam into the workpiece.

Adaptation of multiple processing also requires a thorough understanding of the allowable variations in the process parameters for the process under consideration. These include the tolerances for focal position, energy (power), and beam diameter and divergence. This permits the selection and design of the system to accommodate variances in workpiece geometry as well as component replacement. For example, if the process permits, it is desirable to use longer-focal-length lenses, thereby accommodating both focal position shifts of the workpiece and the tolerance variability of the lens focal length.

Illustrations of Systems

Most laser and systems manufacturers can design and provide sharing systems to enhance the efficiency and productivity of their systems. Examples of commercially available systems are illustrated schematically in Figures 12 through 14.

A commercial utilization of the beam-division principle is illustrated in Figure 12. Mirror M2 is used to intercept and independently direct a portion of the laser's output beam to one fiber while the remainder of the beam is directed by M3 to the second fiber. Each fiber output is then directed to separate locations on the workpiece. A telescope is included to assist in system alignment. Although the figure illustrates two-beam generation, up to four modules can be incorporated to obtain four separate beams. The fiber within each module homogenizes each beam during transit through the fiber to produce a circular spot of uniform intensity at the workpiece. Each skimming mirror location can be adjusted to provide either four beams of equal intensity for multiple processing or a preselected set of values (such as 40%:30%:20%:10%) to meet certain specific process requirements.

Figure 13 illustrates the use of a multiposition optical switch in a fast time-share distributor system. A galvanometer-controlled mirror, M2, is used to direct the laser beam output to any of up to eight fibers in response to an electrical signal that is provided by a system controller. The switching action can be accomplished

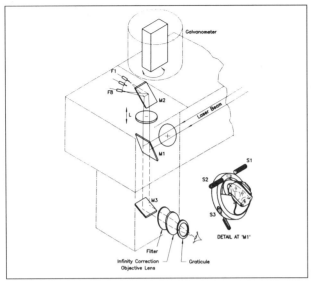

Figure 13. Schematic representation of a fast time-share beam distributor system (courtesy of GSI Lumonics Inc.).

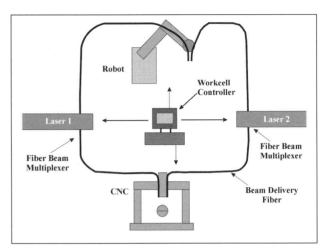

Figure 15. Schematic representation of a prototype distributed laser processing system that is operated under computer control.

between the pulses of a laser operating at rates up to 40 Hz. The controller switches the beam in response to process system needs (e.g., part-is-in-position) allowing random access to the fibers; that is, the switching from fiber to fiber need not be in numerical sequence.

Figure 14 shows an industrial fiber optic laser system that illustrates the building block capability and performance flexibility of fiber optic modules. When these types of fiber optic configurations are implemented, they provide system flexibility and versatility to accommodate changing process requirements. The fiber system pictured in Figure 14 has a combination dual and quad beam capability. The flexibility of multiple beams in combination with system controllers, as discussed previously, can be extended to include a multiplicity of lasers and workstations. A prototype system incorporating dual lasers and workstations, with the laser output coupled to the workstations through fibers, was developed by AT&T under the auspices of the National Center for Manufacturing Sciences (NCMS) to identify and demonstrate the essential concepts of a distributed laser processing system under computer control (2). The prototype distributed laser processing System (DLAPS) is schematically shown in Figure 15.

The DLAPS development program demonstrated that implementation of a flexible manufacturing system requires a computer control system to realize its full potential. The computer control system is employed to control the particular part programs, the laser parameters for processing, and the switching of fibers as well as to run a scheduling model that simulates the operation of the system. This model, developed in the program, determines the sequence of jobs to be processed, based on the process time and priority of each job in order to minimize the time required. A simulated test demonstrated an improvement in utilization of approximately 32%.

References

1. T. R. Kugler and T. J. Culkin, "Nd:YAG Advances Aid Production," *Photonics Spectra* **143,** November, 1989.
2. R. S. Armington, R. J. Coyle, A. Kestenbaum, P. P. Solan, and L. S. Watkins, *Research Program to Develop a Distributed Laser Processing System,* NCMS Report TA1677.N358, National Center for Manufacturing Sciences, Ann Arbor, MI, May 1993.
3. D. B. Veverka, "Implementing Laser Robotic Welding," *Industrial Laser Review* **19,** January 1996.
4. R. Cunningham, "Delivering Nd:YAG Laser Beams the Easy Way," *Lasers and Optronics* **9,** 59, September 1990.
5. R. J. Coyle, R. Webb, and P. P. Solan, "Matched Laser Spot Welding Using Dual Fiber Optic Delivery," *Power Beam Processing,* E. A. Metzbower and D. Hauser, eds., ASM International, 149, 1988.

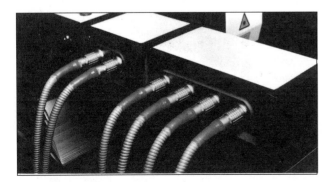

Figure 14. Example of an industrial multiple-beam fiber optic system that can be configured to accommodate changing process requirements (courtesy of Lasag Corporation, Arlington Heights, IL).

RICHARD J. COYLE
RONALD M. GAGOSZ

Chapter 2

Lasers for Materials Processing

2.0 Introduction

Many different types of lasers have been operated but only a relatively small number of them are useful for materials processing. This chapter will describe those lasers, their properties, and their capabilities relevant to materials processing.

The two types that have been used for the longest period of time and most often used are the carbon dioxide laser and the Nd:YAG laser. Much of this chapter will be devoted to these two types. But, in recent times, a number of other laser types have been developed to a level of maturity so that they are also useful; these types too will be discussed.

2.1 Carbon Dioxide Lasers

2.1.1 Basic Principles

General Capabilities

Carbon dioxide (CO_2) lasers offer the highest average power for materials processing. CO_2 lasers with output power capability of 1000 W or less are considered low-power systems. High-power systems with average power capability to 50 kW are available, but most systems in industrial use are under 15 kW, with the majority under 3 kW. Compared to other lasers, the higher power capability of CO_2 lasers allows their use for processing heavier-gauge materials and/or for processing at faster rates in many industrial applications. For this reason, they are often the laser of choice for automotive and other steel parts manufacturing operations.

Laser Excitation

Excitation of carbon dioxide lasers results from an electric discharge maintained in a gas mixture of carbon dioxide, nitrogen, and helium. The exact mixture depends on the laser design, operating pressure, and operating mode (continuous or pulsed), with the volumetric concentration ranging from 2–5% CO_2, 10–60% N_2, and 40–90% He. The pressure in the discharge chamber is usually in the range of 10–100 Torr, depending on the type, size, and operating mode of the laser. Pulsed lasers usually operate at higher pressures than continuous-wave (CW) lasers, with some pulsed laser pressures as high as 1 atm. However, relatively few of these higher-pressure systems are currently used in industrial processing operations. Because of the low-pressure operation of most CO_2 laser systems, good vacuum integrity of the laser enclosure with very low leak rate is essential to prevent contamination of the laser gas mixture and associated degraded performance. Likewise, it is essential that materials used inside the laser, whether by design or for special tests, be carefully selected to avoid contamination by outgassing.

The discharge systems in CO_2 lasers are either pure DC or high-frequency AC, usually RF. The DC systems require the least expensive and easiest to maintain power sources, but the AC units offer advantages in improved discharge stability, "electrodeless" discharges (insulated metallic electrodes not exposed to the discharge), and pulse-control capability. For most applications it is desirable that the carrier frequency be sufficiently high so that the output power is not modulated by the carrier. However, with these high-frequency lasers, the carrier can be modulated by the control systems to provide pulsed output that may be desirable or required for a specified application.

Power Extraction

Power is extracted from the excited laser medium by means of an optical resonator (oscillator), which consists of at least two mirrors aligned to face each other with the excited medium in the cavity between them, as shown in Figure 1. The purpose of the resonator is to build up an intense optical flux at the lasing wavelength within the cavity to assure that excited molecules in the medium are deactivated by stimulated emission (lasing) before they decay (lose their optical energy) by collisions with other molecules or with the cavity walls. The other essential feature is that one of the cavity mirrors allow some of the optical flux to escape from the cavity in the form of a well-defined laser beam. This type of power extraction is most notably obtained by using a partially transmitting mirror as one of the cavity mirrors. The power transmitted through the mirror is the laser beam. The selection of the proper transmissivity of the mirror is a critical factor affecting the efficiency of the laser. There are other types of optical resonators and cavity configurations that are used in the CO_2 lasers. These are described in more detail in Section 2.1.3.

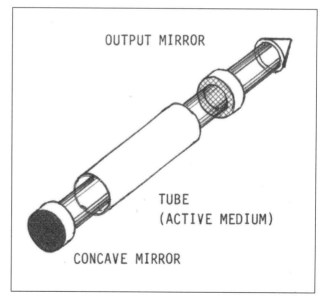

Figure 1. Basic tube laser with stable resonator formed between a concave mirror and a partially transmitting output mirror.

The salient feature of every laser beam is its coherence, which relates directly to its capability to be propagated with low divergence and to be focused to a small spot by a lens or mirror. Techniques have been developed to measure the beam quality, which is essentially the actual focusability compared to that of a theoretically perfect Gaussian beam. This quantity is expressed in terms of M^2, with $M^2 = 1$ being a perfect Gaussian beam. The parameter M^2 is described in more detail in Section 3.4. When selecting a laser it is useful to compare the M^2 values quoted for different lasers as a comparison guide.

Some representative values of M^2 for continuous CO_2 lasers are presented in Table 1. These values were derived from the literature of laser manufacturers. The value of M^2 tends to increase with increasing output power. At any particular power level, the values of M^2 vary from one laser model to another; the ranges given in the table cover typical CO_2 laser models.

Table 1. M^2 Values for Continuous CO_2 Lasers

Output power (W)	M^2
< 500	1.1–1.2
800–1000	1.2–2
1000–2500	1.2–3
5000	2–5
10,000	10

Before one selects a laser, one should carry out performance tests on the intended process operation because in some cases there is a variation in quoted values of M^2. Also, surprisingly in other cases, lasers with higher M^2 values have exhibited better overall performance for some other processes. This latter effect is usually related to difference in beam intensity distribution and/or the peak intensity.

Laser Cooling

The biggest enemy of CO_2 lasers is heat, or more exactly, high temperature. As more power is deposited in the medium by the discharge, the attendant increase in medium temperature causes a more rapid decay of the excited molecules and an associated decrease in extraction efficiency. Thus effective cooling of the laser medium is essential to stable and efficient laser operation. Lasers are often categorized by their method of cooling, namely, (1) diffusion-cooled, in which heat is conducted out of the medium by diffusion of molecules to the laser tube walls; or (2) convection-cooled, in which heat is removed by the high flow rate of laser gases through the active medium. In either case, auxiliary cooling of critical components such as cavity walls and gas/liquid heat exchangers, respectively, are required to remove waste heat. In this regard, it should be noted that the overall (wall plug) efficiency of CO_2 lasers is less than 10%, and usually less than 5%. Therefore, most of the power deposited in the laser system must be removed in the form of waste heat. In high-power systems, a chilled water supply with well-regulated water temperature is an important auxiliary equipment requirement.

Wavelength Effects

The wavelength of the CO_2 beam is 10.6 micrometers (μm), well into the infrared. At this wavelength, most materials that we consider transparent, such as glass, are in fact opaque. Thus required transmitting elements, such as windows, partial reflectors, and lenses, must be made from less conventional materials such as zinc selenide (ZnSe) or gallium arsenide (GaAs). Potassium chloride (KCl) and sodium chloride (NaCl) crystals also transmit well at 10.6 μm, but they are hygroscopic and generally considered to be too fracture sensitive for use in commercial laser systems. ZnSe has been the substrate of choice for most transmitting elements, but it must be antireflection coated to prevent excessive power loss by reflections from both surfaces.

Other implications of the long wavelength of the CO_2 laser are the high reflectivity of most metals, a factor that can reduce the effectiveness of metal processing; and the high absorption coefficient of the plasma that forms on a workpiece, as during welding. The adverse effect of high reflectivity is usually not a severe problem when the intended process requires a penetration of the material, because the hole formed becomes an effective absorber. On the other hand, the plasma absorption problem requires the use of special dissipative means to quench the plasma. Thus the proper design and use of a gas jet (usually helium) for plasma suppression is a critical requirement for laser welding. The requirement for effective plasma suppression increases with laser irradiance and is also dependent on the workpiece material characteristics.

2.1.2 Laser Configurations

Basic Features

Most CO_2 laser incorporate either a cylindrical tube or rectangular cross-section discharge chamber. Historically, early model lasers used cylindrical tubes because of the ready availability of pyrex or quartz tubes and the ease of generating a stable discharge in a tube. As lasers were scaled to higher power levels, larger discharge volumes and improved cooling techniques were required. This led to the use of rectangular discharge chambers, as shown in Figure 2. To further increase power capability some lasers use combinations of the basic cylindrical tubes or rectangular channels arranged in different types of geometrical arrays.

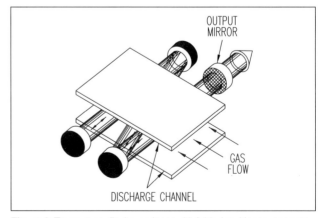

Figure 2. Transverse discharge laser with folded multipass resonator.

In addition to the distinguishing configurational features, lasers are defined by their method of heat removal, their mode of electrical excitation, and orientation of the electric discharge in the flow. In sealed lasers (laser tube charged with an appropriate gas mixture and hermetically sealed) and in slow-flow lasers (a small amount of gas is continuously purged through the laser to stabilize the mixture and/or control the pressure), heat removal from the laser medium is primarily by diffusion of molecules to the laser chamber walls. In these diffusion-cooled lasers, the effectiveness of heat transfer is directly related to the area of the conducting walls, usually the electrodes, and inversely proportional to the characteristic diffusion length in the medium. These types of lasers, characterized by the lower-power waveguide lasers and the higher-power version slab lasers, utilize large-area electrodes spaced close together, typically a few millimeters, to enhance heat transfer and thereby increase power capability.

The other technique of removing heat from the laser medium is the use of a high flow rate of gas mixture through the laser tube or channel. These convection lasers have a larger cross-sectional area than the conduction-type lasers, and they require the use of a pump or blower system to circulate the gas mixture through the laser chamber and associated heat exchangers.

Axial-Flow Lasers

Axial-flow lasers derive their name from the common axis of the flow and the optical resonator, with the active medium contained in a cylindrical tube or array of tubes, as shown in Figure 3. In DC-excited systems the discharge is usually also maintained along this common axis, whereas in high-frequency AC-excited lasers the discharge is maintained transverse to the axis by means of electrodes located on diametrically opposite sides of the tubes. Power is coupled into the tubes capacitively, and the voltage requirement is significantly lower than with the DC system because of the relatively close spacing of the electrodes.

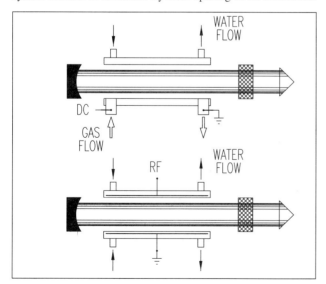

Figure 3. Water-cooled tube laser showing a DC excitation scheme (upper) and an RF excitation scheme (lower).

In low-power axial-flown systems, the gas flow rate is low, and the gas mixture is purged through the system and exhausted. Because waste heat is removed by conduction (via diffusion) to and through the tube walls, in all but the very low power systems double-walled tubes are used to form annular passages for coolant flow, usually water. The diameter of the inner discharge tube is typically 10 mm or less, which is also the approximate size of the output beam that is generated between the two mirrors located at the ends of the discharge tube. As with all resonator designs, the support structure that holds these mirrors in proper register for lasing is a critical component. Often this structure is made of a low-expansion material such as invar or quartz to minimize thermal distortions. Stable resonators (Fig. 1) that generate high-quality, single-mode output beams are used almost exclusively in these slow-flow systems.

Fast axial-flow lasers, as shown in Figure 4, produce power levels into the kilowatt regime by using high flow rates of the laser gas mixture. Tube diameters up to 75 mm have been employed in these designs, but most industrial systems are in the 30 to 50 mm diameter range. These larger diameters provide a method of power scaling by increased discharge volume. Also, the low aspect ratio (L/D) of these tubes provides a relatively low flow-impendence path for the circulating gases so that the pressure head requirements for the gas-circulating pumps can be kept in a reasonable range. However, because of the mechanical loads imposed on the system by the circulating pump(s), effective mechanical isolation and vibration damping means must be employed so that the optical alignment and laser stability are not adversely affected.

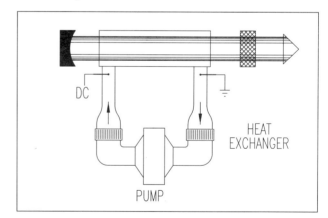

Figure 4. Closed-cycle, fast-axial flow laser with DC excitation. Circulating pump and heat exchangers depicted.

In both the slow-flow and fast-axial flow systems, higher output power levels are achieved by using multiple discharge tubes as shown in Figure 5. In the multiple-tube systems arrays are often stacked side by side to reduce the overall length of the system. These stacked arrays require the use of additional flat mirrors to connect all the tubes in series optically to form a single resonator path (optical axis). In the fast-axial flow systems the tubes are connected in parallel flow-wise to minimize the overall flow impedance (pressure drop).

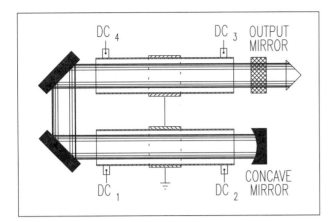

Figure 5. Multitube laser with folded resonator.

The relatively low aspect ratio of the fast-axial flow systems, even in the stacked arrays, results in a high optical Fresnel number (radius^2)/(wavelength × optical cavity length). Because stable resonators require a low Fresnel number to produce a single-mode Gaussian beam (optimum beam quality with $M^2 = 1$), most of these systems produce a multimode or higher-order mode output beam, and M^2 is significantly higher than 1. For this reason, the larger-diameter resonators often employ an unstable resonator to produce a single-mode output. However, the annular form of the unstable resonator beam also has $M^2 > 1$, but usually not as high as that of the multimode stable resonator. Salient features of these resonators used in CO_2 lasers are outlined in Section 2.1.3.

Transverse-Flow Lasers

Transverse-flow lasers use a large volume discharge maintained in a rectangular flow channel (Fig. 2). The discharge is maintained across the height of the channel, essentially transverse to the flow, by sets of electrodes exposed to the flow in DC discharge systems and by electrodes embedded in or on the outside of the top and bottom walls of the channel in the RF discharge systems. Power is extracted by means of a resonator system with mirrors located on the sides of the channel, so that the three axes, flow, discharge, and optical, are mutually orthogonal.

Large-volume discharges are inherently less stable than those maintained in cylindrical tubes, with a greater tendency toward nonuniformities and an associated transition from a stable glow to a constricted arc. The arc produces no laser excitation. However, with careful attention to flow and discharge uniformity in the design of these large-volume systems, good discharge stability can be achieved, and such systems now provide the highest output power available in industrial laser systems, upwards of 50 kW.

Because of the large cross-sectional flow area, the pressure loss in these lasers is usually considerably less than that in the fast-axial-flow lasers. Therefore, as shown in Figure 6, higher flow fans can be used to provide the high rate of gas flow required to remove waste heat, and the gas flow velocity itself has a stabilizing influence on the glow discharge. Operating pressure levels up to 100 Torr (about 1/8 atm) are typical. For a given flow velocity the cooling rate increases directly with pressure. Thus the selection or development of an appropriate circulating fan or blower is a critical part of the laser design.

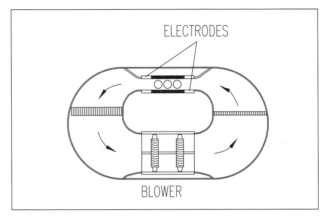

Figure 6. Closed-cycle transverse discharge laser showing circulating blower and heat exchangers. Optical passes are orthogonal to discharge and flow.

Because of the rectangular cross section of the active medium, efficient power extraction requires the use of multiple passes, a folded resonator, to assure that the resonator cavity fills the active medium. The use of multiple passes also provides a higher optical gain, which also contributes to improved extraction efficiency.

As with the fast-axial-flow lasers, the highest output power levels are achieved by using multiple arrays of discharge channels (Fig. 7) connected in parallel but with the optical paths in series. Also, as with the fast-axial-flow systems, the Fresnel number of the resonator is quite high. Thus multimode output is usually obtained with the use of a stable resonator, and therefore use of an unstable resonator, described in Section 2.1.3, can provide improved beam quality (focusability).

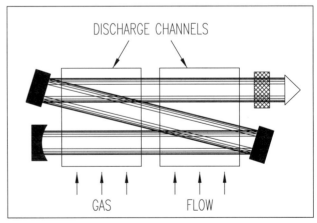

Figure 7. Multichannel transverse discharge laser with folded resonator.

Waveguide Lasers

Waveguide lasers have a rectangular cross-section discharge chamber formed between two rectangular electrodes spaced quite close together, several millimeters, so that diffusion to the water-cooled electrode walls is enhanced to provide effective conduction cooling. Because of the geometry, RF excitation is used almost exclusively. The name, waveguide laser, derives from resonator design in which the upper and lower channel walls form a waveguide to contain the beam within the resonator. Such lasers usually have a very low flow rate of gas purged through the system, or they are sealed with no flow. In the latter case, catalytic materials are often used inside the laser to maintain a proper gas composition.

Because of the rectangular cross section of the active medium, it is necessary to use a folded path resonator to effectively fill the medium. The multiple passes and small beam diameter provide a low Fresnel number so that a single-mode Gaussian beam can be produced. However, the many optical passes necessary to fill the active medium limit the practical size, and therefore, the output power of such lasers, usually to 50 W or less. Use of a hybrid resonator such as employed in the slab laser, described below, permits a substantial increase in output power. The slab laser is essentially a larger version of the waveguide laser, differing primarily in the optical extraction scheme.

Slab Lasers

The essential features of the slab laser are shown in Figure 8. Similar to the waveguide laser, it incorporates cooled rectangular RF electrodes to form the top and bottom walls of the discharge chamber. The spacing of the electrodes is similar to or only slightly larger than the waveguide laser to enhance the diffusion-cooling process. However, the area of the electrodes is much larger than that in the waveguide system. This provides the slab with a much higher power capability, with output power levels now in the 3 kW range. Power is extracted using a special resonator design such as that depicted in Figure 8. In this type of resonator the output beam has a rectangular cross section, and it must be transformed to a near-circular cross section to be of practical use in most industrial applications. This transformation is accomplished by using a specially designed beam-forming module located in the output beam just outside the laser.

Very important benefits of the slab laser are the low (or zero) gas consumption and the elimination of the need for a gas-circulating fan or blower. With no requirement for a circulating fan, the laser can be packaged in a very compact module.

Pulsed Lasers

Pulsed output from most of the previously described CO_2 lasers may be obtained by pulsing the applied voltage. The output is essentially a modulated power output with relatively low peak power (1 to 3 times the average power) and corresponding low pulse energy. In order to generate more intense pulses, the input electrical pulse must be enhanced by providing a significant overvoltage to the discharge electrodes. To accommodate this overvoltage the electrodes must be designed to prevent unwanted electrical breakdown. Not all laser system electrodes can accommodate this type of operation.

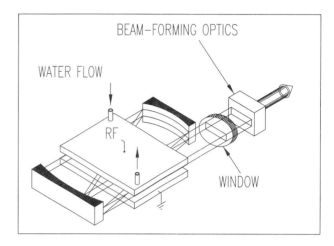

Figure 8. RF-excited slab laser with hybrid resonator, also showing output window and external beam-forming optics.

Two different types of pulsed lasers that are in common use are the superpulsed laser and the TEA (transversely excited atmospheric pressure) laser. Both types are established in tube geometries (Fig. 1) and provide repetition frequencies ranging from a few to a few hundred hertz. Average power is low, limited primarily by electrical charging times, so that fast axial flow is not required. Most of these lasers provide pulse energies from a fraction of one J to about 20 J, but some superpulsed systems can provide hundreds of J.

The superpulsed laser uses a basic DC electrode configuration as shown in Figure 3. Pressure is maintained in a moderate range from ten to a few hundred Torr to limit the voltage required for the rather long electrode separation. Voltages from 10,000 to over 100,000 volts are used to generate the intense pulses. However, at the lower pressures the pulse duration is increased. Pulse durations from under 100 microseconds to over a millisecond are typical. Some CW axial-flow lasers also have the capability to operate in this mode.

TEA lasers are uniquely pulsed lasers because of their high operating pressure of 1 atm or above. The electrodes in a TEA lasers are a multiplicity of diametrically opposed pin electrodes arranged along the length of the tube. Preferably the electrodes are arranged in a spiral array along the length of the tube to provide on average a more uniform active medium that that of a straight-line array. The short radial spacing between opposing pins keeps the voltage in a reasonable range; and the high pressure results in short pulses, submicrosecond to tens of microseconds. In commercial systems pulse energies range from 1 to about 20 J.

2.1.3 Optics

Resonators

The standard of beam quality against which all other laser beams are compared is the Gaussian beam, which is the fundamental mode of a stable resonator. One example of a stable resonator is depicted in Figure 1; when the concave reflecting mirror is aligned with the partially transmitting output mirror, the optical flux trapped between the cavity mirrors does not geometrically couple out of the cavity. Power is lost from the cavity by diffraction, mirror absorption, and transmission out of the cavity in the form of a laser beam. It is apparent that efficient power extraction requires that the transmission loss be a substantially higher loss than all others combined. Generation of a Gaussian mode (TEM_{00}) beam in a stable resonator requires that the Fresnel number, (internal aperture radius)^2/(cavity length x wavelength), of the optical cavity be quite low, approximately $1/\pi$, in order to discriminate against the production of higher-order modes. Higher-order or multiple modes produced with higher Fresnel numbers have a substantially degraded beam quality ($M^2 > 1$) with an attendant loss in beam focusability. Except for some of the lower-power CO_2 lasers with small beam modes, the low Fresnel number condition cannot be achieved. For this reason, higher-power lasers with stable resonators often have M^2 values as high as 8–10. These high values can still provide a useful, but limited, focusability in higher-power lasers. However, some improvement is usually possible with the use of an unstable resonator.

The basic features of a typical unstable resonator are depicted in Figure 9. In the version depicted, the cavity mode is established between a concave and a convex cavity mirror; and a hole coupler (or scraper) mirror located in front of the convex mirror reflects the outer annulus of the beam from the cavity to provide the output beam. The output beam need not be reflected out at 90 degrees as shown but can be directed as desired by the laser designer. In some designs the output beam is directed back across the chamber at a low angle relative to the cavity axis.

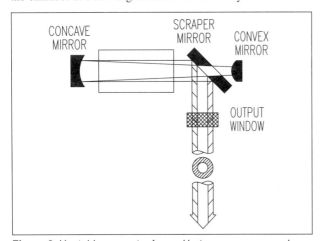

Figure 9. Unstable resonator formed between concave and convex mirrors with a hole-coupling (scraper) mirror to produce an annular beam. The output window is also shown.

Two important features of unstable resonators that make them especially desirable for high-power lasers are (1) single-mode operation can be achieved in higher Fresnel number systems, and (2) all the resonator mirrors can be directly water-cooled, because a partially transmitting mirror is not required. This latter mirror is one of the more vulnerable elements used in laser systems and requires frequent replacement in high-power systems. A shortcoming of the unstable resonator is the annular output beam, which reduces the beam focusability.

From a laser marketing standpoint, the name unstable resonator is quite unfortunate. In this configuration the term unstable does not imply any lack of stability in the usual sense. Rather, the term derives from the basic design feature of the resonator in which a light ray launched close to and parallel with the optical axis undergoes multiple reflections and moves radially outward until it geometrically couples out of the resonator. Some diffraction and mirror absorption losses also occur, but the primary loss of power from the cavity is the geometric output coupling. The effective output coupling (transmission) is a function of the cavity design and is related directly to the resonator magnification, M_R (not to be confused with M in M^2, the measure of beam quality). For a confocal resonator, the type most commonly employed, M_R is the ratio of the outside diameter (D_o) to the inside diameter (D_i) of the beam. In CO_2 lasers, values of M_R range from 1.5 to 5.0.

Because M_R influences both the output coupling and beam focusability, the selection of M_R is not arbitrary. Beam focusabilty increases with M_R, but so does output coupling. If coupling is too high, the intracavity flux is not maintained at a high enough level for efficient power extraction. With the gain conditions that prevail in high-power CO_2 lasers, M_R values in the 2.0 to 4.0 range offer a good compromise. These values provide a theoretical M^2 of approximately 4 and 3, respectively. Considering other beam-degrading effects that can occur in laser cavities, more realistic values of M^2 are 7 and 6, respectively. These values offer some improvement over the higher-order-mode stable resonator beams.

In addition to the standard stable and unstable resonators described, there are hybrid resonators such as that used in the slab laser shown in Figure 8. Typically, this hybrid is a stable-unstable resonator with the short dimension (chamber height) governed by stable resonator conditions, and the lateral dimension governed by unstable resonator conditions. The output beam is usually rectangular in cross section, and therefore requires external processing to provide a nearly axisymmetric beam.

Mirrors

Mirrors are, of course, a critical part of a laser resonator. In low-power lasers most mirror substrates are silicon or germanium, and the reflecting surfaces are multilayered dielectrics that provide a very high reflectivity at the CO_2 wavelength of 10.6 μm. Except at the lowest power levels, most mirrors are indirectly cooled by cooling plates on their backs or edges.

In high-power lasers silicon or metal mirror substrates are used, and the latter are often directly water cooled. The reflecting surfaces are usually protected copper, silver, or gold, which also provide high reflectivity in the visible so that a visible laser, such as HeNe, can be used effectively to align the cavity. Enhanced coatings, which provide higher values of reflectivity at 10.6 µm, and therefore higher laser extraction efficiency, have been developed. Some of these coatings, however, have a shorter useful life than the metal reflectors when used inside the laser. The degradation is caused by chemical reactions, electrical conduction, ultraviolet irradiation, and/or thermal stressing. Newer coatings appear to have effectively dealt with these problems; so the enhanced coatings can now be used to increase output powers.

The most vulnerable mirror in lasers that employ a stable resonator is the partially transmitting output mirror. In most cases this window is a zinc selenide (ZnSe) substrate with a specified reflectivity (and/or transmissivity) on the cavity side and an antireflection coating on the outside. Although these mirrors are now quite reliable, they do degrade with time and require replacement periodically. The lifetime depends on the incident intensity and the size of the mirror. Because these mirrors must be egde-cooled, smaller mirrors can be cooled more effectively.

Output Windows

The output window used on most CO_2 lasers is a zinc selenide (ZnSe) substrate with antireflection coating on both surfaces. If adequately protected from atmospheric contamination, the ZnSe window is less vulnerable to degrading factors than a ZnSe partial reflector. However, the window, which is also edge-cooled, is one of the elements that requires periodic maintenance.

Edge cooling is not completely adequate at power levels in the higher kilowatt range because thermal variations that occur in the window because beam power absorption causes a lensing effect. One solution to this problem is face-cooling. This can be accomplished by means of a device (Fig. 10) that incorporates two ZnSe windows with provision for cool gas flow (usually helium) between the windows. The system is completely sealed, and the gas is continuously recirculated and cooled. It is also possible to use this device to provide a combination partial reflector (inner element) and output window. One shortcoming of this device is that window servicing requires replacement of two windows.

Another very successful device that also eliminates the window replacement problem is the aerodynamic window, depicted in Figure 11, which eliminates the physical window altogether. This window, which is quite trouble free, is ideally suited for high-power systems. It uses a source of high-pressure dry air in a special supersonic flow nozzle to provide a curtain of air that supports atmospheric pressure on the outside and approximately 1/10 atmosphere on the inside. In fact the device can be set to pump gas out of the laser to assure that no air leaks into the system. This window is mounted on the laser with an intermediate valve, so that the valve provides the vacuum seal when the laser is in standby operation.

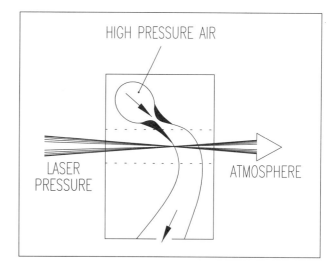

Figure 11. Aerodynamic window that uses a supersonic flow of dry air to form an atmosphere-supporting air curtain across the output aperture. The laser beam is focused through the window aperture.

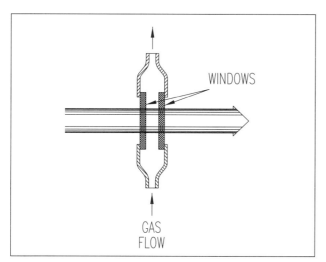

Figure 10. Face-cooled output window assembly which uses a high flow of cooled gas between a dual-window arrangement.

Although aerodynamic windows work very reliably and do not noticeably degrade or change the laser beam as solid windows sometimes do, their initial cost is higher than other windows because of the requirement for a high-pressure dry-air supply and additional optical components. The latter are required because the aperture in the window is kept small to minimize the airflow requirement. Aperture sizes are usually in the range of 1 to 2 cm. Thus the beam must be focused through the window and then recollimated on the atmospheric side.

2.1.4 Power Sources, Accessories, and Controls

DC Power Systems

Lasers with a DC discharge require a current-controlled DC power supply and a resistive ballast network. Control of laser power is by feedback control of the discharge current that is compared to a current command signal. If the laser has a continuous power monitor option, the power is controlled directly by comparing the monitored power signal to a control command signal and adjusting the discharge current accordingly.

The ballast network is a very important feature of the discharge system. Parallel ballast circuits connected to multielement electrodes are required to establish a uniform discharge. This requirement is especially critical in transverse flow systems with their large area discharges. The addition of ballast also helps to reduce laser power fluctuations induced by power supply ripple.

Some DC-powered lasers can produce a repetitively pulsed output. In these lasers the power supply must be capable of rapid modulation. This capability is more readily achieved in the switch-mode power supplies that are employed in many lasers. The switch-mode supplies offer advantages over the older SCR-controlled units because the switch modes are much smaller in size and have a faster frequency response. Even so, most DC-power lasers do not produce high-energy pulses but rather provide a means to modulate the output power.

RF Power Systems

Most high-frequency AC lasers are fact in the RF regime. RF power supplies are more complex and costly than DC supplies, but RF discharge systems can provide superior discharge stability and a more extensive modulation and control capability. For example, some RF lasers do not use a beam shutter to control the beam output, because the power can be readily turned on and off by the power supply control.

In addition to the basic power supply, RF discharges require a matching network to assure safe and efficient power transfer to the discharges. Without a matching network much of the power supplied to the laser would be wasted and, in fact, radiated from the system. Today's RF lasers employ effective matching devices that assure safe and efficient transfer of power over the full range of laser operation.

Accessories

Especially in the higher-power laser systems special accessories are often required or desirable for industrial production processing. The most commonly used accessories are summarized in the following list.

Power meter (usually standard) – direct readout of laser power, except when the laser beam is transmitted out of the laser enclosure.
Continuous power monitor – provides power readout even when the beam is transmitted out of the laser enclosure.
Beam viewer – displays visual profile of beam intensity distribution.
Beam shutter – Controls transmission of beam out of laser enclosure. Used in process control. Typical response time – 0.1 sec.
High-speed shutter – Fast-acting process control shutter with response time of 10 msec or less.
Safety shutter – Backup shutter located after main shutter and controlled by interlocks in a workstation. Provides an additional safety factor to protect against inadvertent exposure to the beam.
Manual lockout – Heavy-duty shutter that can be manually closed and locked by service personnel to assure the beam cannot be transmitted into a workstation.
Visible alignment system – Visible beam such as HeNe or diode laser that can be used to check cavity alignment and/or external beam propagation path.
Beam switch (shuttle) – Actuated mirror system that can direct the output beam in at least two different directions. Used to share the laser beam alternately between two or more workstations.

Controls

A wide variety of laser controls are in use today ranging from hard-wired relay circuits with push-button actuation in the simplest systems to programmable logic controls (PLC) to computer (PC) controls. The latter two connect to a man-machine interface (MMI) to provide a user-friendly operator control and function monitor. In all the systems, programming in relay ladder logic is preferred by most users. The large high-power systems usually have the biggest and most sophisticated control systems. From the user's standpoint the direct control and monitoring of system functions are the essential features of the control system. However, other important features include fault detection and warning as well as component calibration features.

It is important to note that even in the PLC and PC control systems, hard-wiring of safety circuits is required to assure fail-safe operation of these components.

2.1.5 Lifetime, Care, and Maintenance

The overall lifetime of CO_2 lasers is indefinitely long. Some CO_2 lasers have been in service for well over 10,000 h. Although many of the lasers utilize glass tubes, the tubes are well protected and isolated within the laser enclosures so that tube breakage is very rare. Almost all CO_2 lasers have some fragile components, but these components can be replaced in most systems. The higher-power industrial systems are more like rugged machine tools rather than sensitive laboratory prototypes. Nevertheless, care and maintenance is required to assure good performance and long useful lifetime.

In many lasers, especially the smaller units and those that are hermetically sealed, service by the user cannot be performed, except to assure that the outside of the output window is clean. These systems must be returned to the supplier to have the output window replaced, to have the mirrors refurbished, to be evacuated and recharged, and for other routine service. The user should, however, follow the supplier's guidelines and use common sense in the installation and use of these lasers. Although most industrial systems continue to operate dependably under adverse conditions, in some factory environments, cleanliness and controlled moderate humidity contribute to more dependable long-term operation. Also, an adequate supply of good-quality cooling water is essential to maintain good performance.

Most of the higher-power systems can be serviced by the user. In addition to routine changes of items like air and water filters, periodic service or replacements of windows, mirrors and electrodes (DC discharge systems) is required. The frequency of service depends on the hours of operation and the level of operation. When operated at rated power, service of these items should not be required more frequently than 500 h, which is typical for some electrode cleaning. Optical component service should be in the thousand-hour range or higher. Usually optical components, such as focus head elements, in the associated processing station, require much more frequent inspection and service because of contamination from fumes and spatter.

JACK DAVIS

2.1.6 Laser Gases for CO_2 Laser Resonators

Mostly, laser gas for a CO_2 laser is a mixture of

- carbon dioxide (1–9% of the gas mixture),
- nitrogen (10–55% of the gas mixture) and
- helium (balance of the gas mixture).

Carbon dioxide is the actual lasing gas, nitrogen is used to excite the carbon dioxide molecules more efficiently, and helium supports the laser process by emptying the lower carbon dioxide energy level and conducting heat out of the resonator.

In some cases small amounts of carbon monoxide or oxygen are added to the laser gas.

Because the gas is a critical component for the laser process, gas impurities are one source of power losses and optical degradation of laser systems. Therefore, laser manufacturers normally specify the required gas purity.

Required Gas Purity

Table 2 presents the gas purity for different laser resonators as specified by some laser manufacturers. Some laser systems mix the gas themselves, others require a gas premix. In this case, the gas supplier has to guarantee that all components stay within the mixture tolerance given by the laser manufacturer.

Laser gases are derived from different sources

- Nitrogen is separated out of the atmosphere.
- Helium is extracted from natural gas.
- CO_2 is manufactured from the waste products of the combustion of carbon compounds, i.e., natural gas in oxygen.

Table 2. Recommended Gas Purity for Different Laser Systems (1, 2)

Laser	Gas		
	Helium	Nitrogen	Carbon dioxide
Rofin Sinar	99.995	99.995	99.99
Trumpf	99.995	99.99	99.998
Fanuc	99.99	99.99	99.99
PRC	99.995	99.7	99.5
Convergent Prima	99.995	99.995	99.995
Panasonic	99.995	99.995	99.99
Mitsubishi [a]	99.99	99.99	99.99
Wegmann Baasel	99.995	99.995	99.995

[a] Uses CO in the gas mixture.

Because the atmosphere and natural gases (i.e., methane) are the main resources for all CO_2 laser gas, impurities such as moisture, oxygen, and hydrocarbons are most likely to be present and are discussed below.

Effects of Gas Impurities on Laser Performance

The effects of gas contamination on the laser performance have been studied thoroughly by laser and gas companies (3). The sensitivity of the laser system for gas contamination certainly depends on the particular resonator and may be the reason for the different requirements in Table 2. The kind of excitation (DC-excited using electrodes inside the cavity exposed to the laser process or RF-excited using electrodes outside the cavity) and the type of gas circulation (no circulation in case of diffusion-cooled or sealed systems, slow-axial-flow, fast-axial-flow, or transverse-flow circulation) influence the sensitivity of the system for impurities.

The effect of oxygen as one possible impurity was studied by adding it to the helium resonator gas. As shown in Figure 12, addition of 100 ppm results in a slightly increased absorptivity of the output coupler.

The negative effect of oxygen contamination on the optics can be explained by additional ozone created by reaction of oxygen atoms coming from the dissociation of CO_2 and O_2 molecules. Ozone can cause erosion of the optics. The coatings for most optics used in CO_2 laser resonators are composed of stacks of alternating high- and low-index dielectric material, such as ZnSe, ThF_4, ZnS, and Ge. The ozone attacks each of these differently by cracking and flaking the coatings. The absorptivity increased with increasing oxygen. Energy-dispersive electron spectroscopy analysis of the output couplers showed an erosion like surface damage (see Fig. 13).

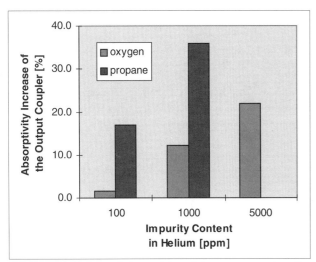

Figure 12. Increase of absorptivity of the output coupler after 3 h run time with impure helium. End mirror and bending mirrors also show increased absorptivity, which leads to reduced laser output power (3).

Besides oxygen, hydrocarbons were investigated. As shown in Figure 12, small amounts of hydrocarbons increase the absorptivity significantly. The surfaces of the optics are not damaged by erosion but by small carbon flakes. Both mechanisms will lead to significant laser power losses and shorten the lifetime of the resonator optics.

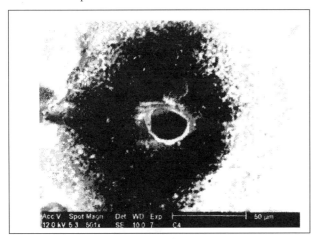

Figure 13. Eroded surface of the output coupler after running the laser for 3 h with 5000 ppm oxygen in helium (3).

It must also be noted that moisture can support the same degradation mechanisms. In addition, moisture can react with decomposed laser gas molecules in the resonator and form ions such as H^-, OH^-, and H_3O^+. The presence of negative ions is particularly critical for the operation of high-power CO_2 lasers because they affect the growth rate of the thermal instabilities in the gas plasma of the electrical discharge. Therefore, moisture should be kept low by the gas supplier and not permeate into the gas supply system. Because the laser is an expensive tool, one should know and reduce those impurities that influence the laser performance and damage the optical components of the laser system. It has been proven in recent investigations that moisture and hydrocarbons cause the most significant damage of the expensive optics. A general purity requirement of 99.99% still allows 100 ppm impurities without specifying whether these are moisture or hydrocarbons or other impurities. Therefore, a maximum amount of moisture and hydrocarbons should also be specified.

Gas Supply Systems

Whenever high purity is required by the laser manufacturer it is advisable to pay attention to a properly installed gas supply system. A leaking gas supply system can contribute to the contaminations of the laser gas or waste expensive gases. A prospective laser user can guarantee the quality of the gas supply by enlisting people with professional experience in high-purity gases to help with the design and installation of the gas supply system.

It is important to know that commonly used hose materials allow different diffusion rates and are not as gas tight as metal tubing (see Fig. 14). The diffusion rates of oxygen, nitrogen, and moisture penetrating the different hose materials were obtained by running helium through a 10-m-long line made of different materials and analyzing the amounts of impurities at the end of the line. Because diffusion is controlled by the partial pressures of the gas components, this process is possible even if the total pressure of gas inside the hose is above atmospheric pressure.

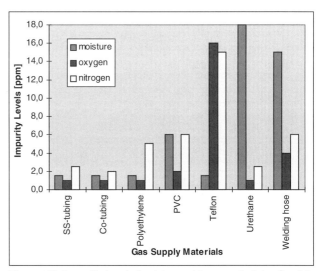

Figure 14. Impurity levels for tube and hose materials after 6 h flushing with helium.

For example, if a hose is used to supply a laser gas mix of 80% He, 14% N_2, 5% CO_2, and 1% O_2 at 3 bar (45 psi) to the laser resonator, the partial pressure of oxygen within this mixture is close to zero and the partial pressure of nitrogen is 0.45 bar. In contrast, the partial pressures of oxygen and nitrogen in the atmosphere are $p_{O2} = 0.21$ bar and $p_{N2} = 0.78$ bar. This means that both oxygen and nitrogen will diffuse through the walls of the hose into the laser gas mixture. Because helium, on the other hand, is not a major component of the atmosphere but a major component of the laser gas mixture, inside the hose it may permeate to the outside so that the ratio of helium in the gas mixture will decrease and the expensive gas is wasted.

The following rules should be applied during installation of high purity gas supply systems:

- Polyethylene appears to be the first choice for hose material and should be used inside and outside of laser machining systems.
- In the case of a central gas supply or long supply distance, hard plumbing made of stainless steel or copper should be preferred to decrease the amount of impurity diffusion, leakage of helium, and to avoid the risk of hose fracture.
- Stainless steel tubing can be TIG-welded, copper tubes can be connected by brazing. In both cases inert backing gas inside the tubes avoids the formation of oxide particles, which can later damage the laser or lead to leakage of the regulators (creeping). As a third method, compression fittings or similar products may be used.
- High-purity gas regulators should have stainless steel diaphragms to avoid diffusion within the regulator.
- Automatic switch-over features, including purge valves, guarantee an uninterrupted operation and avoid moisture coming into the system. These features are available as standard solutions today and should be considered an important component of the laser processing system.
- If possible the gas system should be installed by trained people.

The investment costs for a gas system for high-purity gases are higher than for an ordinary system. Investigations that compare the savings for one set of resonator mirrors and reduction of downtime show that the payback time for the gas system is less than one year, even if the uptime of the laser system increases only by as little as a few percent.

Besides being contaminated during production or within the gas supply system, the gas can be contaminated by material outgassing in the gas cavity itself. Today the laser manufacturers select their materials carefully according to high standards to guarantee minimal contamination. The same is true for the gas supply companies delivering high-purity gases and assisting during installation of the gas supply system.

References
1. G. Broden, 1989: *Laser Gases for CO_2 Lasers,* Report AGA Gas, Inc., GIW-89010.
2. *Facts About: Laser Resonator Gases,* information from AGA Gas, Inc.
3. C-J. R. Hsu, 1996: *The Influence of Foreign Gaseous Impurities on the Performance of an Industrial CO_2 Laser,* Dissertation, The Ohio State University.

JOACHIM BERKMANNS

2.2 Nd:YAG Lasers

2.2.1 Basic Principles

The Nd:YAG laser is the most prevalent high-power, solid-state laser in use today. Its lasing action is developed in the Nd^{3+} ion. It is based on a four-level system of electron energy level changes within the ion. Figure 1 shows the energy levels and laser transitions of this type of laser.

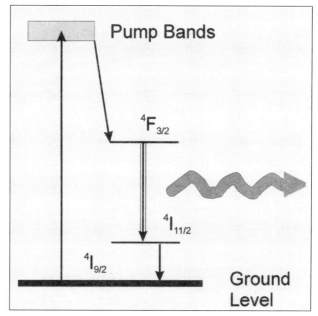

Figure 1. Basic energy-level diagram for Nd:YAG laser.

YAG is the host for the Nd ion. YAG stands for yttrium aluminum garnet ($Y_3Al_5O_{12}$). Neodymium is doped into the YAG crystal, taking the place of yttrium in the crystal as it is grown via the Czochralski method. Typical doping levels are between 0.5% and 1.1% Nd. After crystal growth is completed, the rough crystal or boule has several rods or slabs cut from it. The ends are polished and coated with an antireflection coating at 1.064 µm. YAG is chosen as the host for the Nd^{3+} ion because of its thermal, optical, and mechanical properties. YAG is a very strong crystal even when distorted by the addition of the slightly larger Nd. It can withstand very high internal stresses produced from optical pumping and cooling at the outer diameter. YAG is optically transparent to both the pump wavelengths and the laser wavelength, and it can take a very high-grade optical polish.

The YAG material is placed within a housing that provides a mechanical mounting, provisions for cooling, and optical alignment with laser mirrors and the pumping source. For lamp-pumped systems, the lasing material is placed within a reflective shroud that directs the lamp light to the lasing medium, usually with a gold-plated reflector or special ceramics that naturally reflect pump light. Deionized (DI) water is used to cool the YAG material and the lamps in lamp-pumped systems to remove up to 97% of the pump energy that does not create laser light. Diode-pumped systems will use some water cooling depending upon the power level.

Nd:YAG lasers are optically pumped lasers that require intense light to populate the upper laser transition levels. In the case of Nd:YAG the main pump band is at approximately 810 nm. For most lasers this light is provided by Kr and/or Xe lamps, which emit a typical blackbody light output but with some localized output peaks, one of which covers the 808 nm laser pump band (see Fig. 2). For more efficient pumping of YAG lasers, a laser diode that emits only in the 808 nm pump band can be used to produce lasers with 25% to almost 50% efficiency.

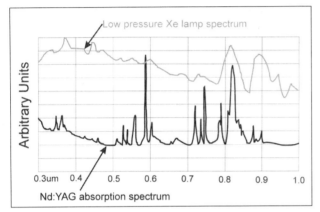

Figure 2. Relative pump output and crystal absorption for Nd:YAG. Note the 808 nm pump band and enhanced lamp output in the pump band.

With the high energies used in lamp-pumped systems, the heat load on the lasing medium creates an optical distortion of the laser light. Because only the outer surfaces of the rod or slab are cooled by DI water, the center of the crystal is at a higher temperature. This thermal gradient from center to edges creates a mechanical stress that results in the optical distortion termed thermal lensing, whereby the laser crystal acts as a positive lens with shorter focal length at higher powers. This lensing results in poorer laser beam quality at higher powers and, unlike gas lasers, a laser that has changing beam quality with average power.

Lamps and their associated power supplies are designed for their mode of operation, i.e., pulsed or CW. Lamp dimensions, electrode shapes, and gas fill pressure are optimized for the power supply and laser pumping chamber.

2.2.2 Laser Configurations

There are many variations of laser crystals and/or pump sources to produce laser beams of the required average power and beam qualities.

Cylindrical Rod

The most typical design for lasers of 600 W and less is a single cylindrical laser rod with one or two pump lamps in a double elliptical reflective cavity. This is shown in Figure 3. Rod diameters vary from 2 to 10 mm and lengths from 50 to over 200 mm. In general, the larger rods produce more laser power but at poorer beam qualities. The laser designer chooses the correct size to fulfill the specification targets.

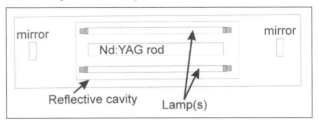

Figure 3. Basic layout of single laser rod resonator.

Multirod

Laser rods longer than 250 mm are very expensive to produce and have optical design limitations; so, for lasers of higher average powers, multiple rods are required. The most typical design is a design termed a periodic resonator illustrated in Figure 4. The spacing between rods is determined by the thermal lensing of the rods and the front and rear mirrors are located at half the rod face-to-rod face distance. Power per rod is additive so these lasers easily scale up in power with the addition of laser rods. For example, a 600-W single rod laser could be expanded into a 1200-W laser with the addition of a second rod in a periodic resonator. Units with power to 4000 W are available.

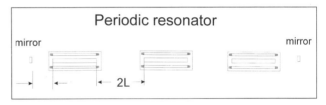

Figure 4. Three-rod periodic resonator showing spacing between mirrors and rods, where L is the length of the rod.

Slab

Cylindrical rod lasers have beam-quality limits determined by thermal lensing. One way to drastically reduce this effect is to have the laser beam pass through the lasing medium in a diagonal, zig-zag path so that the thermal lensing gradient in the crystal cancels itself as it crosses the axis of the crystal. While this is not possible in a cylindrical crystal, it can be done in a crystal with square or rectangular cross section, called a slab. The zig-zag path is made possible by using total internal reflection (TIR) within the crystal. To eliminate reflection losses at the ends of the slab, the ends are cut and polished at the Brewster angle so p-polarization can pass between mirrors and through the crystal without loss. Figure 5 depicts the slab laser configuration.

A rectangular cross section is typically used so that there is more volume in which the thermal gradient is across the thin section of the slab. These lasers are usually pumped from the large faces in a reflective cavity and produce beam qualities about 10 to 20 times better than rod-type lasers. They are expensive, however,

Chapter 2: Lasers for Materials Processing

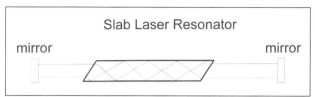

Figure 5. Basic slab laser resonator showing total internal reflection of laser light within the slab. Note the Brewster angle facets polished on the slab ends for *p*-polarization transmission.

because of the large crystal, the very flat and parallel polishing required on the slab flats, and the difficult water sealing required on the rectangular end faces. The slab laser can be more efficient for diode pumping because diode bars are more easily coupled into the large rectangular side faces of the slab.

Diode-Pumped

Diode-pumped lasers often employ very different optical pumping scenarios and, therefore, deserve some separate discussion of their special configurations.

Laser diodes have a very asymmetric output in their beam quality. Their small rectangular resonators generate beams with highly elliptical divergence. It is an optical and engineering challenge to deliver this beam efficiently into a cylindrical laser rod and have the pump light fill the space evenly. This task is made much more difficult by the fact that for high-average-power diode sources, a series of separate diodes in a long matrix, called a diode bar, is used. These diode bars are a long rectangle with evenly spaced individual lasers each emitting its characteristic elliptical beam.

Low-power diode lasers can use a few laser diodes and inject the pump light into the end of the rod. Special optics such as aspheric lenses can be used to better fill the round rod face, but the basic layout is shown in Figure 6. These are termed end-pumped lasers. Coatings on the mirrors are transmissive at the pump laser wavelength, but reflective at the Nd:YAG laser wavelength, so as to allow amplification of the laser light.

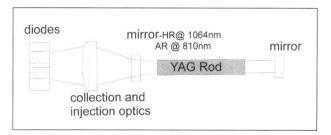

Figure 6. Typical end-pumped laser schematic.

For higher-power lasers and more efficient coupling of diode bars into the laser medium, the use of side-pumped resonators is most common. This scheme can be as simple as placing the diode bars around the laser rod so that their pump output has diverged to a size similar to the rod diameter. Two, three, or more radially symmetric layouts can be used. Flats can be ground into the rod for more even coupling. When slabs of laser material are used, the entire flat surface of the slab can be used to accept the diode laser pump energy. For small slabs the spacing of the diode bar and laser resonator can be designed so that the pump diodes are placed at the position in the slab where the laser light is undergoing each of its TIR reflections for better efficiency.

MOPA or Osc-Amp

Another laser resonator configuration is the master oscillator-power amplifier (MOPA) or more commonly termed an oscillator-amplifier (osc-amp) design. The most common reason to employ an osc-amp configuration is improved beam quality at high power. Large laser crystals produce poor-quality laser oscillators (resonators), but are required to produce high laser energies. Also, the alignment between components and the mechanical tolerances that exist can also introduce aberrations into the laser beam, reducing its quality. For this reason a simple oscillator is designed to produce the beam quality required. This oscillator is then sent through a series of laser rods or slabs called amplifiers making a single pass through each of them. Pumping occurs at the amplifier crystals, and each one will amplify the beam produced by the oscillator without adding much aberration to the original "seed" beam. The optical alignment is less critical in the amplifier because no feedback is required in the single pass through these stages. This scheme has a number of variations such as a two-rod system with a 500-W oscillator and a single amplifier rod producing 1-kW output power or a small mJ oscillator with kJ-level amplification for laser fusion research. Some laser systems even use multirod oscillators with multirod amplifiers.

Q-Switched Lasers

For very high-peak-power pulses from solid-state lasers, the use of a Q-switch introduces another laser configuration. The Q of a laser is the ratio of energy stored in the resonator to the power dissipated per optical cycle from the resonator. If one introduces an optical element in the oscillator that causes a misalignment or opacity, the laser crystal will be completely pumped to full energy storage with no energy lost via the output beam. If the laser resonator is then very quickly realigned or made transparent, the laser crystal will dump its excess laser photons from all the metastable atoms. This pulse lasts from a few nanoseconds to a few hundred nanoseconds, depending upon Q-switch type and resonator design. The Q switch must be located in the resonator (between the laser mirrors) and can be used with a pulsed or CW laser. Two types of Q switches are used: acousto-optical (AO) or electro-optical (EO).

The AO Q switch employs a block of fused silica with a piezoelectric oscillator bonded to it. The piezoelectric oscillator is driven by an RF power supply and produces standing acoustic compression waves in the silica that act as a diffraction grating, deflecting a portion of the laser beam away from the optical axis. This loss of intracavity laser intensity effectively misaligns the laser cavity, producing enough energy loss to spoil the Q of the cavity. When the RF supply is energized, it misaligns the cavity. When it is turned off, the cavity is realigned (see Fig. 7). A laser with an AO Q switch will produce its highest peak power pulses at frequencies below the repopulation rate of the laser. For Nd:YAG lasers, this is about 3 kHz. Frequencies higher than 3 kHz will produce lower peak power pulses, but average power will continue to increase until full average power is achieved, about 10 kHz. Lasers that use the AO Q switch are CW pumped and the Q switch is usually used to produce pulses from about 1 kHz to over 50 kHz. A 50-W CW laser, when Q-switched, will produce more than 25 kW peak power.

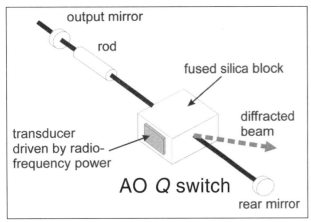

Figure 7. Acousto-optic Q switch employed in a CW-pumped Nd:YAG laser (1).

There is a limit to the AO Q switch in terms of the laser power that it can spoil. For low-power CW lasers (< 100 W), the AO Q switch can hold off or spoil all laser action. However, the AO Q switch diverts only a fraction of the laser beam, and if the laser's average power is too high, the undiverted laser light is sufficient to sustain lasing action regardless of the Q switch's induced loss. For higher average powers, multiple synchronized Q switches might be required, and they must operate at higher and higher repetition rates, so that the energy stored in the laser crystal(s) and resonator does not exceed the lasing threshold before the next pulse is generated. These types of lasers have been configured with up to 2 kW output power.

EO Q switches, usually Pockel's cell Q switches, can hold back very high peak powers; however, their repetition rate is limited to a few pulses per second in Nd:YAG lasers, and they are rather expensive. EO Q switches work using the electro-optic effect in solid crystals. An electric field applied to an electro-optic crystal, such as KDP (potassium dyhydrogen phosphate), will alter the polarization of a transmitted light beam. When one adjusts the voltage on the crystal, the linearly polarized input beam can be changed to circularly polarized light, or, at a different voltage, the output beam can remain linearly polarized, but the plane of polarization is rotated by 90 degrees. In Nd:YAG lasers either method can be used. To illustrate the latter method, the EO Q switch is placed in the cavity between a pair of crossed polarizing filters. Linearly polarized light from the first filter will not be transmitted by the second until the Q switch voltage is set to rotate the plane of polarization of the laser light by 90 degrees (see Fig. 8). The EO Q switch attenuates light by at least an order of magnitude more than an AO Q switch. This allows much higher-energy pulses to be created. Therefore, EO Q switches are normally used with pulsed solid-state lasers producing nanosecond-level pulses with up to multimegawatt peak powers. However, the drawbacks are that the voltages required are on the order of 3 to 15 kV, and they must be switched very quickly. Also, the laser must be operated at low average power, usually less than 20 W, to reduce depolarization of the beam in the crystal. Maximum repetition rates used are approximately 100 Hz, and the maximum energy per pulse is about 0.2 J. The EO Q switches can be used in an oscillator with one or more amplifier stages for higher energies, if required.

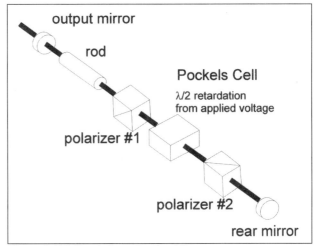

Figure 8. EO Q-switch application (1).

Harmonic Generation

Harmonic generation can also be called frequency doubling, tripling, or quadrupling as it applies to Nd:YAG lasers. It results in a single harmonic of shorter wavelength than the fundamental 1.06-μm output. This expands the capability of the laser source and involves using a special crystal called a nonlinear optical material to generate these harmonic frequencies. Nonlinear optical effects are described in more detail in Section 2.5.6.

In simple terms, inside these nonlinear crystals, the laser beam's fundamental frequency couples into a separate electromagnetic wave at a frequency of two times the fundamental. This higher frequency propagates out of the crystal. For Nd:YAG this is a 532 nm wavelength (green) output from the 1064 nm infrared input.

Efficient harmonic generation requires the fundamental laser to have very high spectral brightness. This means a high power density, low beam divergence, and small spectral linewidth (2).

If a laser with these characteristics is used with a good nonlinear crystal, then conversion efficiencies up to approximately 60% of the fundamental are possible. Typical systems available today range from 10 to 50%. Often AO Q-switched lasers are used because their high peak powers improve the efficiency.

Harmonic generation can be accomplished outside the laser or inside the laser resonator. The latter approach is termed intracavity frequency doubling. This approach is typical because the power density inside the resonator is approximately $1/T$ that of the output beam, where T is the transmission of the front mirror. Special dual-wavelength coatings are used to develop the output (see Fig. 9).

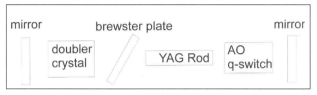

Figure 9. Typical intracavity second-harmonic generation scheme.

Tripling involves using some unconverted fundamental to mix with the doubled wavelength to produce output at one-third the fundamental wavelength, or 355 nm. Quadrupling uses multiple harmonic crystals or multiple passes through a crystal to produce output at 266 nm in the ultraviolet. This wavelength is of great interest due its photoablative effect on many materials; so it can process materials without heat input in the same way an excimer laser interacts with matter.

There are a multitude of crystals available for harmonic conversion, and the choice of crystal depends upon damage threshold, ease of handling, power capacity, and efficiency. Choices include KDP, $LiNbO_3$, barium sodium niobate, lithium iodate, KTP, and beta-barium borate.

2.2.3 Pump Sources

Flashlamps (Pulsed)

As discussed in Section 2.2.1, the Nd:YAG laser absorbs light energy in the 810 nm region to produce the 1064 nm laser output. For pulsed Nd:YAG lasers, the flashlamps are specifically designed for the typical repetitive high-peak-current electrical pulses that create the laser pulses. For Nd:YAG lasers the typical gas fill for the lamps is krypton (Kr) or xenon (Xe). Both Kr and Xe lamps produce a typical blackbody light output when pulsed but with a peak of light energy that covers the 810 nm pump band of the laser. This factor improves the laser's efficiency. The choice of gas fill is determined by their output of light in the pump bands for the peak currents delivered by the power supply.

Because of the high peak currents in the lamp during a pulse, these flashlamps have special design features to improve their reliability and life. Wall thickness is optimized for the high-pressure spikes; the electrodes are shaped for repeatable arc production; and the mass and placement of the electrodes is optimized for minimal thermal stresses where the metal electrode is sealed to the glass envelope. The gas fill pressure and the lamp's internal bore diameter must be carefully engineered to match the impedance of the lamp to the impedance of the power supply to get maximum power transfer of electrical energy to the lamp with minimal reflected electrical energy (ringing). The electrodes, especially the cathode, are designed with specific shapes and alloy contents to optimize their operation and minimize sputtering of metal from their surfaces during operation. Great care is taken during manufacturing to eliminate impurities in all components.

Arc Lamps (CW)

Lamps for CW lasers employ similar gas fills of Xe and Kr; however, the continuous mode of operation of these lamps results in slightly different designs. A laser operating in the CW mode can often require much higher pumping energy because of lower photon flux in the laser, and the lamps must be able to withstand the higher average power delivered to them. Cooling must be optimized for the high-power operation, but the high-pressure spikes of pulsing lamps are not a concern for CW lamps. Therefore, the lamp jacket walls can be thinner, but the electrode size must be increased for better cooling. Lamp impedance values are just as important for efficiency of this style of lamp.

Lamp Aging and Failure

Aging and failure of lamps is a concern because the lamp is a consumable item. Lamp aging is the reduction in pump power delivery to the laser crystal over time. Almost all aging can be attributed to sputtering of metal from the cathode onto the lamp envelope or from impurities in the lamp. The buildup of metal vapors and particles on the envelope result in lower transmission of pump light from the plasma. Special low-sputter metallurgies are used to reduce this effect as well as to minimize high-energy spikes from the laser power supply. As a lamp ages, the pump light, and therefore the laser output, will diminish. Additional current can be delivered by the power supply to bring the laser output back to its nominal value; however, there is a point at which the power supply reaches maximum output and the lamp must be replaced. This aging mechanism is typical in all types of laser lamps with typical lifetimes of 400–1500 h for CW lamps and 5–200 million pulses for pulsed lasers, depending upon the laser's operating parameters as compared to the maximum rated output.

Lamp failure can occur via a destructive mode. For example, the laser flashlamp can become weakened by excessive heating because of absorption by deposits and pressure spikes can cause explosive failure at these areas. Lamps can also lose their glass-to-metal seal at the electrodes, releasing their gas charge, which, in effect, causes the lamp to stop conducting. Rarely, if ever, do these failures result in any damage to the laser but do require a few minutes for removal of lamp debris during the lamp replacement procedure.

Laser Diode Pumping

Laser diodes for optical pumping of solid-state lasers are a special adaptation of the standard single laser diode used for many different applications from pointers to compact disk reading. The 808 nm pump band of the Nd:YAG laser is best suited to being pumped by diode lasers such as GaAlAs diode lasers. These diode lasers are usually manufactured in linear arrays of multiple diode lasers in a single package that can be several centimeters long, called diode bars. Typical laser diode output powers of 10 to 50 W per bar are required for Nd:YAG laser outputs in the 2–20 W range. High power density in a small package does require very good cooling of the diode bars for satisfactory operation and diode laser life. One drawback of diode pumping is matching the diode wavelength output to the rather narrow 808 nm pump band for Nd:YAG. Only about 20 Å in variation is permissible in the laser diode output wavelength before the pump light falls outside the pump band. The diode output can vary by 3 Å/°C. Careful manufacture of the diode bars to ensure they have output energy in the proper spectral range and very good temperature control of the diode bars are essential in diode pumping. Diode pumping does offer substantial advantages in terms of increased efficiency, reduced cooling, and smaller size and weight as compared to lamp pumping. Many commercial models of diode-pumped Nd:YAG lasers have become available.

2.2.4 Power Control

Output power is determined by the pump power to the lasing medium. There are two basic types of power supplies, pulsed power supplies and CW power supplies.

Pulsed lasers require that the power supply produce very high-current pulses (up to several hundred amps) to a gas-filled flashlamp. The voltage is rather low, usually from 400 to 800 V. To achieve the high peak powers, this type of power supply must store some energy between pulses or the current draw at the mains will be excessive. Older-style power supplies simply charged a capacitor bank and discharged it through a pulse-forming network of inductors and capacitors. This approach is very inefficient and has a low repetition rate and poor pulse-to-pulse control. Modern pulsed power supplies employ switched-mode DC first stages and transistor-controlled lamp drivers to develop and deliver the energy efficiently and with a very high degree of control. Closed-loop feedback and microprocessor control are also typical. Lasers in the 350 to 550 W output range require an electrical pump power of about 10 kW.

CW power supplies employ all the same modern electrical components as pulsed supplies, but the peak currents are much lower. These supplies will deliver comparable total electrical energy, but the lamp driving stage will be designed for constant output of a few hundred amps at about 400 V.

Most crucial to laser power control are microprocessor control and laser power feedback. Most lasers have a photodiode that samples the laser output power for display on the control but also is used by a closed-loop output power control. The laser controller can be programmed to deliver a certain pulse energy or average power. With feedback from the power monitor, the laser power supply will be automatically controlled to maintain the laser's output as the lamps age or the main voltage changes.

2.2.5 Lifetime, Care, and Maintenance

Nd:YAG lasers require very little maintenance, but the standard planned maintenance (PM) schedule should be followed diligently. Lamps should be changed at the proper intervals determined by the manufacturer to reduce the chance of lamp breakage. DI water filters and particle filters must be changed at the proper intervals to maintain good water quality. Water conductivity meters will sound alarms when water conditions have degraded, but it is best to change filters during the allotted PM time slot.

Chilled water delivered to the laser should meet the manufacturer's specifications at all times, and closed-loop systems should have chemical additives to prevent bacteria and algae growth. Filters should be used with tower water systems and city water to eliminate heat-exchanger fouling. If over-temperature conditions begin to occur, the cause should be found and corrected.

As with any high-power laser, the maintenance should be performed by trained personnel who follow the correct procedures for both repair and safety. Nd:YAG lasers are one of the most reliable laser systems in use today because of the simplicity of the solid-state laser. There are industrial systems in use today with well over 60,000 h of operation, and there is no reason they cannot be used for another 100,000 hours or more. History has shown that the lifetime is not limited by any component but by the availability of spare parts and knowledgeable service personnel.

2.2.6 Output Beam Quality

Unlike gas lasers, the Nd:YAG laser crystal is optically active in the resonator. This means that its optical characteristics vary with the laser parameters, affecting the output beam quality. As discussed previously, the YAG crystal acts as a positive lens when it is pumped because of the higher temperatures at the center, because cooling water is in contact only with the rod's outer surface. This thermal lensing of the rod increases with increasing pump power in a rather linear fashion.

Beam quality can be discussed in terms of the M^2 value (see Section 3.4) or another value, called the diameter-divergence product, in units of millimeter-milliradians (mm mrad).

Large-diameter laser rods produce the most laser power but have the poorest beam quality because of higher temperature gradients in the rod. Similarly, short laser resonators produce higher average power because of the increased mode volume in the resonator, but short resonators also produce poorer beam quality because higher-divergence light is still amplified. Laser designers must find a compromise between average power, beam quality, and optical complexity. In general, welding lasers can employ poorer beam quality because larger focus spots improve weld strength and tolerance to joint position. Fine cutting and drilling lasers often require much better beam quality because the cut width is directly related to beam quality and wide cut kerfs greatly increase heat input into the part. Figure 10 shows the typical beam quality output from a typical 400 W pulsed welding Nd:YAG laser. Note the increasing diameter-divergence product for increasing power in a linear fashion.

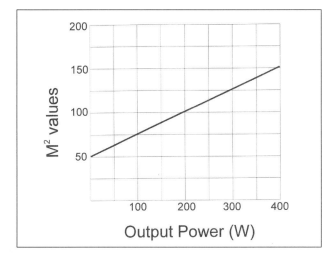

Figure 10. Typical output beam quality versus power for a 400 W pulsed Nd:YAG laser.

One way to improve the beam quality from this laser is to lengthen the resonator, the distance between the front and rear mirrors. This requires a much more stable resonator, but functions well for low powers. At higher powers the highly focused light rays in the resonator begin to focus on the mirror surface and at higher pump powers actually focus before the mirror and diverge out of the resonator, causing a severe power loss (see Fig. 11).

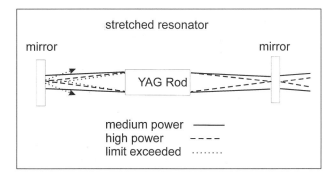

Figure 11. Schematic diagram of increasing beam divergence with increasing power. With a stretched resonator, the beam will focus onto the mirrors or even before them at higher powers.

Another method of beam-quality improvement is to place an aperture in the resonator to eliminate highly divergent light from being amplified. This practice is wasteful of laser power, however. A 6 mm rod with a 2 mm aperture in the cavity has an effective power output equal to the area of the rod face open to the resonator, which in this case is $2^2/6^2$, or 1/9 of the output of the laser without an aperture (see Fig. 12).

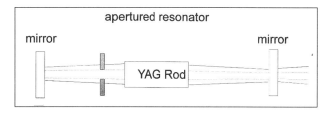

Figure 12. Improving beam quality with an aperture but with very high power losses because of lost rod volume for amplification.

Using a mirror with a convex surface or a laser rod with a convex-ground end surface will act to counter the positive focusing of the rod. This will result in a laser with much better beam quality but a laser that might not begin to lase until the pump power produces enough thermal lensing to counter the diverging optical surfaces. A laser with no output at the low range is a result of this type of system (see Fig. 13).

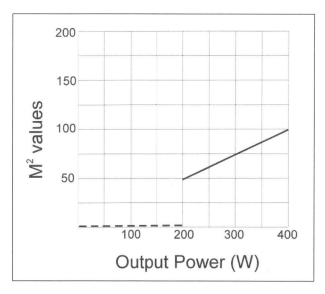

Figure 13. Negative rear mirror and/or curved rod resulting in no output at low powers but improved beam quality at higher power.

Using a negative lens in the resonator will greatly improve beam quality, but the rod needs to be pumped at a predetermined value so that the thermal lensing of the rod matches the negative value of the lens. This has the advantage of allowing very good beam quality while using the entire rod volume for laser generation as shown in Figure 14.

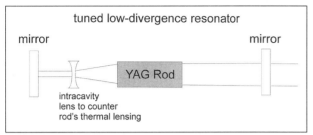

Figure 14. Schematic diagram showing the use of a negative lens in the resonator to produce very good beam quality at high average power.

In general the laser's beam quality will increase with average power until the laser output reaches approximately 500 to 700 W. At that point multiple rods are employed in a periodic resonator or oscillator-amplifier configuration with similar beam qualities above 700 W of output power. Table 1 shows some representative values of M^2 for pulsed and CW Nd:YAG lasers. Their values were derived from the literature of laser manufacturers. At any particular power level, the values of M^2 vary from laser model to another. Because of the 10 times shorter wavelength of Nd:YAG lasers, they will produce similar focus spot sizes to a CO_2 laser of 10 times better M^2 value. A value of $M^2 = 100$ for Nd:YAG is similar to $M^2 = 10$ for CO_2.

Table 1. M^2 Values for CW and Pulsed Nd:YAG Lasers

Output power (W)	M^2
0–20	1.1–5
20–50	20–50
50–150	50–75
150–500	75–150
500–4000	75–150

Reference
1. W. Koechner, 1988, *Solid State Laser Engineering*, Springer-Verlag, New York, Chapter 8.
2. W. Koechner, 1988, *Solid State Laser Engineering*, Springer-Verlag, New York, Chapter 10.

THOMAS R. KUGLER

2.3 Other Solid-State Lasers

This section describes many types of solid-state lasers that may prove useful to the materials-processing community in coming years. While lamp-pumped Nd:YAG lasers predominate in the market today, it is thought that refined methodology requiring additional flexibility in power, wavelength, and pulse format may be needed to address the needs of each specific application. With the emergence of practical diode array pumps to replace the lamps that currently service the community today, as well as allow the deployment of new laser materials, many new viable solid-state lasers can be expected to become commonplace in the next decade (1). Table 1 summarizes a possible list of lasers that might prove valuable to materials processing. The list is by no means intended to represent the entirety of solid-state laser laser development (2), but instead is a judgment of what is mostly likely to be embraced within the next few years. Noted in Table 1 are the gain medium, output wavelength, preferred/typical pump source, thermal shock parameter (suggestive of resistance against thermal fracture under load), and the most common operational modes.

Table 1. Summary of Solid-State Laser Technologies That May Have a Growing Role in Materials Processing in the Future

Laser type	Wavelength (μm)	Pump source	Thermal shock R_T (W/cm)	Operational modes
Nd:YLiF$_4$	1.047, 1.32	lamps, diodes	–	Continuous, Q-switched
Nd:YVO$_4$	1.06, 1.34	diodes	–	Q-switched
Nd:glass	1.05	lamps, diodes	1.0	high energy, short-pulse
Alexandrite	0.7–0.82	lamps	20	high-power
Cr:LiSAF	0.78–1.01	lamps, diodes	0.8	short-pulse, Q-switched
Ti:Sapphire	0.66–1.2	Nd:YAG, Ar$^+$	31	short-pulse
Tm:YAG	2.0	diodes	6.5	CW, pulsed
CTH:YAG	2.1	flash lamps	6.5	pulsed, Q-switched
Ho:YAG	2.1	lamps	6.5	pulsed, Q-switched
Er:YAG	2.94	diodes	6.5	CW, pulsed
Yb:YAG	1.03	diodes	6.5	high-power, Q-switched
Yb:SiO$_2$	1.0–1.2	diodes	31	CW, medium power
Doubled Nd:YAG	0.53	lamps, diodes	6.5	Q-switched

Nd:YLiF$_4$ (neodymium-doped yttrium lithium fluoride or YLF) and Nd:YVO$_4$ (neodymium-doped yttrium vanadate) represent alternate hosts for the Nd^{3+} ion. They have similar characteristics to Nd:YAG. Both have been used for material processing applications.

Nd:glass lasers are based on the use of phosphate glass host material, in which 2–4% Nd doping is added. The crucial advantage of Nd:glass over other materials is that it can be fabricated in very large sizes, as large as 80 cm in length. Furthermore, Nd:glass has a reduced gain cross section compared to Nd:YAG (4×10^{-20} versus 28×10^{-20} cm^2, respectively); so it is possible to store far more energy in a large optical element than for Nd:YAG, while averting the onset of parasitic oscillations. On the other hand, the thermal conductivity and thermal shock parameter are lower than those of most other materials (3). In short, Nd:glass functions best in circumstances where high pulse energy is needed at a moderate repetition rate. In order for a laser of this type to offer the highest average power (i.e., repetition rate), techniques such as phase conjugation and the slab geometry are sometimes used. A recent flashlamp-pumped Nd:glass slab laser of this nature is shown in Figure 1. It was possible to generate 30 J/pulse at 6 Hz, with high beam quality (using phase conjugation) (4).

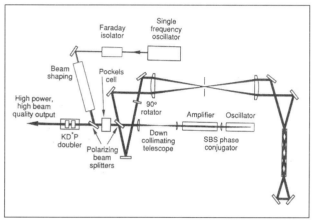

Figure 1. Schematic layout of a 30-J, 6-Hz flashlamp-pumped Nd:glass laser with high beam quality, incorporating the use of zigzag slab gain modules and phase conjugation (4).

Nd:glass lasers have also been useful as femtosecond ultrashort pulse oscillators, where they are mode locked by the Kerr lens effect. Pulse durations < 200 fsec have been achieved, at an average power level of < 1 W (5). These systems are compact, can be pumped by laser diodes, are robust, and may potentially prove useful for materials processing. In cases where ablative materials processing is needed at low power, the fsec diode-pumped Nd:glass laser may prove ideal.

Alexandrite lasers entail the material Cr-doped BeAl$_2$O$_4$, and offer very robust performance (6). The host medium is thermomechanically robust, and the chromium luminescence does not quench significantly even at 100°C. Alexandrite lasers operate near 0.8 µm, are tunable, and can be Q switched (at somewhat reduced average power). The material is generally pumped by CW or flashlamps, although diode pumping may become practical in the future. Average power levels close to 100 W have been reported. The shorter wavelength compared to Nd:YAG (0.8 versus 1.06 µm) may be important for certain applications, arising from the absorption characteristics of the substrate. Alexandrite laser rods are commercially available with high optical quality.

Cr:LiSAF (chromium-doped lithium strontium aluminum fluoride) does not have the thermomechanical robustness of alexandrite, but can be readily pumped by present laser diode technology, thereby offering a direct means by which to generate laser pulses < 50 fsec in duration (5). While the average power is generally < 1 W, this type of laser could be an economical means of generating ultrashort pulses. Flashlamp-pumped tunable Cr:LiSAF lasers are also practical at the 1–10 W level, and can be readily Q switched (7). The absorption and emission spectra of Cr:LiSAF in Figure 2 indicate the spectral pump and gain regions.

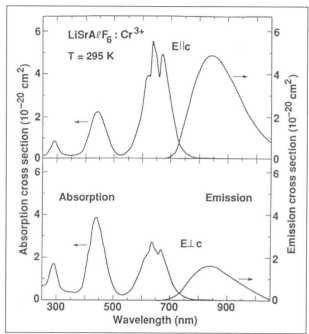

Figure 2. The absorption and emission spectra of Cr:LiSAF, indicating the spectral pump and gain regions.

The discovery of titanium-doped sapphire (Al$_2$O$_3$) is one of the great accomplishments of modern solid-state laser research, because it can be operated in a wide range of different configurations. Ti:Sapphire can be pumped by Ar$^+$ lasers as well as by doubled Nd:YAG lasers (in both cases near ~ 0.5 µm). The host medium is very robust and has a high thermal conductivity, allowing operation at several tens of W. In addition, Ti:Sapphire offers a very broad bandwidth, which permits an extended tuning range and the routine generation of ultrashort pulses of < 50 fsec (< 10 fsec in special systems). The use of the very short-pulse Ti:Sapphire lasers for materials processing will be discussed further in Section 2.5.9. Ti:Sapphire also may be configured in several amplifier stages, so that higher power levels can be achieved, even with femtosecond pulses. One promising approach is to employ doubled Nd:YAG lasers as the pump sources (e.g., diode-pumped intracavity-doubled modules). This architecture for an ultrashort-pulse Ti:Sapphire laser system operates at > 10 W of average power.

Some materials processing applications may require laser systems that operate in the mid-infrared, in order to be appropriately tailored to the absorption of the workpiece. The Tm, Ho, and Er lasers mentioned in Table 1 can provide this opportunity, as they lase at 2.0, 2.1, and 2.94 µm. As also noted, the host material is YAG, or $Y_3Al_5O_{12}$, a crystal that is particularly useful because it incorporates rare earth ions and is relatively robust (although not as robust as Al_2O_3 or $BeAl_2O_4$, which, however, cannot dissolve rare earth ions). The 2.01 µm Tm:YAG, pumped at 0.78 µm by laser diodes, is the most efficient of these laser materials in the CW mode (8). Much of the advantage of this laser crystal is derived from the unique cross-relaxation process that the Tm ions experience, whereby two nearby ions (one excited at 0.78 µm, one in the ground state) are converted to two ions capable of lasing at 2.01µm. Unfortunately the low gain cross section renders it problematic to lase Tm:YAG efficiently in the Q-switched mode. Figure 3 shows a plot of the CW output power of a Tm:YAG laser pumped by a 23-bar stack of laser diode bars and using a silicon microchannel heat sink (9).

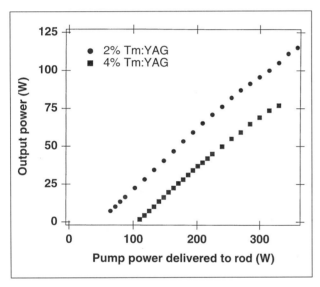

Figure 3. Plot of the CW output power of a Tm:YAG laser end-pumped by a 23-bar stack of laser diode bars (8).

The Cr,Tm,Ho:YAG laser crystal (CTH:YAG) is co-doped with three ions, so that Cr is first pumped by the flashlamps, transfers its energy to Tm, which then undergoes the "2-for-1" cross relaxation, before passing the energy on to the Ho ions. This laser crystal presents different opportunities for laser operation, in particular permitting more effective Q-switching schemes (as a consequence of ~3x greater gain cross section of Ho). Nanosecond pulses in the 2.1-µm range, where water absorbs to some extent, allow for more impulsive heating of the material, perhaps leading to chemical changes or fast boiling. CTH:YAG lasers can provide additional flexibilty to the materials-processing community (10). Work on the related doubly doped material Tm,Ho:YAG demonstrates that direct diode pumping of the Tm ions is also a viable path to a robust laser design (11).

The diode-pumped Er:YAG laser offers the longest wavelength available in a commercial laser as the direct output (i.e., not nonlinearly frequency-converted), at 2.94 µm. Interestingly this wavelength is strongly absorbed by water and hydroxyl ions, with a penetration depth of only several micrometers. The Er:YAG laser is a viable laser, but has only experienced limited exposure outside the experimental laser community. CW and quasi-CW operation are well known, but Q-switching methodology is not well developed. Watt-level CW or quasi-CW powers have been demonstrated for Er lasers (12).

Yb:YAG lasers are another technology that is rapidly growing in sigificance, by virtue of their ability to operate at high average power (13, 14). CW power levels of 1 kW and Q-switched power of > 280 W have been reported (Fig. 4), using laser diode pumping. And importantly, Yb:YAG lasers are capable of higher beam quality than Nd:YAG lasers because about 1/3 of the thermal load is generated. The special requirement of Yb:YAG lasers is that they must be pumped by very bright laser diode arrays, capable of producing power levels of ~20 kW/cm². The potential future dominance of Yb:YAG over Nd:YAG does significantly depend on progress in the laser diode array industry.

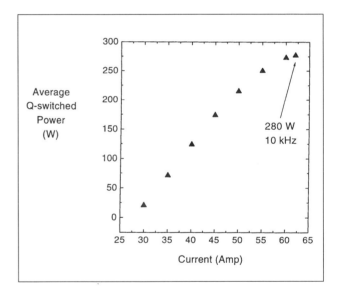

Figure 4. Output power of a diode-pumped Yb:YAG laser Q switched at 10 kHz (13).

A recent addition to the field of high-average-power, solid-state lasers is diode-pumped fiber lasers, in particular Yb:SiO$_2$. These lasers can produce power as high as 100 W. One of the key technologies is the cladding-pumping technique, where, although the fiber core (of several micrometers) is doped with Yb, the inner cladding region (of several hundred micrometers) serves as a waveguide for the pump light from which the light becomes absorbed into the doped core over an appropriate length. Even though the effective absorption coefficient is diminished by the ratio of the areas of the two regions, the diode brightness is suitable for laser operation. The diode-pumped cladding approach is an effective means of converting the low beam quality of a diode bar into a TEM$_{00}$ CW laser source for precision cutting.

While Nd:YAG lasers have long been regarded as the "workhorse" solid-state laser, only recently has it been shown it is possible to efficiently and reliably double a repetitively Q-switched power oscillator (10–30 kHz) using an intracavity frequency-conversion crystal at high average power. In fact, in comparing the doubled 0.53 µm output level to that which is achievable at 1.06 µm with optimized output coupling, > 50% conversion to the green is possible. The point is that lasers operating with high-average power at 0.53 µm are nearly available for experimentation; a typical set of performance parameters might be 100 W, 30 kHz, and 100 nsec. Figure 5 displays data involving 0.53 µm output of a diode-pumped KTP-doubled Nd:YAG laser module.

This discussion has not mentioned the ruby laser, operating at 0.694 µm. The ruby laser, the first laser ever to be operated, was used in many early materials-processing operations, but its limitations (especially its high threshold pumping energy) lead to low pulse repetition rate and low average power. Thus ruby lasers have not been used much in recent times.

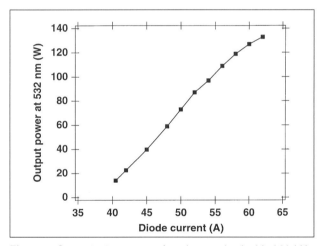

Figure 5. Green 0.53 µm output from intracavity doubled 30-kHz diode-pumped Nd:YAG laser.

References
1. S. A. Payne et al., "Diode arrays, crystals, and thermal management for solid-state lasers," *IEEE J. Selected Topics in Quantum Electronics* **3**, 71–81 (1997).
2. J. A. Caird and S. A. Payne, "Crystalline paramagnetic ion lasers," in *Handbook of Laser Science and Technology. Supplement 1: Lasers*, ed. M. J. Weber, CRC Press, Boca Raton, Florida, 1991, 1–99.
3. S. A. Payne et al., "Laser properties of a new average-power Nd-doped phosphate glass," *Appl. Phys. B* **61**, 257–66 (1995).
4. C. B. Dane et al., "Design and operation of a 150 W near diffraction-limited laser amplifier with SBS wavefront correction," *IEEE J. Quantum Electronics* **31**, 148–63 (1995).
5. Ursula Keller, "Materials and new approches for ultrashort pulse lasers," *Current Opinion in Solid State and Materials Science* **1**, 218–24 (1996).
6. J. C. Walling et al., "Tunable alexandrite lasers," *IEEE J. Quantum Electronics* **16**, 1302–15 (1980).
7. M. Stalder, B. H. T. Chai, and M. Bass, "Flashlamp pumped Cr:LiSAF laser," *Appl. Phys. Lett.* **58**, 216–18 (1991).
8. E. C. Honea et al., "115-W Tm:YAG diode-pumped solid-state laser," *IEEE J. Quantum Electron.* **33**, 1592–600 (1997).
9. R. Beach et al., "Modular microchannel cooled heatsinks for high average power laser diode arrays," *IEEE J. Quantum Electron.* **28**, 966–76 (1992).
10. S. R. Bowman et al., "Laser and spectral properties of Cr,Tm,Ho:YAG at 2.1 µm," *IEEE J. Quantum Electron.* **27**, 2142–49 (1991).
11. T. T. Fan, R. L. Byer, and P. Mitzscherlich, "Spectroscopy and laser diode-pumped operation of Tm,Ho:YAG," *IEEE J. Quantum Electron.* **24**, 924–33 (1988).
12. R. H Page et al., "1-watt composite-slab Er:YAG laser," in *OSA Trends in Optics and Photonics, Vol. 10, Advanced Solid State Lasers*, C.R. Pollack and W.R. Bosenberg (Eds.), Optical Society of America, Washington, D.C. 1997, 214–16.
13. C. Bibeau et al., "CW and Q-switched performance of diode end-pumped Yb:YAG laser," in *OSA Trends in Optics and Photonics, Vol. 10, Advanced Solid State Lasers*, C. R. Pollack and W. R. Bosenberg (Eds.), Optical Society of America, Washington, D.C. 1997, 276–79.
14. E. Honea et al., High Power Dual Rod Yb:YAG Lasers, *Opt. Lett.* **25**, 805–7 (2000).

Dominic, et al., "110 W Fiber Lasers," *Proceedings of Conference on Lasers and Electro-Optics*, Baltimore, MD, paper CPD11-1, May 23–28, 1999.

STEPHEN A. PAYNE

2.4 Excimer Lasers

2.4.1 Basic Principles

Excimer lasers are pulsed gas lasers that use a mixture of gases to provide emission at a series of discrete wavelengths in the ultraviolet region of the spectrum (1). The word *excimer* is a contraction of the term "excited dimer," which refers to a diatomic molecule bound in its electronically excited upper state but repulsive or only weakly bound when in the lower ground state. Excitation of the laser gas mixture is usually by means of a fast electric discharge with a duration of a few tens of nanoseconds. This causes the formation of the excited molecule appropriate to the mixture of gases selected. Laser action takes place as a result of the transition of this short-lived species back to the repulsive ground state, where the atoms recombine to their original individual components, enabling the process to be repeated.

The mixture of laser gases is confined within a pressure vessel, usually at a total pressure between 3000 and 5000 millibar. The electrodes used in the excitation process are typically between 50 and 100 cm long and between 1 and 2 cm wide, to provide an adequate gain volume, and are separated from each other by a centimeter or more. The resultant laser beam is rectangular in cross section with an aspect ratio between 1 and 3. A typical dimension for such an excimer laser beam would be 1 x 2.5 cm.

All excimer lasers use a noble gas, a halogen gas, and an inert buffer gas whose function is to transfer energy efficiently to the excited dimer molecules composed of one noble and one halogen gas atom. In a typical gas mixture, approximately 2% of the gas will be the noble gas, 0.2% will be the halogen gas, and the balance of several thousand millibars the buffer gas, usually helium or neon. Neon is often preferred, despite its higher cost, because it is the more efficient in transferring energy from the discharge to the lasing molecule.

2.4.2 Wavelengths

The wavelength emitted depends upon the selection of rare and halogen gas mixture. The most commonly used rare gases are argon, krypton, and xenon and the halogen gases fluorine or chlorine (supplied in the form of HCl). The halogen gases are usually supplied diluted by the buffer gas in concentrations of between 5 and 10%.

Table 1 shows the most commonly used combinations of excimer laser gases and outlines the practical attributes of each transition. Other gas mixtures exist but are used infrequently. Krypton-chloride mixtures emit at 222 nm, but the advantages of this wavelength are not compelling, and the efficiency and lifetime of the laser gas mixture are mediocre when compared to KrF. Molecular fluorine, F_2, will lase at 157 nm but is a very inefficient laser medium, delivering energies of only a few millijoules per pulse. The short wavelength is very attractive from a materials absorption standpoint but the difficulty of transmitting it to the workpiece and the short operational lifetime of this gas mixture means that very few such lasers are used in practical tasks.

Typical operating parameters of an excimer laser are given in Table 2.

Table1. Excimer Laser Wavelengths

Gas	Wavelength	Comments
ArF	193 nm	Requires high operating voltages to transfer energy to the discharge efficiently. The laser beam is absorbed by O_2 molecules in air so beam path requires N_2 flush for efficient propagation. Usually the shortest absorption depth in organic materials of all excimer wavelengths.
KrF	248 nm	Generally the best combination of power and lasing efficiency. The most commonly utilized transition for machining polymers because of the combination of its absorption characteristics in plastics and overall average power from the laser.
XeCl	308 nm	Very long lived gas lifetimes. Longer absorption lengths in polymers can lead to higher etch rates than KrF but lower average powers generate slower rate of material removal overall. Often used for marking applications.
XeF	351 nm	Lower absorption in polymers often make this a less attractive wavelength for machining tasks.

Table 2. Typical Excimer Laser Parameters

Parameter	Value
Wavelength (nm)	193, 248, 308 or 351
Pulse energy (mJ)	400–500
Repetition rate (Hz)	100–200
Average power (W)	40–100
Pulse duration (nsec)	15–30
Peak power (MW)	10–30
Peak fluence (mJ/cm^2)	100–200
Beam divergence (mrad)	1–3
Beam size (mm)	8–15 x 25–30

2.4.3 Resonator Configurations

Most excimer lasers are used with stable resonators, usually with plano-plano high reflector and output coupler mirrors. The resonator mirrors are normally attached to the laser pressure vessel and form part of the gas seal. The high gain of the excimer medium requires output coupling reflectivities of 10–30 % for most efficient energy extraction. Typical beam divergences are then of the order of 3 mrad (50% energy points).

When lower divergence is required, excimer lasers may be equipped with unstable resonators with a high magnification (up to 10X) to take account of the relatively few number of round trips that the discharge duration will support. This will reduce the beam divergence to a value between 200 and 400 microradians in a beam with 60–70% of the energy obtained with a conventional, stable resonator (2).

For some applications, line-narrowed operation is required. In this case, windows are used to seal the laser pressure vessel and dispersive elements (etalons, diffraction gratings, or both) are inserted between the laser resonator mirrors. Using this technique, stable linewidths of the order of 1 pm can be realized. The principal applications of line-narrowed excimer lasers are lithography and LIDAR.

2.4.4 Optical Configurations

With a stable resonator, the typical beam divergence of an excimer laser is approximately 3 mrad. For conventional, focused spot machining, this would represent a poor beam for producing small or precise features. However, excimer laser machining is normally performed by illuminating an aperture with the laser beam and forming a demagnified image of the aperture on the workpiece to achieve the desired feature size and the laser fluence needed to ablate material from the workpiece. In such an optical system, the beam divergence has lesser importance providing it is sufficient for the laser energy to be captured by the finite aperture of the final imaging lens.

Figure 1 shows schematically the principal elements of a simple excimer laser imaging system for ablative machining. See Chapter 15 on image micromachining for more details.

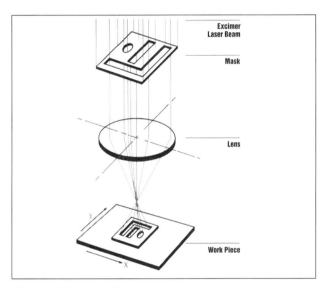

Figure 1. Schematic of an excimer laser imaging system for ablative machining.

In such a simple optical system, the ability to illuminate the mask with a uniform fluence relies entirely upon the uniformity of the laser beam itself. Most excimer laser beams exhibit a reasonably flat topped profile in their long axis but a more peaked distribution in the short one. The effects of beam inhomogeneity at the workpiece will be determined by the power dependence of the material being processed. In cases where the uniformity is critical, external beam homogenizers are included in the optical beam delivery. A wide variety of such devices exists, including fly's eye lens arrays, crossed cylindrical lens arrays, and prismatic beam folding optics. Using these devices, spatial uniformity can normally be improved to within a few percent. Invariably, these homogenizing devices cause a significant increase in the divergence of the laser beam and require subsequent optical elements to be large enough to collect this more divergent beam for efficient utilization of the laser energy.

2.4.5 Power Sources

Excimer lasers are energized by the deposition of charge stored in a capacitor array into the volume of gas between the main laser electrodes. To ensure that a glow discharge is achieved between the main electrodes, a preionization discharge provides ultraviolet photons to initiate photoionization of the laser gas between them. Usually, this takes the form of a spark discharge between an array of small, secondary electrodes that run the full length of the main electrodes.

Switching of energy from the main storage capacitor into the discharge has often been effected by a hydrogen thyratron. In early excimer lasers, the fast discharge with its associated high peak currents and current reversals caused these thyratrons to have a life limited to few tens of millions of pulses. This formed a major component of the cost of operating an excimer laser. More advanced circuit designs, including the use of saturable magnetic materials, pulse compression stages, and suppression of reverse currents, have extended thyratron lifetimes into the region of several billion pulses, with a consequent reduction in operating costs.

Recently, solid-state switching devices (SCRs) have been used in conjunction with multiple stages of magnetic compression of the current pulse to provide the source for energizing the excimer laser gas. This increases the lifetime substantially.

2.4.6 Lifetime, Care, and Maintenance

There are three main, elements in the lifetime and maintenance of excimer lasers. They are:

- Laser gas
- Laser optics
- High-voltage discharge components

Laser Gas

Excimer lasers are not sealed-off devices. The laser gas deteriorates with use, and therefore the laser is normally left connected to gas bottles that are used to replenish the laser gas fill in its entirety once its performance is no longer adequate.

Two separate mechanisms explain the deterioration of the laser gas with usage (3). In the first mechanism, gaseous impurities evolve within the laser and reduce the laser output by absorbing laser light within the pressure vessel. In the second, removal of halogen by interaction with the material of the vessel causes its concentration to fall below the optimum value. The net effect of both is to reduce laser efficiency over time.

To compensate for this, excimer lasers generally contain a system that continuously monitors the level of laser output and adjusts the power input to the laser to maintain constant optical output as the gas fill ages. Simultaneously, the laser control will introduce small quantities of halogen gas ("injections") to the gas mix as a software algorithm predicts its depletion.

In all modern excimer lasers, careful selection of materials, particularly the elimination of organic materials used as insulators, seals, or lubricants, minimizes these effects. Additionally, cryogenic gas processing may be used to remove gaseous impurities by selectively freezing them into a solid form in an external gas processing system from which they can later be removed. In combination, these techniques now make it possible to operate an excimer laser for intervals in excess of 100 million pulses between exchanges of laser gas.

Optics

As the laser operates, small particles are generated inside the pressure vessel by sputtering of material from the main discharge and preionization electrodes. These particles can settle on the laser optics, where they will cause loss of efficiency and output. The laser manufacturers use a number of techniques to minimize this effect, including electrostatic gas filtration (4) and control of gas flow near the laser optics. Despite this the laser optics must be removed periodically and cleaned. A typical optic cleaning interval would normally be in the region of 50–100 million pulses. Excimer lasers designed for industrial use now contain valves that seal the pressure vessel and retain the gas fill while optics are removed for cleaning. This minimizes the time taken for cleaning and also provides protection for the operator from egress of halogen gas while the optics are removed.

Optics for KrF, XeCl, and XeF laser operation will normally require replacement after 500 million pulses. ArF optics degrade more quickly, because of color center formation at the shorter operating wavelength, and require replacement at more frequent intervals.

High-Voltage Discharge Components

High-voltage components suffer wear in use and eventually require replacement. Of these, the laser vessel represents the most significant work and cost to replace. Its replacement is dictated by erosion of the main discharge and preionization electrode structures with use. The lifetime of a laser vessel is typically of the order of $(1–3) \times 10^9$ pulses, depending upon the transition and energy at which the laser is operated. The thyratron switch will typically have a lifetime of 2×10^9 pulses.

Table 3 summarizes the typical maintenance operations on a high-energy KrF excimer laser over each period of operation of 10^9 pulses.

Other components in the discharge circuit (triggering components, high-voltage power supplies, control electronics) are subject less to systematic wear than to statistical failure and will typically demonstrate lifetimes of $(2–10) \times 10^9$ pulses before requiring replacement.

Table 3. Typical Maintenance Operations for a KrF Laser

Interval	Action
Each 100 million pulses	clean optics
	exchange gas fill
At 500 million pulses	replace rear optic
	replace front optic
	replace beamsplitter
At 1 billion pulses	replace laser vessel assembly
	replace rear optic
	replace front optic
	replace beamsplitter
	maintain gas processor pump
	replace gas particle filter
	replace gas scrubber
	replace vacuum pump oil

References
1. J. J. Ewing, *Physics Today* **31** (5), 32, May 1978.
2. T. J. McKee and G. T. Boyd, *Appl. Optics* **27,** 1840, 1988.
3. G. M. Jursich, W. A. Von Drasek, R. K. Brimacombe, and J. Reid, *Appl. Optics* **31** (12), 1975, April 1992.
4. U.S. Patent No. 5,319,663, Reid et al., June 1994.

JAMES HIGGINS

2.4.7 Gas for Excimer Lasers

The laser gas for an excimer laser consists of a mixture of:

- The halogen gas (0.1–0.5% of the gas mixture)
- The rare gas (5–10% of the gas mixture)
- The buffer gas (balance)

By choosing different combinations of rare gas atoms and halogen atoms, a different wavelength of the ultraviolet radiation can be obtained, as shown in Table 4. The buffer gas can affect the laser power. Neon will produce somewhat higher laser powers than argon.

Table 4. Gas Mixtures for Excimer Lasers

Rare gas	Halogen gas	Wavelength
xenon	fluorine	351 nm
xenon	chlorine	308 nm
xenon	bromine	282 nm
xenon	iodine	253 nm
krypton	fluorine	248 nm
krypton	chlorine	222 nm
krypton	bromine	206 nm
argon	fluorine	193 nm
argon	chlorine	175 nm
fluorine	fluorine	158 nm

Chapter 2: Lasers for Materials Processing

Required Gas Purity

The values listed in Table 5 represent the purities required by the well-known excimer laser manufacturers.

Table 5. Recommended Gas Purity for Different Excimer Laser Systems (1, 2)

Gas	Purity (%)
halogen gas	99.8 or better
rare gas	99.99–99.995
buffer gas	99.99–99.9999

At present, excimer laser gas lifetime is the most important operating cost parameter (see Fig. 2). The gas lifetime is limited mainly because of two processes. First, the halogen component of the laser gas is slowly depleted because of reactions with the construction materials of the laser. Second, impurities that are generated by the electrical discharge poison the laser gas and quench laser action.

Effects of Gas Impurities on Laser Performance

It is well known that impurities in the laser gas mixture can decrease the performance of the excimer lasers. This can occur in various ways. The impurities can absorb the laser radiation or they can quench the excited rare gas/halogen molecules before they can emit laser radiation. Furthermore, air contamination can distort the spatial intensity profile of the laser beam. A uniform intensity profile is important for some excimer applications such as eye surgery and microlithography.

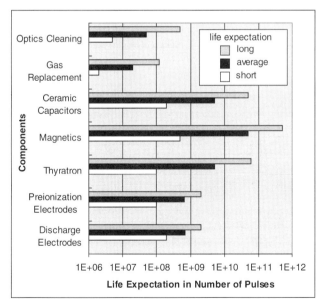

Figure 2. Component life of KrF excimer laser (5).

There are different sources of the impurities that are present in the gas mixture inside the laser resonator. Some impurities come from the cylinder gases themselves, for example, O_2, N_2, H_2O, and HF. HF impurities are, of course, mainly found in fluorine mixtures. Air contamination such as N_2, O_2, and H_2O can arise from leaks in the gas supply system or if the gas lines have not been purged sufficiently.

When the excimer laser is in operation, the impurity levels will gradually increase. At the same time the halogens react with the wall material of the laser cavity. Both processes, the increase of the impurities and the halogen depletion, result in a lower laser power as demonstrated in Figure 3.

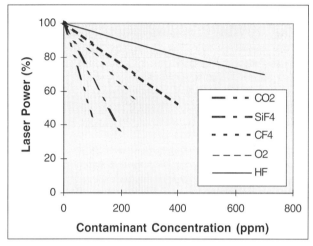

Figure 3. Effect of contaminations on the laser energy.

In order to extend the lifetime of the gas fill in the laser vessel, some measures can be taken:
- Injection of a small volume of the halogen to compensate the halogen depletion in the laser gas mixture.
- Replacing a fraction of the gas fill with fresh laser gas mixture.
- Cryogenic laser gas processing to trap impurities. (This is a continuous flow process in which the laser gas mixture is cooled to condense away volatile impurities. Before the purified gas is returned to the laser resonator, it can be passed through a particle filter so that the interval between optics cleanings will be extended.

Gas Supply Systems

The requirements of the gas supply system for excimer lasers are extremely high (6). The main reasons for this are:
- The required gas purity is very high (higher, for example, than the purity required for a CO_2 gas laser).
- The halogen gases are highly toxic.
- The halogen gases are highly corrosive in combination with moisture.

The following rules should be obeyed during installation of high-purity gas supply systems (6):
- To avoid poisoning of people and corrosion, it is important to have a gas-tight and sealed gas supply system with a leakage rate of less than 10^{-7}–10^{-9} cm^3 helium per second. This is best accomplished with orbital welded stainless steel supply sys-

tems. (Corrosion may produce microparticles in the supply system. These particles may cause damage to the laser and get caught on the inside of the regulator. The resulting increase in delivery pressure and the disability to obtain tight closure is a failure commonly known as "regulator creep."

- In the halogen lines the tubes should be electropolished, whereas for the other gases it is sufficient to use cleaned stainless steel tubes. The cleaning should be made with a chemical solvent to remove dirt and grease. Regulators may also be electropolished using membranes out of nickel-base alloys (i.e., Hastalloy).

- As shown in Figure 4, the halogen supply is installed in a ventilated cabinet. It is equipped with a facility for purging the halogen lines and the laser resonator. Since helium is part of the gas mixture or can be considered as a harmless impurity, it is used as purge gas. (Purging is necessary before replacing a halogen cylinder so that the operators will not be exposed to the halogen gas that remains in the gas line between cylinder valve and the regulator! Purging should also be carried out after the new halogen cylinder has been connected to flush out air that has entered the gas line during the cylinder change.)

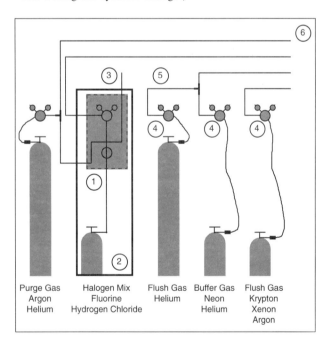

Figure 4. Gas supply system for excimer laser
(1 halogen gas panel with TIG welded SS components,
2 ventilated cabinet, 3 halogen scrubber,
4 gas supply unit for one cylinder,
5 stainless steel pipe 1/4" cleaned,
6 compression fitting stainless steel, welded SS-Tee).

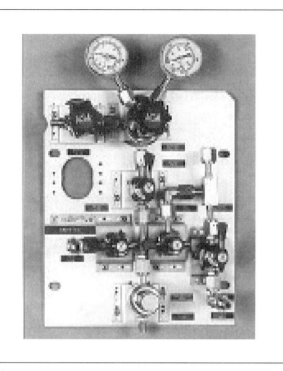

Figure 5. Halogen panel, detail out of Figure 4.

Figure 5 shows details of the halogen panel.

References
5. S. Metev and G. Sepold, 1993, *Excimer Lasers and New Trends in Laser Microtechnology*.
6. *Facts about: Excimer Lasers,* Information AGA Gas, Inc.

JOACHIM BERKMANNS

2.5 Other Lasers

2.5.0 Introduction
This section describes several diverse types of lasers that have been used for materials processing, or that are under development and are of potential application in laser materials processing. These lasers are not yet in widespread use as are the carbon dioxide, solid-state, and excimer lasers discussed in earlier sections. They have the potential for increased application in the future.

2.5.1 CO Lasers
Carbon monoxide lasers have been used in materials processing in a limited way. Compared to CO_2 lasers, CO lasers, operating near 5 μm, offer the advantages of higher absorption (see Chapter 5) and the capability of being focused to a smaller spot

diameter, leading to higher irradiance. Additionally, CO laser light can be delivered through special optical fibers at moderate power levels (under 100 W).

The oscillations between the vibrational - rotational energy levels in a CO molecule produce a number of laser lines in the 5 μm band (1). A number of these lines will be present simultaneously in the output of a CO laser, unless a wavelength-selecting element is inserted into the laser to restrict operation to a single line.

CO lasers are quite similar to CO_2 lasers in that laser operation can be generated by with slow axial flow, fast axial flow, or transverse flow systems. The output power per unit volume of gas is almost equivalent to that of a CO_2 laser, and the highest output power of the CO laser compares well with that of a CO_2 laser of similar size. Prototype CO lasers have achieved power outputs up to 20 kW (2).

Despite the advantages of their shorter wavelength, CO lasers have not become widely used in industrial materials processing applications. Compared to the CO_2 laser, the CO laser has two shortcomings:

1. The gas must be maintained at a low operating temperature because for temperatures 77 K and above, the lower the gas temperature, the higher the power output. To obtain low gas temperatures, the gas is either cooled aerodynamically (3) or with a coolant, such as liquid nitrogen (4). Although recent efforts have succeeded in producing high output power at ambient temperatures, the output power remains undesirably sensitive to the operating temperature (5, 6).

2. The gas is unstable during operation, being decomposed into C and O by the electric discharge. However, the accumulation of carbon can be prevented by mixing O_2 with gas. Of course, there will be an increase in CO_2 until there is a balance with CO according to

$$CO + (1/2) O_2 \rightleftharpoons CO_2$$

Thus for long-term operation, a flowing gas system must be used. A sealed system is not feasible at present. This is the greatest hurdle to be overcome in the commercialization of the CO laser.

The use of CO lasers for cutting will be described in Section 12.2.7.

References
1. C. K. N. Patel, *Appl. Phys. Lett.* **7,** 246 (1995).
2. S. Kuribayshi et al., *Mitsubishi Juko Giho* **31,** 1 (1994).
3. F. Maisenhalder, *Proc. LAMP '92* **1,** 43 (1992).
4. S. Sato et al., *J. Appl. Phys.* **58,** 3991 (1985).
5. M. Uehara and H. Kanazaw, *Appl. Phys. Lett.* **65,** 22 (1994).
6. S. Sato, et al., *Optics Lett.* **19,** 1 (1994).

TOMOO FUJIOKA

2.5.2 Metal Vapor Lasers

Metal vapor lasers utilize a metallic vapor at high temperature as the active medium. Because of the difficulties of working with a high-temperature metallic vapor, such lasers have developed relatively slowly, but have now reached the point where they can be considered for selected materials-processing applications. For some applications, they offer decided advantages. The two most common of these lasers are the copper vapor laser, operating at wavelengths near 511 and 578 nm, and the gold vapor laser, operating near 628 nm. The discussion will emphasize copper vapor lasers. The characteristics of the other types of metal vapor lasers are similar.

Principles

The copper vapor laser (CVL) was first demonstrated in 1966 (7). Much of the early development of CVLs was a result of their use in atomic vapor laser isotope separation (AVLIS) for the production of uranium reactor fuel. Subsequently, their widespread use in high-speed photography and flow visualization resulted in further development as an applied engineering tool (8). As a consequence of this development work and the unique characteristics of this laser type, the copper laser is being employed in a number of micromachining applications.

The copper laser consists of a refractory ceramic tube containing elemental copper and a buffer gas (see Fig. 1). The tube is heated by an electrical discharge, pulsed at multikilohertz frequencies, running between electrodes at each end of the tube. The heat generated by the discharge raises the tube temperature to 1400–1500°C. Approximately 1% of the copper is converted to a vapor state. Laser action results from the interaction of the electrical discharge with the copper vapor.

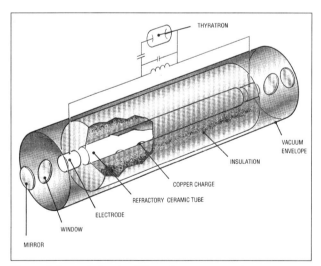

Figure 1. Layout of major CVL system components.

The upper laser levels are populated by single-step electron "impact" excitation from the ground state (see Fig. 2). The electrons are provided directly by the laser discharge current. The high efficiency of this excitation process, together with the favorable quantum efficiency, makes the CVL the most efficient visible laser system. Other metals including gold, lead, and manganese can also be made to lase. However, the differences in their structures (operation on any one transition) make them far less efficient than copper.

Because copper atoms in the lower laser level require a relatively long time to relax to the ground state, the population inversion, and hence laser output, cannot be sustained on a continuous basis. Therefore, the laser output is inherently pulsed, with all the power of the laser contained in very short, high-peak-power pulses at high repetition frequencies.

Table 1 presents typical specifications for a CVL laser.

Table 1. CVL Specifications

Specifications	
Wavelength	510.6, 578.2 nm
Average power	20–120 W
Pulse duration	15–60 ns
Pulse repetition rate	4–30 kHz
Peak power	100–400 kW
Amplitude stability	5% RMS for 10^5 pulses
Divergence	2X diffraction limit
Services	
Power consumption	4–15 kW
Water supply	4 L/min
Gas supply	99.995% neon
Gas consumption	0.5 liter atm/h

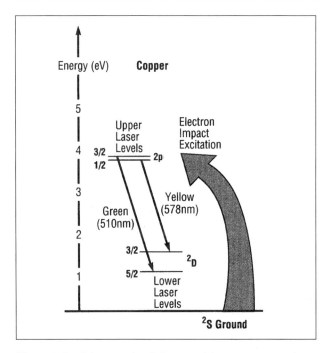

Figure 2. Partial energy-level diagram of the copper atom, showing excitation mechanism.

The copper laser possesses a combination of characteristics that make it unlike any other laser source (visible wavelength, short pulse width, high repetition rate, and high peak power with near-diffraction-limited beam quality). These unique attributes make the CVL ideal for micromachining applications.

Repetition Rate

The repetition rate and average power of the laser determine the rate of material removal or process speed. For micromachining applications, the copper laser is pulsed at a rate of 5 to 20 kHz with powers ranging from 10 to 200 W. The CVL has the highest pulse repetition frequency-average power product for any visible laser.

Wavelength

The wavelength of the light emitted from a laser determines the type of material interaction, whether primarily thermal or ablative and the amount of energy absorbed. In the case of metals, the reflectivity in the infrared from CO_2 or Nd:YAG lasers is typically greater than 90%, and the process requires a high thermal load to melt the material. This produces a substantial heat-affected zone (HAZ). The molten metal is removed by high-pressure gas jets, making micrometer-scale features difficult.

For the ultraviolet wavelengths of an excimer laser, 80% of the energy is absorbed, although only to a depth less than 0.5 μm. As such, excimers are typically used for large area etching and are not well suited for direct drilling or deep cutting.

A single CVL laser pulse removes material to a depth on the order 10 μm. This combined with the high pulse repetition frequency, results in a higher material removal rate compared to an excimer in direct-write applications such as deep hole drilling and high-aspect-ratio slot production. Furthermore, the visible wavelength, aided by the short, high-peak-power pulse, results in a "cold cut" or ablative process with a precision that cannot be matched by infrared lasers.

Pulse Width

To minimize the HAZ, it is necessary to deliver the laser energy in high-intensity, short bursts to allow vaporization of the material to be removed and little heat to transfer to the host material. This requires an intensity 10^8 to 10^9 W/cm^2 and short pulse durations are needed to achieve these peak powers (9). The short pulse width (30 ns) and high peak power of the CVL produces very little HAZ, less than 500 nm thick in many metals.

Beam Quality

The minimum size, d_{min}, to which a laser beam may be focused to is determined by its wavelength and the beam quality. The minimum beam size is given by

$$d_{min} = 4M^2 f \lambda / \pi D$$

where M^2 is the beam quality factor, f the focal length of the lens, λ the laser wavelength, and D the diameter of the beam at the lens. The CVL has significant advantages over CO_2 and

Nd:YAG lasers in terms of the minimum spot size to which it may be focused. Whereas the CO_2 laser is similar to the copper laser in that it can produce high power with near-diffraction-limited output, the CO_2 laser's wavelength is 20 times greater than that of the CVL. For Nd:YAG lasers at high powers, thermal distortion of the laser crystal degrades the beam quality to several times the diffraction limit.

References
7. W. T. Walter et al., *Bull. Am. Phys. Soc.* **11**, 113 (1966).
8. D. C. Hogan, *Applications of copper vapor laser lighting to high speed motion analysis*, SPIE Proceedings of Ultra-high and High-speed Photography, Videography, Photonics and Velocimetry '90, San Diego, 1990.
9. G. Herziger, *The Industrial Laser Annual Handbook 1996*, PennWell Books, Tulsa, OK, 108–15, 1996.

RICHARD SLAGLE

2.5.3 Ion Lasers

Basic Principles

Ion lasers are typically continuous-wave (CW) lasers that provide emission at a series of discrete wavelengths from the infrared to the ultraviolet regions of the spectrum, but are most commonly used in the visible. Ion lasers are a subset of the broader classification gas lasers and are distinguished by the ionic state of their gaseous gain medium. Most commercially available ion lasers are of the noble gas variety using argon (Ar), krypton (Kr), or a combination thereof (mixed gas) as the fill gas.

The low-pressure fill gas is usually excited by a continuous electric discharge. High-energy electrons in the discharge collide with the neutral fill gas atoms, ionizing them with the initial collisions. The resulting ions are then excited to higher energy levels by subsequent collisions with electrons. Laser action takes place as a result of the transitions of the excited ions to lower energy states. It is this plasma of ions that distinguishes the ion laser from neutral atom or molecular gas lasers.

Wavelengths

The wavelengths emitted by an ion laser depend on the type of fill gas and on the spectral characteristics of the mirror coatings. Argon and krypton ions each have lasing transitions capable of providing useful output beams with wavelengths from the infrared to the ultraviolet. Commercial CW argon ion, krypton ion, and mixed-gas ion lasers come in a variety of sizes from small air-cooled models with output powers of tens of milliwatts, to much larger water-cooled systems capable of tens of watts. Tables 2 and 3 list the most commonly used wavelengths and their corresponding output powers from several sizes of commercially available argon and krypton ion laser systems.

Table 2. Typical Wavelengths and Output Powers from Commercial Argon Ion Lasers[a]

λ (nm)	Ion	Output power (W)			
		SP 163D[b]	CR Ent.[c]	SP 2060[d]	SP 2080[e]
275.4	Ar III	–	–	–	0.360
300.3	Ar III	–	–	–	0.500
305.5	Ar III	–	–	–	0.450
333.6	Ar III	–	–	–	0.420
334.5	Ar III	–	–	–	0.840
335.8	Ar III	–	–	–	0.840
351.1	Ar III	–	–	0.190	1.500
351.4	Ar III	–	–	0.060	0.500
363.8	Ar III	–	–	0.250	2.000
379.5	Ar III	–	–	–	0.420
454.5	Ar II	–	–	0.160	0.800
457.9	Ar II	0.003	0.080	0.550	1.500
465.8	Ar II	–	–	0.240	0.800
472.7	Ar II	–	–	0.320	1.300
476.5	Ar II	–	–	1.000	3.000
488.0	Ar II	0.025	0.200	2.500	8.000
496.5	Ar II	–	–	1.000	3.000
501.7	Ar II	–	–	0.640	1.800
514.5	Ar II	0.015	0.350	3.200	10.000
528.7	Ar II	–	–	0.550	1.800
1092.3	Ar II	–	–	0.100	–

[a]The manufacturers and models listed here are presented for purposes of specificity and do not represent an endorsement of the manufacturers as compared to other manufacturers.
[b]Air-cooled laser operating TEM_{00} ($M^2<1.1$). Specifications taken from Spectra-Physics, Inc., data sheet dated 6/96.
[c]Water-cooled laser with 1-ft plasma tube operating TEM_{00} ($M^2<1.2$). Specifications taken from Coherent, Inc., data sheet dated 3/96.
[d]Water-cooled laser with 2-ft plasma tube operating TEM_{00} ($M^2<1.1$). Specifications taken from Spectra-Physics, Inc., data sheet dated 7/96.
[e]Water-cooled laser with 4-ft plasma tube operating TEM_{00} ($M^2<1.1$). Specifications taken from Spectra-Physics, Inc., data sheet dated 7/96.

The singly ionized species, Ar II and Kr II, account for the majority of the infrared (752–1092 nm) and visible (454–676 nm) transitions producing relatively high powers, most notably the 514.5- and 488.0-nm Ar II transitions. The less probable doubly-ionized species, Ar III and Kr III, are the sources of the ultraviolet (275–386 nm) transitions (10). Because the ultraviolet transitions originate from doubly ionized species with relatively high current density thresholds, these wavelengths are usually available only on larger, more powerful water-cooled systems. In addition, deep ultraviolet (229–264 nm) can be produced through intracavity doubling of the stronger visible lines in water-cooled systems. Table 4 lists the wavelengths and corresponding output powers from a commercially available, intracavity doubled argon ion laser.

Table 3. Typical Wavelengths and Output Powers from Commercial Krypton Ion Lasers[a]

λ (nm)	Ion	Output power (W)		
		CR Ent.[b]	CR I300[c]	CR Sabre[d]
350.7	Kr III	0.040	0.250	0.800
356.4	Kr III	–	0.120	–
406.7	Kr III	–	0.200	0.900
413.1	Kr III	0.040	0.300	1.800
415.4	Kr III	–	0.050	0.280
468.0	Kr II	–	–	0.500
476.2	Kr II	–	0.050	0.400
482.5	Kr II	–	0.030	0.400
520.8	Kr II	0.010	0.070	0.700
530.9	Kr II	–	0.200	1.500
568.2	Kr II	0.010	0.150	1.100
647.1	Kr II	0.010	0.800	3.500
676.4	Kr II	–	0.150	0.900
752.5	Kr II	–	0.100	1.200
799.3	Kr II	–	–	0.300

[a]The manufacturers and models listed here are presented for purposes of specificity and do not represent an endorsement of the manufacturers as compared to other manufacturers.
[b]Water-cooled laser with 1-ft plasma tube operating TEM_{00} ($M^2 < 1.2$). Specifications taken from Coherent, Inc., data sheet dated 3/96.
[c]Water-cooled laser with 2-ft plasma tube operating TEM_{00} ($M^2 < 1.1$). Specifications taken from Coherent, Inc., data sheet dated 3/95.
[d]Water-cooled laser with 4-ft plasma tube operating TEM_{00} ($M^2 < 1.1$). Specifications taken from Coherent, Inc., data sheet dated 1/96.

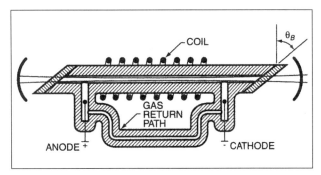

Figure 3: Schematic diagram of an ion laser.

Table 4. Typical Wavelengths and Output Powers from a Commercial Intracavity-Doubled Argon Ion Laser[a]

λ (nm)	Ion	Output power (W)
		CR I300[b]
229.0	Dbld. Ar II	0.010
238.3	Dbld. Ar II	0.030
244.0	Dbld. Ar II	0.100
248.3	Dbld. Ar II	0.030
257.3	Dbld. Ar II	0.100
264.4	Dbld. Ar II	0.020

[a]The manufacturer and model listed here are presented for purposes of specificity and do not represent an endorsement of the manufacturer as compared to other manufacturers.
[b]Water-cooled laser with 2-ft plasma tube and BBO intracavity doubling crystal. Specifications taken from Coherent, Inc., data sheet dated 7/93.

For completeness, Table 5 lists additional specifications from the various sizes of commercially available ion lasers for comparison of their performance, size, weight, and power requirements.

Ion Laser Construction

Plasma Tubes. Most commercial ion lasers have the same general linear cavity construction illustrated in Figure 3. The fill gas is contained in a tube (plasma tube) of suitable bore diameter (typically a few millimeters) that is sealed at each end by optical windows inclined at Brewster's angle θ_B (Brewster windows) to minimize reflection losses at the surfaces. Spherical mirrors, or a combination of a spherical and planar mirror, are generally used to form the optical cavity.

Some plasma tubes are sealed at one or both ends, depending on the application, directly by the mirrors themselves to minimize the number of intracavity optical surfaces, such as the Brewster windows, that may be subject to power-reducing contamination. However, direct exposure of the mirror coatings to the intense vacuum ultraviolet radiation (resulting mostly from depopulation of the lower levels by spontaneous emission to the ion ground state) emitted by the plasma may cause premature mirror damage. A few centimeters of air space between the Brewster window and mirror is sufficient to absorb most of this vacuum ultraviolet radiation. In most cases, this intracavity air space is sealed and lined with an active catalyst (e.g., silver mesh) to eliminate ozone buildup, which can cause detrimental thermal lensing effects.

Plasma tubes are generally constructed of either glass, with a continuous beryllium oxide bore liner, or ceramic, with a segmented bore of tungsten disks and copper heat webs. Because of the high current density, there is a migration of ions toward the cathode, and a return path, as shown schematically in the figure, is provided to compensate for this. In ceramic tubes, the return path is through holes in the copper heat webs. Glass tubes with

Chapter 2: Lasers for Materials Processing

Table 5. Typical Specifications from Commercial Ion Lasers[a]

Specification	Laser model			
	SP 163D[b]	CR Ent.[c]	SP 2060[d]	SP 2080[e]
Beam diameter (mm)[f]	0.72	1.0	1.7	1.9
Beam divergence (mrad)[f]	0.95	0.70	0.45	0.45
Polarization	>100:1	>100:1	>100:1	>100:1
Optical Noise[g]	<0.50% rms	<1.00% rms	<0.15% rms	<0.20% rms
Power stability	±1%	±1%	±0.3%	±0.3%
Beam pointing stability (mrad/°C)	<10	<5000	<5	<5
Input power type	1-phase	1-phase	3-phase	3-phase
Input voltage (Vac)	110	208	208	480
Input current, maximum (A/∅)	20	34	60	73
Cooling water flow rate (lpm)	n/a	8.0	11.3	18.9
Head size, l×w×h (cm)	31.0×13.3×15.9	76.2×18.5×19.2	127.0×24.1×23.0	188.1×24.1×23.0
Head weight (kg)	6.1	32.0	66.0	100.0
Power supply size, l×w×h (cm)	28.5×22.1×14.5	50.2×43.8×19.2	63.5×42.5×37.2	63.5×42.5×37.2
Power supply weight (kg)	11.5	39.0	79.5	79.5

[a]The manufacturers and models listed here are presented for purposes of specificity and do not represent an endorsement of the manufacturers as compared to other manufacturers.
[b]Air-cooled laser. Specifications taken from Spectra-Physics, Inc., data sheet dated 6/96.
[c]Water-cooled laser with 1-ft plasma tube. Specifications taken from Coherent, Inc., data sheet dated 3/96.
[d]Water-cooled laser with 2-ft plasma tube. Specifications taken from Spectra-Physics, Inc., data sheet dated 8/97.
[e]Water-cooled laser with 4-ft plasma tube. Specifications taken from Spectra-Physics, Inc., data sheet dated 8/97.
[f]Specification for 514.5 nm.
[g]Typically measured in a 10-Hz to 2-MHz bandwidth.

their continuous bores usually provide more output power per foot of length than the ceramic tubes; however, the glass tubes are generally not as long lasting, rugged, or reliable. For these reasons, most tubes manufactured today are of the ceramic type.

In the case of the higher-power water-cooled systems, there is a water-cooled electromagnet surrounding the plasma tube that provides a magnetic field to reduce the drift rate of electrons to the walls of the bore. This serves to increase the plasma density, which, in turn, improves the laser efficiency, especially when operating in the shorter wavelengths of the doubly ionized species.

Ion lasers are relatively inefficient devices with overall efficiencies of $< 10^{-3}$. Most of the excess energy is given off as waste heat by the plasma tube and power supply. Lower-power (< 100 mW) plasma tubes with heat loads of < 2 kW are usually cooled by forced air and are equipped with cooling fins attached directly to the plasma tube. Higher-power tubes with heat loads of > 4 kW are usually cooled with water. Water is first circulated through the power supply to cool the dissipative components, and then through the electromagnet and around the plasma tube. In some cases where the available water is of questionable quality, closed-loop water-to-water heat exchangers are employed to ensure a clean, constant-temperature supply to the laser.

Resonators. The resonator structure serves to provide the laser with dimensional stability in the presence of large thermal loads, mechanical stresses, and vibrations. Dimensional stability is critical to maintaining laser alignment, power stability, and beam pointing stability (i.e, directional stability of the output beam).

There are two general types of ion laser resonators in use today. The first type of resonator utilizes the plasma tube itself, as in the case of most air-cooled systems, the magnet, or an additional thermally conductive supporting member, such as a piece of aluminum angle, as the resonator structure to which the mirror plates are directly attached. Because of its high thermal conductivity, this type of resonator exhibits relatively good angular stability, but no length stability. Most air-cooled and low-cost water-cooled systems use this type of resonator, because it is relatively inexpensive, compact, lightweight, and rugged. However, systems with this type of resonator typically exhibit only mediocre beam pointing (> 7 mrad/°C) and power stability (> ±1%) performance, require a relatively long time to warm up (> 30 min.), and in the case of water-cooled systems, have higher optical noise (> 0.5% rms), mostly because of microphonic vibrations from the cooling system.

The second type of resonator commonly used in more expenpsive water-cooled systems provides both angular and length stabil-

ISBN 0-912035-15-3

ity. This type of resonator usually consists of three carefully matched low-expansion rods supported by a thermally conductive structure. The low-expansion rods are attached directly to thermally compensated mirror plates providing the length stability. Angular stability is provided by the thermally conductive supporting structure. This type of resonator design is inherently more stable (especially longitudinally, which is critical for single-frequency operation to be discussed later), resulting in significantly better beam pointing and power stability, shorter warm-up times, and less optical noise. However, systems with this type of resonator are relatively expensive, and are larger and more fragile than comparable systems with the first type of resonator. An active resonator stabilization device (11) is commercially available that significantly improves system stability. This device monitors the beam position with an extracavity quadcell detector and adjusts the output mirror angle (via a three element piezoelectric stack attached to the mirror) to correct for any beam drift due to resonator instability. With this simple strategy, the beam pointing is improved to < 5 mrad/°C and the warmup time reduced to only a few minutes. When used in parallel with the laser's light control (i.e., automatic adjustment of the tube current to compensate for power fluctuations), this type of stabilization also improves the power stability to < ±0.3%.

Power Sources. Inside the power supply, there are transformers and rectifiers that produce the dc voltages required by the laser. There are usually also logic cards that control interlocks, start up, and operation of the laser. The primary function of the power supply is, however, to provide high-voltage dc to the plasma tube.

The incoming ac line is converted to high-voltage dc by rectifiers. The operating voltage range of the plasma tube is determined by the tube length and operating fill gas pressure. The high-voltage dc goes from the rectifier to a passbank that controls the current to the plasma tube over the operating voltage range.

There are generally two types of ion laser power supplies, linear-passbank and switched-resistor, each referring to the particular method of current regulation. The linear passbank design uses hundreds of transistors mounted on a cold plate to control the dc current to the plasma tube. Although a relatively low-noise dc source, linear-passbank power supplies are generally relatively large, expensive, and unreliable because of the many active components of the passbank.

Switched-resistor power supplies, on the other hand, achieve power regulation with much fewer (on the order of nine) power semiconductors. Although they introduce small amounts of switching noise into the system, switched-resistor power supplies have a wider regulation range, are inherently more compact, and because they have fewer active components, tend to be more reliable than linear-passbank designs.

In addition to the dc current supplied to the plasma tube, the power supply also provides dc current to the electromagnet and ac current to the cathode filament. In some commercial systems, transformer taps are used to set the magnet and filament currents proportional to the incoming line voltage. This works well in areas of the world with constant line voltage. However, for those areas where significant fluctuations in line voltage are common, it is advisable to have a power supply with magnet and filament current regulation capabilities. Regulation of the magnet current is important, because the magnetic field directly influences the power output, stability, and lifetime of the system. Likewise, proper regulation of the ac filament current is required to avoid overheating the cathode, which may cause it to sag into the beam resulting in premature failure of the plasma tube.

Optical Configurations

The optical configuration determines, in part, the wavelength output and beam characteristics of the laser. The mirror curvatures, cavity length, and bore diameter define the beam size, divergence, and mode quality. Fine tuning of these parameters is usually achieved with a fixed or adjustable intracavity aperture. In general, opening of the intracavity aperture allows multiple transverse cavity modes to oscillate simultaneously resulting in higher power, higher divergence, and a larger beam diameter. Closing down the intracavity aperture ultimately restricts oscillation to the lowest-order transverse cavity mode, designated as TEM_{00}, resulting in somewhat lower power and the minimum divergence and beam size for the prescribed mirror curvatures.

Mode quality is usually characterized by the M^2 value of the beam (12). The M^2 value indicates the transverse mode content of the beam, where the minimum theoretical M^2 value of 1 represents a beam consisting purely of the TEM_{00} mode. Commercial ion lasers operating in TEM_{00} mode have M^2 values on the order of 1.05. The setting of the intracavity aperture depends on the requirements of the application. A beam with a low M^2 value focuses more tightly than a beam of the same wavelength with a greater M^2 value. However, those applications not requiring a tight beam focus would most likely open the aperture to take advantage of the higher power output.

Cavity mirror coatings are usually designed for optimum performance over a particular band of the available wavelengths. For argon and krypton ion lasers, these bands are generally defined as deep-ultraviolet (275–306 nm), ultraviolet (334–379 nm), visible (407–676 nm), near-infrared (752–799 nm), and infrared (1094 nm). Maximum power output is obtained when operating the laser in broadband mode within the particular band. Broadband mode refers to when all the available wavelengths in the selected band are lasing simultaneously, each contributing in a cumulative manner to the overall power of the beam. Most thermal processing applications, such as cutting, would use the laser in this mode.

Single-Line Operation

For applications requiring a particular wavelength within a band, such as lithography, a dispersive prism element in either an intracavity or extracavity arrangement is commonly used to select and isolate the required wavelength. With an intracavity prism, the desired wavelength is selected by a prism located inside the laser cavity, resulting in what is referred to as single line operation. This arrangement is the simplest and most convenient, because the resulting beam maintains the original path of the broadband beam. The disadvantage is that the reflection and absorption losses introduced in the laser cavity usually result in less output power compared to an external cavity prism arrangement. However, in the case of the stronger visible wavelengths, this effect is minimal and the convenience of the intracavity prism makes it the preferred arrangement for most applications.

With an extracavity prism, the laser runs in broadband mode while a prism located outside the laser cavity disperses the different wavelengths. Because the prism is outside the laser cavity, the effects of reflection and absorption losses on the performance of the laser are minimized, making the external prism the preferred arrangement for the weaker transitions. The disadvantage is that the extracavity prism arrangement adds complexity to the beam train and, in the case of a krypton ion laser, competition between the many wavelengths present in broadband mode may reduce the performance of the one selected (10).

There are sophisticated narrowband output mirror coatings now available that enable the selection of a single wavelength without the use of a prism. These mirrors provide more power and are inherently more stable than either prism arrangement, but are only available for select spectrally isolated lines, for example the argon ion lines at 514.5, 488.0, and 363.8 nm.

Single-Frequency Operation: When operating an ion laser in single-line mode, there are many longitudinal cavity modes oscillating simultaneously within the gain bandwidth of the particular transition. As a result, the laser linewidth approximates the gain bandwidth, which for water-cooled systems operating in the visible, is on the order of 5–10 GHz. However, some applications, such as those based on holography or interferometry, require even narrower linewidths. By inserting an etalon into the laser cavity, an ion laser operating in single-line mode can be forced to oscillate on only one of the longitudinal cavity modes. The laser would then be operating in what is commonly referred to as single-frequency mode. Typical conversion efficiencies (i.e., single-frequency power/single-line power) are typically on the order of 50–70% depending on the wavelength.

The actual single-frequency linewidth of an ion laser is usually determined by the envelope of the frequency jitter caused by microphonic vibrations stemming from the cooling system. This frequency jitter results in typical single-frequency linewidths of 10–15 MHz for a water-cooled system. A unique frequency jitter reduction device is commercially available that is capable of reducing the frequency jitter and narrowing the laser linewidth by more than a factor of 5. This device derives an error signal by sampling the output beam with a high-resolution 2-GHz confocal interferometer and drives a three-element piezoelectric stack on the output mirror (the same stack described earlier in relation to beam pointing stabilization) according to the error signal. The piezoelectric stack rapidly moves the output coupler along the cavity axis, counteracting the resonator vibrations and reducing the jitter-induced linewidth to less than 2–3 MHz.

Single-frequency applications usually require long-term frequency stability. In an unstabilized system, the cavity and etalon optical lengths may change during warm up or as the cooling water and/or ambient temperatures change. If the cavity and etalon optical lengths change in unison, the output frequency of the laser will drift accordingly, but if the cavity and etalon optical lengths change relative to each other such that the selected longitudinal mode drifts away from the etalon loss minimum, a mode hop will occur as the laser frequency hops to the adjacent longitudinal cavity mode.

Long-term frequency stability requires minimization of frequency drift and elimination of mode hops. This can be achieved by first having a resonator with very good length stability, and second by either using the etalon as a reference and locking the cavity length to the etalon, or using the cavity as a reference and locking the etalon length to the cavity. Because the etalon is compact, it is much easier to isolate from ambient temperature changes and, therefore, makes a better reference.

There is a frequency stabilization device (13) commercially available that slaves fine adjustment of the cavity length to the optical length of the etalon, which is mounted in a constant temperature oven. Fine adjustment of the laser cavity length is accomplished with the same three-element piezoelectric stack on the output mirror described earlier in relation to beam pointing stabilization and frequency jitter reduction. With this type of stabilization, mode hops are completely eliminated and frequency drift is reduced to < 30 MHz/°C.

Intracavity Doubling: As mentioned earlier, deep ultraviolet (229–264 nm) can be produced through intracavity doubling of the stronger visible lines in water-cooled systems. Intracavity doubling is achieved by placing a temperature-stabilized nonlinear crystal (BBO, see Section 2.5.6) into the laser cavity where circulating powers on the order of 200 W greatly enhance the power-dependent doubling process. A small portion of the fundamental wavelength (typically 5–7% based on output power) is converted by the crystal to the second harmonic at one-half the wavelength of the fundamental. Note, however, that the relatively expensive doubling crystals used in these systems are prone to optical damage in the presence of such high CW intracavity power and, as a result, tend to be relatively short-lived. Unfortunately, there are few practical alternatives available for CW deep-ultraviolet emission.

Lifetime, Care, and Maintenance
Lifetime: Ion laser lifetime, which for modern lasers is synonymous with plasma tube lifetime, can vary widely depending on the wavelength, power level, and end-of-life definition of the application. For example, it is not unusual to get more than

10,000 hours out of a water-cooled plasma tube running continuously at a visible wavelength and a moderate tube current, while the same tube running continuously at an ultraviolet wavelength and maximum tube current may last less than 3000 h.

Plasma tube lifetime is primarily related to erosion of the plasma tube bore diameter by sputtering. As the bore diameter increases, the plasma density decreases reducing the efficiency of the laser, especially for the ultraviolet wavelengths, for the given maximum tube current. In addition, sputtered material from the bore redeposits elsewhere in the tube, trapping fill gas atoms in the process. This fill gas consumption is most evident during the initial hours of operation when the bore erosion rate is highest, and tapers off as the tube bore approaches an equilibrium shape. The bore erosion and gas consumption rates are proportional to the current density and inversely proportional to the fill gas pressure.

Because air-cooled lasers typically have a finite-volume gas reservoir at one end, end of life is determined by when the gas pressure reaches the minimum required for acceptable output power. On the other hand, most commercially available water-cooled systems have automatic gas fill systems. The tube pressure is monitored by reading the voltage across the plasma tube, which is directly proportional to the tube pressure for a given tube current. When required, a metered amount of gas is injected into the plasma tube from a higher-pressure reservoir. In this way, the tube pressure is always kept at an optimum level. With the high-pressure reservoir, it is rare that water-cooled tubes run out of gas. End of life is more likely determined by loss of power due to bore enlargement or optical surface contamination.

Maintenance: Periodic maintenance of an ion laser may be required, especially if the laser cavity is not hermetically sealed or the tube has a manual gas fill system. Any of the optics and Brewster windows may require cleaning to remove accumulated dust or other contaminants. The cleanliness of the intracavity surfaces is especially critical to the laser's performance. The frequency of cleaning depends on the cleanliness of the environment in which the laser is operating. Typically a drop in laser performance will indicate a need for servicing. In addition, if the tube does not have an automatic gas fill system, the tube voltage must be routinely monitored and fills manually administered as required. Running a tube for any significant amount of time at low pressure may cause irreparable damage.

Once the plasma tube has reached its end-of-life condition, it will have to be replaced. This procedure may be quite simple, as in the case of most prealigned air-cooled systems, or more involved, requiring special training to handle a complete realignment of the resonator.

For water-cooled systems, the cleanliness of the cooling water is critical to the cooling efficiency of the laser system. Dissolved minerals and debris in the water can accumulate on internal surfaces, greatly reducing thermal conduction to the cooling water. This can create hot spots and eventually lead to a cracked plasma tube. In areas with poor water quality, it is recommended to filter the water and/or use a closed-loop water-to-water heat exchanger that circulates clean, conditioned water through the laser.

References

10. M. J. Weber (Ed.), 1982: *CRC Handbook of Laser Science and Technology: Vol. II Gas Lasers*, CRC Press, Inc., Boca Raton, FL, Section 2.
11. S. C. Guggenheimer and D. L. Wright, *Review of Scientific Instruments* **62**, 2389–93 (1991).
12. M. W. Sasnett, in: *The Physics and Technology of Laser Resonators*, D. R. Hall and P. E. Jackson (Eds.), Adam Hilger, New York, NY, 1989, 132–42.
13. J. Ekstrand and S. C. Guggenheimer, in: *Frequency Stabilized Lasers and Their Applications*: SPIE Proceedings Vol. 1837, Y. C. Chung (Ed.), Hyperion, Inc., Cambridge, MA, 58–67 (1993).

KURT G. KLAVUHN

2.5.4 Diode Lasers

Introduction to Diode Lasers

The first diode lasers were operated in the early 1960s. They required cryogenic working temperatures and only allowed pulsed operation. In 1970, the first CW diode laser was operated at room temperature, emitting only a very low laser power in the milliwatt range (14). Since then, the power has increased dramatically, resulting in coherent, diffraction-limited laser light output of several hundreds of milliwatts. These lasers are mainly used for telecommunication applications such as broadband optical fiber transmission. For material processing purposes, the structures of these diode lasers are modified to yield higher output power, sacrificing a high degree of coherence.

Beam Characteristics of Diode Lasers

Diode lasers are extremely interesting because they convert electrical current directly into laser light. Thus, the efficiency of such lasers is typically in the range of 30–50%.

The wavelength of a diode laser is determined by its bandgap energy E. Upon de-excitation of an exited electron from the conduction band into the valence band of a diode laser, a photon may be emitted with a high probability. Its wavelength λ_0 is determined according to

$$E = h\nu = h c_0/\lambda_0$$

where h is Planck's constant and c_0 the speed of light. By means of the combination of different semiconductor materials, it is possible to create several bandgap energies with corresponding wavelengths. A list of common semiconductor materials and their wavelength ranges are shown in Table 6.

Table 6. Typical Compounds Used for Diode Lasers (15)

Material	Wavelength (µm)
$In_{1-x}Ga_xAs_yP_{1-y}$	1.2–1.6
$GaAs_xSb_{1-x}$	1.2–1.5
$InAs_xP_{1-x}$	1.0–3.1
$(Al_xGa_{1-x})_yIn_{1-y}As$	0.9–1.5
$Al_xGa_{1-x}As$	0.7–0.9
$GaAs_{1-x}P_x$	0.6–0.9
$In_xGa_{1-x}As$	0.55–3.0
$(Al_xGa_{1-x})_yIn_{1-y}P$	0.55–0.8
CdS_xSe_{1-x}	0.5–0.7
$Cd_xZn_{1-x}Se$	0.3–0.5
AlGaInN	0.2–0.64

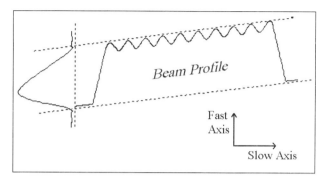

Figure 5. Near-field beam profile of a diode laser bar.

The laser radiation is diffraction-limited in the fast axis, which means that the beam parameter product assumes a minimum value given by:

$$(\theta w_0)_{TEM_{00}} = \frac{\lambda}{\pi}$$

with λ being its wavelength. Thus a diode laser oscillates in a transverse single mode in the fast axis, and the beam intensity distribution is Gaussian (see Fig. 5).

In the slow axis a high-power diode laser commonly oscillates in a transverse multimode. The coherence is low and the beam parameter product indicates a beam far from the diffraction limit. The near-field profile of the single laser emitter is close to a top-head shape. The superposition of these individual lasers can be seen in Figure 5. The far field of a high-power diode laser exhibits a double-lobed profile with a relative minimum in the middle of the intensity distribution.

The spectral width of the radiation is typically in the range of 2 nm, which is relatively high compared to other laser types. This means that many longitudinal modes oscillate in a high-power diode laser resonator.

The radiation of a diode laser is considerably different from the radiation of conventional high-power lasers such as Nd:YAG or CO_2 lasers (see Fig. 4). The beam parameters θ (angle of divergence) and w_0 (beam waist) are different for the two main axes of the diode laser. This results in an unsymmetrical beam.

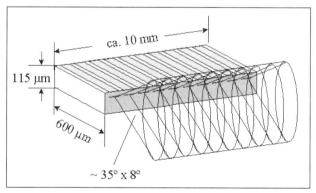

Figure 4. Radiation of a diode laser bar.

The axis perpendicular to the *p-n* junction is called the *fast axis*, and the axis parallel to the *p-n* junction the *slow axis*. Typical values for the divergence angle of the beam in the fast axis are 35° (FWHM), whereas the angle in the slow axis is only in the range of 8° (FWHM) (see Fig. 4). The lateral extension shows a different situation. The fast axis exhibits a smaller extension of about 1 µm, whereas the slow axis shows a width of 100 to 500 µm for a single emitter and up to 15 mm for a whole diode laser bar. A bar width of approximately 10 mm has become the most common standard in recent years.

Electronic Properties of Diode Lasers

To make laser action possible in a diode laser, three mechanisms must be included. First, there is the resonator, which is realized by the cleaved end facets of the semiconductor material. Second, there has to be an active medium, and third, a pump mechanism must be present. The latter two are discussed in more detail in this section.

In order to understand the way a diode laser works, it is advantageous to start with a simple *p-n* junction of a diode. Initially, a *p-n* junction in equilibrium is considered. Figure 6a shows its energy-level diagram in space coordinates.

On the left side, a *p*-doped semiconductor is shown and on the right side an *n*-type semiconductor. The straight lines mark the edges of the valence and the conduction band. The dashed lines give the position of the acceptors (in the *p*-type semiconductor) and the donators (in the *n*-type semiconductor). The dotted line marks the Fermi level. In a simplified definition it can be said that the Fermi level is the energy level up to which the electronic states are occupied. That means all levels above the Fermi level are empty and all levels below the Fermi level are occuped with electrons.

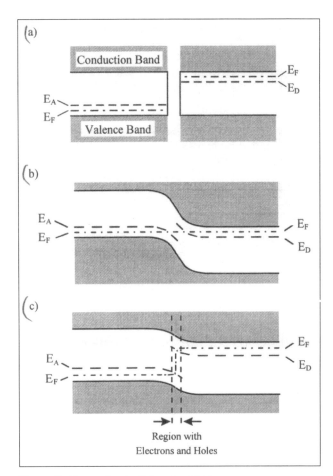

Figure 6. Energy levels of a *p-n* junction.

In fact, the first semiconductors that demonstrated laser action were composed of a simple *p-n* junction of direct semiconductor materials. However, in order to breach the threshold for laser action, a very high current density of up to 50×10^3 A/cm^2 is necessary (17). Thus the first diode lasers were only operated at low temperatures and with a low duty cycle.

In order to decrease the current applied across the junction, a mechanism is employed that confines the area in which recombination of the carriers takes place to a small region. So-called heterojunctions are used to create a potential barrier for the carrier. In Figure 7 a double heterostructure diode laser is shown.

The active region exhibits the smallest band gap of the three-layer system, and thus the recombination of the carriers only takes place here. The adjacent layers are designed in such a way that they represent a potential barrier for the negative and the positive carriers, respectively.

The term *homojunction* is used for two materials adjacent to the interface that are made of the same material but differently doped. A heterojunction incorporates two different materials on both sides of the interface. The materials belong to the same material system, such as $Al_xGa_{1-x}As$. Here *x* takes on a value between 0 and 0.42, where 0 represents the GaAs compound without any aluminum content. An *x* value of 0.42 marks the transition of $Al_xGa_{1-x}As$ from a direct semiconductor to an indirect semiconductor (16).

Now if these two semiconductors are electrically connected, the energy levels of the two semiconductors shift relative to each other in such a way that the Fermi level in both parts is at the same level (see Fig. 6b). Therefore, the edges of the valence and the conduction band are now at different levels.

Finally, the *p-n* junction is extremely forward-biased. Figure 6c shows that the Fermi level is bent according to the bias level. In a very small region that is only a few micrometers in width, there are occupied states of the conduction band facing empty states of the valence band (see Fig. 6c) (15). In this small region a situation is created equal to a population inversion. Thus one important prerequisite of a laser is fulfilled.

For actual laser action to take place, more conditions have to be matched. First, the de-excitation of the electron from the conduction band to the valence band has to emit a photon. This only occurs under a sufficient probability in a *direct* semiconductor such as GaAs and InP (16). Semiconductor materials commonly used for electronic diodes such as Si or Ge are *indirect* and thus not suitable for diode lasers since a de-excitation under emission of a photon is very unlikely.

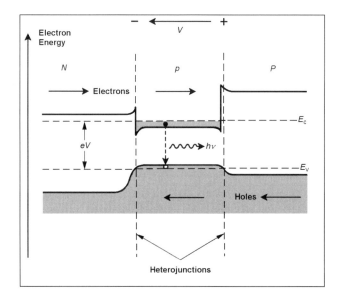

Figure 7. Energy levels of a double heterostructure DL.

In order to compensate the resonator losses of the diode laser and start the laser action, a certain threshold of injection current I_{th} has to be reached. Below this threshold, no stimulated emission is observed, and the only light produced is because of spontaneous emission. Thus below the laser threshold the diode laser works as a light-emitting diode (LED). The output power is low.

Upon breaching the threshold I_{th}, laser action takes place and the output power P increases significantly with the injection current I (see Fig. 8). A linear dependency between the current I and the output power P is observed.

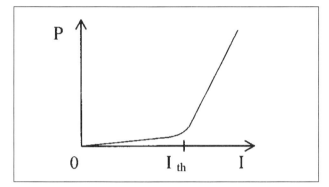

Figure 8. Dependence of the laser intensity from the injection current.

Today's high-power diode laser bars exhibit a laser threshold of typically 6 to 20 A depending on the packaging density and the structure of the individual emitters. The CW-output power of such bars has reached values of 80 W and more. For efficient heat removal they are mounted on water-cooled microchannel heat sinks (18).

Optical Wave Guiding in Diode Lasers

The shape of the resonator in a diode laser is somewhat different from that of gas lasers or conventional solid-state lasers such as Nd:YAG. First, the length of the resonator is considerably shorter, typically a few hundred micrometers. Second, the out-coupling mirror has a much lower reflectivity. The mirrors are composed of cleaved surfaces of the semiconductor material. A reflective coating is applied on one side and the other is left uncoated. The high index of reflection of GaAs (3.6), for example, is sufficient to produce a Fresnel reflection of approximately 32%. Third, the shape of the transverse modes in a diode laser is determined by the step in refractive index of the active zone to the adjacent layers. This produces mode patterns similar to that of a waveguide rather than those of free-space propagation as in most other lasers.

The third point requires more discussion, because it represents a major difference between diode lasers and other lasers. The laser light in the semiconductor material is mainly guided using total internal reflection. Figure 9 is a schematic of the situation. In the case of the $Al_xGa_{1-x}As$ system, the active region contains less aluminum than the surrounding layers and thus has a higher refractive index (the less aluminum the compound contains, the higher its refractive index).

The width of the active region has to be chosen to match the extension of a propagating optical wave. It is usually designed to only let the fundamental transverse mode to propagate free of major losses. Thus the out-coupled wave of such an optical guide is a TEM_{00} mode and exhibits a Gaussian shape, as indicated in Figure 9 on the left side.

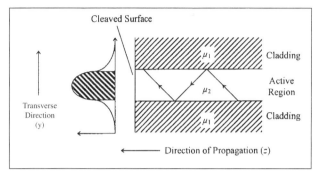

Figure 9. Optical guiding and near field in the fast axis.

Since the wavelength of high-power diode lasers is in the range approximately 0.8 to 1.0 µm, the active region is accordingly narrow. The light wave diverges strongly at angles of typically 35° (FWHM) upon exiting the waveguide.

Figure 10 compares the energy band structures, the index of refraction of the layers, and the extension of the optical mode of a homojunction and a double-heterostructure diode laser. The improved confinement of the optical mode is shown.

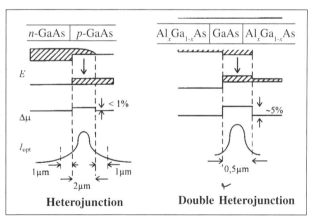

Figure 10. Comparison of a simple homojunction and a double-heterojunction diode laser structure.

Newer designs of high-power diode lasers employ a so-called quantum-well structure, in which the carriers are confined to a much smaller layer than in the conventional double heterostructure. A typical layer thickness of a quantum well is in the range of only a few nanometers. This layer is too thin to contain the optical mode. However, to prevent the optical mode from extending far into the semiconductor, a further layer design is employed to achieve the wave guiding. These structures are called separate-confinement heterostructures (SCH), because two different pairs of layers achieve carrier confinement and optical confinement (19).

The optical guiding in the slow axis, on the other hand, is accomplished differently. The so-called *gain guiding* structure is employed for high-power diode lasers mainly for cost reasons, because it requires fewer processing steps during the manufacturing process. In the slow axis there is no structure except for the very top layer, the contact film. It consists of either highly doped semiconductor material, which is then bonded to a metal contact, or an oxide layer, which prevents electrical conduction into the layers below it.

Figure 11 shows a schematic drawing of the layer structure. The active region shows a uniform structure, and the width of the mode is determined by the extension of the area containing pumped laser medium. A laser mode is only amplified in these regions. Any mode extending beyond this region does not experience optical amplification. The broad pumped area is responsible for the fact that the laser beam in the slow axis is a multimode beam. The coherence of the laser beam in the slow axis is low, because the individual modes of its multimode beam exhibit a low correlation.

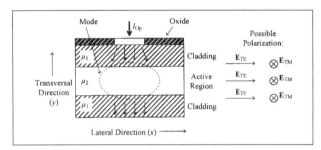

Figure 11. Optical guiding in the slow axis.

The output of diode laser is commonly polarized to a high degree of approximately 95%. The direction of polarization can be determined through the design of the semiconductor structure. The most common polarization is the TE mode, where the electric field vector of the modes is oriented parallel to the layer interfaces.

References
14. M. B. Panish, I. Hayashi, and S. Sumski, *Appl. Phys. Lett.* **16**, 326 (1970).
15. G. P. Agrawal, and N. K. Dutta, 1993: *Semiconductor Lasers*, 2nd Ed., Van Nostrand Reinhold, New York.
16. C. F. Klingshirn, 1997: *Semiconductor Optics*, 2nd Ed., Springer Verlag, Berlin.
17. R. N. Hall, G. E. Fenner, J. D. Kingsley, T. J. Soltys, and R. O. Carlson, *Phys. Rev. Lett.* **9**, 366 (1962).
18. T. Ebert, H.-G. Treusch, P. Loosen, and R. Poprawe, *Proc. SPIE* **3285**, 25 (1998).
19. N. W. Carlson, 1994: *Monolithic Diode Laser Arrays*, Springer Verlag, Berlin.

BODO EHLERS

High-Power Diode Lasers for Materials Processing
Remarkable advances in semiconductor laser technology have been one of the most important commercial developments in laser technology during the past ten years. Semiconductor laser diodes can be used directly in laser materials processing applications or they can be used in place of arc lamps to pump solid-state lasers, so-called diode pumped solid-state lasers (DPSSLs).

Semiconductor laser diodes are of interest because of (1) their unparalleled efficiency, typically above 35–40% and reported as high as 66% in champion devices, (2) their reliability, typically near 10,000 h for high-power, multiwatt devices, in well-developed materials packaged in rugged configurations, (3) their compactness, typical 20 W average power diodes being approximately 100 μm by 400 μm by 1 cm and supported on a package or submount of somewhat larger dimensions for heat removal and for ease of maintenance, and importantly (4) their low cost. In terms of dollars per watt, semiconductor laser arrays are already very low cost and their cost continues to drop year by year. It is the belief of many proponents of the technology that increases in manufacturing volume alone will be sufficient to drive prices to ten dollars per watt and lower for high-power CW laser arrays. Already it is possible to purchase low-duty-cycle (ca. 1%) diode arrays for ten dollars per peak watt or less.

Semiconductor laser diodes are fabricated in a broad range of III–V and II–VI materials spanning the electromagnetic spectrum from the visible to the middle infrared. Typically the high-power laser diode arrays used for materials processing are in the near-infrared region of the electro-magnetic spectrum and are based upon the materials systems AlGaAs, InGaAs, and the rapidly emerging InGaAsP. The wavelengths of the first two systems span the range from roughly 0.77 μm to slightly longer than 1 μm.

The operation of a diode laser is based upon the recombination of carriers and holes in forward-biased *p-n* junctions. This recombination spontaneously emits a photon and, because of the densities of carriers and holes and the cross sections involved, results in very high-gain, roughly 1000 cm^{-1}, structures. A typical semiconductor laser cavity, defined by physical cleaving of an epitaxially grown semiconductor laser wafer, is about 400 μm in length, with a cavity width, defined lithographically, of from a few to approximately 50 μm, and a thickness, defined by the region or distance from the *p-n* junction over which carrier-hole recombination takes place, being about 1 μm. This structure, a laser diode, typically delivers about 5 mW/μm of lithographically defined cavity width or about 250 mW for a 50-μm-wide laser diode cavity. A laser diode bar is formed by cleaving the epitaxially grown laser wafer into a cavity length of about 400 μm and a bar width of about 1 cm, on which are typically arranged 100 laser cavities all parallel to each other and separated by about 50 μm from diode to diode. Using the above figures, such a bar would be capable of emitting 25 W of CW radiation. A laser diode bar is usually also referred to as an edge emitter, because the optical radiation is emitted from the edge of the cleaved bar. Laser diodes may also be fabricated to be surface emitters, in which the radiation is emitted normal to the broad surface of the semiconductor wafer. This can be accomplished using micromirrors, gratings, and other methods. These devices are not yet broadly available commercially and are not as mature technologically as edge emitters and are therefore not covered in the remainder of this short review.

The radiation emitted from a single diode laser is generally diffraction limited in the plane perpendicular to the laser diode junction. The radiation emitted parallel to the junction in so-called broad stripe diode lasers (as in the above example with a 50-μm-wide photolitho-graphically defined stripe) is many times diffraction limited since such a broad cavity is multimode. Thus the perpendicular axis, also known as the fast axis, even though diffraction limited has a beam divergence of about 1 rad, because the gain thickness as described above is about 1 μm. The parallel axis, also called the slow axis, usually has a beam divergence of usually many degrees. A laser diode bar can be organized such that the collection of laser diodes emit independently without any influence on each other, or they can be organized to be coupled due to a process whereby evanescent waves from each diode cavity are allowed to leak into nearest-neighbor cavities. In general, while in principle it is possible to organize a bar so that all laser diodes on a bar emit their radiation coherently, in reality it is not yet practical nor easily manufacturable. One bar structure that is simple to manufacture in which the individual diodes are coupled to each other is one in which each diode emits out of phase with its nearest neighbor, resulting in the well-known rabbit ear structure of a simple diode laser bar. The emission pattern for this structure becomes two lobes in the far field angled from each other by many degrees, with each having a slow-axis divergence of many degrees and a fast-axis divergence of a radian.

Laser diode bars can be stacked on top of each other to form two-dimensional diode arrays. These two-dimensional (2D) arrays can be used to pump solid-state lasers or can be used directly in laser materials processing applications. The stacking density of bars to form 2D arrays is called the stacking pitch and is typically from one to a few bars per centimeter. Figure 12 summarizes the geometries of laser diodes, bars, and laser diode array stacks or 2D arrays fabricated from edge-emitter components.

To operate a laser diode bar, typically 2 V or slightly more of forward-bias is applied with approximately 1 A required per watt of emitted optical radiation. One-centimeter-wide bars operating to about 20 W per centimeter can be cooled by attaching the bars to large heat-conductive fins, which are in turn convectively cooled by fan-circulated air. Water cooling in a variety of configurations can be used to cool bars operating at higher power. Support utilities for diode lasers are modest in size and complexity.

To summarize, diode lasers are very efficient, reliable, compact, and low-cost devices that are rapidly evolving. Their pulse length

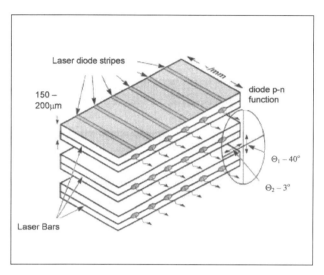

Figure 12. Two-dimensional diode arrays can be fabricated by stacking edge-emitting, laser-diode consisting of rows of individual diode lasers on a bar of dimensions nominally 200 μm X 400 μm X 1 cm.

and shape can be controlled nearly arbitrarily. Their single detracting feature for materials processing applications is that in order to scale to very high power, the output of many individual diode lasers, usually operating incoherently, must be coupled optically prior to delivery to the workpiece. This coupling can be complex, expensive, and inefficient, and still may result in a beam of limited depth of focus and relatively high divergence.

Many design approaches for using laser diode arrays for materials processing have been proposed and utilized (20). The most obvious is to use the diode arrays as pumps for solid-state lasers, which convert the output of many independently emitting diode lasers into a single coherent beam at some addition to system cost and complexity and typically a factor of three to five (or more) loss in system efficiency. Optical designs using fibers and micro-optics have also been employed with considerable success.

The beam intensity on each laser diode array emitting facet is typically about 2 MW/cm^2. The intensity requirement of laser surface processes ranges from 10^3 to 10^{10} W/cm^2. One example of the use of fibers to combine a large number of individual laser diodes to produce intensities of 10 kW/cm^2 at a numerical aperture of 0.2 is taken from Reference 21. A 20-W laser diode bar consisting of nineteen 1 x 150 μm emitters with individual beam divergences of 10 x 40 deg is first collimated by a single cylindrical microlens along the fast axis. A linear array of fibers of NA 0.11 matching each diode lateral divergence and the diode spacings on the bar collects the output. The linear array of fibers at the receiving end is collected into a bundle of fibers at the opposite end. This procedure can also be carried out for three (or more) diode bars, resulting (in the case of three bars) in a 1.91-mm circular output at NA of 0.11 with 45 W CW power. This output can be reimaged to a brightness of 4 x 10^4 W/cm^2-sr and an intensity of 10 kW/cm^2 at NA of 0.4. While this brightness is two orders of magnitude below that of an individual diode array facet, it is high enough to perform a number of laser processes, such as surface melting, alloying, cladding, vapor deposition, transformation hardening, and so forth.

Applications

Careful analysis shows that high-average-power incoherent two-dimensional arrays can be condensed by practical optical systems to intensities no greater than 100 kW/cm^2 at present, thereby making their direct use most important in the areas of melting or sintering, transformation hardening, and possibly deep penetration welding.

Beckett et al. (22), argue that the ability to transport diode near-infrared radiation through glass fibers and the effective absorption of this radiation by metallic surfaces, coupled with the many advantages cited above, will combine to give an increasingly important role to laser diodes in the soldering of electronic components. The reduction in the size of electronic interconnects, the increasing pin counts per chip, and the availability of laser diode units have now made these systems economically viable for electronic manufacturers.

The University of Hull in Hull, England, has conducted experiments to evaluate the soldering of fine-pitch components, with an example shown in Figure 13.

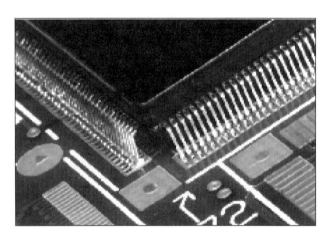

Figure 13. Typical laser-soldered 208-pin 0.020-in.-pitch package.

Roychoudhuri and colleagues at the University of Connecticut in Storrs have used fiber-coupled arrays of the type described above to perform rapid prototyping by sintering of metal powders. The optical system is described in Reference 23.

Laser sintering of most metal powders to create "net shape objects" (solid, free-form formation, SFF) can be achieved with laser power densities as low as 10 kW/cm^2; 50 kW/cm^2 is more than enough power for most applications. Commercial fiber-coupled CW high-power diode arrays are now easily available to deliver such power densities (see Chapter 16 for more detail on sintering).

The potential applications of microscopic semiconductor laser diodes for surface hardening, soldering, marking, sintering, etc., have been reviewed in References 24 and 25.

A final example of the direct use of laser diodes in manufacturing is the recent work of Pflueger, et al. in the transformation hardening of machine tool steel (26).

References

20. W. Chen, C. Roychoudhuri, and C. Banas, *Opt. Eng.* **33** (11), 3662–69 (1994).
21. Product Catalog, Opto Power Corporation (1994).
22. P. Beckett, A. Fleming, R. Foster, J. Gilbert, and D. Whitehead, *Op. and Quantum Electron.* **27,** 1303–11 (1995).
23. W. Chen, C. Roychoudhuri, and C. Banas, Design Approaches for Laser Diode Material Processing Systems, *Opt. Eng.* **33** (11), 3662 (1994).
24. C. Roychoudhuri, Manufacturing with High-Power Diode Lasers, *Encyclopedia of Electronics,* Section #3807, J. Webster (Ed.), Wiley, New York (1999).
25. C. Roychoudhuri, Desk-Top Manufacturing Using Diode Lasers, *SPIE Proceedings* 3274, SPIE, Bellingham, WA (1998).
26. S. Pflueger, Fraunhofer Resource Center, Univ. of Michigan, Ann Arbor, private communication (1996).

RICHARD W. SOLARZ

2.5.5 Iodine Lasers

Lasers based on emission from iodine have been considered attractive because of their potential scalability to very high power outputs at a relatively short wavelength (1.3 µm). This section discusses two approaches to iodine lasers, the chemical oxygen-iodine laser (COIL) and the photolytic iodine laser (PIL).

Iodine-based laser technology is less mature than that of lasers such as CO_2 and Nd:YAG.

The Chemical Oxygen Iodine Laser (COIL)

Coil was invented in 1977 at the Air Force Phillips Laboratory and is the shortest wavelength (1.315 µm), high-power chemical laser ever developed. Figure 14 illustrates the major components and processes of a COIL.

Gaseous chlorine reacts with an aqueous mixture of hydrogen peroxide and potassium hydroxide to produce singlet delta oxygen, an excited molecular state of oxygen. The singlet delta oxygen gas flows through a mixing nozzle, where molecular iodine is combined with the flow. Some of the energy in the oxygen dissociates the molecular iodine, creating a gas mixture of atomic iodine and singlet delta oxygen. Energy is transferred to the atomic iodine, which is resonant with the oxygen. The gas flow passes through a laser resonator, which extracts laser light at 1.315 µm wavelength. The exhaust gas is then cleaned by a chemical scrubber to remove the iodine and residual chlorine, producing easily disposable waste products such as oxygen, water, and salts.

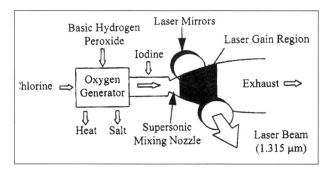

Figure 14. Block diagram of major COIL systems.

COIL has several characteristics that make it useful for high-power applications. First, the COIL wavelength of 1.315 μm allows it to couple well with metal, which gives it an advantage in materials processing speed over an equivalent sized CO_2 laser. This wavelength also has low absorption in standard fused silica optics, which allows its use at high powers without active cooling and makes it possible for low-loss transmission through commercially available fiber optics. Based on demonstrated power densities and a review of available fibers, as much as 25 kW can be transmitted through a single, 1500-μm core fiber optic.

Next, the scalability of COIL has been demonstrated by the Phillips Laboratory's RotoCOIL device, which produced 39 kW of continuous-wave power. Long run-time operation was demonstrated in Japan with the operation of a 1 kW subsonic gas flow COIL for 2 h. The Phillips Laboratory demonstrated 10 kW for 2 min with a supersonic COIL. A comprehensive list of references on COIL development in the United States is given by Truesdell et al. (27), with additional references on the theoretical operation of COIL given by Avizonis and Truesdell (28).

References
27. K. A. Truesdell, C. A. Helms, and G. D. Hagar, 25th Plasmadynamics and Lasers Conference, AIAA-94-2421 (1994).
28. P. V. Avizonis and K. A. Truesdell, 25th Plasmadynamics and Lasers Conference AIAA-94-2416 (1994).

WILLIAM P. LATHAM
ARAVINDA KAR

Photolytic Iodine Lasers

The photolytic iodine laser system (PILS) provides a unique very small, high-intensity processing beam for materials processing versus other laser processing equipment due to its performance capabilities. The PILS very high power density and very small beam size is due to its 1.3 μm wavelength and almost diffraction-limited beam, making it ideal for many precision materials processing applications. The measured spot size for the CW PILS is 20 μm, using a 5-in. standard focus lens (f/7.5), which is 3–8 times smaller than typical Nd:YAG and CO_2 laser technologies. The power density, at 20 W, is in the vaporization mode at approximately 10^7 W/cm², considerably higher than other laser systems. Only the PILS and other iodine lasers such as the COIL operate in this mode with continuous-wave (CW) operation. These features of the PILS enable faster feed rates and finer feature sizes with less adjacent material thermal damage. The very high intensities and minimal materials damage also provides the PILS with the potential ability to process materials not traditionally done by laser processes. The PILS will compete with slower and more expensive nonlaser technologies, such as electric discharge machines (EDM) in the metal industry and etching and electron beam machines (EBM) in the electronics industry and others, where current laser technology is not satisfactory.

A commercial photolytic iodine laser system has been in development since 1994 and is undergoing expanded commercialization.

The modern PILS is a simple, reliable laser system using a high-molecular-weight gas, C_3F_7I, which flows in a closed-loop cycle similar to some CO_2 lasers. The gas has thermal and physical properties similar to refrigerants such as R-114, but is heavier. The gas used is nontoxic, nonflammable, is not an ozone-depleting compound, and is environmentally benign. It can be shipped unregulated in DOT-approved bottles on common shipping carriers, including aircraft.

The gas flow system is most similar to an ammonia refrigeration system, with a liquid phase section in the cycle. The system has two moving parts, reducing complexity and increasing reliability and service life. A mechanical refrigeration system cools the condenser, which condenses the gas. An evaporator boils the liquid to provide gas flow to the laser's gain cell. The second moving part, a liquid gear pump, helps move the liquid between the condenser and the evaporator as shown in Figure 15.

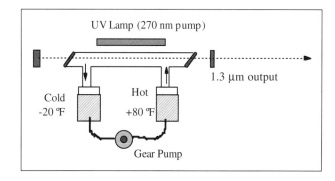

Figure 15. Functional diagram of modern photolytic iodine laser system (PILS) pumping C_3F_7I.

The C_3F_7I gas, when exposed to intense ultraviolet radiation in the 260–300 nm band, creates an excited iodine atom, the same as generated in chemical oxygen iodine lasers, which provides the laser's gain medium (29).

$$C_3F_7I \longrightarrow C_3F_7 + I^*$$

After photon extraction, the two radicals recombine to reform the parent gas molecule in the closed-loop cycle. This gain medium can provide high gains (gains of 4–6% per cm) sufficient to operate unstable resonators. It is one of a family of compounds, e.g., CF_3I, C_2F_5I, C_4F_9I, etc., which lase strongly but have different thermal and physical properties.

A unique feature of the PILS is that it can be operated in the continuous-wave mode or in the pulsed mode with small hardware changes. The fuel system, resonator optics systems, controls, and optical beam delivery system are common to both types of lasers. The source of the ultraviolet pumping radiation is different for the two types of lasers.

For CW PILS operation, ultraviolet radiation is provided by electrodeless plasma lamps driven by microwave radiation. Based on commercially available microwave-driven plasma lamps, microwave power supplies and S-band (2450 MHz) magnetrons and waveguide hardware, the CW systems are very hardy, simple to operate, and provide many hours of CW processing time for cutting, welding, and other applications.

For pulsed PILS operation, commercial electroded ultraviolet plasma lamps are driven by traditional electric discharge-driven systems very similar to those used for solid-state lasers. These will provide high-repetition-rate, low-pulse energy, short-time-length pulses similar to diode-pumped, solid-state laser systems. Pulse rates up to 100–300 Hz, 10–20 µsec pulse lengths, and energies of 0.5–1 J/pulse are suitable for many materials drilling and machining operations because of their focused 10^8-10^9 W/cm^2 irradiance. High-energy, low-repetition-rate pulsed PILS (70 J/pulse) have been tested and can be fabricated for industrial percussion hole drilling applications where a single pulse processing is desired (29).

The high-power pulsed PILS has been successfully doubled in frequency with high efficiencies using several types of commercial doubling crystals. The resultant highly focused, almost diffraction-limited 658-nm output beam delivers very high irradiance at a visible wavelength, very useful for high-precision laser processing, particularly micromachining and cutting of electronics and semiconductor components. High-beam-quality, high-power beams at ultraviolet wavelengths can also be obtained using commercially available optical crystals for tripling and quadrupling of the PILS output beam.

Comparison tests on focal spot size have been made using commercial Nd:YAG and CO_2 lasers; the output beam of the PILS is much smaller than that of these lasers using the same focusing optics. The PILS-focused beam is 20 µm in diameter, which is 3–5 times smaller than good Nd:YAG lasers and 5–10 times smaller than CO_2 lasers, using the same 5-in. focusing lens (f/7.5). These very small spots provide very high irradiance, 10^7 to 10^8 W/cm^2, in CW operation. These valves of irradiance are similar to those in drilling applications using high-energy, pulsed Nd:YAG lasers.

Because of the high irradiance resulting from the tightly focused PILS beams, materials processing results and parameters are expected to be different from typical laser processing. For example, there is less thermal damage with the high-quality, high-intensity beam. The heat-affected zone (HAZ) is smaller than for parts processed by Nd:YAG and CO_2 lasers. Most processing appears to be in the vaporization mode, since little melt and slag is observed.

Another aspect of processing with almost diffraction-limited beams is that as beam quality improves, the depth of focus (Rayleigh range) increases. With almost-diffraction-limited beams, the depth of focus was on the order of 0.5–0.7 mm with a 5-in. FL focusing lens (f/7.5) for the PILS. This assists processing with varying thickness of materials; often no focus height adjustment was necessary. With short 1.5-in. FL optics (f/2), focal spots are possible having approximately 6 mm diameter with 54 mm depth of focus, suitable for microelectronics and micromachining applications. With higher power, very fine cutting and welding is possible for thicker section materials normally encountered in the traditional metals industries.

Beam quality of the PILS was determined from traditional burn pattern measurements. A layer of 25-µm-thick aluminum on silicon was removed by incident beams of the PILS. The round 20-µm-diameter holes in the aluminum were considered to be approximately the $1/e^2$ point in irradiance distribution. Estimates of beam quality indicate an essentially diffraction-limited beam output from the laser, with $M^2 = 1.1$.

Output Power to Date

The PILS has generated 50-W output beams of CW radiation using a stable resonator with a 55% transmissive outcoupler. Using a high-quality negative branch unstable resonator, magnification $M = -2$, output power of 38 W of diffraction-limited output was obtained. Outputs are expected to increase as modifications in the laser's ultraviolet pumping radiation system are improved from the prototype system, where considerable losses have occurred.

Reference

29. L. A. Schlie and R. A. Rathge, *IEEE J. Quant. Electron.* **QE-31,** 1069 (1995).

PHILIP R. CUNNINGHAM
L.A. (VERN) SCHLIE

2.5.6 Nonlinear Optical Effects in Crystals

Nonlinear optics (NLO) is a powerful tool to generate coherent sources that may not be readily available through the lasing action in a medium. Many types of lasers are commercially available, offering a wide variety of different output wavelengths. However the number of different wavelengths available that are suitable for materials processing is somewhat limited.

For example, there are not many solid-state laser sources in the visible region, only the ruby laser operating at 649.3 nm. The Nd:YAG laser is one of the most well-developed industrial lasers, operating at 1064 nm in the near infrared region. The use of nonlinear-optical effects allows this laser wavelength to be halved, so as to generate coherent radiation at 532 nm (in the green). The 1064 nm wavelength can be further subdivided to produce one-third wavelength (355 nm) or one-fourth wavelength (266 nm) or to produce tunable visible coherent radiation. This wavelength shortening offers the advantage of reduced focal diameter, increased irradiance, and possibly higher absorption coefficient.

This section offers a brief introduction to nonlinear optics and also describes how nonlinear optics can be used to increase the range of possible laser wavelengths for materials processing.

The electric field, $\mathbf{E}(t)$, of electromagnetic radiation interacts with the electrical field within the molecules of a crystalline medium. It polarizes the atoms by slightly displacing the electrons along the direction of the field. At low intensities, the induced polarization, $\mathbf{P}(t)$, follows, with some phase retardation, the sinusoidal oscillation of a monochromatic wave. The temporal variation of the electric field is

$$\mathbf{E}(t) = \mathbf{E}_o \sin(\omega t)$$

Maxwell's electromagnetic wave equations describe the linear-optical effects in the medium, and the response

$$\mathbf{P}(t) = e_o \chi \mathbf{E}_o \sin(\omega t + \Theta)$$

where e_o denotes the electric permeability of vacuum, and χ and Θ are frequency-dependent material constants, referred to as the magnitude and phase of the electric susceptibility of the medium. This linear relationship between P and E generally fails to give an accurate description of the medium polarization for strong external electric fields $E \gg 1$ kV/cm, such as those that are present in laser radiation. Lasers are the only radiation sources capable of producing sufficiently high electric fields to induce an appreciable nonlinear response in crystals.

Since its discovery by Peter Franken (1961) and his group, the field of nonlinear optics has established itself as an important research tool, benefiting several areas of science and technology. The most important practical implications of NLO arise from the possibility of converting coherent laser radiation to new frequencies. Thus frequency conversion in a suitable medium (dielectric solids or gases) allows researchers to develop coherent sources of wavelengths that are wanted, with a broad tuning range, and/or at frequencies where coherent laser sources are simply not available. For example, for underwater laser communication between two submarines, a coherent source at 532 nm (where water is most transparent) is required. This is achieved by frequency doubling an Nd:YAG laser operating at 1064 nm, in a crystal of potassium titanyl phosphate (KTP), or similar NLO medium.

For photon energies much smaller than the energy gap between populated and the lowest unpopulated excited states, the polarization response of these materials can be written as:

$$\mathbf{P}(t) = e_o \{\chi_1 \mathbf{E}(t)^1 + \chi_2 \mathbf{E}(t)^2 + \chi_3 \mathbf{E}(t)^3 + \cdots\}$$

This expression is valid for weak nonlinearities, i.e., at moderate field strengths. The contributions to the induced polarization rapidly decrease with increasing order of nonlinear susceptibility χ_n ($n > 2$). The second-order term gives rise to second-harmonic generation (SHG), the third-order term gives rise to third-harmonic generation (THG), and so on.

Crystal Media for Nonlinear Optics

All piezoelectric crystals exhibit an electro-optic (EO) effect as well as a nonlinear optical (NLO) effect. A good NLO crystal must be anisotropic, that is, the properties depend upon the direction of propagation in the crystal. Whether a crystal is isotropic or anisotropic, and in the latter case, whether it is uniaxial (one optic axis) or biaxial, is determined by the crystal symmetry. Thus crystals with a cubic symmetry are always isotropic. All others are anisotropic. Crystals with trigonal, tetragonal, and hexagonal symmetries are always uniaxial; and crystals with orthorhombic, monoclinic, and triclinic symmetries are always biaxial. For an NLO crystal device to work well without degradation of performance over the lifetime of its assignment, it must meet a number of criteria.

1. Reliable crystal growth techniques for adequate size
2. NLO susceptibility coefficient
3. Birefringence ($n_o - n_e$) and optical dispersion
4. Moderate to high transparency
5. Good optical homogeneity
6. Good mechanical strength
7. Chemical stability
8. Ease of polishing and antireflection coating
9. Low linear and nonlinear absorption
10. Temperature phase-matching bandwidth
11. Fracture toughness
12. Damage threshold
13. Nonlinear index of refraction
14. Brittleness

Recent efforts in molecular engineering are making progress in growing crystals such as barium borate (BBO), lithium borate (LBO), and cesium-lithium borate (CLBO).

The terms that are often used in connection with NLO work are:

1. *Ordinary ray (O ray)*—optical ray that obeys Snell's law.

2. *Extraordinary ray (E ray)*—ray that does not obey Snell's law. The phase velocity of this ray depends upon the direction of polarization.

3. *Birefringence*—the double refraction in a crystal forms an E-ray and an O-ray, and its value is $(n_o - n_e)$.

4. *Beam walkoff*—the angular deviation between the O-ray and the E-ray as they propagate through the crystal. Along the optic axis, it is zero as the two rays propagate with equal velocity and $n_o = n_e$.

5. *Phase-matching (PM) condition*—expressed by the law of conservation of momentum, and given by $K_{\omega_1} + K_{\omega_2} = K_{\omega_3}$.

6. *Second-harmonic generation (SHG)*, also called frequency doubling—a special case of mixing of two waves of the same frequency (ω_1) to obtain a wave of double the frequency ($\omega_2 = 2\omega_1$) or half the wavelength.

Other terms similar to this are sum frequency mixing (SFM) and difference frequency mixing (DFM), used for mixing of two waves of different frequencies ($\omega_1 + \omega_2 = \omega_3$) or subtracting these two waves ($\omega_1 - \omega_2 = \omega_3$) to generate a third frequency. The SHG or SFM process combines two low-energy photons into a high-energy photon of the third frequency, at a lower wavelength (downconversion). In the case of DFM, one low-energy photon is taken away from a high-energy photon to generate a third low-energy photon in the infrared (upconversion).

In the case of SFM, the final wavelength, governed by the law of conservation of energy, is given by the equation:

$$\frac{1}{\lambda_1} + \frac{1}{\lambda_2} = \frac{1}{\lambda_3}$$

The PM angle condition that must be satisfied is given by the equation:

$$\frac{n_{\omega_1}}{\lambda_1} + \frac{n_{\omega_2}}{\lambda_2} = \frac{n_{\omega_3}}{\lambda_3}$$

DFM is expressed by a similar equation.

7. *Critical phase matching (CPM)*—in SHG, the NLO process is most efficient when the ω_1 and ω_2 phase velocities are made equal by choosing the internal crystal angle between the input plane of polarization and the optic axis of the crystal. This is called critical phase matching or sometimes angle phase matching or angle tuning (AT). Both conservation of energy and conservation of momentum must be satisfied.

8. *Noncritical phase matching (NCPM)*—when this angle is set at 90°, it may be possible to make ΔK [given by $K_{\omega_3} - (K_{\omega_1} + K_{\omega_2})$] vanish in some crystals by taking advantage of their thermal birefringence. When ω_1 propagates normal to the optic axis, the output beam ω_2 is also normal to it and all the rays (inside and outside the crystal) are collinear (zero beam walkoff). This is called noncritical phase matching or sometimes temperature tuning (TT). This is preferred because it produces the highest efficiency possible from the NLO material.

9. *Type I phase matching process*—cases (7) and (8) fall in this category, where the input plane of polarization is perpendicular to the plane containing the optic axis. This is also called an oo-e interaction for a negative ($n_e < n_o$) uniaxial crystal, or an ee-o interaction for a positive crystal (see Fig. 16A).

10. *Type II phase matching*—it is also possible to angle phase match when the plane containing the optic axis is rotated by 45°, so that two rays (one an E ray and the other an O ray) enter the crystal and the third (mixed) frequency ray is an E ray. This is called an eo-e interaction. Type II angles usually need numerical calculations. For biaxial crystals, such as KTP, LBO, or $KNbO_3$ (potassium niobate), these calculations are quite involved (see Fig. 16B).

11. *Optical parametric oscillation (OPO)*—an NLO process where the crystal is placed in a resonator and pumped by high-energy radiation (ω_3) to generate two frequencies called signal (ω_1) and idler (ω_2). A high-energy photon is split into two low-energy photons and in a degenerate case, by choice of a proper angle, $\omega_1 = \omega_2$, and the output frequency is one-half the input frequency; thus the wavelength is doubled by this process (see Fig. 17A).

12. *Intracavity frequency doubling*—an NLO crystal is placed inside the laser cavity, where the circulating powers are high, to obtain high efficiency in a CW laser (see Fig. 17B).

13. *Angular acceptance width*—the angular radiation that can be accepted by the crystal. Similar terms are spectral acceptance width and temperature acceptance width, and each NLO crystal has a unique property.

14. *Figure of merit*—the ratio d^2/n^3, where d is the nonlinear susceptibility coefficient and n is the refractive index. The converted SHG output is higher when this figure is larger.

15. *Efficiency of conversion*—in the case of SHG, it is the ratio of power at ω_2 to that at ω_1.

16. *Damage threshold*—a property of the crystal to withstand the laser radiation without damage.

17. *Deuterated crystal*—crystal such as KDP (potassium dihydrogen phosphate) grown in deuterium oxide (heavy water) and called D-KDP or KD*P, (deuterated KDP or potassium dideuterium phosphate).

18. *Coherence length*—that length over which the two waves (ω_1 and ω_2) remain in a constant phase relationship.

Chapter 2: Lasers for Materials Processing

Most important selection rules for the NLO crystal are:

1. High NLO coefficient and large figure of merit.

2. Phase matchability and excellent transmission over the region of interest.

3. Large angular, spectral, and temperature acceptance widths.

4. Large damage threshold.

5. Large size with optical homogeneity.

For example, KDP crystal frequency doublers, grown for laser fusion, are 750x750 mm² in cross section with a length of 500 mm, while the largest KTP, BBO, or LBO crystal size is about 15 x 15 x 20 mm³. KDP-type crystals are grown near room temperature, while BBO type crystals are grown at about 900°C.

Second Harmonic Generation

The simplest case of NLO mixing is that of SHG. The second-harmonic (SH) power generated by a single mode, Gaussian beam of angular frequency ω_1, and power P incident along the principal axis of a plane parallel crystal rod of length L is given by

$$P_{\omega_2} = \frac{J(P_{\omega_1})^2 L^2 d^2 \sin^2 \Theta}{W_0} \left(\frac{\sin^2 x}{x^2} \right)$$

where $x = \Delta K L / 2$

and the efficiency of conversion is given by the ratio $P_{\omega_2} / P_{\omega_1}$. Here J is a crystal dielectric constant at ω_1, d is the effective

Table 7. Parameters and Typical Performance of Some Nonlinear Crystals

Material	Refractive index			Nonlinear susceptibility		Nominal damage threshold		Linear absorption	Temperature acceptance	Angular acceptance	Length used	Typical SHG efficiency
	λ (nm)	n_o	n_e	$d \times 10^{12}$ d_{14}	m/volt d_{36}	t_p (ns)	(GW/cm²)	(% per cm)	$\Delta T \cdot d$ (°C cm)	$\psi \cdot d$ (mrad cm)	(cm)	(%)
ADP	347	1.55	1.50						0.8	32.0	6.0	23
	530	1.53	1.48									
	694	1.52	1.48	0.48	0.49			3%				
	1060	1.51	1.47	0.55	0.56	60.0	0.5					
KDP	347	1.54	1.49						3.5	1.0	2.5	20
	530	1.51	1.47			0.2	17.0					
	694	1.51	1.47	0.47	0.47	20.0	0.4	2.4%				
	1060	1.49	1.46	0.49	0.47	0.2	23.0	3%				
KD*P	347	1.53	1.49									
	530	1.51	1.47					0.6%				
	694	1.50	1.46	0.46	0.50				6.7	1.7	3.8	25
	1060	1.49	1.46	0.50	0.50	10.0	0.5	0.6%				
RDP	347	1.53	1.50					1.5%				
	530	1.51	1.48								2.0	20
	694	1.50	1.47			10.0	0.2	1%				
	1060	1.50	1.47	0.56	0.48	12.0	0.3	4%				
RDA	347	1.60	1.55					5%	3.3	40.0	2.0	25
	694	1.55	1.50		0.42	10.0	0.35	3.5%				
CDA	347	1.60	1.57									
	530	1.57	1.55									
	694	1.56	1.54						5.8	70.0	3.0	22
	1060	1.55	1.53		0.43	10.0	0.5	4%				
CD*A	347	1.59	1.57									
	530	1.57	1.55					0.4%				
	694	1.56	1.54						6.0	70.0	3.0	30
	1060	1.55	1.53		0.43	12.0	0.36	0.6%				

ISBN 0-912035-15-3

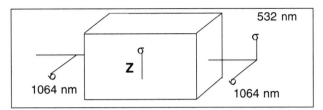

Figure 16A. Type I noncritically phase-matched (NCPM) crystal D-CDA (deuterated cesium dihydrogen arsenate) for efficiently doubling of 1064 nm radiation to 532 nm, with temperature tuning at 110°C.

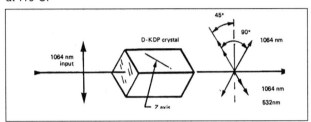

Figure 16B. Type II angle-phase-matched (angle tuned) crystal D-KDP for doubling 1064 nm radiation to 532 nm.

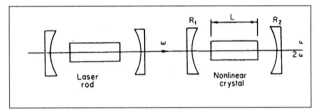

Figure 17A. Optical parametric oscillator (OPO) where a proper NCPM or CPM crystal is employed in a resonator with specially coated (reflective) mirrors. For an NLO application, a large number of parameters of the laser as well as those of the crystal must be taken into account. Also, tuning a crystal requires special skills and equipment, mounts, and a great deal of attention to detail to obtain fruitful results, unlike tuning a station on the radio dial. A number of questions need to be answered to succeed in the experiment.

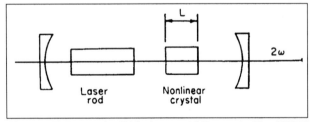

Figure 17B. Intracavity SHG where an NLO crystal, either NCPM or CPM Type I or Type II, is employed.

SHG coefficient depending upon the NLO susceptibility, W_0 is the minimum beam waist, and Θ is the angle between the crystal optic axis and the plane of polarization of ω_1. Because of dispersion, there is usually a wave vector mismatch ΔK between ω_1 and ω_2. For a fixed ΔK, the function $\sin^2 x/x^2$ undergoes oscillation as a function of crystal length with a period $2\pi/x$. Half this distance is called the coherence length and is the distance from the input at which the SH power is a maximum. Typical values range from a few millimeters to several centimeters. For normal incidence, the coherence length is given by $L_{coh} = \lambda_1 / 4 (n_{\omega_2} - n_{\omega_1})$, where λ_1 is the fundamental wavelength.

Phase-Matching Angles

The phase-matching angles for Type I (Θ_1) and Type II (Θ_2) can be calculated. For negative uniaxial NLO crystals, such as KD*P, CD*A, BBO, or $LiIO_3$ these are given by

Type I PM angle:

$$\sin^2\Theta_1 = \{ [n_{o\omega_1}]^{-2} - [n_{o\omega_2}]^{-2} \} / \{ [n_{e\omega_2}]^{-2} - [n_{o\omega_2}]^{-2} \}$$

Type II PM angle:

$$\left[\frac{\cos^2\Theta_2}{(n_{o\omega_2})^2} + \frac{\sin^2\Theta_2}{(n_{e\omega_2})^2}\right]^{-1/2} = \frac{1}{2}\left[(n_{o\omega_1}) + \left\{\frac{\cos^2\Theta_2}{(n_{o\omega_1})^2} + \frac{\sin^2\Theta_2}{(n_{e\omega_1})^2}\right\}^{-1/2}\right]$$

Inorganic NLO Materials

Visible and New Infrared Materials: Crystals of the KDP family have a transmission range from 220 to 840 nm (90% inclusive of Fresnel losses). These crystals are fairly easy to grow in a crystallizer by dropping the temperature of a solution of KDP salt in water. For materials grown in heavy water, transmission is from 220 to 1240 nm. There are seven members, KDP, ADP (ammonium dihydrogen phosphate), RDP (rubidium dihidrogen phosphate), ADA (ammonium dihydrogen arsenate), KDA (potassium dihydrogen arsenate), RDA (rubidium dihydrogen arsenate), CDA, and seven other deuterated isomorphs, KD*P, AD*P, RD*P, AD*A, KD*A, RD*A, and CD*A. The chemical formula for KDP is KH_2PO_4 and that for KD*P is KD_2PO_4. In the case of ADA, it is $NH_4H_2AsO_4$. These crystals are commonly used as they have broad angle of tunability; a ± 5° angle change tunes the wavelength from 600 to 800 nm in Type I KDP. When a crystal KDP is angle phase matched, that is, oriented at the proper PM angle, a 30-mm-long rod can produce SHG efficiency of 10 to 20% with a dye laser, since the d_{eff} coefficient is small. These crystals have similar values of nonlinearity within 20% of each other, and therefore these produce about the same efficiency under similar conditions. Crystal ADP angle phase matched at 600 nm (angle 61.5°) will produce slightly better results than a crystal KDP angle phase matched at 600 nm (angle 60°). However, if it is possible to find an NCPM crystal at 600 nm, higher efficiencies up to 30% are achievable. Fortunately, crystal ADA can be temperature tuned (NCPM) at 68°C for SHG at 600 nm.

Table 7 shows typical performance and parameters of some of these crystals.

Figure 18 shows the Type I angles for phase matching for some of these crystals as well as for $LiIO_3$ (hexagonal, 320 to 3800 nm), BBO (trigonal, 200 to 2000 nm), and LBO (orthorhombic, 200 to 2200 nm) crystals.

The important feature is that these crystals operate in an NCPM mode over a narrow range; for example, crystal ADA will produce excellent SHG efficiency (without beam walkoff) from 585

Chapter 2: Lasers for Materials Processing

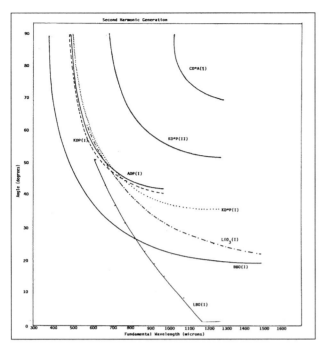

Figure 18. Tuning angles versus wavelengths for selected crystals.

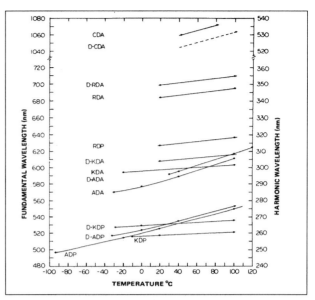

Figure 19. Temperatures for NCPM versus wavelength for KDP materials.

to 620 nm over the temperature range +25 to +125°C. For a rod length of 30 mm, the SHG efficiency is about 20–40%. Crystal RDA is an NCPM doubler for ruby (PM temperature of 92°C) and CD*A is an NCPM doubler for Nd:YAG (PM temperature of 110°C). The efficiency of RDA is 30–40% and that of CD*A is 50–60%. The peak power damage threshold of these crystals is about 250 MW/cm². The fluence damage threshold is 10 J/cm².

For NCPM crystals, the angular acceptance is large; so it is customary to use a 50-cm focal length lens and to place the crystal halfway between the lens and the focus. To increase the power density, a beam reducer is sometimes employed. If the power density is too high, a beam expander is required. Since these are hygroscopic materials, the crystal rods must be protected with antireflection (AR) coated windows in a hermetically sealed housing. The maximum safe operating temperature for NCPM is about 120°C. These crystals need special care in handling (use of gloves), storing, polishing, and AR coating, because they can crack from thermal shock (rate of temperature rise > 5° / min).

BBO and LBO crystals are excellent harmonic generators for Nd:YAG, Ti:Sapphire, and alexandrite lasers because of their high damage threshold and ultraviolet transmission. With a BBO rod 7 mm in length, cut at an angle 31° (Type 1), 32% conversion efficiency is achieved in the ultraviolet (378 nm). With a high-average-power (100 W) Nd:YAG laser (100 mJ, 14 ns, 1000 Hz), 37% efficiency is obtained (extracavity) without thermal detuning. Crystal LBO, operated (NCPM) intracavity, produces 50% SHG efficiency in a diode-pumped Nd:YAG (100 W) laser. Figure 19 shows the NCPM temperatures for various wavelengths for KDP-type crystals. Figure 20 shows the Type II phase-matching angles for various wavelengths for KDP, BBO, and LBO crystals.

Mid-Infrared Materials: There are many crystals that are useful in the mid-IR range from 2 to 5 μm. These crystals are

1. Lithium niobate, $LiNbO_3$ (trigonal, 420 to 4500 nm)

2. Potassium niobate, $KNbO_3$ (orthorhombic, 450 to 5000 nm)

3. Barium sodium niobate, $Ba_2Na(NbO_3)_5$, also known as banana (orthorhombic, 460 to 5000 nm)

4. Potassium titanyl phosphate, KTP (orthorhombic, 420 to 4500 nm).

Banana is now replaced for SHG at 1064 nm by KTP, or MgO-doped lithium niobate (LN). MgO-doped (5%) LN has a higher damage threshold.

There are many homologs of KTP available, such as KTA, RTA, and CTA. These have similar properties with slight variations. While LBO and BBO are grown by the flux method at temperatures around 1000°C, niobates are grown by the Czochralski method at 1400°C. KTP crystals are grown by either the flux method or the hydrothermal method. All crystals grown by the flux method tend to have inclusions and defects that lower the damage threshold. BBO and LBO are hygroscopic and suffer from degradation of polished faces.

ISBN 0-912035-15-3

Table 8. Properties of Nonlinear Optical Materials, Part A

Unixial crystals	KD*P	ADP	CD*A	BaB$_2$O$_4$	LiNbO$_3$	LiIO$_3$
Refractive index						
n_o	1.4931	1.5087	1.5500	1.6551	2.2322	1.8567
n_e	1.4582	1.4680	1.5431	1.5425	2.1560	1.7168
Transparency (μm)	0.18–1.8	0.184–1.5	0.27–1.66	0.198–2.6	0.35–5	0.31–5 ;c
						0.34–4 ⊥c
Nonlinear susceptibility (pm/V)						
$d_{21}=d_{16}$	0	0	0	-2.3	-2.1	0
d_{22}	0	0	0	2.3	2.1	0
$d_{14}=d_{25}=d_{36}$	0.37	0.47	0.3	0	0	(0)
$d_{31}=d_{15}$	0	0	0	0.1	-4.3	4.4
$d_{32}=d_{24}$	0	0	0	0.1	-4.3	4.4
d_{33}	0	0	0	0	-27	4.5
Thermo-optic coefficient (10^{-6} K^{-1})						
dn_o/dt	-30	-52	-25	-17	5	-89
dn_e/dt	-20	0	-16	-9	38	-75
Noncritical wavelength (μm)						
Type 1	0.519	0.524	1.045	0.409	1.062	0.378
Thermal Conductivity (W/m K)						
k_{11}	1.86	1.26	(1.5)	0.08	(5.6)	(1.47)
k_{33}	2.09	0.71	—	0.8	—	
Phase matching			T_{pm} = 112°		T_{pm} = 107°	
Type	II	II	I I	I II	I I	I
θ	54	62	82 90	23 32	77 90	30
φ	—	—	— —	— —	— —	—
Nonlinear susceptibility						
d_{eff} (pm/V)	0.35	0.39	0.30 0.30	1.9 1.6	5.1 4.7	1.8
C^2 (GW^{-1})	1.0	1.2	0.62 -0.63	22 16	70 59	13
Angular acceptance						
(mrad cm) critical						
(mrad cm) noncritical	2.3	2.2	7.2 51	0.53 0.80	1.2 33	0.34
Walkoff angle						
$ρ_ω$ (deg)	1.3	1.2	0 0	0 3.8	0 0	0
$ρ_{2ω}$ (deg)	1.4	1.5	0.26 0	3.2 3.9	1.0 0	4.3
Temperature bandwidth (°K cm)	12	2.1	3 3.3	51 37	1.0 0.75	23
Wavelength bandwidth (nm cm)	5.6	26	2.5 2.5	2 2.1	0.31 0.31	0.82
Threshold power P_{th} (MW)	30	27	3 NA	21 13	0.70 NA	66
Resonant SHG P_{50} (W)	120	210	46 26	3.6 5.8	0.38 0.05	6.6
Maximum drive C^2I_{dam} (cm^{-2})	5(1 ns)	7(15 ns)	0.15 0.16 (12 ns)	297 216 (1 ns)	700 590	26 (1 ns)
Thermal dephasing $η/δ_{th}$	5 x 10^{-4}	8 x 10^{-6}	5 x 10^{-4} - 7.4 x 10^{-4}	0.01 x 10^{-3} - 4 x 10^{-3}	0.1 0.4	0.05
Thermal focusing f_{th} (cm W)	-3.9	-0.13	-6.8	-3.8	47	-12
Surface damage intensity (GW/cm^2)	5(1 ns) >8(0.6 ns, 0.53 μm)	6(15 ns) >8(0.6 ns, 0.53 μm)	0.25(12 ns)	13.5(1 ns) 23(14 ns) 32(8 ns, 053 μm)	10(1 ns) 0.3(10 ns)	2(1 ns) 1(0.1 ns, >0.53 μm)

Chapter 2: Lasers for Materials Processing

Table 8. Properties of Nonlinear Optical Materials, Part B

	AgGaS$_2$	AgGaSe$_2$	ZnGeP$_2$	Bixial crystals	KTP	KNbO$_3$		LiB$_3$O$_5$	
	2.3472	2.5912	3.0728	Refractive index					
	2.2934	2.5579	3.1127	n_x	1.7367	2.1194		1.5649	
				n_y	1.7395	2.2195		1.5907	
				n_z	1.8305	2.2576		1.6052	
	0.5–13	0.78–18	0.74–12	Transparency (µm)	0.35–4.5	0.4–5.5		0.16–2.3	
				Nonlinear susceptibility (pm/V)					
	0	0	0	$d_{21}=d_{16}$	0	0		0	
	0	0	0	d_{22}	0	0		0	
	@17.5	33	69	$d_{14}=d_{25}=d_{36}$	0	0		0	
	(11.2 10.6 µm)	(10.6 µm)	(10.6 µm)	$d_{31}=d_{15}$	2.0	-11.3		-0.67	
	0	0	0	$d_{32}=d_{24}$	3.6	-12.8		0.85	
	0	0	0	d_{33}	8.3	-19.5		0.04	
	0	0	0						
				Thermo-optic coefficient (10^{-6} K^{-1})					
	154 (10.6 µm)	70 (3.39 µm)	150	dn_x/dt	11	60		-1.9	
	155 (10.6 µm)	40 (3.39 µm)	170	dn_y/dt	13	22		-13	
				dn_z/dt	16	-35		-8.3	
				Noncritical wavelength (µm)					
	1.8, 11.2	3.1, 12.8	3.2, 10.3	Type I	—	0.860		0.554	
						0.982		1.212	
	(11.5)	(1)	(35)	Type II	0.990	—		1.19	
					1.081				
				Thermal conductivity (W/m K)					
	I	I	I	k_{11}	2	—		(3)	
	31	52	56	k_{22}	3	(5.6)		—	
	—	—	—	k_{33}	3.3	—		—	
				Phase matching type		T$_{pm}$=183°		T$_{pm}$=148°	
	10.4	28	70		II	I	I	II	I
	14	81	292	θ	90	71	90	70.1	90
				ϕ	23	90	90	90	0
				Nonlinear susceptibility					
	3.7	6.0	5.0	d_{eff} (pm/V)	3.2	-11	-13	0.69	0.85
	0	0	0.65	C^2 (GW^{-1})	47	312	390	3.2	4.6
	1.2	0.64	0	Angular acceptance (mrad cm)					
				critical					
	50	50	40	noncritical	9	0.24	13	9.4	72
	11	22	20	Walkoff angle					
	4.3	0.25	0.069	ρ_ω (deg)	0.20	0	0	0.33	0
	6.9	0.58	0.68	$\rho_{2\omega}$ (deg)	0.27	2.5	0	0	0
				Temperature bandwidth (K cm)	17	0.5	0.3	6.2	3.9
	0.4 (10 ns)	3 (10 ns)	15	Wavelength bandwidth (nm cm)	0.46		0.12	4.6	3.6
			(25 ns)	Threshold power P_{th} (MW)	0.029	4.0	NA	1.7	NA
	0.15	0.14	13	Resonant SHG P_{50} (W)	0.28	0.24	0.01	17	8.6
				Maximum drive $C^2 I_{dam}$ (cm^{-2})	470	2200	2730	4.5	6.4
	13	1.5	1.0		(1 ns)	(1 ns)		(12 ns)	
	0.025 (10 ns)	0.01 0.04	0.05 (25 ns,	Thermal dephasing η/δ_{th}	0.9	0.07	0.6	0.1	0.2
		(50 ns, 2 µm)	2 µm)	Thermal focusing f_{th} (cm W)	36	22		-440	
	0.5 (10 ns, bulk)	0.02 0.03		Surface damage intensity (GW/cm^2)	9-20 (1ns)	7 (ns)		25 (0.1 ns)	
		(10 ns, 10.6 µm)	1 (2 ns, 10.6 µm)						

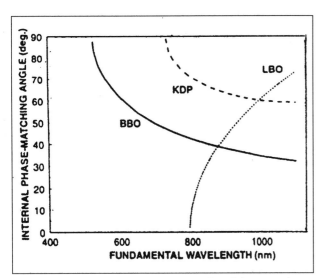

Figure 20. Type II PM angles versus wavelength for several non-linear crystals.

Both materials are difficult to AR coat. Niobates and KTP are easy to AR coat, and their polish does not degrade. Crystal lithium iodate (LI), (hexagonal, 320 to 3800 nm) is also usable in the midinfrared range. It is grown by dropping the temperature of the solution of the salt in water and the crystal polished faces degrade with time even at low relative humidity. It is, however, easy to AR coat with magnesium fluoride.

Far-Infrared Materials: There are three popular materials:

1. Crystal silver gallium sulfide, $AgGaS_2$ (tetragonal, 500 to 13,000 nm)

2. Silver gallium selenide, $AgGaSe_2$ (tetragonal, 780 to 18,000 nm)

3. Zinc germanium phosphide, $ZnGeP_2$ (tetragonal, 740 to 12,000 nm).

Their NLO properties, as well as those of other materials, useful in the near and mid-IR are given in Table 8. All data are for room temperature and 1.06 μm, unless otherwise noted.

For frequency conversion of a CO_2 laser, a few other crystals besides the three mentioned in Table 8 are available. These are crystals of proustite ($AgAsS_3$) and TAS (Tl_3AsSe_3). Conversion efficiency of 40% is achievable in crystal TAS at 10 MW/cm² and of 60% is achievable in silver gallium selenide at 12 MW/cm². Both crystals have low absorption, high damage threshold, and moderate d_{eff}. The selenide is limited by the surface damage threshold, although the bulk damage is higher by one order of magnitude. These crystals are used in an OPO pumped by a Nd:YAG laser (1340 nm) or by Ho:YAG (2050 nm). These crystals can produce frequency doubling of 4000 nm radiation.

Third Harmonic Generation (THG) and Sum Frequency Mixing (SFM)

For a Ti:Sapphire laser, LBO Type I (31.8° at 800 nm) is used as a doubler and BBO type II (55.2°) is used as a tripler to generate 266 nm. The residual 800-nm radiation coming out of a doubler is mixed with 400-nm radiation in a tripler. The tripler can be a Type I crystal (44.3° angle); however, a wave plate is needed to rotate the plane of polarization of the 800-nm radiation to coincide with that of the 400 nm. This process is also called sum frequency mixing (SFM, mixing of 800 and 400 nm). SFM of two dye lasers has generated 197-nm radiation in a BBO crystal. Similarly it is possible to generate fourth-harmonic (quadruple, 266 nm), as well as fifth-harmonic (quintuple, 212.8 nm) radiation from a Nd:YAG laser in a BBO crystal (by mixing the fourth harmonic with the fundamental [4 + 1] radiation). The only crystal phase matchable for fifth-harmonic generation is BBO. It is difficult to generate ultraviolet below 200 nm because good optical-quality NLO crystals are not yet available.

Since BBO and LBO crystals are expensive in large sizes, a popular method of Nd:YAG laser tripling is to use Type I NCPM CD*A as a doubler and Type II KD*P as a tripler.

Optical Parametric Oscillator (OPO)

The OPO process is an NLO process in which a high-energy pump photon (ω_3) propagating in an NLO crystal spontaneously breaks down into two low-energy photons ($\omega_1 + \omega_2$) with the total photon energy conserved (i.e., $\omega_3 = \omega_1 + \omega_2$). The gain mechanism is based upon the stimulation emission process. The rate of emission through the NLO parametric process is proportional to the photons present. OPO is an inverse process of SFM. An NLO crystal is placed in a cavity formed by two mirrors. For a fixed pump wavelength, many signal and idler wavelengths

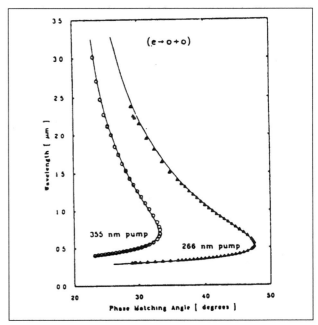

Figure 21. Tuning curves for an OPO based on BBO.

Chapter 2: Lasers for Materials Processing

can be generated by tilting an NLO crystal. BBO, KTP, LBO, and $AgGaSe_2$ are good NLO crystals for achieving efficiencies greater than 30–40%.

Figure 21 shows tuning curves for Type I, 355 nm pumped BBO OPO.

Figure 22 below shows a typical experimental setup.

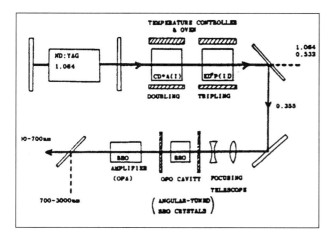

Figure 22. Typical arrangement for an OPO.

Wavelengths for Materials Processing

Materials processing is the broad field of cutting, drilling, welding, and otherwise modifying industrial materials and includes both metals and nonmetals. CO_2 and Nd:YAG lasers are by far the most widely used. Both CW and pulsed lasers are used, depending upon the application. Recently, solid-state diode lasers (emitting 809 nm radiation) have been used to pump Nd:YAG rods at the absorption peak. This improves the optical pump efficiency of Nd:YAG lasers as compared to the krypton lamp pumped lasers. For example, to achieve 50 W 1064 nm output, the electrical power to the diode lasers is about 240 W, whereas for the same output, a flash lamp consumes about 19 times more power. This new advancement has made Nd:YAG lasers more attractive than CO_2 lasers.

During the laser processing of materials, the conversion of the laser radiation into material removal can be significantly more efficient in the visible and ultraviolet regions than in the infrared. For this, 532, 355, and 266 nm are generated using NLO methods in a Nd:YAG laser. In a CW acousto-optically Q-switched Nd:YAG laser, a NCPM LBO crystal is used at a temperature of 149°C, and 50 W of green (multimode) or 8 W of TEM_{00} mode is available in a standard commercial laser. Crystal LBO is seven times more damage resistant than crystal KTP. Two other crystals, MgO-doped lithium liobate and potassium niobate, will generate 532 nm at NCPM temperatures of 107 and 200°C, respectively. However, these also have lower damage thresholds.

Third-harmonic 355 nm can be produced by using Type I LBO (in place of CD*A) and Type II LBO (in place of KD*P). Again 266 nm is produced in LBO (Type I) by mixing (3 + 1) or in crystal BBO (Type I) by doubling 532-nm radiation. There are advantages of reliability in using an all-solid-state system (as compared to excimer lasers). One can obtain with average powers up to 1 W in the ultraviolet for semiconductor and microelectronics manufacturing industries.

A harmonic frequency conversion flow chart for generating many typical wavelengths is shown in Figure 23.

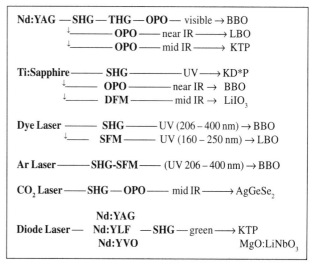

Figure 23. Harmonic frequency generation flow chart.

In an NLO system design, there are many variables that must be considered to optimize the efficiency. NLO crystals play an essential role for the generation of coherent sources in spectral ranges where useful levels of direct output from existing lasers cannot be achieved for materials processing applications.

References

R. S. Adhav and R. W. Wallace, *IEEE J. Quant.Electron.* **QE-6**, 793 (1970).

Y. R. Shen, *The Principles of Nonlinear Optics*, John Wiley and Sons. (1984).

A. Yariv and P. Yeh, *Optical Waves in Crystals*, John Wiley and Sons (1984).

H. Rabin and C. Tang, *Quantum Electronics, Volume I, Part B, Nonlinear Optics*, in *Methods of Experimental Physics*, Academic Press (1975).

G. A. Rines, et al., *IEEE J. Quant. Electron.* **31** (1), 50 (April 1995).

H. Komine, et al., *IEEE J. Quant. Electron.* **31** (1), 44 (April 1995).

Quantum Technology, Inc., data sheets No. 701 to 716.

RATAN S. ADHAV

2.5.7 Free-Electron Lasers

Free-electron lasers (FEL) employ a beam of relativistic electrons as the active medium. These electrons travel at a velocity that approaches the velocity of light. The FEL directly converts the kinetic energy of the electron beam into light. An FEL can be designed to operate at any wavelength and has potentially high power and efficiency.

The structure of an FEL uses a series of magnets called wigglers, so that the electron beam travels through an alternating magnetic field. Figure 24 shows a schematic diagram of a typical FEL structure. The electron beam is introduced into the laser cavity by magnets. The electrons radiate laser light by stimulated emission, and the light emerges through the output mirror.

A number of factors determine the wavelength of the FEL. The wavelength depends on the velocity of the electron beam, the spacing of the wiggler magnets, and the magnetic field. The wiggler spacing is fixed, but the laser wavelength may be tuned by varying the velocity of the electron beam and the magnetic field. Operation of FELs at wavelengths from the ultraviolet to the millimeter wave region has been demonstrated at a number of laboratories throughout the world.

Free-electron lasers have a number of important properties. They have an essentially unlimited range of operational wavelengths. The output power can potentially be scaled to high values. There is no material medium to be damaged.

FELs do require a high-quality beam of relativistic electrons, with low angular spreading and very little variation in electron velocity. These sources are large and expensive. In the past, it has required substantial resources to build and operate a FEL. Thus FELs have not been used for industrial materials processing.

In recent work (30), relatively inexpensive compact free electron lasers have been demonstrated. Although the output power of these devices has been low so far, it is possible that further advances may lead to FELs suitable for materials processing applications.

Reference
30. *The Industrial Physicist,* p. 18, February, 1999.

JOHN F. READY

2.5.8 X-Ray Lasers

Principles

The emitting medium is a hot plasma produced by cylindrical focusing of high-power pulsed infrared-laser radiation on a solid target (31). The principle of the system is represented in Figure 25, which shows the plasma column formed close to the target.

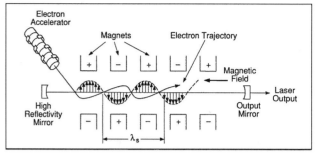

Figure 24. Schematic diagram of free-electron laser. (From J. F. Ready, *Industrial Applications of Lasers,* Second Edition, Academic Press, San Diego, 1997.)

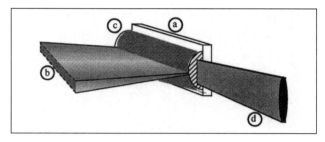

Figure 25. Principle of soft X-ray amplifying plasma column production: (a) solid target; (b) pumping infrared laser beam; (c) hot plasma; (d) soft X-ray laser beam.

The infrared pulse duration is 0.1-1 ns. Laser-plasma interaction raises the temperature to the value that makes the main plasma components to be neonlike ions (10 bound electrons) and free electrons. This temperature ranges from 200 to 800 eV according to the atomic number of the target element. Because free electron heating is a very fast process as compared with atom ionization, the electron temperature may largely exceed the equilibrium temperature of the neonlike plasma during the leading pulse slope. The departure from equilibrium generates population inversions between the $3p$ and $3s$ levels of neonlike ions. A simplified diagram of the pumping scheme is displayed in Figure 26.

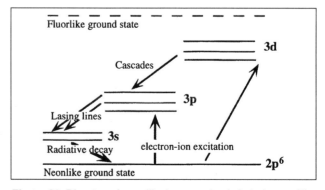

Figure 26. Diagram of neonlike ion pumping in hot plasma. The $2p$ ground-state excitation to the $3p$ and $3d$ levels is due to plasma free-electron collisions with ions. Population inversions occur between the $3p$ and $3s$ levels.

This so-called collisional pumping (32) produces soft X-ray lasing lines with large gain coefficient (3-10 cm^{-1}). The X-ray pulses last only 50–200 ps. A similar process is demonstrated for the $4d$-$4p$ lines of nickel-like ions (28 bound electrons). Pumping improvement by using a nanosecond infrared-pulse followed by a picosecond one is under investigation (33).

Figure 27 displays laser wavelengths against atomic number for the two ion species. Neonlike argon, in the left part of the figure, is a unique case where collisional pumping is produced in gaseous electrical discharge. Table 9 gives the accurate wavelengths of the three main lasing lines of the neonlike ions for which strong lasing has been experimentally achieved and are of practical interest for X-ray lasers in the present state of the art. All lines correspond to $3p$-$3s$ transitions. $J = 0$-1, etc. mean transitions that take place between levels of total angular momentum 0 (upper level) and 1 (lower level), etc.

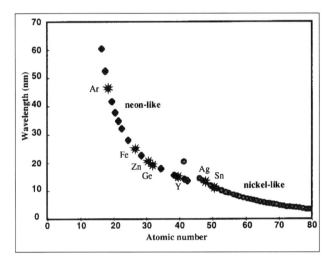

Figure 27. Lasing line wavelengths of elements versus atomic numbers. For each element the selected value corresponds to the $J = 0$ to $J = 1$ transition. The star symbols point to wavelengths for which high laser intensity is already tractable.

Table 9. Important Neonlike Lasing Lines

Z	Ion	Wavelengths (nm)		
		$J = 0$-1	$J = 2$-1	$J = 2$-1
18	Ar^{8+}	46.88		
22	Ti^{12+}	32.65	45.94	47.21
26	Fe^{16+}	25.50	34.04	34.79
30	Zn^{20+}	21.22	26.23	26.72
32	Ge^{22+}	19.61	23.22	23.63
34	Se^{24+}	18.25	20.64	20.97
39	Y^{29+}	15.50	15.50	15.71
47	Ag^{37+}	12.30	9.94	10.04

X-ray Laser Configurations

All lasers of very high brightness are neonlike ion based at the present time. The characteristics of the pumping laser, the target material, the choice of a particular line in the lasing spectrum, as well as other possible experimental peculiarities, lead to various X-ray laser configurations. For instance, according to the available pumping power, the energy (0.5–20 kJ) is conveyed to the target by one or by several optical beams. Targets are thin foils, thin layers deposited on thick supports, massive matter slabs. The target length is 2–3 cm. Configurations that illustrate some of these characteristics are shown in Figure 28a and b.

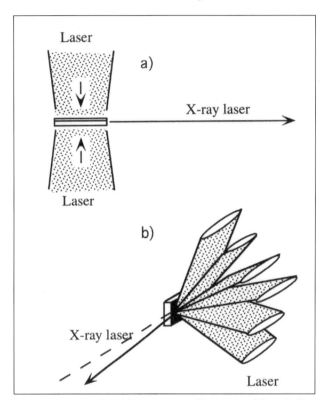

Figure 28. Examples of X-ray laser configurations: (a) exploding foil technique making use of two opposite pumping beams and a thin foil target; (b) massive target technique with six pumping beams.

Because of the fast plasma expansion from target to vacuum, strong density gradients appear in the plasma volume. The refractive-index gradients that follow from them lead to curvature of the X-ray path. So the laser beam may emerge from the narrow amplified channel before reaching the plasma end. Then the laser output decreases. Various techniques are used either to compensate for refraction or to smooth plasma density gradients. As an example, Figure 29 shows a double-target configuration in which the deviation at the exit of the first plasma is approximately compensated by the shifting of the turned-back second target (34). Some refraction correction can also be provided by using a slightly curved target (35).

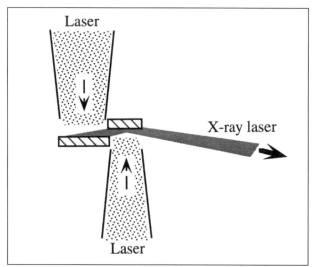

Figure 29. The figure shows the X-ray laser beam diverging from the amplification axis because of refraction inside the plasma. The two-target configuration makes it possible to increase the amplifying length by balancing the deviations.

Density gradient smoothing is achieved by using a prepulse technique. A few nanoseconds before the main infrared pulse, a small prepulse (10^{-3} - 10^{-2} times the main pulse energy) is sent to the target. A cold dense plasma, which expands before the main pulse arrival, is produced. So the density gradients are partially relaxed before plasma heating (36). This technique must especially be applied to the lines of the column $J = 0$ - $J = 1$ in Table 9, for which the amplifying channel is very narrow (~50 µm wide). The best value of the prepulse energy, as well as the temporal delay, depends on the target element and must be experimentally determined.

Standard laser cavity operation cannot be achieved yet with X-ray lasers because the amplification does not last much longer than a single pass of radiation through the plasma column. However, a multilayer mirror at one of the plasma ends, as shown in Figure 30, improves the intensity and optical coherence of the beam.

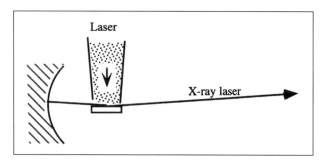

Figure 30. Sketch of a half-cavity. The multilayer mirror, in the left part of the figure, yields a laser beam double-pass through the plasma.

Though the reflection coefficient of the mirror is generally less than 50%, this "half-cavity" enhances the laser brightness by 2–3 orders of magnitude. This is because the same propagation path is used in two opposite directions, which strongly reduces the ratio between refractive deviation and effective path length. It also appreciably reduces the beam divergence as well as the source size. Systems combining these various techniques, as shown in Figure 31, have been successfully tested.

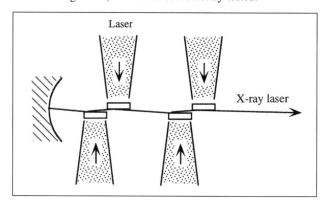

Figure 31. Combination of multiple-target and half-cavity techniques.

Achievements

Characteristics of X-ray lasers at saturation intensity are presented in Table 10. The pulse-averaged power is tens of megawatts. Characteristics of two other laboratory sources - high harmonic generation (HHG) and synchrotron radiation - are given for comparison. Because of their large power and strong directionality, X-ray lasers exhibit far greater spectral brightness than other X-ray sources (7–8 orders of magnitude difference). However, their repetition rate, which is controlled by the pump laser cooling time, is very low: the interval between shots is 20 min for the zinc laser and 2–3 h for the yttrium laser. The current working mode involves single-shot experiments, for which there is no great difficulty on account of the large photon number per pulse. New laser techniques, such as pumping diodes and disk amplifiers, could considerably reduce the time interval between shots in the future.

The X-ray laser is not monomode, neither spatially nor temporally. Nevertheless the number of photons per mode, N, depends on the spectral brightness, B, according to the relation (in units used in Table 10)

$$N = 3.7 \times 10^{-11} \lambda^3 B$$

which shows N to be of the order of 10^9. This very large number makes feasible single shot experiments with coherent optics.

Applications

The X-ray laser may be used for situations that require extremely intense monochromatic soft X-ray flashes. Typical examples are interferometric studies of dynamical processes for which two

Chapter 2: Lasers for Materials Processing

Table 10. Main Characteristics of X-Ray Laser Emission

Element	$Zn^{20+}(J_{0-1})$	$Ge^{22+}(J_{0-1})$	$Y^{29+}(J_{2-1})$	HHG - Ar 27th	Ondulator
	(LULI-Fr)	(DRAL-GB)	(LLNL-US)	(CEA-Fr)	(ALS, US)
Pump laser energy	0.4 KJ (600 ps)	0.15 KJ (75 ps)	4 KJ (600 ps)		
Prepulse	0.1 %	~1 %	0		
Wavelength	21.2 nm	19.6 nm	15.5 nm	31 nm	Tunable
$\lambda/\Delta\lambda$	~10^4	~10^4	~10^4	3×10^2	10^3
Photons/pulse	~1×10^{14}	~9×10^{13}	~7×10^{14}	10^9	10^6
X-UV energy	~1 mJ	~0.9 mJ	~10 mJ	5 nJ	0.1 nJ
Pulse duration	80 ps	40 ps	200 ps	50 fs	50 ps
Power	~12 MW	~20 MW	~45 MW	100 kW	2 kW
Solid angle (steradian)	2.5×10^{-5}	1.8×10^{-4}	2×10^{-4}		
Spectral brightness (W/cm²/steradian/10^{-4}BW)	1×10^{16}	7×10^{14}	2×10^{15}	10^8	10^8

Table 10 exhibits the emission parameters of three soft X-ray lasers and, by comparison, similar quantities for other important sources, i.e. high harmonic generation (HHG) and synchrotron radiation (ondulator). In the second line, the prepulse percentage is the prepulse-to-main-pulse energy ratio. In the last line, the spectral interval, given as 10^{-4} BW (bandwidth) as is usual for synchrotron radiation, fits the X-ray laser line widths (~0.02 nm).

types of interferometers are in use. (1) The Mach-Zehnder type in which multilayer beam-splitters are necessary to divide the X-ray beam into two. (2) The Fresnel bimirror, which consists of two grazing incidence mirrors arranged as a ridged roof (37). In the first case a sophisticated technique is necessary for making the beam-splitters. Electronic density maps of dense plasmas have been investigated by this method (38). The second system is based on conventional techniques, but it requires more spatial coherence than the previous one. As an illustration of bimirror capability, Figure 32 shows the single shot interferometric footprint of an electric-field induced defect zone on a polished metal surface.

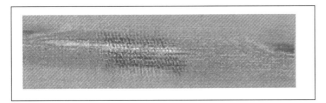

Figure 32. Electric-field-induced defect on a polished niobium surface revealed by X-ray laser interferometry. Such an image is obtained by making the pixel-to-pixel difference between perturbed and unperturbed interferograms. Holographic reconstruction shows the defect "depth" to be of 10–20 nm. The transverse size of the perturbed zone is about 500 μm. X-ray laser enables the defect evolution to be observed in an electric field. In the case of the figure the field was near 35 Mv/m.

It is worthwhile mentioning that because X-ray laser radiation is not subject to "skin" absorption in matter, surfaces are not damaged by the beam.

Other applications are thin foil radiography, crystal fluorescence at very large excitation intensity, and, generally speaking, soft X-ray interaction with matter at large flux. A future X-ray laser application may be semiconductor lithography.

X-ray lasers have not been used for industrial materials processing. As the size of very high power Nd: glass lasers used for producing the high-temperature plasmas shrinks to table-top size, it is possible that materials processing applications may become feasible.

References

31. Exhaustive information is to be found in:
    a) *"International Colloquium on X-ray Lasers"* P. Jaeglé and A. Sureau, (Eds.), Editions de Physique, Les Ulis, Fr., 1986.
    b) *"X-ray Lasers 1990"*, G. J. Tallents (Ed.), Institute of Physics Conference Series n° 116, IOP Publishing, Bristol, G.B.
    c) *"X-ray Lasers 1992"*, E.E. Fill (Ed.), Institute of Physics Conference Series n° 125, IOP Publishing, Bristol, G.B.
    d) *"X-ray Lasers 1994"*, C. C. Eder and D. L. Matthews (Eds.), IAIP Conference Proceedings n° 332, American Insitute of Physics, Woodbury, NY, USA.
    e) *"X-ray Lasers 96"*, S. Svanberg and C-G. Wahlström (Eds.), Institute of Physics Conference Series n° 151, IOP Publishing, Bristol, G.B.
32. D. L. Matthews, P. L. Hagelstein, M. D. Rosen, M. J. Eckart, N. M. Ceglio, A. U. Hazi, H. Medecki, B. J. MacGowan, J. E. Trebes, B. L. Whitten, E. M. Campbell, C. W. Hatcher, J. H. Scofield, G. Stone, and T. A. Weaver, *Phys. Rev. Lett.* **54**, 110 (1985).
33. P. V Nickles, V. N. Shlyaptsev, M. Kalachnikov, M. Schnürer, I. Will, and W. Sandner, *Phys. Rev. Lett.* **78**, 2748 (1997).
34. D. Neely, C. S. L. Lewis, D. N. O'Neill, J. Uhomoibhi, M. H. Key, S. J. Rose, G. J. Tallents, and S. A. Ramsden, *Opt. Commun.* **87**, 231 (1992).
35. R. Kodama, D. Neely, Y. Kato, H Daido, K. Murai, G. Yuan, A. MacPhee, and C. L. S. Lewis, *Phys. Rev. Lett.* **73**, 101 (1994).
36. J. Nilsen, J. C. Moreno, *Phys. Rev. Lett.* **74**, 337 (1995).
37. F. Albert, et al., *Optics Commun*, 1997.
38. L. B. Da Silva , et al., *Phys. Rev. Lett.* **74**, 15 (1995).

PIERRE JAEGLÉ

2.5.9 Ultrafast Lasers for Materials Processing

A new type of materials processing is enabled with ultrashort (< 10 psec) laser pulses. Cutting, drilling, sculpting of all materials (biological materials, ceramics, sapphire, silicon carbide, diamond, metals) occurs by new mechanisms that eliminate thermal shock or collateral damage. High-precision machining to submicrometer tolerances is enabled, resulting in high surface quality and negligible heat-affected zone.

Much of this work has been done with Ti:Sapphire lasers, which are covered in Section 2.3.

The depth of material removed at the optimum fluence with ultrashort-pulse lasers is limited to ≈0.5 µm per laser pulse for both dielectrics and metals. Hence, the rate of material removal scales essentially linearly with the repetition rate of the laser system. Since the optimum fluence is fixed by the material to be machined and the aspect ratio of the feature of interest, the area that can be machined per laser pulse is set by the energy of the pulses. Combining these features, the volumetric machining rate scales linearly with the average power of the laser.

Ultrashort-pulse lasers are based on the concept of chirped-pulse amplification described for lasers by Fisher and Bischel (39). This technique was first realized to produce picosecond pulses in a solid-state laser system by Strickland and Mourou (40, 41). Since the first demonstration, dramatic improvements in laser architecture, laser materials, and technology have led to compact systems producing terawatt and even petawatt pulses (42, 43). These relatively high pulse energy systems are of limited use for machining applications. Instead, high-repetition-rate systems with only modest pulse energy 1–20 mJ are required. These systems are almost all based on titanium-doped sapphire as the laser material. Commercial systems designed for scientific research are available at the 1 W level (1 mJ per pulse at 1 kHz repetition rate) and 2 W custom systems have been produced. Table 11 shows some properties for a commercial system.

Table 11. Typical Properties of Commercial Ultrafast Ti:Sapphire Lasers

Wavelength (nm)	800
Mode	TEM_{00}
Pulse energy (nJ)	1000
Pulse duration (fs)	100
Pulse repetition rate (Hz)	1000
Average power (W)	1
Beam divergence (mrad)	1.5

The first true machining system for use in industrial production was recently developed at Lawrence Livermore National Laboratory. The system is based on Ti:Sapphire as the laser material and produces 1.5 mJ pulses with a duration of 120 fsec and diffraction-limited beam quality. In order to achieve high machining speed, the repetition rate of the system is 10 kHz, resulting in an average power of 15 W. The system is fully computer controlled and is designed to be operated by a machininst. The system is modular in design and completely self-contained. Individual modules can be removed and replaced on the line to minimize any down time for maintenance.

Although Ti:Sapphire based ultrashort-pulse lasers can be scaled in average power up to ≈100 W, the complexity of these systems will limit their use. This complexity arises from the short upper-state lifetime ($\tau \approx 2$ µsec) of the laser material itself. The short energy storage time requires that the Ti:Sapphire be pumped by a second laser system. This laser-pumped laser requirement leads to a complex system where industrial quality standards of availability and ease of use will be difficult to achieve (particularly beyond the ≈20 W level). This complexity can be substantially reduced by the use of new laser materials that offer both broad bandwidth (necessary to produce the short pulse) and a long upper-state lifetime, enabling direct diode pumping. Such systems offer the promise of kilowatt-class average power in a simplified, compact package. The first of these new direct diode-pumped systems is currently in development.

The use of ultrashort-pulse lasers allows materials processing of practically any material (diamond, SiC, teeth, stainless steel, explosives, TiC, etc.) with extremely high precision and minimal collateral damage. Advantages over conventional laser machining (using pulses longer than a few tens of picoseconds) are realized by depositing the laser energy into the electrons of the material on a time scale short compared to the transfer time of this energy to the bulk of the material (either by electron-phonon coupling or thermal diffusion). The process forms a critical density plasma, which then expands away from the surface following the laser pulse. High ablation efficiency is achieved with negligible energy deposition to the remaining material either by heat or shock. As a result, high-speed machining of materials to the micrometer scale can be realized.

References

39. R. A. Fisher and W. Bischel, *Appl. Phys. Lett.* **24**, 468 (1974); *IEEE J. Quantum Electron.* **QE-11**, 46 (1975).
40. D. Strickland and G. Mourou, *Opt. Comm.* **56**, 219 (1985).
41. P. Maine, et al., *IEEE J. Quantum Electron.* **24**, 398 (1988).
42. M. D. Perry and G. Mourou, *Science* **264**, 917 (1994).
43. G. Mourou, C. P. Barty, and M. D. Perry, *Physics Today*, p. 22, January (1998).

M. D. PERRY
B. C. STUART
P. S. BANKS
M. D. FEIT
J. A. SEFCIK

2.6 Water Chiller Considerations for Laser-Cooling Applications

2.6.0 Introduction
Most industrial lasers require cooling water for optimum performance. A plant water supply will be adequate for some of these requirements. Many times, other factors rule out the use of plant water. Some of these factors are:

- Water is not available at required location.
- A suitable drain is not available.
- Environmental regulations prohibit dumping the water.
- The water quality is poor.

Poor water quality can encompass a variety of factors. It can refer to unsuitable temperature conditions. The temperature could be fluctuating, or it could be too high, so that the water does not provide adequate cooling, or it could be too low so that condensation results. Poor water quality could arise from impurities in the water, such as minerals, solids, or sulfur. It could also arise from lack of adequate pressure.

It is often advantageous to install a chiller to provide a continuous water supply at constant temperature, constant pressure, and constant quality. Many factors must be taken into consideration when selecting a chiller for installation on a laser system.

There are two basic types of lasers that require different cooling specifications for chilled water applications. The first type has an internal water recirculation and purification system. These units use a water to water heat exchanger to carry away the generated heat. This is illustrated in Figure 1a.

The second type of laser requires a water chiller to recirculate directly through such items as resonators, optics, and controls to carry away the generated heat. This situation is illustrated in Figure 1b.

Common types of chiller concerns for both systems will be covered.

2.6.1 Capacity of Cooling System
The heat removal capacity of the chiller, in either BTU/h or kW, is normally specified by the laser manufacturer. It includes resonator heat, control panel heat, and heat removal from the beam delivery system.

Water temperature and temperature stability must also be specified. Many times the resonator is cooled at a lower temperature than the control panel and beam delivery system.

A rising plant temperature can also affect the rated load of the laser. A rise in temperature will cause the entire laser to absorb more heat, which will be transferred to the chiller. The chiller must be selected with these "worst-case" conditions taken into consideration.

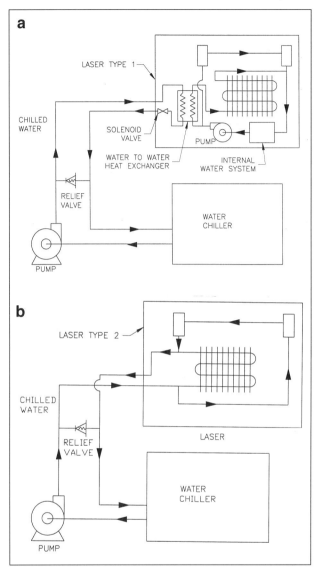

Figure 1. (a) Indirect cooling system. (b) Direct cooling system.

2.6.2 Power Requirements
Power requirements for the chiller are very important. One must consider the distance from the power source to the chiller when selecting wire sizes.

Chillers in the United States are normally rated in BTU/h output or kW with a 60 Hz power source. When chillers designed for 60 Hz power are used with 50 Hz power, output capacity is reduced 17%. Water pressure and flow on centrifugal and turbine pumps can be reduced as much as 40%. The manufacturer must be consulted to ensure that adequate flow and pressure are available.

ISBN 0-912035-15-3

2.6.3 Chiller System Components

The chiller system is comprised of a number of major components, which will be discussed.

Compressor

The compressor is the heart of the refrigeration system. It must continually pump the refrigerant through the condenser and to the evaporator. There are a number of compressor types that can be specified:

Hermetically Sealed Compressors. These normally operate at 3450 RPM. They are manufactured in higher volumes and hence are usually lower in cost than the other types. They are also quieter with lower sound pressure levels. They are the most common type used, and can be either a reciprocating or scroll design.

Semihermetic Compressors. These compressors operate at 1750 RPM. They are more costly than the hermetic type and are usually noisier. They are commonly found in heavy industries. They are also field serviceable, and can be rebuilt.

Open-Type Compressors. The motor and compressor are mounted separately. They operate at 1750 RPM. They are the most expensive type and they are not very common except in the automotive industry. There is also a potential for leaks at the shaft seal.

Condenser Considerations

Air-Cooled Condensers. The heat of rejection of the condenser is equal to the heat being absorbed by the chiller, plus 25% heat of compression. A laser that has a 20-kW heat load would require a chiller that rejects 25 kW into the space where it is located. The air that moves over the condenser rises about 20 to 30°F, at a flow rate of 170 CFM per kW of heat removal.

This discharge heat can cause worker discomfort and heat buildup in the area where the chiller is located, and it will add to the cooling load of an air conditioned plant.

Chillers are commonly rated at a specific capacity when operating in 95°F ambient. If the plant temperature exceeds 95°F, the chiller capacity must be reduced 6% for each 10°F rise over 95°F.

Air-cooled units are available in four basic configurations:

1. Self-contained propeller fans
2. Self-contained heat reclaim type suitable for ducting
3. Remote located air-cooled condenser
4. Outdoor chiller

1. The self-contained propeller fan condenser (see Fig. 2) is designed to reject heat into the space where the chiller is located.

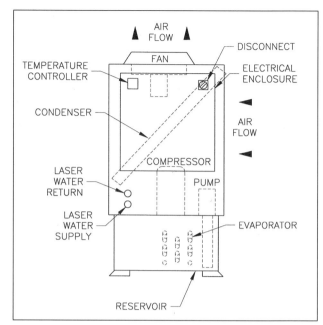

Figure 2. Self-contained propeller fan condenser.

The advantages of the self-contained propeller fan condenser are:

a. All components are in one package.
b. Most commonly used in industry.
c. Lowest cost to purchase and install.

The disadvantages of self-contained air cooled condensers are:

a. Heat removed from the process is discharged into the work area.
b. Air sound pressure levels can be objectionable.
c. Increased air conditioning load.
d. Condenser coils can be blocked by dirty plant air.

2. The self-contained heat reclaim type (see Fig. 3) is designed with fans (usually blower style) of suitable capacity to reject the condenser heat outdoors through ducting. It is normal to do this in the hot summer months and then to direct it indoors (reclaim the heat) in the winter months when heating is required.

The advantages of heat reclaim type systems are:

a. All components are in one package.
b. Discharge heat can supplement the plant heating system.
c. Lower sound pressure level.

The disadvantages of heat reclaim type systems are:

a. Higher purchase price.
b. Higher current draw of fan motors.

Chapter 2: Lasers for Materials Processing

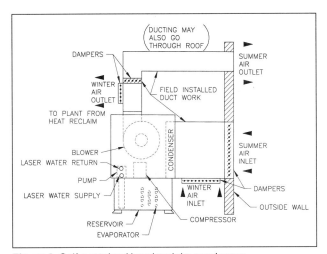

Figure 3. Self-contained head reclaim condenser.

c. Expensive installation costs.

3. The remote located air-cooled condenser (see Fig. 4) is where the air-cooled condenser is split from the rest of the chiller package and set outdoors. This is very similar to a household-type central air conditioner installation.

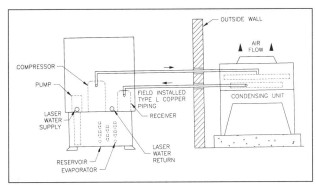

Figure 4. Remote located air-cooled compressor.

The advantages of remote condensing are:

a. Heat removed from the process is discharged outdoors.
b. Fan noise is not in the work area.
c. The indoor part of the package is more compact, requiring less floor space.

The disadvantages of remote condensing are:

a. Higher equipment cost.
b. Higher installation cost—interconnecting wiring and refrigeration must be done by outside contractors—more plumbing, wiring, and refrigerant are required.
c. Functional reliability is reduced.
d. Service is more difficult.

If the chiller is built as a split system with the air-cooled condenser being located outdoors, other factors must be considered.

a. Again, maximum outdoor ambient temperature
b. Low ambient conditions for winter operation – possibility of freezing
c. Prevailing wind direction
d. Sun loads
e. Proximity to a saw mill, foundry, generating plant or other dust-creating conditions that can block the coil
f. Location on the roof or on a slab

4. Outdoor Chillers. The outdoor chiller method requires many design considerations such as low ambient temperature controls, antifreeze additives, preheating capabilities, remote controls, etc.

Water-Cooled Condensers. The other type of condenser that can be used on some applications is the water cooled type (see Fig. 5). This is a good design selection when a cooling tower or pond supply of water is available. This design requires 3 GPM per 12,000 BTU/h of chiller capacity.

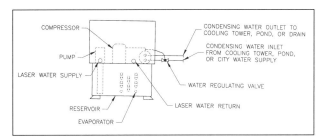

Figure 5. Water-cooled compressor.

City water requirements, providing that the temperature is not over 75°F, are 1-1/2 GPM per 12,000 BTU/h of chiller capacity.

City water is usually prohibitive to use from the standpoint of cost, environmental, or municipal restrictions.

The advantages of water-cooled condensing are:

a. Lower initial equipment cost.
b. Lower electrical energy cost.
c. Lower sound level (no air movement).
d. Smaller equipment package.

The disadvantages of water cooled condensing are:

a. Cost of water.
b. Environmental constraints of using water.
c. Additional plumbing required.

Evaporator (Heat Exchanger)

This is the portion of the system that absorbs the heat of the laser cooling water. There are three common types of evaporators:

ISBN 0-912035-15-3

Table 1. Friction Loss of Water in Feet per 100 Feet Length of Pipe, Based on Williams & Hazen Formula Using Constant 100 Sizes of Standard Pipe in Inches.

Flow U.S. Gals. Per min.	½" Pipe		¾" Pipe		1" Pipe		1 ¼" Pipe		1 ½" Pipe		2" Pipe	
	Vel. Ft. per Sec.	Loss In Feet	Vel. Ft. per Sec.	Loss In Feet	Vel. Ft. per Sec.	Loss In Feet	Vel. Ft. per Sec.	Loss In Feet	Vel. Ft. per Sec.	Loss In Feet	Vel. Ft. per Sec.	Loss In Feet
2	2.10	7.4	1.20	1.9								
4	4.21	27.0	2.41	7.0	1.49	2.14	0.86	0.57	0.63	0.26		
6	6.31	57.0	3.61	14.7	2.23	4.55	1.29	1.20	0.94	0.56	0.61	0.20
8	8.42	98.0	4.81	25.0	2.98	7.8	1.72	2.03	1.26	0.95	0.82	0.33
10	10.52	147.0	6.02	38.0	3.72	11.7	2.14	3.05	1.57	1.43	1.02	.50
12			7.22	53.0	4.46	16.4	2.57	4.3	1.89	2.01	1.23	.79
15			9.02	80.0	5.60	25.0	3.21	6.5	2.36	3.00	1.53	1.08
18			10.84	108.2	6.69	35.0	3.86	9.1	2.83	4.24	1.84	1.49
20			12.03	136.0	7.44	42.0	4.29	11.1	3.15	5.20	2.04	1.82
25					9.30	64.0	5.36	16.6	3.80	7.30	2.55	2.73
30					11.15	89.0	6.43	23.0	4.72	11.0	3.06	3.84
35					13.02	119.0	7.51	31.2	5.51	14.7	3.57	5.10
40					14.88	152.0	8.58	40.0	6.30	18.8	4.08	6.6
45							9.65	50.0	7.08	23.2	4.60	8.2
50							10.72	60.0	7.87	28.4	5.11	9.9
55							11.78	72.0	8.66	34.0	5.62	11.8
60							12.87	85.0	9.44	39.6	6.13	13.9
65							13.92	99.7	10.23	45.9	6.64	16.1
70							15.01	113.0	11.02	53.0	7.15	18.4
75							16.06	129.0	11.80	60.0	7.66	20.9
80							17.16	145.0	12.59	68.0	8.17	23.7
85							18.21	163.8	13.38	75.0	8.68	26.5
90							19.3	180.0	14.71	84.0	9.19	29.4
95									14.95	93.0	9.70	32.6
100									15.74	102.0	10.21	35.8
110									17.31	122.0	11.23	42.9
120									18.89	143.0	12.25	50.0
130									20.46	166.0	13.28	58.0
140									22.04	190.0	14.30	67.0
150											15.32	76.0

ISBN 0-912035-15-3

2 ½" Pipe		3" Pipe		4" Pipe		5" Pipe		6" Pipe		Flow
Vel. Ft. per Sec.	Loss In Feet	Vel. Ft. per Sec.	Loss In Feet	Vel. Ft. per Sec.	Loss In Feet	Vel. Ft. per Sec.	Loss In Feet	Vel. Ft. per Sec.	Loss In Feet	U.S. Gals. Per min.
										2
										4
										6
0.52	0.11									8
.65	.17	.45	.07							10
.78	.23	.54	.10							12
.98	.36	.68	.15							15
1.18	.50	.82	.21							18
1.31	.61	.91	.25	.51	.06					20
1.63	.92	1.13	.38	.64	.09					25
1.96	1.29	1.36	.54	.77	.13	.49	.04			30
2.29	1.72	1.59	.71	.89	.17	.57	.06			35
2.61	2.20	1.82	.91	1.02	.22	.65	.08			40
2.94	2.80	2.04	1.15	1.15	.28	.73	.09			45
3.27	3.32	2.27	1.38	1.28	.34	.82	.11	.57	.04	50
3.59	4.01	2.45	1.58	1.41	.41	.90	.14	.62	.05	55
3.92	4.65	2.72	1.92	1.53	.47	.98	.16	.68	.06	60
4.24	5.4	2.89	2.16	1.66	.53	1.06	.19	.74	.076	65
4.58	6.2	3.18	2.57	1.79	.63	1.14	.21	.79	.08	70
4.91	7.1	3.33	3.00	1.91	.73	1.22	.24	.85	.10	75
5.23	7.9	3.63	3.28	2.04	.81	1.31	.27	.91	.11	80
5.56	8.1	3.78	3.54	2.17	.91	1.39	.31	.96	.12	85
5.88	9.8	4.09	4.08	2.30	1.00	1.47	.34	1.02	.14	90
6.21	10.8	4.22	4.33	2.42	1.12	1.55	.38	1.08	.15	95
6.54	12.0	4.54	4.96	2.55	1.22	1.63	.41	1.13	.17	100
7.18	14.5	5.00	6.0	2.81	1.46	1.79	.49	1.25	.21	110
7.84	16.8	5.45	7.0	3.06	1.17	1.96	.58	1.36	.24	120
8.48	18.7	5.91	8.1	3.31	1.97	2.12	.67	1.47	.27	130
9.15	22.3	6.35	9.2	3.57	2.28	2.29	.76	1.59	.32	140
9.81	25.5	6.82	10.5	3.82	2.62	2.45	.88	1.70	.36	150

Table 2. Water Friction in 100 Feet of Smooth-bore Hose

For various flows and hose sizes, this table gives velocity of water and feet of head lost in friction in 100 feet of smooth-bore hose. Sizes of hose shown are actual inside diameters.

Flow in (U.S. Gal /Min)	Velocity (Feet /Sec.)	Friction Head in Feet	Velocity (Feet /Sec)	Friction Head in Feet	Velocity (Feet /Sec)	Friction Head in Feet	Velocity (Feet /Sec)	Friction Head in Feet	Velocity (Feet /Sec)	Friction Head in Feet	Velocity (Feet /Sec)	Friction Head in Feet
	5/8"		3/4"		1"		1 1/4"		1 1/2"		2"	
1.5	1.6	2.3	1.1	.97								
2.5	2.6	6.0	1.8	2.5								
5	5.2	21.4	3.6	8.9	2.0	2.2	1.3	.74	.9	.3		
10	10.5	76.8	7.3	31.8	4.1	7.8	2.6	2.64	1.8	1.0	1.0	.2
15	2 ½"		10.9	68.5	6.1	16.8	3.9	5.7	2.7	2.3	1.5	.5
20	1.3	.32			8.2	28.7	5.2	9.6	3.6	3.9	2.0	.9
25	1.6	.51	3"		10.2	43.2	6.5	14.7	4.5	6.0	2.5	1.4
30	2.0	.70	1.4	.3	12.2	61.2	7.8	20.7	5.4	8.5	3.1	2.0
35	2.3	.93	1.6	.4	14.3	80.5	9.1	27.6	6.4	11.2	3.6	2.7
40	2.6	1.2	1.8	.5			10.4	35.0	7.3	14.3	4.1	3.5
45	2.9	1.5	2.0	.6			11.7	43.0	8.2	17.7	4.6	4.3
50	3.3	1.8	2.3	.7			13.1	52.7	9.1	21.8	5.1	5.2
60	3.9	2.5	2.7	1.0			15.7	73.5	10.9	30.2	6.1	7.3
70	4.6	3.3	3.2	1.3					12.7	40.4	7.1	9.8
80	5.2	4.3	3.6	1.7	4"				14.5	52.0	8.2	12.6
90	5.9	5.3	4.1	2.1	2.3	.5			16.3	64.2	9.2	15.7
100	6.5	6.5	4.5	2.6	2.5	.6			18.1	77.4	10.2	18.9
125	8.2	9.8	5.7	4.0	3.2	.9					12.8	28.6
150	9.8	13.8	6.8	5.6	3.8	1.3					15.3	40.7

1. Submersed coil
2. Shell and tube
3. Brazed plate

Usually, the chiller manufacturer selects the type of evaporator to be used. However, certain types lend themselves to particular applications.

Submersed coils are common on nonferrous systems but are not normally used where a high level of resistivity is needed, like in a deionized water system.

Shell and tube type and brazed plate exchangers can be easily packaged into a sealed water system for maintaining water purity.

Reservoir

Open Atmospheric. Open atmospheric reservoirs are usually fabricated from plastic or stainless steel. These are common on most chilling systems, especially where lasers have their own internal water system.

Sealed Pressurized. These are usually cylindrical and fabricated from stainless steel or polyester. These are used when high-purity or deionized water is needed to circulate through the laser.

Pumps

End Suction Centrifugal. These are most common. Materials are brass or stainless steel, and they can maintain pressures of 75 to 80 PSI (5 bar). The centrifugal pumps are the most reliable. They normally operate at 3450 RPM and are usually close coupled to a pump motor.

Turbine Pumps. These are used where higher pressure over 100 PSI (6 bar) and lower flows are needed. The turbine pump impeller spins against a pressure plate. Clearance between the impeller and pressure plate is held to a very tight tolerance, allowing for high discharge pressures.

Vane Pumps. These pumps will operate at pressures up to 200 PSI (13 bar) and flows to 4 GPM. The vane type pump can deliver high pressures but at low flow rates.

The pumps on the chiller are designed for continuous operation when the laser is powered. Many of the lasers that are cooled with an indirect heat exchanger incorporate a solenoid valve to control system temperature tolerance. On/off action of water solenoid valves on the laser can cause severe water hammer. To prevent water hammer or pump damage, a bypass relief valve or a bypass line is required.

Some laser systems require dual circuit water delivery for the addition of a cooling loop for the laser optics. This design allows the resonator cooling circuit to operate with circulating water below the dew point. If this same water is circulated through the optics, it could cause condensation. This condensation can damage the optics. Therefore, it is necessary to deliver higher-constant-temperature water to the optics. This requires a separate pump and a temperature control for the optics. Operating temperature must be specified.

The laser manufacturer must specify minimum water flow and pressure drop requirements across the laser system for the complete resonator circuit and the optics circuit (if one is utilized).

2.6.4 Water Issues

Temperature Stability

The closer the temperature of the cooling water is maintained, the more consistent the beam quality of the laser.

It is normal to require ±1°F or better for chiller performance. This close temperature control is obtained by unloading the chiller with a hot gas solenoid and a large reservoir so that the compressor does not cycle too frequently, causing premature wear.

Water Quality

This is an important issue and the source of much misunderstanding. On systems where the chilled water circulates directly through the resonator and optics, attention to water quality is more important. Laser manufactures will normally suggest water guidelines such as:

- Use of a filter (usually 50 μm) and periodic system flushing
- Use of an inhibited glycol at a certain percent concentration to prevent bacteria growth
- Use of biocides without glycol
- Use of water maintained at a high level of resistivity. This normally requires all 316 stainless steel construction and continuous deionization of the water circuit

On systems with indirect cooling, the issue of water quality is much less of a concern.

In general, it is always good practice to use nonferrous materials for the construction of the wetted surfaces in the cooling system. It is also necessary to provide some means of controlling bacteria growth.

Equipment Location

The distance between the laser and the chiller should be kept as short as possible to prevent excessive pressure drop and line temperature losses to ambient. These lines are normally hoses, PVC piping, or copper piping.

The user should refer to piping or hose tables, in order to correctly size the lines for water carrying capacity.

Tables 1 and 2 present the water velocity and friction loss (in feet of head) for a 100-ft length of standard pipe and smooth bore hose, respectively. The tables present the values for various water flow rates and for various inside diameters. The tables may be used to estimate the distances that may be tolerated between laser and chiller.

TERRY L. ARMBRUSTER

Notes

Chapter 3

Optics and Optical Systems

3.0 Introduction

Optics and optical systems have two primary uses with lasers. First, the laser beam is generated by the combination of a lasing medium, which is the energy source for the laser, and an optical resonant cavity, which forms the laser output beam into a highly directional and coherent light source. Second, the laser beam is delivered to the workpiece by an optical system, which includes lenses, mirrors, and/or optical fibers. This chapter discusses the optical properties of laser beams and optics and optical systems for the generation and delivery of laser light in laser materials processing. The emphasis in this chapter is mainly on optical principles relevant to laser beams and their propagation. Specific components are mentioned or described briefly as necessary to understand these principles, but more detailed discussion of specific components will be deferred to Chapter 4.

3.1 Properties of Laser Beams

There are several basic properties of lasers that make them useful for a number of applications including materials processing. These include directionality, monochromaticity, coherence, and brightness (or radiance). Another characteristic that can affect laser materials interaction is the polarization state of the laser electromagnetic field. The primary operational characteristic of a laser is its extreme coherence. The electromagnetic field created through the lasing process is very nearly monochromatic. This property ensures that the laser beam can be focused to an extremely small spot, which contains a major percentage of the total laser output power or energy. High brightness and directionality of a laser enable remote delivery of a large amount of optical energy in the laser beam to a small spot on a material to cause melting and vaporization of the material. These unique properties of lasers are utilized in laser materials processing, where the quality and repeatability of a given process depend largely on the optical quality of the beam and the properties of the material being processed.

3.1.1 Monochromaticity

Lasers are highly monochromatic because of the fundamental physics involved in the production of the laser beam. There are two types of physical interactions in the laser cavity: (1) the interaction between the resonant electromagnetic radiation with the gain in the lasing material, and (2) the interaction between the laser light and the resonant cavity formed by the mirrors. Lasing is the equilibrium condition that is established when the energy gained within the lasing medium from stimulated emission is equal to the energy lost from the optical cavity because of outcoupling at one of the mirrors. Because the electromagnetic field that is produced by the lasing process must satisfy the boundary conditions at the mirrors, the optical resonant cavity produces oscillation at characteristic frequencies only. The longitudinal or axial modes of a laser cavity are given by $\omega_q = 2\pi cq/2nL$, where c is the speed of light in vacuum, q is an integer, n is the index of refraction in the gain medium, and L is the mirror separation. For a Fabry-Perot resonant cavity in which both of the two mirrors are flat, the longitudinal modes are the resonant eigenfrequencies of the cavity. In a more general resonator case, the eigenfrequencies are slightly shifted from these frequencies. Amplified spontaneous emission within the lasing medium broadens the laser line, so that the linewidth is finite and the field is not exactly monochromatic. The finite laser linewidth is related to the temporal coherence length of the laser, and this relationship is given later. In many cases, the laser linewidth is so small that it is practically unmeasurable. Empirically determined linewidths near 1 kHz have been demonstrated. Because of this extremely narrow linewidth, the laser is nearly monochromatic. Lasers are used for interferometry, holography, velocimetry, isotope separation, and communications, applications in which the narrow frequency range of the laser is very important.

Although the focal length of a lens is a constant determined by the materials properties of the lens, the focal distance also depends on the wavelength of the incident radiation, and therefore the monochromaticity of a laser enables it to be focused to a very small transverse region. This property is used in laser materials processing to deposit a large amount of energy on the workpiece surface.

3.1.2 Directionality

For a conventional light source, light emanates outward from the source in all directions equally. A conventional light source therefore cannot be pointed in a specific direction and cannot be focused to a small spot, because it disperses too rapidly. On the other hand, a laser is very directional and can be pointed and focused to a small spot. A measure of the directionality of a laser beam is the beam divergence, which is defined as the diffractive spread of the beam. Diffractive spread is a physical property of light that is determined by the ratio of the wavelength of the field and the size of the laser. The average wavelength of the laser can be used to determine the beam divergence, since a laser is nearly monochromatic. A definition of the beam divergence as a measure of the diffractive spread is the ratio of the average wavelength λ to the half-size of the laser beam. In this case, we use the full angle θ, and not the half-angle $\theta_{1/2}$. The beam divergence for various laser wavelengths is given in Figure 1. This figure allows one to determine the beam divergence angle, given the laser size, s, and the wavelength, λ. The abscissa represents either the size, in which case one uses the curve for the proper wavelength, or the wavelength, in which case one uses

ISBN 0-912035-15-3

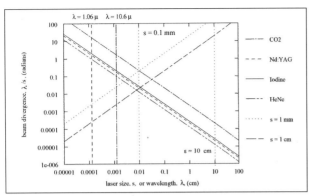

Figure 1. Divergence versus laser size or λ. s is width or length for a rectangular beam; $D/1.22$ for a circular beam of diameter D, πw_0 for a Gaussian beam of waist size w_0.

the curve for the proper size. In the figure, the four vertical lines represent, from left to right, $\lambda = 1.06\ \mu m$, $\lambda = 10.6\ \mu m$, $s = 0.1$ mm, and $s = 10$ cm. The two lines running upward from left to right represent $s = 1$ mm (upper) and $s = 1$ cm (lower). The four curves running downward left to right represent the wavelengths of the various lasers identified at the right of the figure. The beam divergence depends on the geometry, circular or rectangular, and the properties of the laser that generates the light. Equations for the beam divergence for various cases are listed in Table 1.

The second expression in the table is commonly employed to estimate the beam divergence angle for specific lasers. Experimentally, the focused spot diameter or spot width can be measured for a given laser. An empirical beam divergence is defined to be the ratio of the spot diameter or spot width to the distance between the focal plane and the lens. For a collimated beam incident on the focusing lens, the distance to the focal plane is the same as the focal length of the lens, f. If the measured diameter or full beam width is d_s, the empirically measured beam divergence, θ_m, is given by $\theta_m = d_s/f$. This form of the beam divergence gives a simple but meaningful definition that can be used for all lasers. Note that θ_m can be easily modified for cases where the focal plane does not occur at f. For most cases, measuring the laser beam divergence as an indication of laser optical quality is a necessary step in increasing the understanding of laser operation. However, if a more complete description of laser performance is required, other optical quality parameters must be defined.

When the geometry of the beam is known, the beam divergence and lateral coherence width can be directly related to the spot size, which is measurable in many cases. For a uniformly illuminated circular aperture of diameter, D, the first zero in the far-field pattern occurs at a radius r_0, which is related to the beam divergence angle θ_c by

$$r_0 = 1.22 f \lambda / D = 0.61 f (\theta_c/2) \qquad (1)$$

For the Cartesian coordinate case, with diffraction through a rectangular aperture, the first zero in the x direction is related to the appropriate beam divergence angle θ_x by

$$x_0 = f \lambda / D = f (\theta_x/2) \qquad (2)$$

An analogous definition holds for the y coordinate with x replaced by y. For the lowest-order Gaussian beam, the far-field spot radius at the $1/e^2$ irradiance point is

$$r_0 = f \frac{\lambda}{\pi \omega_o} = f \frac{\theta_g}{2} \qquad (3)$$

where θ_g is the beam divergence angle for the Gaussian beam.

Table 1. Beam Divergence Angles

Expression	Description
Beam Divergence:	
$\theta_i = 2\lambda/D_i$	Divergence angle in the ith direction, $i = x$ or y, for the fundamental mode (TEM_{00} mode) due to a plane wavefront incident upon a rectangular aperture of dimension $D_x \times D_y$. About 81% of the total energy is contained in a rectangular spot defined by these divergence angles.
$\theta_c = 2.44\lambda/D$	Divergence angle for TEM_{00} mode due to a plane wavefront incident upon a circular aperture of diameter D. About 84.5% of the total energy is contained in a circular spot defined by this divergence angle.
$\theta_g = D_l/f = 2\lambda/\pi w_0$	Divergence angle for TEM_{00} mode in the far field of a circular Gaussian beam of waist radius w_0. About 86.5% of the total energy is contained in a spot defined by this divergence angle. θ_g is measured at the beam waist.
$\theta_{gl} = 2w_0/f = 4\lambda/\pi D_l$	Divergence angle for TEM_{00} mode of a circular Gaussian beam. θ_{gl} is measured at the focusing lens.
$\theta_{gi} = D_{li}/f = 2\lambda/\pi w_{0i}$	Divergence angle in the ith direction, $i = x$ or y, for TEM_{00} mode in the far field of a rectangular Gaussian beam. θ_{gi} is measured at the beam waist.
$\theta_{gli} = 2w_0/f = 2\lambda/\pi D_{li}$	Divergence angle in the ith direction, $i = x$ or y, for TEM_{00} mode of a rectangular Gaussian beam. θ_{gli} is measured at the focusing lens.
$\theta_m = d_s/f$	Divergence angle for any laser beam. d_s is the measured spot size and f is the focal length of the focusing lens.
$\theta_h = M \theta_g$	Divergence of a higher-order mode. Here θ_g (see above) is the divergence of the TEM_{00} Gaussian mode that is the fundamental mode for the higher-order mode of interest. See Section 3.4 for M.

Chapter 3: Optics and Optical Systems

Notice that all these values of far-field beam sizes, that is, spot radii, are directly proportional to the focal length f of the focusing lens and the beam divergence half-angle $\theta_a/2$, for $a = c, x, y,$ or g.

For a higher-order-mode Gaussian beam, the measured beam divergence angle, θ_m, is related to the spatial structure of the beam, and therefore, it can provide a measure of the laser optical quality. The diameter of a multimode beam will be larger than the diameter of a TEM_{00} Gaussian beam, that is, the lowest-order mode, produced by the same laser cavity. The extent by which a multimode laser beam deviates from a Gaussian beam can be expressed as a ratio of the beam sizes or divergence angles of these two types of beams. The beam divergence of a higher-order beam, θ_h, is proportional to the beam divergence of the lowest-order Gaussian mode, θ_g (see Table 1).

3.1.3 Coherence

Laser optical quality is directly related to the coherence properties of the laser. Laser coherence is divided into two categories: temporal or longitudinal coherence and spatial or transverse coherence. Since the laser linewidth is extremely narrow, the laser temporal coherence length is generally very long, which means that lasers are very monochromatic and can be well represented by a single-frequency, monochromatic, electromagnetic field or a finite set of multiple-discrete-frequency fields. This approximation can be applied to continuous-wave lasers as well as pulsed lasers with pulse lengths as short as picoseconds. For shorter pulsed lasers, such as femtosecond lasers, the pulse width may determine the temporal coherence length, and the monochromatic field approximation is generally not valid.

The two physical characteristics that result because of the extreme coherence of the electromagnetic field produced by a laser are diffraction and interference. A physical estimate of the extent of the diffraction for a collimated light source in one dimension is the beam divergence full angle, which is a ratio of the wavelength (λ) to the size (s) of the diffracting source, $\theta = 2\lambda/s$. At a distance z away from the diffracting source, the new diffracted beam size s_d would be

$$s_d = s + \theta z.$$

The extent of the diffraction and the beam size define a one-dimensional distance within which the light interferes with itself. This distance is the lateral coherence width. These spatial interactions occur within a field that has a long coherence length.

Temporal Coherence Length

The temporal coherence length L_c is the length over which a beam of light interferes with itself along the propagation direction of the light beam. It is given by the coherence time T_c, speed of light c, laser linewidth $\Delta\lambda$, average laser wavelength λ, laser frequency spread $\Delta\nu$, and laser wavelength spread $\Delta\lambda$ (see Table 2). The second equality in the first equation is exact only for a rectangular lineshape. There is an additional constant in the expression for other lineshapes such as the Lorentzian lineshape. Since the coherence length is inversely proportional to the frequency width (laser linewidth), which is very narrow for a laser operating on a single homogeneously broadened gain line, extremely long coherence lengths are encountered in such lasers. If the laser has different saturation characteristics, the coherence length is somewhat shorter. The study of laser temporal coherence characteristics is directly related to the study of laser gain media saturation characteristics and transverse and longitudinal mode structure. The coherence time T_c, which is related to the coherence length, as indicated in the first expression in Table 2, is the time period over which the light beam is coherent.

Table 2. Coherence

Coherence Parameter	Expression	Beam Cross Section
Temporal coherence length	$L_c = cT_c \approx c/\Delta\nu = \lambda^2/\Delta\lambda$	
Spatial coherence width		
Linear distance	$L_{wi} = 2f\lambda/D = f\theta_i$, $i = x$ or y	Rectangular
Radial distance	$L_w = 2.44 f\lambda/D = f\theta_c$	Circular
Coherence area		
Rectangular area	$A_c = L_{wx}L_{wy} = f^2\theta_x\theta_y$	Rectangular
Circular area	$A_c = (\pi/4)L_w^2 = (\pi/4)f^2\theta_c^2$	Circular
Coherence volume		
Rectangular volume	$V_c = A_c L_c = (\lambda^2/\Delta\lambda) f^2\theta_x\theta_y$	Rectangular
Cylindrical volume	$V_c = A_c L_c = (\lambda^2/\Delta\lambda)(\pi/4)f^2\theta_c^2$	Circular

Spatial Coherence Width

The spatial coherence width L_w at a distance z away from a laser source is defined to be the one-dimensional size of the coherence area from a source of area A_s. L_w is the length within which the laser beam interferes with itself. The physical meaning of L_w is that it defines a one-dimensional transverse or lateral distance over which the laser beam is spatially coherent. Since lasers are very coherent, this lateral cross section contains most of the laser energy. It is given by the second and third expressions in Table 2. In these equations, D is the width or diameter of the laser beam, f is the distance between the source plane (e.g., the plane of the focusing lens with F number $F = f/D$ and focal length f) and observation planes (e.g., focal plane). $\theta_i = 2\lambda/D$, with $i = x$ or y, or $\theta_c = 2.44 \lambda/D$ is the beam divergence of the laser with rectangular or circular geometry, respectively. If a laser could produce a perfect plane wave, the lateral coherence widths, L_w in Table 2 would be equal to the width or diameter of the focal spot of a rectangular or circular beam, respectively.

Coherence Area

In the more general case, when the laser spatial profile is not a plane wave, the lateral coherence width L_w can be calculated using the Van Cittert-Zernike theorem, since the electromagnetic field produced by a laser always satisfies the quasimonochromatic assumption. The far-field beam spot diameter or spot widths can usually be measured. The spatial coherence area A_c represents a spatial area transverse to the propagation direction in which the light beam is coherent with itself and contains most of its energy. A_c is a useful beam characteristic because it can always be calculated when the output irradiance distribution is measured, and under certain assumptions it enables one to calculate the laser far-field irradiance, which is an important parameter in laser materials processing. Empirically, the coherence area can be taken as the product of the spot widths for rectangular cross sections or π times the square of the spot radius for circular cross sections as given in Table 2. L_{wx} and L_{wy} are spatial coherence widths in the x and y directions, respectively, and θ_x and θ_y are the corresponding beam divergence angles.

Coherence Volume

The coherence volume V_c represents a volume in space in which the electromagnetic field of the laser interferes with itself and is thus coherent. It is given by the expressions in Table 2. It should be noted that the size of the coherence volume is a phenomenological estimate in terms of the basic coherence parameters L_c and L_w. To more accurately define this volume, an empirical measurement of the light source is needed to determine L_c and L_w. The experimental determination of L_c is outlined above. L_w is measured by interfering adjacent pieces of a laser beam.

3.1.4 Brightness

There are many definitions of brightness (also called radiance) within the laser and optics community. The term *brightness* has been applied to thermal incoherent broadband blackbody sources and to very directional and coherent laser sources. The definition of the brightness may be different for different applications. Also, the terminology for incoherent and coherent laser sources may not be the same. For a coherent laser source of output area A_s and total power P, the brightness B is generally given by the first expression in Table 3, where Ω is the solid angle subtended by the coherence area in the far field or observation plane a distance f from the laser source, and the solid angle is given by

$$\Omega = A_c/f^2 = \lambda^2/A_s.$$

Brightness has units of watts per steradian per unit cross-sectional area.

Table 3. Brightness

Brightness Parameter	Expression
Brightness	$B = P/(A_s \Omega) = P/\lambda^2$
Total brightness	$B_t = P/\Omega = PA_s/\lambda^2$
Spectral brightness	$B_v = P/(\Omega \Delta v) = PT_c/[(A_c/D^2)/F^2]$ and $B_\lambda = P/(A_s \Omega \Delta\lambda)$

For a blackbody source, the radiance of the source is defined in units of watts per steradian per unit cross-sectional area. The irradiance is defined in units of watts per unit cross-sectional area, while the radiant intensity is defined in units of watts per steradian. It appears that brightness B in Table 3 also refers to the radiance of a blackbody.

Another useful definition of brightness is the total brightness of the source rather than the brightness of a single point on the source. If the output aperture is assumed to be uniformly illuminated, the total brightness can be obtained by multiplying the single point brightness by the area of the source, so that B_t in Table 3 is the total brightness, which is defined in units of watts per steradian. B_t also refers to the radiant intensity of a blackbody source. Both brightness and the total brightness are proportional to the inverse square of the average wavelength. They are also related to the far-field peak irradiance I_0. I_0 is equal to the total laser power (P) times the area of the source (A_s) divided by the product of the squares of the wavelength (λ) and source distance (f); that is,

$$I_0 = PA_s/(\lambda^2 f^2) = B_t/f^2$$

where the area of the source is

$$A_s = D_x D_y, \; A_s = \pi (D^2/4), \; A_s = \pi w_0^2/2$$

for rectangular, circular, and Gaussian beams, respectively.

Finally, the spectral brightness of a laser source is defined as the power output per steradian of solid angle per hertz of bandwidth. The spectral brightness B_v is defined in Table 3. A laser of high power density, small beam divergence, and narrow linewidth is desired for most applications in materials processing. To express these properties of the laser by a single parameter, the spectral brightness is also defined as

$$B_v = P/(\lambda^2/A_s) \Delta v = PA_s/\lambda^2 \Delta v$$

when the definition of the solid angle is used. Using the coherence time, $T_c = 1/\Delta v$, and the focal length (f) to beam diameter (D) ratio, that is, $F = f/D$, B_v can be written as

$$B_v = PT_c / [(A_c/D^2)/F^2]$$

which states that brightness is the laser energy per unit normalized spatial coherence area produced by a lens of F number F. The brightness in this form depends on the power, the focusing lens, and both the temporal coherence and the spatial coherence. Notice that the dependence of brightness on wavelength is the same in all expressions for brightness. For a thermal source, the meaning of the bandwidth Δv is clear. For a single line (single-mode laser), the bandwidth is the laser linewidth, Δv. For pulsed lasers, the meaning of the bandwidth may be ambiguous. In some cases, the coherence length might be determined by the pulse width. However, one might define a peak brightness and/or an average brightness to describe more accurately the performance of a particular pulsed laser.

Polarization

The color of light is characterized by the length of a light wave, that is the wavelength. Polarization is characterized by the direction of vibration of the electric field of the light wave. It indicates the direction of motion of the end of the electric field vector on a plane that is transverse to the direction of propagation of the electromagnetic radiation. A light beam is said to be polarized if the electric vectors of the electromagnetic waves are oriented in a given direction in space. Polarization affects the absorptivity of a given material, that is, the coupling of laser energy with the workpiece. The electric field of the incident light wave can be parallel or perpendicular to the plane of incidence. The parallel component is referred to as the transverse magnetic (TM) mode, or p-polarization, which comes from the German word "parallel." The perpendicular component is called the transverse electric (TE) mode, or s-polarization, which comes from the German word "senkrecht," meaning perpendicular.

WILLIAM P. LATHAM
ARAVINDA KAR

3.1.5 Stable Resonator Modes

Stable laser resonators can operate in a variety of electromagnetic modes, much as waveguides do. Different modes result in different irradiance (power per unit area) distributions across the wavefront. The lowest-order mode for any stable laser resonator is the Gaussian mode (TEM_{00}) (see Fig. 2). This mode provides the optimum irradiance distribution for minimizing divergence due to diffraction. The far-field half-angle divergence for a Gaussian laser beam is given by

$$\theta = \lambda/(\pi w_0)$$

where w_0 is the radius of the beam waist measured to the point at which the irradiance has dropped to $1/e^2$ of the peak irradiance. Eighty-six percent of the beam's power is contained in a circle of this radius. Hence, the larger the beam waist radius, the smaller the far-field divergence. Through collimation, a new larger, or smaller, waist can be produced thereby changing the far-field divergence angle. An interesting, and important, characteristic of stable resonator modes is that they do not change form over distance like electromagnetic radiation from waveguides, antennae, or unstable laser resonators, which have different patterns in the near and far fields.

Lasers, especially high-power ones, tend to operate in higher-order modes or even multimode. These modes may have either rectangular or circular symmetry ideally. In reality, they may be mildly to extremely distorted because of thermal optical effects, gas flow nonuniformities, or a myriad of other causes. Figure 3 shows a computer plot of a rectangular TEM_{12} mode. TEM stands for transverse electromagnetic. The subscripts 1 and 2 mean that there is one node in one direction and two parallel ones orthogonal to it. A node is a place of zero amplitude, therefore zero irradiance. Circular modes have circular as well as straight diagonal nodes.

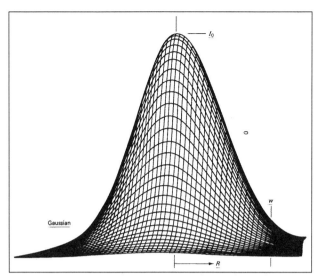

Figure 2. Computer-generated Gaussian irradiance distribution.

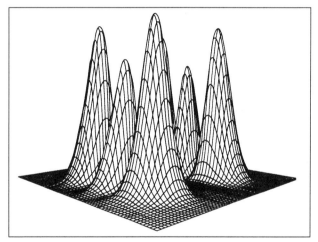

Figure 3. Computer plot of rectangular TEM_{12} mode.

One can see that this beam is made up of six Gaussian-like spots. The divergence due to diffraction for this beam will be larger than a Gaussian beam of about equivalent size because the effective spot size is now approximated by the size of the individual spots, not the overall beam size. In general, the divergence of higher-order beams is greater than that of lower-order beams for this reason. This is somewhat compensated by the fact that higher-order modes usually occur in high-power lasers, which have larger output beam diameters. For calculational purposes, the difference between the actual mode and the Gaussian mode is accounted for by a quantity called the *beam* or *mode quality factor*, M^2, (see Section 3.4). The value of this quantity for the Gaussian mode is 1. The higher the value of M^2, the higher the mode(s) and the lower the beam quality with respect to divergence and focusing. The value of M^2 for a given laser is the amount by which the actual far-field divergence angle exceeds that of a Gaussian mode for that laser.

3.1.6 Polarization

It is natural for the output of a laser to be linearly polarized. The electromagnetic field associated with an individual photon oscillates parallel to a unique direction that is perpendicular to the direction of propagation. If that photon stimulates the emission of another photon, the second photon must have the same polarization as the first. Because lasers are not absolutely coherent, because the radiation has its origin from different initializing photons at different times, the direction of polarization may change rapidly, leading to what is called *random polarization*. From the standpoint of the way the light interacts with matter, it is effectively the same as unpolarized light.

With the development of extremely precise optical elements and lasers that are both mechanically and thermally very stable, it is possible for the direction of polarization to remain fixed, either permanently or for long periods of time. This may cause problems in cutting and welding applications. The reason that the polarization state affects laser material processing applications is that absorption and reflection of light is dependent on the angle between the direction of polarization and the surface upon which the light is incident. When one cuts thick materials with a CO_2 laser, high absorption at the front edge of the cut is desirable, whereas high reflection is preferred on the sides. If the beam is polarized parallel to the cut direction, maximum absorption occurs at the leading edge of the cut, resulting in the optimum cutting rate and narrowest kerf. As the direction of polarization changes relative to the direction of cut, the cut quality diminishes and the rate of cutting decreases. A linearly polarized beam cannot be used effectively for cutting patterns in thick metal. Linearly polarized light also has a deleterious effect on quality in deep penetration welding for the same reasons that it does in cutting.

Strangely enough, to eliminate the potential problems associated with a linearly polarized beam, it is necessary deliberately to linearly polarize the output of the laser. This is done to ensure that the output is linearly polarized parallel to a precisely known direction. This is accomplished by incorporating a dichroic coating on an internal mirror, which absorbs components of the radiation parallel to a known direction. This does not affect the output power of the laser; it just forces it to operate in a fixed polarization state. With the direction of polarization precisely known, an external optical system can be used to convert the linearly polarized beam to a circularly polarized beam. This means that the direction of the electric field vector is actually rotating with an angular frequency equal to the frequency of the light. The optical device used to achieve this for CO_2 lasers consists of a system of mirrors in which one or more have coatings that act as a quarter-waveplate, a device routinely used to convert linearly polarized light to circularly polarized light. For material processing purposes, circularly polarized light has the same effect as unpolarized or randomly polarized light (see Section 12.1 for more detail).

References

S. S. Charschan (Ed.), 1993: *Guide to Laser Material Processing*, Laser Institute of America, Orlando, FL.

J. T. Luxon and D. E. Parker, 1992: *Industrial Lasers and Their Applications*, Prentice-Hall, Englewood Cliffs, NJ.

JAMES T. LUXON

3.2 Beam Delivery Before Focusing

3.2.0 Introduction

This section deals with optical systems for delivering the beam from the laser to workpiece, excluding the optics for focusing the beam. It covers conventional beam delivery devices, fiber optic transmission, and robotic applications.

This section provides a general review of beam delivery methods. Details of specific components are given in Section 4.1.

3.2.1 Conventional Beam Delivery

Beam Size

There are a number of considerations such as the size of the beam required at the workpiece and the polarization of the beam that dictate the beam delivery size and the choice of optics. Before selecting the size of the beam delivery, one must know the largest beam diameter that will pass through the components. It is imperative that the smallest inside diameter of any of the components in the system be at least 1.5 times the $1/e^2$ diameter of the beam.

Polarization

Polarization of the beam as it leaves the laser must be known so that optics such as splitters, phase retarders, and anti-back-reflection optics can be used properly. Orientation of the polarization of a laser beam is sometimes specified by the manufacturer of a laser, but often this information must be requested. Because of the property of cavity mirrors called preferential reflection, the output beam is most always linearly polarized in either a vertical or horizontal plane, depending on the relative number of cavity mirrors reflecting up or down between lanes of glassware in the resonator. Some resonator designs polarize the beam randomly and do not work with conventional optics unless they are first linearly polarized with one of several methods.

Beam Tubing

All high-powered laser beams over a few milliwatts must be isolated from human contact and also from atmospheric contamination. This is usually done with some form of tubing as shown in Figure 1.

Tubing is the equivalent of guards on industrial machinery and often provides the support structure for the components of the system. Figure 1 shows larger-diameter tubing, which is designed to isolate vibrations between the laser and the rest of the beam delivery, to provide added volume of air space for high-powered

Chapter 3: Optics and Optical Systems

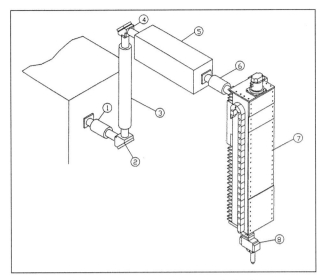

Figure 1. Typical beam delivery system. 1, 3, 6 – beam protection tubing; 2, 4 – 90° beam bender with quick-remove mirror; 5 – collimator with reflective ratio of 1:1 or 1.5; 7 – Z axis focus slide, 36" range, motorized, with 90° beam bender; 8 – reflective focus module with 250 mm f.l. off axis parabolic mirror with cutting nozzle.

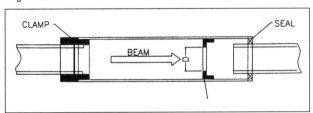

Figure 2. Beam protection tube cross section.

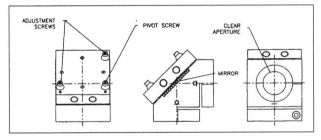

Figure 3. Beam bender with mirror.

beams, and to prevent thermal expansion and contraction from affecting beam alignment. Sometimes an aperture is added inside the tube as shown in Figure 2 to absorb diffracted light energy, which tends to cause unwanted reflections at the focusing optics.

Beam Benders

Laser beams will travel in a straight line unless turned by some form of mirrored surface, which must be optically flat within a few wavelengths to avoid dispersion of the beam. A typical beam bender as shown in Figure 3 consists of the supporting block, a mirror, and an adjustable mirror mounting plate to steer the beam.

Beam steering is commonly done with fine-pitch adjustment screws in the mirror mounting plate that tilt the mirror about a corner screw, thereby moving the reflected beam in the x or y plane. The beam position is detected by placing a cross-hair in the next bender or component downstream from the bender being adjusted. A short burst of the laser beam will burn an impression of the cross-hair on a target material such as wood or acrylic.

Mirrors are made of glass, silicon, or metal depending on the power of the laser beam and the wavelength of the laser. The reflecting surface is the front surface of the mirror to eliminate refraction effects. Laser beams therefore will follow the basic law of reflection (the angle of incidence equals the angle of reflection). Table 1(1) compares the types of mirror materials, their reflectivity, the laser damage thresholds, and the amount of phase shift introduced into the beam, for mirrors typically used in industry (1).

Table 1. Materials and Parameters Used in Bender Mirrors

Substrate	Surface	Reflectivity[a] (%)	Laser[b] Damage Threshold MW/mm²	Phase Shift (°)
Silicon	Dielectric	99.7	1.5	4–8
Cu/Ni	Gold Plate	99.0	2	0.5–1
Cu	Gold Evap	99.0	≤ 1	0.5–1
Cu	Gold Plate	99.0	10	0.5–1
Cu	Bare Metal	97–99	2–18	0.5–1
Cu/Au	Dielectric	99.7	4	2–4
Cu/Au	Dielectric	99.5	4	90 ± 10
Mo	Bare Metal	98.0	2	0.5–1
Al	Bare Metal	98.0	?	?
Al	Gold Plate	99	?	?

[a]Reflectivity is a typical value.
[b]CW use, an average figure.

Precautions

Mirrors are usually held in place with a retaining ring and a spring to keep consistent pressure and limit movement. If the mirror mounting plate is not perfectly flat, the spring can exert sufficient force to warp the mirror. The result is beam distortion, which affects the ability to focus properly.

Mirrors are generally coated with a dielectric coating to eliminate phase shifting. This coating is only a few micrometers thick and is easily damaged during cleaning. Mirrors should be regularly cleaned with acetone and lens tissue to avoid buildup of contamination. If contamination is allowed to build up, the resultant heat absorption will distort and ultimately destroy the mirror.

Other Optics

Mirrors can also be coated with multilayer dielectric coatings, which effectively rotate the polarization of the laser beam by 90°.

This is often referred to as a quarter-wave phase retarder and is used to circularly polarize a linear polarized beam. Circular polarization is necessary for bidirectional cutting or welding so that the beam creates a consistent kerf width in all directions of travel.

A second optic used in beam benders is an anti-back-reflection mirror. The coating on this mirror is designed to absorb one component of a linear polarization and totally reflect the orthogonal component. This optic is used in the beam delivery (always with a phase retarder) to absorb reflected energy, which may otherwise travel back to the laser and damage the laser resonator. The anti-back-reflection mirror is the first optic after the laser, before the phase retarders and mirrors, so that the proper alignment with laser polarization can be controlled.

Reference
1. M. Wilkinson, Laser Mirrors—Technology and Applications, *Engineering Lasers*, February, 1991.

DANIEL A. BAKKEN

3.2.2 Fiber Optic Beam Delivery: Diode Lasers

Fiber optic beam delivery technology, in conjunction with the commercialization of high-power diode lasers, is about to bring major changes to the manufacturing shop floor, as well as to business planning. Laser-assisted manufacturing processes such as cutting, drilling, welding, surface hardening and cladding of metal parts, laser-assisted machining, solid free-form fabrication (or SFF) by sintering metal powders, soldering, marking, engraving, cutting cellulose materials, etc., will find major cost reduction through flexible fiber delivery technology. This advance will bring system flexibility, miniaturization, and computer automation so that customization of parts will be at a cost comparable to volume production (2).

Since laser material processing requires very high irradiance, from 10^3 to 10^8 W/cm^2 at 10^0 to 10^4 watts of average power, our focus will be on fiber coupling of high-power lasers. Our discussion will also focus on coupling high-power lasers into multimode fibers, in contrast to single-mode fibers, because of high coupling efficiency and high damage threshold (3–6). Further, the emerging low-cost, high-power diode lasers are essentially multi-spatial mode and require multimode fibers for any practical coupling. The importance of diode lasers comes from (1) their high efficiency (50%) compared to other lasers, (2) their compact size (shoebox size for a kilowatt system), (3) wavelength diversity (0.64 to 1.55 μm now and 0.4 to 5 μm in the future), (4) direct electrical control from DC to GHz, (5) least electrical hazard in operation (requires 2 V), (6) very high reliability (5000 h or more with good cooling), and (7) potentially the least expensive in large volume. Since diode lasers are manufactured from semiconductor wafers, somewhat like computer chips, we expect a great reduction in the price of diode lasers compared to mature, big and bulky lasers such as: CO_2, Nd:YAG, excimer, Ar-ion, etc. This is why diode lasers and diode-laser-pumped fiber lasers will eventually replace most of the other high-power lasers, except where unique wavelengths, such as ultraviolet and infrared, are essential for certain material processing applications.

Intensity Requirements

Different laser material processing applications require different irradiance, usually from 10^3 W/cm^2 for soft and absorbing materials to 10^9 W/cm^2 for hard and partially absorbing materials. *Soft* and *hard* in this case refer to weakness or strength, respectively, of atomic or molecular binding forces in the materials undergoing processing. Table 2 shows the irradiance that may be transmitted for laser power from 1 to 1000 W through a single mode (typically 5 μm core diameter) or a set of multimode fibers (typically 100 to 1000 μm core diameter). Continuous wave (CW) irradiance much above 10^6 W/cm^2 through a single fiber should be avoided for the sake of safety and reliability because any impurity or imperfection on the fiber facet could create damaging heat-generating sites (assuming that the fiber core quality, like fused silica, is excellent). Processes requiring irradiance much higher than 10^6 or 10^7 W/cm^2 should utilize optical image size reduction techniques to achieve the higher intensity, as shown in Figure 4a and b.

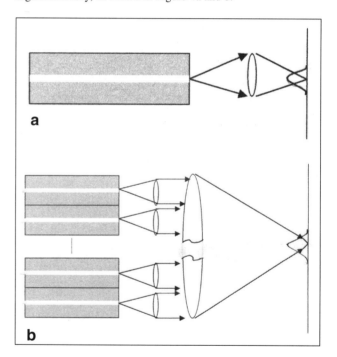

Figure 4. Optical arrangement to achieve irradiances on workpiece higher than the fiber facet can withstand or deliver (a and b). Fig. 4b also allows transporting higher total power than a single fiber is capable of. The lens also helps protect the fiber facet from the debris generated during laser material processing.

Demagnification in Figure 4a would imply a larger numerical aperture (sin θ) of the focused beam and a shorter distance to the workpiece. This imaging approach is suitable when the desired laser spot size for a particular material processing application should be smaller than the core diameter of the fiber providing the power. The restrictions in the above approach can be relieved by using a bundle of fibers (Fig. 4b) to divide the power carrying load, followed by a micro-optic lens array and a large focusing lens to achieve higher intensity with a longer working distance. The approach of Figure 4b is also suitable for cases where individual fibers, because of limitations in the source laser, cannot carry sufficient total (CW or average) power for the particular material processing application. In some commercial systems, delivering 50 to 100 W or more power, the end of the multi-fiber bundle is imaged onto another single-strand multimode fiber for further transportation and convenience of machining. In general, using a focusing lens at the delivery end of the fiber is also desirable to protect the fiber facet from debris generated during material processing.

Plastic fibers, usually multimode, although less expensive than high-quality glass fibers, are not suitable for transporting high laser power because of absorption and poor optical quality. High-quality (pure fused silica) glass fibers have a negligible absorption over the few meter path that is necessary in a laser processing setup. The absorption and scattering loss is about 2 dB/km at 0.8 µm and 0.2 dB/km at 1.55 µm (7).

Single-Mode Fibers

Single-mode fibers require stringent optical conditions for efficient power coupling. They are suitable for transporting power from lasers emitting a uniphase (or fundamental) mode beam (usually a Gaussian amplitude envelope with a uniform coherent phase front). Lasers like Ar-ion, high-quality Nd:YAG, high-quality laser amplifiers, or single-mode fiber lasers themselves fall in this category. In most cases of laser material processing, the state of polarization of the optical beam is not important. Normal fibers are not designed to preserve polarization even though most lasers are usually polarized. So this is normally not an important issue. In some cases, where a specific state of polarization is important, one must resort to using expensive, polarization-preserving single-mode fibers. Multimode fiber cannot preserve polarization; it scrambles the laser beam into randomly polarized multiple spatial modes resembling a typical laser speckle pattern.

Multimode Fibers

Multimode fibers are the workhorse for transporting high-power beams from the visible through near-infrared lasers. Fiber materials for ultraviolet lasers (like the excimer laser) and infrared lasers (like the CO_2 laser) are not yet well developed for commercialization, although intense research work is continuing. Because of a larger core diameter and their capability of accepting optically incoherent and multiphase wavefronts, the coupling optics are simple and the coupling efficiency, particularly for multimode diode lasers, can be as high as 80% in many commercial systems. One of the drawbacks of a multimode fiber is in the reduction in the intensity as shown in Table 2 because of large core diameters. Higher brightness and/or smaller spot size can be achieved using the focusing arrangement of Figure 4. A possible second drawback of broadening of the laser pulse comes from the intrinsic property of modal dispersion of all multimode fibers. However, this will be relevant only for laser processing where pulses in the domain of nanoseconds or shorter are important. Modal dispersion, extensively studied in the field of high-speed fiber optic communications, depends upon the numerical aperture (accepting beam angle, shown in Figure 4) and the length of the fiber used. The physics is simple to appreciate; an optical ray entering at a steep angle into the fiber will be delayed in arrival at the other end by a longer time than that ray traveling collinear to the fiber core axis. The relative delay is, of course, larger for a longer fiber.

Table 2. Irradiance Transmitted through Different Fiber Diameters

Laser Wattage	Irradiance (W/cm²)				
	Single-mode core 5 µm	Multimode core diameter			
		100 µm	200 µm	500 µm	1 mm
1	5.1×10^6	1.3×10^4	3.2×10^3	5.1×10^2	1.3×10^2
10	5.1×10^7	1.3×10^5	3.2×10^4	5.1×10^3	1.3×10^3
100	5.1×10^8	1.3×10^6	3.2×10^5	5.1×10^4	1.3×10^4
1000	5.1×10^9	1.3×10^7	3.2×10^6	5.1×10^5	1.3×10^5

Coupling Nd Lasers to Fibers

High-power Nd lasers, pumped by either lamps or diode lasers, even when operating multimode, produce fairly low divergent beams (a few times diffraction limited). So these beams are coupled by a simple focusing lens into multimode fibers, usually of 500 µm core diameter. Heavy-duty cutting and welding laser machines usually use 2 kW or less CW or quasi-CW power, giving rise to 1 MW/cm² irradiance at the fiber facet. The machining on large workpieces is done by articulating the fiber end, which is imaged by another lens on to the workpiece. At 1 MW/cm² irradiance, the fiber ends must be well protected from any contamination.

The drilling applications of many aerospace parts typically require 20 kW peak power pulses (average power 100 W) delivered into a spot size of 100 µm. So the required irradiance is too high for fiber delivery through 100 µm core fiber. But these aerospace parts are usually small and are articulated for machining directly under the laser beam, eliminating the need of fiber delivery.

Coupling Diode Lasers to Fibers

Ar-ion (usually single mode) and Nd:YAG (sometimes low-order multimode) lasers produce high-brightness beams because of their low beam divergences. Such beams are easy to couple to multimode fibers by assuring the focused laser spot size and the numerical aperture are smaller than that of the multimode fiber core. Unlike with single-mode fibers, no stringent mode matching is required.

The situation is very different for current commercial high-power semiconductor diode lasers, called edge-emitting Fabry-Perot lasers. Over 65,000 microscopic (200 x 600 μm) lasers can be produced by cleaving a 4-in. diameter laser wafer (crystal). These wafers are grown epitaxially to create a p-n junction (that provides laser gain through electrical pumping) and optical waveguides (that provide laser cavities).

Each of the microscopic elements can be designed as a single-stripe (3 μm wide), single-mode device (Fig. 5a) to emit 5 to 30 mW CW power or a multistripe, multimode device to emit power as high as 20 W or more (Fig. 5b). The material composition can be altered to produce various wavelengths like GaAlAs (0.8 μm), GaAsSb (0.98 μm), InGaAsP (1.55 μm), etc. To achieve electrical pumping efficiency as high as 50% requires an extremely thin (1 μm) optical waveguide embedding an even thinner p-n junction. This also creates the key optical engineering problem if one wants to utilize the diode laser beam for material processing. The beam divergence, perpendicular to the p-n junction, is almost 60° with an equivalent numerical aperture (NA) of 0.5 (sin 30°). It is difficult to produce high-quality optical fiber with such a large NA to couple the diode directly to the fiber. Fibers of NA up to 0.37 (θ = 22°) are commercially available. Thus efficient coupling requires using a miniature cylindrical lens to reduce the large beam divergence to match that of the fiber core. This is one of the most critical elements that keeps the price of high-power diode lasers as high as other lasers. Figure 5c shows the coupling of a 20 W (200 μm) wide multimode laser stripe into a 200 μm core multimode fiber (3, 4). This will give about 50 kW/cm^2 irradiance at the output end of the fiber, assuming an 80% coupling efficiency, a value that may now be achieved commercially. Fewer than 65 such modules can deliver a total CW power of 1 kW from a 65-fiber bundle. The imaging arrangements shown in Figure 4b can then be used to obtain higher irradiance and smaller spot size for heavy-duty laser material processing.

One of the next generation high-power DLs to be commercialized employs the geometry shown in Figure 6. This DL emits light vertically through the wafer surface by virtue of second-order Bragg gratings. The emission cross section can be very wide, for example, 15 x 200 μm instead of 1 x 3 μm as in an edge-emitting Fabry-Perot laser. This broader source size provides a much higher brightness source because of the lower divergence and is capable of giving an irradiance of 1 MW/cm^2 or higher at a focused spot. A multimode fiber can be directly coupled to such devices without any collimating optics for efficient power coupling. A monolithic 2D array of such lasers will eventually replace most of the current lasers for laser materials processing.

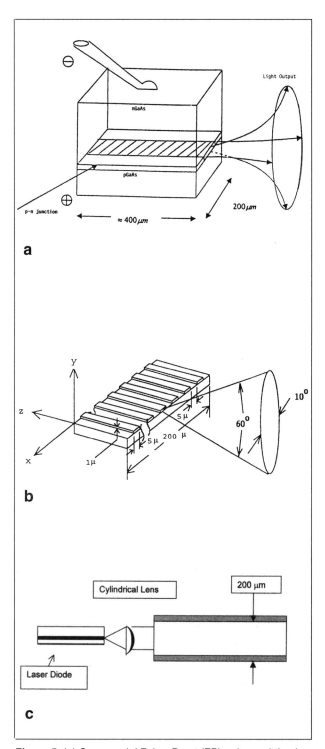

Figure 5. (a) Commercial Fabry-Perot (FP), edge emitting laser diodes have almost 60° (full angle) beam divergence, creating difficulty in fiber coupling; (b) A 200 micrometer bar containing a monolithic array of such FP lasers can emit 20 W CW power; (c) a short focal length cylindrical lens can help couple this 20 W power into a 200 micrometer core multi mode fiber.

ISBN 0-912035-15-3

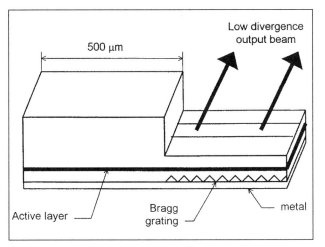

Figure 6. Grating coupled surface emitting lasers (GCSEL) will be the next generation high-power diode lasers. Because of their low beam divergence, they are capable of providing focused high-intensity spots up to 1 MW/cm² or higher with low cost fiber optical system.

References

2. M. Steen, *Laser material processing* (2nd ed.), Springer 1998. This is an excellent comprehensive introductory text on the subject but not meant for fiber coupling.
3. W. Chen, C. Roychoudhuri, and C. Banas, "Design approaches for laser-diode materal processing systems using fibers and micro-optics," *Optical Engineering* **33** (11), 3662 (1994).
4. N. G. Muller, R. Weber, and H. P. Weber, "Output beam characteristics of high power continuous wave diode laser bars," *Optical Engineering* **34** (8), 2384 (1995).
5. J. G. Endriz et al., "High power laser diode arrays," *IEEE Jour. Quant. Electron.* **28** (4), 952 (1992).
6. D. Mehuys and D. Evans, "High power diode lasers tune into diverse applications," *Laser Focus World*, p. 117, May 1995.
7. D. Derickson (Ed.), Fiber Optics Test and Measurement, Prentice Hall, 1998.

CHANDRASEKHAR ROYCHOUDHURI

3.2.3 Fiber Optic Beam Delivery: Nd:YAG Lasers

General Considerations

Fiber optics are an attractive alternative to conventional beam delivery because of the ability of a glass fiber to flex (within the limits of specified bend radii for the fiber bundle). Glass is essentially pure silica and is very transmissive to wavelengths between 400 and 1200 nm or so. Fiber optics are generally not very efficient in the ultraviolet range wavelengths (below 400 nm) and would be destroyed by carbon dioxide lasers at 10,600 nm. Bulk transmission efficiencies greater than 99% are possible with silica fibers at 1.064 nm (the Nd:YAG wavelength). It is important to note that plastic fibers are often used with visible wavelength lasers but do not work as well with Nd:YAG lasers because of transmission losses and lower damage thresholds.

Perhaps the major advantage of fiber optics over conventional beam delivery components is the ability to transmit laser beams over long distances, up to 50 m, and around curves. A second difference from conventional optics is that fibers and focusing modules are compact and easily moved so that the beam can be manipulated about a fixed workpiece. Overall losses in fiber optic systems are comparable to conventional systems because of the reflective loss of about 4% at each end of the fiber, internal losses, and reflective losses at the protective glass window beyond the lens. Total losses can be around 10–15%.

Construction

A glass fiber by itself is not very strong and therefore must have a protective coating of a polymer for distribution of stress and tensile strength. There is normally a second polymer layer for abrasion resistance. The coated fiber is then enclosed by an armored cable for industrial durability.

Fiber Sizes

The diameter of the transmissive silica core of a fiber optic cable varies depending on the power of the laser and the desired spot size. Generally, the range is between 0.2 and 1.0 mm (see Table 3).

Table 3. Laser Power vs. Diameter and Minimum Bend Radius

Laser Power (maximum) (W)	Core Diameter (mm)	Minimum Bend Radius (mm)
0–20	0.20	25–60
20–50	0.40	100–120
50–100	0.60	150–180
100–200	0.80	200–240
200–400	1.00	250–300

Laser Input Assembly

In order for light to be transmitted into the fiber, the laser beam must be focused into the end of the fiber cable very accurately. The ends of the fiber bundle must be highly polished and perpendicular to the axis so the entering beam can enter efficiently. The focal spot diameter should generally not exceed 80% of the core diameters listed in Table 3. The minimum bend radii listed in Table 3 represent a range of values for silica fibers that assure long life of the fiber.

Most Nd:YAG (solid-state) lasers have output beams roughly the same diameter as the laser rod and are highly divergent (M^2 = 20 to 200 X diffraction-limited divergence, depending on the power of the laser). Fiber optic cables therefore require an input and output housing that can focus the beam into the fiber and recollimate the beam as it leaves the fiber before the final focus lens (see Fig. 7 next page) (8).

The input housing consists of a collimating beam expander and a refocusing lens. The focusing lens focal length can be calculated if the numerical aperture (NA) of the fiber cable is known. Pure silica usually has an NA around 0.22, but values as high as 0.48 are possible with special cladding. The formula for acceptance angle θ (the maximum angle of the focused beam at which all the laser beam energy will be contained within the silica fiber) is the numerical aperture.

$$NA = \sin 2\theta$$

For NA = 0.22, θ = 12.7°, which is the half-angle of the beam from the focusing lens to the fiber input face. From this angle, one can select a value of focusing lens that will have a cone angle of about 70% of 2θ, and a spot size less than 80% of the fiber diameter. Care must be taken not to focus the beam waist inside the fiber to avoid potential damage to the fiber material. Focus slightly in front of the fiber face, but close enough so that the beam does not exceed 80% of the fiber diameter.

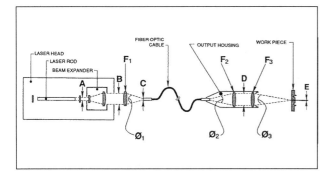

Figure 7. Fiber optic focus system.

The output module of the fiber is very much like the input in that it usually has both a collimating lens and a focusing lens. The angle of the beam cone as it leaves the fiber is roughly the same as the entering beam, but the diameter will be slightly larger because the beam has completely filled the fiber at the exit.

It is possible to use only a single focusing lens if it is located beyond the focal distance to refocus the beam. A single lens configuration is rarely used because of the resulting large beam spot diameter. A rule of thumb is that the collimated beam diameter should never be greater than half the focal length of the focusing lens because of spherical aberrations of short-focal-length lenses.

The damage threshold of silica fiber material is of the order of 1-5 X 10^9 W/cm². Safe operating practice says that laser power density should be less than 10% of the threshold value. Nd:YAG laser manufacturers claim to have transmitted up to 6 kW through fibers without damage as long as the minimum bend radii and acceptance angles are not exceeded.

Beam Splitting

Because the mode of the output beam from a fiber is almost homogenized and round regardless of the shape of the input beam, it is possible to share a single beam with half-round mirrors that "scrape" off part of the beam and divert the remainder to a second focusing module, thereby splitting the beam. Splitting can also be done with conventional splitter optics if the beam from the laser is polarized.

Time sharing occurs when the beam is switched from one focus module to another with a mirror on a precision slide or with a galvanometer mirror. In this case, the entire energy of the beam is directed into each fiber as the mirror is moved. There should be an interlock to prevent laser beam damage as the mirror is being moved.

Comparisons with Conventional Optics

An important characteristic of all Nd:YAG lasers is that the beam divergence changes with the average power output. With fiber optics, the core diameter and the focal length of the final focus lens determines the spot diameter, which is independent of power. With a fiber optic system, it is necessary to change the focal length of the lens for a different spot size. A longer lens focal length will increase spot size, and a shorter focal length (faster) lens will decrease spot size.

With conventional optics, the spot size varies directly with divergence angle and therefore gets larger as laser power increases. It may be desirable to change the spot size for different tasks. With conventional beam delivery, it is as simple as changing the average power by varying the cycle rate. It would also be possible to change the beam size with the aid of a beam telescope. The size of the focal spot is inversely proportional to the beam diameter at the focusing lens.

An analogous technology for CO_2 lasers is called totally reflective waveguides (see Fig. 8). Waveguides are small-diameter tubes (typically stainless steel) that have approximately 1 mm diameter. They are lined with a silver or sapphire-based material that is deposited in a thin layer for total reflection of the beam. Transmission losses are quite high (10–25% or more), depending on bend radius, and tubes are not available longer than about 2 m. Severe degradation of the fundamental mode is usually seen in the output beam. Cooling of the waveguide is also required. As with fiber optics, it is necessary to focus the input beam into the guide and recollimate the output beam. This technology is in its infancy and has some severe problems to overcome at this time.

3.2.4 Robotic Applications

General Considerations

Both conventional and fiber optic beam delivery can be used with robots to do complex tasks in laser processing. The simpler method is to use fiber optics. This limits the laser choice to an Nd:YAG. In almost all industrial applications, other visible wavelengths are not used. Robots with conventional optics (for CO_2 lasers) require optical beam benders that must have extreme precision and be very robust to maintain alignment with

Chapter 3: Optics and Optical Systems

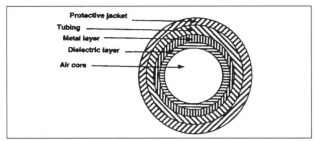

Figure 8. Waveguide cross section.

wear. Conventional optics are very expensive when compared to fiber optic systems. The range of motion with the two systems depends on the bend radius of the fiber, the number of swivel mirrors in conventional optics, and the configuration of the robot itself.

Accuracies

Robotic systems are generally not as accurate as fixed-beam, moving workpiece systems, but are sometimes the best choice when process accuracy is not precise, such as welding. When part geometry is complex and the process requires three-dimensional motion, robots offer the least expensive and most versatile approach. Cutting high-tolerance parts may be possible with robots, but this application usually requires an end effector to maintain a close standoff distance to parts. Table 4 compares the advertised accuracies of several major robot manufacturers. This table mentions several companies for illustrative purposes only and does not represent an endorsement of these companies.

The term *accuracy* is not the same as *repeatability* in Table 4. Repeatability is approximately one-half the positional accuracy (9) when the reversal error due to backlash in the system is considered. Standards for accuracy of machines varies according to the country of manufacture of the robot. The major stan-

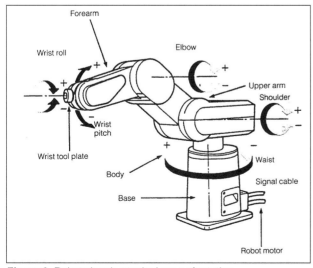

Figure 9. Robot showing typical axes of rotation.

Table 4. Comparison of Robot Parameters

#	Company Name	Model Number	Number of Axes	Nominal Payload (lbs)	Reach (ft/in.)	Repeatability (± in.)
1	Staublie	RX 60	6/5/4	5.5	2'2"	±0.0008
2	Staublie	RX 90	6/5/4	13	3'3"	±0.0008
3	Staublie	RX 90L	6/5/4	8	3'11"	±0.001
4	Staublie	RX 130	6/5/4	26	4'6"	±0.0012
5	Staublie	RX 130L	6/5/4	13	5'5"	±0.0014
6	Staublie	RX 170	6/5/4	66	6'	±0.0016
7	Staublie	RX 170L	6/5/4	44	7'	±0.002
8	Fanuc	ARC Mate 100i	6	13	4'6"	±0.004
9	Fanuc	ARC Mate 120	6	26	5'3"	±0.004
10	Fanuc	ARC Mate mini	5	7	3'6"	±0.004
11	Fanuc	LR Mate 100i	5	11	2"	±0.002
12	Fanuc	M-6i	6	13	4'6"	±0.004
13	Fanuc	P-200	6	33	9'2"	±0.020
14	Fanuc	S-12	6	26	5'3"	±0.004
15	Fanuc	S-500	6	33	8'12"	±0.0100
16	Kuka	KR 6/1	6	13	5'2"	±0.004
17	Kuka	KR 15/1	6	33	5'2"	±0.004
18	Kuka	KR 30/1	6	77	6'8"	±0.006
19	Kuka	KR 30L 15/1	6	33	10'1"	±0.006
20	Motoman	SK 16	6	35	5'1"	±0.004
21	Motoman	SK 6	6	13	4'4"	±0.008
22	Motoman	SK 45	6	99	5'10"	±0.006
23	Motoman	K10A	6	4.4	5'1"	±0.004
24	Panasonic	VR-008A	6	18	4'10"	±0.004
25	Panasonic	AW-005A	6	11	3'4"	±0.004
26	Panasonic	AW-005AL	6	11	4'5"	±0.004
27	Panasonic	AW-005C	6	11	3'4"	±0.004
28	Panasonic	AW-005CL	6	11	4'5"	±0.004
29	Panasonic	AW-010C	6	22	5'4"	±0.004
30	Panasonic	AW-006A	6	13	4'5"	±0.004
31	Panasonic	AW-010A	6	13	5'4"	±0.008
32	Panasonic	AW-006AL	6	22	5'11"	±0.004
33	Nachi	SC15	6	11	?	±0.004
34	Nachi	SC50	6	33	?	±0.012
35	Nachi	SC151	6	22	?	±0.010
36	ABB	IRB 1400	6	11	4'9"	±0.004
37	ABB	IRB 2400L	6	11-15	5'11"	±0.004
38	ABB	IRB 4400	6	99	6'5"	±0.006
39	ABB	IRB 510	6	11	8'6"	±0.12
40	ABB	IRB 5002	6	11-22	9'4"	±0.008
41	ABB	IRB 5003	6	11-22	13'1"	±0.008
42	JMC	TRICEPT	6	132	?	±0.0008
43	Mitsubishi	RV-N4	6	9	2'12"	±0.002
44	Mitsubishi	RV-N10	6	22	4'5"	±0.004
45	Mitsubishi	RV-N12	6	26	5'1"	±0.004

ISBN 0-912035-15-3

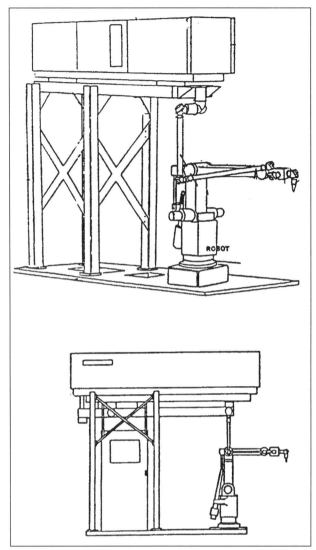

Figure 10. Robot with laser and conventional beam delivery.

cally have capability for an additional 4–8 axes of motion control. Robots generally have a "teach" control to eliminate the need for complex programming of positions. The robot is jogged to critical inflection points on the workpiece and the control memorizes the position and will traverse a straight line in between.

Robots can be integrated with conventional beam delivery as shown in Figure 10. The delivery system consists of bender-tube sections swiveling via precision bearings. The bearings must be very rigid to prevent beam misalignment from wear. The beam path is always constant in length (as with fiber optics), which assures consistent spot size at any position.

Robots have been designed with reflective mirrors built into the arms of the robot. These have proven to be difficult to align and very expensive. The advantage is that fewer optics are used, which reduces losses (approximately 2% per mirror for metal mirrors).

Fiber optics are easily adapted to almost any type of robot with a relatively simple bracket. Alignment is always maintained, and spot size is not subject to bearing wear. Focus modules are light weight compared to CO_2 benders and tubes. The cost of fiber optic components is a fraction of CO_2 optics. The laser may be across the room from the robot with fiber optics, and a single laser may service several robots. These and many other reasons make robots and fiber optics an ideal combination.

References
8. Thomas R. Kugler, Fiber Optic Beam Delivery for High Powered YAG Lasers, Lumonics Industrial Products Division, ICALEO 11/5/90.
9. James J. Childs, "All Accuracies Are Not the Same," *American Machinist,* September, 1991.

DANIEL A. BAKKEN

3.3 Focusing and Depth of Focus

3.3.1 Focusing
In most materials processing operations, one focuses the laser beam onto the workpiece. Frequently one desires a small focal area. One cannot focus the beam to an infinitesimal point. There is a minimum spot size that is determined by diffraction.

If the original divergence of the beam was determined by diffraction at the aperture of the laser, then the minimum spot radius r_s that can be obtained when the beam is focused by a lens with focal length F is

$$r_s = F\theta \qquad (1)$$

where θ is the beam divergence angle. This equation is commonly used as a convenient approximation for estimating minimum focal size.

dards are NMTBA in the United States, VDI/DGQ in Germany, JIS in Japan, and ISO230-2, which is rapidly becoming the worldwide standard (9). They differ primarily in the number of target points, runs, direction of approach, and the method of calculation. The ISO standard is very close to and was developed from the German VDI standards.

Accuracy of standard two-axis machine tool tables is on the order of 0.0005–0.001 in. per foot of travel. The robots in Table 4 have accuracy approximately 0.002–0.02 in. or more depending on the reach. When part-to-part inaccuracies are considered, the combined tolerances almost always require an end effector such as a capacitive autofocus unit that controls the position of the focus lens in either conventional or fiber optic systems.

Figure 9 shows a typical configuration for a five-axis robot without beam delivery. The controllers supplied with robots typi-

Because the diffraction-limited beam divergence angle is approximately $\theta = \lambda/D$, where D is the diameter of the limiting aperture, one has (assuming that the beam fills the lens aperture)

$$r_s = F\lambda/D = \lambda\, F\# \tag{2}$$

where $F\#$ denotes the F-number of the lens. Because it is impractical to work with F numbers much less than unity, the minimum value of the spot size is of the same order of magnitude as the wavelength. Thus it is often said that laser light can be focused to a spot the size of its wavelength.

This value of focal spot size represents an ultimate limit that is set by diffraction. It applies only if the spatial distribution in the beam is Gaussian. If the beam contains higher-order modes, the focal spot size will be larger.

This discussion also neglects the effect of lens aberrations, which will increase the focal spot size, especially as the focal length of the lens becomes very short. To produce a small focal area, one must use a lens with a short focal length, according to Equation 1. But as the focal length becomes short, lens aberrations become more important. For a collimated monochromatic laser beam incident along the axis of the lens, most of the aberrations considered in elementary optics may be neglected.

The most important aberration is spherical aberration. With spherical aberration the light rays from a point source entering the lens at different distances from its axis are focused to a blurred circle, rather than to a point. Spherical aberration sets a practical lower limit to the focal length that can be used, and hence to the focal spot size.

One may reduce the effects of spherical aberration by using best-shape lenses, by using compound (multielement) lenses or by using aspheric lenses with specially ground shapes. In the visible or near-infrared portions of the spectrum, a planoconvex lens, with the convex side toward the laser, is the best shape, producing the minimum spherical aberration. In the far-infrared spectrum, the optimum lens shape is a meniscus (concave-convex) lens, also with the convex side toward the laser. The choice of multielement lenses or ashperic lenses will be discussed further in Section 4.2.1.

Summarizing methods for focusing the beam to the minimum focal area, one must use a laser with a Gaussian beam profile. One should choose a lens with as short a focal length as possible, consistent with the desired depth of focus and the lens aberrations. The shape of the lens should be chosen to give minimum spherical aberration, that is, planoconvex in the visible and near infrared and meniscus in the far infrared. Alternatively, one should consider use of multielement lenses or aspheric lenses, especially in cases where the focal length is small.

JOHN F. READY

3.3.2 Depth of Focus

The depth of focus of a laser beam depends on the modal structure of that beam. A general expression for the depth of focus of a general laser field does not exist. However, some understanding can be obtained by considering the depth of focus for the lowest-order Gaussian mode. Within this section, the term *Gaussian beam* refers to the lowest-order Gaussian mode, TEM_{00}.

When a Gaussian beam is focused with a lens, the size of the beam becomes minimum at the focal plane of the lens. This minimum size is referred to as the *beam waist*. Because of diffraction, the focused laser beam spreads and does not remain focused as it propagates away from the beam waist in free space. The radius of a Gaussian laser beam, $w(z)$, at any distance z from the axial location of the beam waist measured along the beam axis, is given by

$$w z^2 = w_o^2 [1 + (\lambda z / \pi w_o^2)^2] \tag{3}$$

where λ is the wavelength of the laser and w_o is the radius of the beam waist. Although the beam diverges as it propagates from the waist, there is a small region on either side of the waist over which the beam radius, $w(z)$, changes slowly, and therefore, the intensity of the laser beam is nearly constant. Letting $w(z) = \xi w_0$ at $z = \pm d_f$ Equation 3 can be written as

$$d_f = \pm \frac{\pi w_o^2}{\lambda}(\xi^2 - 1)^{1/2} \tag{4}$$

The physical significance of this expression is that at a distance d_f on either side of the beam waist, the intensity of the laser beam decreases to $1/\xi^2$ of its maximum value because the beam radius increases to ξ times its minimum value.

One possible definition (1) of the depth of focus, d_f, is the distance on either side of the beam waist over which the laser intensity $I(0,z)$ drops to half the peak value $I(0,0)$, that is $I(0,z)/I(0,0) = 1/2$ at $z = \pm d_f$, where $I(r,z)$ represents the laser intensity at any radial and axial locations r and z, respectively, from the axis of the laser beam. According to this definition,

$$\xi = \sqrt{2}$$

and the depth of focus is given by

$$d_f = \pm \frac{\pi w_o^2}{\lambda} \tag{5}$$

At this point the beam radius $w(z) = \sqrt{2}\, w_o$; the laser intensity $I(0,z)$ decreases to 50% of $I(0,0)$ and the beam radius increases by 41.42% of the beam waist.

Another more frequently used definition (2) of the depth of focus is the distance on either side of the beam waist at which $\xi = 1.05$, which yields the following expression for the depth of focus,

$$d_f \pm 0.32 \frac{\pi w_0^2}{\lambda} \pm \frac{w_0^2}{\lambda} \tag{6}$$

ISBN 0-912035-15-3

At this point the laser intensity $I(0,z)$ decreases to 90.87% of $I(0,0)$ and the beam radius increases by 5% of the beam waist. Equation 6 is the most widely accepted definition for the depth of focus. According to Equation 6, if the beam is focused to a spot size equal to the wavelength, the depth of focus is also equal to the wavelength. This means further that the workpiece surface must be positioned accurately to within one wavelength of the desired position.

The depth of focus as given in Equation 5, that is,

$$d_f = \pm \frac{\pi w_o^2}{\lambda} \quad (5)$$

is known as the Rayleigh range, which is denoted by z_R. A parameter $b = 2z_R$ is referred to as the *confocal parameter*. The Rayleigh range z_R is a measure of the length of the waist region over which the spot size does not change significantly. For a smaller Rayleigh range, the growth of the beam radius from the waist is more rapid. In practical applications, care must be taken to maintain an optimum Rayleigh range. As the structure of the laser beam fluctuates, the Rayleigh range also fluctuates. These changes modify the penetration depth of the laser beam into the workpiece and affect the quality and repeatability of the process.

Reference
1. J. F. Ready, *Effects of High-Power Laser Radiation*, Academic, New York, 19–20, 1971.
2. S. S. Charschan (Ed.), *Guide to Laser Materials Processing*, Laser Institute of America, Toledo, OH (1977).

WILLIAM P. LATHAM
ARAVINDA KAR

3.4 Mode Quality

One measure of laser mode quality is the focusability of the laser beams. If the laser output field is measured, the focusability of the field can be readily predicted using diffraction theory. Both optical imperfections in the optical cavity and the optical beam train and nonuniformities in the gain medium can change the laser mode or output field and thus change the laser focusability. Measures of optical quality are divided into two categories. The first category is empirical quantities or measureables, such as total laser output power or energy, laser linewidth, focal spot size, far-field peak irradiance, and encircled power or energy in the focal spot. Also included in this category are parameters that are directly calculated using these measured values, such as beam divergence, coherence length, coherence width or area, and brightness. These parameters quantify the lasers performance empirically without comparison to a standard. A second category involves relative parameters, which compare the focusability of an actual laser beam to the focusability of an ideal standard laser beam. Some of these relative parameters are beam quality, mode quality, and Strehl ratio. Table 1 lists a summary of these parameters. Definitions of some of the parameters have been presented in Table 1 of Section 3.1.

Many materials processing applications utilize high-power lasers. For some of these lasers, the ideal standard is taken to be the lowest-order Gaussian mode (TEM_{00}). For lasers that employ an unstable resonator, the standard for comparison is usually a uniformly illuminated plane wave in the output aperture. The basic parameters of interest for the focused laser field are the far-field peak irradiance and the spot size. When these two parameters are measured and the parameters of the laser and the focusing lens are given, the beam divergence and brightness of the laser can be calculated (see Section 3.1).

Table 1. Optical Quality

Optical Quality Parameter	Expression
M and M^2 factors $M = \theta_h/\theta_g$	$M = (2p+l+1)^{1/2}$ for circular TEM_{pl} mode
	$M_x = (2m+1)^{1/2}$ in the x direction for rectangular TEM_{mn} mode
	$M_y = (2n+1)^{1/2}$ in the y direction for rectangular TEM_{mn} mode
Gaussian beam quality	$\beta_g \approx M$
	M^2 = beam quality factor
Strehl ratio	$S = I_m/I_0 = \exp[-(2\phi/\lambda)^2]$
Strehl ratio beam quality	$\beta_s = 1/S^{1/2} = \exp[+(\phi/\lambda)^2]$
Encircled power ratio in a circle of radius r_c	$\beta = (p_{ideal}/p_{act})^{1/2}$
Total beam quality	$\beta_t = \Pi_i \beta_i$

The Strehl ratio is the ratio of the far-field peak irradiance of an ideal standard laser beam to the actual far-field peak irradiance. It should be noted that the term *irradiance* is also referred to as power density, or the radiant-flux density. The Strehl ratio is useful in determining the effects of optical aberrations on laser performance and is generally used within the optics community to evaluate the performance of optical systems.

Another measurable is the encircled energy or encircled power within a small area around the focal spot. This gives a more complete understanding of the far-field performance than peak irradiance, because it depends on the distribution of irradiance in this area rather than at a single point. The encircled power can be used to determine the beam quality or M^2 factor of the laser, which compares the actual laser performance to an ideal standard for laser encircled power. Because the ideal standard is compared to the mode of the laser, the beam quality is some times referred to as the mode quality of the laser.

Beam Quality, M^2, or Mode Quality

The primary measurable quantity that determines laser performance is the encircled energy or power in a small region around the focal spot. By using a circular or rectangular aperture with a power meter, the encircled power can be readily measured to determine what fraction of the total laser output power is delivered by the laser into a small disk. The disk radius, half-width, or Gaussian radius is usually taken to be at the first zero in the far-field diffraction pattern for a uniformly illuminated or lowest-order Gaussian beam-illuminated output aperture. These sizes are given in Equations 1–3 in Section 3.1. If the power or energy measured in the small area around the focal spot is P_s and the total laser output power or energy is P, the fraction of power or energy delivered by the laser to the focal spot is $p = P_s/P$. The fractional power, p, or energy in the far-field focal spot is a readily measurable and meaningful quantity. If the laser is operating in a single lowest loss mode, the fractional power can be near the maximum obtainable for some ideal standard waveform. For a uniformly illuminated circular aperture, $p \approx 0.84$. For a rectangular beam geometry, $p \approx 0.81 = (0.90)^2$. For the lowest-order Gaussian beam, $p \approx 0.86$. The beam quality β is defined as the square root of the ratio of the fractional power p_{ideal} in the far-field spot for an ideal standard beam to the fractional power p_{act} in the actual laser beam, that is, $\beta = (p_{ideal}/p_{act})^{1/2}$. When the laser operates in the lowest loss mode, the value of β is almost unity. If the actual beam has exactly the same profile as the ideal standard, the beam quality would be exactly one, that is, $\beta = 1$. The physical mechanism that determines the mode structure of the laser beam and the focused beam spread is diffraction. When $\beta = 1$, the laser is said to be "diffraction limited"; that is, its performance is limited only by diffraction. When the laser beam is not ideal, the laser is said to be β times diffraction limited. The beam quality β has this specific meaning in optics terminology. The Strehl ratio (S) can be related to a beam quality (β_s) by $\beta_s = (1/S)^{1/2}$. When S and β_s are equal to 1, the optical system, in this case the optical resonator, is said to have diffraction-limited performance; that is, the only phenomenon that limits the performance of the laser is diffraction, since the optical aberrations have been reduced to zero.

The bare cavity modes of a stable resonant cavity are Gaussian modes. For a single higher-order Gaussian mode, the beam waist is M times the beam waist for the lowest loss Gaussian beam, that is, the TEM_{00} mode. For a single higher-order Gaussian mode, the far-field peak irradiance and the power within a small area around the focal spot having radius or half-width given by Equation 3 in Section 3.1 is reduced by a factor of M^2; that is, the Gaussian beam quality β_g is related to M^2 by $\beta_g = (M^2)^{1/2} = M$. M^2 or β_g provides a meaningful measure of the optical quality when the beam structure consists of some combination of the Gaussian modes. The fractional power or energy transmitted to a small area around the focal spot can always be determined. The beam quality or M^2 factor can be useful to analyze laser focusability by relating the actual laser performance to an ideal standard, which is the lowest-order Gaussian mode. Tables of typical values of M^2 for CO_2 lasers and Nd:YAG lasers have also been presented in Sections 2.1 and 2.2, respectively.

If there are several sources of aberration or beam degradation, the total beam quality is equal to a product of all individual contributions, so that

$$\beta = \prod_i \beta_i$$

Finally, by noting that the beam quality factor is the ratio of actual peak irradiance to ideal peak irradiance, a single figure of merit for the focusability of the laser system can be expressed by the reduced brightness (B_β) as $B_\beta = (1/\beta^2)(PA_s/\lambda^2) = f^2 I_r$. B_β/f^2 yields an estimate of the actual reduced far-field peak irradiance I_r. Therefore, B_β is extremely useful for estimating the materials processing capability of a laser. Various expressions for brightness are summarized in Table 3, in Section 3.1.

Some representative values of M^2 for continuous CO_2 lasers are presented in Table 2. These values were derived from the literature of laser manufacturers. The value of M^2 tends to increase with increasing output power. At any particular power level, the values of M^2 vary from laser model to another, the ranges given in the table cover typical CO_2 laser models.

Table 2. M^2 Values for Continuous CO_2 Lasers

Output (W)	Power/M^2
< 500	1.1–1.2
800–1000	1.7–2
2500	2–3
5000	3–5
10,000	10

Strehl Ratio

The Strehl ratio (S) is commonly used in the analysis of optical system performance. For a laser, it can be helpful in evaluating degradations to optical performance of the laser resonator and the optical beam train, which directs the laser beam to the material external to the resonant cavity. In the presence of optical aberrations, mirror distortions, gain medium imperfections, and/or beam jitters, the far-field peak irradiance is reduced or degraded. If these optical distortions are small, the ratio of the actual or aberrated far-field peak irradiance (I_m) to the ideal or unaberrated peak irradiance (I_0) is the Strehl ratio, given in Table 1. The aberration ϕ is the magnitude of the distortion of the wavefront measured in wavelengths, and I_m refers to the measured peak irradiance. When ϕ is a small fraction of the wavelength, the Strehl ratio gives a good estimate in the degradation of the far-field peak irradiance. This approach is very useful when there is one dominant distortion causing the degradation.

The Strehl ratio can readily be modified to include multiple aberrations, but the specific form depends on whether or not the aberrations are correlated with one another.

The Strehl ratio has the advantage that it is simple and can be useful in troubleshooting laser optical performance problems or during laser design when a particular distortion will potentially be introduced by the system. An empirical form of the Strehl ratio is given by measuring the actual far-field peak irradiance (I_a) and calculating the ideal peak irradiance (I_0) from the laser output power. By the central ordinate theorem, the centroid of the far-field irradiance distribution is related to the output area of the laser, so that I_0 can be calculated from the laser output power. Thus $I_0 = PA_s/(\lambda^2 f^2) = P/A_c$ (see the discussion on brightness in Section 3.1). This can be used as the ideal standard peak irradiance with the measured far-field peak irradiance to determine the Strehl ratio. The Strehl ratio in the empirical form then depends only on three measurable quantities: the parameters of the focusing lens, the measured total laser output power, and the measured far-field peak irradiance.

WILLIAM P. LATHAM
ARAVINDA KAR

Notes

Chapter 4

Components for Laser Materials Processing Systems

4.0 Introduction

This chapter describes various components and different types of accessory equipment that are commonly used as part of a complete system designed for materials processing. These devices represent separate fields of technology, some of which were well developed before the advent of lasers. Because these components are necessary for a complete system to perform a processing application, a complete description of laser materials processing includes discussion of these related components. Because these technologies are well developed in their own right, the description in this chapter will necessarily be somewhat abbreviated.

Specific components used in a laser processing system include beam delivery components, lenses, mirrors, infrared transmitting materials, photodetectors, beam profilers, power and energy meters, gas nozzles, and a variety of other devices.

4.1 Components for Beam Delivery Systems

Optical principles relevant to laser beam delivery to a workpiece have been described in Chapter 3. This section emphasizes the components used in beam delivery systems.

4.1.1 General Remarks on Beam Delivery Systems and Design Criteria

The beam delivery system represents one of the most important parts of a laser material processing system, because it influences dramatically the quality of the achievable processing results. The initial laser beam quality at the laser output is also very important, but only a few applications can use the laser beam as it emerges from the laser. For laser material processing either the workpiece or the laser beam (or both) have to be moved in order to perform the requested process. During this movement temporal and spatial changes of the available laser beam at the tool center point (TCP) may occur. It is the function of the beam delivery system, if properly designed, to avoid or reduce (compensate) the influence of disturbing external parameters or physical intrinsic laser beam propagation properties.

Such a design has to take into consideration:

- The laser type
- The type of laser resonator
- The laser beam quality
- The laser output power
- The type of application; workpiece geometry
- The processing speed
- The necessary handling/maintenance requirements
- The length of the beam delivery system
- The necessary variation of the length of the beam path
- The beam shape at the TCP
- The beam polarization at the TCP
- The necessary adjustment requirements

Specific safety requirements also have to be observed and properly implemented.

Complete systems for laser material processing available on the market at present offer answers for all these questions. It is very difficult to compare such systems, because they have different specifications. The following sections are intended to answer and explain the background of several of the questions mentioned.

The following sections deal with specific CO_2 laser beam delivery components and systems, but also present some general aspects of laser material processing. Some other sections will present typical solid-state laser (Nd:YAG) components and solutions for existing problems.

A good laser beam quality represents only the starting point for continuously good and reliable work results. In order to maintain good beam quality, the beam delivery system has to be properly designed dependent on the criteria mentioned earlier. On the other hand, the beam delivery system can be designed in such a way that it becomes more tolerant to the variation of several important parameters. This is indispensable for the design of the standard laser material processing machinery supposed to keep the promised specifications, possibly independent of the laser choice.

Another aspect should also be considered during the development of the system design specifications: the amount of necessary flexibility for present and future system options or applications (a good example here is represented by the integration of sensors and monitoring devices into a running system).

The most trivial fact about laser beams is their divergence. It is measured in mrad and represents the angle described by the raw laser beam from the laser. This value is mode dependent and has the smallest value for TEM_{00}. Typical values for industrial CO_2 lasers are smaller than 3 mrad and for Nd:YAG lasers smaller than 15 mrad. Also the divergence may show an important temporal variation because of the thermal load of several system components during operation. Under thermal load beam-bending effects also may occur. Another sort of laser beam deformation may occur because of beam diffraction effects, if the laser beam accidentally touches scattering objects not supposed to interfere with the beam. The most common example is a laser beam delivery tube having too small an inner diameter compared with the laser beam diameter at any place along the tube (the inner diameter of the tube should be at least 1.6 times larger than the raw beam diameter at any place along the tube).

For measuring the high-power laser beam diameter, adequate devices are available on the market, but it is important to verify the definition of the measurement, because not all devices use identical definitions. Normally the envelope surface of a laser beam including 95% of the locally measured laser power, cut with a plane perpendicular to the beam axis, will deliver a curve, which is not necessarily a circle, considered to be the "laser beam diameter."

In case of elliptical curves, the larger diagonal has to be considered for the design of the beam delivery system.

Another laser beam specific property is the beam polarization (circular or linear, polarization degree and angle). There are only a few devices available on the market for the measurement of the beam polarization. It is difficult to define the reference coordinate system for the "polarization angle" measurement in case of linearly polarized laser beams, so that normally the "polarization angle" has to be observed with respect to the cutting or welding direction. Because of the polarizing effects of most reflective optical components, it is important at least to know the orientation of the resulting linear polarization with respect to the cutting or welding direction at the TCP. Especially in the case of 2D processing (e.g., cutting of diverse shapes) a circularly polarized beam is necesary. In such cases it is also possible to use linearly polaized laser beams, but the polarization orientation has to be controlled in real time to keep a constant angle relationship with the cutting path.

Figures 1 and 2 show the results of different laser beam polarization effects.

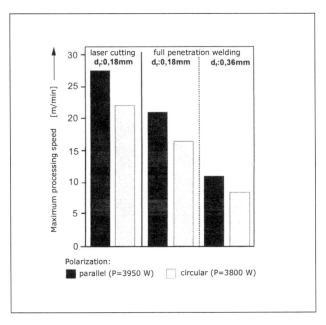

Figure 2. Effect of circular versus linear polarization on maximum processing speed.

4.1.2 Components for Beam Delivery

Telescopes (Collimators)

Some basic facts about the divergence of a laser beam are mentioned in Chapter 3. Figures 3 and 4 show the typical development of the laser beam diameter along the optical axis of the beam delivery system. From these curves it is clear that the beam divergence has to be compensated, at least for the following applications:

- Beam delivery paths longer than 15 m,
- Beam delivery systems with "flying optics," where the length of the beam delivery system varies more than 3 m.

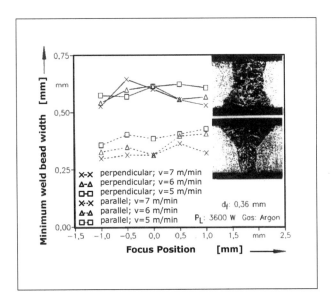

Figure 1. Influence of the orientation of the polarization in tailored blank welding.

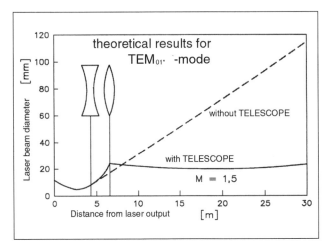

Figure 3. Laser beam diameters change along the beam path.

ISBN 0-912035-15-3

Chapter 4: Components for Laser Materials Processing Systems

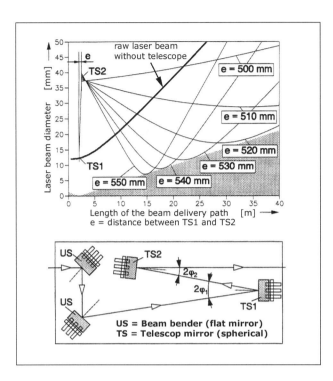

Figure 4. Design of an adjustable coaxial telescope.

Figures 3 and 4 also show how the beam divergence can be compensated with a telescope, substantially reducing the beam diameter at large distances from the laser. Figure 3 shows a simple two-lens design for a collimating telescope. Figure 4 includes the design of an adjustable collimating telescope.

Figure 5 shows typical telescope configurations, both using mirrors (Figs. 5A–D) and lenses (Figs. 5E–G).

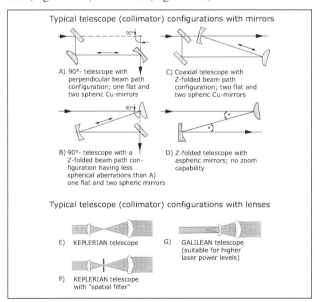

Figure 5. Design concepts for typical telescopes.

The simplest telescope consists of two lenses (see Figs. 5E–G). The types E and F can only be used at low power levels (< 1 kW CW) because of the high power density within the focus between the lenses. The maximum power that can be handled by the type G depends on the effectiveness of the cooling system for the two lenses (power levels up to 5 kW have been reported).

The advantages and disadvantage of the lens-based collimators are:

Advantages
- Coaxial design
- Good adjustability
- Light weight
- Reasonable prices
- Small aberrations

Disadvantage
- The thermal lens deformations have to be considered

For high power levels reflective telescopes with water-cooled mirrors are needed. Some of the currently used concepts are presented in Figures 5A–D. The simplest divergence compensation consists of one focusing mirror with a long focal distance (no drawing). Such a solution can be used only in case of a determined, unchangeable beam delivery system length. The aberrations generated by such an off-axis focusing mirror might be important and very sensitive to thermal load (direct water cooling indispensable). A common telescope (Fig. 5D) built with two off-axis aspheric mirrors delivers a parallel beam with the input and has three major disadvantages:

- Difficult alignment and adjustment
- Design has to match the beam quality
- Design sensitive to aberrations (also thermally induced)

Two slightly different "90°-telescope" concepts including spherical mirrors are presented as Figures 5A and B. The 90° concept simplifies the alignment and adjustment capability. Also the amount of aberration is smaller than D. On the other hand, the amount of aberration is expected to be larger for A than for B.

The best technical concept is presented in Figures 4 and 5C. It has a coaxial design, which assures the best alignment and adjustment capability, but for best results two mirrors have to be moved (second US-flat mirror and TS1 in Fig. 4) for adjustment. These linear movements can also be motorized in order to be remotely controlled.

Adjustable telescopes can also be designed by taking adaptive mirrors into consideration. Adjustable telescopes are useful for the following reasons:

- Variable length of the beam path (more than 3 m)
- Long beam delivery paths (more than 15 m)
- Beam switching between processing stations
- Compensation of large undesired thermally induced changes of the beam divergence

ISBN 0-912035-15-3

One of the most important characteristics of a telescope to be specified is the magnification of the diameter of the raw laser beam. The other characteristics to be specified are the beam power, the beam quality (divergence), the free beam aperture input/output, and the distance to the laser beam output.

Beam Bending Units for CO_2 Laser Beams

Beam bending units are often considered to be simple components so that many machine manufacturers of laser material processing systems produce their own beam bending units and purchase only the Cu mirrors from suppliers.

The small, but important, details of the beam bending units represent the subject of this section. It is not possible to present beam bending units without discussing the Cu mirrors themselves. For low power levels indirectly water cooled mirrors are used. For high power levels the mirrors are directly cooled, usually with water flowing through coolant channels, which are buried within the Cu mirror body.

From the thermal point of view, the necessary cooling water flow rate for both types of mirrors is as low as 1–2 L/min at a temperature of 20 to 24°C (68–75°F). In practice much higher cooling water flow rates are used, because of improper cooling channel design and the resulting unacceptable mirror deformation under thermal load. Higher water flow rates can be achieved by increasing the water pressure. Especially in the case of directly cooled mirrors, water pressure values higher than 5 bar will lead to additional unacceptable mirror surface deformations, so that such pressures should be avoided. The most common water cooling channel design consists of parallel nuts, which are interconnected at their ends. Under thermal load this design will always lead to a slight heat-dependent bending effect. This effect can be neglected for short beam delivery systems with large free laser beam apertures.

Better results (lower mirror deformation under thermal load) can be obtained with spiral-shaped coolant channels. Thermal deformations will then lead to slight changes of the mirror curvature, because the spiral starts in the middle of the mirror and ends at its circumference and so a radial temperature (positive or negative) gradient will occur under thermal load. This means that such a mirror becomes slightly divergent if the cold cooling water is connected in the middle of the mirror, and slightly convergent, if the cold cooling water is connected at the circumference of the mirror. The best results can be obtained with double-spiral-shaped coolant channels. The cooling water flows through the two spiral-shaped coolant channels in alternate directions, and the resulting thermal load deformation is a parallel translation of the mirror surface. This design starts to become necessary for laser power levels higher than 12 kW CW or for the case that the lowest possible wave front deformation is requested.

Other sources of mirror deformations are:

- Shipment of improperly packed single mirrors
- Improperly mounted mirrors (unbalanced or too great mounting force) (see Fig. 6)

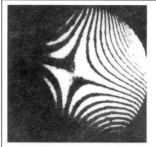 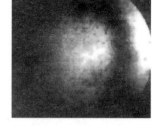

a) Interferogram of a flat Cu-mirror with ø 100 mm disadvantageously (too tight) mounted on holder

b) Interferogram of the same flat Cu-mirror as a), correctly mounted on holder

Figure 6. Influence of the metallic mirror mounting force on mirror surface deformation.

Both problems can be solved if the mirrors are not mounted directly onto the beam bending unit, but first onto a stiff mirror holder plate. Then the mirror and holder plate are treated as one entity (see Figs. 7 and 8). This procedure has another important advantage, because no additional readjustment of an exchanged mirror unit (premounted mirror onto holder plate) will be necessary.

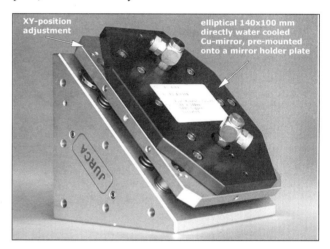

Figure 7. Beam bending unit with a free beam aperature of 100 mm.

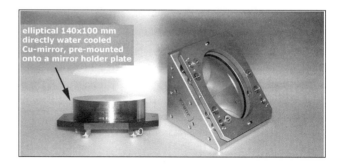

Figure 8. Beam bending unit with a free beam aperature of 100 mm, disassembled.

Because of safety requirements for the beam bending units, each mounted mirror has to be sensed by a microswitch or a similar device. This switch should be wired as an interlock switch within a laser material processing system.

The cleaning process for the mirrors integrated into the beam bending units usually takes place according to a specific experience-based time schedule. This procedure has to be done very carefully, because just opening the beam delivery tube might lead to a swirling motion of the dirt particles deposited within the beam delivery system and consequent contamination of the mirrors surfaces. A very simple device can help to avoid opening the beam delivery system just for a visual inspection of the beam bending mirror surfaces. It is a device capable of measuring the temperature difference between the cooling water input and output of each single mirror of a beam delivery system.

An increased mirror absorption due to a contaminated mirror surface leads to a higher temperature reading. A microprocessor-based processing unit can handle up to five temperature difference measuring modules and generates an alarm signal when preset limits will be exceeded.

A further step for higher system efficiency and improved handling of the beam delivery system is motorizing the beam bending units. The typical resolution in the X or Y direction is 1.15×10^{-6} degree of mirror inclination. Such a device can be combined with a laser beam position detector within the beam delivery system in order to build an on-line or off-line auto-alignment system. This might save hours and days of adjustment/alignment work (see Fig. 9). For the adjustment work a remote terminal with a keypad and a small graphic display is available.

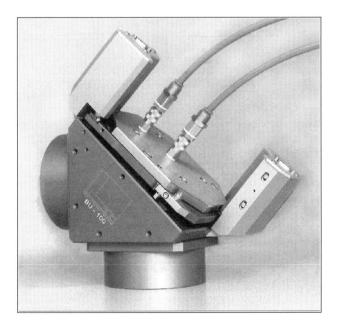

Figure 9. Motorized beam bending unit.

Usually the beam delivery system has to be sealed in order to allow a slight purge gas pressurization with dry and absolutely clean air, especially free of oil. This means that the beam bending units have to have seals between their housings and the mirror body.

Adaptive Mirrors

Adaptive mirrors are flat or spherical mirrors that can change surface curvature in response to an input signal. Adaptive mirrors are usually required in laser material processing systems in order to control the propagation of the raw beam through the beam delivery and guiding system by compensating the axial shifts of the focal position due to the thermal load of the optical components. Correspondingly the focal position of the entire laser material processing system can be kept in a constant position or changed according to the necessary position of the focal point. Adaptive optics are particularly important for applications with "flying optics," where the varying distance between laser source and focusing head causes important changes of the beam diameter. If one uses an adaptive mirror within a beam expander located near the laser source, the beam diameter on the focusing optics can be kept constant for a large working area. Also thermal deformation of the mirrors as part of the beam path and thermal blooming may be prevented by use of closed-loop control systems and defined variation of the optical behavior.

Additionally the adaptive control of the focal position, dependent on external sensors, can track workpiece height tolerances in a range up to 10 mm in real time without any other moving axis than the adaptive mirror. For focal position control the adaptive mirror can be integrated into the beam delivery system or into the focusing head itself.

Usually adaptive mirrors may have almost any radius as the nominal curvature radius, because they are manufactured at a certain customer-specified water pressure. From this nominal radius positive and negative deformations are possible. The total deformation is relatively small, but large enough for most industrial applications. On the other hand, too-large deformations can diminish the laser beam quality.

Most common implemented deformation control principles for adaptive mirrors can be listed as follows:

Hydraulic deformation is based on the principle of deformation of a circular plate under hydrostatic pressure. Usually in high-power material processing applications, all bending and focusing mirrors are copper mirrors with internal water cooling. The pressure that will force the deformation of the mirror is applied by the cooling water, which is circulating on the backside of the mirror.

The cooling water pressure is controlled with analog electromagnetic valves. The resulting deformation has a nearly parabolic characteristic (see Figs. 10–12). A major disadvantage of the hydraulic principle is its limited control frequency.

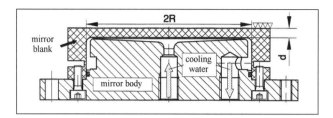

Figure 10. Sectional drawing of a typical adaptive mirror.

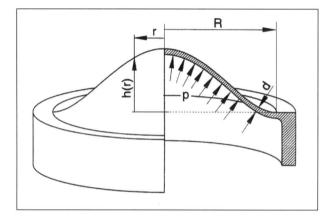

Figure 11. Schematic drawing showing the working principle of a hydraulic adaptive mirror.

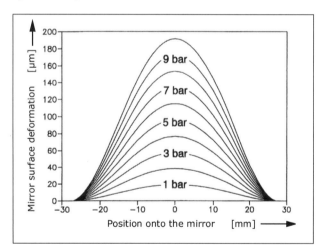

Figure 12. Mechancial deformation of the mirror surface for various values of the water pressure.

Piezoelectric deformation also acts on the backside of the mirror by direct force of one or more piezoelectric actuators. As a result of the working principle, a high reaction frequency is possible. With a special copper material for the mirror, a bandwidth up to 1000 Hz is available. The range of variation of the refractive power or focal length can be shifted from - 40 m to -3 m. For large deformations the mirror surface may lose its spherical shape. For the best possible spherical deformation, the laser beam diameter should not be larger than 50% of the total mirror diameter. This limitation applies also for the hydraulic deformation-based adaptive mirrors.

Figure 13 shows one typical application of an adaptive mirror, which represents a real-time closed-loop workpiece height tracking system. For this application a plasma sensor delivers the information concerning the optimum focal position.

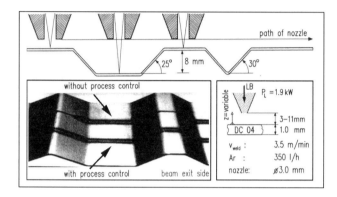

Figure 13. Compensation of workpiece height variation with an adaptive mirror.

4.1.3 Adjustment/Alignment of Beam Delivery Systems

This section will cover the adjustment and alignment of mirror-based beam delivery systems. It will also describe typical alignment procedures and available tools.

Theoretically once a beam delivery system is aligned and adjusted, it should not generate any additional readjustment needs. But usually the beam comes at different positions and at different angles out of the laser. There are also exceptions, but for the machine builder it is better to assume such behavior in order to provide sufficient adjustment space for the beam bending units. Also depending on the design of the beam delivery components, small readjustments might be necessary after changing mirrors. Usual multimirror beam delivery systems have to be realigned two to five times per year. The typical time necessary for realignment is between 2 hours and 2 days.

One of the best-known alignment methods is based on the use of a visible HeNe laser already integrated within the laser itself. For all alignment methods based on the HeNe laser pointer, a perfect prealignment of the HeNe laser beam precisely onto the optical axis of the high-power laser beam is necessary. This should be checked from time to time. Figure 14 shows a typical mirror-based focusing head with a horizontal path. The focusing mirror assembly has been removed and exchanged with an adjusting mirror assembly. The adjusting mirror is precisely preadjusted with its surface perpendicular to the optical axis of the focusing head. This mirror reflects the HeNe laser beam precisely back into the beam delivery system.

ISBN 0-912035-15-3

Chapter 4: Components for Laser Materials Processing Systems

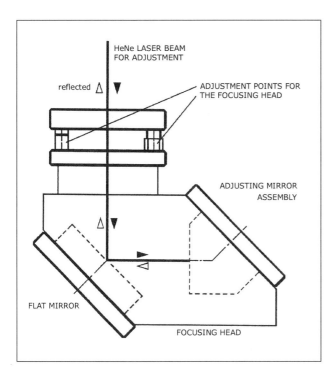

Figure 14. Typical placement of the adjusting mirror assembly.

Figure 15 shows how to evaluate the position of the reflected HeNe laser beam between the laser output and the machine.

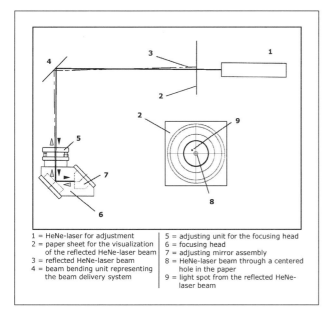

1 = HeNe-laser for adjustment
2 = paper sheet for the visualization of the reflected HeNe-laser beam
3 = reflected HeNe-laser beam
4 = beam bending unit representing the beam delivery system
5 = adjusting unit for the focusing head
6 = focusing head
7 = adjusting mirror assembly
8 = HeNe-laser beam through a centered hole in the paper
9 = light spot from the reflected HeNe-laser beam

Figure 15. Sketch showing the optical adjustment procedure.

This alignment method is very reliable and simple and needs only one optical component, the adjusting mirror assembly. Another advantage is the fact that the HeNe laser beam passes two times through the beam delivery system, so that all angular misalignment of the mirrors within the beam delivery system will be amplified by two.

Another alignment method is based on the fact that the focusing head is the most precise and best preadjusted component within a laser beam delivery system. Again removing the focusing mirror assembly and coupling a preadjusted visible laser beam precisely into the optical axis of the focusing head makes a "backward" adjustment of the entire beam delivery system possible. Another advantage is that the machine builder in this case is independent of the HeNe laser integrated into the high-power laser.

In combination with a HeNe laser beam XY-position detector, which can be placed sequentially into the beam bending units, all mirrors can be precisely readjusted step by step. This procedure can also be automated by motorizing the adjustment mechanism of the beam bending units and closing the loop with the position detector. Such systems are feasible at moderate prices, but they remain off-line working systems based on a different laser beam as the working beam.

In principle it is possible to build such an automatic beam alignment system, which can also work on-line based on the position detection of the main high power laser beam during operation (see Fig. 16).

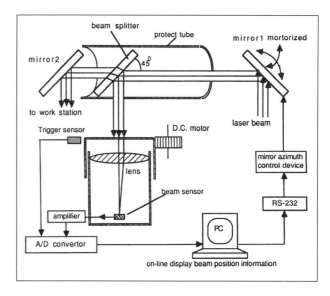

Figure 16. Laser beam position detection using a rotating beam.

Based on present estimates, such systems are not really necessary for beam delivery path lengths within the range up to approximately 20 m (depending on the laser source and beam path length variation during operation), because the lasers are sufficiently stable for such an operation. Larger machines will profit from this technology within the next few years.

MARIUS JURCA

4.2 Focusing Optics

4.2.0 Introduction
Section 3.2 covers beam delivery up to the point of the final optical element that focuses the laser beam onto the workpiece. This section is concerned with the focusing elements, which includes lenses, mirrors, and diffractive optical elements.

4.2.1 Lenses
The most common optical elements used for focusing laser beams are lenses.

Design

The performance of a lens is closely related to the way the manufacturer makes it. The designer needs to keep in mind the end use and cost factors for his design. Therefore, the designer needs to work closely with the manufacturer's optical engineers in deciding the tradeoff among image quality, number of lens elements, and cost. Using fewer elements and flatter lens surfaces allows more lenses to be placed on a single polishing block. The selection of the material used can also dramatically affect the end cost.

Because of the potentially high power levels associated with laser material processing, the designer needs to be familiar with the absorption in an optic. This is a rather complex subject because of its varied origins. Absorption problems may originate in the base material, the coating materials and processes, the interfaces, inclusions in the coatings, and surface contamination. Each material has its own characteristic absorption coefficient. However, different production techniques lead to large variations from vendor to vendor.

The effects of absorption can be optical distortion, which causes the optical performance of the lens to become distorted, and thermal runaway, when heat builds up in the optic faster than it can be conducted away, resulting in catastrophic damage.

Since there is no universal best lens material, it is important for the designer to optimize each different type of optic for its particular laser type and application.

Simple Lenses

A simple lens is a one-element optic, usually with a focal length less than 254 mm. Simple lenses can be meniscus, plano-convex/concave, or aspheric.

Plano-convex lenses are the industry's choice for focusing many laser beams and are used for the widest variety of laser processing applications, including cutting, welding, heat treating, scribing, and selective removal in a broad range of metals, plastics, and composites. Plano-convex lenses utilize one spherical convex surface and one flat surface. They combine the advantages of precision focusing and low spherical aberration in the visible and near-infrared regions with cost effectiveness and maximum process tolerance (see Fig. 1).

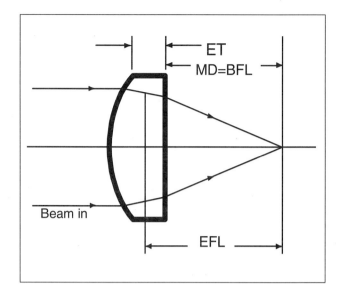

Figure 1. Plano-convex lens.

Positive-meniscus lenses (concave-convex) offer minimum spherical aberration in the far-infrared and are used for high-precision material processing applications, such as ceramic scribing and machining (see Fig. 2), fine metal cutting, high-accuracy material removal, and paper and plastic cutting. Positive-meniscus lenses achieve the smallest focal spot sizes for infrared lasers to produce the minimum heat-affected zone in the laser processed material. These lenses are manufactured with the highest-quality, low-absorption coatings and materials matched to requirements of the laser application, operating environment, and service life. Lens materials for infrared application include zinc selenide (ZnSe), gallium arsenide (GaAs), and germanium (Ge).

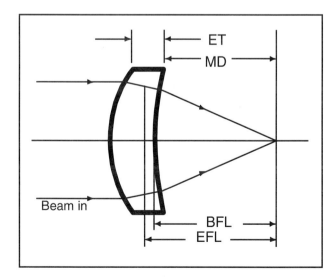

Figure 2. Positive-meniscus lens.

The *effective focal length (EFL)* of a lens can best be described by imagining that all the focusing action of the lens takes place not at the two surfaces, but rather at one plane surface. An incoming ray is drawn straight to that plane, and then straight to the focal point as if all the "effective" power of the lens were in that plane. EFL is the physical distance along the optical axis from the plane to the focal point. It is this distance that is calculated from the lensmaker's equation, and that should be used in various theoretical calculations, such as spot sizes. (See any elementary optics text for the lensmaker's equation.)

Back focal length (BFL) is the physical distance between the surface of the lens closest to the work and the focal plane. Because this reference surface closest to the work is flat for plano-convex lenses, the back focal length is equal to the *mounting distance (MD)*. Since positive-meniscus lenses use two curved surfaces, the back focal length for these lenses is not equal to the mounting distances. The mounting distance is also known as the working distance.

Edge thickness (ET) is an important factor in determining the mechanical strength of the lens. As the edge thickness increases, the ability of the lens to handle assist gas pressures associated with the process also increases.

Compound Lenses

A compound lens is one made of two or more separate lenses. Compound lenses have shapes that when put together, reduce spherical aberration, which is inherent in a simple single lens. Generally for laser systems they take the form of either double lenses (doublets) or triple lenses (triplets) (see Figs. 3 and 4).

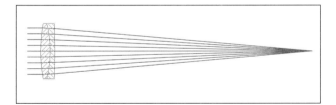

Figure 3. Doublet lens.

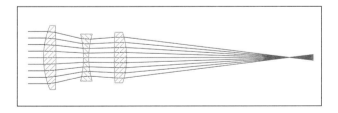

Figure 4. Triplet lens.

Aspheric Lenses

Aspheric lenses are simple one-component lenses designed to reduce spherical aberration. In general, the correction is accomplished by diamond turning one surface of the lens to a calculated aspheric curve. As a result, the aspheric lens provides the tightest focused spot and highest power density possible. However, aspheric lenses are generally higher in cost than those with spherical surfaces.

For many applications, such as thin section cutting or drilling, the higher the irradiance at the focus, the faster the processing speed. Irradiance can be increased by increasing power laser or by decreasing the focal length of the lens. The diameter of the minimum focused spot is proportional to the focal length; hence the area is proportional to the focal length squared. For example, decreasing the focal length by a factor of 2 (e.g., from 127 to 63.5 mm), decreases the spot diameter by 2, but the irradiance increases by a factor of 4.

In this way, short-focal-length aspheric lenses produce very high irradiance, but may be limited in their application because of a shallower depth of focus.

Consequently, the higher irradiance must be traded off against a decrease in depth of focus which is proportional to the square of the focal length. Therefore, aspheric lenses are appropriate for use with thin materials and in high-speed operations where the material can be held within the tolerances of the depth of focus of the lens.

Materials for Infrared Transmitting Lenses

Lenses used for applications in the visible spectrum employ glass. But glass does not transmit in the infrared region.

Depending on the application and laser type, there are basically three usable wavelength regions within the infrared spectrum. These regions are defined by the transmission of the atmosphere. At other infrared wavelengths the atmosphere is absorbing. The first region is in the near-infrared from 0.8 to 2.4 µm, the second region is in the mid-infrared from 3 to 5 µm, and the third is the far-infrared from 8 to 12 µm. The optical materials that transmit in these wavelengths are referred to as IR materials.

Germanium (Ge) has evolved as an important infrared material. Originally developed as a semiconductor material, Ge is used in the far-infrared wavelength region, mainly in forward-looking infrared (FLIR) systems, thermal imaging systems, and CO_2 laser processing. The metallic element Ge is not found in nature but is almost always recovered from processing residue of other materials such as copper and zinc. Ge is opaque in the visible region, which makes it difficult to align Ge optics. The refractive index of Ge is 4.0 at 10.6 µm, which would cause high reflection loss, but if one coats germanium with an anti-reflection (AR) coating, the reflectance per surface becomes less than 0.25%.

Germanium has high mechanical strength, which makes it less susceptible to breakage than other infrared materials. It has an excellent hardness, which helps in achieving a quality polish.

Because of the relatively large absorption coefficient of Ge, which causes a buildup of heat energy, a Ge lens will show rapid deterioration because of temperature increase. Therefore, a Ge lens cannot be used with high-power lasers.

Silicon (Si) is the most economical infrared material available because of its abundance on earth. Like germanium, Si is mainly used in the semiconductor industry. Because of its limited transmission range, the only wavelength region where Si could be used as a transmissive optic is in the 3–5 μm region. Therefore, Si is most often used as a CO_2 laser mirror because of its excellent thermal conductivity, hardness, and chemical durability.

Zinc selenide (ZnSe) has been used as an infrared material for several decades. Until the early 1970s, ZnSe was known as Irtran 4, a polycrystalline hot-pressed material. Since that time, chemically vapor deposited (CVD) ZnSe has become available and has now all but replaced Irtran 4. Most properties of Irtran 4 and CVD ZnSe are nearly identical except that Irtran 4 has unacceptable absorption for laser applications. ZnSe is used primarily in FLIR windows and CO_2 components. It can also serve for chromatic correction in predominantly germanium FLIR lens systems.

Because the low absorption coefficient of ZnSe significantly reduces the chances of thermal runaway, it has found use in high-power HF-DF lasers and high-power CO_2 lasers. ZnSe has less thermal focusing problems than the other materials and is used for partial reflectors, output couplers, and lenses. Because of its relatively high refractive index of 2.403 at 10.6 μm, ZnSe needs to be AR coated for efficient operation. The cost of ZnSe optics increases very rapidly as their size increases.

Zinc sulfide (ZnS) is also produced by a CVD process, which is very similar to the one used to produce ZnSe. Like ZnSe, ZnS is a polycrystalline zinc chalcogenide. ZnS has better mechanical strength, however, and is thus better suited to serve as a window material for high-speed aircraft. It also provides better rain erosion resistance. Because of its higher absorption and reduced optical transmission at 10.6 μm, ZnS is typically used for windows and domes in FLIR systems.

Clear or multispectrum zinc sulfide can be fabricated by subjecting ZnS to thermal treatment under significant pressure. This causes the material to become clear and transparent in the visible wavelength region while maintaining the infrared transmission properties of the standard CVD process ZnS. This clear ZnS has been successfully tested as an aspheric focusing lens as an alternative to the traditional optics in high-power Nd:YAG laser systems.

Gallium arsenide (GaAs) is a binary compound resulting from the chemical combination of gallium and arsenic. GaAs is another semiconductor material, with some properties superior to those of silicon. Only a small percentage of GaAs is used for optoelectronic devices such as diode lasers and infrared detectors. An even smaller percentage is specifically grown for use as infrared materials for CO_2 optics.

Gallium arsenide can be used as an alternative to ZnSe in high-power CO_2 lasers. It can sometimes handle high irradiance better than ZnSe optics; however, thermally induced optical distortion is worse. Although the absorption coefficient for GaAs is about ten times higher than for ZnSe, the nearly three times greater thermal conductivity offsets this sufficiently. Sometimes GaAs can outperform ZnSe in high-power CO_2 systems, but there is no cost advantage in choosing GaAs over ZnSe.

There are many other infrared transmitting crystals. Some are not of commercial value, although they are of great interest to researchers.

Heavy metal salts such as silver chloride (AgCl), silver bromide (AgBr), and thallium bromide (KRS-5) transmit well into the infrared. They are quite soft and easily hot pressed. Their softness makes them difficult to polish. Heavy metal salts have a tendency to darken upon exposure to light because of a photochemical reaction. For these and other reasons heavy metal salts are not useful in laser or thermal imaging optics.

Cadmium sulfide (CdS) and cadmium telluride (CdTe) are useful infrared materials, although their use has somewhat declined over the years. Optical-grade CdTe has been used as a window or output coupler for low-power CO_2 lasers.

Sapphire is aluminum oxide (Al_2O_3). Single-crystal sapphire can be produced in commercial quantities and sizes. It is a very hard material and can be used in the short-wavelength infrared regions.

Diamond is also an excellent infrared material. It is the hardest material in nature. This makes it hard and expensive to polish. Also it is very expensive and traditionally only available in very small sizes. However, new CVD diamond has become available recently and is finding applications in certain high-power CO_2 lasers, where high irradiance limits the performance of ZnSe.

Spectral transmission curves plus other physical and optical data for these and other materials are presented in Section 4.3.6.

Damage Thresholds

The point at which optics begin to fail due to exposure to laser radiation is called the *damage threshold* (see Section 1.2.4). For cw laser beams the damage threshold depends on the material, cooling method, beam diameter, mode structure, and total power in the beam. In other words, there is no one number that determines the damage threshold. For example, many waveguide CO_2 lasers operate with cw irradiance of up to 50 kW/cm^2, but most optics would be damaged severely if there actually were 50 kW of total power in a one square centimeter area. Although the optics can withstand the peak value, the heat load from 50 kW total power would be excessive. Most important, for cw beams it is not damage, but rather optical distortion that limits the performance of optics and causes mode problems, loss of laser power, and/or focusing problems. This occurs at power levels significantly lower than the level that produces damage. Therefore, for the cw lasers we generally discuss power-handling capability rather than damage threshold. Damage threshold is meaningful for short pulse lasers such as CO_2 TEA lasers or Q-switched Nd:YAG lasers.

The following information and examples are provided as general guidelines for power-handling capability of substrate and coatings.

In waveguide CO_2 lasers, inside cavity power densities of up to 50 kW/cm² in 2-mm-diameter beams are possible with the proper heat sinking and low-absorption coatings.

Typical industrial CO_2 lasers, emitting 500-2000 W and having 10–15 mm-diameter beams, and circulating power 1000–4,000 W, have average power densities 1–4 kW/cm². Note that peak power in a TEM_{00} mode is twice the average power density.

Larger industrial lasers, emitting 5000 W, have 10-kW circulating power in a 4-cm-diameter beam, so that the average power density is less than 1 kW/cm². If the same laser has a 2.5-cm-diameter beam, the average power density would be 2 kW/cm². With a 1.3-cm-diameter beam, the average power density would be 7.5 kW/cm².

Studies performed by Los Alamos National Laboratory in the 1970s showed the following for TEA CO_2 lasers.

In the pulse-length regime characteristic of TEA CO_2 lasers, approximately 1–200 ns, the energy density damage threshold scales with the square root of the pulse length; so if the threshold is known at one pulse length, it can be calculated for other pulse lengths.

For moderate lifetime (say 1,000–10,000 pulses) the energy density must be a factor of 4 below the single pulse energy damage threshold. For long lifetime (say 10,000 pulses and up) the factor has to be 10.

For a 1 ns pulse energy the damage threshold was in the 0.5–1.0 J/cm² range for common ZnSe and Ge optics.

Absorption

The absorption of an optical element depends on the material, the antireflection or partial reflection coating, and the contaminants deposited on the surface during routine materials processing or laser use.

Absorption in an optical element is a rather complex subject because of its varied origin. The base material has its own characteristic absorption coefficient (i.e., bulk absorption for zinc selenide is typically in the range between 0.0005 and 0.0006 cm⁻¹).

The excess heat generated by too much absorption leads to physical changes in the properties of the optical element that degrade its performance. This can manifest itself in a phenomenon called *optical distortion*. This happens when the center of the element (where most of the laser beam's energy hits) expands relative to the cooler material around it.

The result depends on the type of optical element, but in a focusing lens, for example, this causes a shortening of the focal length, which can lead to severe process problems. If this heat buildup happens very fast, the optic might experience thermal runaway, at which point catastrophic damage may occur (see Fig. 5).

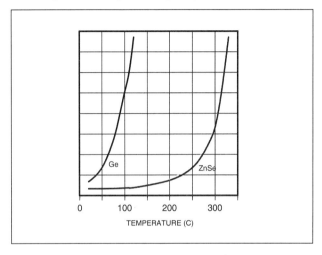

Figure 5. Rapid increase in absorption in a CO_2 optic can lead to thermal runaway, rendering the optic useless. The y-axis gives the Absorption Coefficient, starting at zero and increasing in units of 0.001 cm⁻¹.

The figure shows the temperature dependence of the absorption coefficient β of two infrared transmitting substrate materials. When the temperature is such that β is in a steeply rising portion of the curve, thermal runaway sets in. Then the optic is absorbing laser energy at a high rate, which further increases the temperature, and therefore β, so that the rate of absorption increases still further. This process continues until the optic melts, burns, or fractures from the large stress created by thermal expansion of the heated material against cooler material near the periphery.

Fortunately, before an overheated optical element enters this stage, the optical distortion usually so affects the system performance that in most cases the laser is shut down before damage occurs. The way in which optical distortion affects performance depends not only on the degree of distortion, but also on the use of each particular distorted optic. A window used to extract energy from an unstable resonator cavity may withstand a great deal of distortion before performance suffers because it does not form part of the resonator, whereas a Brewster window internal to the cavity may affect laser performance when distortion is minimal. Perhaps the components most sensitive to optical distortion are output couplers because they must serve both as cavity reflectors and also as beam transmitters. In reflection they affect laser performance as total reflectors may, while in transmission they affect beam focusability.

Thus the best way to extend the lifetime of an optical element is to keep the absorption level as low as possible. The first step in extending operating life is to start with an element that has the lowest initial absorption possible.

The next step is regular optics maintenance. Even though the amount of contaminants deposited on an element varies depending on the laser process performed and the air quality surrounding the laser, regular cleaning can extend the optics lifetime. Make sure to handle each optical element carefully, following the cleaning instructions provided by the manufacturer.

Lens Protection Techniques

Windows may be used to protect the lenses from laser plume and splatter from the process. The window is generally installed in front of the lens either by mounting together with the lens or using a cartridge-style lens holder that can be interchanged quickly in the event the window is damaged. This technique can increase the lifetime of more expensive lenses; however, it can also introduce distortion, which can negatively affect the laser processing.

Cover gases are used for a variety of reasons in laser welding. These include protection of focusing optics, control of weld plasma, and protection of the weld bead from contamination and oxidation.

There are several ways of applying the cover gas. A flow of gas coaxial with the laser beam prevents smoke and mild splatter from depositing on the focusing optics. However, this type of cover gas arrangement will not prevent violent splatters from reaching the final focusing lens or mirror, even for relatively long focal lengths, such as 25 cm. To stop or minimize the damage to optics from violent ejection of molten material, a strong crossflow of air is frequently employed. This technique must be applied carefully to avoid disruption and contamination of the weld bead by the airflow.

The gas jet manifold provides a means for primary gas to be introduced through the tip and secondary gas around the tip for gas-assisted laser processing and lens protection. The gas jet as shown in Figure 6 provides minimal jet turbulence and maximizes the effect of laser cutting processing. The gas jet tip is usually a separate and easily removable copper piece held in place by a tip retainer nut.

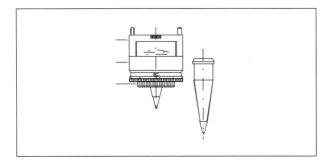

Figure 6. Sample of a gas jet manifold and nozzle.

Cooling Techniques

Cooling of lenses is accomplished by heat sinking the lens in the mount which in turn is in contact with a massive metal structure that may be water cooled. Sometimes a thicker lens is used to allow greater surface contact to the heatsink to minimize thermal distortion. However, the finite thermal conductivity of ZnSe fundamentally limits the heat flow rate and, therefore, the power levels at which this material can be used. Large thermal gradients in the lens create local distortion of the beam in the center of the optic and also increase the "hoop stress" at the edges, leading to microfracture propagation and early thermal stress failures.

Heat generated in the lens moves from the center to the edge and into the optical mount, where the heat is dissipated (see Fig. 7). The flow of heat is in the radial direction, creating both a significant radial thermal gradient and a rise in the absolute temperature of the lens. As the power load from the laser increases, the temperature (and, consequently, the structural forces) near the center of the lens increase as well, finally resulting in significant stress as well as thermal distortion. Since material stress is one of the primary causes of failure, heating of the lens in this fashion may contribute to shortened lifetimes, in addition to poor performance.

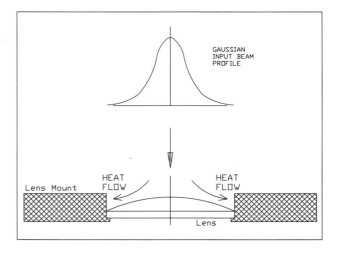

Figure 7. Schematic diagram of a normally cooled lens to a lens mount. Heat flow is radial from the center to the edge of the optic when a Gaussian beam is used.

In order to overcome the seemingly insurmountable thermal distortion and spherical aberration limitations, an optical configuration that avoids using edge-cooled optics was designed. The natural alternative to edge cooling is face cooling. While most face-cooling techniques, however, are naturally inefficient because of weak thermal coupling to the optical cooling surface, one optics manufacturer employs a novel cooling approach using two lenses in an "air-spaced doublet" arrangement that removes heat axially in a very efficient manner. In this design, a turbulent cooling gas (normally air, but also helium or nitrogen for special applications) is injected at high flow rates into the space between the two lenses. Because the thermal path is considerably shorter in the axial direction, the absolute temperature of the optics is much lower, resulting in a significant lowering of both the internal "lifetime-reducing" stresses and the hoop stress at the edge. The radial thermal gradient is also greatly reduced, virtually eliminating temperature-induced spherical aberration.

With these improvements, ZnSe can be used at much higher power levels than can a normal single lens, while still providing diffraction-limited performance.

Lens Performance

A lens is said to be "diffraction limited" when the aberration contribution from the lens is very small, and the performance is primarily governed by diffraction. This is true when the calculated geometric spot size is much smaller than the diffraction spot size. The diffraction-limited spot size is proportional to the beam quality factor (M^2). The more a beam deviates from TEM_{00}, the higher the M^2 value will be, and the larger the minimum obtainable spot size will be (see Section 3.4). A beam is generally considered diffraction limited when the wavefront error is less than 0.25λ.

Higher-order modes are more complex spatial energy distributions than defined by the TEM_{00} mode. Higher-order modes are associated with higher M^2 values and, therefore, create larger focal spots than those obtainable with a perfect Gaussian TEM_{00} beam.

The smallest possible attainable spot size is given by the diffraction limit (down to about twice the wavelength). The diffraction-limited spot diameter for a laser is given by:

$$d_{dl} = 1.27\lambda M^2 (f/BD)^2$$

where $BD = 1/e^2$ x beam diameter at the lens; f, the effective focal length of the lens; λ, the usage wavelength; and M^2, the laser beam quality constant. Note that the beam diameter at the lens should be at least 1.5 m smaller than the clear aperture to avoid truncation effects.

If the lens is diffraction limited, the geometric aberration content is negligible and the spot size is given by the preceding formula. For lenses that are not diffraction limited, the spot size may be estimated by adding the geometric spot to the diffraction spot diameter as given.

As long as the lens focuses to a diffraction-limited spot, the focal spot size is linearly dependent on the focal length, as seen in the equation above. Since power density is proportional to the inverse square of the focal spot size, it is also proportional to the inverse square of the focal length. For example, a doubling of focal length results in one-fourth the power density.

It may be possible to increase the focal length of a lens and still get the same focused spot size. The diffraction-limited spot size varies with $f/\#$, so that if the focal length gets longer, the beam diameter must also get larger to maintain the same $f/\#$ and, therefore, diffraction-limited spot size.

The depth of focus is defined as the axial distance from the focus where the focal spot grows to 1.1 times the diameter at the focus (see Section 3.3.2).

$$Depth\ of\ focus = \pm\ 1.27\lambda M^2 (f/BD)^2$$

If the beam diameter is held constant, then, as the focal length gets shorter, the depth of focus also becomes shorter. All else being constant, the change in depth of focus (*DOF*) can be related as follows:

$$DOF_2 = \left(\frac{f_2}{f_1}\right)^2 DOF_1$$

where f_2 and f_1 are the associated focal lengths.

However, in choosing lenses for applications, a plano-convex lens should be used rather than a meniscus when spherical aberration is not a major concern, or when the $f/\#$ is sufficiently large so as to cause a plano-convex lens to perform as diffraction limited. For ZnSe at 10.6 µm, a good rule of thumb for the $f/\#$ at which there is not much difference between performance of a plano-convex lens and a best-form meniscus lens is at around $f/5$ or $f/6$, in other words, when the focal length is 5 or 6 times the beam diameter or more. Generally, a plano-convex lens is the optic of choice when the beam diameter is small and the focal length is long.

An aspheric focusing lens should be used rather than a best-form meniscus lens when a best-form meniscus lens cannot provide desired diffraction-limited performance. For ZnSe at 10.6 µm, this generally occurs when the $f/\#$ is small (less than around $f/3$) and the input beam quality is very good (i.e., $M^2 \approx 1$).

For high-pressure cutting, it is best to use a lens with the appropriate thickness to handle the required pressure. An equation used to estimate the minimum thickness requirement is that for an unclamped window, using a safety factor of 4. It is as follows:

$$T_{min} = 1.06D(P/F_a)^{1/2}$$

where T_{min} is the minimum lens thickness; F_a, the apparent elastic limit/rupture modulus (7500 psi for ZnSe); P, the pressure (psi); and D, the diameter.

This equation should be considered as an "indicator only," especially at higher powers, since it does not take into account the additional stresses caused by the heated central part of the lens expanding against the cooler periphery of the lens.

The following are factors that degrade the focusing performance of lenses. For laser applications, the most significant is spherical aberration. Spherical aberration is the condition where different radial zones of an axial input beam are focused to different positions along the optical axis. With ordinary spherical lenses (plano-convex and meniscus) the rays near the outer edge of a collimated input beam (marginal rays) are focused closer to the lens than those near the center (paraxial rays). The sketch below further illustrates this concept.

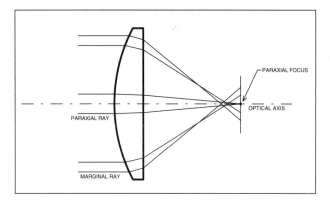

Figure 8. Example of spherical aberration.

A second factor, chromatic aberration, causes the focal length to change with "color" (wavelength). This is caused by the index of refraction of a material changing with wavelength. Generally, shorter wavelengths focus closer to a lens than do longer wavelengths. Chromatic aberration is not generally a problem when focusing a single monochromatic beam.

However, it could be a problem for a laser lens when the intent is to use different wavelength beams with the same lens. One example of this is the case of medical lasers where a HeNe beam is used for alignment purposes, and the CO_2 beam is used for the actual work. In this case, the HeNe beam will focus closer to the lens than the CO_2 beam.

A factor called thermal focusing also affects lens performance. As the lens heats up, the shape and index of refraction change. This shortens the focal spot's position and increases its size.

Finally, in high-power systems that preclude the use of transmissive optics, or in any system where chromatic aberration is to be completely avoided, reflective optics (mirrors) should be used instead of lenses. Focusing with mirrors is covered in the next section.

References
R. Kingslake, *Lens Design Fundamentals*, Academic Press, New York, (1978).
H. Karow, *Fabrication Methods of Precision Optics*, Wiley, New York, (1993).
G. H. Sherman, Electro-Optical System Design **June** (1982).
D. Van Wijk, *Laser Power Focal Point* newsletter **3**, 2 (1997).

J. Evanecky, F. Foote, and T. Von Der Ahe, 1996: *Turbo-Cooled® Optical Assemblies: A New Transmissive Optical Design for Very High Power Industrial CO_2 Lasers*, Laser Power Optics, San Diego, CA.

DANIEL L. SHERMAN

4.2.2 Mirrors

Design

Mirror design for industrial lasers requires the designer to have knowledge of the materials used in fabrication of the mirrors. This implies knowledge of the substrate material, thermal properties, physical properties, the power of the laser, and the cost. Most commonly used materials for either intracavity mirrors or external beam delivery mirrors are silicon and copper.

As to which material is better, there is no single correct answer for all situations because copper and silicon each have their advantages and disadvantages, and both are used in high-power CO_2 lasers depending on the application. Several key factors determine the choice of material for high-power laser mirrors. Engineering tradeoffs between the material's thermal properties, mechanical properties, and cost determine the ultimate choice of substrate material.

Silicon is generally favored for most lasers because of its lower cost compared to copper mirrors. This is particularly true for most cutting systems that utilize 1–2-kW lasers. However, as thermal loading increases, copper tends to dominate because of the ease of machining water cooling channels directly into the copper. Table 1 presents relevant mechanical and thermal properties for copper and silicon.

Table 1. Mechanical and Thermal Properties of Copper vs. Silicon (1)

Parameter	Cu	Si	Units
Specific heat	380	678	J/kg/K
Thermal conductivity	0.941	0.20	Cal/cm^2/cm/s/°C
Mass density	8.96	2.33	g/cm^3
Hardness	3.0	7.0	Mohs

Mirrors are generally coated with a thin film coating to increase the reflectivity and lower the absorbed power from the incident laser beam. The mirror substrate acts as an efficient heat sink to prevent distortion of the mirror surface and deterioration of the laser beam quality. Copper has 2.5 times the thermal conductivity of silicon, which means it conducts the absorbed heat from the coating more effectively than silicon. However, this is offset by the fact that copper has 6.5 times the thermal expansion coefficient of silicon and the surface distorts more for a given increase in temperature. Thus silicon is more thermally stable than copper, resulting in less thermally induced distortion.

Compared to silicon, copper is much easier to machine, making it the material of choice when water cooling passages are required. With internal water cooling close to the mirror surface where the heat is being generated in the coating, the distortion of the copper surface can be kept very low even at power levels in excess of 10 kW. A limitation is that copper is a soft metal that is easier to scratch and is more demanding to polish. This is why copper mirrors are frequently diamond turned. Diamond turning allows for machining of complex shapes such as parabolic focusing mirrors or annular cavity mirrors.

Copper requires extra care in handling and mounting because it is soft and malleable and more easily deformed by mechanical stress. It is also heavier than silicon and requires stronger mechanical mounts, which may add cost to the system.

Spherical Mirrors

Spherical mirrors are used either within a laser cavity as rear mirrors or folding mirrors, or external to the laser as bending mirrors to deliver the beam to the workpiece. Standard laser mirrors are round, square, or rectangular. They may be flat or may have radii machined into the surface. In the case of copper mirrors, they may have water-cooling channels to allow their use in higher-power lasers.

Cylindrical Focusing Mirrors

Cylindrical focusing mirrors are copper mirrors that focus a beam into a line at a 90 degree angle to the incoming beam. They can be useful in surface hardening and surface cladding applications. When they are used in combination with a ring-shaped beam produced with an axicon, a very high uniform intensity profile at the focus can be achieved (see Fig. 9).

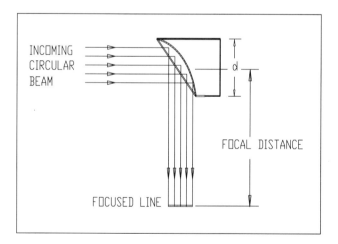

Figure 9. Example of a cylindrical focusing mirror.

Parabolic Focusing Mirrors

A parabolic focusing mirror is a 90 degree off-axis parabola produced by single-point diamond turning of copper. A perfectly aligned incoming beam will be focused to a diffraction-limited spot at 90° from the incoming beam (see Fig. 10).

Since parabolic focusing mirrors are hard to keep aligned and are very sensitive to angular beam shifts, an alternative technology has been developed. The axially cooled assembly, described in Section 4.2.1, overcomes these limitations, providing a potential alternative to parabolic focusing mirrors in certain applications.

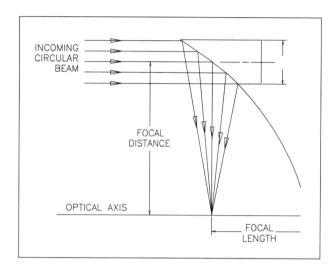

Figure 10. Example of a parabolic focusing mirror.

Coatings

No matter what the substrate material, one usually has a coating on it for surface protection, reflectivity enhancement, and/or polarization control purposes.

A standard total reflector has a coating that should not affect the polarization of the incoming laser beam (see Fig. 11). A reflective 90 degree phase retarder, also commonly called a circular polarizer, has a special coating to transform the linearly polarized beam into a usable circularly polarized beam (see Fig. 12). The notation for S and P polarization is illustrated in Figure 13.

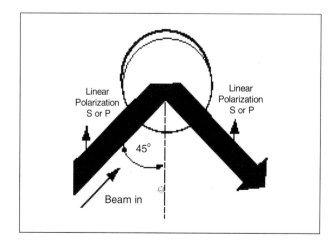

Figure 11. Total reflector coating does not affect polarization or phase as long as input polarization is all S or all P.

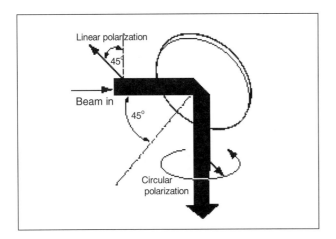

Figure 12. The 90° phase retarder coating turns linear polarization into the needed circular polarization. Input polarization should be half S and half P.

Table 2 (below) presents some values of reflectance at specified angles for some common coatings for CO_2 lasers.

Figure 13 illustrates polarization components, and the related notation follows.

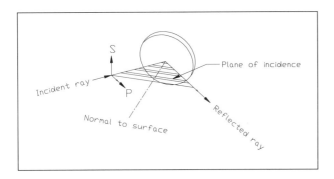

Figure 13. Polarization components illustrated.

S is S polarization, perpendicular to the plane of incidence; P is P polarization, parallel to the plane of incidence; U stands for unpolarized; and the plane is the plane defined by the incident ray and the normal to the surface.

Laser optics manufacturers design innovative coatings to help original equipment manufacturers and laser users solve problems inherent to certain laser applications. For example, it is well known (but rarely discussed) that back (or retro) reflections off the workpiece may upset the laser's intra-cavity conditions, destroying mode quality and power stability. Many process quality problems can be traced to this phenomenon.

One way of dealing with this phenomenon is to use a special coated optic known as an isolation reflector (IRC). This optical element replaces a standard S-polarization oriented 90 degree bending mirror. It absorbs the back-reflected P-polarized component of the laser beam, while passing the outgoing S-polarized component, which contains the laser's processing power (see Fig. 14).

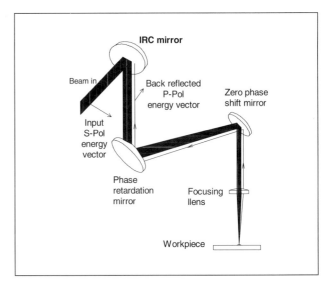

Figure 14. The isolation reflector (IRC) absorbs the back-reflected P-polarized laser beam before it can upset the laser performance.

Table 2. Common Coating Performance References for CO_2 Lasers

COATING DESCRIPTION	Coating Designation	% Reflectance at 10.6 microns				% R at .6328um 45° U	10.6μm phase retardation at 45° equal S&P or Circular	10.6μm phase retardation with zero phase formulation	Comments
		0	45° S	45° P	45° U				
Highly Enhanced Reflectance, Hard	HH	99.75	99.85	99.64	99.75	45	7.7° ± 1°	0 ± 1°	Specially formulated to withstand harsh environment inside laser cavities; harder surface enhances cleanability
Highly Enhanced Reflectance, Proprietary	HP (HC on Cu)	99.82	99.92	99.67	99.79	85 ± 10	8.0° ± 2°	0 ± 2°	Proprietary industrialized coating formulation which combines the best properties of silver (high reflectance) and gold (robustness) and eliminates worst properties of silver (peeling, tarnishing) and gold (low reflectance, high cost)
Enhanced Reflectance, Proprietary	EP (EC on Cu)	99.70	99.84	99.53	99.69	85 ± 10	7.4° ± 2°	0 ± 2°	
Protected Silver	PS	99.3	99.5	99.1	99.5	98	-4.8° ± 1°	NA	Industry standard, best visible performance
Quarterwave Retardation RR Series	90	99.5	99.1	98.1	98.8	70 ± 20	90° ± 2°	NA	Converts linear polarization to circular polarization

A typical application of the IRC mirror is presented here. The incoming S-polarized laser beam strikes the mirror surface at the proper 45° angles so virtually all the power is reflected from the IRC mirror while only a small fraction is scattered or absorbed. After the beam is circularly polarized, it is focused onto the workpiece. When the returning beam energy encounters the circular polarizing mirror, it again becomes linearly polarized light, but with its polarization in the P direction. Returning along the beam path, when it strikes the IRC mirror, it is absorbed based on the reflectance values specified. Virtually none of the reflected beam reaches the laser cavity from the workpiece, thereby minimizing stability problems, power fluctuations, etc.

Mounting

Generally all industrial laser manufacturers have standard internal and external mounts for either copper or silicon mirrors. However, most optics manufacturers have available many different mounts for external use in laser beam trains. Beam bender blocks, cutting heads, welding heads, boring heads, automatic tracking heads, and many other types of delivery mounts are available. See Figure 15 for an illustration of a beam bender block.

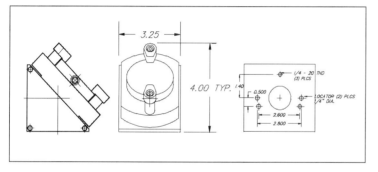

Figure 15. Sample of a beam bender block.

Reference

Laser Power Optics 1995: *High Performance Replacement Optics for Industrial CO_2 Lasers and Systems*, Laser Power Optics, San Diego, CA, 5–11.

DANIEL L. SHERMAN

4.2.3 Diffractive Optics

A diffractive optical element uses diffraction to focus/control the wavefront, whereas an ordinary lens operates under the principle of refraction. One kind of diffractive optical element is known as a "kinoform" (see Fig. 16). This is a diamond-turned surface-relief diffractive optic made up of several zones typically spaced to cause modulo 2π phase jumps. While the cross-section often resembles a Fresnel lens, the zone spacings on a Fresnel lens are much larger than those of a diffractive optical element, so that refraction (rather than diffraction) is really the primary operating mechanism for a Fresnel lens.

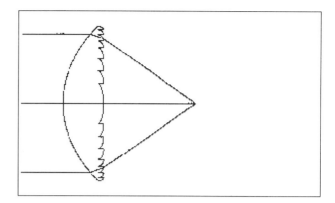

Figure 16. Cross section of kinoform.

Unlike binary optics, which are stepwise approximations to the ideal phase profile, the diamond turning allows the continuous machining of the aspheric profile within each zone. Consequently, this manufacturing technique is able to come very close to the ideal profile, resulting in higher-efficiency optics.

The surface relief (on the order of a few wavelengths) is controlled by the precision of the CNC diamond turning lathe. Although best suited for longer infrared wavelengths, like 8–12 µm, diamond turning has yielded diffractive optics for certain applications for near-infrared and visible wavelengths.

Diffractive optical elements can be used for aberration correction, wavefront shaping, and scanning, as well as for beam focusing, collimation, and deflection. The technology of diffractive optics is not nearly as mature as that of refractive optics or reflective optics, but it is developing rapidly.

DANIEL L. SHERMAN

4.2.4 Focusing Head and Integrated Actuators

The focusing head represents one of the most critical components of a beam delivery system. The quality of the laser processing depends strongly on the focusing head performance. The user of the laser technology desires to have the simplest possible focusing head without any actuators or sensors. On the other hand, considering the technology accepted on the market, most users are prepared to take a risk, if a better and more efficient technology becomes available. So the trend in this field is toward more complex, but application-specific, products. Key words include integrated sensors and actuators, closed-loop systems, self-learning or self-adapting systems. This section will present some of the newest available technologies in this field.

Figure 17 shows three possibilities for off-axis heads, which build rotary axes into focusing heads for increased flexibility. The first rotary axis (called the *C* axis) can be very useful in the case of the integration of seam tracking devices. The combination of the two axes (*C* and *A* axis) offers the advantage of being able to achieve the necessary inclination of the laser beam onto the workpiece surface. However, the additional components and sensors increase the weight (higher mechanical inertia) of the focusing heads. On the other hand, because of the continuously improving laser beam quality, a general market demand can be observed to increase the processing speed. These contradictory trends can only be solved satisfactorily, if completely adapted sensors and additional components are delivered as pretested single complex items having the lowest possible overall weight and the highest possible stiffness to the customers. Such complex focusing heads have to be specified at a certain acceleration value.

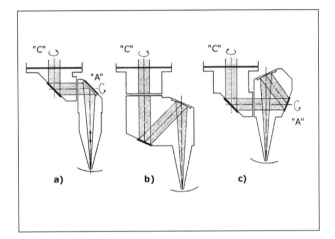

Figure 17. Typical layout of off-axis focusing heads.

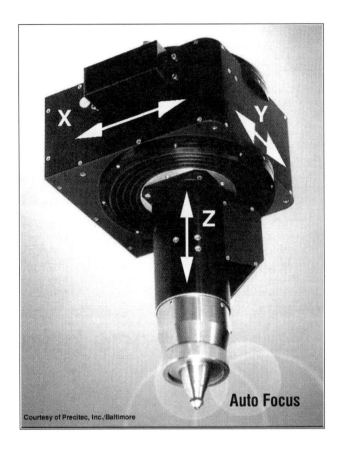

Figure 18. Three-axis robotic motion subsystem for 3D Nd:YAG laser cutting.

Another example of integrated moving axes is presented in Figure 18, where for a robotic Nd:YAG laser cutting application, the focusing head not only includes the vertical acting autofocus axis, but also a small XY table capable of cutting any off-line preprogrammed shape with a superior precision to most available five- or six-axis robots. The XY table covers 55 x 55 mm and the Z axis ± 15 mm. A fiber-optic collimator with a maximum diameter of 2 in. fits into the system.

In another example the focusing head may include an adaptive mirror (see Section 4.1.2.) for automatic focus position control and compensation of the thermal drift of the beam delivery system. Such a focusing head configuration can even be used to weld corrugated sheet steel without any additional vertical moving axis. Up to 10-mm workpiece height variations can be compensated in real time at usual welding speeds.

Another group of focusing heads, which are used for 3D-robotic applications, include devices supposed to assure the right working distance and clamp the usual overlap joint. These devices (see Figs. 19 and 20) have been integrated into car-body production lines.

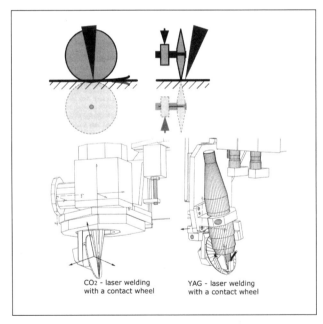

Figure 19. Contact wheel focusing head for Nd:YAG laser.

Chapter 4: Components for Laser Materials Processing Systems

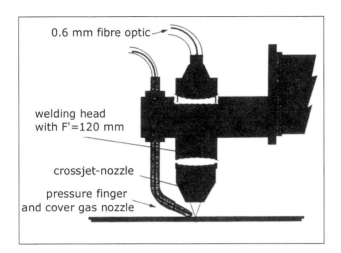

Figure 20. Focusing head with pressure trigger.

Another distinct group of special focusing heads include the so-called dual-spot-focusing heads. They represent another contribution for better efficiency and higher flexibility.

In principle there are three major possibilities to combine two laser beams:

(1) superposition (addition),

(2) tandem (one behind the other), or

(3) parallel (side by side).

For 2D or 3D applications, dual-spot focusing heads with setups (2) and (3) have to be oriented parallel with the tangent at the processing path within the TCP. Of course, it is also possible to modify the relative position of the two foci in conformity with the direction change of the processing path within the focusing head, but this is usually too difficult to be implemented.

The dual-spot technology has the following advantages:

- It implements the addition of two different laser beams having different properties.
- The geometry of the weld profile can be varied within a large range (depth/width ratio).
- In the case of tailored blanks welding, joints with gap sizes of 0.3 mm can be welded.
- The dual-spot technology is applicable for all laser types.

Figure 21 shows the layout of a mirror-based focusing head for CO_2 lasers and Figure 22 a focusing head for the same technology, but for fiber-optic beam delivery, for Nd:YAG lasers.

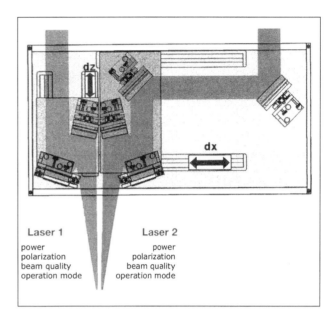

Figure 21. Focusing head for the combination of two CO_2 laser beams.

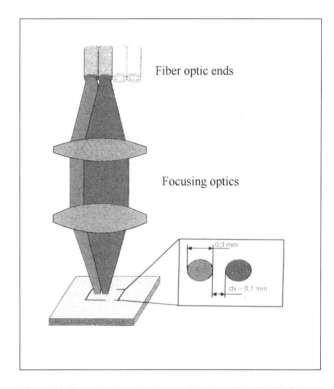

Figure 22. Focusing head for the combination of two Nd:YAG laser beams.

MARIUS JURCA

4.3 Other Optical Components

4.3.1 Beam Shaping Optics

Quite often the high-power/energy laser beam needs to be of a special shape to be compatible with particular applications. Typical shapes include circular, annular (i.e., ring or donut), rectangular, square, hexagonal, and solid lines. For materials processing applications the irradiance distribution within the beam is often of importance. Various techniques are used to produce these shapes, while controlling the irradiance distribution or uniformity on the surface being processed.

Integrators

Perhaps the oldest method used to shape and produce a uniform intensity profile for laser materials processing is the kaleidoscope integrator. This device, similar to a waveguide or light pipe, is an optically polished inside hollow tube, typically square or rectangular in shape. In the case of a square shape, a converging or diverging circular beam, either Gaussian or of nonuniform random irradiance distribution, would enter one end of the square hollow tube, reflect off the walls of the tube a multiple number of times, and produce a square image with a relatively uniform intensity profile near the exit of the tube. In lieu of the beam converging or diverging, in some applications the integrator can have tapering sidewalls (see Fig. 1). The uniform output image can often be reimaged to other locations and increased or decreased in size with conventional optics, but it cannot be recollimated. One of the drawbacks of this type of integrator is that it absorbs some of the beam on every reflection, inside the tube, and therefore suffers relatively large losses of radiant power. It has also been observed that some of these integrators lose 20–30% power from polarization absorption effects.

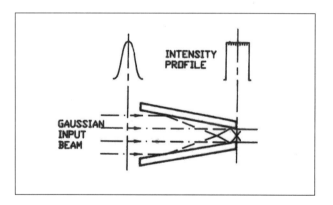

Figure 1. Kaleidoscope integrator with tapering sidewalls.

Other integration techniques have included strips of mirrors, similar in shape to venetian blinds, with flat or curved optical surfaces (see Fig. 2). The beam reflects off these strips of mirrors and forms a line or rectangular image, or other shape if each strip has its own curvature. This type is integrated in one axis only. To integrate in two axes, a second set of similar mirrors would be positioned 90° to the first set of mirrors. This approach can produce rectangular or square images.

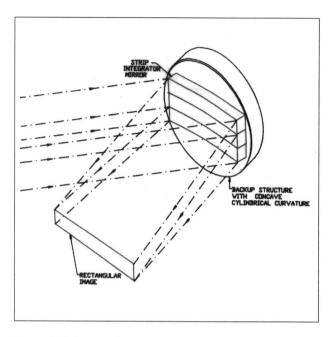

Figure 2. Strip mirror integrator.

A technique using a segmented mosaic array of square optical surfaces has become popular for producing various shapes and sizes of uniform intensity profiles (see Fig. 3). This technique has been used with both reflective and transmissive optical elements. The segmented optical array concept is a passive device that dissects, in two axes, the incident laser beam into an array of small sections and superimposes those sections on top of each other at a precise image plane (see Fig. 4). The reflective devices (discussed below) can be used with a broad range of wavelengths, but the transmissive type is often restricted to a narrow spectral transmission bandwidth of the optical material used. The transmissive segmented array typically is a solid lens with a multitude of small flat facets on one side (see Fig. 5). Each flat facet is in itself an optical surface. Each flat facet is immediately adjacent to another facet, thereby forming the mosaic array. The optical axis of each facet is tipped, respective to each other, thereby directing the dissected segment of the beam to a common image plane (see Fig. 6). The introduction of lenses can increase or decrease the image size. Diffracted optical surfaces have also been produced that achieve similar results.

Segmented Mirror

The segmented mirror optical integrator (U.S. Patent No. 4,195,913) is a mosaic array of individual mirrors mounted adjacent to each other on a common curved surface backup structure (see Figs. 3 and 4). The backup structure curve can be concave or convex. The surface of each segment mirror facet can be concave, convex, spherical, or cylindrical. The physical shape of each segment can be square, rectangular, or hexagonal. These combinations of variations can produce integrated images that are square, rectangular, hexagonal, or solid lines, in a large variety of sizes and aspect ratios. The segmented mirror integrator has been used for lasers producing in excess of 250 kW of power.

Chapter 4: Components for Laser Materials Processing Systems

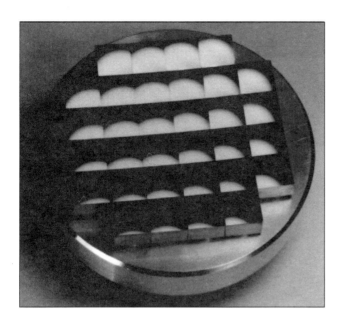

Figure 3. Segmented aperture integrator.

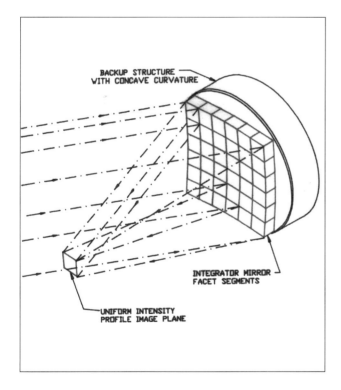

Figure 4. Superimposed segment images.

The reflective integrator has also been produced in replicated, molded, and electroformed versions. All the beam integration techniques mentioned are subject to diffraction and optical interference effects, which can dominate the irradiance profile at the image plane, when the laser light is monochromatic. These effects are illustrated in the "typical output intensity profile" in Figure 7. For this reason segmented faceted integrators are often custom designed for particular applications. Typical theoretical irradiance uniformities are ±4%, but in practice values are closer to ±10% about the average. This is generally acceptable for materials processing of metallic surfaces.

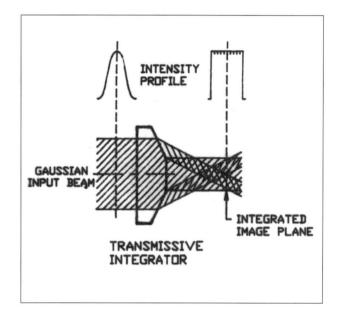

Figure 5. Transmissive integrator.

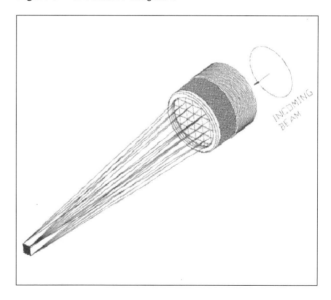

Figure 6. Lens integrator illustration (Courtesy of Laser Power Optics).

When the material being processed does not have sufficient thermal diffusion properties to integrate the high irradiance zones, which are produced from diffraction and optical interference effects (see Fig. 7), then the integrated beam image can be scanned (see Section 4.3.2).

ISBN 0-912035-15-3

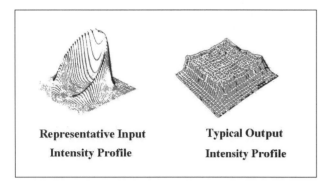

Figure 7. Typical uniformity profile.

Conics

Axicon and waxicon optical surfaces have unique influences on light beams that are useful in materials processing applications. The waxicon (Fig. 8A) typically has solid mirrored surfaces, whereas axicons can be either mirrors or lenses (see Fig. 8). Waxicons can either produce a hole in the center of a solid beam or remove an existing hole. The waxicon can reflect the beam back toward the direction of origin (Fig. 9) or pass through on axis (Fig. 10). Axicon lenses are used in the same basic manner, but the lens has added features of simplicity. Figure 11 illustrates typical capabilities for conic optical elements.

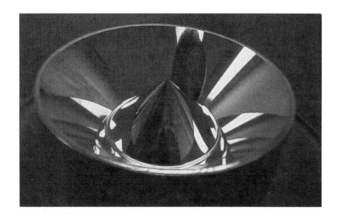

Figure 8A. Waxicon in metal substrate.

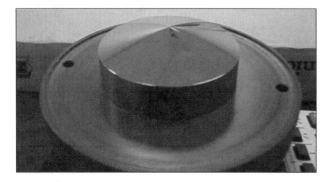

Figure 8B. Axicon in metal substrate.

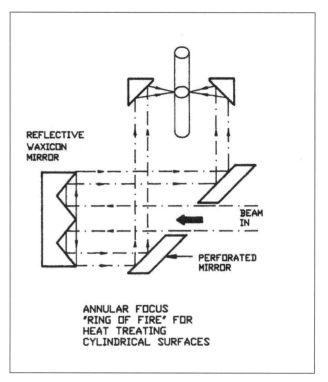

Figure 9. Waxicon "ring-of-fire" system.

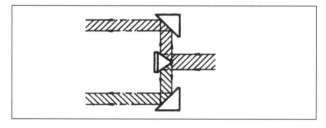

Figure 10. Pass-through waxicon.

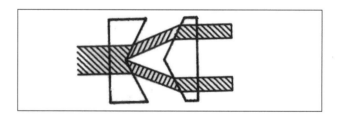

Figure 11. Beam expander/reducer with lens axicons.

4.3.2 Scanners

Materials processing optical scanners are used to move the laser beam across the surface of the material being processed. Scanner mirrors are typically rotating polygons or mirrors that rotate, pivot, or oscillate about an axis in or near the plane of the mirror surface. Such scanners are used for welding, heat treating, glazing, cladding, cleaning, paint stripping, engraving, and component formation.

Scanners can operate at speeds from near zero to 10^6 cycles per second (Hz). The speed is limited by the size of the mirror or aperture required. Larger laser beams require larger mirrors, and therefore larger mass and moments of inertia. Precise speed and acceleration/deceleration controls are required reliably to repeat laser materials processing applications. Mirrors that scan by continually rotating or spinning about a central axis are difficult to water cool for very high-power laser applications. The oscillating scan mirror is usually used when water cooling is required. Oscillating scanners typically have a sinusoidal waveform, exhibiting a dwell time at the end of each scan sweep. The dwell is from the angular acceleration/deceleration time periods caused by direction-reversing forces. This dwell deposits a higher thermal load at that location, which may cause overheating and be detrimental in some applications. The dwell can be very small and relatively indistinguishable, such as with a near triangular wave device. Figure 12A illustrates the comparative heat load on the target with a sinusoidal wave (dwell time) and a triangular wave (no dwell time) scanned profile. Figures 12B and 12C are photographs of plastic burn samples produced with sine wave and near triangular wave scanners. Figure 13 is a near triangular wave scanner for a 25 kW laser. Mirror scanners that rotate at constant speeds to form circular scans do not suffer from dwell times because the beam is moving continuously in a nonchanging arc (see Fig. 14).

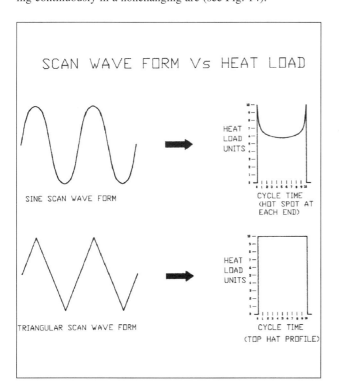

Figure 12A. Scan waveform vs. heat load.

Polygon scanners exhibit the reverse of a dwell at the ends of each sweep. Lower irradiance at the ends comes from the beam transitioning from one polygon mirror facet to an adjacent facet. During that transition, the beam, not being infinitely small, is dissected at the corner between facets. The dissection forms two separate beams. One of the dissected portions is near the end of the sweep when the other dissected portion is at the other end beginning a new sweep. Once the entire beam is located on the facet, it scans as a uniform unit until it starts transitioning to the next facet. A means of turning the beam off, or the use of beam stops, is utilized to control the reflected energy distribution profile during the facet to facet transitioning period. Figure 15 is a polygon scanner system with drive motor.

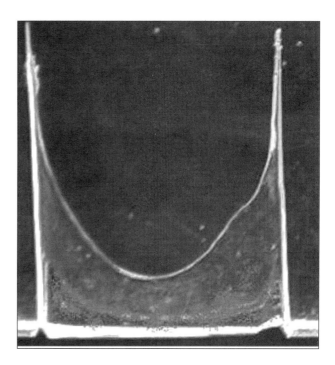

Figure 12B. Sine wave plastic burn.

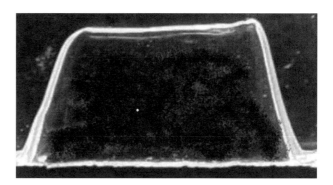

Figure 12C. Near trianglular wave plastic burn.

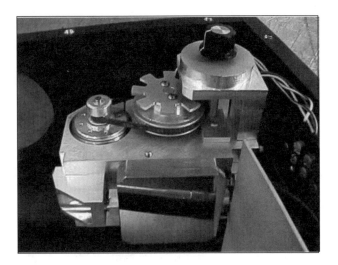

Figure 13. Triangle wave scanner for 25 kW laser.

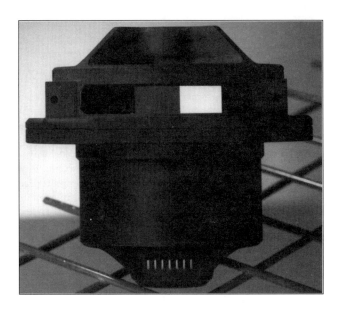

Figure 15. Polygon scanner assembly (Courtesy of Lincoln Laser).

4.3.3 Beam Splitters

A beam splitter is an optical element that splits a light beam into multiple beams. It can be either a reflective or transmissive element. A transmissive element is simply a partial reflective mirror, where a percentage of the beam reflects off the front surface and the remaining percentage passes through. The absolute percentage reflected off the front surface can be accurately controlled by the vacuum-deposited coating applied to the surface. A typical transmissive element will maintain the same energy distribution profiles in both the reflected and transmitted beams (see Fig. 16A). Some materials processing applications have used transmissive beam splitters to simultaneously time share one laser beam source with two separate workstations. Reflective beam splitters are simply total reflective mirrors that cut off and reflect a section of the beam. They can be single edge scrapers (Fig. 16B), single hole scrapers (Fig. 16C), multiple hole scraper mirrors, or combinations of these. Reflective beam splitters do not maintain the same energy distribution profiles in both the transmitted (or uninterrupted) and reflected beams.

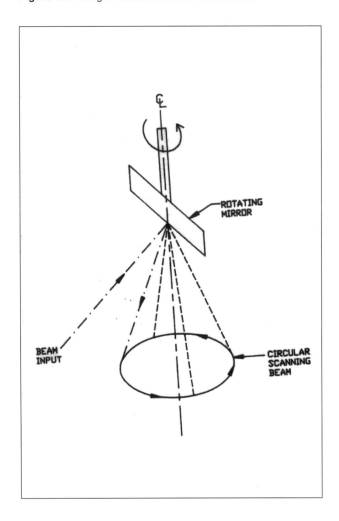

Figure 14. Circular scan illustration.

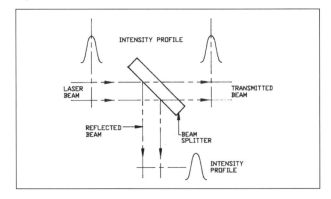

Figure 16A. Transmissive beam splitter.

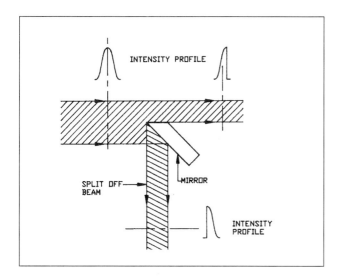

Figure 16B. Single-edge reflective beam splitter.

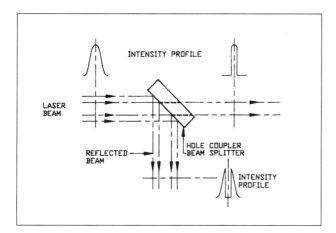

Figure 16C. Single-hole coupler/beam splitter.

4.3.4 Polarizers

In the late 1970s and early 1980s laser beam polarization and its effects on materials processing came to the forefront in the industrial laser community. It was found that beam polarization had a dramatic effect on deep penetration welding, cutting, and scribing on materials including metals and ceramics.

Laser beam polarization is plane, random, or circular. The polarization of a laser beam is primarily dependent on its resonator design. If desired, a laser's natural polarization can be changed by use of optical components outside of the resonator.

It was found that a plane-polarized beam could cut faster, weld deeper, or scribe faster in one axis than in another. A circularly polarized beam could perform equally well in either the X or Y axis. A randomly polarized beam gave variable results. It was clear that a circularly polarized beam was best for the vast majority of material processing applications.

The definition of a circularly polarized laser beam is as follows: A circularly polarized laser beam is a waveform of electromagnetic radiation in which the electric field vector rotates about the propagation axis by one revolution per wavelength.

Most industrial lasers produce a beam that has plane polarization. Circular polarization is created by retarding the phase of one component of the laser beam's electric field by 90° (one-quarter wave), behind the other orthogonal component. This can be done external to the laser resonator in either of two ways:

1. Transmitting a plane-polarized beam through a birefringent crystal, a ¼ waveplate, that retards the phase of one component of the electric field of the laser beam by 90° relative to the other orthogonal component.
2. Reflecting a plane-polarized beam with a properly designed mirror that provides a 90° phase shift between the s and p components of the beam's polarization. This mirror is usually the last 90° (aligned at a 45° angle to the axis of the beam) folding mirror in the beam delivery system.

4.3.5 Isolators

An isolator is a device that will limit or totally eliminate return reflections along an optical beam transmission path. When a high-power laser beam interacts with a target, such as a metal surface, scattered back reflections along a 180° return path could cause damage to optical components of the laser resonator and/or beam delivery system. To prevent this from occurring, devices such as a pinhole spatial filter or a Faraday rotator are incorporated into the beam delivery system.

A Faraday isolator allows light to propagate through it in one direction, but not in the opposite direction. It uses a rotation of the polarization of light by means of the Faraday magnetooptic effect, which occurs in certain materials. Incident light has its plane of polarization defined by an initial polarizer. A magnetic field is applied to the material by means of a coil of wire. The direction of polarization is rotated by 45° as it emerges from the magnetooptic material, and the light will pass through a second polarizer oriented at 45° to the first polarizer.

Light incident from the opposite direction passes through the second polarizer and has its direction of polarization defined by that polarizer. As it passes through the magnetooptic material, the direction of polarization will be rotated another 45° so that it is now polarized 90° to the pass direction of the first polarizer, and the light will not pass through that polarizer. Thus the device acts as a one-way valve. The rotation θ is given by

$$\theta = VBL$$

where V is a constant of the material, called the Verdet constant, B is the magnetic field, and L is the length of the magnetooptic material. The length of the material and the magnetic field are selected so that the total rotation is 45°. For the visible spectrum, the magnetooptic materials are glasses with Verdet constants around 0.1–0.2 min/cmG. For reasonable values of magnetic field, the isolator material has dimensions of centimeters. In the near-infrared region, materials include yttrium iron garnet and bismuth-substituted rare earth iron garnet, with Verdet constants up to 800 min/cmG. These materials can have submillimeter length. Optical isolators are available commercially with extinction ratio (ratio of the intensity of the light transmitted in the two opposite directions) greater than 40 dB.

4.3.6 Infrared and Ultraviolet Transmitting Materials

Properties of the most common infrared and ultraviolet transmitting materials are given below, including transmission range, physical and chemical properties, and any unusual properties. The data represent "typical values." Information about factors affecting the choice of some of these materials has been presented in Section 4.2.1.

Barium Fluoride (BaF$_2$)

Barium fluoride is used for optical windows, lenses, and prisms, particularly when transmission into the ultraviolet is desired. The transmission range is from 0.2 to 11 μm. Transmission in the vacuum-ultraviolet region is degraded by prolonged exposure to a moist atmosphere, but it is not significantly degraded by exposure to high-energy radiation.

Barium fluoride is less resistant to attack by water than calcium fluoride. Pronounced water attack occurs at 500°C, but the material can be used at temperatures up to 800°C dry. Barium fluoride is the most resistant fluoride to high-energy radiation but does not have the vacuum-ultraviolet transmission of other types. The material is relatively hard but is very sensitive to thermal shock. Figure 17 shows the spectral transmission of barium fluoride, and Table 1 presents data on its refractive index. This transmission curve and following transmission curves are relevant to thin samples, one or a few millimeters thick.

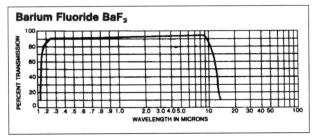

Figure 17. Transmission of barium fluoride.

Table 1. Barium Fluoride Refractive Index vs. Wavelength

λ (μm)	n	λ (μm)	n	λ (μm)	n
0.26	1.51	3.24	1.46	9.20	1.41
0.30	1.50	5.14	1.45	9.80	1.40
0.36	1.49	6.50	1.44	10.6	1.39
0.48	1.48	8.00	1.43		
0.85	1.47	8.60	1.42		

Borosilicate Crown Glass (BK7)

Borosilicate crown glass is used for windows, lenses, and prisms where transmission in the range 0.4 to 1.4 μm is desired. The refractive index varies from about 1.53 to 1.50 through this range. It is used for thermally noncritical applications. Figure 18 shows its spectral transmission, and Table 2 presents data on its refractive index.

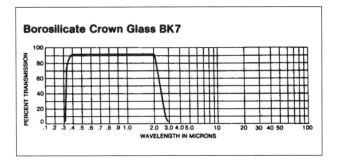

Figure 18. Borosilicate crown glass BK7.

Table 2. BK-7 Glass Refractive Index vs. Wavelength

λ (μm)	n	λ (μm)	n	λ μm	n
0.37	1.535	0.63	1.515	2.00	1.495
0.40	1.530	0.84	1.510	2.30	1.490
0.43	1.525	1.06	1.505	2.60	1.485
0.52	1.520	1.60	1.500		

Cadmium Telluride (CdTe)

Cadmium telluride is chiefly used as a filter substrate in the 12 to 25 μm region, where many other infrared materials have absorption bands. It is also used in CO_2 laser systems, particularly as output couplers, but only when the power level is low (time-averaged power below several hundred watts) since its absorption is as low as that of ZnSe (≤ 0.0015/cm) but its thermal conductivity is one-third that of ZnSe. The useful transmission of CdTe extends from about 1 to more than 25 μm. Its index varies from about 2.7 to 2.4 in this range (n=2.67 at 10.6 μm). Figure 19 shows the spectral transmission of cadmium telluride.

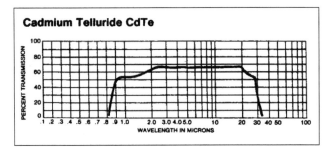

Figure 19. Cadmium Telluride CdTe.

Calcium Fluoride (CaF₂)

Calcium fluoride is used for optical windows, lenses, and prisms in the transmission range 0.15 to 9 μm. The refractive index varies from about 1.7 to 1.3 in this wavelength range. Calcium fluoride is particularly popular for high-power laser optics in the infrared at wavelengths less than 6 μm because of its low absorption. Degradation due to moisture in the atmosphere is minimal, and polished surfaces may be expected to withstand several years of exposure to normal atmospheric conditions. Because of its low refractive index, calcium fluoride can be used without an antireflection coating.

Calcium fluoride is attacked by atmospheric moisture at 600°C, where it begins to soften. The top use temperature is 800°C, when moisture is not present. Irradiation of calcium fluoride causes some loss in UV transmission. The material is sensitive to thermal shock. A vacuum-ultraviolet grade is available. Figure 20 shows the spectral transmission of calcium fluoride, and Table 3 presents data on its refractive index.

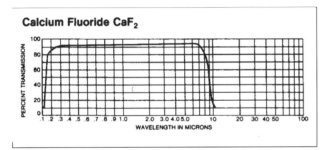

Figure 20. Spectral transmission of calcium fluoride.

Table 3. Calcium Fluoride Refractive Index vs. Wavelength

λ (μm)	n	λ (μm)	n	λ (μm)	n
0.19	1.51	0.33	1.45	5.80	1.39
0.20	1.50	0.41	1.44	6.20	1.38
0.21	1.49	0.88	1.43	6.70	1.37
0.22	1.48	2.65	1.42	7.00	1.36
0.25	1.47	3.90	1.41	7.50	1.35
0.27	1.46	5.00	1.40	8.22	1.34

Fused Silica

Fused silica, or fused quartz, is used for windows, lenses, and prisms in the transmission range 0.16 to 2 μm. Its refractive index varies from 1.53 to 1.43 through the transmission range. It is less dispersive than cultured quartz, and it is not birefringent. It is available in infrared and ultraviolet, grades depending upon the transmission needs. Figures 21 and 22 show spectral transmission curves for the infrared and ultraviolet grades, respectively. Table 4 presents data on the refractive index.

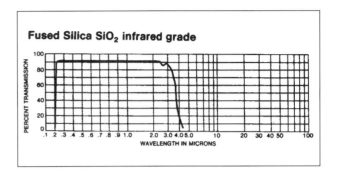

Figure 21. Fused silica infrared-grade spectral transmission.

Table 4. Fused Silica Refractive Index vs. Wavelength

λ (μm)	n	λ (μm)	n	λ (μm)	n
0.22	1.53	0.33	1.48	2.44	1.43
0.23	1.52	0.40	1.47	3.00	1.42
0.24	1.51	0.55	1.46	3.35	1.41
0.26	1.50	1.05	1.45	3.70	1.40
0.29	1.49	1.81	1.44		

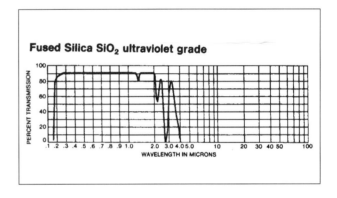

Figure 22. Fused silica SiO₂ ultraviolet-grade spectral transmission.

Gallium Arsenide (GaAs)

Gallium arsenide is an excellent optical material for high-power lasers, either as windows or lenses. In its properties of inertness and mechanical ruggedness it is like germanium. The absorption is lower than that of germanium and it does not show the phenomenon of thermal runaway until 250°C. Its thermal conductivity is more than 2½ times that of ZnSe. Its useful transmission range is from about 2.5 to 16.5 μm depending on sample thickness. Its refractive index varies between 3.3 and 2.6 in this range. Figure 23 shows the spectral transmission of gallium arsenide, and Table 5 presents data on its refractive index.

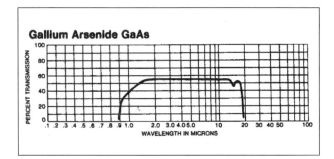

Figure 23. Spectral transmission of gallium arsenide.

Table 5. Gallium Arsenide Refractive Index vs. Wavelength

λ (μm)	n	λ (μm)	n	λ (μm)	n
8.0	3.34	13.7	2.90	19.0	2.41
10.0	3.14	14.5	2.82	21.9	2.12
11.0	3.05	15.0	2.73		
13.0	2.97	17.0	2.59		

Germanium (Ge)

Germanium is used widely for lenses and windows in infrared laser systems. Its high index of refraction (greater than 4) makes it of particular interest. Its useful transmission range is from 2 to 12 μm. Germanium is opaque in the visible.

Germanium has the property of thermal runaway; that is, the hotter it gets, the more the absorption increases. It is the most widely used material for infrared lasers. Figure 24 shows the spectral transmission of germanium, and Table 6 presents data on its refractive index.

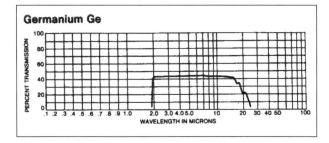

Figure 24. Germanium (Ge).

Table 6. Germanium Refractive Index vs. Wavelength

λ (μm)	n	λ (μm)	n	λ (μm)	n
2.06	4.10	3.00	4.05	8.66	4.00
2.15	4.09	3.42	4.03	9.72	4.00
2.44	4.07	4.26	4.02	11.04	4.00
2.58	4.06	6.24	4.01	13.02	4.00

Irtran 2 (ZnS)

Irtran 2 is a hot-pressed form of ZnS used for windows and lenses in the 2-12 μm range. It is similar in density but has a higher modulus of elasticity and is even harder than CVD ZnS. Figure 25 shows its spectral transmission, and Table 7 presents data on its refractive index.

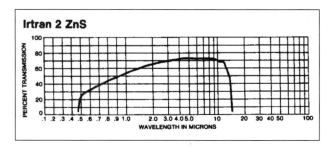

Figure 25. Irtran 2 ZnS.

Table 7. Irtran 2 Refractive Index vs. Wavelength

λ (μm)	n	λ (μm)	n	λ (μm)	n
1.00	2.29	5.75	2.24	10.5	2.19
1.24	2.28	7.00	2.23	11.3	2.18
1.50	2.27	8.20	2.22	12.0	2.17
2.25	2.26	9.00	2.21	12.5	2.16
4.00	2.25	9.80	2.20	13.0	2.15

Lithium Fluoride (LiF)

Lithium fluoride is used for windows, lenses, and prisms in the vacuum ultraviolet, ultraviolet visible, and infrared where transmission in the range 0.104 to 7 μm is desired. The refractive index varies from about 1.6 to 1.25 in this range. Modest precautions should be taken against moisture and high-energy radiation damage.

LiF is attacked by atmospheric moisture at 400°C, and softens at 600°C. LiF is sensitive to thermal shock. Irradiation produces color centers. The material can be cleared. A vacuum-ultraviolet grade is available. This is the best vacuum-ultraviolet transmitter available. Figure 26 shows its spectral transmission, and Table 8 presents data on its refractive index.

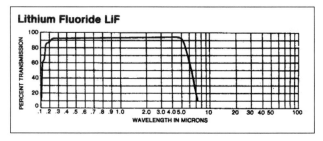

Figure 26. Lithium Fluoride (LiF).

ISBN 0-912035-15-3

Table 8. Lithium Fluoride Refractive Index vs. Wavelength

λ (μm)	n	λ (μm)	n	λ (μm)	n
0.20	1.44	0.29	1.41	1.75	1.38
0.22	1.43	0.39	1.40	2.75	1.37
0.24	1.42	0.60	1.39	3.40	1.36

Magnesium Fluoride (MgF$_2$)

Magnesium fluoride is used for optical elements in the infrared where extreme ruggedness and durability are required. Its useful transmission range is from 0.11 to 7.5 μm. The single crystal exhibits slight birefringence through its useful transmission range and its birefringence in the infrared could be useful. The refractive index varies from about 1.4 to 1.3. The difference n_e-n_o is 0.012 at 0.6 μm for the birefingent single crystal.

Magnesium fluoride is similar to calcium fluoride in its resistance to water. The material is sensitive to thermal shock but does not cleave. Irradiation does not lead to color centers. Figure 27 shows its spectral transmission, and Table 9 presents data on its refractive index.

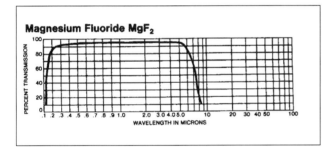

Figure 27. Magnesium fluoride (MgF$_2$).

Table 9. Magnesium Fluoride Refractive Index vs. Wavelength

λ (μm)	n_e	n_o	λ (μm)	n_e	n_o
0.20	1.43	1.42	0.34	1.40	1.39
0.23	1.42	1.41	0.56	1.39	1.38
0.27	1.41	1.40			

Potassium Chloride (KCl)

Potassium chloride is used for infrared windows, lenses, and prisms when transmission in the range 0.3 to 20 μm is desired. Its transmission extends beyond that of sodium chloride. The refractive index ranges from about 1.6 to 1.4 in this wavelength range. Potassium chloride is soluble in water, and polished surfaces must be protected from moisture. Maximum use temperature is 400°C. Figure 28 shows its spectral transmission, and Table 10 presents data on its refractive index.

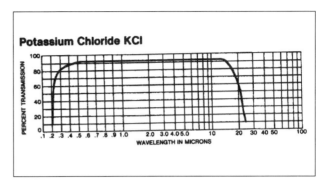

Figure 28. Spectral transmission of potassium chloride.

Table 10. Potassium Chloride Refractive Index vs. Wavelength

λ (μm)	n	λ (μm)	n	λ (μm)	n
0.40	1.51	11.7	1.45	20.2	1.39
0.47	1.50	13.5	1.44	21.0	1.38
0.59	1.49	15.0	1.43	22.8	1.37
0.98	1.48	16.7	1.42	23.4	1.36
5.30	1.47	18.1	1.41	24.3	1.35
8.90	1.46	19.1	1.40		

Quartz (SiO$_2$)

Cultured quartz is a crystal used primarily for prisms, but also for windows and lenses, in the ultraviolet. Its useful transmission range is 0.15 to 3.6 μm. Cultured quartz exhibits birefringence. Its refractive index varies from about 1.7 to 1.5 through the transmission range. Orienting the optical axis along the crystal *c* axis produces higher vacuum-ultraviolet transmission. The spectral transmission is shown in Figure 29, and Table 11 presents data on its refractive index.

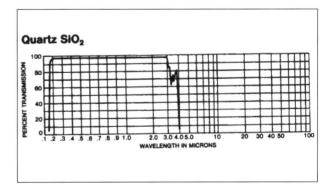

Figure 29. Spectral transmission of quartz.

ISBN 0-912035-15-3

Table 11. Quartz Refractive Index vs. Wavelength

λ (μm)	n_e	n_o	λ (μm)	n_e	n_o
0.20	1.66	1.65	0.31	1.59	1.58
0.21	1.65	1.64	0.33	1.58	1.57
0.22	1.64	1.63	0.38	1.57	1.56
0.23	1.63	1.62	0.49	1.56	1.55
0.24	1.62	1.61	0.77	1.55	1.54
0.25	1.61	1.60	1.30	1.54	1.53
0.27	1.60	1.59	2.05	1.53	1.52

Silicon (Si)

Silicon is used as a high-reflectivity mirror for lasers. It is used for windows and lenses in the 1 to 7 μm range. The refractive index is near 3.4 throughout the range. Silicon is also useful as a transmitter in the 20 to 300 μm range. Its high thermal conductivity and low weight are attractive features in some applications.

Because of the strong absorption at 9 μm, silicon is not suitable for use with CO_2 lasers as a transmitting optic but is widely used for CO_2 mirrors. The density of silicon is only half that of germanium, gallium arsenide, and zinc selenide. Figure 30 shows its spectral transmission, and Table 12 presents data on its refractive index.

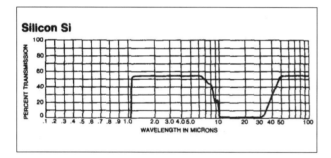

Figure 30. Silicon (Si).

Table 12. Silicon Refractive Index vs. Wavelength

λ (μm)	n	λ (μm)	n	λ (μm)	n
1.40	3.49	1.82	3.46	3.30	3.43
1.50	3.48	2.05	3.45	6.00	3.42
1.66	3.47	2.50	3.44		

Sodium Chloride (NaCl)

Sodium chloride is used for windows, lenses, and prisms where transmission in the range 0.25 to 16 μm is desired. The refractive index varies from about 1.6 to 1.4 in this range. Because of its low absorption, sodium chloride is used in high-power laser systems. Polished surfaces must be protected from moisture by exposing them to only a dry atmosphere or by using a heating element to maintain the temperature of the sodium chloride part above the ambient temperature.

Sodium chloride can be used to a temperature of 400°C. The material is sensitive to thermal shock, and irradiation generates color centers. Figure 31 shows its spectral transmission, and Table 13 presents data on its refractive index.

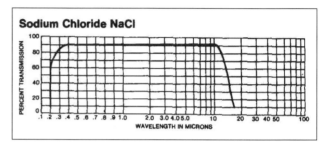

Figure 31. Sodium chloride (NaCl).

Table 13. Sodium Chloride Refractive Index vs. Wavelength

λ (μm)	n	λ (μm)	n	λ (μm)	n
0.35	1.58	1.25	1.53	12.0	1.48
0.37	1.57	4.50	1.52	13.1	1.47
0.46	1.56	7.30	1.51	14.2	1.46
0.51	1.55	9.50	1.50	15.1	1.45
0.68	1.54	10.6	1.49	16.0	1.44

Zinc Selenide (ZnSe)

Zinc selenide is used for infrared windows, lenses, and prisms where transmission in the range 0.58 to 22 μm is desired. The refractive index is near 2.4. Zinc selenide has a very low absorption coefficient and is used extensively for high-power infrared laser optics. It is nonhygroscopic.

Zinc selenide is a relatively soft material and scratches rather easily. The low absorption of the material avoids the thermal runaway problem of germanium. Zinc selenide requires an antireflection coating because of its high refractive index if high transmission is required. Figure 32 shows its spectral transmission, and Table 14 presents data on its refractive index.

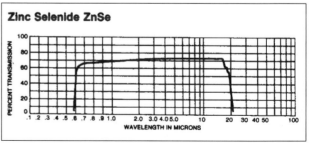

Figure 32. Zinc selenide (ZnSe).

Table 14. Zinc Selenide Refractive Index vs. Wavelength

λ (μm)	n	λ (μm)	n	λ (μm)	n
2.75	2.44	12.5	2.39	17.8	2.34
5.00	2.43	13.5	2.38	18.5	2.33
7.50	2.42	15.0	2.37	19.3	2.32
9.50	2.41	16.0	2.36	20.0	2.31
11.0	2.40	16.9	2.35		

Zinc Sulfide (ZnS)

Zinc sulfide is used for windows and lenses in the 0.7 to 12 μm range. The refractive index is near 2.2. Zinc sulfide is particularly hard and is used for infrared windows for high-speed aircraft. It is also available in a water-free form with transmission from 0.35 to 12 μm. This type of ZnS does not have absorption in the 6-μm region, as is found in regular CVD-type material. Figure 33 shows its spectral transmission, and Table 15 presents data on its refractive index.

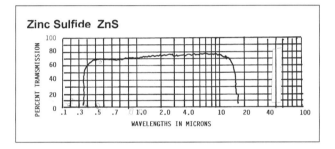

Figure 33. Zinc sulfide (ZnS).

Table 15. Zinc Sulfide Refractive Index vs. Wavelength

λ (μm)	n	λ (μm)	n	λ (μm)	n
1.00	2.29	5.75	2.24	10.5	2.19
1.24	2.28	7.00	2.23	11.3	2.18
1.50	2.27	8.20	2.22	12.0	2.17
2.25	2.26	9.00	2.21	12.5	2.16
4.00	2.25	9.80	2.20	13.0	2.15

WALTER J. SPAWR

4.4 Photodetectors

4.4.1 Basics of Photodetectors

Frequently in laser materials processing, a photodetector is used to monitor the laser power reaching the workpiece. This section will discuss some of the basic considerations regarding photodetectors.

Optical detectors may be considered in two broad classes, photon detectors and thermal detectors. Photon detectors detect quanta of light energy that interact with electrons in the detector material and produce free electrons. The quanta must have sufficient energy to release an electron. The wavelength response of photon detectors has a long-wavelength cutoff. If the wavelength is longer than the cutoff wavelength, the photon energy is too small to release a free electron, and the response of the detector drops to zero.

Thermal detectors employ a temperature-dependent effect, like a change of electrical resistance. They respond to the heat energy delivered by the light. Their response is independent of wavelength.

Figure 1 shows the general shape of the output of photon detectors and thermal detectors as a function of wavelength. Figure 1 does not give quantitative values; these vary from material to material. The purpose of the figure is to compare the general spectral dependence of the response for the two types of detectors. The output of photon detectors increases with increasing wavelength at wavelengths shorter than the cutoff wavelength. At the cutoff wavelength, the response drops rapidly to zero. The output of thermal detectors is independent of wavelength, and extends to longer wavelengths than the response of photon detectors.

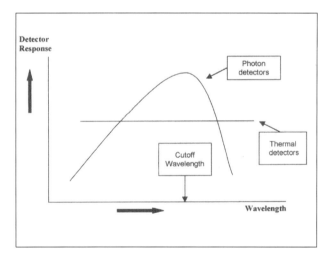

Figure 1. Schematic diagram showing the relative response as a function of wavelength for photon detectors and thermal detectors.

Photon detectors utilize several different types of physical effect to produce the detector response. Some important classes of photon detectors include:

- Photoconductive effects. Light produces free electrons inside the detector material. These electrons carry electrical current so that the electrical conductivity of the detector material, usually a semiconductor, changes as a function of the intensity of the incident light. Photoconductive detectors are fabricated from materials like silicon.

- Photovoltaic effects. These detectors are fabricated with a *p-n* junction in a semiconductor material. A voltage is generated when optical energy is absorbed near the junction.

- Photoemissive effects. These detectors rely on the photoelectric effect. Incident light releases electrons from the surface of the detector material, which is in a vacuum environment. The free electrons may be collected in an external circuit by application of a voltage between electrodes.

Before discussing these effects in more detail, we shall define some important detector characteristics.

Detector Characteristics

The performance of optical detectors is characterized by a number of different parameters, sometimes called figures of merit. The manufacturers of detectors usually describe the performance of their detectors in these terms.

Some of the figures of merit were developed to describe the performance of detectors responding to a small signal in the presence of noise. These figures of merit may not be highly relevant for laser materials processing applications, because there is no question of detection of a small signal in a background of noise. The laser signal is far larger than any noise source that may be present.

Responsivity

The first term that we will define is *responsivity*, a term that is relevant in laser materials processing. Responsivity is the detector output per unit of input power. The units of responsivity are either amperes/watt (alternatively milliamperes/milliwatt or microamperes/microwatt, which are numerically the same) or volts/watt, depending on whether the output is an electric current or a voltage. The responsivity is usually specified by the manufacturer. The responsivity allows the user to determine how much detector signal will be available for a specific application, or to determine the laser power from the detector output.

Detector Response Time

Another important detector characteristic that the user should know is the speed of the detector response to changes in light intensity. If a light source is instantaneously turned on and irradiates an optical detector, it will take a finite time for voltage or current to appear at the output of the device and for the response to reach a steady value. If the source is turned off instantaneously, it will take a finite time for the response to decay to zero. The term *response time* refers to the time it takes the detector output to rise to a value equal to 63.2% of the steady-state value, which is reached after a relatively long period of time. The recovery time is the time it takes for the response to fall to 36.8% of the steady-state value when the light is turned off instantaneously.

Another important term, the *rise time*, is also used to describe the speed of detector response. Rise time is the difference between the time when the detector has reached 10% of its peak output and the time at which it has reached 90% of its peak response, when a very short pulse of light strikes it. Fall time (also called decay time) is the time between the 90% point and the 10% point on the trailing edge of the pulse. The fall time may differ numerically from the rise time.

Because short pulses of light energy are often used in laser materials processing, these time constants are important in monitoring processing applications.

Linearity

Another important characteristic of optical detectors is their linearity. Over some range, detectors are characterized by a response in which the output is linear with incident power. The response may be linear over a broad range, perhaps many orders of magnitude. Noise will determine the lowest level of incident light that is detectable. The upper limit of the input/output linearity is determined by the maximum current or voltage that the detector can produce without becoming saturated, a condition in which there is no further increase in detector response as the input light is increased. When the detector becomes saturated, its output can no longer represent the input faithfully. In a laser materials processing operation, for which power levels are often high, the user must ensure that the detector is operating in the range in which it is linear.

Manufacturers of optical detectors often specify a maximum continuous light level. Light levels above this maximum may cause undesirable effects, including saturation, hysteresis, and permanent damage to the detector. If the detector views a very short pulse, one may exceed the continuous rating by some factor (perhaps as much as 10 times) without damage or noticeable changes in linearity.

Noise Equivalent Power

Another figure of merit, one that does depend on noise characteristics, is the *noise equivalent power* (NEP). NEP is often specified by the manufacturer, but is not often of importance for laser materials processing. NEP is defined as the optical power that produces a signal voltage (or current) equal to the noise voltage (or current) of the detector. The noise depends on the bandwidth of the measurement, so that bandwidth must be specified. The equation defining NEP is

$$\text{NEP} = IAV_N/V_S(\Delta f)^{1/2}$$

where I is the irradiance incident on the detector of area A, V_N is the root-mean-square noise voltage within the measurement bandwidth Δf, and V_S is the root-mean-square signal voltage. The NEP has units of $W/(Hz)^{1/2}$, usually called watts per root hertz. It is apparent that the lower the value of the NEP, the better are the characteristics of the detector for detecting a small signal in the presence of noise.

Detectivity

Detectivity is a very important characteristic for many applications, but again is not often critical for materials processing applications. It is derived from the NEP. The NEP of a detector depends on the area of the detector. Detectivity is a figure of merit that is dependent on the intrinsic properties of the detector, not on how large it happens to be. Detectivity is represented by the symbol D^*, pronounced "D-star." It is defined as

$D^* = A^{1/2}/NEP$

Since many detectors have NEP proportional to the square root of their area, D^* is independent of the area of the detector. Detectivity gives a measure of the intrinsic quality of the detector material itself.

When D^* for an optical detector is measured, it is usually measured in a system in which the incident light is modulated at a frequency f so as to produce an AC signal, which is then amplified with an amplification bandwidth Δf. These quantities must also be specified. The notation expressing the dependence of D^* on the wavelength λ, the frequency f and the bandwidth Δf is $D^*(\lambda, f, \Delta f)$. The reference bandwidth is often 1 Hz. The units of $D^*(\lambda, f, \Delta f)$ are cm Hz$^{1/2}$/W. A high value of $D^*(\lambda, f, \Delta f)$ means that the detector is suitable for detecting weak signals in the presence of noise.

We now return to the discussion of different types of detectors and present more detail on the various available optical detectors.

Photon Detectors

Photovoltaic detectors. The photovoltaic effect is produced at the *p-n* junction in a semiconductor. At the junction, there is an internal electric field because of a change in the level of the conduction and valence bands. This change leads to electrical rectification. It also causes the generation of a voltage when light is absorbed near the junction. The photovoltaic effect is measured using a high-impedance voltage measuring device, which determines the open-circuit voltage produced at the junction.

When no light is present, there is no open-circuit voltage. When the junction is irradiated by light with wavelength shorter than the cutoff, it is absorbed and produces free hole-electron pairs. The electric field at the junction separates the electrons and holes moving the electrons into the *n*-type region and the holes into the *p*-type region. This produces the open-circuit voltage, which is be measured externally. The open-circuit voltage generated in the photovoltaic effect may be detected directly with no bias voltage required.

If the junction is short circuited by an external load resistance, then current will flow in the circuit. One may measure either the open-circuit voltage or the short-circuit current. Either of these quantities can give a measure of the light falling on the junction.

Photoemissive Effect

The photoemissive effect is the emission of electrons from a surface irradiated by quanta of light energy. The cathode of a photoemissive detector is coated with a material that emits electrons when light of wavelength shorter than the cutoff wavelength is present. The electrons are accelerated by a voltage to an anode, where they produce a current in an external circuit. The detectors are enclosed in a vacuum environment to allow free flow of electrons. These detectors are available commercially from a number of manufacturers. They represent an important class of detectors for many applications.

Some spectral response curves for photoemissive cathodes are shown in Table 1. The cathodes often contain mixtures of alkali metals, like sodium and potassium, which emit electrons easily.

Table 1. Characteristics of Photomultiplier Tubes

Designation	Cathode type	Spectral range (μm)	Peak photocathode responsivity (mA/W)	Current gain (cathode to anode)
4516	Bialkali	300–660	70	5.2×10^5
8644	Multialkali	300–820	50	4.3×10^5
C83051	High temperature bialkali	220–640	62	2×10^5
S83063	Multialkali	300–880	78	5×10^5
S83068	Bialkali	300–660	100	5×10^6
C83050	Bialkali	300–660	82	1.8×10^6
903	Multialkali	300–820	68	5.2×10^5
C31000M	Bialkali	185–660	60	1.6×10^7
8852	Extended red multialkali	260–920	30	6×10^5
C7164R	Extended red multialkali	300–880	50	5×10^5
S83006E	Bialkali	300–660	100	6.7×10^4
C31034A	GaAs	185–930	94	6×10^5
4832	GaAs	200–930	64	1.3×10^5

Based on information from Burle Industries, Inc.

ISBN 0-912035-15-3

Table 2. Characteristics of Representative Infrared Photon Detectors

Detector type	Operating mode	Temperature (K)	Wavelength range (μm)	Wavelength of peak detectivity (μm)	Peak detectivity (cm Hz$^{1/2}$/W)
InAs	Photovoltaic	77	1.8–3.8	3.1	6 X 10^{11}
$Hg_{0.61}Cd_{0.39}Te$	Photoconductive	77	1.5–4.8	3.8	1.5 X 10^{11}
InSb	Photovoltaic	77	1.5–5.5	5	10^{11}
$Hg_{0.73}Cd_{0.27}Te$	Photoconductive	77	1.5–5.5	5.2	7 X 10^{10}
$Hg_{0.8}Cd_{0.2}Te$	Photoconductive	77	2–15	12	2 X 10^{10}
Au-doped Ge	Photoconductive	60	3–11	6	8 X 10^9
Cu-doped Ge	Photoconductive	4.2	2.5–30	25	1.5 X 10^{10}
Zn-doped Ge	Photoconductive	4.2	2–40	35	10^{10}

At wavelengths longer than about 1000 nm, no photoemission is available. The user can select a device with a cathode with maximum response in a selected wavelength region.

An important variation of the photoemissive detector is the photomultiplier. This device has a photoemissive cathode and a number of secondary emitting stages called dynodes. Electrons from the cathode are accelerated by an applied voltage to the first dynode, where their impact causes emission of numerous secondary electrons. The dynodes are arranged so that electrons from each dynode are delivered to the next dynode. These electrons are accelerated to the next dynode and generate even more electrons. Finally, electrons from the last dynode are accelerated to the anode and produce a large current pulse in the external circuit. The photomultiplier is packaged as a vacuum tube.

The result of the process is a large value of current gain, which is the ratio of anode current to cathode current. Values of current gain may be in the range 100,000 to 1,000,000. Thus 100,000 or more electrons reach the anode for each photon striking the cathode. The high-gain process means that photomultiplier tubes offer the highest available responsivity in the ultraviolet, visible, and near-infrared portions of the spectrum. But their response does not extend to wavelengths longer than about 1000 nm.

Table 1 shows some characteristics of representative photomultiplier types. In the table, the short-wavelength limit for the response is determined by the transmission of the window on the photomultiplier tube. Photomultiplier tubes are available from a number of sources; values for the parameters may vary from one manufacturer to another.

Photoconductivity

A semiconductor in thermal equilibrium contains a relatively small number of free electrons and holes. The number of electrons and holes is changed when light is absorbed by the semiconductor, provided that the light has photon energy large enough to excite free electrons within the material. The increased number of charge carriers leads to an increase in the electrical conductivity of the semiconductor. This increase in conductivity is called *photoconductivity*. A photoconductive detector is used in a circuit with a bias voltage and a series load resistor. The change in electrical conductivity leads to an increase in current flowing in the circuit, and hence to a change in the voltage drop across the load resistor.

Photoconductive detectors are most widely used in the infrared region, at wavelengths where photoemissive detectors are not available. There are many different materials used as infrared photoconductive detectors. Some characteristics, including detectivity (in cm Hz$^{1/2}$/W) for some photoconductors operating in the infrared are shown in Table 2, along with characteristics for other detectors. The exact value of detectivity for a specific photoconductor depends on the operating temperature and on the field of view of the detector. Most infrared photoconductive detectors operate at a cryogenic temperature (frequently liquid nitrogen temperature, 77 K) which may involve some inconvenience in practical applications.

There are many manufacturers of infrared detectors. The values in Table 2 may be considered representative, but the exact values will vary from one manufacturer to another.

Photodiodes

The photovoltaic effect, for which no bias voltage is required, has been described earlier. One may also use a *p-n* junction to detect light if one does apply a bias voltage in the reverse direction, that is, the direction of low current flow with the positive voltage applied to the *n*-type material. A *p-n* junction detector with bias voltage is termed a *photodiode*.

Figure 2 shows the current-voltage characteristics of a photodiode. This figure is intended to illustrate the general operation of a photodiode, and does not show quantitative values, which vary with material. The curve marked dark is the current-voltage relation in the absence of light. It shows the rectification characteristics of a semiconductor diode. The other curves show the current-voltage characteristics when different light levels strike the device. The photovoltaic detector, which has zero applied voltage, is represented by the intersections of the different curves with the vertical axis.

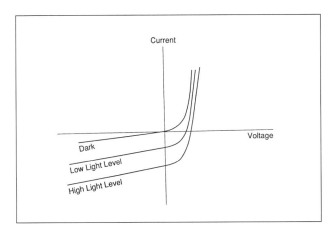

Figure 2. Photodiode current–voltage characteristics.

Photodiode detectors operate in the lower left quadrant of this figure. The current that may be drawn through an external load resistor increases with increasing light level. Generally one measures the voltage drop appearing across the resistor.

A number of different semiconductor materials are in common use as photodiodes. They include silicon for use in the visible, near ultraviolet, and near infrared, germanium and indium gallium arsenide in the near infrared, and indium antimonide, indium arsenide, mercury cadmium telluride, and germanium doped with elements like copper and gold in the longer-wavelength infrared.

Silicon photodiodes are frequently encountered. Silicon photodiodes respond over the approximate spectral range of 400–1100 nm, covering the visible and part of the near-infrared regions. The spectral responsivity (in A/W) of typical commercial silicon photodiodes is shown in Figure 3. The responsivity reaches a peak value around 0.7 A/W near 900 nm, decreasing at longer and shorter wavelengths. Optional models provide somewhat extended coverage in the infrared or ultraviolet regions. Silicon photodiodes are useful for detection of many of the most common laser wavelengths, including argon, AlGaAs, Nd:YAG, and doubled Nd:YAG.

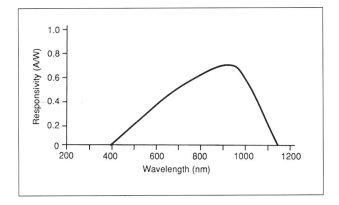

Figure 3. Spectral responsivity of a typical commercial silicon photodiode.

In practice silicon photodiodes have become the detector of choice for many laser materials processing applications using lasers with wavelengths within their spectral range. They represent a well-developed technology and are relatively inexpensive.

Table 2 presents values of D^* (or detectivity) for a number of commercially available detectors operating in the infrared spectrum. The table includes both photovoltaic detectors and photoconductive detectors. The choice of detector for an infrared application at a wavelength past the cutoff of a silicon detector will depend on the wavelength region that is desired. For example, for a laser operating at 5 mm, an indium antimonide photovoltaic detector would be suitable.

A variation of photodiode structure is the so-called PIN structure. This structure was developed to increase the frequency response of photodiodes. A PIN photodiode has a layer of nearly intrinsic semiconductor material bounded on one side by a relatively thin layer of highly doped p-type semiconductor, and on the other side, by a relatively thick layer of n-type semiconductor. Hence it is called a PIN device.

Light absorbed in the intrinsic region produces free electron-hole pairs, provided that the photon energy is high enough. These carriers are swept across the region with high velocity and are collected in the heavily doped regions. The frequency response of PIN photodiodes can be very high, of the order of 10^{10} Hz. This is higher than the frequency response of photodiodes without the intrinsic region. PIN photodiodes are useful for detection of short laser pulses.

Another variation of the photodiode is the avalanche photodiode. The avalanche photodiode offers the possibility of internal gain. The most widely used material for avalanche photodiodes is silicon, but they have been fabricated from other materials, such as germanium.

An avalanche photodiode has a large internal electric field that produces multiplication of the number of charge carriers through ionizing collisions. The signal is increased, to a value perhaps 100–200 times greater than that of a nonavalanche device. Avalanche photodiodes cost more than conventional photodiodes, and they require temperature compensation circuits to maintain the optimum bias, but they provide very high responsivity and represent an attractive choice when high performance is required.

Thermal Detectors

The second broad class of optical detectors is *thermal detectors*, which respond to the heat energy delivered by a laser beam, regardless of its wavelength. Thermal detectors do not have a long-wavelength cutoff, as photon detectors do. The values of responsivity and of D^* do not vary with wavelength. Thermal detectors often do not have as rapid a response as photon detectors. For many applications, thermal detectors are often not used in the wavelength region in which photon detectors are most effective (≤ 1.55 μm). They are often used at longer wavelengths, where some of the best photon detectors no longer respond.

Bolometers and thermistors: Probably the most common manifestation of thermal detectors uses an element whose properties change with temperature as an absorber for the incident light. Absorption of the light energy heats the element, and some change in its properties is sensed. The temperature-measuring elements include bolometers and thermistors. Bolometers and thermistors employ the change in electrical resistivity that occurs as temperature rises. Bolometers use metallic elements; thermistors use semiconductor elements. The bolometer or thermistor is in series with a voltage source, so that current flows through it. As the resistance changes, the voltage drop across the element changes. The magnitude of the voltage drop gives a measure of the light intensity.

Thermocouples: In a thermocouple detector light is absorbed by an element to which a thermocouple is attached. The thermocouple is a device formed of two dissimilar metals joined at two points. Thermocouples may be fabricated from wires, but for detector applications they are often thin films. The thermocouple, as it is heated by the light energy, generates a potential difference, which is a measure of the temperature difference between the two points. One point is at a constant reference temperature. The second point is in contact with the absorber. The light energy heats the absorber and the thermocouple junction in contact with it. This causes the voltage generated by the thermocouple to change, in turn providing a measure of the temperature rise of the absorber and of the incident light energy.

Often there are a number of thermocouples in series, perhaps as many as 100. This enhances the performance of the device. The "hot" junctions are all attached close together. This type of device is called a *thermopile*.

Pyroelectric Detectors: The pyroelectric detector is another common type of thermal detector. Pyroelectric detectors respond to the change in electric polarization that occurs in certain classes of crystalline materials (like lithium tantalate) as their temperature changes. The change in polarization is called the *pyroelectric effect*. It may be measured as an open-circuit voltage or as a short-circuit current. Because they respond to changes in temperature, pyroelectric devices are useful as detectors only for pulsed or chopped radiation. The response of pyroelectric detectors is fast, faster than that of other thermal detectors, like thermistors and thermopiles. Pyroelectric detectors are fast enough to monitor very short optical pulses.

The spectral detectivity D^* of pyroelectric detectors tends to be higher than the detectivity of thermistor or thermopile detectors. Pyroelectric detectors are frequently encountered in laser materials processing applications, such as those using short-pulse carbon dioxide lasers.

Table 3 shows values of some characteristics, including values of detectivity, for some thermal detectors, including thermistors, bolometers, thermocouples, thermopiles, and pyroelectric detectors. The values of detectivity are independent of wavelength.

In the visible and near infrared, the values of detectivity for thermal detectors are usually lower than for good photon detectors, but the response does not decrease at long wavelength.

Table 3. Characteristics of Representative Thermal Detectors

Detector type	Operating temperature (K)	Useful wavelength range (μm)	Typical detectivity (cm $Hz^{1/2}$/W)
Pyroelectric	300	0.4–35	8 X 10^8
Bolometer	300	0.8–40	5 X 10^9
Thermocouple	300	0.8–20	1.5 X 10^8
Thermopile	300	0.8–35	5 X 10^9
Thin film thermopile	300	0.8–35	1.7 X 10^8
Thermistor	300	0.4–30	3 X 10^8

The values presented in the table may be considered representative of what is easily available, but there are numerous manufacturers of these detectors, and the exact characteristics may vary from one manufacturer to another.

JOHN F. READY

4.4.2 Commonly Used Detectors

Most sensors successfully used for process monitoring are of the light-sensitive type. Table 4 (next page) shows some of the most commonly used sensors, including some important characteristics and descriptions of their operating principles. The list presented here, while not complete, offers an overview of the detectors most commonly used in laser material processing devices.

MARIUS JURCA

4.5 Beam Monitoring and Measurement

4.5.1 Beam Samplers

In most materials processing applications, a portion of the beam is sampled to monitor the laser output and to control the operation. Many techniques have been used to extract the power (or energy) to be sampled.

Real-time operation and pulsed-laser compatibility require a real sampler as opposed to a time sampler, since the latter provides only average values. A sampler is designed to extract a small

ISBN 0-912035-15-3

Table 4. Commonly Used Detectors

Sensor	Measuring Range*	Description
Bolometer	Wavelength: 0.001–>300 µm Bandwidth: cw–10^2 Hz Responsivity: up to 2×10^3 V/W	Electrical monitoring of the change in electrical conductivity induced by the change of the temperature of the sensing element as a consequence of thermal radiation absorption
Thermocouples Thermopiles	Wavelength: UV to FIR Bandwidth: cw–10^3 Hz Responsivity up to 10^3 V/W	Heating a junction of two dissimilar materials will generate a voltage across the two open leads according to the thermovoltaic effect. A thermopile consists of several thermocouples. Typical detector materials: metallic joints of Sb/Bi or Si/Au, etc.
Pyroelectric detectors	Wavelength: 0.0001–100 µm Bandwidth: 0.1 Hz–70 MHz Responsivity: up to 10^5 V/W	A thermal gradient in the crystalline structure of a pyrodetector induced by absorption of thermal radiation changes the loal electrical balance of the crystal according to the pyroelectric effect. Usually such materials are also sensitive to mechanical stress and vibrations according to the piezoelectric effect, which generates a similar voltage across the crystalline structure. For correct measurements the thermal radiation flux to be detected has to be "mechanically" interrupted by a chopper. Typical detector material: $LiTaO_3$
Photodetector (photovoltaic effect)	Wavelength: 0.3–12 µm Bandwidth: 0.1 Hz–100 MHz Responsivity: up to 10^8 V/W	A semiconductor *p-n* structure produces an output voltage dependent on the number of incident photons. Typical detector materials: Si (0.3–1.3 µm), Ge (0.8–1.8 µm), InAs (1–3.6 µm), InSb (1–5.5 µm), HgCdZnTe (2–12 µm)**
Photodetector (photoconductive effect)	Wavelength: 1–24 µm Bandwidth: 0.1 Hz –10 MHz Responsivity: up to 10^6 V/W	Incident photons are absorbed at the surface of the detector material and free charge carriers are generated. This effect changes the electrical conductivity of the detector material. Typical detector materials: PbS (1–3.5 µm), PbSe (1–5 µm), HgCdTe (2–24 µm)**

*Data dependent on detector type, material, window, and electronics. **Thermoelectric or LN_2 (liquid nitrogen) detector cooling necessary.

but representative part of the laser beam without inducing any perturbation to the main beam. Such a sampler should have the following properties: insensitivity to polarization, very low sampling factor, high damage threshold, insensitivity to vibration, temperature, and humidity, preservation of a Cartesian beam, virtually no losses, and preservation of the spatial profile of the beam. Many approaches have been considered to create a beam sampler, with desirable combinations of properties. These approaches have included the following:

- Low-reflectivity dielectric coatings (R_{min}) may be used on both faces of a wedge. Such an element will yield two well-separated weak reflections. However, this method is expected to be sensitive to environmental conditions and vibrations.
- The leakage from a high-reflectivity mirror (R_{max}) could also be used to sample a laser beam. In this case, questions arise about the light-polarization sensitivity, the reproducibility of low sampling factor, and the environmental condition (temperature and humidity) sensitivity.
- The use of Fresnel reflection from two cascaded wedges makes the sampling factor insensitive to polarization, but such a scheme has large unusable losses.

- Frustrated total internal reflection (FTIR) offers the advantage of an adjustable sampling factor by changing the gap between two prisms. However, this scheme is very sensitive to incident beam polarization, temperature variation, and vibration.
- Diffractive elements use a periodic structure to produce a replica of the main beam. The large number of samples produced by the hole grating along with its relatively low design versatility makes this technique unattractive.
- Holographic samplers. These devices, discussed in detail below, present an attractive combination of desirable properties.

Table 1 (next page) summarizes these methods and the properties from the list of desirable properties that they possess. The presence of a dot in a box indicates that the method possesses the specified property.

Holographic Beam Sampler

Relief holograms etched directly on highly transparent substrates can sustain a high power level. For example, high-quality fused silica can be used from the near-ultraviolet through near-infrared. The fabrication process starts with a photoresist-coated fused-silica substrate, in which the desired pattern is recorded.

Table 1. Comparison of Different Sampling Methods
(The dots indicate that the particular method has the specified desired property.)

Property \ Method	R_{min} method	R_{max} method	Holographic sampler	Diffractive grating	FTIR method	Cascaded wedge
Polarization insensitive	•		•	•		•
Low sampling factor	•		•		•	•
High damage threshold	•	•	•	•	•	•
Vibration insensitive			•	•	•	
Environmentally insensitive			•			•
Cartesian main beam		•	•	•	•	
Weak unusable losses	•		•	•	•	
Spatial profile reproduction	•	•	•	•	•	•

After development, the pattern is transferred to the fused-silica substrate through an etching process, producing the thin surface-relief phase hologram required for this application.

A holographic sampler offers several advantages. Among them are ease in obtaining a low sampling ratio, a very high damage threshold, production of calibrated replicas of the main beam, and a low sensitivity to environmental conditions, vibrations, and light polarization (at low diffraction angle). The operation of a holographic beam sampler is sketched in Figure 1.

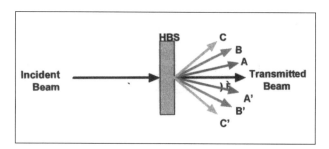

Figure 1. Schematic of a holographic beam sampler.

Holographic sampling is a very attractive and versatile technology for laser control (power and energy monitoring, beam profiling, M^2 measurements, etc.) This author's company produces a complete line of HBS in fused silica for wavelengths from 308 nm to 2.1 µm, which can attain 80 J/cm² of damage threshold. For the far ultraviolet, HBSs are recorded in MgF_2. Fused silica has strange behavior at those wavelengths. The only drawback of this material is that it tends to degrade with time in a nondry environment, unless it is completely coated. For the far infrared (CO_2 lasers), ZnSe may be used for the sampler. These are unfortunately limited by a lower damage threshold (around 900 W/cm²) and higher prices.

Some applications of the HBS are:

- Power and energy measurement (see Section 4.5.4)
- M^2 characterization
- Wavefront analysis
- Wavelength measurement or detection
- Simultaneous near-field and far-field profiling
- Feedback loops

All HBSs are recorded at one precise wavelength with a precise first-order sampling ratio and diffraction angle. For example, 1.000% ratio, at 10°, for 1.064 µm. This does not mean that this particular HBS cannot be used at different wavelengths. The only effect will be a slight change in both the ratio and the angle, which can be expressed as:

New ratio R_2: $\quad R_2 = R_1 (\lambda_1^2/\lambda_2^2)$

New angle θ_2: $\quad \theta_2 = \sin^{-1}[\lambda_2/\lambda_1 \sin \theta_1]$

4.5.2 Energy Meters

An Overview

Joulemeters (energy meters) are made of electroded pyroelectric material (ceramic or crystal), coated with a thin layer of light-absorbing material and bonded to a heatsink. The energy of the light pulse to be measured is absorbed and transferred to the pyroelectric material as a heat pulse. Figure 2 shows the construction of a joulemeter.

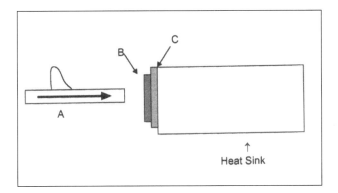

Figure 2. Joulemeter construction. A: light pulse; B: light-absorbing material; C: pyroelectric material.

The pyroelectric material contains oriented permanent dipoles that are temperature sensitive. Rapid temperature variation in the material alters the dipole orientation, thus changing the internal electrical field. The return to electrical equilibrium of the material produces a charge transfer between its electrodes. This charge then flows through a load resistor, connected to the electrodes, and generates a voltage variation with a peak value proportional to the applied energy.

Figure 3 shows a typical joulemeter output pulse. To obtain a calibrated peak voltage response from a joulemeter, the applied light pulse width must be shorter than the detector's rise time (10% to 90%). Longer pulses will not be fully integrated and the peak voltage for very long pulses will become proportional to peak power rather than pulse energy.

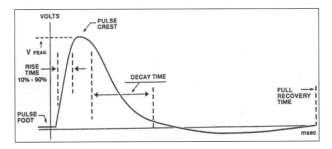

Figure 3. Typical joulemeter response.

The detector rise time is mostly influenced by the thermal time constant of the absorber and the pyroelectric material, but is also sensitive to the electrical time constant and thus to the load resistor value.

Its decay time is mostly influenced by the electrical time constant of the pyroelectric material and thus to the load resistor value. This decay time has the most influence on the detector's maximum repetition rate capability. It can be changed to increase the maximum repetition rate with a corresponding decrease in output sensitivity.

The joulemeter's full recovery time is mostly influenced by the thermal time constant of the pyroelectric material. If the monitoring does not take into account the zero offset value, the resulting maximum repetition rate is limited by this time if measurement accuracy is to be maintained.

If energy is measured at repetition rates higher than that determined by the full recovery time, a rate-related DC offset will occur (see Fig. 4). This DC offset must be excluded from the measurement.

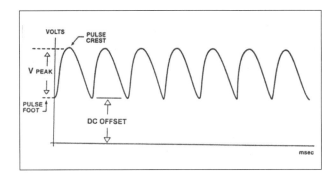

Figure 4. Repetition-rate-related DC offset.

An important limitation while measuring at high repetition rate is the average power impinging on the detector. Table 2 indicates some examples of energy versus maximum repetition rates for some of the detectors manufactured at the author's company.

Table 2. Effect of Pulse Energy on the Maximum Repetition Rate for Joulemeters

Detector	Energy per pulse (J)	Maximum repetition rate (Hz)
A	1	10
A	0.5	20
A	0.14	70
B	1	5
B	0.5	10
B	0.025	200
C	0.1	1.5
C	300 µJ	500

4.5.3 Power Meters

Low Power

In low-power measurements, the method used is a planar thermopile mounted on a massive aluminum heat sink, which generates a Seebeck effect voltage when heat flows through it. Optical radiation is converted into heat by the absorbing material applied to the sensor element. This generates a proportional output voltage. This planar thermopile technology has the great advantage of being insensitive to beam position and diameter. There is no critical alignment of the detectors, allowing for fast setup and extremely flexible operation. The problem of these planar elements is heat dissipation. This is why only low-power meters are constructed in this way.

Typically, a coating is applied on the thermopile. This coating has very fast response time, but has limited damage threshold. There are two families:

1. For high average power density (small beams), a surface absorbing material is placed in front of the thermopile. It helps for high average power density, but cannot survive at high peak power or at high energy density. This author's company has a unique surface absorber that tolerates up to 50 kW/cm^2 of average power density.

2. For high peak power or high energy density, volume absorbers (usually different types of glass) are used. Because of their nature, they do not cool efficiently, making them inefficient at high average power.

A built-in calibration heater bonded to the thermopile surface allows for an electrical equivalence calibration capability. When a DC voltage is applied to this coil, heat is generated and sensed by the detector. The response of the detector is the same whether the heat is generated electrically or by the absorption of a laser beam. The amount of electrical heat is easily determined from voltage and current measurements. This allows easy calibration of the detector response.

High Power

Calorimetric methods of measuring high power are defined as those in which radiant energy is absorbed and converted into heat, thus creating a rise in the absorber temperature. The energy absorbed can then be measured by monitoring a temperature change. High-power sensors are continuous-flow calorimeters that measure power by sensing the temperature gradient created by means of a radial thermopile deposited on the rear of the detecting surface. Since the thermopile is deposited in such a way that the hot junction is oriented toward the middle of the thermopile, at a small radius r, and the cold junction is at a radius R (on the outside edge of the disk), the output is proportional to the temperature difference between R and r, and hence to the incident radiant power. Because the radiation is absorbed within a radius r, the beam shape and position do not affect significantly the measurements.

The response time of calorimeters is mostly determined by the thermal resistance, the thermal capacities, and the geometrical sizes of the disk. Response times, while good, are not as fast as with the planar thermopiles used for low power measurement.

Power meters may be supplied with an "intelligent" connector. This connector contains programmable read-only memory with a calibration factor for the detector head in use. This connector allows a power monitor to adjust its characteristics automatically to the power sensor being connected. Thus no calibration procedure is required when installing the power heads, allowing rapid setup.

4.5.4 Optimizing Meters

Configuring a Reference System

Several examples exist to prove that many power and energy meters are selected for their peak performances in one particular application, but these detectors are deficient in other applications. So several sensors have to be purchased in order to have high performance everywhere. That is usually a high-cost solution. A lower-cost, longer-term solution is available to optimize both the accuracy and the peak performance of power and energy meters.

The most efficient approach is to build, with the assistance of the detector manufacturer, one's own standard for power and energy measurement while still using high-performance but low-cost devices. This system is then used to calibrate lower-cost instruments or detectors for a specific demanding requirement, such as high power or energy levels, high irradiance, very broad dynamic range, and high speed. The standard requires sufficient versatility to permit use for all calibration needs of the user, and should be adequately characterized and documented to allow correction or compensation, at nonoptimum operating conditions, of any response deviation of the detector being calibrated.

An example of a common standard application is the integration of a photodetector assembly into a laser system to monitor the absolute output power. This type of situation dictates that each laser system include a calibrated photodetector to produce an accurate measurement. Thus the cost of this detector becomes critical.

The global requirement for low cost and accuracy can be fulfilled with both a holographic beam sampler (HBS) and a broadband power meter as standard. The holographic device, described in Section 4.5.1, allows sampling of different beam orders and covers a very broad attenuation range. The HBS is supplied with an optical calibration of the power ratio between the first diffractive orders and the zero order. Also available is an optical calibration of the power ratio between the second diffractive order and the zero order. The power meter reference standard has its own stand-alone calibration. The power meter is then used to monitor the zero-order absolute signal while a laser-system photodetector monitors, via either the first or second diffracted order, the attenuated signal.

The simultaneous monitoring of both power meter and photodetector output signals calibrates the photodetector output, which is traceable to the laser power meter manufacturer's standard. This maker's standard should itself be traceable to an absolute NIST standard.

In the case in which the laser beam power in the transmitted, or zero, order is too high for the power meter reference standard, the device can be placed in one of the first orders while the photodetector is located in the other. Both first orders have exactly the same sampling ratio; thus the power in both is identical. The diffractive-element insertion losses, which can be as low as 0.6% in an HBS, can thus be characterized so that the output signal of different detectors can be directly related to the incoming power.

The HBS can also act as a wavelength selector for use with power and energy meters without selective antireflection coating and can provide one calibration per wavelength. Therefore, from the individual first-order diffracted beams, it is possible to monitor the multiple harmonic generator efficiencies using a single optical component and broadband low-cost power or energy meter. Figure 5 illustrates the use of the HBS for determining multiple parameters.

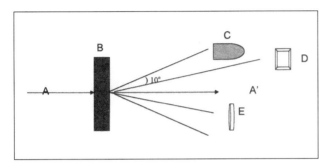

Figure 5. Multiple parameter analysis. A: incident laser beam; A' : unpertubed transmitted laser beam; B: calibrated holographic beam sampler; C: photodetector to monitor stability; D: thermopile power meter for on-line power measurements; E: CCD camera for on-line profile analysis. Angles between each set of lines: 10°.

Measurements of the laser-beam profile and other beam parameters can be performed simultaneously, because the diffracted beam samples are identical, except for intensity, to the incoming beam. This approach leads to the possibility of using multiple low-cost detectors (photodetectors, for example) having acceptable measurement uncertainty once they have been calibrated against a single standard reference unit. The high damage threshold of the HBS, combined with a standard-reference power meter, provides a standard reference having both high damage threshold and high measurement accuracy.

FRANCIS AUDET

4.5.5 Positioning of Power Monitors
An on-line power measurement within a laser material processing system is very useful as it offers a status display of the system at any time. It is very important to place this measurement device as close as possible to the TCP (tool center point) in order to measure all possible power diminishing factors along the beam delivery path, independent of workpiece laser power reflections. From this point of view the ideal location of such a power meter will always be the focusing head.

Most lasers available on the market have an integrated power meter. The readout of this power meter can only offer the user an off-line indication of the available laser power. For production laser systems this kind of measurement is often not sufficient.

In addition, most laser beam power measuring devices integrated in lasers do not completely suppress the laser power reflected from the processing point (TCP) into the laser, so that during the processing no correct laser output power measurement can be effected.

In practice there are two kinds of laser material processes: continuous and piece by piece. For continuous welding (or cutting) purposes a laser power measuring device is necessary to measure the laser beam power independent of the reflected laser power from the workpiece. This can be achieved with a transparent beam splitter or with a grating mirror (or lens) separating in direction the part of the laser beam to be measured from the workpiece reflections.

Such a separating component (beam splitter, grating mirror, or holographic transmitting element) is also useful in case of a piece-by-piece laser material process, but in this case there is also another possibility: a stationary thermal laser power probe at the "home" position of the movement system. This kind of measurement is not useful during the material processing, but it is not expensive and measures the entire laser and the beam delivery system. For an adequate specification of such a home-measuring power meter, it is necessary to know the exact beam diameter and also to consider the actual laser power distribution at the measuring point for the calculation of the maximum allowable peak power density on the power meter surface.

These considerations are independent of the laser type (CO_2 or Nd:YAG). For CO_2 lasers most of the power meters utilized are of the bolometer or thermopile type. They also can be integrated into calorimetric power meters. The sensing elements for Nd:YAG laser power meters are usually Si photodiodes.

Additionally devices for measuring the laser power of the raw beam are available. They are usually combined with a laser beam power distribution measurement. There are three different (but similar) working principles of such power distribution measuring devices for CO_2 laser beams: (1) flying needle, (2) flying detector, and (3) spatial filter. Such power meters can be installed in welding or surface treatment systems, but not in cutting systems because of diffraction effects.

MARIUS JURCA

4.5.6 Beam Profilers
Beam profilers provide easy and rapid characterization of laser beams. They are used to determine mode structure, beam spatial profiles, beam quality information, beam divergence, astigmatism, asymmetry, and beam diameter at any position along the beam. Such information is needed for many materials processing applications.

Two common approaches are used to determine the profile of a beam. One may direct the beam into a large area detector and then scan an opaque mask through the beam. Masks have included a knife edge, slits, or pinholes. The variation in signal is measured as the mask is scanned. A computer then determines the intensity profile. The second approach is to use a camera consisting of a large array of small area detectors. The detectors are often charged-coupled devices (CCDs).

The resulting signals are processed to obtain the beam profile and power distribution, which are presented on a display. The display make take a variety of formats, including two dimensional plots, isometric three dimensional plots, or cross sectional profiles. Commercial beam profilers are available covering the spectral range from the ultraviolet to the infrared.

The devices with scanning masks may be used with continuous lasers or lasers with high pulse repetition rates. Their resolution can be in the submicrometer regime, so that they can deter-

Table 3. Select Laser Beam Diagnostics Instruments* and Their Characteristics

Company and product name	Wavelength range (type of detector)	Type of applicable laser	Laser power range	Pixel details on the camera	Laser beam size limits	Techniques and other comments
Spiricon-beam propagation analyzer	350 nm – 1.1 µm	Continuous wave and pulsed	Damage total power: 1 W over entire array Damage threshold: 1 W/cm^2 Pulsed laser, 1 to 10^5 Hz, 1 ps to 4 ms, Damage threshold: 1mJ/cm^2	Element spacing: 100 x 100 µm; Active area: (12.4 mm)^2 Number of elements: 124 x 124		Solid state pyroelectic camera Large area Si camera 10^4 greater intensity than CCD cameras
Coherent mode master propogation analyzer	0.22 – 0.688 µm (Si) 0.34 – 1 µm (Si) 0.80 – 1.80 µm (Ge) 1.80 – 15 µm (pyroelectric IR solid state)	Continuous wave or pulsed	7.5 mW – 10 W 2.5 mW – 25 W 2.5 mW – 2.5 W 400 mW – 20 W		12 – 25 mm 12 – 25 mm 12 – 15 mm 12 – 45 mm	
Coherent multiaxis knife edge scanning beam analyzer/ profiler	400 – 1100 nm (Si) 800 – 1800 nm (InGaAs)	Continuous wave and pulsed	10 µW – 1 W (Si) 10 µW – 5 mW (InGaAs) 0.1 µW resolution		3 µm – 9 mm (Si); 3 µm – 3 mm (In GaAs) 1 µm beam size resolution; 0.1 µm for laser beam with size < 100 µm	Two orthogonal knife edges or slits to scan the beam profile
Photon beam profiler	190 nm – 30 µm	Continuous wave and pulsed	CW CO$_2$: few µW to 100 W	(a) 7 µm (b) 0.14 to 14 mm	a. 80 µm – 4.5 mm b. 5 µm – 25.4 mm	(a) CCD-photodiode detector array and (b) pinhole slit method (beam scan method)

*Representative measurements systems – not an exhaustive list

ISBN 0-912035-15-3

mine profiles near the beam focus. Profilers based on detector arrays can perform single shot profiling for single laser pulses.

Their resolution is determined by the number of detectors in the array. Two dimensional arrays with hundreds of detectors in each dimension are available.

Table 3 presents information about the characteristics of some commercial instruments. This information is presented for illustrative purposes to show the types of capability that are available; it does not represent an endorsement of the companies named.

The following are some of the representative beam properties that can be measured or analyzed for: M^2, waist diameter, divergence angle, waist location, astigmatism, asymmetry ratio, beam mode patterns.

Over the wavelength range 190 – 1100 nm, a silicon CCD array is the best choice.

Three physical sensor properties are important to the beam imaging process: number of pixels, sensor area, and pixel spacing. The maximum surface area that can be imaged by any camera depends on the vertical active area dimension.

JOHN F. READY
KARTHIK NAGARATHNAM
JYOTI MAZUMDER

4.6 Components for Motion Systems

4.6.1 Basic Considerations

In laser materials processing, one must often be able to position components, including the workpiece, very precisely. One must also be able to move the components from one position to another. This section describes some of the basic components used for micropositioning, with emphasis on what is commonly available commercially.

Degrees of Freedom

Micropositioning equipment can accurately position a component in space. The positioning is usually described in terms of six degrees of freedom, three translational and three rotational. The three translational degrees of freedom describe the position in terms of location along three orthogonal axes. The three rotational degrees of freedom describe the orientation of the component with respect to rotation about three orthogonal axes.

According to the application, it is possible that a micropositioner can position a component in any number of these degrees of freedom, from one to six. Thus one may employ devices that have only translational capability, in one, two, or three axes. There are devices that control the orientation of a part by rotation about one, two, or three axes, and there are devices that combine translation and rotation.

Definitions

A number of terms are commonly used in connection with micropositioning equipment. The following list defines some important concepts.

Accuracy is the maximum difference between the actual position and the desired position for a component.

Precision is the average difference between the desired position and the actual position when a number of measurements are made for the position. It is also called repeatability.

Resolution is the minimum controllable motion that the system can produce.

Backlash is the motion that is lost when the direction of a driving element is reversed. The effect of backlash can be eliminated by always approaching a position from the same direction.

Environmental Considerations

Environmental considerations that affect the performance of micropositioning equipment include temperature and vacuum.

Temperature changes can cause changes in the size and shape of micropositioning equipment. The coefficient of thermal expansion for stainless steel is lower than that of aluminum so that stainless steel components may be preferred under conditions where the temperature may vary. In conditions of nonuniform temperature distributions, the higher value of thermal conductivity of aluminum may lead to aluminum components being preferred.

In any case, it is desirable that the temperature be stable when one uses micropositioning equipment. Changes in temperature can lead to dimensional inaccuracies and to bowing and twisting of the positioning equipment.

If micropositioning equipment is to be used in a vacuum environment, special lubricants often will be required. The equipment may have to be baked before use; it must be tolerant of the baking temperature. Motors with performance usually specified at atmospheric pressure may have to be derated for vacuum operation because the motor cannot dissipate heat by convection.

Manufacturers of micropositioning equipment offer versions of micropositioning devices suited for vacuum operation.

4.6.2 Guiding Methods

A positioner uses a drive device, like a motor, to drive a lead screw that controls the position of the stage. The motion is controlled by a guidance system. Commercial devices are commonly classified according to the guidance method.

Micropositioning equipment uses four main methods for guiding movable platforms on which components are mounted. These methods include dovetail guidance systems, ball bearing slides, crossed roller bearings, and flexure devices.

Dovetail slides have two flat surfaces sliding against each other. They use a fan-shaped tenon that interlocks into a corresponding mortise. They are the most simple of the guidance methods and provide moderate performance at low cost.

Ball bearing slides use balls held in guideways by hardened metal rods. The motion of the device over its range of travel is controlled by the rods. This method produces very low friction.

Crossed roller bearings use a series of cylindrical roller bearings held in a cage. Successive bearings are arranged to be at right angles to each other. They replace the point contact of a ball bearing with the line contact of a roller bearing, so that the load capacity is higher.

A flexure device uses elastic deformation of a structure to produce motion. Such devices completely eliminate friction, but their range of travel is limited.

Table 1 compares the relative characteristics of these four guidance methods. The user can choose a device with characteristics matched to a specific application.

For any of the guidance methods, there is a tradeoff between the total range of motion and the resolution that can be achieved. For longer ranges of travel, the resolution becomes worse (larger) than for shorter ranges of travel. Table 2 summarizes the tradeoff for common commercial units.

Table 1. Comparison of Guiding Methods

Method	Dovetail	Ball bearing	Crossed roller bearing	Flexure
Cost	Low	Moderate	High	High
Friction	High	Low	Low	Zero
Range of motion	Large	Moderate	Moderate	Small
Load capacity	High	Low	High	High
Precision	Moderate	High	Very high	Very high

Table 2. Typical Resolution for Various Ranges of Motion

Translational Units

Range of motion (mm)	Resolution (µm)
20	0.1
100	1
250	10
1000	100

Rotational Units

Range of motion (degrees)	Resolution (degrees)
45	$10^{-3} - 10^{-2}$

The load capacity of the device is an important consideration. Excessive loads can deform the units, degrading their performance and increasing the force required to make a movement. Commercial units have ratings for maximum load capacity. The load capacity is specified for loads located at the center of the stage. If the load is off center, the load capacity should be derated.

Many translational and rotational stages are available commercially, with a wide range of characteristics, including number of degrees of freedom, range of travel, load capacity, etc.

4.6.3 Drive Units

A variety of drive types are available to move the stage to its desired position, including manual and motorized actuators. The user may choose a drive that meets the needs of a specific application.

Manual drives are basically micrometers, with high-precision lead screws actuated by turning a knurled knob. They provide low-cost operator-controlled positioning capability. But when rapid or repetitive positioning is required, motor-driven actuators are required.

Motors used in micropositioning equipment are usually either DC motors or stepping motors. The DC motor contains a rotor in a magnetic field. The field causes the rotor to rotate when current is applied to the motor windings. DC motors provide smooth motion, high speed, good efficiency, and a high power/weight ratio.

Stepper motors have a rotor and several windings. When current flows in the windings, a magnetic field is generated, which causes the rotor to turn. Stepper motors move in a continuous fashion from one point to another. Thus they are well suited to repetitive micropositioning applications. At a stop position, stepper motors maintain position without application of power.

Stepper motors are controlled by applying voltage to the windings in a sequential fashion, which makes the rotor move to various positions in a stepwise fashion. This is called a full step. The distance between two stable positions of a stepper motor is a full step. The minimum resolution of the stepper motor is determined by the size of the step.

The minimum resolution of a stepper motor may be reduced by balancing currents so that the rotor may assume any angular position. This essentially divides the full step into a number of smaller discrete steps, frequently around ten. These motors are called ministepping motors. A variety of different commercial models are available.

Electrostrictive actuators are another type of drive unit. They use ferroelectric materials that change dimension when an electric field is applied to them. They provide very precise motion, but the range of travel is limited. They are preferred to piezoelectric actuators because piezoelectric devices exhibit larger hysteresis.

Table 3 provides information about the minimum resolution that may be obtained with easily available models of the different types of drive units.

Table 3. Typical Minimum Resolution for Drive Units

Drive	Resolution (μm)
Electrostrictive	0.02
Micrometer	0.25
Stepper motor	0.07
DC motor	0.03

For the driver units, there is a tradeoff between speed and resolution, with units having higher speed tending to have poorer (larger) minimum resolution. Table 4 provides typical ranges for the resolution available for various speeds.

Table 4. Tradeoff between Resolution and Speed

Translational Units

Resolution (μm)	Maximum speed (mm/sec)
0.1	0.02
1	2
5	10
10	20

Rotational Units

Resolution (degrees)	Maximum speed (degrees/sec)
0.001	2
0.01	20
0.05	100

There are many models of drivers available commercially with a wide range of characteristics.

JOHN F. READY

4.7 Controllers

4.7.1 Laser and Motion Control

In the simplest form an industrial laser processing system consists of a laser, beam delivery system, motion mechanism, and ancillary equipment related to the process. Under the category of ancillary equipment items such as fixtures, clamps, sensors, and a gas delivery system would be found. Also for most laser processing systems some type of heat exchanger would be necessary to remove the excess heat from the laser. To ensure that the laser process operates consistently and reliably, some form of system control is needed.

Many lasers and laser systems now have self-monitoring systems that can maintain the commanded power even as the laser resonator optics or arc lamps degrade. Messages come up on the controller screen showing which maintenance items need to be either cleaned or replaced prior to their failure. Some lasers have modem connections so that a remote service technician can analyze a problem and give advice over the phone, instructing the user on the proper repair procedure or how to determine if a component needs replacement. High-speed height sensors that maintain the nozzle standoff distance for cutting and seam tracking devices that control path position for welding are commonly incorporated into laser systems to improve process reliability. Part nesting programs are often used in cutting systems to improve material usage and minimize scrap (1). These features greatly improve the overall process quality and reliability and improve the operating costs of laser systems.

The motion controller's primary function is to maintain the path accuracy and the commanded travel speed. Additionally, the motion controller may control the movement of an indexing device, safety and programming-related features, and be the storage device for the part programs. It may also have the capability of controlling other ancillary devices necessary for the laser process.

4.7.2 Laser System Control

The function of a system controller is to provide communication and control over the various functions of the laser system. Many systems have been designed with a single integrated controller that controls all the functions of the system. Other systems will have both a motion controller and a laser controller. As stated previously, the laser controller will monitor and control laser functions such as power output, operating temperature, and general degradation of key components. The motion controller will control path accuracy, travel speed, and possibly the ancillary equipment. Normally under this condition the motion controller will be the primary controller and the laser will be the secondary controller. Communication between the various devices is normally handled by using input and outputs (I/O). The controller can command and/or monitor such functions as part presence, closing clamps, indexing parts, laser power, and shutter control and gas assist control. More complex systems where communication goes beyond the laser cell may require a main computer or programmable logic computer (PLC).

The broad range of controls offered by laser and system manufacturers are dependent on process, material geometry, laser and motion type. It is important that the end user understand the requirements of the process and determine the features necessary for the application. Several trade journals annually list companies that manufacture lasers and laser systems (2) (3). This is a good starting point to begin an evaluation process. Most laser or laser system manufacturers will evaluate applications and make recommendations. By contacting several suppliers and going through a review process, the customer can get a clearer picture about which features are required for the process and the strengths and weaknesses of each supplier. In general, laser systems have been designed to accommodate a wide range of features that may be necessary for a particular application. It then becomes a matter of cost and the number of options that a customer needs or can afford. The end user will take on more risk by acting as the system integrator, incorporating the major components together and dealing with communication and safety issues associated with a laser system.

4.7.3 Programming

There are two basic programming methods for generating a motion path. Some systems use computer numeric control (CNC) or numeric control (NC). Others use a direct-entry teaching method. The type of process, part geometry, and motion type will normally determine which type of programming method is most commonly used (4).

CNC Programming

In general 2D and simple 3D part processing that uses rectilinear motion to generate the process path employs either NC or CNC programming. These parts are normally made from drawing information that contains the X, Y, and Z dimensional information necessary for part programming. Depending on the information on the drawing, the program can either be done using absolute or incremental code (5). If there is a 0,0,0 datum position related to the part, it may be easier to use an absolute programming method in which all the program positions are listed by their relationship to the 0,0,0 position. If the drawing information is in the form of distance in X, Y, and Z from point to point, incremental programming may be easier. Both types have their advantages and disadvantages, and most parts can be successfully processed using either method.

Direct Entry Teaching Method

Large parts or stampings that are processed using multiaxis articulated robots or other similar devices normally use a direct entry teaching method. Typically a master part with a scribed process path is positioned on a fixture and the robotic device is maneuvered along the path. As the part programmer moves either the cutting or welding head along the process path, the positional information is entered into the program via a teach pendant. A visible low-power beam on-axis with the high-power processing beam is normally used as an alignment aid for the programmer. Some system suppliers have software features that make common shape generation easy by requiring that only the center location be programmed. Other software features allow the part programmer to easily maintain true perpendicularity of the process head to the part, enhancing programming efficiency (5) (6).

4.7.4 CAD/CAM and Off-Line Programming

In order to justify the cost of a laser system, up time has to remain high and production rates have to be met. Off-line programming and CAD/CAM software packages are sometimes necessary to meet these goals.

There are several factors that can affect the decision to use either direct teaching or CAD/CAM programming method (4). The CAD data may not be available or in a format that is useful to a particular system. Some prototype parts may not have completed CAD data available because of design changes. The cost of an off-line CAM/CAM software package may not be justifiable in all cases. The number of parts to be cut may favor using the direct teaching method over CAD programming because of time constraints. In addition, the skill level required to generate a CAD/CAM program is normally higher than required to generate a direct teaching program. However, the most important reason to use off-line programming is that it frees up the laser processing system so it is not being used to generate taught programs. Figure 1 shows a decision-making flow chart that can be used to determine if teaching or CAD/CAM should be used to generate part programs (4).

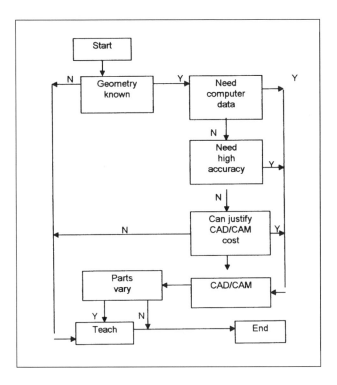

Figure 1. Decision-making flow chart to determine whether to use teaching or CAD/CAM programming method.

Many laser cutting systems have software packages that allow the part programmer to work off-line and then download the part information to the laser system. However, many other systems do not have this capability. There are many companies that manufacture software packages for off-line programming with varying capabilities and costs (7). Three steps are involved in generating a part program from a drawing file. The first step involves translating DXF (drawing interchange file) or IGES (initial graphics exchange standard) formatted part files into a graphical display (8). Once the part program has been generated using CAD, it has to be translated using CAM to the program language specific to the machine that will process the part. Finally the part program can be run. Modifications may be made depending on the complexity and repeatability of the part and the accuracy requirements.

Nesting software optimizes the part or parts orientation and then determines the quantity of material required to make the production run (9). Many times these types of software packages are used to estimate part cycle time accurately and to identify potential interference problems with fixture clamps and other devices that may lie in the program path. Part orientation and system component layouts can be evaluated and optimized prior to actual system construction. Job shops that use laser cutting systems use their CAD/CAM or off-line programming capabilities to determine cost per part information. In a very real sense the cost of these software packages can often be justified by reduced operating costs and reducing delivery time.

References
1. D. Lichtenwalner, *The Fabricator*, Vol. 27, No. 7, 59–61 (1997).
2. *The Fabricator*, Vol. 27, No. 5, 67–86 (1997).
3. *The Fabricator*, Vol. 27, No. 12, 54–62 (1997).
4. T. VanderWert, *The Fabricator*, Vol. 23, No. 7, 34–40 (1993).
5. Manual, Laserdyne™ System 94 Laser Process Control Software and Hardware Features (1996).
6. Manual, FANUC Robotics Laser Shape Generation Software (1997).
7. *The Fabricator*, Vol. 28, No. 2, 62–74 (1998).
8. C. Grosso, *The Fabricator*, Vol. 26, No. 3, 86–9 (1996).
9. Vicki Wei Sun, *The Fabricator*, Vol. 27, No. 6, 38–41 (1997).

DAVID B. VEVERKA

4.8 Process Gas Nozzles

4.8.0 Introduction
Unlike other thermal cutting methods (oxy-fuel and plasma), the laser beam does not produce its own gas jet with which to blow away the molten material and plasma that it generates. Thus an auxiliary gas jet must be provided from a pressurized source through a suitable nozzle. The shape, orientation, alignment, and standoff distance of this nozzle, as well as the gas pressure that drives it, have important consequences upon the resulting laser cut. In particular, the nozzle plays a key role in the ability of the assist gas to eject molten material effectively, which is then reflected in the amount of dross formed, the maximum cutting speed, and the overall cut quality (for any laser power level).

4.8.1 Nozzle Configurations

Sonic Nozzles
The great majority of laser cutting is now done using simple coaxial gas nozzles, in which both the laser beam and the gas jet exit from the same orifice in the cutting head and impinge coaxially upon the workpiece. The nozzle, which may be of either the sonic or supersonic type (Fig. 1), is governed by the principles of gas dynamics (1).

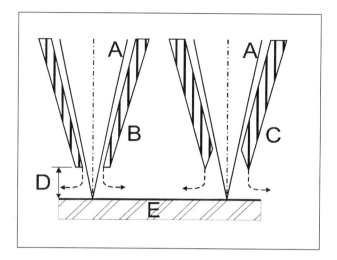

Figure 1. Diagram of sonic and Laval laser cutting nozzles. A: laser beam, B: sonic nozzle, C: Laval nozzle, D: standoff distance, E: workpiece.

Simple *sonic* nozzles are used almost universally, in which the nozzle converges to a minimum area or throat at its outlet. If the cutting gas pressure just upstream of the nozzle is more than about twice that of the atmosphere, the gas speed will be sonic at the nozzle throat. Still higher gas pressures lead to supersonic flow after the nozzle exit. The resulting gas jet from the nozzle impinges upon the workpiece, causing a high local pressure near the laser beam focus. Since the pressure below the workpiece is atmospheric, a pressure gradient is created that drives a gas flow along the kerf leading edge, ejecting the melt from the bottom of the kerf.

Laval Nozzles
At least for inert assist gases, increasing the gas pressure upstream of the nozzle usually facilitates faster and cleaner laser cuts. However, for gas pressures several times that of the atmosphere, a complex supersonic jet with strong internal shock waves impinges upon the workpiece. This can cause the cut quality to be very sensitive to the small changes in nozzle standoff distance that can occur in normal cutting practice. In these high-pressure cases a converging-diverging or *Laval* nozzle design (Fig. 1) is more advantageous.

The Laval nozzle avoids this problem by expanding the gas flow after the nozzle throat so that a better match with atmospheric pressure is produced at the nozzle exit. For each Laval nozzle design (characterized by its exit-to-throat area ratio), however, there is an optimum upstream gas pressure to achieve this match (1). Moreover, severe geometric design constraints are placed on a Laval nozzle for laser cutting: It must pass the laser beam unobstructed through its throat, and the combined lengths of the nozzle divergent section and standoff distance are then limited by the distance from throat to laser focus. This distance is short when the laser beam has a small f number. Thus a rapid conically divergent section is usually the best nozzle design compromise.

Despite these constraints, Laval nozzles outperform sonic nozzles in terms of cut quality, maximum cutting speed, and insensitivity to standoff distance when cutting with high assist-gas pressure. Limits on this pressure eventually occur due to the strain placed upon the laser optics and the eventual occurrence of flow separation at the kerf leading edge due to shock waves inside the kerf (2).

The cross-sectional shape of a coaxial nozzle, like that of the laser beam itself, should normally be round. Lobed cross sections and other complex shapes have been tried, but there appears to be no gas-dynamic justification for them. An oblong nozzle exit shape might gain some advantage by conforming to the kerf if oriented along the cutting direction, but this would sacrifice the omnidirectional cutting advantage of the round coaxial nozzle.

Off-Axis Nozzles

Once the assist-gas jet is moved to an axis different from that of the laser beam, the new variables of jet angle ϕ and jet target point arise (Fig. 2). Experience shows that such an off-axis jet should follow rather than lead the cutting head, and that angles ϕ in the range of 20-45 degrees yield maximum cutting speeds up to 50% better than that of a coaxial nozzle (2). The off-axis nozzle type, whether sonic or Laval, has a comparatively small effect. In fact, crude off-axis nozzles are sometimes simply made from copper tubing. The target point of the off-axis jet should normally lie at the laser focus or at some small distance beneath it inside the kerf. In one example (inert gas cutting of mild steel at 6 atm nozzle gage pressure) an off-axis nozzle at ϕ = 30 degrees produced a much cleaner cut edge than did a coaxial nozzle (2).

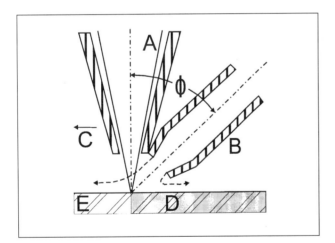

Figure 2. Diagram of an off-axis laser cutting nozzle installation. A: laser beam, B: off-axis nozzle, C: cutting direction, D: kerf, E: workpiece, ϕ: jet angle.

The advantages gained by an off-axis nozzle appear to stem from the alleviation of shock-wave-induced flow separation at the kerf leading edge. The off-axis nozzle also decouples the assist gas from the laser optics of the cutting head, and allows greater head standoff distance, which improves damage resistance. However, one must weigh against these advantages the added complexity and alignment difficulty of the off-axis nozzle and the loss of omnidirectional cutting capability. For these reasons, off-axis nozzles are used far less often than coaxial nozzles in routine laser cutting.

References
1. J. E. John, 1984: *Gas Dynamics*, 2nd ed., Prentice Hall, Paramus, NJ.
2. A. D. Brandt, and G. S. Settles, *J. Laser Applications* **9**, 269–77 (1997).

GARY S. SETTLES

4.8.2 Nozzle Selection

A variety of gas nozzles and shields are generally used in laser beam welding, depending on the need in each case. It is, therefore, important to note that this section describes only general guidelines and thus they may be insufficient to a specific situation, and if so, some modification or improvement should be made accordingly.

The need to use gas nozzle and shield depends on the heat input, which is a function of power input and welding speed. Therefore, the level of power and the welding speed have to be chosen first, and then what type of nozzle and/or shield to use can be determined. The following suggests nozzle and/or shield according to power levels used for a given speed. Although irradiance is the more appropriate quantity, power level serves as a simple, convenient guideline.

Low-Power Laser Beam Welding

At low power levels, it may not be necessary to use a nozzle and/or shielding device. Examples are: (1) pulsed solid-state laser spot welding, and (2) single-pulse, solid-state laser welding. However, if tolerance of the weld quality is stringent, shielding gas with an appropriate nozzle and/or shield should be used. For example, in overlapping spot welding with a pulsed laser, a shielding gas with a nozzle is recommended (3).

Moderate-Power Laser Beam Welding

In pulsed or moderate power CO_2 laser welding, a coaxial nozzle is used where He or Ar gas flows along the laser beam axis to the laser-material interaction zone, as shown in Figure 3.

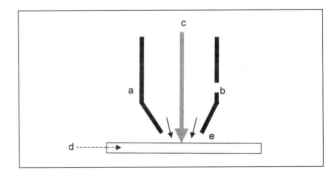

Figure 3. Schematic diagram of a gas feed system: Coaxial nozzle (a), gas inlet (b), laser beam (c), workpiece (d), and gas jet (e).

Chapter 4: Components for Laser Materials Processing Systems

High-Power Welding

For high-power CO_2 welding or pulsed laser beam welding with irradiance above 10^6 W/cm² where keyhole penetration occurs, it is strongly recommended that both shields to protect the hot weld, and a nozzle to suppress plasma be used. However, if atmospheric contamination is minimal and can be tolerted without compromising the mechanical properties, a simple gas nozzle may be used, as shown in Figure 4.

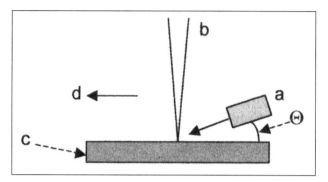

Figure 4. Schematic diagram of a simple gas nozzle (a) parallel to the welding direction (d) at a certain angle from the workpiece (c) and laser beam (b).

For example, with the nozzle 55° from the workpiece, full penetration welds in 1-in.-thick A-38 mild steels were achieved with 10 kW power, 25.4 cm/min (10 ipm), speed and a He gas flow rate of 14,158 cm³/min (30 cubic feet per hour) (4). Note that this is an example, and 55° may not be the optimum angle for all situations. Therefore, adjust the angle experimentally to get the best value.

When both good quality of the weld surface (oxidation free) and sufficient penetration are desirable, shielding fixtures (Fig. 5) are used with a combination of shields covering the entire weld and a nozzle for plasma suppression.

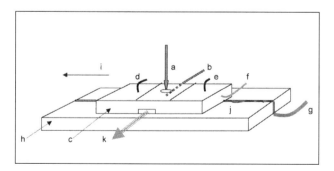

Figure 5. A schematic shielding device showing the laser beam (a), a transverse plasma suppression nozzle (b), frame of the shields (c), lead (d), trail (e), trail-trail (f), and bottom shielding (g). Also shown are the workpiece (h), welding direction (i), solidified weld beads (j), and plasma suppression gas outflow (k).

There are four shielding gas flows in the illustrated shielding device, where the lead is in front of the interaction zone (or molten weld pool); the trail is behind the molten pool; the bottom covers the bottom of entire weldment; and the trail-trail protects the area behind the trail being solidified. A plasma suppression gas nozzle is directed horizontal (parallel to the work) and perpendicular to the welding direction to blow away the plasma plume as shown in Figure 5. The height of the shield has to be adjusted so that suppression gas aims at the center of the plasma mass. The plasma plume was blown away from the beam pass without disturbance to the molten pool, resulting in formation of pretty beads. This shielding fixture was used at the Naval Research Laboratory to laser weld successfully half-inch-thick plates of HY-80, HY-100, HY-130, A-36, HSLA-80, and HSLA-100 in the 10–15 kW range.

A similar shielding device to that in Figure 5 is introduced in Figure 6 for a case where deeper penetration is desirable. A gas nozzle is directed to the interaction area of the laser beam and the workpiece along the direction of welding, as opposed to the transverse direction in Figure 5. The gas jet not only suppresses the plasma above the molten pool but also suppresses the molten surface, contributing to additional penetration.

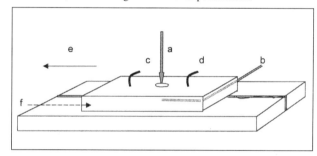

Figure 6. A shielding device showing laser beam (a), a plasma suppression gas nozzle parallel to the welding direction (b), shielding gas supplies (c,d), welding direction (e), and a shielding box (f).

References
3. The ASM Committee on Laser Beam Welding, ASM Metals Handbook, ninth edition, Vol. 6, p. 659.
4. ASTM A-38 mild steels were laser welded in 1981 at the Naval Research Laboratory.

D. W. MOON

4.8.3 Process Gas Nozzles for Cutting

Gas Flow from Nozzles

The gas flow from laser cutting nozzles is, under practical cutting conditions (for metals), almost always supersonic. This means that shocks that can be present in the flow can affect the cut quality and cutting speed if the nozzle standoff is too large (5). The flow is supersonic if the nozzle pressure is above 1.9 bar (absolute pressure) with oxygen, nitrogen, or a mixture (air) as assist gas. The flow rate, in liters/min, is (6):

flow rate = $10pd^2$

where d is the nozzle exit diameter in mm and p the applied pressure in bar (absolute pressure).

Types of Nozzle

Laser cutting nozzles are generally manufactured out of copper, having a threaded end for easy replacement. Whereas early laser cutting nozzles merely had a conical shape, current designs have been optimized for good cutting performance. This includes accurate manufacturing and optimum external tip shape and internal profile.

Two types of laser cutting nozzle exist: conical nozzles and Laval nozzles (see Fig. 7.).

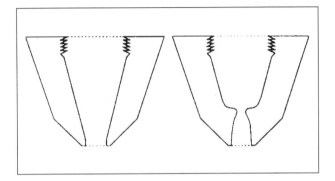

Figure 7. Conical laser cutting nozzle (left) and Laval laser cutting nozzle (right).

Conical nozzles are used the most, and are fitted as standard on almost every laser cutting machine. This nozzle has a conical internal shape with a short parallel exit hole. Conical nozzles must be used close to the surface to be cut (gap less than about 1 mm) in order to obtain a high cutting pressure and to avoid difficulties associated with shocks. Conical nozzles are cheap to manufacture and can be used over a wide range of gas assist pressure to suit the specific application.

A Laval nozzle has a more complicated internal shape, resulting in a more even gas flow without significant shock waves in the supersonic flow, so that these nozzles can be used at much larger standoff, up to several mm. This has the advantages of the nozzle tip being less prone to damage from sputter and collision, and the capability to cut into corners of 3D shaped components. On the other hand, Laval nozzles are more expensive than conical nozzles and can be used at one specific pressure only, for which the internal profile is designed.

Since the narrowest section (the throat) of a Laval nozzle is not at the tip but some way inside the nozzle, alignment of this type of nozzle with the laser beam (see below) is slightly more tricky than with conical nozzles. The variable d in the approximation for flow rate given above refers to the smallest diameter of a Laval nozzle (its throat), and not the diameter of the exit.

Nozzle Pressure and Gas Supply

Laser cutting uses assist gas pressures up to 20 bar, depending on the material species and thickness being cut. The highest pressures are normally used when cutting stainless steel with nitrogen if a dross–free cut and unoxidized cut edge is required. Care should be taken when using high-pressure assist gas on a cutting system not designed for it. An upgraded nozzle assembly and a special, thicker lens may be have to be fitted first.

The gas pressure setting at the regulator is not necesarilly the same as the pressure inside the nozzle, especially if the pressure is high or the flow rate large (large nozzles). Significant pressure losses can occur in the gas lines toward the nozzle. This is not a problem, so long as the same gas line is used all the time once the optimum gas pressure setting on the regulator has empirically been established. A gas pipe of adequate diameter will avoid the problem altogether. If a gas pipe of 6 mm (or 1/4 in.) internal diameter is used, then the pressure loss over a length of 10 m is no more than about 5%.

Coarse Nozzle Alignment

The gas jet must be accurately aligned with the focused laser beam. This can be facilitated either by moving the lens or by moving the nozzle, both by means of adjustment screws. It is better to move the nozzle than to move the lens, because moving the lens may cause the incident laser beam to be no longer in the center of the lens. Coarse alignment can be done with a piece of polycarbonate, held well below the nozzle and exposed very briefly with the laser beam. The resulting burn mark will indicate if the laser beam is clipping the edge of the nozzle (assuming that all other lenses and mirrors are properly aligned). Once it has been established that the whole of the beam goes through the nozzle exit, fine adjustment must be carried out to align the laser beam with the gas jet.

Fine Nozzle Adjustment

Fine adjustment is critical to the laser cutting process. Good laser cutting cannot be achieved with only a coarsely adjusted nozzle, which would result in drossy cuts, low cutting speed, or burning (unless the user is lucky). The laser beam should traverse the center of the nozzle exit to within 50 µm or better. While this adjustment sounds difficult to do, it is not. One method uses a small amount of thick black grease applied to the surface to be cut, which is exposed briefly to the gas jet and a low power pulse of the laser. The radial pattern in the grease, caused by the gas jet, accurately defines the center of the jet, and the mark by the laser pulse shows any misalignment that may be present. Figure 8 shows several examples.

The black grease method is also a very sensitive indicator of nozzle damage (see Fig. 9). Even microscopic blemishes on the nozzle tip edge have a marked effect on the gas flow pattern, and therefore on the laser cut quality. So it is important to protect the nozzle from collisions, and to replace it regularly.

Pressure Sensor

Another method for precise alignment, suitable for thin sheet of up to about 2 mm, uses a simple pressure gauge mounted on a hand–held clamp as shown in Figure 10. First, the sheet is pierced with the laser in the normal way, and then (with the laser off) the pressure gauge is applied and the assist gas turned on. If the laser beam and the gas jet are aligned, the pressure read on the gauge will be at a maximum, and if not the nozzle can be adjusted to reach the maximum. If the nozzle cannot be adjusted but the lens instead, then this method can of course not be used.

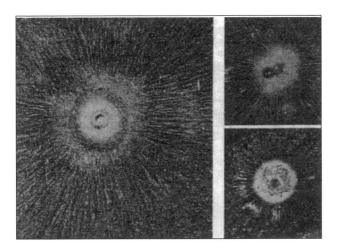

Figure 8. Grease marks of properly aligned laser and nozzle (left) and misaligned laser and nozzle (top and bottom right).

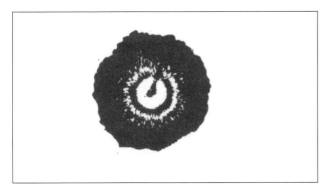

Figure 9. Grease mark from nozzle with very slight tip damage, showing large deviations from symmetric flow.

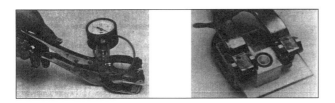

Figure 10. Simple tool for centering the laser beam and nozzle.

Nozzle Standoff and Nozzle Diameter

The gap between nozzle and workpiece should be kept constant and small (for conical nozzles). Nearly all commercial laser cutting machines are fitted as standard with a mechanical or capacitive height sensor so that the gap can be held constant very precisely. Almost all materials that can be cut by laser need the same standoff distance so that this dimension need be set once and can (almost) be forgotten.

The diameter of the nozzle is determined largely by the thickness of the material to be cut. For thin sheets (less than 2 mm) a nozzle exit diameter of 1.0 mm is mostly used. For thicker sections, progressively wider exits are used, up to 2 mm. Larger nozzles have a better tolerance to misalignment, but use much more gas.

Figure 11 shows an example of a typical nozzle for CO_2 laser cutting, with the components identified.

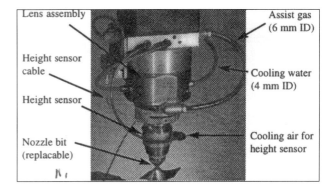

Figure 11. A high-pressure-capoable CO_2 laser cutting head. Photograph courtesy of Quantum Laser Engineering Ltd. Conventry, UK.

References
5. J. Fieret, M. J. Terry, and B. A. Ward, *Aerodynamic interactions during laser cutting,* Proc. SPIE, Quebec, 2–6 June 1986.
6. L. D. Landau, and E. M. Lifshitz, 1982: Course of Theoretical Physics, Volume 6: Fluid Mechanics, Pergamon Press, p. 347–9.

JIM FIERET

4.9 Process Monitoring Systems

Real time sensing methods to perform on-line process monitoring are required to maintain high product quality at high production rates in laser materials processing operations. This section describes some of the methods that have been developed toward achieving this end.

4.9.1 Optical Penetration Sensing

Detection of the degree of penetration during laser welding is an important parameter in quality control. This information can be obtained by looking down the laser keyhole using a scraper mirror in the beam delivery system (1) or by using photodiodes mounted near the focusing mirror (2). When full penetration is required, detectors may be mounted under the workpiece to sense emission from the keyhole as it exits the weld.

Miyamoto and Mori (3) have shown that a comparison of optical emission from the keyhole plasma observed at oblique and near-normal incidence can also be used to monitor penetration depth. The basic measurement in all these systems is that of plasma emission intensity over one or more spectral regions. Changes in integrated intensity averaged over time can then be used to infer welding conditions. With the keyhole closed the keyhole plasma is localized near the entrance and oscillates about this position. As a result, emission from the plasma above the keyhole and that inside it are out of phase, and the plasma is not free to expand toward the closed end of the keyhole. Under full penetration conditions the plasma can expand in both directions, so that plasma emission detected above the inside the keyhole will be correlated. This behavior will be apparent through a variation in fast Fourier transform (FFT) spectra of signals obtained under fully penetrated and nonpenetrated welding conditions. The variation may not be as obvious when one compares emission intensity.

The intensity of plasma emission as recorded by looking down the keyhole or through imaging of the plasma at an angle relative to the laser beam is most useful in detecting weld fault conditions because these commonly involve significant changes in total plasma emission. Analysis of the frequency spectrum of the transients in these signals can provide additional information, but this adds an extra level of complication to the monitoring system.

References
1. D. Maischner, A. Drenker, B. Seidel, P. Abels, and E. Beyer, *Proc. ICALEO* **74**, 150–5 (1991).
2. H. Heyn, I. Decker, and Wohlfahrt, *Proc. SPIE* **2207**, 381–91 (1994).
3. I. Miyamoto, and K. Mori, *Proc. ICALEO* **80**, 759–67 (1995).

W. W. DULEY

4.9.2 Optical Plasma Intensity Monitoring
Monitoring of spectral line emission from a plasma produced during laser cutting and welding is a common method of diagnostics and yields information on the presence of a plasma. The intensity of such a spectral line, when monitored as a function of time, can be used to define a "set point" for the laser condition and for the detection of defects that are accompanied by a change in the intensity of plasma emission. Fast Fourier transform (FFT) techniques when applied to an analysis of the temporal variation of spectral line intensity can be useful in identifying frequency components that are characteristic of specific process faults. A comparison of spectral line intensities provides information on plasma temperature while spectral linewidth can be used to infer plasma electron density. Both of these parameters are important diagnostics of the plasma itself, but may be difficult to relate to process conditions. They are also sensitive to the presence of impurities, particularly elements such as the alkali metals or the alkaline earths with low ionization potentials.

Simultaneous measurement of spectral line emission from the plasma together with infrared radiation from the fusion zone itself provides a way to relate changes in plasma characteristics to the size and temperature of the weld pool in laser welding. The reliability of this technique may be compromised by the fact that infrared emission from the plasma is also present, making it difficult to separate infrared signals emitted from the plasma from those arising at the surface of the weld pool. In addition, the thermal time constant for temperature changes in the weld pool can be much longer than plasma fluctuation time scales.

The spatial extent and brightness of the plasma generated during laser processing can also be observed via direct imaging using a CCD camera. The low framing rate (30 Hz) of standard cameras makes such monitoring of limited value, but higher framing rates when combined with image analysis algorithms can yield useful diagnostic information.

Table 1 summarizes the response of plasma emission detectors to various fault conditions during laser welding.

Table 1. Detector Response for Various Defects and Faults in Laser Welding

Error	Detector Response
Gaps/displacement	Reduction in signal
Keyhole failure	UV, IR decrease
Surface defect	UV, IR decrease
Humping/penetration	UV, IR oscillate
Edge misalignment	Enhanced near IR
Pits	Difference between keyhole and plume plasma signals decreases
Underfill	Difference between keyhole and plume plasma signals increases

If one uses a fast detection system, fluctuation in the coupling of laser radiation to the workpiece can be minimized. This is the basis for the plasma shielding control (PSC) system developed by Seidel et al. (4) and Otto et al. (5). With PSC, the intensity of one or more spectral lines emitted by the plasma is monitored and used as a diagnostic of plasma conditions. When a threshold emission is reached, a correction signal is generated that acts to interrupt the laser intensity. The plasma then dissipates and the laser intensity is then allowed to increase again. This technique has been shown to provide more uniform weld penetration as well as a reduction in the consumption of shield gases.

References
4. B. Seidel, J. Beersick, and E. Beyer, *Proc. SPIE* **2207**, 290–300 (1994).
5. A. Otto, G. Deinzer, and M. Geiger, *Proc. SPIE* **2207**, 282–8 (1994).

W. W. DULEY

4.9.3 Acoustic Sensing

A noticeable characteristic of laser cutting and welding is the acoustic emission that accompanies these processes, particularly when a plasma is present. The range of frequencies emitted includes those in the audible range (20 Hz–20 kHz) so that an experienced operator may monitor optimal processing conditions by listening to the tones emitted. Essentially, this process consists of Fourier transformation of the acoustic wave intensity, followed by application of an algorithm that compares the amplitude within a range of detected frequencies to an expert database. Simulation of this procedure using an acoustic detector (other than the ear) offers the possibility of process diagnostics and control.

A number of physical processes contribute to the emission of acoustic energy during laser cutting and welding, but because of strong coupling to the ambient gas, keyhole oscillations, vaporization, and plasma heating/expansion are dominant contributors to airborne acoustic signals. These signals may also be detected via transducers attached to the workpiece, but in practice contact sensors are used only in the detection of acoustic emission accompanying solidification and cracking.

The spectrum of acoustic emission during laser processing can extend to MHz frequencies, but useful information can be obtained from spectra recorded over a much smaller range (≤ 100 kHz). This is particularly true under keyhole welding conditions when vaporization and plasma formation are closely related to instabilities and mass motion in the melt surrounding the keyhole. The frequency of oscillations characterizing these processes are typically ≤ 10 kHz so that acoustic spectra in the 100 Hz–20 kHz range will be indicative of keyhole stability and welding conditions.

4.9.4 Neural Networks

Monitoring sensor outputs for changes in signal level or other signal characteristics is the primary activity of any control system. The outputs from these sensors after conditioning can be fed into one or more control loops that act to change process variables so as to maintain operation at optimized locations on the control surface. Operating points are located after a series of trial experiments in which the result of laser welding under the given condition is evaluated. Such closed-loop operating systems are capable of maintaining optimized welding but are often inflexible and do not always respond to changes in an intelligent manner.

A more flexible approach is to superimpose a diagnostic level that evaluates the sensor outputs in an intelligent way and provides supervisory control. This diagnostic level contains a separate feedback loop that compares observed inputs to a database and optimizes the output response. One logical framework for such an intelligent control system has been described by Steen (6).

In physical systems where complex ill-defined processes are encountered and the knowledge available is often imperfect or incomplete, information processing is best carried out using an artificial neural network to classify and evaluate the information that is available. Such fuzzy or imprecise information contains details about the behavior of the system at hand, but this information is not compatible with specific mathematical algorithms relating input and output variables. This situation is encountered frequently during laser materials processing, particularly in laser welding.

Some advantages of neural networks have been identified by Farson et al. (7). These include:

1. Ability of network to generalize principles from incomplete data
2. Ability to deal with complex classification tasks
3. Fast computation
4. Relatively low cost
5. Elimination of the need for procedural programming or knowledge from experts or end users

Figure 1 illustrates the structure of a neural network.

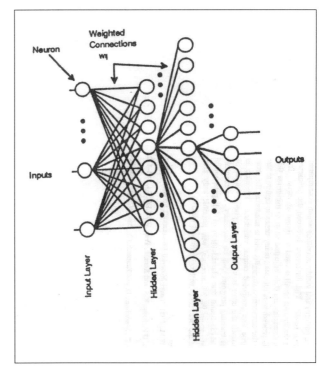

Figure 1. Neural network structure (8), best read by rotating 90° clockwise.

The neural network is based on an architecture that contains one or more hidden layers. Each input is connected to each "neuron" in the hidden layer, but these connections are weighed via a connection strength. The number of neurons in the input layer is determined by the number of input variables, while that in the output layer is equal to the number of output variables. As an example, the input variables could include the filtered output of an optical or acoustic signal measured from the workpiece after FFT processing, with individual spectral components assigned to specific input neurons. The output variable is typically weld penetration depth. This output can then be used to derive a control system based on fuzzy logic principles which outputs to the motion control system or to laser power. Evaluation of the output variable by the fuzzy logic controller results in the optimal change in weld speed or laser power to maintain correct welding conditions. The input to such systems can be obtained from an acoustic monitor but could also involve plasma, optical, or CCD signals. The connection strengths between neurons are obtained by a "back propagation" technique, whereby the input layer is given a specific set of inputs (i.e., a pattern) and yields an output that is compared to the known result.

The difference between the predicted output and the known result is used to assign an error. The connection strengths are then adjusted so as to minimize this error. This procedure is repeated many times to optimize the values for the connection strengths and to minimize the error between true and predicted output variables. Iteration is continued until the error is within an acceptable range. A substantial training program may be necessary: For example, Beyer et al. (8) found that classification of full penetration welds with up to 98.5% accuracy was possible only after training of the neural net with 60 different welds.

References
6. W. M. Steen, 1991 *Laser Material Processing*, Springer Verlag, New York.
7. D. F. Farson, K. S. Fang, and J. Kern, *Proc. ICALEO* **74**, 104–12 (1991).
8. E. Beyer, D. Maischner, and C. Kratzsch, *Proc. ICALEO* **79**, 51 (1994).

W. W. DULEY

4.9.5 Seam Tracking

Basic Considerations

The ability of a welding system to follow the seam between two components is crucial to successful welding operations. In principle, seam tracking is not required when the seam position in space is known, and this information can be programmed into a CNC system, which moves the welding head along this trajectory. This is generally the case in simple linear welds in tailored blanks where the position of the seam is carefully controlled and care is taken to maintain this geometry by clamping during welding. In many other practical applications of laser welding, however, the position of the seam is either not constant because of motion of the part during welding, or cannot be predicted with sufficient accuracy. The extent of this problem is evident when one realizes that a drift of ≤ 0.2 mm may be all that is required to go from satisfactory to unsatisfactory welding conditions.

Seam tracking can be carried out in two general ways. In the first method, some aspect of an acoustic, optical, or plasma signal that reflects seam geometry is monitored and is used to control the position of the laser beam relative to the seam. The second technique uses a vision sensor to monitor the seam position either by projection of light from one or more auxiliary laser beams, or by CCD imaging of the workpiece together with data processing of the image to extract seam position.

With signal processing from an optical or acoustic sensor, the primary difficulty is in assigning an observed change in signal to a specific directional change in the system, that is, to distinguish "left" from "right". Generally this is not possible through monitoring of plasma or acoustic emission from a single detector even after application of pattern recognition algorithms. Exceptions to this rule may occur in welding of dissimilar materials where spectral features attributable to specific elemental components may be distinguished. An example of this approach has been discussed by Mueller et al. (9) in a study of seam detection in butt welds between Cu and steel and mild/stainless steel.

Vision-based seam trackers yield seam accuracies as good as ± 0.1 mm and have been adapted to robotic laser welding. Operation is at scanning rates up to 50 Hz, permitting integration into laser welding systems at speeds in excess of 10 m/min.

References
9. R. E. Mueller, J. A. Hopkins, V. V. Semak, and M. H. McCay, *Proc. ICALEO* **81**, B86–95 (1996).

W. W. DULEY

Evaluation of Seam Tracking Methods

Most of the available systems are opto-electronic. An overview of the most common methods for acquiring the joint geometry data is shown in Figure 2. The methods include image processing approaches and scanning methods.

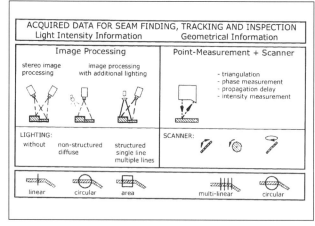

Figure 2. Schematic diagrams of seam tracking methods.

Table 2 presents an evaluation of the data acquisition methods illustrated in Figure 2 taking various practical considerations into account. It assigns weighting factors *W* to these considerations. The boxes in the table provide evaluation numbers *f* for

Chapter 4: Components for Laser Materials Processing Systems

the advantage of each measurement method with respect to each practical consideration. The products *Wf* are summed to provide a relative result for each method.

Table 2. Evaluation of Seam Tracking Methods
Legend: + = advantageous (f = +1); O = neutral;
− = disadvantageous

Criteria	Weighting factor W	Measuring method				
		Scanning triangulation	Stereoscopic measurement	Image proc. with a CCD-line camera	Split-beam method	Multi split-beam method
Surface sensitivity	4	+	−	−	−	−
High measuring rate	4	+	−	+	+	+
Usable as distance measurement	3	+	O	−	+	+
Overall sensor sizes	2	−	+	O	O	−
Mechanical reliability	2	−	+	+	+	+
Laser safety aspects	2	−	+	O	O	O
Complexity of the data processing	1	O	−	+	O	−
RESULTS Σ (wf)		+5	−3	0	+5	+2

The scanning triangulation method and the split beam image processing methods have the highest scores

Table 3 presents features for three seam tracking systems and criteria to be considered in the choice of a seam tracking device.

Figure 3 (next page) shows drawings defining the three scan tracking systems.

Table 4 (page 165) shows the advantages and disadvantages of the three systems.

Other Important Measuring Principles for Seam Tracking
According to Table 2, the most suitable measuring methods are the scanning/triangulation and the split-beam method. However, there are two more measuring methods to be considered because of the their low cost and high realiability: a) inductive eddy-current probe and b) a mechanical contact probe. Both methods have a similar lateral precision of about 0.1 mm and a two-axis control capability: Y (lateral position, perpendicular to the weld) and Z (height). Figure 4 (next page) shows a diagram of inductive seam tracking.

Table 3. Seam Tracking Systems*

	SYSTEM 1: ST-CCD attached to the FH with a solid bracket	SYSTEM 2: ST-CCD attached to the FH over an additional LA	SYSTEM 3: ST-CCD attached to the FH over an additional RA
Key-words description	• Simple implementation (retrofit possible) • Low cost level • Limited dynamic resolution • Limited operation speed • Best application: quasi-linear welds	• Moderate complex implementation (retrofit possible) • Fair cost level • Medium dynamic resolution • Medium operation speed • Track capability for larger direction changes as SYS1 • Best application: quasi-linear welds up to 2D-welds	• Complex implementation (retrofit not possible) • Moderate high cost level • High dynamic resolution • High operation speed • Track capability for larger direction changes as SYS2 • Best application: up to 3D-welds
MAIN FEATURE: Lateral TCP-"Y" position control	No supplementary axis is required.	Short supplementary LA moves for tracking the ST-CCD perpendicular to the welding direction.	RA moves for tracking the ST-CCD around the FH-axis.
	According to the measured joint position change a TCP-position change is calculated in real-time. The TCP-position change can usually be performed by the corresponding welder axis. If the welder controller has no TCP-position correction input, not sufficient real-time capability or such an interface becomes too expensive, a supplementary axis carrying the FH and the ST-CCD can perform the necessary TCP-position correction in real-time. Such an axis is shown in the principle system drawings ("C"-axis).		
ADDITIONAL FEATURE: Height TCP-"Z" position control	For all systems an additional height control function can be implemented since the height information is independently available from the lateral position information at any time. The corresponding Z movement of the FH can be performed over the Z-axis of the welder or over an additional Z-axis-LA on which the entire FH is build on.		
ST-CCD mounting location	ST-CCD is mounted onto the FH and measures ahead the position of the joint at a distance D from TCP	ST is mounted onto the a.m. LA which is mounted onto the FH and measures ahead the position of the joint at a distance D from TCP.	ST is mounted onto the a.m. RA which is mounted onto the FH and measures ahead the position of the joint at a distance D (=radius of the rotary movement) from TCP.
Conditions for use	The lateral FOV of the ST-CCD must be larger than the maximum expectable joint position variation (no more than approx. 60% of the FOV should be used). For large changes of the welding direction not usable (max. tolerable change in welding direction 3.5° within typical D= 50 mm and for a ST-CCD- FOV of 10 mm). An improvement of the system dynamic can be achieved if the FH is oriented along the welding path according to the CAD welding path design data.	The length of the LA must be larger than the maximum expectable joint position variation (no more than approx. 60%). For large changes of the welding direction not usable (max. tolerable change in welding direction dependent on the dynamical properties of the supplementary axis). An improvement of the system dynamic can be achieved if the FH is oriented along the welding path according to the CAD welding path design data.	The ST precision and operation speed are highly dependent on the dynamic properties of the RA. This should be as fast as possible (small weight of the ST-CCD), but the FH needs also a special design, which allows the fast movement of the RA without uncontrolled TCP-position changes induced by the RA movement.
	No TCP-position encoder is necessary.		A TCP-position encoder is necessary.

*FH – focusing head, FOV – field of view, PU – processing unit, ST – seam tracker, TCP – tool center point, X – welding direction, Y – correction direction, perpendicular to X, Z – height (vertical axis), LA – linear axis, RA – rotary axis, C – rotary axis of the FH, WPP – weld path planning

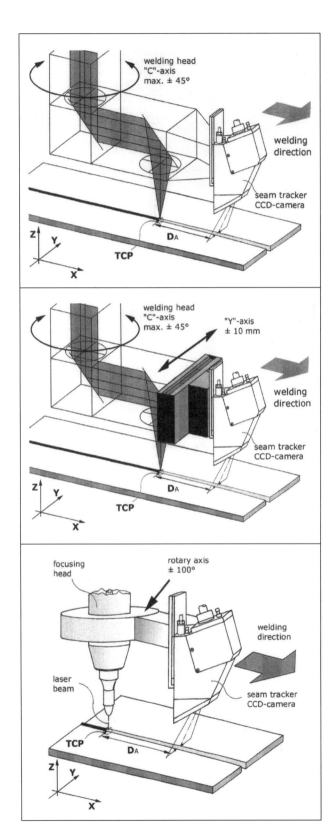

Figure 3. Diagrams of three seam tracking systems, from top to bottom, systems 1, 2, and 3.

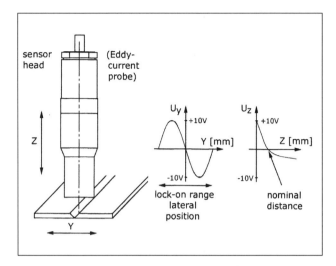

Figure 4. Inductive seam tracking illustrated.

This kind of sensor can detect all known weld and joint geometries. It can measure diverse materials (ferrous and nonferrous) and is insensitive to all kinds of contamination agents such as fumes, steam, oil, spatters, electromagnetic fields, or water.

The measurement is instantaneous so that the operation speed of the welder using such a device depends only on the reaction time of the positioning slides. Table 5 presents some features of this device.

Table 5. Characteristics of an Inductive Seam Tracker

Accuracy	± 0.1 mm
Sensor diameter	20 mm
Nominal distance	6 mm
Lock-on range	30 mm
Operating-temp.	60° max. (or, air cooled: 350 °C)

A mechanical seam tracker, as illustrated in Figure 5 (next page), uses a two-dimensional contact probe.

The contact probe is held at an angle of 45° toward the metal sheet so that it can measure the height and the lateral position of the joint edge.

The contact probe touches the joint edge only 2–3 mm ahead of the TCP. This fact allows one to build a very simple seam tracking system.

This sensor can also be used for the TEACH prodecure in case of 3D robotic applications.

Chapter 4: Components for Laser Materials Processing Systems

Table 4. Advantages and Disadvantages of Three Seam Tracking Systems

System	1	2	3
Advantages	Reasonable prices, simple to build, it needs no position encoder, can be used as an inspection device without the tracking function, if the tracking function is enabled only one axis in **Y** direction has to be steered. The interface with the welder and welder controller is very simple. Such a system can be retrofitted in almost any welder.	The additional costs of the **Y-LA** are generally not comparable with the advantages of this set-up. Due to the additional axis a **WPP** can be performed. This allows higher resolution and operation speed. The interface with the welder and welder controller has an acceptable complexity. Such a system can be retrofitted in almost any welder.	The additional costs of the **RA** is generally not comparable with the advantages of this set-up. Due to the additional axis a **WPP** can be performed faster. This allows larger joint direction changes, a higher resolution and operation speed. The interface with the welder and welder controller has an acceptable complexity. If the **ST**-sensor can detect the orientation of the **FH**-axis onto the object surface (multiple line projection or circular scanner), this can also be controlled in real-time.
Disadvantages	Since the entire **FH** has to be moved, due to its important weight only slow **TCP-Y** (or **Z**-) positions corrections can be performed at a reasonable precision. If the joint to be tracked disappears from the **ST-CCD FOV** the welder has to stop. In order to avoid this the **FOV** is usually relatively large, which reduces the achievable resolution.	The additional costs of the **Y-LA**. Most linear axes available on the market cannot be used for such an application. The "right choice" is here very important.	The additional costs of the **RA**. Most rotary axes available on the market cannot be used for such an application. The "right choice" is here very important. The **ST** system according to the concept **SYS3** represents a part of the **FH** and has to be considered correspondingly.

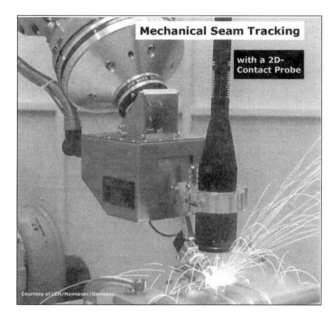

Figure 5. Mechancial seam tracking.

Table 6 presents some features of a mechanical seam tracking system.

Table 6. Characteristics of a Mechanical Seam Tracker

Accuracy	< 0.1 mm
Distance range	± 5 mm
Max robot. speed	12 m/min
Max. acceleration	3.4 m/s^2
Max correction v:	1 m/min
Look-ahead dist.	2–3 mm

MARIUS JURCA

4.9.6 Measurement of Keyhole Depth

Measurement of keyhole depth provides a direct measurement of the penetration depth during the laser welding process with both Nd:YAG and CO_2 lasers. This measurement is based on the fact that the laser power is absorbed at the walls of the keyhole by multiple reflection. The laser power that has not been absorbed within the keyhole is reflected out of it along the axis of the keyhole under a small solid angle. The measurement of this reflected laser power is dependent on the aspect ratio of the keyhole, (depth/diameter), which is mainly dependent on the penetration depth.

For the measurement of the reflected laser power a detector is used. The detector is sensitive to the wavelength of the laser. The detector has to be positioned on the optical axis of the keyhole. For small welding speeds, the keyhole inclination is not large so that the reflected laser power will be intercepted by the focusing element. It has to be selectively separated from the beam delivery path (beam splitter, slightly transparent mirror, diffracting elements, or holes in a nontransparent mirror).

For large welding speeds, the keyhole inclination becomes important and the reflected laser power can only be measured by an off-axis detector looking into the keyhole. Of course the inclination of the keyhole depends on many factors, such as: material, laser power, welding speed etc. This leads to the necessity of positioning the detector in the right position depending on the application.

The use of an optical integrating element (lens) to cover a larger solid angle with the detector will not improve the measurement results. In this case the detection will be independent of the inclination of the keyhole, but the integrating element amplifies disturbing noise within the solid angle corresponding with the diameter of the detector focusing lens.

Because of the exponential dependence of the absorbed laser power on the keyhole depth, this kind of measurement is useful for depths up to 5–6 mm in the case of welding steel with CO_2

lasers and up to 3 mm in the case of Nd:YAG lasers. The resolution of the measurement is better by about 0.1 mm for superficial welds up to 60% of the above limits and decreases near these limits. The above limits are caused by optical noise generated by scattered and/or diffuse reflected laser light from the keyhole neck and/or from the vapor cloud above the weld pool.

The difference between the higher absorption of the Nd:YAG laser compared with the CO_2 laser can be better understood by comparing the relative amount of reflected laser power for the two different lasers for the same penetration depth.

MARIUS JURCA

4.9.7 Infrared Monitoring

The infrared radiation emitted from the pool of liquid metal associated with a laser welding operation has been used to monitor the welding process. In one example, the photodiode used to monitor the infrared emission was integrated with the beam delivery optics (10).

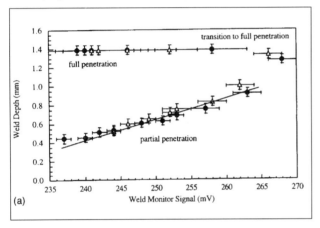

Figure 6. Correlation between dc monitor signal and penetration depth for CO_2 laser bead-on-plate welds in 1020 steel.

The output signal from the monitor increased with weld penetration, until full penetration was approached. An example of the weld monitor signal as a function of weld penetration depth is shown in Figure 6. These results were obtained using a 6-kW CO_2 laser beam incident on 1020 steel. The penetration was varied by changing the travel speed or by varying the power.

When full penetration was approached, the monitor signal dropped. But full penetration could be distinguished from partial penetration by increased variability in the signal near full penetration.

The monitor signal was also sensitive to defects resulting from part misalignment or surface contamination. The monitor signals were repeatable and could be used for online process monitoring.

A variety of other emission monitoring procedures have been developed, including use of multiple infrared sensors on both sides of the workpiece, and the use of a combination of infrared and ultraviolet sensors.

Reference
10. P. G. Sanders, et al., *J. of Laser Appl.* **10,** p. 205 (October 1998).

JOHN F. READY

Chapter 5

Laser-Material Interactions

5.0 Introduction

The ability of a high-power laser to deliver very high values of irradiance to a workpiece leads to many applications involving heating, melting, and vaporization. A conventional thermal source, such as a welding torch, delivers much lower irradiance, and the energy input cannot be localized as well as a laser beam. The total power is not necessarily as important as the ability to focus to a small spot, producing high irradiance.

This chapter describes the physical processes that occur during the interaction of high-power laser radiation with materials. Knowledge of these processes is important for understanding the capabilities and limitations of laser-based materials processing. These interactions are the basis for laser applications in material processing. The chapter includes information about the relevant properties of the workpiece, especially reflectivity and absorptivity, and how they affect the ability of the laser light to couple to the surface. It also describes the basic processes involved, including the flow of the energy that is coupled to the workpiece, the changes of phase, and the generation of laser-supported absorption waves. These phenomena affect the result of the processing.

In following chapters, results of materials processing by laser beams will be described, including important factors such as penetration, processing rates, etc. These results are strongly dependent on the phenomena described in this chapter.

The results of a materials processing operation also depend strongly on a wide variety of factors, like workpiece surface condition, the beam profile at the surface, the flow of gas around the surface, and the like. These factors are not always described fully. Thus it is sometimes difficult to reproduce quoted results, not knowing the exact conditions under which they were obtained. The tabulations of results like penetration, coverate rate, etc. are presented not so much to provide exact values, but rather to indicate ranges of results that may reasonably be obtained in laser processing.

5.1 Materials Characteristics

This section presents basic information on optical and thermal properties that affect the results of a laser materials processing operation.

5.1.1 Optical Properties

When light passes from an optically "thin" into an optically dense medium, one observes that in the dense medium, the *angle of refraction* β (i.e., the angle between the refracted light beam and a line perpendicular to the surface) is smaller than the *angle of incidence*, α. This phenomenon is used for the definition of the *index of refraction* of a material:

$$\frac{\sin \alpha}{\sin \beta} = \frac{n_{med}}{n_{vac}} = n, \quad (1)$$

where the subscripts med and vac refer to the dense medium and vacuum, respectively.

See Table 1 for a tabulation of basic optical properties. The *refraction* is caused by the different velocities, c, of the light in the two media

$$\frac{\sin \alpha}{\sin \beta} = \frac{c_{vac}}{c_{med}}. \quad (2)$$

The magnitude of the refractive index depends on the wavelength λ of the incident light (see Table 2). This property is called *dispersion*. In metals, the index of refraction varies in addition with the angle of incidence. This is particularly true when n is small.

Metals damp the intensity of light in a relatively short distance. Thus, to fully characterize the optical properties of metals, an additional material constant is needed, namely the *damping constant, k*, which is contained in the wave equation:

$$E = \text{Damped amplitude} - \text{Undamped wave}$$
$$= E_o \exp\left[\frac{2\pi k}{\lambda} z\right] - \exp\left[\frac{2\pi ci}{\lambda}\left(t - \frac{zn}{c}\right)\right] \quad (3)$$

Equation 3 indicates that the electric field strength, E, decreases exponentially with increasing distance, z, from the interface between vacuum and matter, as schematically shown in Figure 1. Characteristic values for k are given in Table 2 as a function of λ. In Equation 3, E_0 is the electric field at the surface.

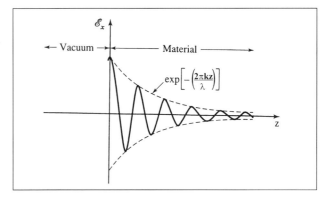

Figure 1. Damped light wave. The electric field strength decreases exponentially. The field strength indicated here is the x component, denoted E_x.

Table 1. Fundamental Optical Properties

Symbol	Definition	Property	Comment	SI units
λ	Wavelength of light	Depends on light source	Visible range between 400 and 800 nm	nanometer (nm) or micrometer (μm)
c	Speed of light	2.998×10^8 (m/s)	Value is for vacuum	meters per second
α	Angle of incidence	Angle between incident light beam and line perpendicular to surface		deg
β	Angle of refraction	Angle between refracted light beam and line perpendicular to surface		deg
n	Index of refraction	$\sin\alpha/\sin\beta = n_{med}/n_{vac}$ $= n = c_{vac}/c_{med}$	See Table 2: in metals n varies with the angle of incidence	Unitless
	Refraction	The property of light to change its direction when crossing the boundary between two media whose optical densities are different	Mathematically expressed by Snell's law (see "index of refraction")	Unitless
k	Damping constant	The property of light to decrease its intensity when entering an optically dense medium, see Figure 1	Also occasionally called "attenuation index" or "extinction coefficient"; for values, see Table 2	Unitless
R	Reflectivity	Ratio between reflected intensity and impinging intensity $R = I_R/I_0$	Reflectivity of a material depends on the wavelength of light; see Table 2	Percent
T	Transmissivity	Ratio between transmitted intensity and impinging intensity $T = I_T/I_0$	Wavelength dependent	Percent
W	Characteristic penetration depth	Distance at which the intensity of light in a medium has decreased to $1/e$ or to 37%	$W = \lambda/4\pi k$; see Figure 2	nanometer (nm) or micrometer (μm)
a	Absorbance	$a = 1/W = 4\pi k/\lambda$	Sometimes called (exponential) attenuation	cm^{-1} or when multiplied by 4.3 in decibels (dB) per centimeter
ε_2	Absorption (or absorption product)	$\varepsilon_2 = 2nk$	Imaginary part of the complex dielectric constant	Unitless
ε_1	Polarization	$\varepsilon_1 = n^2 - k^2$	Real part of the complex dielectric constant	Unitless

The field strength E is hard to measure. Thus the intensity, I, which can be measured easily with light-sensitive devices (such as a photodetector) is commonly used. The intensity is proportional to the square of the field strength. Thus the damping term in Equation 3 may be written as

$$I = E^2 = I_0 \exp\left(\frac{4\pi k}{\lambda} z\right). \tag{4}$$

where I_0 is the intensity at the surface.

We define a *characteristic penetration depth*, W, as that distance at which the intensity of the light wave, which travels through a material, has decreased to $1/e$ or 37% of its original value, that is, when

$$I/I_0 + 1/e = e^{-1} \tag{5}$$

This definition yields in conjunction with Equation 4

Chapter 5: Laser-Material Interactions

Table 2. Optical Properties of Silver, Copper, and Nickel

λ (nm)		Ag			Cu			Ni		
		n	k	R (%)	n	k	R (%)	n	k	R (%)
2	Ultraviolet	0.997	2.69×10^{-3}	4×10^{-4}	0.997	6.3×10^{-4}	2.3×10^{-4}	0.997	5.2×10^{-4}	2.3×10^{-4}
5		0.989	3.5×10^{-3}	3×10^{-3}	0.980	1.9×10^{-2}	1.9×10^{-2}	0.982	8.1×10^{-3}	9.9×10^{-3}
10		0.926	6.22×10^{-3}	0.15	0.966	5.1×10^{-2}	9.7×10^{-2}	0.955	4.1×10^{-2}	9.7×10^{-2}
20		0.881	0.211	1.6	0.965	0.107	0.33	0.964	0.112	0.36
50		0.906	0.522	7.2	0.96	0.396	4.0	0.91	0.421	4.8
80		1.202	0.691	9.7	0.981	0.695	11.0	1.01	0.687	10.5
100		1.308	0.581	7.6	1.09	0.128	11.0	1.07	0.711	10.7
200		1.072	1.24	26.5	1.0	1.45	34.4	1.0	1.54	37.2
300		1.51	0.902	15.1	1.41	1.68	34.6	1.74	2.00	39.5
400	Visible	0.173	1.95	86.6	1.18	2.21	51.0	1.61	2.36	48.0
500		0.130	3.0	94.9	1.13	2.55	59.0	1.68	2.98	58.2
600		0.128	3.70	96.6	0.35	3.01	87.1	1.88	3.56	64.1
700		0.144	4.65	97.5	0.213	4.15	95.4	2.19	4.07	64.1
800		0.144	5.31	98.0	0.24	4.31	95.2	2.48	4.38	68.3
1000	Infrared	0.266	6.99	98.2	0.41	7.51	97.2	2.82	5.01	71.6
2000		0.650	12.2	98.3	0.85	10.6	97.0	3.78	8.20	83.2
3100		1.387	18.8	98.4	1.59	16.5	97.7	3.84	11.4	90.0
4133		2.446	25.1	98.5	2.59	22.2	97.9	4.19	15.0	93.3
5166		3.732	31.3	98.5	3.81	27.5	98.0	4.16	18.4	95.4
8266		9.441	47.1	98.4	8.57	42.6	98.2	5.45	30.6	97.8
9919		13.11	53.7	98.3	10.8	47.5	98.2	6.90	36.2	98.0

$$z = W = \frac{\lambda}{4\pi k}. \quad (6)$$

as the value of the penetration depth.

Figure 2 presents values for W for some materials at various wavelengths.

The inverse of W is sometimes called the (exponential) *attenuation* or the *absorbance*, which is, making use of Equation 6

$$a = \frac{4\pi k}{\lambda}. \quad (7)$$

It is measured in cm^{-1}, or when multiplied by 4.3, in decibels (dB) per centimeter (dB = $10 \log_{10} I/I_0$).

The ratio between reflected intensity I_R and incoming intensity I_0 of the light serves as a definition for the *reflectivity*

$$R = \frac{I_R}{I_0}. \quad (8)$$

Similarly, one defines the ratio between the transmitted intensity, I_T, and the impinging light intensity as the *transmissivity*

$$T = \frac{I_T}{I_0}. \quad (9)$$

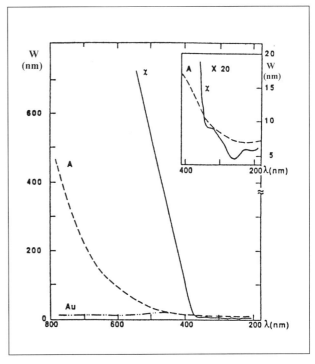

Figure 2. Mean penetration depth of light, W, for crystalline (χ) and amorphous (A) silicon and for gold, as a function of wavelength of light.

Experiments have shown that for insulators, R depends solely on the index of refraction. For perpendicular incidence one finds

$$R = \frac{(n-1)^2}{(n+1)^2}. \qquad (10)$$

For materials for which $k \neq 0$ (metals, semiconductors, etc.) Equation 10 needs to be modified and reads:

$$R = \frac{(n-1)^2 + k^2}{(n+1)^2 + k^2} \qquad (11)$$

This is called the Beer equation. The reflectivity is a unitless material constant and is often given in percent of the incoming light. R is, like the index of refraction, a function of the wavelength of the light. See Table 2 for values for several metals.

The reflectivity is a complicated function of the real and imaginary parts of the complex dielectric constant, ε, that is, of ε_1 (polarization) and of ε_2 (absorption), with ε_1 and ε_2 the real and imaginary parts of ε, respectively.

Table 3. Fundamental Thermal Properties

Symbol	Definition	Property	Comment	SI units
E	Energy	Energy, work, and heat are equivalent	Thermal energy and mechanical energy are equivalent	J = kg m²/s²
W	Work		Mechanical work (friction), electrical work (resistive heating) radiation, contact	J = kg m²/s²
Q	Heat		1 J= 0.239 cal	J = kg m²/s² (formerly "cal")
T	Temperature			°C or K
C'	Heat capacity	Amount of heat, dQ, transferred to a substance to raise its temperature by a certain interval	Heat capacity at constant volume $C'_v = (\partial E/\partial T)_v$; also used: heat capacity at constant pressure C'_p	J/K
c	Specific heat capacity	Heat capacity per unit mass	$c = C'/m$	J/g K
C	Molar heat capacity	Heat capacity per mole	$C = c M$ (M = molar mass)	J/mol K
θ_D	Debye temperature	Temperature at which C_v has reached 96% of its final value		K
J_Q	Heat flux	Heat that flows through a cross section of a bar per time and area		J/m² s
K (or λ)	Thermal conductivity or heat conduction	A constant that describes the amount of heat flux in a material	$J_Q = -K\, dT/dx$	J/m s K (or W/m K)
α_L	Linear expansion coefficient	A constant that describes the amount of linear expansion when increasing the temperature	$\Delta L/L = \alpha_L \Delta T$	K⁻¹
α_{th}	Thermal diffusivity	A constant that describes the time dependence of the spatial distribution of the temperature	$\alpha_{th} = K/\rho C_p$	m²/s

ISBN 0-912035-15-3

Chapter 5: Laser-Material Interactions

$$R = \frac{\sqrt{\varepsilon_1^2 + \varepsilon_2^2} + 1 - \sqrt{2(\sqrt{\varepsilon_1^2 + \varepsilon_2^2} + \varepsilon_1)}}{\sqrt{\varepsilon_1^2 + \varepsilon_2^2} + 1 + \sqrt{2(\sqrt{\varepsilon_1^2 + \varepsilon_2^2} + \varepsilon_1)}} \quad (12)$$

where

$$\varepsilon_1 = n^2 - k^2 \quad (13)$$

and

$$\varepsilon_2 = 2nk. \quad (14)$$

Finally, the reflectivity is related at large wavelengths (infrared spectral region) to the conductivity, σ, of the material by

$$R = 1 - 2\sqrt{\frac{c}{\sigma\lambda}} \quad (15)$$

This is called the Hagen-Rubens relation. As σ becomes large, R approaches unity. In other words, materials having a large electrical conductivity are good reflectors in the infrared. This is also indicated by the values in Table 2.

5.1.2 Thermal Properties

An increase in thermal energy can be achieved by mechanical work (friction), electrical work (resistive heating), radiation, or by direct contact with a hotter medium. *Energy, E, work, W*, and *heat, Q*, have the same unit, namely the joule (J) or the now-obsolete calorie (cal), where 1 cal = 4.184 J. The temperature, T, of a material is given in degrees centigrade (°C) or in kelvin (K). Table 3 summarizes some important thermal properties.

Different substances need different amounts of heat to raise their temperature by a given temperature interval. For example, it takes 4.18 J to raise the temperature of 1 g of water by 1 K. But the same heat raises the temperature of 1 g of copper by about 11 K. In other words, water has a larger *heat capacity* compared to copper. The heat capacity, C', is the amount of heat dQ that needs to be transferred to a substance in order to raise its temperature by a certain temperature interval. Units for the heat capacity are J/K (or cal/K).

The heat capacity is not defined uniquely; that is, one needs to specify the conditions under which the heat is added to the system. Even though several choices for the heat capacities are possible, one is generally interested in only two: the *heat capacity at constant volume* C'_v and the *heat capacity at constant pressure* C'_p. The former is the most useful quantity because C'_v is obtained immediately from the energy of the system. The heat capacity at constant volume is defined as

$$C'_v = \left(\frac{\partial E}{\partial T}\right)_v. \quad (16)$$

On the other hand, it is much easier to measure the heat capacity of a solid at constant pressure than at constant volume. Fortunately, the difference between C'_p and C'_v for solids vanishes at low temperatures and is only about 5% at room temperature. C'_v can be calculated from C'_p if the volume expansion coefficient, α, and the compressibility, κ, of a material are known, by applying

$$C'_v = C'_p - \frac{\alpha^2 TV}{\kappa}, \quad (17)$$

where V is the volume of the solid.

The *specific heat capacity* is the heat capacity *per unit mass m*

$$c = \frac{C'}{m}. \quad (18)$$

It is a material constant and is temperature dependent. Characteristic values for the specific heat capacity (c_p) are given in Table 4.

The *thermal energy* (or heat) that is transferred to a system equals the product of mass, increase in temperature, and specific heat capacity:

$$\Delta E = Q = m\Delta T c_v \quad (19)$$

A further useful material constant is the heat capacity *per mole* (i.e., per amount of substance of a phase, n). It compares mate-

Table 4. Experimental Thermal Parameters of Various Substances at Room Temperature and Ambient Pressure

Substance	Specific heat capacity (c_p) (J/g K)	Molar (atomic) mass (g/mol)	Molar heat capacity (C_p) (J/mol K)	Molar heat capacity (C_v) (J/mol K)
Al	0.897	27.0	24.25	23.01
Fe	0.449	55.8	25.15	24.68
Ni	0.456	58.7	26.8	24.68
Cu	0.385	63.5	24.48	23.43
Pb	0.129	207.2	26.85	24.68
Ag	0.235	107.9	25.36	24.27
C (graphite)	0.904	12.0	10.9	9.20
Water	4.184	18.0	75.3	

rials that contain the same number of molecules or atoms. The *molar heat capacity* is obtained by multiplying the specific heat capacity c_v (or c_p) by the molar mass, M.

$$C_v = \frac{C'_v}{n} = c_v \cdot M \quad . \tag{20}$$

Table 4 shows that the room temperature molar heat capacity at constant volume is approximately 25 J/mol K. The experimental molar heat capacities for some materials are depicted in Figure 3 as a function of temperature. We notice that some materials, such as carbon, reach the upper limit of 25 (J/mol K) only at very high temperatures. The temperature at which C_v has reached 96% of this upper limit is called the Debye temperature, θ_D (Table 5).

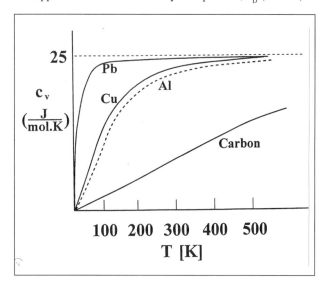

Figure 3. Temperature dependence of the molar heat capacity, C_v, for some materials.

Table 5. Debye Temperatures of Some Materials

Substance	θd(K)
Pb	95
Au	170
Ag	230
W	270
Cu	340
Fe	360
Al	375
Si	650
C	1850
GaAs	204
InP	162

Heat conduction (or *thermal conduction*) is the transfer of thermal energy from a hot body to a cold body when both bodies are brought into contact. Consider a bar of a material of length x whose ends are held at different temperatures. The heat that flows through a cross section of the bar divided by time and area, (i.e., the *heat flux*, J_Q) is proportional to the temperature gradient dT/dx. The proportionality constant is called the *thermal conductivity*, K. We thus write

$$J_Q = -K \frac{dT}{dx}. \tag{21}$$

The negative sign indicates that the heat flows from the hot to the cold end (Fourier Law). Figure 4 and Table 6 give some characteristic values for K. The thermal conductivity decreases slightly with increasing temperature. For example, K for copper decreases by 20% within a temperature span of 1000°C. In the same temperature region K for iron decreases by 10%.

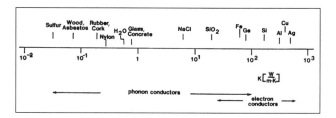

Figure 4. Room temperature thermal conductivities for some materials.

Table 6. Thermal Conductivities at Room Temperature[a]

Substance	K(W/m K) = (J/s m K)
Diamond type IIa	2.3×10^3
SiC	4.9×10^2
Silver	4.29×10^2
Copper	4.01×10^2
Aluminum	2.37×10^2
Silicon	1.48×10^2
Brass (leaded)	1.2×10^2
Iron	8.02×10^1
GaAs	5×10^1
Ni-silver[b]	2.3×10^1
Al_2O_3 (sintered)	3.5×10^1
SiO_2 (fused silica)	1.4
Concrete	9.3×10^{-1}
Soda-lime glass	9.5×10^{-1}
Water	6.3×10^{-1}
Polyethylene	3.8×10^{-1}
Teflon	2.25×10^{-1}
Snow (0°C)	1.6×10^{-1}
Wood (oak)	1.6×10^{-1}
Sulfur	2.0×10^{-2}
Cork	3×10^{-2}
Glass wool	5×10^{-3}
Air	2.3×10^{-4}

[a] See also Figure 4.
[b] 62% Cu, 15% Ni, 22% Zn.

Near the right side of the figure, for high values of conductivity, the process is dominated by electrons; at the left side, conduction is dominated by phonons. The length L of a rod increases with increasing temperature. Experiments have shown that in a relatively wide temperature range the *linear expansion* ΔL is proportional to the increase in temperature ΔT. The proportionality constant is called the *coefficient of linear expansion* α_L.

$$\frac{\Delta L}{L} = \alpha_L \Delta T \qquad (22)$$

Experimentally observed values for α_L are given in Table 7.

Table 7. Linear Expansion Coefficients α_L for Some Solids Measured at Room Temperature

Substance	α_L (10^{-5} K^{-1})
Hard rubber	8.00
Lead	2.73
Aluminum	2.39
Brass	1.80
Copper	1.67
Iron	1.23
Glass (ordinary)	0.90
Glass (pyrex)	0.32
NaCl	0.16
Invar (Fe–36% Ni)	0.07
Quartz	0.05

The expansion coefficient has been found to be proportional to the molar heat capacity C_v; that is, the temperature dependence of α_L is similar to the temperature dependence of C_v.

The *thermal diffusivity*, α_{th}, describes the time dependence of the spatial distribution of the temperature, according to

$$\frac{\partial T}{\partial t} = \alpha_{th} \frac{\partial^2 T}{\partial x^2} \qquad (23)$$

Equation 23 is equivalent to Fick's second law for non-steady-state diffusion. It is defined as

$$\alpha_{th} = \frac{K}{\rho C_p}, \qquad (24)$$

where K is the thermal conductivity (see above), C_p is the molar heat capacity (see above), and ρ is the molar density, given in mol/m^3. This yields the unit m^2/s for α_{th}. It plays the role of a diffusion constant for heat energy.

References
R. E. Hummel, *Electronic Properties of Materials*, 2nd Ed, 1993, Springer-Verlag, Berlin, Heidelberg, New York, Chapter 10.
R. E. Hummel, *Optische Eigenschaften von Metallen und Legierungen*, 1971, Springer-Verlag, Berlin.

ROLF E. HUMMEL

5.2 Laser Characteristics

A laser is a unique device that allows the user to utilize its energy in the form of light in distinct ways. Consider that a 100-W light bulb and a 100-W laser both have the same power. If we surround both the light bulb and the laser in a sphere 1 m in diameter, the power density of the light bulb on the inside of this sphere is about 8×10^{-4} W/cm^2. On the other hand, if the laser exits with a diameter of 1 cm, the power density on the sphere is 127 W/cm^2. Assuming that each beam can then be focused to a spot size of 0.01 cm, the laser beam then has a power density of 1.3×10^6 W/cm^2, which is about the power density to form a keyhole weld in steels. Taking the 8×10^{-4} W that strike the sphere and focusing that to 0.01 cm gives a power density of about 10 W/cm^2 for the light bulb. 10 W/cm^2 may be enough to burn one's hand, but is insufficient to process materials.

5.2.1 Important Laser Properties

The characteristics of laser radiation that are dependent on the wavelength of the laser beam and are significant in materials processing are:
  monochromaticity,
  coherency,
  radiance,
  low beam divergence,
  ability to focus to a small spot size,
  depth of focus, and
  absorption.

Some of the characteristics are interrelated, as will be explained. Several books (1–3) give good explanations of the characteristics of lasers relevant to materials processing.

Monochromaticity

Most lasers are tuned in their optical cavity to produce a single wavelength; for example, an Nd:YAG laser has a wavelength of 1.06 µm, whereas a CO_2 laser has a wavelength of 10.6 µm. Dye lasers are the exceptions to this in that they can be tuned to several wavelengths.

Coherency

Laser radiation is coherent in both space and time. Coherency in time is related to monochromaticity. Coherency in space is related to output power in that all the radiation is in phase and the amplitude increases as the laser beam travels through the active laser material.

Radiance

Radiance is a measure of the power per unit area per solid angle, and is inversely related to the square of the wavelength. Lasers have much higher radiance than any other source of light. Raidance has also been called brightness.

Low Beam Divergence

The divergence of a laser beam allows it to propagate over significant distances without changing significantly in diameter. This factor also allows it to be collected and focused easily.

Small Spot Size

A laser beam is capable of being focused to a small spot size. For a circular laser beam of diameter D, focused with a lens having a focal length f and wavelength λ, the minimum spot size (or diffraction-limited spot size) is

$$d = 2.44\, f\lambda / D$$

The ratio f/D is also called the F number of the focusing lens (sometimes written as F#). For a wavelength of 0.5 μm focused with an f:1 lens, this equation predicts a spot size of 1.22 μm. The very small values of spot size lead to very high values of irradiance at the surface of a workpiece. We note that spot size is proportional to wavelength. This means that short-wavelength lasers may be more finely focused than longer-wavelength lasers.

Depth of Focus

The depth of focus of a laser beam is a measure of the range over which the intensity of the laser beam is approximately the same. The depth of focus is a function of the F# of the focusing lens and the wavelength of the laser beam and can be expressed as

$$z = 1.48\, F^2\, \lambda$$

Absorption

The absorption of the laser beam by a material is a function of the wavelength of the laser beam. For a given material, a shorter wavelength usually means greater absorption at room temperature. Absorption is also a function of the temperature of the material.

At low intensity, the laser beam may be almost completely reflected from a reflective material. As the intensity increases, melting will occur and absorption will increase. At greater intensities, a vapor column will form and keyhole welding becomes possible. At even greater intensities, the vapor from the keyhole will become ionized, forming a plasma. This plasma is itself a very good absorber of laser energy and can decouple the laser from the material. See Section 5.4.3 for a further discussion of the variation of reflectivity during irradiation and Section 5.7 for more information on plasma shielding.

5.2.2 Pulsed versus CW Characteristics

In a continuous wave (CW) laser, the output power (W) of the laser is constant with time. During CW laser beam welding, the beam forms a stable molten weld pool as long as the beam is on. The heat input to the material during the processing is then the power divided by the processing speed (m/s) and is expressed as J/m.

In a pulsed laser the output laser energy is expressed in J. A pulsed laser may have a short pulse length and high peak power at relatively low average energy. In laser pulsed welding, a series of overlapping pulses is used to form the weld. The laser pulse energy determines the amount of melting per pulse. Thus it is possible that the material may not heat up as much when processing with a pulsed laser as opposed to a CW laser. On the other hand, the thermal shock delivered by each pulse may be sufficient to cause cracking in materials that are sensitive to sudden changes in temperature. Control of the total amount of energy delivered to the material during processing is a very important consideration in deciding the type of laser to use.

5.2.3 Focusing Characteristics

The focusing characteristics of a laser beam are primarily a function of the wavelength of the beam and the expression that has been stated above for the diffraction-limited spot size or the minimum laser spot size. That expression is for a single-mode laser. A multimode laser can be focused to a slightly greater spot size (2).

5.2.4 Irradiance

Irradiance is a measure of the power density (W/cm^2) on the material. Irradiance is very important in keyhole welding in that a power density of about 2×10^6 W/cm^2 is required to initiate a vapor column or keyhole in steels. If the irradiance is less than about 1.0×10^6 W/cm^2, only melting will occur. For aluminum alloys a power density of about 3.5×10^6 W/cm^2 is required. The alloying elements in aluminum alloys are very important in determining the required irradiance.

References

1. W. W. Duley, *Laser Processing and Analysis of Materials*, Plenum Press, New York, 1983, Chapter 1.3.
2. W. M. Steen, *Laser Material Processing*, 2nd Ed., Springer-Verlag, London, 1998, Chapter 2.
3. J. F. Ready, Industrial Applications of Lasers, 2nd Ed., Academic Press, San Diego, 1997, Chapter 2.

E. A. METZBOWER

5.2.5 Important Lasers for Materials Processing Applications

Many different types of lasers have been developed, but only a small number are useful for materials processing. The leading contenders are listed in Table 1. CO_2 and Nd:YAG lasers have long dominated laser materials processing. Many established materials processing applications use one of these two types. Ruby and Nd:glass lasers have been used in applications where a small number of pulses of relatively large energy are required. Excimer lasers have become well established because of the high absorption of their ultraviolet wavelengths. The availability of the short wavelengths also offers the advantage of being able to focus to a smaller spot size. Applications of the other lasers in the table are developing.

For CO_2 and Nd:YAG lasers, the two leading types, Tables 2 and 3 provide information about applications that have become common. The tables also identify power levels used in typical applications, for metals and nonmetals, respectively. The tables represent an applications matrix, indicating lasers that are commonly employed for selected applications.

Chapter 5: Laser-Material Interactions

Table 1. Lasers for Materials Processing

Laser	Wavelength (μm)	Operating regimes	Typical applications
CO_2	10.6	Continuous, pulsed, TEA	Welding, heat treating, marking, drilling
Nd:YAG	1.06, 0.532	Continuous, pulsed	Welding, trimming, marking, drilling
Ruby	0.6943	Pulsed	Spot welding, drilling
Nd:glass	1.06	Pulsed	Spot welding, drilling
Diode	0.8	Continuous	Heat treating, micromachining
Copper vapor	0.511, 0.578	Pulsed	Drilling
Excimer	0.249	Pulsed	Micromachining, ablation, photolithography, marking
Argon	0.488, 0.5145	Continuous	Semiconductor processing

Table 2. Lasers for Processing Metals

Laser	Heat treat	Weld	Drill	Cut	Mark
Med-power CO_2 (200–900 W)	-	Yes	Yes	Yes	-
High-power CO_2 (> 900 W)	Yes	Yes	Yes	Yes	-
Low/med-power Nd:YAG (< 100 W)	-	Yes	Yes	-	Yes
High-power Nd:YAG (> 100 W)	Yes	Yes	Yes	Yes	-

Table 3. Lasers for Processing Nonmetals

Laser	Drill	Cut	Scribe	Mark
Low-power CO_2 (20–200 W)	Yes	Yes	-	Yes
Med-power CO_2 (200–900 W)	Yes	Yes	-	-
High-power CO_2 (> 900 W)	-	Yes	-	-
Low/med-power Nd:YAG (< 100 W)	Yes	-	Yes	-
Excimer	Yes	-	-	Yes

JOHN F. READY

5.3 Reflectivity and Absorptivity of Opaque Surfaces

Section 5.1.1 describes the basic optical properties of reflectivity and absorbance. The coverage in this section gives more specific information about how these properties affect the intrreraction of laser light with surfaces.

5.3.1 Definitions

When laser irradiation (in the form of *electromagnetic waves* or *photons*) impinges on the surface of a workpiece, a fraction of the energy is reflected at the surface, and a part penetrates into the substrate. A surface cannot absorb or emit photons: Attenuation takes place inside the solid, as does emission of radiative energy (and some of the emitted energy escapes through the surface into the adjacent medium). In practical systems the thickness of the surface layer over which absorption of irradiation from a laser beam occurs is very small compared with the overall dimensions of a workpiece—usually a few nanometers for metals and a few micrometers for most nonmetals. The same may be said about emission from within the solid that escapes into the adjacent medium. Thus, in the case of opaque materials it is customary to speak of absorption by and emission from a "surface," although a thin surface layer is implied.

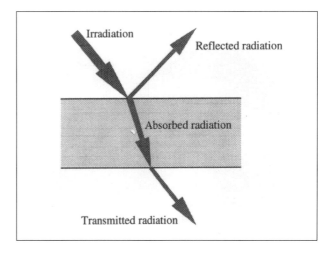

Figure 1. Reflection, absorption, and transmission by a slab.

Consider thermal radiation impinging on a medium of finite thickness, as shown in Figure 1. In general, some of the irradiation will be *reflected* away from the medium, a fraction will be *absorbed* inside the layer, and the rest will be *transmitted* through the slab. Based on this observation three fundamental radiative properties are defined:

Reflectivity, $\rho \equiv \dfrac{\text{reflected part of incoming radiation}}{\text{total incoming radiation}}$,

Absorptivity, $\alpha \equiv \dfrac{\text{absorbed part of incoming radiation}}{\text{total incoming radiation}}$,

Transmisivity, $\tau \equiv \dfrac{\text{transmitted part of incoming radiation}}{\text{total incoming radiation}}$.

Since all radiation must be either reflected, absorbed, or transmitted, it follows that

$\rho + \alpha + \tau = 1.$

If the medium is sufficiently thick to be *opaque*, then $\tau = 0$ and

$\rho + \alpha = 1.$

Note that all three of these properties are nondimensional and may vary in magnitude between the values 0 and 1. An ideal surface that absorbs all incoming radiation is called a "black surface." It follows for such a surface that $\alpha = 1$ and $\rho = \tau = 0$.

All surfaces also emit thermal radiation (or, rather, radiative energy is emitted within the medium, some of which escapes through the surface). Since, at a given temperature, the maximum possible is emitted by a black surface, we define a fourth nondimensional property, the emissivity ε:

$\varepsilon = \dfrac{\text{energy emitted from a surface}}{\text{energy emitted by a black surface at same temperature}}.$

The emissivity can, therefore, also vary between the values of 0 and 1, and for a black surface $\varepsilon = 1$.

All four properties may be functions of temperature as well as wavelength (or frequency). In addition, the absorptivity may be different for different directions of irradiation, while emissivity may vary with outgoing directions. Finally, the magnitude of reflectivity and transmissivity may depend on both incoming and outgoing directions. Thus one distinguishes between spectral and total properties (i.e., an average value over the spectrum), and between directional and hemispherical properties (i.e., an average value over all directions).

It is readily shown that—for any given wavelength and any given direction—$\varepsilon = \alpha$ (known as *Kirchhoff's law*). Thus the radiative characteristics of an opaque "surface" are described by a single independent property, the reflectivity, as

$\rho = 1 - \alpha = 1 - \varepsilon.$

More detail on the various definitions of the radiative properties of materials, and their theoretical and experimental determination, may be found in the textbook by Modest (1).

5.3.2 Predictions from Electromagnetic Wave Theory

The spectral, directional value of the reflectivity of an optically smooth interface is *specular* (i.e., reflects incoming radiation like a mirror into a single outgoing direction), and may be calculated from *electromagnetic wave* and *dispersion theories*. The resulting equations are called *Fresnel's relations* and are fairly involved functions of incidence angle θ and *complex index of refraction*

$m = n - ik,$

where n is the *refractive index* (since it governs the angle of refraction of light across an interface), and the imaginary part k has various names in the literature, but is most aptly called the *absorptive index* (since it governs internal absorption as described in Section 5.4). It was called the damping constant in Section 5.1. For normal incidence ($\theta = 0$) onto a material adjacent to a gas or vacuum Fresnel's relations give for the normal reflectivity ρ_n.

$$\rho_n = \frac{(n-1)^2 + k^2}{(n+1)^2 + k^2} \tag{1}$$

If the complex index of refraction of the material is known, Equation 1 may be used not only for normal incidence but, as an estimate, for a large range of incidence directions ($\theta \leq 60°$).

5.3.3 Reflectivities of Metals

Metals are, in general, excellent electrical conductors because of an abundance of free electrons. The dependence of radiative properties on the ability to conduct electromagnetic waves (and, thus, on free electrons) has led to several theoretical descriptions.

Directional Dependence

The reflectivity of metals is governed by the complex index of refraction as it appears in Fresnel's relations. For metals both n and k are relatively large, and Fresnel's relations for directional reflectivity simplify to

$$\rho_\| = \frac{(n\cos\theta - 1)^2 + (k\cos\theta)^2}{(n\cos\theta + 1)^2 + (k\cos\theta)^2}, \tag{2a}$$

$$\rho_\perp = \frac{(n - \cos\theta)^2 + k^2}{(n + \cos\theta)^2 + k^2}, \tag{2b}$$

Chapter 5: Laser-Material Interactions

$$\rho = \frac{1}{2}(\rho_\parallel + \rho_\perp), \qquad (2c)$$

where $\rho_\parallel$ and $\rho_\perp$ are the reflectivities for parallel- and perpendicular-polarized light, and ρ is the average value for *unpolarized* as well as for *circularly polarized* light (see also Section 5.3.5 on polarization effects). Here parallel and perpendicular mean that the electric field vector is parallel or perpendicular to the plane formed by the beam direction and the surface normal. Figure 2 shows experimental data for the directional dependence of the reflectivity for platinum at $\lambda = 2$ µm, together with results from Fresnel's relations, Equation 2, with $m = 5.29 - 6.71i$. The figure shows typical directional behavior for the reflectivity of metals in the infrared: The reflectivity tends to be high at normal incidence, with very weak directional dependence up to angles of incidence of 60° or more, followed by a sharp drop (due to the contribution of $\rho_\parallel$), before becoming perfectly reflective at grazing angles. Note that this "typically metallic behavior" is generally observed only for relatively long wavelengths (with different thresholds for different metals). At shorter wavelengths (YAG laser, visible lasers) the directional behavior of metals usually resembles that of nonconductors, as described in the following section.

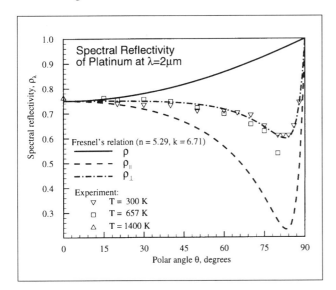

Figure 2. Spectral, directional reflectivity of platinum at 2 µm.

Wavelength Dependence

The complex index of refraction in Fresnel's relations depends on a number of thermophysical properties of the metal and, as such, is wavelength dependent. For long wavelengths ($\lambda \geq 10$ µm) the *Hagen-Rubens relation* postulates that

$$n \approx k \approx \sqrt{30\lambda\,\sigma_{dc}} \gg 1, \quad \lambda\,\sigma_{dc} \text{ in } [\Omega^{-1}], \qquad (3)$$

where σ_{dc} is the *dc conductivity* of the material. Substituting Equation 3 into 2 leads to

$$\rho_n \approx 1 - \frac{2}{\sqrt{30\lambda\,\sigma_{dc}}} + \frac{1}{\sqrt{15\lambda\,\sigma_{dc}}}, \quad \lambda\,\sigma_{dc} \text{ in } [\Omega^{-1}], \qquad (4)$$

that is, for metals the absorptivity for normal incidence, $\alpha_n = 1 - \rho_n$, is small for large wavelengths, and tends to decrease as $1/\sqrt{\lambda}$. These trends are shown in Figure 3 for extremely carefully prepared (vapor-deposited) metal surfaces, together with results from the Hagen-Rubens relation as well as from the more sophisticated *Drude theory*. The Hagen-Rubens relation is seen to predict the trends well for $\lambda > 10$ µm, and may—at least qualitatively—also be used for somewhat shorter wavelengths, in particular for less clean and smooth metal surfaces.

The high value of reflectivity at long infrared wavelengths has an important practical effect involving the choice of lasers for processing metals. The high reflectivity of wavelengths near 10 µm means that much of the incident power is reflected and not absorbed by the surface. Thus CO_2 lasers may have difficulty performing some functions unless the power is very high. This statement is especially true for conductive metals, like aluminum and copper, for which the reflectivity is very high near 10 µm. For such metals, it may be better to employ an Nd:YAG laser, for which the reflectivity will be lower. At shorter wavelengths, the absorptivity, equal to $1 - \rho$, is much higher than at long infrared wavelengths. For example, the factor $1 - \rho$ for steel is about 0.35 at 1.06 µm, about 7 times higher than its value at 10.6 µm. This means that at least initally, 7 times more light is absorbed from an Nd:YAG laser than from a CO_2 laser for equal irradiance. Often it will be easier to carry out welding with a shorter-wavelength laser because of the increased coupling of light into the workpiece.

For ferrous metals, the conductivity is not so high, and thus the reflectivity will be somewhat lower. For those metals there may be enough absorption to break down the surface and increase the coupling above its initial value. A description of the decrease in reflectivity during irradiation is described in Section 5.4.3.

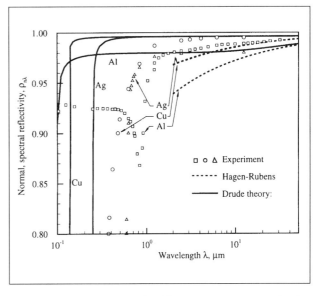

Figure 3. Spectral, normal reflectivity at room temperature for aluminum, copper, and silver.

ISBN 0-912035-15-3

Temperature Dependence

The Hagen-Rubens relation, Equation 4, predicts that the spectral, normal emissivity of a metal should be proportional to $1/\sqrt{\sigma_{dc}}$.

Since the electrical conductivity is approximately inversely proportional to temperature, the spectral emissivity should, therefore, be proportional to the square root of absolute temperature for long wavelengths. This trend should also hold for the spectral, hemispherical emissivity (i.e., averaged over all directions). Experiments have shown that this is indeed true for many metals. A typical example is given in Figure 4, showing the spectral dependence of the hemispherical emissivity for tungsten for a number of temperatures (2). Note that the emissivity for tungsten tends to increase with temperature beyond a *crossover wavelength* of approximately 1.3 µm, while the temperature dependence is reversed for shorter wavelengths. Similar trends of a single crossover wavelength have been observed for many metals.

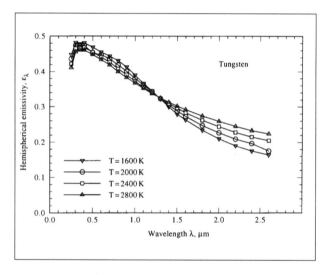

Figure 4. Temperature dependence of the spectral, hemispherical emissivity of tungsten.

5.3.4 Reflectivities of Nonconductors

Electrical nonconductors have few free electrons and, thus, do not display the high reflectivity/opacity behavior in the infrared as do metals.

Wavelength Dependence

Reflection of light by insulators and semiconductors tends to be a strong, sometimes erratic, function of wavelength. Crystalline solids generally have strong absorption-reflection bands (large k) in the infrared commonly known as *Reststrahlen bands*, which are due to transitions of intermolecular vibrations. These materials also have strong bands at short wavelengths (visible to ultraviolet), due to electronic energy transitions. In between these two spectral regions there is a region of fairly high transparency (and low reflectivity), where absorption is dominated by impurities and imperfections in the crystal lattice. As such, these spectral regions often show irregular and erratic behavior. Defects and impurities may vary appreciably from specimen to specimen and even between different points on the same sample. As an example, the spectral, normal reflectivity of silicon at room temperature is shown in Figure 5 [redrawn from data collected by Touloukian and deWitt (3)]. The strong influence of different types and levels of impurities is clearly evident. Therefore, looking up properties for a given material in published tables is problematical unless a detailed description of surface and material preparation is given.

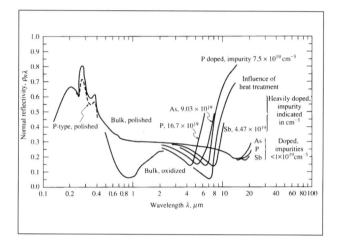

Figure 5. Spectral, normal reflectivity of silicon at room temperature (3).

In spectral regions outside Reststrahlen and electronic transition bands the absorptive index of a nonconductor is very small, typically $k < 10^{-6}$ for a pure substance. While impurities and lattice defects can increase the value of k, it is very unlikely to find values of $k > 10^{-2}$ for a nonconductor outside the Reststrahlen bands. This implies that Fresnel's relations can be simplified significantly, and the spectral, normal reflectivity may be evaluated as

$$\rho_n = \left(\frac{n-1}{n+1}\right)^2$$

Therefore, for optically smooth nonconductors the radiative properties may be calculated from refractive index data. Refractive indices for a number of semitransparent materials at room temperature are displayed in Figure 6 as a function of wavelength (4). All these crystalline materials show a similar spectral behavior: The refractive index drops rapidly in the visible region, then is nearly constant (declining very gradually) until the midinfrared, where n again starts to drop rapidly. This behavior is explained by the fact that crystalline solids tend to have an absorption band due to electronic transitions near the visible, and a Reststrahlen band in the infrared. The first drop in n is due to the tail end of the electronic band; the second drop in the midinfrared is due to the beginning of a Reststrahlen band.

Chapter 5: Laser-Material Interactions

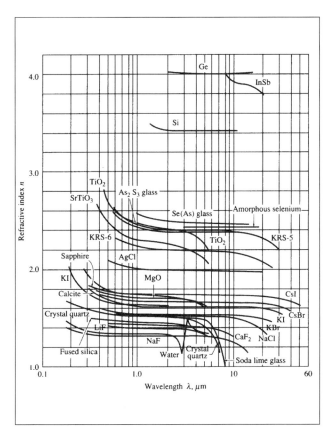

Figure 6. Refractive indices for various semitransparent materials (1, 4).

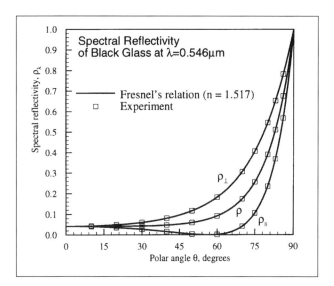

Figure 7. Spectral, directional reflectivity of blackened glass at room temperature.

Directional Dependence

For optically smooth nonconductors, for the spectral region between absorption-reflection bands, experimental results have been found to closely follow Fresnel's equations of electromagnetic wave theory. Figure 7 shows a comparison between theory and experiment for the directional reflectivity of glass (blackened on one side to avoid multiple reflections) for polarized, monochromatic irradiation (5). Because $k^2 \ll n^2$, the absorptive index may be eliminated from Fresnel's relations, and the relations for a perfect dielectric become valid. For unpolarized light incident from vacuum (or a gas), this leads to

$$\rho_\lambda = \frac{1}{2}(\rho_\parallel + \rho_\perp) \qquad (5)$$

$$= \frac{1}{2}\left[\left(\frac{n^2 \cos\theta - \sqrt{n^2 - \sin^2\theta}}{n^2 \cos\theta + \sqrt{n^2 - \sin^2\theta}}\right)^2 + \left(\frac{\cos\theta - \sqrt{n^2 - \sin^2\theta}}{\cos\theta + \sqrt{n^2 - \sin^2\theta}}\right)^2\right].$$

Comparison with experiment agrees well with electromagnetic wave theory for a large number of nonconductors.

Temperature Dependence

The temperature dependence of the radiative properties of nonconductors is considerably more difficult to quantify than for metals. Infrared absorption bands in ionic solids due to excitation of lattice vibrations (Reststrahlen bands) generally increase in width and decrease in strength with temperature, and the wavelength of peak reflection/absorption shifts toward higher values. The reflectivity for shorter wavelengths largely depends on the material's impurities. Often the behavior is similar to that of metals; that is, the emissivity increases with temperature for the near infrared, while it decreases at shorter wavelengths. As an example, Figure 8 shows the normal emissivity for zirconium carbide (6). On the other hand, the emissivity of amorphous solids (i.e., solids without a crystal lattice) tends to be independent of temperature.

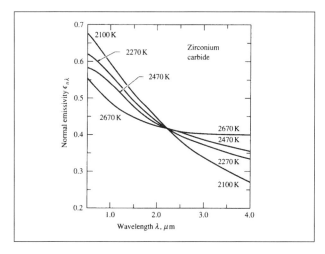

Figure 8. Temperature dependence of the spectral, normal emissivity of zirconium carbide (6).

ISBN 0-912035-15-3

5.3.5 Polarization Effects

Wavelength, direction of propagation, and energy content do not completely describe the nature of a laser beam. Every train of electromagnetic waves has a property known as the *state of polarization*. Polarization effects are generally not very important to the heat transfer engineer since emitted light generally is randomly polarized; that is, there is no relationship between the planes formed by the electric field vectors of the individual waves making up a wavetrain. Laser sources, on the other hand, tend to be strongly polarized, either *linearly polarized* (also called *plane* polarized), or *circularly polarized* (1). In the case of optically smooth surfaces the state of polarization has a strong impact on the material's reflectivity and vice versa.

A polarized laser beam impinging on a surface can be decomposed into parts: a parallel component (the electric vector lies in a plane parallel to the plane formed by the beam's direction of propagation and the surface normal) and a perpendicular component (normal to the parallel component). According to Fresnel's relations, each component is reflected to a different extent, as given by Equation 2 for metals and Equation 5 for nonconductors. Simple averaging gives the overall reflectivity for circularly polarized light, while more complicated formulae must be applied for more general states of polarization. Figures 2 and 7 show the behavior of platinum (a metal) and glass (a nonconductor), respectively. It is observed that the parallel components of reflectivity, $\rho_{\parallel}$, have a sharp minimum at large angles. For a perfect dielectric ($k = 0$) this minimum is zero; that is, the material is a perfect absorber for parallel-polarized light at an irradiation angle of

$$\theta_p = \tan^{-1} n,$$

known as *Brewster's angle* or as the *polarizing angle* (since at that angle of incidence any reflected light—regardless of the incident polarization—will be completely polarized). In laser processing applications this sharp minimum in reflectivity (and, therefore, strong maximum absorptivity) is sometimes exploited by using oblique laser irradiation at that angle (note, however, that this diminishes the incident energy per unit area—as compared to normal incidence—by a factor of cos θ, i.e., absorbed energy *density* is always highest at normal incidence). Note also that—since perpendicularly polarized light is reflected more strongly—the state of polarization of the reflected beam is always different from the state of polarization of the incident beam.

Due to the dependence of reflectivity on polarization, the orientation of the laser beam can have profound effects (desired or undesired) on the groove or cut formed by a scanning laser beam: A linearly polarized laser beam with its electric vector in the plane formed by the scanning laser will be more strongly reflected sideways than backwards along the groove, resulting in a wide and shallow groove. If the electric vector is perpendicular to the scanning direction, there will be little sideways reflection, and a deep and narrow groove develops. If the electric vector is at an angle to the scanning direction, the groove will become asymmetric and has been observed to develop into a "banana shape."

5.3.6 Effects of Surface Conditions

Up to this point the present discussion of reflectivity and other radiative properties has assumed that the material is pure and homogeneous, and that its surface is isotropic and optically smooth. Very few real material surfaces come close to this idealization.

Under intense laser irradiation, causing rapid heating to extremely high temperatures, melting/ablation/decomposition of material, and/or breaking of molecular bonds, even an initially ideal material will have its surface composition and quality altered: Heating of the material may be accompanied by strong oxidation or other chemical reaction, producing an opaque surface layer of a material quite different from the substrate; material removal by whatever mechanism is generally accompanied by a roughening of the surface finish.

In this subsection a brief discussion is given of how surface roughness and surface layers affect the radiative properties of opaque surfaces.

Effects of Surface Roughness

A surface is "optically smooth" if the average length scale of *surface roughness* is much less than the wavelength of the electromagnetic wave. Therefore, a surface that appears rough in visible light ($\lambda \approx 0.5$ μm) may well be optically smooth in the far infrared ($\lambda \approx 50$ μm). This difference is the primary reason why results from electromagnetic wave theory cease to be valid for very short wavelengths.

The character of roughness may be very different from surface to surface, depending on the material, method of manufacture, surface preparation, and so on, and classification of this character is difficult. A common measure of surface roughness is given by the *root-mean-square roughness*, σ_m. The root-mean-square roughness can be readily measured with a *profilometer* (a sharp stylus that traverses the surface, recording the height fluctuations). Unfortunately, σ_m alone is woefully inadequate to describe the roughness of a surface. Surfaces of identical σ_m may have vastly different frequencies of roughness peaks, as well as different peak-to-valley lengths; in addition, σ_m gives no information on second-order (or higher) roughness superimposed onto the fundamental roughness.

In general terms one may state that surfaces will become less reflective, and the behavior of reflection will become less specular and more diffuse as surface roughness increases. This behavior may be explained through geometric optics, by realizing that, for a rough surface, a laser beam hitting the surface may undergo two or more reflections off local peaks and valleys (resulting in increased absorption), after which it leaves the surface into an off-specular direction. Simple models predict sharp peaks in reflection in the specular reflection direction, and less reflection into other directions, with the strength of the peak depending on the surface roughness. This has also been found to be true experimentally for most cases as long as the incidence angle was not too large. For large off-normal angles of incidence, experiments have shown that the reflectivity has its peak at polar angles greater than the specular direction; that is, for larger incidence angles rough surfaces tend to display *off-specular peaks*, apparently due to shadowing of parts of the surface by adjacent peaks.

Effects of Surface Layers and Oxide Films

Even optically smooth surfaces have a surface structure that is different from the bulk material, due to either surface damage or the presence of thin layers of foreign materials. Surface damage is usually caused by the machining process, particularly for metals and semiconductors, which distorts or damages the crystal lattice near the surface. Thin foreign coats may be formed by chemical reaction (mostly oxidation), adsorption (e.g., coats of grease or water), or electrostatics (e.g., dust particles). All these effects may have a severe impact on the radiation properties of metals and may cause considerable changes in the properties of semiconductors. Other materials are usually less affected, because metals have large absorptive indices k, and thus high reflectivities. A thin, nonmetallic layer with small k can significantly decrease the composite's reflectivity (and raise its absorptivity). Dielectric materials, on the other hand, have small ks, and their relatively strong emission and absorption take place over a very thick surface layer. The addition of a thin, different dielectric layer cannot significantly alter their radiative properties.

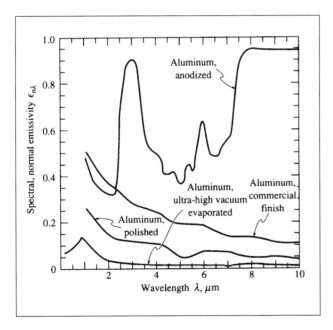

Figure 9. Spectral, normal emissivity for aluminum with different surface finishes (1).

Figure 9 shows the spectral, normal emissivity (or absorptivity) of aluminum for a surface prepared by the ultra-high-vacuum method, and for several other aluminum surface finishes. While ultra-high-vacuum aluminum follows the Drude theory for $\lambda > 1$ μm (Fig. 3), polished aluminum (clean and optically smooth for large wavelengths) has a much higher absorptivity over the entire spectrum. Still, the overall level of absorptivity remains very low, and the reflectivity remains rather specular. As Figure 9 shows, the absorptivity is much larger still when off-the-shelf commercial aluminum is tested, probably due to a combination of roughness, contamination, and slight atmospheric oxidation. Deposition of a thin oxide layer on aluminum (up to 100 Angstroms) appreciably increases the emissivity only for wavelengths less than 1.5 μm. This clearly is not true for thick oxide layers, as evidenced by Figure 9: Anodized aluminum (i.e., electrolytically oxidized material with a thick layer of alumina, Al_2O_3) no longer displays the typical trends of a metal, but rather shows the behavior of the dielectric alumina. The effects of thin and thick oxide layers have been measured for many metals, with similar results. As a rule of thumb, clean metal exposed to air at room temperature grows oxide films so thin that infrared emissivities are not affected appreciably. On the other hand, metal surfaces exposed to high-temperature oxidizing environments (furnaces, laser heating, etc.) generally have radiative properties similar to those of their oxide layer.

While most severe for metallic surfaces, the problem of surface modification is not unknown for nonmetals. For example, it is well known that silicon carbide (SiC), when exposed to air at high temperature, forms a layer of silica (SiO_2) on its surface, resulting in a reflection band around 9 μm. Nonoxidizing chemical reactions can also significantly change the radiative properties of dielectrics. For example, the strong ultraviolet radiation in outer space (from the sun) as well as gamma rays (from inside the earth's van Allen belt) can damage the surface of spacecraft protective coatings like white acrylic paint or titanium dioxide epoxy coating, and similar results can be expected for UV laser irradiation.

5.3.7 Summary

Reflectivity and absorptivity for many materials have been compiled in a number of books and other publications. These tabulations show large amounts of scatter, i.e., radiative properties for opaque surfaces, when obtained from tabulations and figures in the literature, should be taken with a grain of salt. Unless detailed descriptions of surface purity, preparation, treatment, etc., are available, the data may not give any more than an order-of-magnitude estimate. One should also keep in mind that the properties of a surface may change during a process or overnight (by oxidation and/or contamination). A representative list of absorptivities (= 1 − reflectivity) for normal incidence of a laser on the material is given in Table 1 for a number of metals and a few nonmetals (mostly ceramics). Three values are given: for CO_2 laser irradiation (10.6 μm), for Nd:YAG irradiation (1.06 μm), and for short-wavelength lasers, such as frequency-doubled or -tripled Nd:YAG, excimer lasers, etc. (300–600 nm). All values are for room temperature and stated surface conditions: As explained earlier, these values may change significantly with temperature, surface roughness, oxidation, etc.

In summary, radiative properties for opaque surfaces, when obtained from tabulations and figures in the literature, should be accepted cautiously. Unless detailed descriptions of surface purity, preparation, treatment, etc., are available, the data may not

Table 1. Normal, Spectral Absorptivity of Materials at Important Laser Wavelengths

Material	300–600 nm	1.06 μm	10.6 μm
Aluminum, smooth		0.06 – 0.2	0.03 – 0.06
rough		0.2 – 0.4	0.1 – 0.4
Beryllium	0.8	0.5 – 0.8	0 – 0.08
Chromium	0.35 – 0.40	0.3 – 0.4	0.06 – 0.10
Copper, polished	0.05	0.04	0.01 – 0.03
rough	0.05	0.1 – 0.3	0.05 – 0.10
oxidized	0.85	0.5	
Germanium	0.05 – 0.3	0.05 – 0.65	0.6 – 0.7
Gold	0.7 – 0.1[a]	0.02 – 0.04	0.01 – 0.02
rough			< 0.12
Iron, polished	0.37 – 0.40	0.25 – 0.32	0.12
Molybdenum, polished	0.4 – 0.5	0.25 – 0.35	0.05 – 0.15
Nickel	0.5	0.15 – 0.35	0.05 – 0.15
Platinum	0.5 – 0.3[a]	0.25 – 0.30	0.03 – 0.08
Rhodium	0.2 – 0.5	0.15 – 0.25	0.05
Silicon, undoped	0.35 – 0.55[a]	0.7	0.25 – 0.38
doped			< 0.75
Silver	0.95 – 0.03[a]	0.03	0.02 – 0.10
Tungsten	0.5	0.35	0.03 – 0.3
Carbon (graphite)	0.75	0.8 – 0.9	0.7 – 0.9
Alumina (Al_2O_3)		0.05 – 0.1	0.90 – 0.99
Magnesium oxide (MgO)		0.2	0.93 – 0.98
Silica (SiO_2)	transp.	transp.	0.9
Zirconia (ZrO_2)		0.1 – 0.2	0.85 – 0.98
Silicon carbide (SiC)	0.8 – 0.9	0.85 – 0.95	0.8 – 0.9
Silicon nitride (Si_3N_4)	0.6 – 0.7	0.6 – 0.8	0.9

[a]Indicates continuous change with wavelength.

give any more than an order-of-magnitude estimate. And to state it again, the properties of a surface may change during a process or overnight (due to oxidation and/or contamination).

References
1. M. F. Modest, *Radiative Heat Transfer,* McGraw-Hill, New York, 1993.
2. D. R. Lide, (Ed.), *CRC Handbook of Chemistry and Physics,* 70+ ed., CRC Press, Boca Raton, FL, annual.
3. Y. S. Touloukian, and D. P. DeWitt (Eds.), *Thermal Radiative Properties: Nonmetallic Solids,* Vol. 8 of *Thermophysical Properties of Matter,* Plenum Press, New York, 1972.
4. *American Institute of Physics Handbook*, 3rd ed., Ch. 6, McGraw-Hill, New York, 1972.
5. W. M. Brandenberg, "The Reflectivity of Solids at Grazing Angles," in *Measurements of Thermal Radiation Properties of Solids,* J. C. Richmond (Ed), NASA SP-31, 75–82, 1963.
6. T. R. Rietof and V. J. DeSaintis, "Techniques of Measuring Normal Spectral Emissivity of Conductive Refractory Compounds at High Temperatures," in *Measurement of Thermal Radiative Properties of Solids,* J. C. Richmond (Ed.), NASA SP-31, 565–84, 1963.

MICHAEL F. MODEST

5.4 Absorption of Laser Irradiation

Any solid or liquid that allows electromagnetic waves to penetrate an appreciable distance into it is known as a semitransparent medium. What constitutes an "appreciable distance" depends, of course, on the physical system at hand. If a thick film on top of a substrate allows a substantial amount of photons to propagate, say, 100 μm into it, the film material would be considered semitransparent. On the other hand, if heat transfer within a large vat of liquid glass is of interest, the glass cannot be considered semitransparent for those wavelengths that cannot penetrate several centimeters through the glass.

5.4.1 Absorption Coefficients
The transparency of a layer is determined from its *transmissivity* τ

$$\tau = e^{-\kappa L} \tag{1}$$

where L is the thickness of the layer and κ is the material's *absorption coefficient*. For a nonscattering material (i.e., one without defects, inclusions, bubbles) the absorption coefficient is related to the absorptive index k by

$$\kappa = 4\pi k / \lambda. \tag{2}$$

Thus it takes an optical thickness κL of approximately 3 to 5 to constitute an "opaque layer." For metals with values of k of the order of 10, this implies that a layer of L of the order of 100 nm may be considered opaque, while for nonconductors ($k \approx 10^{-6}$ to 10^{-2}) thicknesses of at least 100 µm, and possibly several meters, are required.

Because the behavior of the absorption coefficient is directly linked to that of the absorptive index through Equation 2, which was discussed in detail in Sections 5.3.3 (for metals) and 5.3.4 (for nonconductors), no further discussion is warranted here.

Temperature Dependence

An increase of temperature of the solid is always accompanied by an increase in free electrons. This effect is most pronounced in semiconductors (since metals always have large populations of free electrons, and because thermal energies are generally not strong enough to bridge a dielectric's band gap), with the number of free electrons increasing exponentially with temperature. Thus an increase in temperature results in increased laser absorption and heating, further increasing the absorption coefficient, etc., and may lead to "thermal runaway."

Multiphoton Absorption

While thermal effects are usually insufficient to produce substantial amounts of free electrons in insulators, the high band gap energy of insulators can be overcome through multiphoton absorption, that is, when several photons (whose combined energy exceeds the bandgap energy) are absorbed simultaneously. To date multiphoton absorption effects remain unimportant during laser materials processing, because of the extremely high laser intensities required (i.e., strong, subnanosecond pulses) (1).

5.4.2 Semitransparent Sheets

For an optically smooth semitransparent sheet of a thickness L substantially larger than the laser wavelength, $L \gg \lambda$, the radiative properties are readily determined through geometric optics and raytracing. Accounting for multiple reflections, absorptivity A_{slab}, reflectivity R_{slab}, and transmissivity T_{slab} of an absorbing layer with index of refraction $m = n - ik$ are given by (2).

$$R_{slab} = \rho \left[1 + \frac{(1-\rho)^2 \tau^2}{1 - \rho^2 \tau^2} \right],$$

$$T_{slab} = \frac{(1-\rho)^2 \tau}{1 - \rho^2 \tau^2},$$

$$A_{slab} = \frac{(1-\rho)(1-\tau)}{1 - \rho \tau},$$

and

$$R_{slab} + T_{slab} + A_{slab} = 1,$$

where ρ is the reflectivity of both sheet-air interfaces, and τ is the transmissivity of the sheet, as given by Equation 1 above.

If the thickness of the semitransparent sheet is of the order of the wavelength of the irradiation ("thin film"), interference effects need to be accounted for; that is, phase differences between first-surface and second-surface reflected light make film reflectivity a strongly oscillating function of wavelength (2), with near-zero reflectivity at some wavelengths and very substantial reflectivities in between. This phenomenon is commonly exploited by putting "antireflection" coatings onto laser optics, optimized to minimize the reflectivity of the optical elements at the laser's wavelength.

References

1. M. von Allmen, "Laser-Beam Interactions with Materials," Springer Series in Materials Science, Vol. 2, Springer-Verlag, Berlin, 1987.
2. M. F. Modest, *Radiative Heat Transfer,* McGraw-Hill, New York, 1993.

MICHAEL F. MODEST

5.4.3 Variation During Irradiation

All metals have high reflectivity at long infrared wavelengths. For wavelengths longer than 5 µm, the reflectivity is strongly dependent on electrical conductivity. Highly conductive metals have the highest values of infrared reflectivity. Thus the reflectivity of copper is higher than that of aluminum, which in turn is higher than that of iron alloys.

The absorptivity of a metallic surface is proportional to 1-ρ, where ρ is the reflectivity. At the CO_2 laser wavelength of 10.6 µm, where ρ is close to unity, 1-ρ becomes small. Only a small fraction of the CO_2 laser beam incident on the surface is absorbed and available for heating the workpiece.

For metals like gold, copper, and silver, 1-ρ is about 0.02 at 10.6 µm, whereas for steels it is about 0.05. Steel then absorbs about 2.5 times as much of the incident light as the more conductive metals. Thus steels are easier to process with a CO_2 laser than are more conductive metals, such as aluminum or copper.

But the initially high reflectivity may decrease during the laser interaction. In one experiment (3), an aluminum surface was exposed to a Nd:glass laser pulse with an irradiance of 10 MW/cm^2. The surface had an original reflectivity around 70%. When the laser pulse began, the reflectivity dropped to 20% after 200 msec and then remained fairly constant until the end of the 1-msec pulse. This meant that the laser energy was coupled effectively into the material, since the average reflectivity during the pulse was low.

The high value of surface reflectivity is especially important for processing with CO_2 lasers. High surface reflectivity at 10.6 µm means that the coupling of energy into the workpiece is poor and may lead to difficulties in welding or heat treating with CO_2 lasers. The high reflectivity has been a barrier to the application of CO_2 lasers in welding of conductive metals such as silver or copper. Ferrous metals, like steels, have lower reflectivity (higher absorptivity) at 10.6 μm. Thus they are better candidates for welding with CO_2 lasers than are the conductive metals. Also the decrease of reflectivity that can occur during the laser pulse is beneficial. Because of this decrease, which occurs when a high-power CO_2 laser beam irradiates a surface, CO_2 lasers have been successful for welding of metals like steels.

Figure 1 shows data on the reflectivity of a stainless steel surface irradiated by a CO_2 TEA laser, which delivered an irradiance of 150 MW/cm² to the target (4). The pulse duration was 200 nsec. The reflectivity dropped rapidly for a few hundred nanoseconds. These results show that the reflectivity can decrease during the time that the surface is irradiated so as to increase the effective absorption of the surface. During much of the pulse the reflectivity was substantially lower than its initial value.

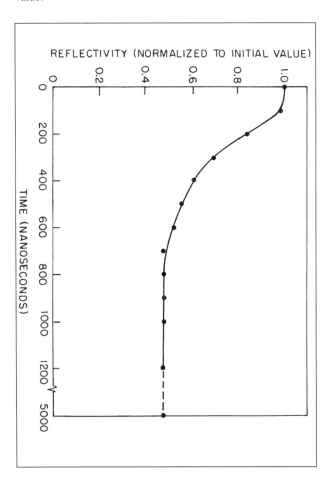

Figure 1. Specular reflectivity at 10 μm as a function of time for a stainless steel surface struck by a CO_2 TEA laser pulse delivering 150 MW/cm² in a pulse 200 nsec long.

To summarize, CO_2 lasers can be effective for welding of ferrous metals, because of the decrease in reflectivity that occurs during irradiation. But for high-conductivity metals, like silver and copper, the coupling of CO_2 laser energy into the surface is very low, and the use of a shorter-wavelength laser, like Nd:YAG, is indicated.

References
3. M. K. Chun and K. Rose, *J. Appl. Phys.* **41,** 614 (1970).
4. J. F. Ready, *IEEE J. Quantum Electron.* **QE-12,** 137 (1976).

JOHN F. READY

5.5 Energy Transport in Laser-Irradiated Materials

5.5.0 Introduction

This section is concerned with the transport of energy within the material. After absorption at or near the surface of a material, the laser energy is transformed into thermal energy, which then is transported through the sample by thermal conduction. This section discusses models for that energy transport, and presents equations and methods for determining factors such as temperature increase, penetration depth, etc., that are of importance in materials processing operations.

This section also emphasizes the importance of mathematical modeling as a tool for understanding and controlling laser-aided processes. It is of a theoretical nature, which makes it unusual with respect to the rest of the handbook.

To facilitate referencing the information in this section, the numbers of the operational equations for a variety of processes are listed in Table 1. Supporting information precedes and follows the key equation in each case. The information in the table will allow the user to locate the key equations relevant to specific processes.

There exist several techniques ranging from simple lumped parameter analysis to complicated numerical procedures to model a variety of laser-aided materials synthesis technology. Analytical techniques are quick but can provide meaningful insight without large resource requirements. These techniques are mostly used for lumped parameter analysis and conductive heat transfer analysis, and are limited by their applicability to real-life situations. On the other hand, numerical techniques do not suffer from these limitations and can closely represent the process physics. Coupled fluid flow, heat transfer, and mass transfer phenomena have successfully been modelled using numerical schemes. Quite often numerical techniques are the only tools available to model the process. Nevertheless, time and resource demands are quite high. Therefore, the choice of solution technique should depend on the process in question and the level of expectations from a model.

Chapter 5: Laser-Material Interactions

Table 1. Summary of Mathematical Models

Model description	Process	Equations	Sources	To solve
Lumped parameter energy balance	Melting and cutting	1, 57	(2), (43)	E, T, P, V_{cut}
1D heat flow, point source, semi-infinite medium, constant properties	Surface hardening and glazing	5, 8, 9, 10	(2), (5), (12)	$T, dT/dt, D_m$
1D heat flow, point source, finite medium, constant properties	Surface hardening and glazing	5, 11, 12, 13	(2), (5), (12)	$T, dT/dt, D_m$
1D heat flow, point source, finite medium, multilayer	Thin-film deposition	5	(15), (16)	$T, dT/dt$
1D heat flow, point source, finite medium, heat generation/sink	Machining	5, 15, 16, 17	(12), (29)	$T, dT/dt, D_e, D_m$
1D conduction, species diffusion, and solidification	Surface alloying and cladding	5, 32, 47, 48	(43)	$T, dT/dt, C_l, C_s$
1D evaporation	Drilling	40, 41	(28), (32)	D_c
2D evaporation	Drilling	42, 43	(30), (31)	T, D_m, D_c
2D heat flow and fluid flow	Laser welding	6, 32, 38, 39	(1), (22), (26)	T, V, D_m
2D heat flow, fluid flow, and mass transfer	Surface alloying	6, 32, 38, 39, 47	(20)	T, V, C_s, C_l, D_m
2D heat flow, fluid flow, and free surface deformation	Welding	6, 32, 38, 39	(1), (24), (25)	$T, dT/dt, V, D_m$
3D heat flow, point source, semi-infinite medium, constant properties, stationary beam	Surface hardening, Alloying	6, 21	(2), (5), (12)	$T, dT/dt, D_m$
3D heat flow, Gaussian source, semi-infinite medium, constant properties, stationary beam	Surface hardening and melting	6, 23	(2), (5)	$T, dT/dt, D_m$
3D heat flow, point source, semi-infinite medium, constant properties, moving beam	Surface hardening and melting	6, 25, 26	(4), (5)	$T, dT/dt, D_m$
3D heat flow, Gaussian source, semi-infinite medium, constant properties, moving beam	Surface hardening and melting	65, 27	(6)	$T, dT/dt, D_m$
3D heat flow, line source, semi-infinite medium, constant properties, moving beam	Keyhole welding	6	(2), (36), (37), (39), (40)	T, D_p, D_m
3D heat flow, Gaussian source, finite depth and width, quasisteady	Surface hardening	6, 28	(11)	$T, dT/dt$
3D heat flow, Gaussian source, finite depth and width, unsteady	Surface hardening	6, 29	(13)	$T, dT/dt$
3D heat flow, Gaussian source, finite medium, variable properties	Laser chemical vapor deposition	6, 30, 31, 47–53	(14), (45)	$T, dT/dt, T_h$
3D heat flow, finite medium, variable properties, melting and solidification, numerical solution	Laser glazing, welding	6, 32, 33, 34, 37	(17), (18)	$T, dT/dt, C_s$
3D evaporation and flow	Keyhole welding	6, 38, 39, 45, 46	(41), (42)	T, V, D_p, D_m
3D heat flow and fluid flow	Welding	6, 38, 39	(1), (21), (23)	$T, V, dT/dt$
3D heat flow, fluid flow, and free surface deformation	Welding	6, 38, 39	(1)	$T, V, dT/dt$
3D evaporation	Cutting	42, 43, 44	(33), (34), (35)	T, D_c

Table 2 provides definitions to allow the ready use of each section's key equations. Table 3 presents the sources for the entries in Table 1.

Table 2. Nomenclature, Symbols, and Units

Symbol	Nomenclature	Units
A	Absorptivity	
c	Speed of light	m/s
C	Concentration of species	wt.%
C_l	Concentration in liquid	wt.%
C_s	Concentration in solid	wt.%
C_p	Specific heat at constant pressure	J/kg K
d	Laser beam diameter	m
D	Depth	m
D_m	Melt depth	m
D_p	Depth of penetration	m
D_c	Depth of crater	m
$\tilde{D}$	Mass diffusion coefficient	m^2/s
E	Energy	joules
f_l	Liquid fraction	
h	Heat transfer coefficient	W/m^2 K
ΔH	Latent heat variable	J/kg
k	Thermal conductivity	W/m K
$\tilde{k}$	Solute partition coefficient	
L_m	Latent heat of melting	J/kg
L_v	Latent heat of vaporization	J/kg
$\mathbf{n}$	Unit normal	m
P	Mean laser power	watts
Pe	Peclet number	
S	Source term	
t	Time	s
t'	Integration variable	s
T	Temperature	K
T_h	Thickness of film	m
T_l	Liquidus temperature	K
T_m	Melting temperature	K
T_s	Solidus temperature	K
U_s	Scanning speed	m/s
U_x, U_y, U_z	Velocity components in x, y, and z directions	m/s
V	Volume	m^3
$\mathbf{V}$	Velocity vector	m/s
V_{cut}	Cutting velocity	m/s
α	Thermal diffusivity	m^2/s
$\mathfrak{R}_1, \mathfrak{R}_2,$ and $\mathfrak{R}_3$	Surface reaction constants	m/s
μ	Viscosity	Pa s
ρ	Density	kg/m^3
σ	Surface tension	N/m
σ_T	Surface tension coefficient	N/m K
γ	Specific-heat ratio	
Γ	Time integral	S
erfc	Error function	

ISBN 0-912035-15-3

Chapter 5: Laser-Material Interactions

Table 3. Sources

Ref.	Title	Author	Publication
1	Overview of Melt Dynamics in Laser Processing	J. Mazumder	*Optical Engineering* **30**(8), 1208–19 (1991)
2	Laser Materials Processing, 2nd ed.	W. M. Steen	Springer-Verlag, London (1998)
3	Numerical Heat Transfer and Fluid Flow	S. V. Patankar	Hemisphere Publishing Corporation, New York (1980)
4	The theory of moving sources of heat and its application to metal treatments	D. Rosenthal	*Trans. ASME.* **68**, 849–66 (1946)
5	Conduction of Heat in Solids, 2nd ed.	H. S. Carslaw and J. C. Jaeger	Oxford University Press, Oxford (1959)
6	Heat treating and melting material with a scanning laser or electron beam	H. E. Cline and T. R. Anthony	*J. Appl. Phys.* **48**, 3895–900 (1977)
7	Transient temperature profiles in solids heated with scanning laser	I. Chen and S. Lee	*J. Appl. Phys.* **54**, 1062–6 (1983)
8	Temperature distributions produced by scanning Gaussian laser beam	D. J. Sanders	*Appl. Optics* **23**, 30–5 (1984)
9	Temperature field with distributed moving heat source	N. Lovov	International Institute of Welding, Study Group 212, Doc. 212-682-87
10	Green's function solution for transient heat conduction problems	J. V. Beck	*Int. J. Heat Mass Transfer* **27**, 1235–44 (1984)
11	Quasi-steady-state three-dimensional temperature distribution induced by a moving circular Gaussian heat source in a finite depth solid	O. Manca, B. Morrone, and V. Naso	*Int. J. Heat Mass Transfer* **38**(7), 1305–15 (1995)
12	Analytical solution for temperature field in laser irradiated materials	A. M. Deus	M. Sc. Thesis, Institute Superior Technics, Lisbon, Portugal (1993)
13	Numerical prediction of the hardened zone in laser treatment of carbon steel	A. Bokta and S. Iskierka	*Acta Mater.* **44**(2), 445–50 (1996)
14	3-D transient thermal analysis for laser chemical vapor deposition on uniformly moving finite slabs	A. Kar and J. Mazumder	*J. Appl. Phys.* **65**(8), 2923–34 (1989)
15	Laser heating of a two-layer system with constant surface absorption: an exact solution	M. K. El-Adawi, M. A. Abdel-Naby, and S. A. Shalaby	*Int. J. Heat Mass Transfer* **38**(5), 947–52 (1995)
16	Temperature field in a multilayer assembly affected by a local laser heating	T. Elperin and G. Rudin	*Int. J. Heat Mass Transfer* **38**(17), 3143–7 (1995)
17	Heat transfer model for CW laser material processing	J. Mazumder and W. M. Steen	*J. Appl. Phys.* **51**(2), 941–7 (1980)
18	Effect of laser processing parameters on the structure of ductile iron	S. P. Gadag, M. N. Srinivasan and B. L. Mordike	*Mater. Sci. Eng.* **A196**, 145–1 (1995)
19	Three-dimensional numerical model for laser transformation hardening of metals	B. Gu, T. Ma, S. K. Brown, and L. Mannik	*Mater. Sci. Tech.* **10**(5), 425–30 (1994)
20	Mass transport in laser surface alloying: Iron-nickel system	T. Chande and J. Mazumder	*Appl. Phys. Lett.* **41**(1), 42–3 (1982)
21	Three-dimensional convection in laser melted pools	S. Kuo and Y. H. Wang	*Metall. Trans.* **17A**, 2265–70 (1986)
22	Thermocapillary convection during laser surface heating	C. L. Chan	Ph. D. Thesis, University of Illinois at Urbana-Champaign (1986)
23	Effect of surface tension gradient driven convection in laser melt pool: Three-dimensional perturbation model	C. L. Chan, J. Mazumder, and M. M. Chen	*J. Appl. Phys.* **64**(11), 6166–74 (1988)

Table 3. Sources (continued)

Ref.	Title	Author	Publication
24	The transient behavior of weld pools with deformed free surface	M. E. Thomson and J. Szekely	*Int. J. Heat Mass Transfer* **32**, 1007–19 (1989)
25	Finite element study on the role of convection in laser surface melting	K. Ravindran, J. Srinivasan, and A. G. Marathe	*Numer. Heat Transfer* **26**(5), 601–18 (1994)
26	Thermocapillary convection during laser surface melting	D. Morvan, F. D. Cipriani, and P. Bournot	*Int. J. Heat Mass Transfer* **37**(14), 1973–83 (1994)
27	Effects of High-Power Laser Radiation	J. F. Ready	Academic Press, New York, London (1971)
28	One-dimensional steady-state model for damage by vaporization and liquid expulsion due to laser material interaction	C. L. Chan and J. Mazumder	*J. Appl. Phys.* **62**, 4579–86 (1987)
29	Laser machining: Theory and Practice	G. Chryssolouris	Springer, New York (1991)
30	Two-dimensional model for laser induced material damage: Effects of assist gas and mulitple reflections inside the cavity	A. Kar, T. Rockstroh, and J. Mazumder	*J. Appl. Phys.* **71**, 2560–9 (1990)
31	Two-dimensional model for material damage due to melting and vaporization during laser irradiation	A. Kar and J. Mazumder	*J. Appl. Phys.* **68**, 3884–91 (1992)
32	Modelling the interaction between laser and target material in laser microspectral analysis	W. Qui, J. Watson, D. S. Thompson, and W. F. Deans	*Opt. Laser Technol.* **26**(3), 157–66 (1994)
33	Effect of variable properties on evaporative cutting with a moving CW laser	S. Ramanathan and M. F. Modest	Heat Transfer in Space Systems, **Vol. HTD-135**, ASME, 924–30 (1990)
34	Three-dimensional conduction effects during evaporative scribing with a moving CW laser	S. Roy and M. F. Modest	*J. Thermoph. Heat Transfer* **4**(2), 199–203 (1990)
35	Three-dimensional, transient model for laser machining of ablating /decomposing materials	M. F. Modest	*Int. J. Heat Mass Transfer* **39**(2), 221–34 (1996)
36	A keyhole model in penetration welding with a laser	J. M. Dowden, N. Postacioglu, M. P. Davis, and P. Kapadia	*J. Phys. D: Appl. Phys.* **20**, 36–44 (1987)
37	A point and line source model of laser keyhole welding	W. M. Steen, J. M. Dowden, M. Davis, and P. Kapadia	*J. Phys. D: Appl. Phys.* **21**, 1255–60 (1988)
38	A numerical model for deep penetration welding process	S. G. Lambrakos, E. A. Metzbower, P. G. Moore, J. H. Hunn, and A. Monis	*J. Materials Eng. Performance* **2**(6), 819–38 (1993)
39	Quasi-steady-state three-dimensional temperature	R. Duchrme, K. Williams, P. Kapadia, J. Dowden, B. Steen, and M. Glowack	*J. Phys. D: Appl. Phys.* **27**, 1619–27 (1994)
40	A model of deep penetration laser welding based on calculation of the keyhole profile	A. Kaplan	*J. Phys. D: Appl. Phys.* **27**, 1805–14 (1994)
41	Mathematical modeling of keyhole laser welding	A. Kar and J. Mazumder	*J. Appl. Phys.* **78**(11) (1995)

Chapter 5: Laser-Material Interactions

Table 3. Sources (concluded)

Ref.	Title	Author	Publication
42	A modeling study on the influence of pulse shaping on keyhole laser welding	P. S. Mohanty, A. Kar, and J. Mazumder	*J. Laser Applications* **8**, 291–7 (1996)
43	One dimensional finite-medium diffusion model for extended solid solution in laser cladding	A. Kar and J. Mazumder	*Acta Metall.* **36**(3), 701–12 (1987)
44	Science and technology of rapidly quenched alloys	M. J. Aziz	Eds. M. Tenhoren et. al, MRS, Pittsburg, PA, p. 25 (1987)
45	Three-dimensional transient mass-transfer model for LCVD of titanium on stationary finite slabs	A. Kar, M. Azer, and J. Mazumder	*J. Appl. Phys.* **69**(2), 757–66 (1991)

5.5.1 Parameters

Laser materials processing involves a wide range of power densities, interaction times, and transport phenomena, and deals with objects of sizes ranging from nanometers to meters. Figure 1 presents a comprehensive picture of the operational regimes and associated transport phenomena for various laser processing techniques (1).

The art of modeling this novel process is to develop a proper understanding in selecting the appropriate transport phenomena, boundary conditions, and solution techniques. A general heat balance principle involved in laser materials processing is presented first. The necessary modifications required for describing a particular process with suitable boundary conditions, solutions, and additional considerations are outlined along with their applicability and limitations.

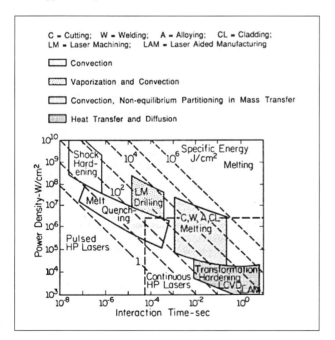

Figure 1. Process map for various laser applications in materials processing (1).

5.5.2 Heat Balance

We next consider generalized principles of heat balance important to laser materials processing. A schematic diagram is presented in Figure 2, which shows heat input Q at the surface, the $z = 0$ plane, with the beam scanning with velocity U_s in the x direction.

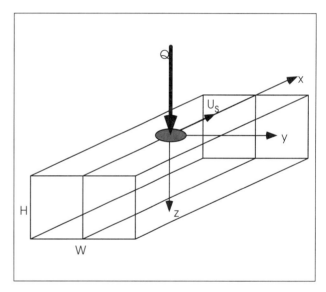

Figure 2. Process schematic.

Upon irradiation, a material absorbs laser light and its temperature increases. If the laser beam has sufficient energy, the material may undergo a change in physical state such as melting and evaporation. A rough approximation of energy required to go through various states can be expressed as

$$\Delta H_t = \rho \, V \left[C_p \, \Delta T_{s \rightarrow l} + L_m + C_p \, \Delta T_{l \rightarrow v} + L_v \right] \quad (1)$$

where, the terms in the equation respectively, account for (1) heating the material from room temperature to melting, (2) the latent heat of melting, (3) heating the melt to the vaporization point, and (4) the latent heat of evaporation. However, the above approximation does not take into account losses, the duration of irradiation, and the distribution of energy in the laser beam. A conservative energy balance should take these factors into account and can be expressed as: heat in minus heat out equals heat accumulated plus heat generated. The governing energy balance equation can be derived following the above principle as in Figure 3.

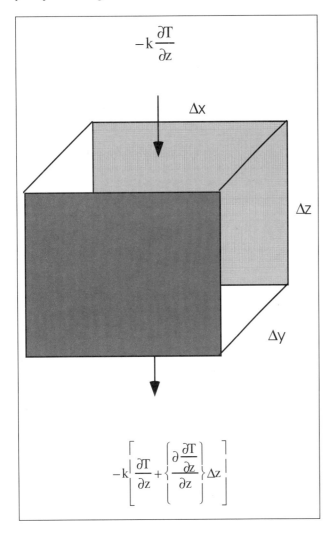

Figure 3. Control volume for energy balance.

The heat flow by conduction in z direction (see Fig. 3), can be expressed as:

$$\left\{-k\frac{\partial T}{\partial z}+k\left[\frac{\partial T}{\partial z}+\left\{\frac{\partial\left(\frac{\partial T}{\partial z}\right)}{\partial z}\right\}\delta z\right]\right\}\delta y = k\frac{\partial^2 T}{\partial z^2}\delta x \delta y \delta z \quad (2)$$

Similarly, heat flow by convection can be expressed as:

$$\rho C_p U_z \delta x \delta y T - \rho C_p U_z \delta x \delta y \left(T+\frac{\partial T}{\partial z}\delta z\right) = -\rho C_p U_z \left(\frac{\partial T}{\partial z}\right)\delta x \delta y \delta z \quad (3)$$

Heat accumulation and generation, respectively, take the following forms:

$$\rho C_p \frac{\partial T}{\partial t}\delta x \delta y \delta z \quad \text{and} \quad \Delta H \delta x \delta y \delta z \quad (4)$$

The total balance is expressed by the following differential form:

$$\rho C_p \frac{\partial T}{\partial t} + \rho C_p U_z \frac{\partial T}{\partial z} = k\frac{\partial^2 T}{\partial z^2} + \Delta H \quad (5)$$

Following the same procedure, the heat balance in 3D can be derived, and the resulting equation is expressed as:

$$\frac{\partial}{\partial t}(\rho C_p T) + \frac{\partial}{\partial x}(\rho C_p U_x T) + \frac{\partial}{\partial y}(\rho C_p U_y T) + \frac{\partial}{\partial z}(\rho C_p U_z T) =$$
$$\frac{\partial}{\partial x}\left\{k\frac{\partial T}{\partial x}\right\} + \frac{\partial}{\partial y}\left\{k\frac{\partial T}{\partial y}\right\} + \frac{\partial}{\partial z}\left\{k\frac{\partial T}{\partial z}\right\} + \Delta H \quad (6)$$

Although, heat transport is the primary transport phenomenon of interest in laser materials processing, quite often, additional transport processes such as fluid flow, diffusion, and evaporation need to be considered, as they become dominant depending on the application. A detailed description of these processes is out of the scope of the present section; however, the appropriate references have been cited in Table 3.

5.5.3 Conduction

Conduction is the predominant heat transport phenomenon at low laser power density applications (see Fig. 1). A typical process application is surface transformation hardening. However, conduction models have often been applied to other processes such as glazing, alloying, welding, cutting and ablation, with limiting assumptions. Some useful solutions to the conduction equation are presented in the following section (2, 4, 5, 12). Also, several sample results have been presented to demonstrate the usefulness of these techniques.

Analytical Solutions
Case: 1D semi-infinite ($0 < z < \infty$) domain, no heat generation, and constant k, ρ, and C_p:

Constant flux q at $z = 0$: $\quad q(t) = \begin{cases} q_o & (t < t_i) \\ 0 & (t > t_i) \end{cases} \quad (7)$

$$T(z,t) = \frac{2q_o}{k}\sqrt{\alpha t}\, ierfc\left(\frac{z}{2\sqrt{\alpha t}}\right) \quad \text{for } t < t_1 \quad (8)$$

$$T(z,t) = \frac{2q_o}{k}\left[\sqrt{\alpha t}\, ierfc\left(\frac{z}{2\sqrt{\alpha t}}\right) - \sqrt{\alpha(t_o-t_1)}\, ierfc\left(\frac{z}{2\sqrt{\alpha(t-t_o)}}\right)\right]$$
$$\text{for } t > t_1 \quad (9)$$

where

$$ierfc(x) = \frac{e^{-x^2}}{\sqrt{\pi}} - x[1 - erf(x)]; \quad \& \quad erf(x) = \frac{2}{\sqrt{\pi}} \int_0^x e^{-\xi^2} d\xi \quad (10)$$

Case: 1D, finite domain ($0 < z < D$), no heat generation, constant k, ρ, and C_p, and constant flux q_0 at $z = 0$:

Case: $q(z = D, t) = 0$

$$T(z,t) = \frac{2q_0}{k}\sqrt{\alpha t} \sum_{n=0}^{\infty}\left[ierfc\left(\frac{2nD+z}{2\sqrt{\alpha t}}\right) + ierfc\left(\frac{2nD+2D-z}{2\sqrt{\alpha t}}\right)\right] \quad (11)$$

Case: $T(z = D, t) = 0$

$$T(z,t) = \frac{2q_0}{k}\sqrt{\alpha t} \sum_{n=0}^{\infty}(-1)^n\left[ierfc\left(\frac{2nD+z}{2\sqrt{\alpha t}}\right) - ierfc\left(\frac{2nD+2D-z}{2\sqrt{\alpha t}}\right)\right] \quad (12)$$

Case: $q(z=D, t) = h(T - T_{med})$

$$T(z,t) = \frac{Dq_0}{k\lambda}\left[1 + \lambda\left(1 - \frac{z}{D}\right) - \sum_{n=1}^{\infty}\frac{2\lambda(\Phi_n^2 + \lambda^2)\cos\left(\Phi_n\frac{z}{D}\right)}{\Phi_n^2(\lambda + \lambda^2 + \Phi_n^2)}e^{-\Phi_n^2 \tau}\right]$$

where $\lambda = Dh$; $\tau = \frac{\alpha t}{D^2}$ $\quad \Phi_n \tan \Phi_n = \lambda$ (13)

Case: 1D, finite domain ($0 < z < D$), with heat generation, constant k, ρ, and C_p, and constant flux at $z = 0$:

Heat generation term:

$$F(z,t) = \begin{cases} F_0 & z < D \\ 0 & z > D \end{cases}; \quad F_0 = \frac{AI}{\delta} \quad (14)$$

With I the intensity and δ the absorption depth.

For $z < D$

$$T(z,t) = \frac{F_0 \alpha t}{k}\left[1 - 2i^2 erfc\left(\frac{D-z}{2\sqrt{\alpha t}}\right) - 2i^2 erfc\left(\frac{D+z}{2\sqrt{\alpha t}}\right)\right] \quad (15)$$

For $z > D$

$$T(z,t) = \frac{2F_0 \alpha t}{k}\left[1 - 2i^2 erfc\left(\frac{D-z}{2\sqrt{\alpha t}}\right) - 2i^2 erfc\left(\frac{D+z}{2\sqrt{\alpha t}}\right)\right] \quad (16)$$

where

$$i^n erfc(x) \equiv \int_x^{\infty} i^{n-1} erfc(\xi) d\xi; \quad n = 1, 2, \ldots \quad (17)$$

$$i^0 erfc(x) = erfc(x)$$

The one-dimensional solutions are reasonably appropriate when the heat source is large compared to the depth considered, or the domain possesses a cylindrical symmetry.

Case: 3D ($\infty < x < \infty$, $\infty < y < \infty$, $0 < z < \infty$), constant k, ρ, and C_p, stationary and instantaneous flux:

Point source:

$$T(x,y,z,t) = \frac{q_o}{4\rho C_p \sqrt{(\pi \alpha t)^3}} e^{\frac{-r^2}{4\alpha t}}; \quad r = \sqrt{x^2 + y^2 + z^2}; \quad (18)$$

$q_o = Apt_i$, with t_i the duration of the irradiation.

Planar source:

$$T(z,t) = \frac{q_o}{\rho C_p \sqrt{(\pi \alpha t)^3}} e^{\frac{-z^2}{4\alpha t}}; \quad q_p = AIt \quad (19)$$

with I the intensity and t_i the duration of the irradiation.

Gaussian source, with radius r_0:

$$T(r,z,t) = \frac{q_g r_0^2}{\rho C_p \sqrt{\pi \alpha t}(4\alpha t + r^2)} e^{\left(-\frac{z^2}{4\alpha t}\right)\left(-\frac{r^2}{4\alpha t + r_0^2}\right)} \quad (20)$$

Where q_g is the Gaussian flux.

Case: 3D ($\infty < x < \infty$, $\infty < y < \infty$, $0 < z < \infty$), constant k, ρ, and C_p, stationary and continuous flux:

Point source:

$$T(x,y,z,t) = \frac{1}{4\rho C_p \sqrt{(\pi \alpha)^3}} \int_0^t q_0(t') e^{-\frac{r^2}{4\alpha(t-t')}} \frac{dt'}{\sqrt{(t-t')^3}} \quad (21)$$

Planar source:

$$T(z,t) = \frac{2q_p}{k}\sqrt{\alpha t}\, ierfc\left(\frac{z}{2\sqrt{\alpha t}}\right) \quad (22)$$

Gaussian source:

$$T(r,z,t) = \frac{r_0^2}{k}\sqrt{\frac{\alpha}{\pi}}\int_0^t q_g(t-t') e^{-\frac{z^2}{4\alpha t} - \frac{r^2}{4\alpha t + r_0^2}} \frac{dt'}{\sqrt{t'}(4\alpha t' + r_0^2)} \quad (23)$$

When, $D \ll 2\sqrt{\alpha t}$, the temperature distribution is independent of the depth. Then the temperature distribution for a Gaussian source can be expressed as:

$$T(r,t) = \frac{q_g \alpha r_0^2}{kD} \int_0^t e^{\gamma^2 t' - \frac{r^2}{4\alpha t} + \frac{r'^2 r_0^2}{4\alpha t(r_0^2 + 4\alpha t')}} \frac{dt'}{(4\alpha t' + r_0^2)} \quad (24)$$

where $\gamma = 2h/D$.

Case: 3D ($\infty < x < \infty$, $\infty < y < \infty$, $0 < z < \infty$), constant k, ρ, and C_p, moving point source:

Rosenthal solution (4):

$$T(\eta, r) = \frac{q_0}{2\pi k R} e^{-\frac{U_s}{2\alpha}(R+\eta)}; \quad R = \sqrt{\eta^2 + y^2 + z^2}; \quad \eta = x - U_s t \quad (25)$$

Carslaw and Jaeger (5):

$$T(x,y,x,t) = \frac{q_0}{\sqrt{\pi^3} kr} e^{\frac{U_s x}{2\alpha}} \int_{\frac{r}{2\sqrt{\alpha t}}}^{\infty} e^{-\Gamma^2 - \left(\frac{U_s r}{4\alpha\mu}\right)} d\Gamma \quad (26)$$

Case: 3D ($\infty < x < \infty$, $\infty < y < \infty$, $0 < z < \infty$), constant k, ρ, and C_p, moving Gaussian source:

$$T(x,y,x,t) = \frac{q_0}{\rho C_p} \int_0^{\infty} e^{-\left(\frac{(x+U_s t')^2 + y^2}{r_0^2 + 4\alpha t'} + \frac{z^2}{4\alpha t'}\right)} \frac{dt'}{\sqrt{\pi^3 \alpha t'}(r_0^2 + 4\alpha t')} \quad (27)$$

Case: Quasisteady, 3D, finite depth and width ($\infty < x < \infty$, $0 < y < W$, $0 < z < D$), Gaussian beam, constant k, ρ, and C_p:

$$T^+(X,Y,Z,l^+,H^+,Pe) = \frac{2\sqrt{\pi}}{H^+ l^+ Pe} \times \sum_{m=0}^{\infty} \sum_{s=0}^{\infty} c_{ms} \cos\frac{2m\pi Y}{l^+} \cos\frac{s\pi Z}{H^+}$$
$$\times \left\{ \exp\left[Pe(1+p_{ms})\left(\frac{Pe}{4}(1+p_{ms}) - X\right)\right] \times \operatorname{erfc}\left[\frac{Pe}{2}(1+p_{ms}) - X\right] \right.$$
$$\left. + \exp\left[Pe(1-p_{ms})\left(\frac{Pe}{4}(1-p_{ms}) - X\right)\right] \times \operatorname{erfc}\left[X - \frac{Pe}{2}(1-p_{ms})\right] \right\} \quad (28)$$
$$\times \int_{Y'=0}^{l^+/2} \exp(-Y'^2) \cos\frac{2m\pi Y'}{l^+} dY'$$

The Peclet number, Pe, is a dimensionless ratio that expresses the interplay between convection and diffusion in viscous fluid flow. As the Peclet number increases, the role of convection increases. The definition of the other terms in the equation and the use of the equation to obtain temperature distributions may be found in Reference 11.

Case: Transient, 3D, finite depth and width ($\infty < x < \infty$, $0 < y < W$, $0 < z < D$), Gaussian beam, constant k, ρ, and C_p:

The solution of the problem has the form:

$$T(x,y,z,t) = \frac{AP}{2\pi\rho C_p} \int_0^t \frac{1}{2\sqrt{\pi\alpha(t-t')}(r^2+2\alpha(t-t'))} \sum_{n=-\infty}^{\infty} \exp\left(-\frac{(z-2nD)^2}{4\alpha(t-t')}\right)$$
$$\times \left\{ \sum_{n=-\infty}^{\infty} \exp\left(-\frac{(x+U_s(t_0-t'))^2 + (y-4nW/2)^2}{2r^2 + 4\alpha(t-t')}\right) F_{1(y)} \right.$$
$$+ \sum_{n=-\infty}^{\infty} \exp\left(-\frac{(x+U_s(t_0-t'))^2 + (y-2(2n-1)W/2)^2}{2r^2 + 4\alpha(t-t')}\right) F_{2(y)}$$
$$\left. + \sum_{n=-\infty}^{\infty} \exp\left(-\frac{(x+U_s(t_0-t'))^2 + (y+2(2n-1)W/2)^2}{2r^2 + 4\alpha(t-t')}\right) F_{3(y)} \right\} dt' + T_{init}$$
$$(29)$$

where t_0 is the time when the coordinate system of the laser and the material coincide, r is the radius of the Gaussian source, $F_{1(y)}$, $F_{2(y)}$ and $F_{3(y)}$ are error functions and their explicit values can be found from Reference 13. Figure 4 presents the transient evolution of the temperature isolines obtained from the above solution.

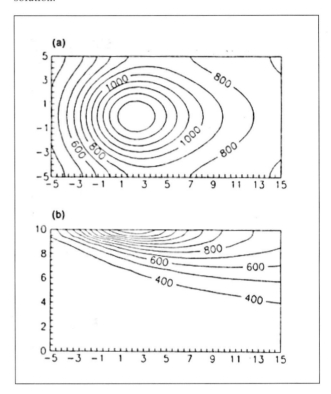

Figure 4. Temperature isoline for carbon steel, $U_s = 0.9$ m/min, $P = 1.5$ kW, $A = 0.7$; (a) surface and (b) longitudinal section (13). The units on the axes are millimeters. The temperatures are K.

Case: Transient, 3D, finite geometry, Gaussian source, variable k:

$$T^* = \frac{1}{(\bar{q}+1)\overline{T}_a^{*\bar{q}}} \left\{ 1 - \overline{T}_a^{*\bar{q}+1} + (\bar{q}+1)T^{'*} \right\} + \overline{T}_a^* \quad (30)$$

where

$$T^*(x^*,y^*,z^*,t^*) = \sum_{l=0}^{\infty} \frac{K_{lx}(x^*)}{N_{lx}} \left[\sum_{m=0}^{\infty} \frac{K_{my}(y^*)}{N_{my}} \times \left(\overline{T}^{iv}(\lambda_{lx}, \lambda_{my}, z^*, t^*) \right. \right.$$
$$\left. \left. + \sum_{n=0}^{\infty} \left[\psi_1(0) e^{-\lambda_{lmn}^2 t^*} + \psi_{20}(t^*) \right] \times \frac{K_{nz}(z^*)}{N_{nz}} \right) \right] - T_c$$
$$(31)$$

The details for each term in Equations 30 and 31 are explained in Reference 14. Figure 5 shows a sample temperature profile obtained from this model.

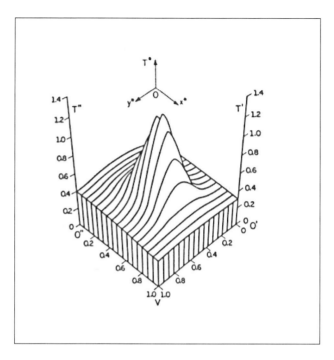

Figure 5. Sample result from variable-conductivity model for a zirconium alloy (14). The units on the *x* and *y* axes are cm. The laser power is 600 W, the beam size 8x2 mm, and the scanning velocity 17 mm/s.

Since Gaussian beams are widely used, a parametric study was carried out using the 3D quasisteady solution, and the following conclusions were derived:

- The temperature field in a solid whose width is far larger than the radius of a Gaussian spot can be assumed to be two dimensional for any thickness of the body.
- In a solid whose thickness is one-tenth the radius of Gaussian spot, thermal gradients along the depth are negligible. Such a body can be considered thermally thin.
- In a solid whose thickness and width are far smaller than the radius of a Gaussian spot the temperature distribution exhibits no maximum.
- In a solid whose thickness and width are thermally finite ($D = l/2 = r$), the maximum midplane temperature is nearly independent of the depth when diffusive contribution to the heat removal is far larger than the convective one (Pe = 0.1). Here D is the thickness, l the width, and r the radius of the Gaussian spot. The maximum temperature on the top surface is much greater than that on the bottom surface when Pe = 10. Therefore, lower Peclet numbers are suitable for processes such as cutting and welding, whereas higher Peclet numbers are suitable for localized heat treatment.

Numerical Solutions

Although analytical methods are quite handy and can lead to meaningful analysis, they are limited by the assumption made to obtain a particular solution. As a result, quite often they deviate from the real situation of a practical problem. These restrictions can be relaxed in a numerical approach to a large extent. Temperature-dependent thermophysical properties, spatial distribution of heat source, radiative and convective heat loss, and the latent heat of transformation can be taken into account. The numerical solutions are obtained either by the finite-element or by the finite-difference method. If melting is involved, then the latent heat can be treated as an equivalent heat capacity (17, 18).

$$\overline{C}_p \Delta T_m = \int_{T_0}^{T_m} C_p dT + \Delta H_m \tag{32}$$

where ΔH_m is the enthalpy of melting.

The other alternative is to express the enthalpy as a function of temperature and dump the evolution into the source term of the governing equation. The enthalpy–temperature relationship is derived from the phase diagram as follows:

$$\Delta H_m(T) = L_m \text{ for } T \geq T_l$$
$$\Delta H_m(T) = L_m(1-f_s) \text{ for } T_l \leq T \leq T_l \tag{33}$$
$$\Delta H_m(T) = 0 \text{ for } T \leq T_s.$$

where f_s is the solid fraction.

$$f_l = \left[\frac{T_m - T_l}{T_m - T}\right]^{1/(1-\bar{k})} \tag{34}$$

Similarly, the absorptivity and conductivty can also be related to the temperature via appropriate relations. See References 3, 17, and 19 for details. The numerical solution process starts with discretizing the domain into small control volumes or elements as shown in Figure 6. The figure defines a midpoint P, an east point E and a west point W. The temperature at the east point is T_E, etc.

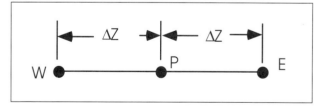

Figure 6. One-dimensional discretization.

The implicit finite-difference form of Equation 5 can be expressed as:

$$\rho C_p \left(\frac{T_p^{t+\Delta t} - T_p^t}{\Delta t}\right) + (\rho C_p U_z)_p \left(\frac{T_E^{t+\Delta t} - T_W^{t+\Delta t}}{2\Delta z}\right) = k\left(\frac{T_E^{t+\Delta t} - 2T_p^{t+\Delta t} + T_W^{t+\Delta t}}{\Delta z^2}\right) + \Delta H \Delta Z \tag{35}$$

By rearranging we obtain the following algebraic equation:

$$(\frac{\rho C_p}{\Delta t} + \frac{2k}{\Delta z^2})T_P^{t+\Delta t} = (\frac{k}{\Delta z^2} - \frac{\rho C_p U_z}{2\Delta z})T_E^{t+\Delta t} + (\frac{k}{\Delta z^2} + \frac{\rho C_p U_z}{2\Delta z})T_W^{t+\Delta t} + \frac{\rho C_p}{\Delta t}T_P^t + \Delta H \Delta z \quad (36)$$

Alternatively,

$$a_p T_P = a_e T_E + a_w T_W + a_p^0 T_P^0 + S \quad \text{where} \quad a_p = a_e + a_w + a_p^0 \quad (37)$$

Here a_p, a_w, and a_E are the coefficients of the algebraic equation derived from Eq. (36), with a_p the coefficient for the midpoint P, a_w the coefficient for the west point W, and a_E the coefficient for the east point E.

Following the same procedure, the equivalent 3D algebraic equation can be derived. There are several well-tested techniques for solving the algebraic equations obtained from the discretization procedure. A detailed discussion is available in Reference 3.

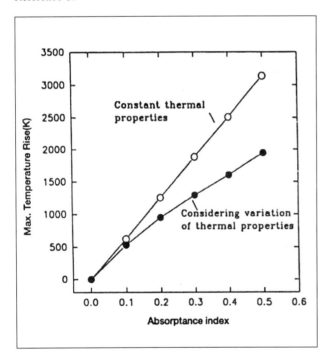

Figure 7. Comparison of constant and temperature-dependent absorptivity for steel (19). The laser beam power is 1500 W, the beam diameter 4 mm, and the scanning velocity 2.5 mm/s.

To demonstrate the flexibility and capability of the numerical technique, Figure 7 presents a comparison of maximum temperature reached on a surface heated by a laser beam, using both constant and variable thermophysical properties. It should be noted that the difference becomes significant at higher temperatures, which cannot be tested by analytical techniques. Analytical techniques lack the flexibility of the numerical technique. On the other hand, a numerical technique is time consuming and resource consuming. Thus the choice of solution technique is very important and should be judged based on the specific problem.

5.5.4 Convection

Convection becomes a dominant transport mechanism when a molten pool is created (1). Surface tension variations arise due to temperature gradients along the interface, and shear stresses acting on the interface induce fluid motions. Convection in the molten pool affects a large number of laser processes such as melt quenching, alloying, and welding. Convection is primarily responsible for mixing in the melt pool and therefore controls the composition during surface alloying (see Fig. 8).

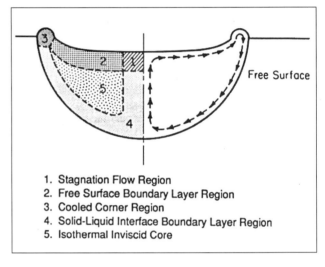

1. Stagnation Flow Region
2. Free Surface Boundary Layer Region
3. Cooled Corner Region
4. Solid-Liquid Interface Boundary Layer Region
5. Isothermal Inviscid Core

Figure 8. General features of convection in the molten pool (1).

Mathematical modeling of convection phenomena is complex, and usually numerical schemes are used for this purpose. Besides the energy equation (Eq. 6), the Navier-Stokes equation, along with a continuity constraint, need to be solved in a coupled manner. The general form of the equations are

$$\nabla V = 0 \quad (38)$$

$$\frac{\partial}{\partial t}(\rho V) + (\rho V \nabla)V = -\nabla p + \mu \nabla^2 V + S \quad (39)$$

The details of the computational procedure are available in References 1 and 21–26. As an example of the type of results that may be achieved, Figure 9 presents the trajectory of a particle injected to the molten pool. It is evident that the particle travels a long path before it solidifies due to the nature of the fluid flow.

Figure 10, presents a plot of the surface temperature for molten steel at 240 W absorbed laser power, 0.55 mm beam radius and 0.012 m/s scanning speed. Figure 11 illustrates the surface deformation due to surface pressure variation.

The following trends are observed from a study of convection processes: Thermocapillary forces drive the surface fluid radially outward at high velocities. These high velocities displace more mass from the central surface region than can be replaced by the recalculating flow, thus causing a depression. The displaced mass builds up at the solid-liquid interface, causing the surface to bulge upward, where it is then forced downward into the melt pool. These modeling efforts involve significant amounts of computational time.

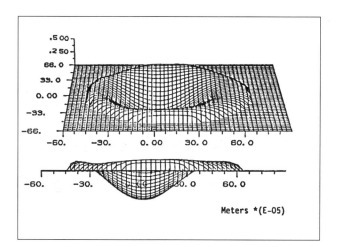

Figure 11. Deformation of liquid surface due to thermocapillary flow for steel (1). The numerical values are in units of 10^{-5} m. The conditions are the same as for Figure 10.

5.5.5 Vaporization

The simultaneous occurrence of convection and vaporization is at the heart of many laser applications, such as welding, cutting, and laser ablation. Depending on the energy density and interaction time, either melting or vaporization may dominate or they may be equally influential. There is very limited understanding of coupled flow behavior and vaporization. As far as modeling is concerned, the major challenge is handling the liquid–vapor boundary, where the interaction is most important. There have been several efforts to do this, ranging from simple volume loss calculations to complicated numerical calculations involving geometry transformation (27, 35).

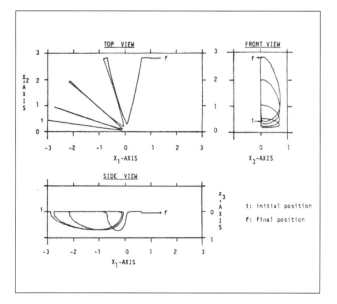

Figure 9. Trajectory of a particle, traced from a flow solution (1). The figure is presented in nondimensional units and is intended to give a qualitative picture of what may happen in the liquid pool.

As an example, a simple volume loss calculation scheme is presented here (32). For a single grid cell, assume that the cell has volume ΔV, which remains in phase 1 at time step t; the net energy into this grid at time step $t+\Delta t$ is Δq. First, the new temperature $T_{ij}^{t+\Delta t}$ is calculated from the heat conduction equation. If $T_{ij}^{t+\Delta t}$ is less than the phase change point, T_v, (i.e., no phase change), the calculation moves to the next grid. Otherwise the partial volume, ΔV_x, of material in phase 2 is determined by

$$\Delta V \rho C_p \left(T^* - T_{ij}^t\right) + \Delta V_x \rho L^* = \Delta q \qquad (40)$$

Second, if $\Delta V_x \leq \Delta V$, the calculation of this grid finishes and moves to the next grid. If $\Delta V_x > \Delta V$, then after the grid has all changed from phase 1 to phase 2, there is still excess energy, $\Delta q'$, which is obtained from:

$$\Delta q' = \Delta q - [\Delta V \rho C_p (T^* - T_{ij}^t) + \Delta V \rho L^*] \qquad (41)$$

This remaining energy will transfer to its downward neighbor cells if phase 2 is gas, and the calculation moves to the next

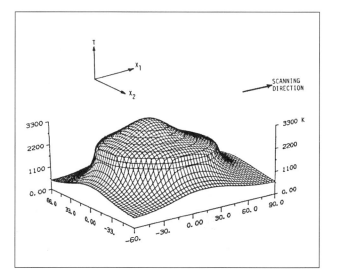

Figure 10. Surface temperature profile obtained from a 3D convective model for steel (1). The numerical values for the x and y axes are in units of 10^{-5} m. The laser power is 240 W, the beam diameter 1.10 mm, and the scan velocity 0.012 m/s.

grid; if phase 2 is liquid, the calculations for the same grid are repeated from the first step, but substituting

$$T_{ij} = T_m, \quad T^* = T_v, \quad L^* = L_v, \quad \Delta_q = \Delta'_q$$

With all x values, the interface at time step $t+\Delta t$ can be drawn. Adopting this tracking method, it was possible to predict the depth of the crater realistically. Figure 12 shows some results that demonstrate excellent agreement with experimental results.

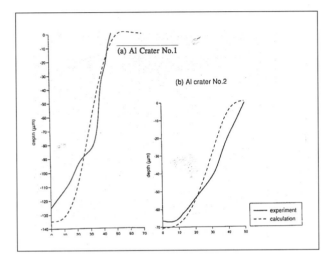

Figure 12. Comparison of vaporization loss for aluminum (32). The x and y axes are in µm. For the (a) curve, the pulse energy was 180 mJ, the pulse duration 320 µs and the beam radius 30 µm. For the (b) curve, the pulse energy was 140 mJ, the pulse duration 350 µs, and the beam radius 30 µm.

In another study (35), it was assumed that the change of phase from solid to vapor occurs in a single step with the rate governed by a simple Arrhenius relation similar to the equilibrium evaporation rate equation originally developed by Langmuir. The governing heat conduction equation takes the form:

$$\text{At} \quad z = S(x,y): \quad AI \cdot n = -n \cdot (k\nabla T) + v_n \rho \Delta h_{re} \quad (42)$$

and the initial conditions as:

$$t = 0: \quad T(x,y,z,0) = T_\infty \quad \text{and} \quad S(x,y,0) = 0. \quad (43)$$

where $S(x,y)$ represents the surface recession, Δh_{re} is the heat of removal, and v_n is the surface recession velocity. The rate of mass loss per unit area is described by

$$\dot{m}'' = \rho C_{1e}^{c_2(1-T_{re}/T)}; \quad C_2 = \Delta h_{re}/RT_{re} \quad (44)$$

where T_{re} is the equilibrium ablation temperature, R is the gas constant, and C_1 is a pre-exponential factor, which may depend on temperature.

The details of the calculation procedure are available in Reference 35. A sample of computational results comparing grooves generated by CW, pulsed, and Q-switched lasers is presented in Figure 13.

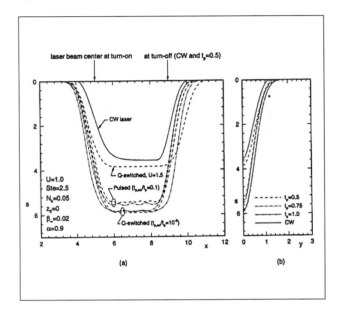

Figure 13. Grooves created by various laser beams (35): (a) the cross section along the center line; (b) the cross section normal to the laser scan direction. The pulse rate was 10 kHz, the average power 30 W, the scan velocity 10 cm/s, and the beam radius 75 µm.

The previous examples neglected any fluid flow. However, at power densities around 10^7 W/cm^2, both convection and evaporation are dominant, and this situation presents a very challenging task for modeling. A typical application is keyhole or deep penetration welding (see Fig. 14). The liquid-vapor interface $z=S_1(r, \theta, t)$, can be determined from the following balance (41)

$$k_l \frac{\partial T_l}{\partial z} + AI = \rho_l L_v \left(\frac{\partial S_1}{\partial t} - u_z \right) \quad (45)$$

and at the solid-liquid interface, $z=S_2(r,\theta,t)$ the following condition satisfies:

$$k_s \frac{\partial T_s}{\partial z} - k_l \frac{\partial T_l}{\partial z} = \rho_s L_m \frac{\partial S_2}{\partial t} \quad (46)$$

The velocity and temperature are determined by the appropriate solution of momentum and energy equations (41). As an example of the results from such modeling, refer to Figure 15 for the effect of different pulse shaping on the depth of penetration for stainless steel for pulses that have the same pulse parameters (duration and peak irradiance), but different temporal shapes.

Chapter 5: Laser-Material Interactions

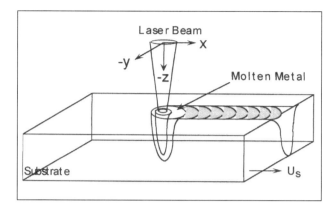

Figure 14. Schematic of keyhole welding process.

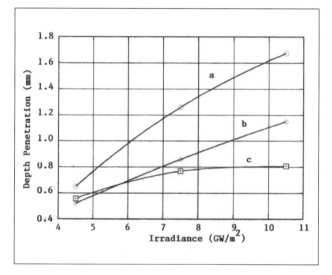

Figure 15. Comparison of penetration depth during keyhole welding (42) versus irradiance for pulses with the same pulse parameters but different temporal shapes. Pulse time: 2.5 ms (a) Ramp-up; (b) Gaussian; (c) Top-hat.

5.5.6 Mass Diffusion

Mass transport plays a considerable role in various laser processing applications. Mass transport can be both convective and diffusive in nature. Convective transport plays important roles in the case of alloying, cladding, and welding. Uniformity of mixing and the resultant average compositions in the liquid state are primarily determined by the nature and level of convection established in the liquid pool. During solidification, the partitioning of alloying elements between solid and liquid also needs to be estimated. Short length scales, unusual phase combinations, and metastable phases are reasons for distinctive behavior and give rise to special considerations for analysis. Mass transport in the gas phase along with chemical reactions are also involved in certain laser processing applications such as laser chemical vapor deposition (LCVD).

The derivation of the diffusion equation follows the same procedure as the energy equation. In one dimension it can be expressed as (20):

$$\frac{\partial C}{\partial t} + U_z \frac{\partial C}{\partial z} = \tilde{D}\left(\frac{\partial^2 C}{\partial z^2}\right) + S \qquad (47)$$

Similarly, the 3D form of the equation can be derived. As mentioned before, convection is coupled with mass transfer, and usually a numerical solution is sought for the problem.

As an example of the results that may be obtained, the effect of laser-substrate interaction time on solute distribution during surface alloying is presented in Figure 16. The average solute concentration increased linearly with increasing interaction time. A change in solute diffusivity by a factor of 10 resulted in only a very small change in the concentration profile, suggesting that convective transport is the dominating mechanism.

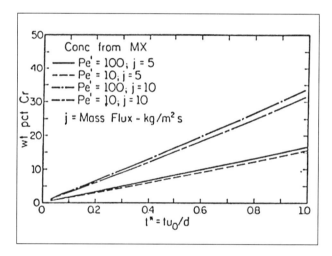

Figure 16. The wt % increase with interaction time during laser alloying. P'_e is the Peclet number. The abscissa is nondimensional. U_0 is the scan velocity. The laser power is 1500 W, the beam diameter 1 mm, and the scan velocity 1.0 cm/sec (20).

Rapid cooling is inherent in the laser processing of materials. During rapid solidification, when growth occurs at rates of the order of 1 m/s, the local equilibrium no longer exists. Interface kinetics models are then needed to predict the kinetic undercooling at the interface and the nonequilibrium solute partitioning coefficient $\tilde{k}$ defined as C_s/C_l, where C_s is the solute concentration in the growing solid and C_l is that in the liquid at the interface (44)

$$\tilde{k}(v) = \frac{v/v_D + \tilde{k}_e}{v/v_D + 1} \qquad (48)$$

ISBN 0-912035-15-3

where $\tilde{k}_e$ is the equilibrium partition coefficient, v interface velocity, and v_D is the diffusion velocity. Figure 17 shows an example of the results. The figure presents the prediction of a coupled heat, mass and solidification solution to demonstrate the effect of nonequilibrium partitioning.

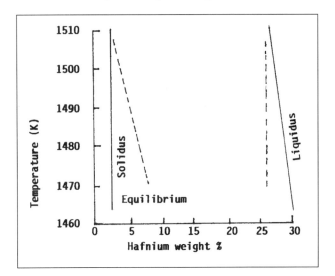

Figure 17. Equilibrium versus nonequilibrium diagram for Ni-Hf (43).

It should be additionally noted that besides heat and mass transfer quite often consideration of chemical reaction kinetics becomes important in modeling certain laser-assisted materials processing such as the laser chemical vapor deposition process. For example, in depositing Ti thin films by LCVD, the following reactions need to be considered (45):

$$\text{TiBr}_4(g) \xrightarrow{\Re_1} \text{TiBr}_2(s) + \text{Br}_2(g), \tag{49}$$

$$3\text{TiBr}_2(s) \xrightarrow{\Re_2} 2\text{TiBr}(s) + \text{TiBr}_4(g), \tag{50}$$

$$4\text{TiBr}(s) \xrightarrow{\Re_3} 3\text{Ti}(s) + \text{TiBr}_4(g), \tag{51}$$

where $\Re_1$, $\Re_2$, and $\Re_3$ are the surface reaction constants with respect to the concentration of TiBr_4, TiBr_2, and TiBr, respectively. The rate of production of various species is a function of the concentration and temperature. An appropriate functional relationship must be chosen to model the process. The reaction constant is related to the temperature by the Arrhenius equation

$$\Re_j = \Re_{0j} exp\{-E_j / [RT(x,y,0,t)]\} \text{ for } j = 1, 2, \text{ and } 3, \tag{52}$$

where $\Re_{0j}$ and E_j are the Arrhenius constant and the activation energy of the jth reaction. Thus the chemical kinetics is coupled to the thermal model. The thickness of the Ti film, T_h, can be calculated as:

$$Th = \dot{r}_4 \gamma_4 \tau \Delta t^* / \rho \tag{53}$$

The cross section of the circular-symmetric film thickness profile obtained from such a model is shown in Figure 18 (45).

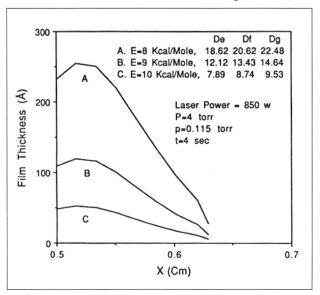

Figure 18. Film thickness at different power. The material is Ti. D_e, D_f, and D_g are the Damkohler numbers for reactions (49), (50), and (51).

See Chapter 27 for more information on LCVD.

5.5.7 Specific Examples

Example 1

Consider the case of drilling a hole in aluminum using a pulsed YAG laser. The aim is to estimate the energy required to drill a hole of 0.1 mm through a 0.5-mm-thick plate. Use the following data for calculation:

C_p = 900 J/kg K, ρ = 2700 kg/m³, T_m = 933 K, T_v = 2723 K, L_m = 0.397 × 10⁶ J/kg, L_v = 9.492 × 10⁶ J/kg, A = 0.3

Following Equation 1,

E_t = 2700 × (π/4) × 0.1 × 0.1 × 0.5 × 10⁻⁹ × (900 × 660 + 0.397 × 10⁶ + 900 × 1790 + 9.492 × 10⁶)

where the underlined groups correspond to the first through fourth terms in the square brackets in Equation 1, and E_t = 111 mj.

Since only 30% of the incident energy is absorbed, the total energy required is equal to 111 mJ/0.3 = 370 mJ.

Example 2

Consider a pulsed laser being used for cutting a material. Estimate the cut velocity for a given laser power, pulse frequency, material thickness, and kerf width. The basic assumption is that cutting occurs only at melting and a gas jet provides forced convection to remove the liquid metal. Following the lumped parameter energy balance principle, we can write:

$$t[AP] = \rho \bar{V} [C_p(T_m - T_{amb}) + L_m] \quad (54)$$

The interaction time can be expressed as;

$$t = \frac{\rho \bar{V}}{AP} [C_p(T_m - T_{amb}) + L_m] \quad (55)$$

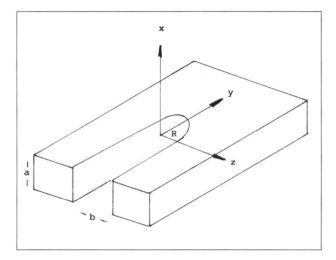

Figure 19. Schematic of cutting process.

The time required for a point source to move a distance R is equal to

$$t = \frac{R}{V_{cut}}$$

and the mass of the material removed is equal to $abR\rho$, where a is the material thickness and b is the kerf width (Fig. 19). Substitution and rearrangement gives

$$V_{cut} = \frac{AP_p P_l P_f}{ab\rho [C_p(T_m - T_{amb}) + L_m]} \quad (56)$$

Using a laser beam with an average power of 800 W and mild steel with $k = 24$ W/m K, $C_p = 400$ J/kg K, $\rho = 7190$ kg/m³, $T_m = 1800$ K, $L_m = 0.272 \times 10^6$ J/kg, $A = 0.18$, $b = 2$ mm, and $a = 3$ mm, V_{cut} is estimated to be around 15 mm/s.

Example 3

For a cladding operation, powder is fed to the laser-target interaction zone. Usually, the cladding powder melts almost instantaneously, as soon as it is exposed to the laser beam. It is assumed that the material reaches a uniform temperature T. Using the lumped parameter energy balance, we can calculate the energy required to melt the cladding powder and raise its temperature to T, which is

$$T = T_{amb} + \frac{1}{C_p}\left[\frac{2PA}{\pi r^2 \rho U_s} - L_m\right] \quad (57)$$

where r, is the radius of the semicylindrical strip of cladding material (see Fig. 20). For a clad layer using a 2 kW laser beam ($r = 1$ mm, $Cp = 400$ J/kg K, $U_s = 9.0$ mm/s, $\rho = 7190$ kg/m³, $A = 0.05$, $L_m = 0.272 \times 10^6$ J/kg), $T = 1783°C$.

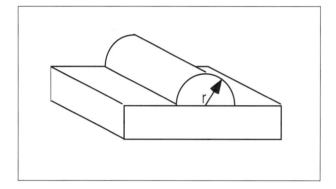

Figure 20. Single clad bead.

Example 4

Consider a uniform distribution of the laser power across the laser beam and one-dimensional heat flow into the workpiece. Our aim is to calculate the maximum local temperature reached during the laser-workpiece interaction, that is, $t = d/U_s$. We will use the following parameters; $P = 1$ kW, $k = 24$ W/m K, $\alpha = 8 \times 10^{-6}$ m²/s, $C_p = 400$ J/kg K, $\rho = 7190$ kg/m³, $A = 0.18$, $d = 2$ mm, and $U_s = 40$ mm/s. Our governing equation and boundary conditions can be expressed as:

$$\rho C_p \frac{\partial T}{\partial t} = k\frac{\partial^2 T}{\partial z^2}; \quad k\frac{\partial T}{\partial z}(z=0) = AP/S; \quad T(z=\infty) = T_0 \quad (58)$$

where S is the area irradiated, d is beam diameter, P is laser power, and U_s is scanning speed. Following Equation 8, the highest temperature profile across the substrate is given by

$$T(z, t=d/U_s) = \frac{8AP}{\pi k d^2}\sqrt{\alpha d/U_s} \times exp\left(-\frac{z}{2\sqrt{\alpha d/U_s}}\right) \quad (59)$$

The maximum temperature at the surface is

$$T_{z=0} = \frac{8PA\sqrt{\alpha d/U_s}}{\pi k d^2} \approx 3020 K \quad (60)$$

Similarly, we can calculate the cooling rate as

$$\frac{dT}{dt} = \frac{4PA\sqrt{\alpha}}{\pi k d^2 \sqrt{d/U_s}} \left[1 - \frac{z}{2\sqrt{\alpha d/U_s}}\right] \times exp\left(-\frac{z}{2\sqrt{\alpha d/U_s}}\right) \quad (61)$$

The cooling rate at the surface, $z=0$, is

$$\frac{dT}{dt}(z=0) = \frac{4PA\sqrt{\alpha}}{\pi k d^2 \sqrt{d/U_s}} \approx 3.02 \times 10^4 \, K/s \quad (62)$$

We also can calculate the maximum depth of the molten zone, without vaporizing the surface material, that is, the maximum depth is attained when the surface reaches evaporation point. Thus

$$z_{max} = 2\sqrt{(\alpha d/U_s) ln(T_v/T_m)} \approx 0.92 \, mm \quad (63)$$

References
The reference numbers are the same as the numbers of the sources in Table 3.

P. S. MOHANTY
J. MAZUMDER

5.6 Phase Changes

Absorption of laser radiation by a solid body results in an increase of the surface temperature and near-surface volume. The temperature field can be described by the standard heat conduction equation (Eq. 1). If the absorbed intensity of the laser beam is high enough, the surface temperature can exceed the melting temperature T_m (Table 1), then melting of the surface occurs. The boundary between solid and the liquid phases, or the melt front, propagates into the bulk of the material. The simplest estimation for propagation of the melting front and increasing mass of the liquid phase can be obtained assuming that the latent heat of melting, L_m (Table 1) (2), is negligible and the location of the front is at the isotherm surface corresponding to $T = T_m$. This approximation is justified in cases when the latent heat of melting, L_m, is significantly smaller than the specific enthalpy of material at the melting point, cT_m, where c is the specific heat.

A more accurate simulation of the melt boundary propagation, known as the "problem of Stefan," is obtained when the heat conduction equation is supplemented with the following boundary condition at the moving front separating solid and liquid phases:

$$k_s \frac{\partial T_s}{\partial n} - k_l \frac{\partial T_l}{\partial n} = V_m \rho L_m \quad (1)$$

where $\partial/\partial n$ is the gradient of the temperature along the normal to the melting front, s and l subscripts correspond to solid and liquid phases, V_m is the velocity of the melting front, k is the thermal conductivity, ρ is the material density, and L_m is the latent heat of melting. This approach disregards phase transition kinetics and does not allow any finite superheating since the latter results in a nonphysical infinite velocity of the melt front propagation. Obviously, the basic assumptions of this approach, that the melting front dynamics are determined by the energy flux only and the melting instantly occurs as soon as the melting temperature T_m is reached, are valid only for slow propagation of the melting front. If the front velocity is high, then melting kinetics must be considered (3). Assuming low superheating, the melt front velocity is proportional to the difference of the chemical potentials of solid and liquid phases, and the expression for front velocity becomes:

$$V_m = V_s \left[\frac{c(T - T_m)}{L_m} + \frac{cT_m \sigma}{\rho L_m^2}(1/R_1 + 1/R_2)\right] \quad (2)$$

where σ is the surface tension at solid-liquid interface, R_1 and R_2 are principal radii of curvature of the melting front, and V_s is an empirical constant close to the speed of sound. Within this approach, which takes into account the melting kinetics, the temperature on the front, T, is no longer assumed to be equal to the melting point, T_m, and the front velocity is proportional to the superheating. The equations above can be used to estimate the depth of penetration of melting in a laser-irradiated sample.

Unlike melting, evaporation occurs at any temperature exceeding 0 K; therefore, laser-induced melting is always accompanied by evaporation. The range of surface temperatures when the evaporation becomes substantial depends on the saturated vapor pressure at the melting point. The evaporation rate is strongly dependent on the temperature (4); thus the thermal field evolution, determined by the thermophysical properties of material and the absorbed laser intensity, is a very significant factor. One can estimate the temperature dependence of the evaporation rate, keeping in mind that the dependence is $\sim exp(-1/T)$ and using the values of melting temperature, saturated vapor pressure at the melting point, and boiling temperature at which the saturated vapor pressure is 1 atm by definition.

Typically laser welding is performed on parts containing metal components with relatively high saturated vapor pressure at their melting points (2), for example, 1 Pa for Fe and Si, 10 Pa for Zn and Mn, 100 Pa for Mg. These materials evaporate readily at the melting point, and their evaporation rate increases as the temperature exceeds the melting point. The thermophysical parameters of those materials and their absorptivities are such that high surface temperature values can be easily achieved.

If a material has low saturated vapor pressure at its melting point, such as Ga, 10^{-35} Pa; In and Sn, 10^{-20} Pa; Al, 10^{-6} Pa; and Cu, 10^{-2} Pa, then substantial superheating must be achieved to produce a relatively high evaporation rate. For example, the absorptivity and thermophysical properties of aluminum are such that, for typical processing conditions, the required overheating

Table 1. Properties of the Elements

Element	M atomic mass	T_m melting temperature (K)	T_v vaporization temperature (K)	L_m latent heat of melting (kJ/mol)	L_v latent heat of vaporization (kJ/mol)
Mg	24.3	923	1380	8.8	128
Al	26.98	933	2333	10.46	291
Si	28.08	1687	2608	50.6	383
Ti	47.9	1998	3533	14.6	426
Cr	51.99	2178	2473	20.9	342
Mn	54.94	1517	2368	14.6	220
Fe	55.84	1808	3003	13.77	340
Ni	58.7	1728	3448	17.15	375
Cu	63.54	1356	2903	13	307
Zn	65.38	692	1203	7.28	114
Ga	69.72	302	2573	5.59	270
Ge	72.5	1231	2973	36.8	328
Mo	95.94	2895	5073	35.6	590
W	183.8	3655	5828	35.1	824
Pb	207.2	575	1730	4.81	178

and, consequently, deep penetration (keyhole) welding can be achieved with moderate laser intensities insufficient to produce highly absorbing plasma.

In contrast, the high reflectivity and thermal conductivity of copper, along with its low of saturation vapor pressure at the melting point, create conditions that require a relatively high beam intensity to be delivered to the surface in order to reach the surface temperature corresponding to a substantial evaporation rate. However, higher laser beam intensities result in the ignition of the near-surface plasma with higher electron concentration and, consequently, higher absorptivity (especially for the CO_2 laser), which can create an impenetrable obstacle preventing the laser beam from producing a keyhole weld in copper.

Since there is no fixed temperature for liquid–vapor transition, the propagation of the evaporation front can not be described, even with a very rough approximation, in terms of the "problem of Stefan." The velocity of the evaporation front propagation can be written as a function of the surface temperature T_s in the form (5):

$$V_v = V_0 \exp(-U/T_s) \qquad (3)$$

where V_v is the evaporation front velocity, $U = ML_v/k_B$, L_v is the latent heat of evaporation, M is the atomic mass, k_B is Boltzmann's constant, and V_0 is a constant with a value close to the speed of sound. Volumetric boiling (vapor bubble formation) does not occur under typical laser interaction conditions (6). Therefore, the evaporating surface is either constant or grows slowly because of keyhole or crater formation. The surface temperature T_s is not limited by the boiling temperature, but instead assumes a value either lower or higher than the boiling temperature depending on the value of the absorbed laser intensity.

References
1. J. F. Ready, *Effect of High-Power Laser Radiation*, Academic Press, New York, 1971.
2. T. Iida, and R. I. L. Guthrie, *The Physical Properties of Liquid Metals*, Clarendon Press, Oxford, 1988.
3. V. I. Motorin, and S. L. Musher, Stability of liquefaction front in fast Joule heating, *Sov. Phys. - Tech. Phys.* **27**, 726 (1982).
4. J. Frenkel, *Kinetic Theory of Liquids,* Dover Publishing, NY, 1955.
5. S. I. Anisimov, Ya. A. Imas, G. S. Romanov, and Yu. V. Khodyko, *Action of High-Power Radiation on Metals*, National Technical Information Service, Springfield, VA, 1971.
6. Yu. V. Afanasiev, and O. N. Krokhin *Sov. Phys. JETP* **25**, 639 (1967).

VLADIMIR V. SEMAK

5.7 Plasma Shielding

5.7.0 Introduction

Plasma shielding generally refers to the fact that once the laser beam breaks down the atmosphere, the light is absorbed in the ensuing plasma, and does not reach the workpiece or other intended target of the beam. Instead, the light is absorbed in the plasma, generally by a process of inverse bremsstrahlung. This absorption of the laser energy into the plasma not only shields the workpiece from the laser beam, but also produces effects in the plasma that have been intensively studied over the past four decades. As pointed out by Radziemski and Cremers (1), plasmas induced by lasers breaking down the atmosphere were demonstrated very soon after the advent of pulsed lasers.

The details of the plasma behavior are determined by the geometry and time dependence of the laser beam, the specific atmosphere (clean air, dirty air, shielding gas, vaporized workpiece material, etc.), and the irradiance (power density) of the laser beam in the region of the plasma. Depending on these conditions, the plasma can simply be sustained in place as long as the laser light is not interrupted, or it can travel back toward the laser.

5.7.1 Atmospheric Breakdown

Laser-Induced Breakdown

Bringing a laser beam to a tight focus in matter (solid, liquid, or gas), if the beam has sufficient power, causes the breakdown of the medium and the evolution of a highly ionized plasma. The initiation of this process, especially in air, has been studied in great detail; a good review of fairly recent work is given by Weyl (2). The breakdown threshold is a strong function of the purity of the medium. The irradiance to break down clean air with CO_2 laser irradiation is between 10^9 and 10^{10} W/cm^2, whereas aerosol-laden air with mean particle size of 30 μm breaks down at irradiances as low as 10^6 W/cm^2.

At a metal surface, the initiation of laser breakdown at the surface is influenced by surface characteristics as well as by the metal itself. Typically plasma initiation at the surface requires irradiances, at 10.6 μm, of the order of 10^6 to 10^7 W/cm^2. One mechanism that has been studied is the initiation of a plasma by a surface flake on aluminum, with the presumption that the more-or-less thermally isolated flake rapidly begins to vaporize when the irradiation commences, and that thermally generated electrons in this vapor initiate the absorption of the laser light and the ensuing cascade of electron absorption via inverse bremsstrahlung.

Laser-Sustained Plasmas

At or near the focus of a CW laser beam, it is possible to continuously maintain a plasma in air or other gaseous media. This laser-sustained plasma, or LSP, is sometimes referred to as a continuous optical discharge. As in all types of laser-supported plasma, the laser energy is absorbed in the plasma, which could result in shielding of the workpiece from the laser irradiation.

These plasmas require initiation, however, as the irradiance, even at focus, of CW CO_2 lasers is insufficient to initiate air breakdown. At 5 kW or higher, plasmas can be initiated at focus by an arc, a pulsed laser plasma breakdown, or by a metallic surface in the focal volume (3). LSP experimental studies have been done primarily at 10.6 μm. Since absorption varies as roughly the square of the laser wavelength, sustaining plasmas with shorter wavelengths requires a great deal more power. Few if any experiments have been conducted at wavelengths below 10.6 μm.

It should be noted that the temperature in LSPs is higher than that in dc arcs or inductively coupled plasmas, giving the LSP a potential for applications where a small, well-controlled continuous plasma is of value.

5.7.2 Laser-Supported Absorption Waves

Laser-supported absorption waves are kindled at the surfaces of absorbing materials. The salient features of a laser-induced absorption wave propagating away from the surface of a material are shown in Figure 1.

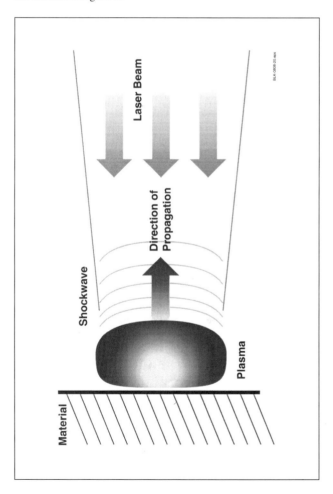

Figure 1. Schematic illustration of the principal features of a laser-supported absorption wave in ambient air.

The hot, high-pressure plasma strongly absorbs the laser energy as it expands, forming a propagating absorption wave. This laser absorption wave (LAW) propagates back along the laser beam toward the laser as long as the beam has sufficient irradiance to sustain the process. The expansion front at higher irradiances propagates at shock velocities as a detonation wave, whereas at lower irradiances it propagates at subsonic velocities and is called a combustion wave. At extremely high irradiances the wave travels as an overdriven shock, and is described as a laser-supported radiation (LSR) wave. Table 1 shows the salient features of laser-supported combustion (LSC) waves, laser-supported detonation (LSD) waves, and LSR waves. In this table typical values of parameters for laser-supported combustion waves, laser-supported detonation waves, and laser-supported radiation waves propagating into ordinary air at laser wavelengths of 1 to 10 μm. Root (4) gives a detailed discussion of the physics of these waves.

Table 1. Laser-Supported Absorption Waves

Wave type	Irradiance (MW/cm^2)	Velocity (cm/sec)	Pressure (bars)	Temperature (K)
LSC	1–10	10^5	50	2×10^4
LSD	10–10^3	10^6	10^2	2×10^5
LSR	10^3–10^4	3×10^6	10^3	10^6

Subsonic – Combustion Waves

LSC waves behave much like chemical deflagration waves, and propagate in air when laser irradiances are of the order of 1 to 10 MW/cm^2. In steady state all the laser energy is absorbed in a zone at the front of the expanding plasma. However, the plasma fills the space between the propagating front and the material surface. This condition is maintained until radial expansion away from the edges of the irradiated area relieves the high pressure and temperature conditions within the plasma. The typical time for this is the time for the rarefaction waves to travel from the outer edges of the laser spot to its center. During this time, shielding of the target from effects of the laser beam has not yet begun. In fact, the hot radiating plasma with its broad-band spectrum of radiation extending into the ultraviolet in many cases provides more effective thermal absorption at the material surface than exists at the single infrared wavelength of the laser beam. This enhanced thermal coupling lasts until the rarefaction waves reach the center of the irradiated spot. The velocities of these waves are of the order of 10^5 cm/sec. Thus for irradiated spots of the order of a few centimeters, this enhanced coupling would persist for times of the order of 10 nsec at irradiances in the range of a few MW/cm^2. Thereafter, the waves would continue to propagate toward the laser, shielding the material from the beam.

Supersonic – Detonation and Radiation Waves

At intermediate irradiances, the shock wave indicated in Figure 1 becomes so hot that it directly absorbs laser radiation. In this case the plasma and the shock wave coalesce, moving at the same velocity, in direct analogy to chemical detonation. These shock velocities are greater than the speed of sound, and the fluid dynamics of shock propagation control the evolution of these waves. Radial expansion in the gas behind the LSD wave does not influence its propagation, because the front is traveling at supersonic velocities. The plasma shields the material very early in the pulse, and the plasma temperature in the expansion fans is too low to effectively transmit thermal energy to the material. Thus the LSD wave is very effective in truly shielding the target material. The wave propagates along the laser beam toward the laser until the irradiance becomes too low to support it or the laser pulse is terminated.

In the case of LSR waves, the plasma radiation is so hot that the ambient gas is sufficiently heated to absorb laser radiation prior to the arrival of the shock wave. These supersonic waves' propagation mechanism is one of plasma radiative transport. The LSR wave converts the absorbed energy into the heating of large amounts of gas, and thus very effectively shields the material from the laser beam. As with the LSD wave, the LSR wave propagates back along the beam until the irradiance becomes too low to support it or the laser pulse is terminated.

5.7.3 Consequences of Plasma Shielding

The presence of plasmas created by the laser beam has significant consequences for the application of lasers. The plasma at lower irradiances can result in higher thermal coupling to a workpiece than would result from optical absorption at the laser wavelength, whereas at higher irradiances the plasma prevents thermal coupling to the material. The pressures in the plasma can produce a mechanical effect on the workpiece, particularly at higher irradiance. In general, the propagation of the absorption waves up the beam carries the laser energy away from the intended point of application, and reduces the desired effect of the beam on the workpiece.

The laser-supported absorption waves are readily controlled. The converging at focus of a strongly focused beam provides a region where the irradiance is appropriate to support a plasma only in a narrow region. The wave is confined to this region, and the optics can be arranged to keep the plasma in a desired location at or near a workpiece. This is essentially what happens in keyhole laser welding.

In many cases, the convergence of the beam alone is not sufficient to confine the plasma to a narrow region, and the plasma tends to travel up the beam as a laser-supported absorption wave. Gas flow across the surface of the workpiece is typically used to prevent the wave from propagating, and the plasma is confined. The gas flow must be at high velocity, high enough to pass across the diameter of the laser-irradiated spot in a time shorter than the time for the wave to propagate far enough from the surface to reduce the coupling.

Part of the reason for the advantage of laser welding as compared to other technologies lies in the fact that the laser-supported plasma is hotter than plasmas found in conventional welding.

The LSD and LSR waves produce shock waves in the material over which they form. In some cases this is a useful effect, as in the shock processing of the surfaces of materials. Shock-hardenable materials have been hardened by the laser-supported absorption waves produced above their surfaces. In fact, a transparent material is often used on the surface of a material being laser shock processed to confine the plasma and enhance the effect.

Finally, LAWs cannot, by definition, take place in a vacuum. They require a material medium in which to propagate. Thus laser processing in vacuum is essentially free of the effects of these waves. However, at very high irradiance, the vaporization of material from the surface provides a medium for the plasma, and the physics of the interaction of the laser energy with this plasma determines the material removal rate and the transfer of thermal and mechanical energy to the target. This is particularly important in the case of the very short, high-power laser pulses provided by the recently emerging femtosecond lasers of petawatt power levels (5) (see Section 2.5.9).

References
1. L. J. Radziemski and D. A. Cremers (Eds.), 1989: Laser-Induced Plasmas and Applications, Marcel Dekker, Inc., New York, NY.
2. G. M. Weyl, Physics of Laser-Induced Breakdown: An Update, Ref. 1, Chapter 1.
3. D. R. Keefer, Laser Sustained Plasmas, Ref. 1, Chapter 4.
4. R. G. Root, Modeling of Post-Breakdown Phenomena, Ref. 1, Chapter 2.
5. B. C. Stuart, M. D. Feit, S. Herman, A. M. Rubenchik, B. W. Shore, and M. D. Perry, *Phys. Rev. B* **53,** 1749–61 (1996).

J. THOMAS SCHRIEMPF

5.8 Regimes of Irradiance and Interaction Time

Various materials processing applications are carried out in different regimes of irradiance and duration of the interaction of the laser light. Figure 1 illustrates typical parameters for some physical phenomena and applications. The figure is representative mainly of metallic samples. The ordinate represents the pulse duration for a pulsed laser or the time that the beam dwells on a spot for a continuous laser. The figure is similar to Figure 1 of Section 5.5, but shows different aspects of the physical processes.

Below the line marked "no melting" the surface is not heated to the melting point. In this region, one may have heat treating applications. Above that line surface melting begins. In the region marked "welding" one obtains a reasonable depth of molten material, and welding applications are possible. To the left of the welding region, the penetration of the fusion front is small because of the short interaction time. To the right of the welding region, the heat spreads over a broad area, and the desirable feature of localized heating is lost. Thus welding operations usually require careful control to remain within this process window.

Below the line marked "no vaporization" the material remains solid or liquid. Above the line marked "surface vaporization" the surface begins to vaporize and welding applications are less desirable. The figure identifies regions useful for cutting, hole drilling, and material removal. For removal of small amounts of material, such as vaporization of thin films, the interaction times are very short.

Above the line marked "plasma production" laser-supported absorption waves develop. The only potential industrial application identified in this region has been shock hardening.

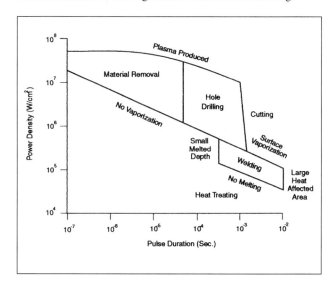

Figure 1. Regimes of laser irradiance and interaction time for materials processing applications.

The regions identified in Figure 1 are not exact, but will vary with target material, laser wavelength, etc. Still they define regions of laser parameters where certain applications are most likely to be productive. The engineer desiring to apply a laser in a specific materials processing application must identify the process parameters suitable for that particular application.

JOHN F. READY

Chapter 6

Hazards and Safety Considerations

6.0 Introduction

Matters of safety involve issues of some subtlety. It is not possible to do justice to the subject within the context of this handbook. At most, this chapter can make you aware of the most common hazards and indicate what is involved in minimizing their risks. This chapter should not be regarded as a safety manual.

Key references to safety standards are included in the text and in Section 6.5. Every laser facility should have copies of the regulations and guidelines available, and administrative controls should be basic to the operation of the facility.

Providing information on laser safety is a primary mission of the Laser Institute of America. LIA provides a number of publications and short courses on this subject. The list of publications include the following concise guides: *LIA Guide for the Selection of Laser Eye Protection* and *LIA Guide to Non-Beam Hazards*. Refer to Section 6.5 for addresses to obtain the referenced material. Abbreviations in this section are either defined at the point of introduction or in Section 6.5.1, *Terms and Abbreviations*.

6.1 Health Hazards and Personnel Safety

Potential optical radiation health hazards include serious eye and skin damage for direct exposure to the beam, laser reflections, secondary emissions from workpiece incandescence, and plasma. All these can exceed personnel viewing exposure standards. Most industrial lasers are far infrared (IR) carbon dioxide lasers and near-infrared (NIR) neodymium-YAG lasers. The IR lasers pose hazards to the cornea of the eye and skin, whereas the NIR lasers pose a potential retinal burn and thermal skin burn hazard. Secondary emissions viewed through properly filtered view ports (1) do not pose a potential for retinal injury within the normal blink response time for the eye. Potentially hazardous actinic ultraviolet emissions are absorbed by the view-port window. Figure 1 illustrates the interaction of radiation of various types with the eye.

6.1.1 Specific Biological Effects
There are at least five separate types of hazards to the eye and skin from lasers and other optical sources, and skin and eye protection must be selected with an understanding of each (2):

1. Ultraviolet photochemical injury to the skin (erythema and carcinogenic effects) and to the cornea (photokeratitis; from 180 to 400 nm) and lens (cataract; about 295 to 325 or even 380 nm). Ultraviolet emissions from laser-induced plasmas require eye protection (3, 4). Whenever a bluish-white light is seen at the laser focal zone, expect UV to be present (Fig. 1, lower left).

2. Thermal injury to the retina (400 to 1400 nm). Normally this type of injury is associated with lasers or from a very intense xenon arc source. The retina is focally photocoagulated at the site of the image. Because a collimated laser beam can normally create a diffraction-limited image on the retina, the optical increase in irradiance from the cornea to the retina is of the order of 100,000! Nd:YAG lasers pose the greatest risk from current material processing lasers (see Fig. 1, lower right).

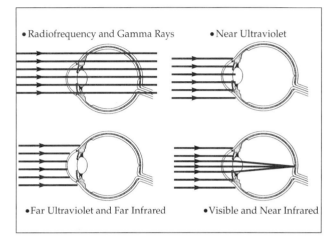

Figure 1. Ocular injury depends upon wavelength.

3. Blue-light photochemical injury to the retina (principally 400 to 550 nm blue light; unless aphakic, 310 to 550 nm); "blue light" photoretinitis, e.g., *solar retinitis*. (Note: Solar retinitis was once referred to as "eclipse blindness" and was associated with "retinal burn." Only in recent years has it become clear that photoretinitis results from a photochemical injury mechanism from retinal exposure to shorter wavelengths in the visible spectrum, i.e., violet and blue light). This hazard can arise from laser-induced plasmas and requires eye protection. Whenever a bluish-white light is seen at the laser focal zone, a blue-light hazard may exist, and wearing conventional approved welding goggles will control this hazard.

4. Near-infrared thermal hazards to the lens (approximately 800 to 3000 nm) with potential for industrial heat cataract. This exposure can come from any molten metal or large, heated surface during treatment. The average corneal exposure from infrared radiation in sunlight is of the order of 1 mW/cm^2 (5). Glass and steel workers exposed to infrared irradiances of the order of 80–400 mW/cm^2 daily for 10–15 years have developed lenticular opacities. These spectral bands include IR-A (700–1400 nm) and IR-B (1.4–3.0 μm). The ACGIH guideline for IR-A exposure of the anterior of the eye is a time-weighted

total irradiance of 10 mW/cm² for exposure durations exceeding 1000 s (16.7 min) (6). Note that this hazard is really only of concern for repeated, chronic exposure day after day.

5. Thermal injury of skin and the cornea and conjunctiva of the eye (limited to approximately 1400 nm to 1 mm for the eye). This type of injury is almost exclusively limited to laser radiation exposure (7). This is the biggest concern driving CO_2 (Fig. 1, lower left) laser safety measures.

The Importance of Wavelength and Time of Exposure
It is important to remember that the thermal injuries (items 2, 4, and 5) can result from very short exposure times, and protection against acute injuries is critical. However, photochemical injuries (items 1 and 3) can result from low dose rates spread over an entire work day. The product of the dose rate and the exposure duration yields a cumulative dose that may be hazardous.

As with any photochemical injury mechanism, one must consider the action spectrum. Safety action spectra are given by the American Conference of Government Industrial Hygienists (6). This describes the relative effectiveness of different wavelengths in causing a photobiological effect. For example, the action spectrum for photochemical retinal injury peaks at approximately 440 nm. Most photochemical effects are limited to a very narrow range of wavelengths, whereas a thermal effect can occur at any wavelength in the spectrum. Hence, eye protection for these specific effects need block only a relatively narrow spectral band to be effective. In contrast, more than one spectral band must be filtered in eye protection for nonlaser sources. Representative laser maximum permissible exposure (MPE) limits are provided in Table 1.

Table 1. Representative Ocular Exposure Limits for Typical Lasers

Type of laser	Principal wavelength(s)	Exposure limit
Argon-fluoride	193 nm	3.0 mJ/cm² over 8 h
Xenon-chloride	308 nm	40 mJ/cm² over 8 h
Argon ion	488 nm, 514.5 nm	3.2 mW/cm² for 0.1 s
Copper vapor	510 nm, 578 nm	2.5 mW/cm² for 0.25 s
Helium-neon	632.8 nm	1.8 mW/cm² for 1.0 s
Krypton ion	568 nm, 647 nm	1.8 mW/cm² for 1.0 s
Nd:YAG	1064 nm 1334 nm	5.0 µJ/cm² for 1 ns to 50 µs No MPE for $t < 1$ ns 5 mW/cm² for 10 s.
Carbon dioxide	10.6 µm	100 mW/cm² for 10 s
Carbon monoxide	~ 5 µm	to 8 h, limited area 10 mW/cm² for >10 s for most of body

All standards/guidelines have MPEs at other wavelengths and exposure durations (1, 6, and 8).

Note: to convert MPEs in mW/cm² to mJ/cm², multiply by the exposure time t in seconds; e.g., the argon MPE at 0.1 s is 0.32 mJ/cm².

Laser Safety Standards
Many nations have published laser safety standards, and most are in accord with the international standard of the International Electrotechnical Commission (IEC). IEC Standard 60825-1.1 (9) applies to manufacturers; however, it also provides limited safety guidance for users. In the United States, the Federal Laser Performance Standard applies (10). The laser hazard classifications described must be labeled on all commercial laser products. A warning label appropriate to the class should appear on all products of Classes 2 through 4. These classes are defined in the following. Figure 2 illustrates typical labels.

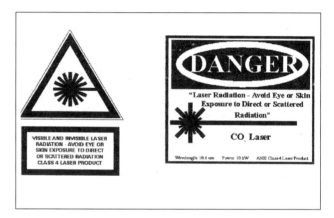

Figure 2. Laser warning labels.

6.1.2 Hazard Classification: Classes of Lasers

The hazard classification system places lasers into four broad categories depending upon their hazard severity potential. Specific details as to how to classify a laser are contained in ANSI Z136.1 (1); these details are beyond the scope of this chapter. Normally a laser system user does not need to determine the laser hazard classification as it is provided by the laser manufacturer. The basic classification system is as follows:

Class 1 lasers are those lasers that do not pose a potential for injury to either the eye or skin. No safety measures are required for Class 1 lasers. A Class 1 laser could also be a higher-class laser that is completely enclosed to prevent personnel exposure to the laser beam.

Class 2 lasers are low-power lasers that produce visible beams that are not considered to pose a significant potential for injury even if the entire beam power entered the eye. Class 2 lasers usually illicit a natural aversion response (or blink response) to the bright laser light. This natural response typically limits the eye's exposure duration to a maximum of about 0.25 s, which is a safe viewing time for a Class 2 laser. Two Class 2 subcategories exist: Class 2 for alignment lasers, which are less than 1 mW, and Class 2a for point-of-sale lasers, where safe levels are not exceeded for 1000 s of viewing.

Class 3 lasers are medium-power lasers that pose a modest potential for injury and the normal aversion response is not sufficiently fast to limit an eye exposure to a safe level. Skin hazards normally do not exist for incidental exposures. Class 3 laser users may be required to follow specific safety precautions and may require the wearing of safety equipment such as laser protective eye wear. Two Class 3 subcategories exist: Class 3a, which is relatively safe with few precautions, and Class 3b, which require further safety considerations.

Class 4 lasers are high-power lasers that pose a serious potential for injury of the eye and skin and require that users follow specific safety precautions and wear laser protective eye wear. Because Class 4 lasers are a significant skin hazard, diffuse-reflection viewing hazard, and a fire hazard, beam termination at the target is usually necessary. Ordinarily personnel are not permitted to make contact with the direct beam, and additional precautions (as given in ANSI Z49.1, 1988) (4) may be necessary to protect personnel skin. Virtually all material processing laser systems for cutting, heat treating, and welding are Class 4 if not enclosed.

6.1.3 Safety Measures

The laser safety classification system greatly facilitates the determination of appropriate safety measures. Laser safety standards and codes of practice routinely require the use of increasingly more restrictive control measures for each higher classification.

In practice, it is always desirable to totally enclose the laser and beam path so that no potentially hazardous laser radiation is accessible. In other words, if only Class 1 laser products are employed in the workplace, safe use without the protective measures may be assumed. In all other cases, worker training in safe use and hazard control measures are required.

Other than the obvious rule not to let a laser beam enter a person's eye, there are no control measures required for a Class 2 laser product. For lasers of higher classes, safety measures are clearly required.

If total enclosure of a Class 3 or 4 laser is not feasible, the use of beam enclosures (e.g., tubes), baffles, and optical covers can virtually eliminate the risk of hazardous ocular exposure in most cases.

When enclosures are not feasible for Class 3 and 4 lasers, a laser controlled area with controlled entry should be established, and the use of laser eye protectors is generally mandated within the nominal hazard zone (NHZ) of the laser beam. Although in most research laboratories where collimated laser beams are used the NHZ encompasses the entire controlled laboratory area, for focused beam applications as is typical in laser material processing, the NHZ may be surprisingly limited and not encompass the entire room. Remember that almost all laser material processing operations—other than microdrilling and microwelding—require radiant powers of Class 4 (whether the beam is totally enclosed and the system becomes Class 1, or the beam is open). Any laser emitting an accessible average power greater than 0.5 W is Class 4.

To ensure against misuse and possible dangerous actions on the part of unauthorized laser users, the key control found on all commercially manufactured laser products, should be secured when the laser is not in use. A laser access protocol should be established, taught, and posted (1).

Special precautions are required during laser alignment, since many serious eye injuries have occurred during alignment and initial setup. Laser workers must be trained in safe practices prior to laser setup and alignment.

Laser Safety Officer

A complete description of Laser Safety Officer (LSO) or Radiation Protection Officer (RPO) duties is beyond the scope of this chapter. However, a brief overview of LSO (RPO implied) duties is provided in the following. Detailed guidance for the LSO are contained in ANSI Z136.1 (1) and other laser safety documents.

For each organization using potentially harmful laser systems, management should assign an individual to serve as LSO to be responsible for their safe use. The LSO requires this authority from management to ensure users maintain safe practices with their equipment. Management may employ an LSO to oversee this responsibility while relying on technical input from an outside expert. The LSO generally receives special safety training and has access to laser safety guidance documents, equipment, and support staff commensurate with the extent of his or her responsibilities.

The LSO determines potentially hazardous areas, degree of hazard, necessary administrative and engineering controls, and necessary safety instructions, and determines appropriate personnel protective equipment such as optical density (OD) for laser protective eyewear. The LSO also maintains an inventory of lasers with detailed information such as: manufacturer, model number, quantity, physical location, user organization, laser active medium, laser radiant power or energy, laser radiant wavelength(s), laser application, and laser hazard category. Other useful information (e.g., history and last maintenance date) may be required by an individual LSO.

There are two general methods to control the safe usage of laser equipment that could pose potential hazards to personnel: engineering controls and administrative controls. Engineering controls are normally preferred as they do not require an action from personnel. Examples of engineering controls include total beam enclosure, electrical door interlocks intended to disable the laser upon entry to an area, warning signs at entrance to laser areas with instructions concerning gaining entry to the area, and warning lights to indicate that the laser is in operation. Often different engineering and administrative controls are needed for laser equipment service or maintenance.

Administrative controls require personnel action, and examples are: preparation and periodic review of safety instructions or safety standard operating procedures (SOP), posting of safety SOP near potentially harmful laser systems, and wearing laser safety eyewear when needed. A guide for selecting laser eye protection is given in Table 7 of Section 6.4.4. The safety SOP should clearly explain the potential hazards posed by the laser equipment and provide detailed control measures and methods for reporting accidents or defective equipment. Safety instructions provided by the laser system manufacturer are normally useful but not complete when preparing a safety SOP.

Training

When investigating laser accidents in both laboratory and industrial situations, a common element emerges: lack of adequate training of the laser operator or accident victim. Laser safety training should be both appropriate and sufficient for the laser operations around which each employee will work. Training should be specific to the type of laser and task to which the worker is assigned.

6.2 Safety with Industrial Lasers

The use of high-power lasers for industrial cutting and welding is becoming widespread in the industrial community. Normal industrial safety practices applicable to arc welding and plasma spray are generally adequate for fixed installations. However, because of the nature of lasers, if collimated laser beams are accessible, conventional safety precautions may not be adequate for these devices. If airborne contaminants are produced, as in welding and cutting, local exhaust ventilation normally must be employed. Users may need to identify additional potential hazards and develop appropriate precautions.

Devices of concern include laser welders, laser heat treaters, laser cutters, and laser punch presses.

6.2.1 Industrial Laser Systems

Enclosed Systems

Many industrial laser systems are "enclosed" and consist of three parts: the actual laser component, a light pipe that carries the laser beam, and an interlocked work enclosure where the beam acts upon a workpiece. Each component encloses the beam so that personnel cannot gain ready access to it. Such systems are classified from a hazard standpoint by ANSI Z136.1 as Class 1 or a safe laser. Personnel are not at any significant risk to primary beam exposure from a Class 1 laser system except perhaps during a malfunction, service, or beam alignment. Service or beam alignment procedures require development of a safety SOP. Only trained personnel should perform these procedures.

Some beam alignment considerations are discussed in more detail in Section 6.3.2.

ANSI Class 4 Industrial Laser Systems

Most laser cutters and punch presses are not entirely enclosed. A small gap may exist, such as where sheet metal can be inserted. Such unenclosed laser systems are normally classified technically from a hazard standpoint by ANSI as a Class 4 or high-power laser. ANSI recommends locating Class 4 lasers in a separate room. Experience indicates that potentially harmful laser emissions do not usually escape at the gap in a laser press. Further measurements may be needed to confirm this for a particular installation, but if the gap is small, the likelihood of dangerous emissions at any visible or infrared laser wavelengths is remote.

6.2.2 Workplace Surveillance

Medical Surveillance

Requirements for medical surveillance of laser workers vary from country to country in accordance with local occupational medicine regulations. At one time, when lasers were confined to the research laboratory and little was known about the biological effects of lasers, it was quite typical that each laser worker was periodically given a thorough general ophthalmological examination with fundus (retinal) photography to monitor the status of the eye. However, by the early 1970s, this practice was questioned by ophthalmologists, since the clinical findings were almost always negative, and it became clear that only acute injury, which was subjectively detectable, needed to be examined. This led the WHO task group on lasers to recommend against such involved surveillance programs and emphasized testing of visual function. Since that time, most national occupational health groups have continuously reduced medical examination requirements. Today, complete ophthalmological examinations are universally required only in the event of a laser eye injury or suspected overexposure, and preplacement visual screening only (screening that is similar to that required when obtaining a driver's license) is generally required, as detailed in ANSI Z136 (1). Additional examinations may be required in some countries.

Laser Measurements

Unlike some workplace hazards, there is generally no need to perform measurements for workplace monitoring of hazardous levels of laser radiation. Because of the highly confined beam dimensions of most laser beams, the likelihood of changing beam paths, and the difficulty and expense of laser radiometers, current safety standards emphasize control measures based upon hazard class and not workplace measurement (monitoring). Measurements must be performed by the manufacturer to assure compliance with laser safety standards to assure proper hazard classification. Indeed, one of the original justifications for laser hazard classification related to the great difficulty of performing proper measurements for hazard evaluation. Because of the concerns regarding reflected beams and other optical radiation emissions from laser welding and cutting, we provide in the next section a synopsis of a study of what one would expect to be one

Chapter 6: Hazards and Safety Considerations

Table 1. Representative Airborne Contaminants Associated with Laser Operations

Contaminant	Probable source	OSHA allowable TWA	OSHA ceiling value
Asbestos	Target backstop	0.1 f[a]/cm^3	———
Beryllium	Firebrick target	0.002 mg/m^3	0.01 mg/m^3
Cadmium oxide fume	Metal target	0.1 mg/m^3	0.3 mg/m^3
Carbon monoxide	Laser gas	35 ppm (25 ppm)	200 ppm
Carbon dioxide	Active laser medium	5000 ppm	30,000 ppm[b]
Chromium metal	Metal targets	0.5 mg/m^3	———
Cobalt, metal fume, and dust	Metal targets	0.1 mg/m^3 (0.02 mg/m^3)	———
Copper fume	Metal targets	0.1 mg/m^3 (0.2 mg/m^3)	———
Fluorine	HF chemical laser	0.1 ppm (1 ppm)	(2 ppm)[b]
Hydrogen fluoride	Active medium of laser	3 ppm	6 ppm[b] (2.3 ppm)
Iron oxide fume	Metal targets	10 mg/m^3 (5 mg/m^3)	———
Manganese fume	Metal targets	1 mg/m^3 (0.2 mg/m^3)	3 mg/m$^{3\ b}$
Nickel and insoluble compounds	Metal targets	1 mg/m^3	———
Nitrogen dioxide	GDL[c] discharge	5 ppm (3 ppm)	9 mg/m^3 (5 ppm)[b]
Ozone	Target & Marx generators	0.1 ppm	(0.1 ppm)
Sulfur dioxide	Laser exhaust	2 ppm	5 ppm[b]
Sulfur hexafluoride	Saturable absorber	1000 ppm	———
Uranium (soluble/ insoluble)	Target	0.2 mg/m^3	0.6 mg/m$^{3\ b}$
Vanadium fume	Target	0.05 mg/m^3	———
Zinc oxide fume	Target	5 mg/m^3	10 mg/m$^{3\ b}$

Values in parentheses denote level recommended by ACGIH (12).
[a]Fibers > 5 mm in length.
[b]Short-term exposure limits.
[c]Gas discharge laser.

of the most hazardous of high-power laser material processing systems: a portable laser system with the laser emitting in the retinal hazard region, where MPEs are low.

Control Measures

Industrial laser systems sold in the United States are required to comply with the safety design features of the Federal standard for laser products contained in 21 CFR 1040 (10). While this assumes safety for Class 1 *products*, the *user* must provide safe operation for Class 4 laser systems. Users should periodically inspect all laser system components (mirrors, view-port windows, light pipe, etc.) for signs of laser beam damage and remove a damaged system from service until it is repaired. Scratched or damaged view-port windows should be replaced only with appropriate materials such as polycarbonate shielding. Personnel who are required to view laser welding operations through unfiltered view-port windows may need to wear electric arc welding eye protection, which affords a comfortable viewing brightness of any secondary emissions such as a plasma.

Associated Hazards

Other associated hazards are addressed in draft ANSI B11.21 (11). Some ancillary hazards are high voltage and toxic materials and vapors. Ventilation of toxic materials may be necessary for the work area to control airborne contaminants as prescribed by an industrial hygienist. Also, high-power lasers are often guided with a coaxial low-power visible laser for alignment. Most low-power alignment lasers do not pose a significant health hazard. Tables 1 and 2 provide examples of airborne contaminants and their permissible concentrations in air. These hazards are covered further in Section 6.4.2.

Ultraviolet radiation and intense visible light are also emitted from the target area, especially if an optical plasma is formed. See Section 6.1.1. Shade filters are required to block ultraviolet and blue light. Table 3 (next page) presents results for blue and ultraviolet light emitted for various laser processing conditions.

Consultants

Technical experts are frequently required to evaluate the potential optical radiation health hazards from an industrial laser system. Laser safety consultants can generally be located in most countries.

Table 2. Main Components of Emissions Generated During Laser Cutting of Plastics[a]

Material processed	First priority	Second priority
Polyethylene	Total particulates	1,3-Butadiene; formaldehyde; acrolein; benzene
Polypropylene	Total particulates	Benzene; formaldehyde; benzo(a)pyrene / PAH
Polystyrene	Total particulates; styrene	Benzene
Polystyrene-butadiene	Total particulates; benzo(a)pyrene / PAH; styrene; 1,3-butadiene	Benzene
Polycarbonate	Total particulates	Benzene; benzo(a)pyrene / PAH; carbon oxide
Polymethylmethacrylate	Total particulates; formaldehyde; methylmethacrylate	Acrolein
Polyamide 6	Total particulates; formaldehyde	Acrolein; 1,3-butadiene
Polyvinyl-chloride	Total particulates; benzene; benzo(a)pyrene / PAH; hydrogen chloride	Formaldehyde; 1,3-butadiene; dibenzoodioxins /-furans

[a]Adapted from Ref. 12.

Table 3. UV and Blue-Light Emissions as Measured at a Distance of 50 cm from the Welding Plasma

Base Metal	Laser power (kW)	Weld speed (mm/s)	Thickness (mm)	Shielding gas (l/min)	UV irradiance (W/cm^2)	t_{UV} (s)	Blue irradiance (W/cm^2)	t_{blue} (s)
Al alloy	4	20	5	Ar 20	7.3×10^{-4}	4.1	1.23×10^{-4}	81
	4	20	5	He 20	3.0×10^{-4}	10.0	4.6×10^{-5}	217
	6	30	6	Ar5/He 15	3.6×10^{-4}	8.3	7.5×10^{-5}	133
	8	40	6	Ar10/He 15	5.4×10^{-4}	5.6	7.9×10^{-5}	127
Mild steel	2.5	20	3	Ar 20	2.5×10^{-4}	12.0	5.7×10^{-5}	175
	2.5	20	3	He 20	2.2×10^{-4}	13.6	4.5×10^{-5}	222
	4	20	3	Ar 20	4.1×10^{-4}	7.3	5.0×10^{-5}	200
Stainless steel	2.5	20	3	He 20	1.3×10^{-4}	23.1	2.5×10^{-5}	400
	2.5	20	3	Ar 20	4.2×10^{-4}	7.1	6.9×10^{-5}	145
	4	20	3	Ar 20	10.8×10^{-4}	2.8	3.38×10^{-4}	30
	8	20	3	Ar 20	19.3×10^{-4}	1.6	5.63×10^{-4}	18

Source: Ref. 13.

References, Cited and Uncited (see Section 6.5 for information on obtaining key references):

1. ANSI Z136.1, 1993: American National Standards Institute, *American National Standard for the Safe Use of Lasers* (NY, NY).
2. D. H. Sliney, *Radiation Safety. The Maximum Permissible Exposure Levels: Our Knowledge of the Hazards*, Optics & Laser Tech. **21** (4), 235–40 (1989).
3. ANSI Z87.1, 1997: American National Standards Institute, *American National Standard for Industrial Protective Helmets* (NY, NY).
4. ANSI Z49.1, 1988: American National Standards Institute, *American National Standard for Safety in Welding and Cutting* (NY, NY).
5. D. H. Sliney, and M. L. Wolbarsht, 1980: *Safety with Lasers and Other Optical Sources*, Plenum, New York.
6. ACGIH, 1997: American Conference of Governmental Industrial Hygienists, TLV's, Threshold Limit Values and Biological Exposure Indices for 1997, American Conference of Governmental Industrial Hygienists (Cincinnati, OH).
7. American Conference of Governmental Industrial Hygienists, 1990, A Guide for Control of Laser Hazards (Cincinnati, OH).
8. A. Duchene, J. Lakey, and M. Repacholi, (Eds.), 1991: IRPA Guidelines on protection against non-ionizing radiation, New York: Pergamon Press.
9. IEC, 1998: International Electrotechnical Commission, *Radiation Safety of Laser Products, Equipment Classification, Requirements and User's Guide*, Publ. 60825-1.1, Geneva, Switzerland.

10. CFR 1040 1995, Title 21 CFR 1040, *Performance Standards for Light Emitting Products*, Center for Devices and Radiological Health of the FDA (Rockville, MD).
11. ANSI B11.21, 1995: American National Standards Institute, *Machine Tools Using Lasers for Processing Materials – Safety Requirements for Construction, Care, and Use* (NY, NY).
12. H. Haferkamp, F. von Alvensleben, D. Seebaum, M. Goede, and T. Püster, 1997: *Air Contaminants Generated during Laser Processing of Organic Materials and Protective Measures*, Proceedings of the 1997 International Laser Safety Conference, Laser Institute of America, Orlando, FL, 209–18.
13. K. Schulmeister, Ch. Schmitzer, K. Duftschmid, G. Liedl, K. Schröder, H. Bursl, and N. Winker, 1997: *Hazardous Ultraviolet and Blue-Light Emissions of CO_2 Laser Beam Welding*, Proceedings of the 1997 International Laser Safety Conference, Laser Institute of America, Orlando, FL, 229–32.

M. Hietanen, A. Honkasalo, H. Laitinen, L. Lindross, L. Welling, and P. von Nandelstadh, Evaluation of hazards in CO_2 Laser Welding and Related Processes, *Ann Occupational Hygiene*, **36** (2): 183–88 (1992).

IEC, 1997: International Electrotechnical Commission, *Safety of Laser Products–Part 4: Laser Guides,* Publ. 60825-4, Geneva, Switzerland.

T. L. Lyon, 1993: *Laser measurement techniques guide for hazard evaluation*, J Laser Appl, [in two parts] **5** (1):53–8 and **5** (2):37–42.

TERRY L. LYON
RODNEY L. WOOD
DAVID H. SLINEY

6.3 Specific Systems and Applications

6.3.1 Portable Laser Welders—An Example

Portable high-power laser welders pose special problems, since they are not used in a fixed installation where doorway interlocks or special enclosures are not feasible. Their use in remote areas or in shipyards for cutting and welding offers the user increased capabilities over conventional arc welding/cutting. To evaluate the potential optical hazards associated with the use of one portable, high-power Nd:YAG laser welder, the authors of this chapter performed laser measurements and evaluated the potentially hazardous optical radiation from one device. The Hobart Laser Products Model MM 1800, portable, high-power Nd:YAG laser welding system was designed to be used in naval shipboard locations and port facilities for laser material processing. At the time of our study, a similar but higher-power (2400-W) model was being planned.

The system was classified as a Class 4 laser product according to the American National Standards Institute (1) and met FDA requirements for a Class 4 laser product prior to the addition of the optical fiber. It had a permanently affixed label with the manufacturer information and warning labels. The laser was heavily interlocked and programmed by a remote controller unit. No spontaneous firing was noted. After final control of the laser was passed by the Laser System Safety Officer (LSSO), who controlled the remote controller, the welding specialist could turn the beam power on and off. The buttons were appropriately labeled. The transmission characteristics of the fiber optic delivery system was specified at 95%. There was no optical viewing instrument associated with the system. Therefore, requirements for built-in protection were not applicable. However, the welder stood behind a welding screen with a viewing window with protective filtration at 1064 nm.

The operators of this laser welder used laser protective goggles that had an OD of 8 at 1050–1400 nm, but also had flip-down shade 6 welders' lenses. A variety of flame-resistant curtain materials that could be used as temporary enclosures around the laser operation had been tried, and the welders had demonstrated that Ametek Siltemp asbestos-free curtains were highly effective in resisting burn through. This material was draped over the laser surfacing operation to terminate the specularly reflected laser radiation from the workpiece.

The laser system had been modified to meet system safety requirements and made more rugged to permit movement to remote locations. The system consisted of a large vibration-isolation-pallet-mounted cooling system, a vibration-isolation, pallet-mounted laser, and a 150-m-long fiber-optic delivery system with remote controller at the beam delivery end. The laser was designed for widespread use for metal cutting and welding and for removing toxic materials from contaminated metal surfaces, etc. The manufacturer-specified parameters are as follows:

Wavelength: 1064 nm
Laser output power (maximum): 1800 W
Pulse duration: Continuous wave (CW)
Beam diameter at $f/16$ focus: 0.04 cm
Beam divergence beyond focal point: 63 mrad (worst case)
Nominal ocular hazard distance (NOHD): 100 m intrabeam
Nominal hazard zone (NHZ): Not specified (diffuse reflection)

Safety Measurements

We were not only interested in measuring reflected laser radiation, but also the visible light produced by the laser-induced plasma. To this end, an International Light Model 1700 Research Radiometer with Actinic Ultraviolet Radiation (UVR), Radiometric, and Blue-Light Detector Heads was used along with a Minolta Spot Photometer to measure luminance. An infrared finder-scope and laser radiometer were used to locate and measure the 1064-nm laser radiation reflected from the workpiece.

With the laser in operation at full power, 1.5 kW was actually delivered to a 0.4-mm-diameter target spot. Measurements were taken of reflected laser radiation and secondary optical radiation emitted from the surface of a rotating 3.5-in. diameter, stainless-steel plunger as it was being surfaced with stellite. The following worst-case measured values were obtained at a reference distance of 100 cm:

- Effective ultraviolet radiation (ACGIH spectrally weighted): 0.1 µW/cm^2
- Effective blue-light irradiance (ACGIH spectrally weighted): 3 µW/cm^2
- Semispecular reflection (maximum toward ceiling): 800 mW/cm^2
- Total infrared irradiance from workpiece immediately after laser shutdown: 10 mW/cm^2
- Luminance of broad-band incandescent radiation emitted from target site: 1.4 X 10^5 cd/m^2 (41,000 ft L) averaged over a 15-mrad spot (0.9-degree spot). This corresponded to 26 cd/cm^2 averaged over α_{MIN} = 11 mrad. Since the luminance exceeded 1 cd/cm^2, comfortable viewing required a dark filter transmitting about 1/26 = 4%. This transmittance corresponds to optical density (OD) of 1.4 and a shade number of 4.3.

Permissible Exposure Durations

At the reference distance of 1 m, the reradiation did not exceed ACGIH threshold limit values (TLVs) for 8-h exposures. However, the specular reflections exceeded the ACGIH TLV and ANSI MPE limit, thus demonstrating the need for laser protective eyewear. The ACGIH TLV for UVR is an effective irradiance of 0.1 µW/cm^2 for 8-h exposure; for blue light, it is 1 µW/cm^2 for 2.8-8 h exposure; and for laser radiation at 1064 nm, it is 5 mW/cm^2 for 10 s, and 1.8 mW/cm^2 for exposures of 1000 s to 8 h. The minimal eye protection for the conditions measured was therefore OD 4. Table 3 in the last Section provides representative UV and blue-light emissions from other welding operations.

Nominal Hazard Zone (NHZ)

The semispecular reflected irradiance will vary with surface finish and shape; however, the process examined here is probably quite representative of nearly worst-case conditions. From a simple inverse-square calculation, the semispecular reflection would reach 5 mW/cm^2 at approximately 12 m. The NHZ is actually only 12 m, and eye protection and other safeguards are only required within this limited area. However, if the laser output cannot be directed downward at the material to be welded, and the beam could continue unterminated by the material being processed, the NHZ is much larger than 12 m. If concern exists that the beam could go beyond the controlled area, then the laser barriers should be used to define the NHZ.

These systems have an NHZ within the immediate area of the operation, but can be used safely when workers in the immediate area wear appropriate laser eye protectors with shade 5 or 6 filters to view the incandescence. Warning signs and portable barriers should be placed around the NHZ, which is normally 12 m in all directions around the workpiece. The laser need not be enclosed unless the NHZ extends to areas that cannot be controlled. In addition, all personnel in the vicinity should wear laser eye protection with a minimum optical density (OD) of 4 at 1064 nm if within the NHZ. These goggles must also have capability for shade 5 or 6 welding filters; laser barrier materials, such as those demonstrated, should be used to terminate the direct beam beyond the workpiece if the direct beam could exit the immediate work area.

Reference

1. ANSI Z136.1, 1993: American National Standards Institute, *American National Standard for the Safe Use of Lasers* (NY, NY).

TERRY L. LYON
RODNEY L. WOOD
DAVID H. SLINEY

6.3.2 Beam Alignment Hazards

Beam delivery provides an example of technical safety issues that may reduce or disable one or more machine functions and as a result may also generate hazardous working conditions. Most of these problems are related to the beam delivery system, its components, and their handling.

For instance, modern CO_2 laser systems include an integrated presence switch for the copper mirror in the beam-bending units. It could be a hazard for the operators and/or for the machine should the mirror not be remounted into the corresponding beam-bending unit before switching the laser beam on (after testing the beam quality). A mirror presence switch will prevent such an occurrence if wired within an interlock circuit. It may be advisable to use low-voltage DC or AC for the interlock circuit instead of the commonly used line voltage.

If a mirror has to be removed from its beam-bending unit for a beam analysis purpose, place a beam dump behind the measuring position into a predetermined position (holder). The dump will absorb the beam power in case no measuring device is in place. The beam dump holder should also be equipped with a presence switch. This switch could then bypass the respective mirror presence switch.

A hazardous condition may occur during the alignment of a multimirror CO_2-laser system using the main laser beam. A mirror might direct the beam onto flammable parts of the beam delivery system, causing fire and dangerous fumes and contaminating mirrors. This condition can be prevented by using a "safety ring." This is a device that includes four temperature sensors in an orthogonal arrangement capable of sensing a significant misalignment of the main laser beam within the beam delivery tube. If this device detects an alarm status (determined by preset signal limits), it can generate an emergency stop signal. Some users prefer to switch off the supply voltage of the machine control in case of an emergency stop.

The processing unit of the "safety ring" memorizes the signals that have generated the emergency stop and displays this after power-on in order to show the operator the direction of the beam misalignment.

Other handling problems related to the beam delivery systems are given in Table 1.

Chapter 6: Hazards and Safety Considerations

Table 1. CO_2 Laser Beam Delivery Hazard Prevention Steps

Cause	Influence description	Possible solution
Presence of laser power absorbing vapors from chemical agents	Due to absorption, the available laser power at the workpiece will be reduced despite the good "in range" output power readout of the laser power meter	Do not use the laser system immediately after "Plexiglass burns;" seal the beam delivery system and use fresh purge air absolutely free of dust and oil
Use of an improper air quality as purge gas	Impurities will burn onto the mirror surfaces; oil will absorb the laser beam power and may finally burn onto the mirror surfaces	Seal the beam delivery system and use fresh purge air absolutely free of dust, oil, and water by an adequate filter system; if not available, use air or nitrogen from a gas bottle having known and acceptable properties
Use of noncopper metallic parts (fittings or metallic tubes) for the cooling water circuit together with copper mirrors	This will produce electrochemical corrosion, which might generate water leaks	All metallic parts having contact with the cooling water should be made of the same metal or alloy
Use of nonfiltered cooling water	Particles and other impurities floating within the cooling water may be deposited within the cooling channels of the copper mirrors, which reduces the water flow rate	A proper filter within the cooling water circuit is necessary in order to collect all particles

In the case of Nd:YAG lasers slightly different problems can be observed because most systems use fiber optics for beam delivery. If mirrors are used within the Nd:YAG laser beam delivery system, the problems will remain similar to CO_2 laser systems.

The cooling water circuit of Nd:YAG laser systems is used mainly for the laser cavities. The circuit has to include a proper filter, one much finer than for the CO_2 laser system. It also should include a device for measuring the degree of ionization of the cooling water. If the water ionization exceeds a certain limit (system dependent), reduced or no laser power will be available.

A major source of possible danger is the fiber optic itself. The mechanical handling of the fiber optic is especially critical. Careless handling can partially destroy the fiber core, resulting in an increased power loss within the fiber optic and leading to the total destruction of the fiber optic and its protective tube. Most of the fiber optic suppliers have integrated monitoring devices into the fiber optic that are designed to prevent the risk of total destruction. There are also some monitoring devices available from independent manufacturers that are capable of being integrated into the beam delivery system. A system is schematically illustrated in Figure 1.

Problems might arise from the applications themselves, as noted throughout this chapter. In the laser welding of highly reflective materials such as copper or aluminum, a large amount of the laser power reflected from the workpiece might be coupled back into the fiber optic. This could overload the fiber optic unless the laser power can immediately be automatically reduced.

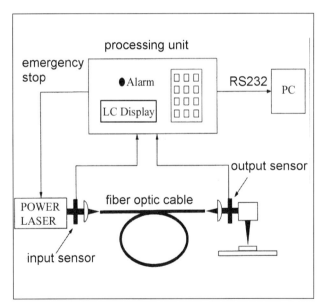

Figure 1. Fiber optic monitoring system.

MARIUS JURCA

6.4 Nonbeam Hazards

6.4.1 Types of Nonbeam Hazards

In addition to the occupational and related production safety concerns that arise from photonics (laser beam) emissions, there are a number of other hazards associated with laser use, that is, nonbeam hazards. Nonbeam hazards constitute the greatest source of noncompliance with United States Federal safety codes. These types of hazards are listed in Table 1. In recent years there has been a steady increase in concerns about these occupational hazards, partly because:

- Such hazards are often difficult to control in the workplace since they require control measures quite diverse and different from those prescribed for lasers or laser systems.
- The laser safety officer (LSO) may have to employ the use of safety and/or industrial hygiene personnel to effect a total laser system hazard evaluation due to the diversity of these hazards.
- Workers can be outside the laser's nominal hazard zone and still be at risk to nonbeam hazards.
- These hazards represent the majority of serious or fatal reported laser accidents.

Table 1. Sources of Nonbeam Hazards

Improper electrical design or use of component, grounding, or shielding
Lack of knowledge for production of laser-generated air contaminants
Unwanted or excessive plasma radiation
Insufficient or inappropriate controls for laser-robotic systems
Excessive noise levels produced by lasers or laser systems
Inadequate or inappropriate ventilation controls for LGAC
Fire hazards
Inadequately controlled waste disposal situations
Inadequately designed, crowded, or inappropriate work space
Improperly handled and labeled compressed gases
Exposure to toxic chemicals and laser dyes
Ergonomic problems arising from repetitive-motion scenarios
Explosion issues from high-pressure tubes
Possibility of electromagnetic/radiofrequency interference issues

As can be seen from Table 1, nonbeam hazards can occur with the use of any laser. However, most are associated with Class 3b and 4 lasers (see Section 6.1.2 for definitions).

6.4.2 Laser-Generated Chemical Hazards

Laser-Generated Air Contaminants

Laser-generated air contaminants (LGAC) may be generated when high-power laser beams interact with matter. While it may be difficult to predict what LGAC may be released in any given interaction situation, target materials such as plastics, composites, metals, and tissues liberate both gaseous and particulate toxic and noxious airborne contaminants. These LGAC may be in the form of aerosols (smokes, fumes, and mists), gases, and vapors. Many LGAC are inhaled into the lower portion of the lungs where the clearance mechanism is least efficient. Unfortunately, information about decomposition byproducts of laser interactions is not normally available, and material safety data sheets may not prove very useful (see Table 1, Section 6.2.1).

In general there are three major control measures available to reduce LGACs; exhaust ventilation, respiratory protection, and process isolation. It is the job of the LSO to ensure that appropriate industrial hygiene characterization of LGAC is effected in accordance with applicable Federal, state, and local requirements.

LGAC from Organic Materials

The cutting, marking, and ablation of organic materials generates aerosols and gases/vapors that, in turn, may partially decompose. Their condensation products may include polycyclic aromatic hydrocarbons that are known to have carcinogenic or toxic properties (see Table 2, Section 6.2.1).

Gaseous byproducts of cutting wood include acrolein and benzene. The former targets the tissues of the lungs, heart, eyes, and skin, while the latter causes leukemia. Exposure criteria are given by OSHA (2) and ACGIH (3).

LGAC from Inorganic Materials

Inorganic materials include metals, glasses, ceramics, and cement. Processing these materials produces airborne fumes containing their respective oxides. In general, inorganics yield dust during processing. Glasses and cement produce aerosol particles. Stainless steel made with chromium and nickel produces contaminants that contain chromium and nickel, both known carcinogens. Control measures applicable to LGAC are shown in Table 2.

Table 2. Control Measures for Laser-Generated Air Contaminants (LGAC)

Irradiance (W cm^{-2})	Potential biological effects	Possible control measures
>10^7	Air contaminants associated with chronic effects	Process isolation Local exhaust ventilation Training and education Limit worker access Robotics/manipulators Housekeeping Preventive maintenance
$10^3 - 10^7$	Air contaminants associated with acute effects; noxious odors; visibility concerns	Local exhaust ventilation Respiratory protection Personal protective equipment Preventive maintenance Training and education
<10^3	Potential for light odors	Adequate building ventilation

Source: ANSI Z136.1-1993 (1).

Chapter 6: Hazards and Safety Considerations

Laser Dyes

Laser dyes are complex fluorescent organic compounds that, in solution with certain solvents, form a lasing medium for dye lasers. Lasers users need to be aware that certain dyes are highly toxic or carcinogenic. Special care must be taken when handling such solutions. Reference to appropriate material safety data sheet (MSDS) is required when working with such compounds.

No toxicity tests have been performed on most laser dyes, but a number are known to be carcinogens or toxic. Prior to mixing, dye powders pose their greatest health risk through inhalation. In solution, the solvents provide a vehicle for transporting dissolved substances through the skin. Ethyl alcohol and ethylene glycol are two of the safest solvents to use with dye lasers.

The Laser Safety Officer (LSO) must consult with an environmental protection professional for guidelines on the proper disposal of dyes and their solvents. The majority of the laser dye solutions can pose fire safety issues.

Laser Dye and Solvent Controls

Standard operating procedures (SOP) must be developed between the LSO and the user. MSDS should be prepared or obtained with information about chemicals, physical properties, hazards, applicable first aid measures, and exposure controls. The SOP should specify protective eyewear and clothing (see Section 6.4.4). Table 3 lists controls for dyes and solvents.

Table 3. Laser Dye and Solvent Controls

Toxic chemicals	Select the least toxic chemicals
Mixing	Use a glove box (not ventilated when weighing and transferring the powder - well ventilated at all other times)
First aid	Emergency eyewashes and showers at hand
Mutagenic dyes	Install enclosed circulation pumps and filters for systems handling. Establish secondary containment beneath reservoirs and pumps in case of leaks. Post work areas where mutagenic dyes are handled

For an effective control system:
- Enclose the source of airborne contaminants.
- Locate the external hood close to laser-target site.
- Place recirculation type systems on a frequent preventive maintenance schedule.

Figure 1 shows the elements of a local exhaust ventilation system.

Compressed Gases

Inert gases such as argon, helium, and nitrogen are often used in material processing as shield gases to inhibit oxidation. However, in some environments there may be gases that can be toxic or corrosive. When handling gases such as chlorine, fluorine, hydrogen chloride, and hydrogen fluoride, standard operating procedures must be developed. In addition, workers need to be aware of hazards associated with the handling and storage of gas containers.

There are the usual hazards associated with gas cylinders (leakage, incorrect labeling, careless handling and improper storage) any of which can lead to flammable and corrosive gas spills, explosion, or asphyxiation (3).

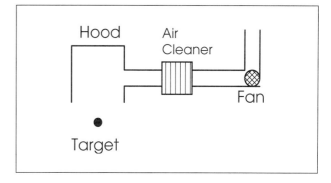

Figure 1. Schematic of a local ventilating system.

For example, the low level of CO in the CO_2 laser equates to 20,000 ppm, well above the danger level of 1200 ppm. Even the inert gases in laser gas mixtures pose an asphyxiation hazard. The inert gases in the CO/CO_2 mixture, nitrogen and helium, when rapidly released pose a threat of asphyxiation (see Table 4).

Compressed Gases Control

Table 4. Compressed Gases Control

Pressure tests	Test all systems at 1.5x maximum allowable pressures.
Leaks	Carry out thorough leak tests.
Gas lines	Test out of service lines with inert gases before reactivating.
Contamination	Install traps or check valves wherever contamination is possible.
Corrosive gases	Tanks of corrosive or reactive gases require a "bonnet" to confine and vent leaking gas to a safe location. Install an orifice to limit the flow rate in case of regulator failure.
Control flow	Downstream valves should be used to control flow.
Cylinder storage	Store in a (vented) gas cabinet.
Toxic gases	Use a toxic gas cabinet (where appropriate); all fittings should be inside the cabinet. Keep gas lines dry by drawing vacuum on them and by cyclically purging with an inert gas.

Standards for gas cabinets and gas delivery systems have been prepared by Semiconductor Equipment and Materials International (SEMI). This information is especially applicable to facilities that use excimer lasers (4, 5).

6.4.3 Physical Hazards

Included in this group are nonbeam radiation hazards and incoherent optical radiation from the target; electrical hazards posed by a laser's energized high voltage components; noise; fire and explosion.

Collateral Radiation

Collateral radiation, that is, radiation other than that associated with the primary laser beam, can be produced by various laser or laser system components. In addition, high-power laser beams, when focused onto a target, can produce a plasma that can also emit collateral radiation. Such radiation may take the form of x-radiation, ultraviolet radiation, visible radiation, infrared radiation, microwave, and radiofrequency radiation (see Table 5).

The U.S. Food and Drug Administration's Federal laser product performance standard (6) refers to collateral radiation as electronic product radiation emitted by any component necessary for the operation of the laser product.

Plasma Radiation

Plasma radiation, also called plume radiation, results from the beam's interaction with matter. Although the visible extent of the plasma is usually millimeters in diameter, it is a source of hazardous UV and blue light radiation (see Table 3, Section 6.2).

Table 5. Possible Health Hazards of Laser Produced Plasma Radiation

Frequency range (nm)	Description	Hazard
180–315	Actinic-ultraviolet	Absorbed by the cornea (photokeratitis & photo-conjunctivitis); erythema (sunburn), skin cancer, accelerated skin aging
315–400	UV-A	Absorbed by the lens (cataracts)
400–780	Visible	Focuses on retina to a spot 10/20 μm in diameter: retinal damage
400–550	Blue light hazard	Long- and short-term exposure, particularly hazardous to retina
700–1000	Near IR	Skin burns, excessively dry skin
780–1400	Near IR	Retinal damage

Nonbeam Radiation Controls

Standard operating procedures must be developed between the LSO and the user. Material safety data sheets should be obtained or prepared with information about materials, radiation sources, hazards, applicable first aid measures, and exposure controls. Other steps include:

- Installing shielding; effectiveness is dependent on shield material and construction for each radiation region.
- Isolating the processing system; locate the processing in a walk-in chamber with interlocks.
- Increasing the distance from the source; distance the work station and control panel from the source.
- Reducing exposure duration; balance the intensity of radiation against time of exposure; increasing the one decreases the other. Post time-averaged exposure guidelines.
- Providing personal protective equipment (PPE) (see Section 6.4.4).

Electric Shock Hazards

Electric shock is a very serious opportunistic hazard, and deaths associated with laser systems have occurred. This type of hazard can occur from contact with exposed utility power utilization, device control, and power supply conductors operating at potentials greater than 50 V. Information about electrical safety requirements can be obtained from the Occupational Safety and Health Administration (7), National Electrical Code (8), and related state and local regulations.

For electric shock hazard control:

1. Limit installation and maintenance to personnel trained in electrical safety.
2. Set up temporary barriers and signs during servicing.
3. Fully discharge storage capacitors before maintenance or service.
4. Use safety grounding rods.
5. Take steps to prevent personnel from being grounded; use insulating floor mats if necessary.
6. When starting a procedure, use one hand only and do not let any other part of the body touch the equipment or a ground.
7. Before making contact with leads or terminals, for extra safety, touch them with the back of the hand.
8. Refer to documents listing equipment's protective controls, interlocks, warning signals, etc. These must be kept on file.

Fire Hazards

The primary causes of laser-system-initiated fires are the ignition of combustible material and the failure of laser equipment. Exposure of various materials to Class 4 laser beams may result in potential fire and smoke hazards if the target is exposed to irradiances exceeding 10 W/cm^2 or beam powers exceeding 0.5 W. However, it is possible to have ignition at lower levels than these, as when, for example, one works in an oxygen-enriched atmosphere.

Controls for Flamable Liquids/Gases

These controls are listed in Table 6.

Table 6. Controls for Flammable Liquids/Gases

Transferring	Areas involved must be well ventilated and away from sources of possible ignition (high voltage, sparks)
Spills	Always employ secondary containment systems
Waste	Store in approved, properly marked containers
Disposal	Check with environmental engineer, chemical safety engineer, or industrial hygienist

Refer to National Fire Protection Association, *Recommended Practice for Laser Fire Protection* (9).

Explosion Hazards

High-pressure arc lamps, filament lamps, and elements of the optical train can shatter during laser operation, creating occupational concerns if appropriate housing enclosures are not used.

Explosion Control

To prevent the more common causes of explosion:

1. Schedule regular replacement and disposal of filters.
2. Schedule regular maintenance of ventilating systems.
3. Limit gas cylinder handling to trained personnel.
4. See that flammable gases or liquids are not in proximity to any possible source of sparks or high heat, or that a leak of either could come within their neighborhood. Stretch your imagination to create any scenario that could produce a lethal combination, no matter how unlikely.

Mechanical Hazards/Robots

In industrial applications, lasers are often used in conjunction with some form of a robot. In these situations several issues must be carefully considered such as the mechanical safety of the robot, the increased effective range in the working envelope of a robot-laser system, and the presence of the worker near the robot.

Noise

Noise levels from certain lasers may be of such intensity that a noise control program may need to be implemented.

6.4.4 Personnel Protective Equipment

Eye Wear

Enclosures, shields, baffles, and door interlocks are more reliable than protective eyewear. Although protective eyewear provides no more than supplementary protection against the effects of laser-produced radiation, safety and administrative controls should require that proper eyewear be used.

Eyewear must be chosen on the basis of wavelengths and have the proper optical density for the intensity of the radiation to be encountered. However, one pair of eyewear may not provide protection from the multiple wavelengths produced by a tunable laser or the combination of beam and nonbeam radiation.

The protective filter can be damaged – crazed, cracked, or shattered – if it absorbs a large fraction of the incident beam that is produced by some high-power lasers. The properties and other characteristics of some filters will change with age. This is especially true of those made of plastic. Visibility and safety will be reduced by some filters; colored warning lights may not be clearly seen. Eye protection should be marked with effective wavelength ranges in nanometers. Because of often discouraging problems they introduce, some workers have failed to wear eye protection that would have protected their sight. With all its limitation, eyewear protection is necessary.

Table 7 provides some basic information on selecting eyewear. *LIA Guide for The Selection of Laser Eye Protection* (10), from which this table was taken, provides more detailed information and lists manufacturer specifications.

Table 7. Simplified Method for Selecting Laser Eye Protection for Intrabeam Viewing: 400–1400 nm.

Q-switched lasers (1 ns to 0.1 ms)		Non-Q-switched lasers (0.4 ms to 10 ms)		Continuous lasers momentary (0.25 s to 10 s)		Continuous laser, long term staring (greater than 3 hrs)		Attenuation	
Maximum output energy (J)	Maximum beam radiant exposure (J/cm^2)	Maximum laser output energy (J)	Maximum beam radiant exposure (J/cm^2)	Maximum power output (W)	Maximum beam irradiance (W/cm^2)	Maximum power output (W)	Maximum beam irradiance (W/cm^2)	Attenuation factor	OD
10	20	100	200	NR	NR	NR	NR	100000000	8
1.0	2	10	20	NR	NR	NR	NR	10000000	7
10^{-1}	2×10^{-1}	1.0	2	NR	NR	1.0	2	1000000	6
10^{-2}	2×10^{-2}	10^{-1}	2×10^{-1}	NR	NR	10^{-1}	2×10^{-1}	100000	5
10^{-3}	2×10^{-3}	10^{-2}	2×10^{-2}	10	20	10^{-2}	2×10^{-2}	10000	4
10^{-4}	2×10^{-4}	10^{-3}	2×10^{-3}	1.0	2	10^{-3}	2×10^{-3}	1000	3
10^{-5}	2×10^{-5}	10^{-4}	2×10^{-4}	10^{-1}	2×10^{-1}	10^{-4}	2×10^{-4}	100	2
10^{-6}	2×10^{-6}	10^{-5}	2×10^{-5}	10^{-2}	2×10^{-2}	10^{-5}	2×10^{-5}	10	1

*NR = Not recommended means that eye protection is not recommended as a control measure at these levels. The calculated levels of output power which would have been listed are above the levels that could damage or destroy the attenuating material used in the eye protection equipment.

Other Protective Gear

Other protective gear includes gloves and gowns, to be used when laser dyes are handled, or to protect the skin from scattering radiation and respirators. The specifications for these items varies according to application; Table 8 provides limited information on glove types.

Table 8. Glove Chart

Type	Application
Natural rubber and natural rubber blends	Bases, alcohol, dilute water solutions; fair for aldehydes and ketones
Polyvinyl chloride (PVC)	Acids, bases, water solutions, alcohols
Neoprene	Oxidizing acids, aniline, phenols, glycol ethers
Nitrile	Oils, greases, aliphatic chemicals, xylene perchloroethylene, trichlorethane, fair for toluene
Butyl	Glycol ethers, ketones, esters
Polyvinyl alcohol (PVA)	Aliphatics, aromatics, chlorinated solvents, ketones (except acetone), esters, ethers
Fluoroelastomer (Viton)	Aromatics, chlorinated solvents, aliphatics, and alcohols
Norfoil (silver shield)	For Hazmat work

If respirators are necessary, Reference 11 requires a program that includes a written plan, hazard evaluation, fire testing, training, and periodic program evaluation. For guidance on establishing a respiratory protection program see References 11–13.

Waste Disposal

Proper waste disposal of contaminated laser material must be handled in conformance with appropriate local, state, and Federal guidelines.

6.4.5 Biological/Medical Hazards

The clinical laser (108–10,000 nm) can produce a chemically hazardous plume from laser-tissue interactions as well as aerosol blood-borne pathogens and viral particles. Beam contact with the polymeric materials that are used in some surgical procedures can lead to fire and the release of gases that are carcinogenic and irritants (i.e., polyvinyl chloride yields benzene and HCl). However, because this handbook does not include the processing of biological materials, we again refer the reader to the *LIA Guide to Non-Beam Hazards* (14) as a starting point.

References

1. ANSI Z136.1 1993 (or latest edition): Standard for Safe Use of Lasers. American National Standards Institute, New York, New York.
2. OSHA, Title 29, CFR Part 1910, Subpart Z, Occupational Safety and Health Administration, Washington, D.C.
3. ACGIH (Booklet) Threshold Limit Values for Chemical Substances and Physical Agents. (Because of more frequent updating, this source is often more up to date than Reference 2.) American Conference of Governmental Industrial Hygienists, Cincinnati, OH.
4. Guidelines for Gas Source Control Equipment (SEMI 13), Semiconductor Equipment and Materials International, Mountain View, CA.
5. Guide for the Design of Gas Source Equipment Enclosures (SEMI 14), Semiconductor Equipment and Materials International, Mountain View, CA.
6. 21 CFR 1040.10, Performance Standards for Light Emitting Products, 1990, Center for Devices and Radiological Health, Rockville, MD.
7. National Electric Code, Occupational Safety and Health Administration (OSHA), Washington, D.C.
8. NFPA 70, National Fire Protection Association, Quincy, MA.
9. NFPA Code #115, Recommended Practice for Laser Fire Protection, National Fire Protection Association, Qunicy, MA.
10. LIA Guide for The Selection of Laser Eye Protection, Laser Institute of America, Orlando, FL.
11. OSHA 29 CFR 1910.134, Occupational Safety and Health Administration, Washington, D.C.
12. ANSI Z88.2, American National Standards Institute, NY, NY.
13. NIOSH, Pocket Guide to Chemical Hazards, National Institute for Occupational Safety and Health, Cincinnati, OH.
14. ANSI Z87.1, 1997: American National Standards Institute, NY, NY.

LIA NONBEAM HAZARD SUBCOMMITTEE
WITH ADDITIONS BY C. EUGENE MOSS

6.5 Laser Safety Standards

Standards that are published by government agencies and by independent and industrial standards organizations place requirements on manufacturers and on users of laser materials processing equipment. This section outlines both types of requirements and provides information on obtaining copies of these standards.

6.5.1 Terms and Abbreviations

ANSI: American National Standards Institute – A U.S. organization that publishes standards for laser users. The ANSI Z136.1 is the general laser safety standard. Other standards in the ANSI Z136 series are intended for specific applications. An ANSI B11 committee publishes standards for machine tool safety.

CDRH: Center for Devices and Radiological Health – An agency within the U.S. FDA that publishes and enforces legal requirements on lasers.

CEN and CENELEC: European equivalents of ISO and IEC. CEN and CENELEC standards are typically European Norms (EN), and many are published in response to directives from the European Commission.

IEC: International Electrotechnical Commission – An organization that publishes international standards on electrical subjects. These are not laws, and the adoption and enforcement of IEC standards are at the discretion of individual nations.

ISO: International Standards Organization – An organization that is equivalent to the IEC, except that the ISO publishes international standards on nonelectrical subjects.

6.5.2 United States Standards

General Laser Safety

Requirements for manufacturers of laser products are published in the Federal Laser Product Performance Standard, 21 CFR 1040, by the FDA Center for Devices and Radiological Health (CDRH). They are legal regulations that require certain product features and labels, manuals and test procedures, and a certification report. The regulations also apply to system integrators who purchase a laser and build it into a processing system for sale, but they do not normally apply to an organization that purchases a laser and assembles a system for its own use.

General safety requirements for users are found in the ANSI Z136.1 *Standard for the Safe Use of Lasers*. It is not a law, but it forms the basis for state and OSHA requirements for laser installations. It specifies requirements for engineering control measures (protective housings, indicators, interlocks, warning signs, etc.) and administrative control measures (limited access areas, standard operating procedures, education and training, etc.). It also defines the responsibilities and training for Laser Safety Officers (LSOs), and it includes procedures for laser hazard evaluation.

Materials Processing Laser Safety

Another ANSI committee has published the B11.21 *Standard for Machine Tools - Machine Tools Using Lasers for Processing Materials - Safety Requirements for Design, Construction, Care, and Use*. The purposes of this document are several: to provide guidance in the design of machine tools for safety; to assist manufacturers in developing equipment suitable for export; to establish a clear distinction between the responsibilities of the manufacturer and the user; and to provide a document that could be used in outlining specifications when purchasing laser systems.

The National Fire Protection Association (NFPA) has issued Document 115, *Recommended Practice for Laser Fire Protection*. This advisory portion of the National Fire Code provides fire protection criteria for the design, manufacture, installation, and use of laser equipment, including suggested criteria for training and responding to fire emergencies involving lasers.

Other Laser Safety Standards

Regulations affect the installation and use of laser materials processing equipment in some states: Texas, New York, Massachusetts, Florida, Arizona, and Illinois. They primarily apply to Class IIIb and Class IV installations and service of enclosed systems containing such lasers.

OSHA Technical Publication 8-1.7 provides guidance to OSHA inspectors in the evaluation of laser hazards. That document was based on an earlier (1986) version of ANSI Z136.1.

Other laser safety standards have been published for fiber optic communication applications (ANSI Z136.2) and for medical installations of lasers (ANSI Z136.3). Standards for use of lasers in educational institutions (ANSI Z136.5) and use of lasers in outdoor applications (ANSI Z136.6) are being published in 2000, and an ANSI standard on laser measurements is being developed.

6.5.3 International Standards

General Laser Safety

The International Electrotechnical Commission (IEC) has published laser safety requirements for product manufacturers (including system integrators) that are similar to those of the CDRH. That standard, IEC 60825-1 *Safety of Laser Products - Part 1: Equipment Classification, Requirements, and User's Guide*, also includes requirements for laser users similar to those in the ANSI Z136.1 document. Standards from the IEC are not laws, but countries can adopt them (or versions of those documents) in any manner that they choose.

Materials Processing Safety

The International Standards Organization (ISO) has teamed with a CEN European standards committee to publish standards specifically for laser materials processing equipment. The ISO 11553 and the CEN 12626 documents have the same title: *Optics and Optical Instruments - Laser and Laser Related Equipment - Safety of Machines Using Laser Radiation to Process Materials*. They are virtually identical, and they resulted from requirements of the Machinery Directive that was published by the European Commission.

These ISO/CEN standards apply only to a machine at the highest level of integration: a ready-to-use installation including materials handling equipment, all guards and controls, and fume extraction provisions in the housing. Where the customer provides the final product integration, it may be the "manufacturer." The hazards involved with the use of the machine must be identified, and safety measures must be instituted to mitigate the effects of these hazards. The standard includes a large number of normative references (European and international documents based on EN 292 and ISO/TR 12100 that become a part of the standard and that provide detailed requirements on safety features.)

Two requirements in the ISO/CEN documents are of particular concern to manufacturers. One is that all systems must be Class 1 during operation, which effectively precludes the use of open sheet cutters. The other is that the manufacturer must specify to the user which materials the equipment is designed to process.

An IEC standard provides requirements on the guards to enclose the process zone of laser materials processing equipment. That document is IEC 60825-4, *Safety of Laser Products - Part 4: Laser Guards*. It covers both passive guards and active guards, but does not apply to the laser head housing or the beam delivery system. The standard discusses how to determine the exposure to laser energy for a guard as installed under reasonably foreseeable conditions. Methods of testing guards are included.

Other Laser Safety Standards

IEC laser safety standards also cover fiber optic communication installations (IEC 60825-2), medical applications (IEC 601-2-22), laser light shows (IEC 60825-3), and visual indicators (IEC 60825-6). Standards are in development for laser measurements and for applications of IR LEDs. Note: The IEC 825 series of laser safety standards were first published as IEC 825-1, IEC 825-2, and IEC 825-3. The current numbering system designates them as IEC 60825-1, IEC 60825-2, etc., as noted above.

6.5.4 European and Other Nations' Standards and Directives

European Norms (EN standards) are documents published by CEN or CENELEC that replace national standards throughout Europe. EN 60825-1 is the European laser safety standard that is the equivalent of IEC 60825-1. As noted above, EN 12626 is virtually identical to ISO 11553.

In order for products to be legally sold in Europe, they must be delivered with a *Declaration of Conformity* that certifies conformance with the health and safety requirements in applicable European Commission directives. They must also display the "CE" mark. EN standards are published for use as one of the means for determining whether the directives are satisfied.

The Machinery Directive includes a requirement that laser energy shall not damage health. The ISO 11553/EN 12626 standards described above were written in response to this directive. The Low Voltage Directive affects all products that operate above 50 VAC. For laser materials processing systems, EN 60204-1, *Safety of Machinery: Electrical Equipment of Industrial Machines: Part 1: General Requirements*, would provide the details for this directive. Also, an EMC Directive specifies requirements for electromagnetic interference and susceptibility that apply to all electronic products.

Australia and New Zealand have adopted IEC 60825-1 as a joint document, AS/NZS 2211.1. Japan uses Japanese Industrial Standard, JIS C 6804-1 - that document includes most of the IEC 60825-1 requirements. Canada has proposed requirements similar to the CDRH and with labels in both English and French, but the proposal is on hold.

6.5.5 Sources

COPIES OF ANSI LASER STANDARDS: Laser Institute of America, 13501 Ingenuity Drive, Suite 128, Orlando, FL 32826, (407) 380-1553, fax (407) 380-5588 or from ANSI in New York, (212) 642-4900, lia@laserinstitute.org, home page http://www.laserinstitute.org.

COPIES OF THE CDRH REGULATIONS: CDRH (HFZ-342), 2098 Gaither Rd., Rockville, MD 20850, (301) 594-4654, fax (301) 594-4672, www.fda.gov/cdrh/radhlth.

COPIES OF THE IEC STANDARDS: International Electrotechnical Commission, 3 Rue de Varemba, CH-1121, Geneva 20, Switzerland, or from ANSI in New York, (212) 642-4900, www.iec.ch.

COPIES OF THE EN STANDARDS: British Standards Institute, 2 Park St, London W1A 2BS, England, fax +44 181 996 7001, www.bsi.org.uk.

COPIES OF THE ISO STANDARDS: International Standards Organization, 1 Rue de Varemba, CH-1121, Geneva 20, Switzerland, www.iso.ch.

OTHER LASER STANDARDS: Status of Laser Safety Requirements, 84–87, Laser & Optronics Buying Guide, September 1996, Cahners, Morris Plains, NJ.

ASSISTANCE WITH CDRH, IEC, ISO, AND EUROPEAN LASER STANDARDS: Contact Bob Weiner, Weiner Associates, 544-23rd St., Manhattan Beach, CA 90266, (310) 545-1190, fax (310) 546-7490, email inerassociates@compuserve.com.

Useful Addresses

American Conference of Governmental Industrial Hygienists (ACGIH), 1330 Kemper Meadow Drive, Cincinnati, OH 45240, (513) 742-2020, fax (513) 742-3355, home page: http://www.acgih.org.

National Fire Protection Association (NFPA), 1 Batterymarch Park, Quincy, MA 02269-9101, (617) 770-3000, fax (617) 770-0700, home page:http://roproc.nfpa.org.

National Institute for Occupational Safety & Health (NIOSH), Department of Health & Human Services, Public Health Service, Centers for Disease Control and Prevention, 4676 Columbia Parkway, Cincinnati, OH 45226-1998, (800) 356-4674, home page: http://www.cdc.gov/niosh/homepage.html.

Occupational Safety & Health Administration (OSHA), U.S. Department of Labor, 200 Constitution Avenue, N.W., Washington, D.C. 20210, (202) 219-9308, home page: http://www.osha.gov.

Semiconductor Equipment and Materials International (SEMI), The Semiconductor Industry Equipment Trade Group, 805 East Middlefield Road, Mountain View, CA 94043-1080, (650) 964-5111, fax: (650) 967-5375, home page: http://www.semi.org.

The following is a list of publications available from the Laser Institute of America, 13501 Ingenuity Drive, Suite 128, Orlando, FL 32826, (407) 380-1553, fax (407) 380-5588, or from ANSI

ISBN 0-912035-15-3

in New York, (212) 642-4900, lia@laserinstitute.org, home page http://www.laserinstitute.org.

American National Standard for the Safe Use of Lasers, ANSI Z136.1-2000.

International Laser Safety Conference Proceedings, 1999.

International Laser Safety Conference Proceedings, 1997.

International Laser Safety Conference Proceedings, 1992.

Laser Safety Guide, 1993.

Regulatory Requirements for Laser Product Manufacturers, U.S. Department of Health and Human Services, Food and Drug Administration, 21 CFR Parts 1000–1040.

Safety with Lasers and Other Optical Sources, D. H. Sliney, and M. L. Wolbarsht, Plenum, New York, 1980.

ROBERT WEINER

Notes

ISBN 0-912035-15-3

Chapter 7

Surface Treatment: Heat Treating

7.0 Introduction

Lasers have been used in a number of ways to modify the properties of surfaces, especially the surfaces of metals. Most often, the objective of the processing has been to harden the surface in order to provide increased wear resistance. This chapter will describe the use of lasers to harden the surface of metals through rapid heating and quenching of a surface layer. This process, termed *transformation hardening*, is applicable to certain types of steel and cast iron. The next chapter will describe several different approaches to surface modification with lasers, including glazing, surface alloying, and cladding.

7.1 Principles of Transformation Hardening

Laser surface transformation hardening, commonly known as heat treating, makes use of the rapid heating and cooling rates produced on metal surfaces exposed to scanning laser beams. Surface mechanical properties (hardness, abrasion, resistance, etc.) and chemical properties, (corrosion resistance, etc.) can often be greatly enhanced through the metallurgical reactions produced during these heating and cooling cycles. Steels and cast irons are particularly good candidates for laser transformation hardening. The process has unique advantages, particularly when used to enhance surface properties in local areas without affecting other areas of the component surface.

Laser heat treating involves solid state transformations, so the surface of the metal is not melted. The fraction of the beam power absorbed by the material is controlled by the absorptivity of the material surface. In many cases this absorptivity is relatively low, especially for CO_2 laser radiation. Special high-absorptivity coatings are applied to the metal surface to increase the power entering the metal when the metal surface absorptivity is low (the reflectivity is high). With the coatings, a very large fraction of the total beam power can be absorbed. Graphite and molybdenum disulfide have been shown to be effective absorption coatings, though a thin layer of paint is often used since most organic materials have a high absorptivity for CO_2 light.

Steels exist in a number of polycrystalline forms depending on chemistry and temperature. At room temperature, plain carbon steels contain a mixture of a body-centered cubic phase (ferrite) and an iron carbide phase. Upon heating to a high enough temperature, the carbides and ferrite dissolve into a single face-centered cubic phase called austenite. The temperatures involved are usually between 750°C and 1000°C depending on the chemistry of the steel.

Scanning laser beams can produce these temperatures in very small fractions of a second. Only the material immediately adjacent to the heated surface is affected, and deeper layers of the material are not heated to the point of forming austenite. The cool material under the heated layer also provides a path for rapid heat transfer by which the heated material is very rapidly cooled. This rapid heating of the surface layer to form austenite, followed by the rapid cooling of the austenite, is characteristic of laser heat treatment, and is somewhat unique to that process. Similar effects can be achieved with induction heating and electron beam heating, but laser heat treating is particularly effective in cost-effective formation of thin-layer heating in localized areas.

Under slow cooling conditions, this high-temperature austenite phase reverts to the ferrite and carbide structure. The rate of cooling affects this reaction. A more finely divided distribution of carbides in ferrite with increased tensile strength is produced as the cooling rate increases. If the cooling rate exceeds a critical value, the reaction to carbide and ferrite is suppressed and austenite is retained down to much lower temperatures. Processes that produce these rapid cooling rates are often called "quenching."

If austenite is retained below a critical temperature, M_s, a structure called martensite is formed. The reaction to form martensite is not time dependent, and depends only the temperature which austenite reaches. The cooler the temperature the greater the percentage of matensite formed. Because martensite is a harder structure than the other crystalline structures, the result of the rapid heating and quenching process is a surface layer with a high value of hardness.

The hardness and tensile strength of martensite increases with increasing carbon content in the range of 0 to 0.6% carbon. Above about 0.1% carbon, the martensite is much harder than the slow-cooled ferrite plus carbide structure.

Time-temperature-transformation (TTT) diagrams shown in Figures 1 and 2 are used to indicate the reaction rates and the transformation products produced.

Figure 1 (next page) is a TTT diagram for 0.8% carbon steel. The two "C" shaped curves represent the time of the beginning and the completion of the reaction of austenite to ferrite and carbide.

In Figure 1, the values of Rockwell C hardness are indicated for the various structures as RC. It is apparent that the martensite has a substantially higher value of hardness than the other crystalline forms.

Addition of alloying chemicals other than carbon to plain carbon steels slows the reaction of austenite to ferrite and carbon. Effectively, these addtions shift the "C" curves to the right, to longer times. Figure 2 (next page) is a TTT diagram for an AISI 4340 steel with nickel, chromium, and molybdenum additions. This

ISBN 0-912035-15-3

shift makes it possible to form martensite with much slower cooling rates. When using alloy steels in laser surface hardening, slower scanning speeds can be used, producing deeper heating. The final result is that martensite can be formed to much greater depth than plain carbon steel.

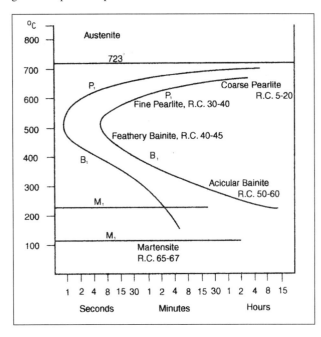

Figure 1. A TTT diagram for 0.8% carbon steel. The values of Rockwell C hardness for the various structures as RC as denoted.

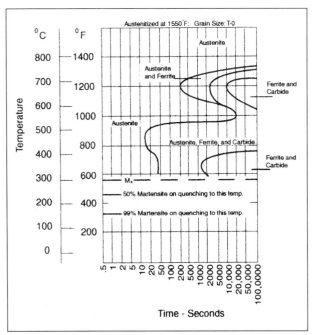

Figure 2. TTT diagram for an AISI 4340 steel: 0.42% C, 0.78% Mn, 1.79% Ni, 0.80% Cr, 0.33% Mo.

Though laser transformation hardening is accomplished with relatively low power density, the cross-sectional area of the beam used to scan the part being heat treated is normally much larger than the focused beams used for welding and cutting. For this reason, relatively high beam power is often required for laser transformation hardening. Traditionally high-power CO_2 laser beams have been used because of the higher power requirements. Unfortunately steels have poor absorptivity for CO_2 laser radiation. This combination of high power requirement and low absorptivity dictates the use of absorptive coatings (see Section 7.3.3).

The power available from Nd:YAG lasers has increased to the degree that they have become more viable candidates for laser transformation hardening. Steels have a much higher absorptivity for Nd:YAG laser beams, making laser transformation hardening practical without absorptive coatings for many applications.

It is important to account for the reflected beam in any laser transformation hardening process, especially if the reflected beam can become a safety hazard. Please see Chapter 6 for details.

References
F. D. Seaman, "Laser Heat Treating," *Industrial Laser Material Processing,* D. Belforte and M. Levitt (Eds.), PennWell Books, Tulsa, OK, 1988.
W. M. Steen, "Laser Cladding, Alloying, and Melting," *Industrial Laser Material Processing,* D. Belforte and M. Levitt (Eds.), PennWell Books, Tulsa, OK, 1988.
C. W. Draper, "The Use of Laser Surface Melting to Homogenize Fe-Al Bronzes," *J. Material Science* **16,** 2774–80, 1981.
C. W. Draper, R. E. Woods, and L. S. Meyer, "Enhanced Corrosion Resistance of Laser Surface Melted Aluminum Bronze," *Corrosion* **36,** p. 405, 1980.

CHARLES E. ALBRIGHT

7.2 Lasers and Optics for Heat Treating

7.2.1 Lasers

Laser transformation hardening is determined by a time-dependent temperature cycle like conventional hardening. The main differences are the much shorter process times involved and the typical properties of the laser beam as a very localized surface heat source. Once the laser energy is transformed into heat, the basic principles of heat transfer in the solid body apply, as described in Chapter 5, and the type and wavelength of the laser are no longer of importance for the actual hardening process.

To decide what type and size of laser might be necessary for the chosen application, several aspects have to be taken into consideration. The weighting of these technical and economical aspects will vary for each application; so no general answer can be given, only suggestions on how to decide in any individual case. Table 1 summarizes some of the more important properties of the laser types that are suitable for hardening applications.

Table 1. Properties of Lasers Suitable for Hardening Applications

	CO_2 laser	Nd:YAG laser		High-power diode laser (HDL)
		lamp pumped (lp)	diode pumped (dp)	
Wavelength (μm)	10.6	1.06	1.06	0.81/0.94
Size: volume (cm³/W)	1000	20	15	1
Available average power (W)	40	5	2	2
Electrical/optical efficiency (%)	5–12	2–4	12–18	20–40
Absorption of iron-based alloys (shiny and clean) (%)	5–15	25–35	25–35	30–40
Investment/cost (laser system) ($/W)	160	240	320	240

CO_2 Lasers

CO_2 lasers are the laser type with the highest available average power. Their conversion of electric power into laser light is quite efficient, more than 10%. At normal incidence, however, the absorption of iron-based alloys is low (see also Chapter 5) and usually not more than 10%.

Nd:YAG Lasers

Because the optical pumping of the Nd:YAG crystal is more efficient when laser diodes are used, diode-pumped Nd:YAG lasers have better beam quality and better overall efficiency. For hardening applications, where good beam quality usually is not required, the savings in energy consumptions of the diode-pumped lasers and the extended maintainance intervals (mainly caused by not having to change lamps) probably justify the higher price of the systems. One main advantage of the Nd:YAG laser is the possibility of transmitting its beam via flexible glass fibers, which facilitates beam handling considerably.

High-Power Diode Lasers (HDL)

The best values for efficiency are offered by HDLs because the electric current in their semi-conductor structure is converted into light by mechanisms with few losses. The absorption of iron-based alloys is also favorable. The small size of the HDL system permits one to mount the whole laser directly onto the machine, saving a beam guiding system. The drawback of HDLs is the limited lifetime of the laser diodes, which means that after approximately 5000 hours of work (usually guaranteed by the supplier) all diodes of the laser system have to be replaced. This exchange of the laser diodes costs roughly two-thirds of the original purchase price of the whole laser system. As soon as the guaranteed lifetime and the exchange intervals of the laser diodes extends to 10,000 hours, HDLs will be the laser of choice. Depending on the current price development and on local energy costs, the use of HDLs instead of Nd:YAG lasers for heat treatment may be more economical.

Considerations for the Choice of the Proper Laser

Mode of Operation: Typically lasers run in the continuous-wave mode for hardening applications. But there are also some reports of successful laser hardening with pulsed Nd:YAG lasers. This seems reasonable for small-volume hardening, like the hardening of needle tips with a single laser pulse. For track hardening, however, pulsed lasers' advantages are not obvious.

Required Surface Condition: The values of the absorptivity that are commonly quoted for most workpieces (see also Table 1) are valid only for smooth and clean surfaces, usually at room temperature and for perpendicular beam incidence. In reality surface and process conditions are different so that the actual coupled fraction of the laser beam is different as well. Depending on the hardening task, you can choose among three general conditions:

- *Shiny surface*: A shiny surface after heat treatment can be obtained by shielding the treated area with inert gas. In this case a Nd:YAG or high-power diode laser can be used. A CO_2 laser can be used only when employing Brewster absorption. Section 5.3 describes the increase in absorptivity, called Brewster absorption, which occurs in the infrared at high values of the angle of incidence.
- *Oxidized surface*: The heat of the process causes an oxidation of the surface. These oxide layers enhance the coupling of the laser beam. For CO_2 lasers coupling rates of 50–60% can be reached in this way. Because of the big difference in energy coupling (a factor roughly 4 to 10 between oxided and nonoxided surfaces) for the CO_2 laser, the process will be unstable, which means that either no hardening or surface melting will occur. Preoxided parts, however, can be treated with CO_2 lasers without any further preparation. For Nd:YAG lasers coupling rates of 70–80% are realistic on oxiding surfaces.
- *Coated surface*: The best coupling rates are obtained when highly absorbing coatings are applied on the workpiece. This means, however, with the removing of the coating, two additional processing steps that require time and incur extra costs. Peak values of 90% absorption are obtained at low intensities and short interaction times. For higher intensities and longer interaction times, as are more typical in real hardening processes, the coating material often degrades and the coupling rate is reduced to values of 60–80% for CO_2 lasers and 70–80% for Nd:YAG lasers. For Nd:YAG lasers the advantages are not so important, and the use of coating material is not recommended. For CO_2 lasers coating is the most common

way to improve the coupling rate to acceptable values. The implications of an additional coating on process control systems are described in the following paragraphs.

Power requirements: As mentioned, the driving force of the hardening process is the heat that equals the coupled laser power. This has to be clearly distinguished from the irradiated power emitted by the laser. Estimating the laser power is shown in this example.

material:	mild steel (similar to AISI 1045)
track width:	10 mm
hardening depth:	1 mm
traverse speed:	200 mm/min

Quite typical for laser-hardened tracks are case geometries like the section of a circle. With this asumption a volume of roughly 22 mm^3 has to be hardened. From the physical properties of the chosen material it can be calculated that an energy of about 6 J/mm^3 is required for the heating of the material to be hardened. In our example 132 W are necessary. As the energetic efficiency of the hardening process is typically between 10% and 20%, a value of 15% is representative. This means that 880 W have to be coupled into the workpiece. Depending on the surface properties of the workpiece, the necessary laser output power can vary between 2950 W [polished surface, CO_2 laser, Brewster angle (70°), 30% absorption at high temperature (1)] and 1260 W (oxided surface, Nd:YAG laser, 70% absorption).

Energy consumption: Assuming a hardening process that requires 600 W of absorbed laser power, where normal beam incidence is necessary and the surface might be oxided or coated, the different energy coupling rates and efficiencies would be as presented in Table 2.

Table 2 shows remarkable differences in the electric power consumption of the different laser types for the same job. Things change, however, if the job changes. Table 3 presents power requirements for a hardening process where no oxidation or coating is allowed.

Depending on the local price for electricity, energy consumption can be a crucial point in the cost of the laser hardening process.

Processing rate: The speed of the hardening process depends on the temperature reached (limited by the melting point) as well as on the metallurgic mechanisms of the martensite formation and therefore on the physical properties of the material. Consequently, the processing rate can be enhanced by going faster only to a very limited extent. The width of the hardened track, however, is not related to these mechanisms and therefore can be controlled independently. The track width is only limited by the heat load of the workpiece that might initiate self-quenching and by the available laser power. If larger areas have to be hardened, wider tracks are advantageous. In some cases a single track produced with a high-power laser might be sufficient instead of multi-pass hardening with a low-power laser, resulting in a much higher processing rate and better properties of the hardened zone (no annealing between passes).

Process control: For laser hardening, usually high temperature levels close to the melting point of the material are employed.

Table 2. Energy Consumption of Different Laser Types Providing 600 W of Absorbed Power at Normal Incidence with an Oxided or Coated Surface

Laser type	Absorbed power	Coupling	Irradiated power	Electrical/ optical efficiency	Electric power consumption	Relative factor
CO_2 laser	600 W	60 %	1000 W	9 %	11,110 W	4.5
Nd:YAG laser (lp)	600 W	70 %	860 W	3 %	28,670 W	11.7
Nd:YAG laser (dp)	600 W	70 %	860 W	15 %	5730 W	2.3
HDL	600 W	70 %	860 W	35 %	2460 W	1

Table 3. Energy Consumption of Different Laser Types Providing 600 W of Absorbed Power without Oxidation or Coating of the Surface

Laser type	Absorbed power	Coupling	Irradiated power	Electrical/ optical efficiency	Electric power consumption	Relative factor
CO_2 laser with Brewster absorption	600 W	15 %	4000 W	9 %	44,440 W	7.8
Nd:YAG laser (lp)	600 W	30 %	2000 W	3 %	66,670 W	11.7
Nd:YAG laser (lp) with Brewster absorption	600 W	45 %	1500 W	3 %	44,440 W	7.8
Nd:YAG laser (dp)	600 W	30 %	2000 W	15 %	13,330 W	2.3
HDL	600 W	30 %	2000 W	35 %	5710 W	1

Chapter 7: Surface Treatment: Heat Treating

To avoid damage to the workpiece by melting of the surface and to ensure the required hardening depth all over the track, process control is highly recommended. This is done frequently by using a pyrometric temperature sensor. The temperature signal then can easily be used to build up a closed-loop control, adjusting the laser power to obtain the set temperature. However, when using a highly absorbing coating material (mostly with CO_2 lasers) on top of the surface, the measured temperature is the temperature of the coating and not the temperature of the workpiece beneath, depending also on the coating thickness. The acquired temperature data can be even more deceptive when the coating material is burning with a bright flame during the process. Much more reliable temperature measurements are obtained using Nd:YAG lasers at surfaces that are only oxided during the process itself.

Conclusion

In principle, the type of the laser is irrelevant when hardening with a laser, as long as the power requirements are met (process rate). The required amount of laser power depends mainly on the surface coupling conditions and the possibility of applying the Brewster effect. The necessary laser power is generated in a different way by each laser system, consuming different amounts of electrical energy. As long as there are no restricting technical reasons (like lack of accessibility, requirement of process control, impossibility to apply a coating and so on), the most economic laser source in terms of coupling *and* efficiency should be chosen. The advantages of beam delivery via flexible fiber, however, cannot be used with the CO_2 laser.

7.2.2 Optics

Beam-shaping optics are used to change the properties of the laser beam to adapt it to the actual working task. Properties that need to be changed are the spot geometry and the intensity distribution within the spot. Interesting for laser hardening are the following spot geometries:

- Circle: Hardening results will be independent of feed direction.
- Line/Area: Advantages in process efficiency and/or speed and in the geometry of the hardened zone.
- Ring: Stationary hardening of items such as valve seat geometries is possible.

Depending on the optics used, the emitted laser mode is preserved within the created laser spot or changed, i.e., usually homogenized. However, special intensity distributions like asymmetric profiles for hardening edges or arm-chair-like profiles for efficient hardening might be required as well. In general, optical elements can be classified according to their properties as transmissive and reflective elements or according to their function as static and dynamic types.

Apart from single exeptions most beam-shaping functions can be realized either with transmissive or reflective elements.

Transmissive Elements (Lenses)

Substrate material: Different transparent optical materials are used for CO_2 lasers and for Nd:YAG or diode lasers. For CO_2 laser processing zinc selenide (ZnSe) is usually used. Gallium arsenide (GaAs) elements are found only rarely. ZnSe can be machined with high accuracy and very good optical quality. It is, however, hygroscopic, and the transmission decays gradually with time. This means that ZnSe optics have to be handled and stored with some care and have to be controlled from time to time. Optics for lasers around 1 µm wavelength consist of "ordinary" optical glasses or fused silica. This means that a huge variety of optical elements can be ordered from many suppliers easily off the shelf at highest quality.

Coating: For high-power applications antireflective coatings are highly recommended to reduce reflection and therefore power losses at the surfaces of the lenses. Such losses also may cause trouble within the optics' housing by extensive heating.

Cooling: Usually transmissive elements are cooled from the rim. However, there are some approaches to cool the surfaces of lenses by a gas stream. Such gas cooling equalizes the radial temperature profile within the lenses (thermal lensing) and so improves the optical quality of the lens. Because very high optical quality usually is not necessary for surface treatment, a sophisticated lens cooling system can usually be avoided.

Reflective Elements (Mirrors)

Basically, either metal mirrors or multi-layer dielectric mirrors are used. For high-power applications mainly gold or copper are used. These mirrors reflect the whole spectrum with virtually no transmission. For high-power CO_2 lasers, diamond-machined copper mirrors are standard. Such mirrors offer the advantage that cooling channels can be machined directly into the mirror substrate. To enhance the reflectivity sometimes copper mirrors are gold coated.

Multi-layer dielectric mirrors can be narrow- or broad-band. These mirror layers can be used to enhance the reflectivity of metal mirrors for the laser wavelength to minimize absorption losses, or (on a transparent substrate) they provide a wavelength-selective mirror such that other wavelengths apart from the laser wavelength can be used for process control or observation. For Nd:YAG lasers dielectric mirrors are always used.

Losses

Highly sophisticated lenses and mirrors can be purchased with initial losses of 0.2% or even less, guaranteed by well-fitted, high-reflective (HR) or antireflective (AR) coatings. In practice, however, losses are usually higher (even 5% or more) due to contamination of the surfaces by spatters or due to scratches or other damage caused, for example, by improper cleaning. These figures show that, depending on the working conditions, the optical elements require some maintainance. The losses of uncoated copper mirrors as are often used with CO_2 lasers, for example, can be kept in the range of 1–2%, even after frequent cleaning procedures.

Static Beam Shaping

In static beam shaping the laser beam is not moved within the contour of the spot. To create the above mentioned spot geometries there are different types of optical systems:

Circular spot: To produce a circular spot a focusing system (lens or mirror) is used. The resulting intensity distribution is the image of the emitted intensity distribution (mode) of the laser source. The diameter of the spot is adjusted by defocusing more or less. For an Nd:YAG laser with a step-index fiber the homogeneous top hat distribution at the fiber outlet can be projected onto the workpiece surface. To do so, the workpiece surface has to be exactly in the image plane of the optical system. This is not necessarily the smallest diameter of the beam, but by arranging the lenses into a telescope, an enlarged image of the top hat distribution can be produced (2). Away from the image plane, the circular laser spot then has a Gaussian-like intensity distribution. Figure 1 shows examples of enlarged images for an Nd:YAG laser beam delivered by a fiber into a telescope.

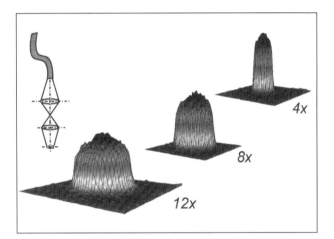

Figure 1. Enlarged images of the top hat distribution (Nd:YAG laser, fiber diameter: 0.4 mm)

Linear/Rectangular spot: The simplest way to produce a linear or rectangular laser spot on the workpiece is just to focus the beam of a line source. This might be the radiation of a single diode bar, of a slab laser, or of a beam with high Hermite mode in one direction. The size of the laser spot is determined by the degree of defocusing, while the intensity distribution is that of the laser source. If no line source is available a beam can be transformed into a more or less linear/elliptic spot using a cylindrical lens/mirror. The structure of the intensity profile, however, is that of the emitted beam. To change both axes of the elliptical spot by defocusing, a second cylindrical lens/mirror can be used for the second axis. With such an astigmatic imaging system, the spot size can be changed widely, but without changing the internal structure of the profile.

Another way to produce a linear, respectively, rectangular laser spot is to use a waveguide or kaleidoscope. A waveguide usually is a tube with highly reflecting internal walls and rectangular cross-section. The laser beam is focused or guided via glass fiber into the waveguide. Figure 2 shows how a kaleidoscope can be used for this purpose.

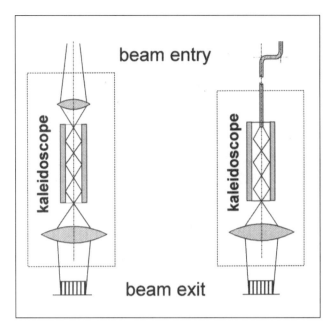

Figure 2. Coupling of the beam into a waveguide/kaleidoscope: via focusing (a) or via fiber (b) (3).

Because of multiple reflections inside the waveguide, the intensity distribution is homogenized. At the outlet of the waveguide, a homogeneous beam profile with the dimensions of the cross-section of the waveguide is available for processing. To make use of it, the workpiece must be very close to the waveguide, in the range of several millimeters. To increase the working distance, an additional imaging optic system can be used. Also, additional optics can be used to change the size of the laser spot. Instead of a hollow tube, a rectangular glass bar or tapered fiber can be used with Nd:YAG lasers as a waveguide for beam-shaping purposes. With CO_2 lasers a linear polarized beam should not be used, because the angles of reflection inside the waveguide are typically in the range of the Brewster angle. Using linear polarized radiation then might cause excessive coupling inside the waveguide, leading to large energy losses or even destruction of the mirror surfaces. Even without polarized radiation, typically 15 to 30% of the laser power is lost inside the hollow waveguide, so that efficient cooling is necessary.

In most cases segmented mirrors or lenses are used to produce a uniform intensity profile with a rectangular shape. The incoming laser beam hits different facets of the mirror or lens. At every facet the beam is reflected or deflected into another direction. The separated single rays are superposed at the workpiece, producing a uniform profile with the size of a single facet. The homogenization effect is better the more facets are irradiated by the incoming beam. The existence of this profile, however, is limited to one working plane. Even small deviations of the working distance may change the profile considerably. To change the size of the laser spot a mirror or lens with another facet size is required or an additional optical system to enlarge the spot or to make it smaller. Figure 3 shows schematically the use of integrators to produce rectangular or line profiles.

Chapter 7: Surface Treatment: Heat Treating

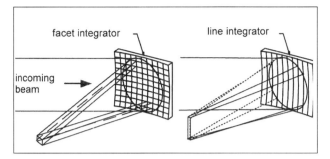

Figure 3. Schematic diagram of segmented mirrors.

With two or more laser sources, the beams also can be superposed to generate an oval or even rectangular laser spot on the workpiece. The best example for the superposition of single laser sources is in the use of diode lasers, which are usually built up in stacks to obtain high power. The size of the common spot can be adjusted by different degrees of defocusing and overlap between the single spots. The variable degree of overlap and the chosen positions of the individual laser beams define the resulting intensity profile. Figure 4 shows a special optic design where the beam of a Nd:YAG laser is split into two rays by a polarizer after being transmitted via glass fiber (4). When the direction of polarization in one branch is rotated 90° and the ray then is joined again at the workpiece with the other branch, the directions of polarization are the same at the workpiece, permitting one to use enhanced Brewster absorption even with Nd:YAG lasers and fiber transmission. The power losses of this splitting and joining of the beam are below 5% and therefore neglectable. One gains advantages like the linear polarized laser beam and the flexibility of the beam combination.

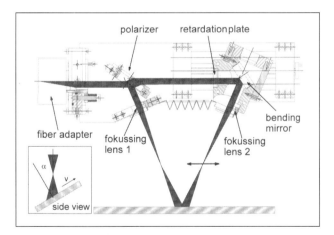

Figure 4. Drawing of a flexible polarization optic for an Nd:YAG laser.

Ring-shaped spot: A beam shape adapted to components such as valve seats is a continuous ring. Such a laser spot can be produced by putting an axicon, a cone-shaped lens structure, into the beam path (4). Because of its unusual properties, an axicon transforms a circular beam into a ring-shaped beam or vice versa. Axicons are sometimes used in lasers with unstable resonators. The advantage of using an axicon for hardening is that the seat geometry can be hardened in just one exposure, without any relative movement between the beam and the workpiece. Also no energy is lost through the centered hole. Since the laser beam is a complete ring without any start or end point, it does not cause tempering and therefore no soft zone. With different angles of the cone and different additional imaging systems (focusing lens/mirror), various combinations of inner and outer diameters of the ring can be realized (5). Figure 5 shows how an axicon can be used.

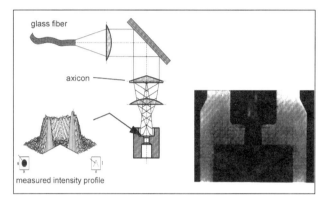

Figure 5. Hardening optic on the base of an axicon and view of the produced ring-shaped spot and related hardened zone.

Others: Another interesting beam profile is the so-called "armchair" profile proposed for efficient line hardening (6). The higher intensity at the front of the profile shortens the heating time. The elevated intensity levels at both sides of the profile are to compensate lateral heat losses. Both effects help to produce a very homogeneous temperature field on the workpiece surface within the irradiated zone, leading to an efficient transformation of the material. Approaches to realize such a profile have been made for CO_2 lasers by using special variable segmented mirrors, holograms (7) or bi-directional scanning (see below). Figure 6 shows such as armchair profile and the resulting burn pattern in plexiglass.

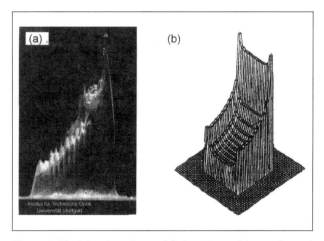

Figure 6. Plexiglass burn from a CO_2 laser beam (a), transformed by a special hologram (7) to obtain a special intensity profile for efficient hardening (b) (6).

A very flexible tool to create specialized spot geometries is the multi-fiber bundle. Independently, whether single fibers are fed by one single laser source or by individual ones, the fiber ends can be arranged as required by the working task. The superposition of all the laser spots generates the desired spot geometry.

Adaptive mirrors are not only used to change the focal length of optics but also for beam shaping. In one application a thin copper mirror is deformed by 19 piezoelectric actuators. A variety of beam profiles can be created and quickly changed (8). The control of this beam-shaping system, however, is very complex.

Difficultly accessible areas, such as openings inside the workpiece contour, can be hardened when optimizing the optics. Even hardening of the inner sides of bores with 10-mm diameters has been demonstrated (9).

Dynamic Beam Shaping

Distinct spot geometries also can be created by quickly moving a laser beam in certain patterns. The repetition rate and the duty cycle have to be high enough that the induced thermal cycles still permit the transformation of the material. Roughly, a repetition frequency of several tens of hertz is required at least. The pattern of the beam motion and frequently a simultaneous power ajustment generate highly flexible intensity profiles in time and geometry. The resulting beam profile is nearly completely independent of the original stationary laser beam. In general, the properties of the generated laser spot often can be varied during the hardening process just by changing some control settings of the beam-shaping system.

Linear spot: A linear laser spot is created by moving a laser beam rapidly in one direction. In contrast to scribing applications, for hardening the focusing lens/mirror (long focal length) is positioned in front of the scanning mirror. Galvanometer drives are used to scan the light-weight mirror. The length of the generated laser line is adjusted by the twisting angle of the mirror. The width is determined by the size of the original spot and usually can be changed by defocusing. A variation of the mirror motion means local variations in interaction time and therefore a special effective intensity distribution. The same effect can be achieved by fast variation of the laser power depending on the actual local position of the beam. An important parameter for the shape of the hardened zone is the ratio between scanning amplitude and beam radius. Figure 7 is a schematic diagram of an oscillating galvanometer-based scanner.

Rectangular spot: When the one-dimensional scanning is extended with a second scanning mirror, rectangular laser spots can also be created.

Ring-shaped spot: A special type of bidirectional scanning is the forming of a ring-shaped spot by harmonizing the two oscillations.

Another way to produce a laser ring is to make use of a trepanning optic. A focusing lens is rotated around an axis that is out of the optical axis in the center of the lens. The diameter of the ring spot is determined by the distance between the optical axis and the axis of the rotation and by the focal length of the lens.

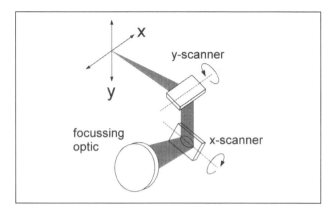

Figure 7. Basic setup of a two-dimensional oscillator system (suitable for CO_2 and Nd:YAG lasers).

A similar effect can be achieved by putting a wedge in the beam path and rotating it. The diameter of the ring spot is determined by the angle of the wedge and the distance between the wedge and the workpiece. The same effect as a rotating wedge can be achieved with a wobble mirror, as shown in Figure 8 (10).

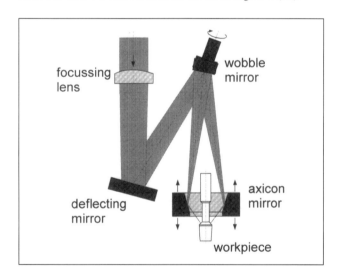

Figure 8. Special optic containing a wobble mirror to harden a surrounding contour quasi-stationary (10).

Instead of rotating the laser beam to produce a ring-shaped spot, the workpiece can be turned. This method is ideal to harden a ring around a workpiece inside a lathe. By rapidly turning the workpiece and irradiating one spot with the laser, one can create a glowing ring as with induction heating. A larger spot size is advantageous to improve the duty cycle. This results from the ratio between spot size and perimeter of the workpiece. After the hardening process, a final cutting process can produce the finished, hardened workpiece (11), (12).

References

1. F. Dausinger, 1995, *Strahlwerkzeug Laser Energieeinkopplung und Prozesseffektivität,* Teubner-Verlag, Stuttgart, Germany.
2. W. Bloehs, and F. Dausinger, Proc. of ICALEO'95, *Beam Shaping Systems for Nd:YAG-Lasers: Examples and Applications*, 1068–77.
3. T. Ishide, M. Mega, O. Matsumoto, S. Ito, and T. Mitsuhashi, Proc. of ECLAT'92: *Kaleidoscope Beam Homogenizer for High Power CO_2 and YAG Laser*, 57–62.
4. W. Bloehs, and F. Dausinger, Proc. of ECLAT'96: *Beam Shaping Systems for Hardening with High-Power Nd:YAG lasers*, 845–52.
5. W. Bloehs, 1997, *Laserstrahlhärten mit angepassten Strahlformungssystemen*, Teubner-Verlag, Stuttgart, Germany.
6. D. Burger, LASER'89: *Optimierung der Strahlqualität bei Laserhärten*, 673–78.
7. C. Haupt, M. Pahlke, C. Budzinski, H. J. Tiziani, and R. Krupka, *Laser und Optoelektronik* **29**, 48–55 (1997).
8. P. Hoffman, S. Schubert, M. Geiger, and C. Kozlik, SPIE Vol. 1834-30: *Process Optimizing Adaptive Optics for Beam Delivery of High Power CO_2 Lasers*.
9. W. Bloehs, and F. Dausinger, Proc. of ISATA'96: *Efficient Hardening with High-Power Solid-State Lasers*, 377–83 (1997).
10. R. O. Lund, and B. Whealon, Proc. of ICALEO'94: *Laser Heat Treating with Rotationally Integrated Beam*, 362–71.
11. M. Wiedmaier, 1997, *Konstruktive und verfahrenstechnische Entwicklungen zur laserintegrierten Komplettbearbeitung in Drehzentren*, Teubner-Verlag, Stuttgart, Germany.
12. H. Hügel, M. Wiedmaier, and T. Rudlaff, *Laser Processing Integrated into Machine Tools - Design, Applications, Economy, Opt. and Quant. Electr.* **27**, 1149–64 (1995).

W. Bloehs, B. Grünenwald, F. Dausinger, and H. Hügel, *J. of Laser Appl.* **1**, 15–23 (1996).

W. Bloehs, B. Grünenwald, F. Dausinger, and H. Hügel, *J. of Laser Appl.* **2**, 65–77 (1996).

WOLFGANG BLOEHS

7.2.3 Optics for Uniform Beam Profiles

Laser surface modification is normally accomplished by scanning a laser beam over the surface of the material to be modified. The power distribution in the beam taken in the scanning direction should be the same for all areas of the beam cross-section in order to expose all areas of the surface equally. This calls for a beam of square or rectangular cross-section with a scanning direction parallel to one of the edges. Since most lasers produce a beam that has a round or other non-rectangular shaped cross-section, the raw laser beam must be modified to achieve the rectangular cross-section with uniform power distribution.

A system known as a beam integrator is shown in Figure 9 (see also Fig. 3, Section 7.2.2). The beam integrator is very effective at producing square, constant power distribution, but is relatively expensive. A less expensive system is the "chimney" shown in Figure 10. A square hole is made in highly reflective polished copper by bolting rectangular blocks together. This system is effective in producing square or rectangular patterns, but appreciable power loss to the system is also experienced.

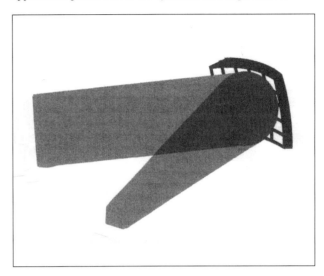

Figure 9. Beam integrator system for creating a square cross-section.

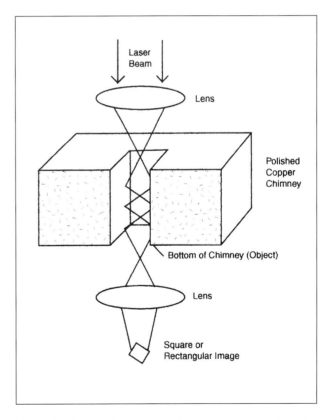

Figure 10. Beam "chimney" for producing a square or rectangular cross-section.

An alternate method of achieving the desired uniform power density is by rapidly scanning with a focused beam. Extremes in surface temperature are avoided by using very rapid traverse speeds. A simple oscillating system with two orthogonal mirrors can be used to produce the raster rectangular pattern. This is shown in Figure 11.

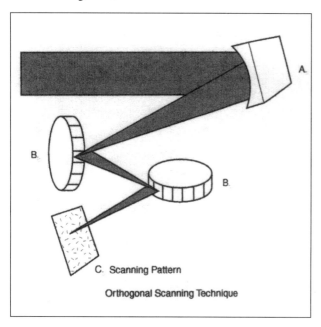

Figure 11. Double segmented rotating mirrors for producing a raster pattern with a focused beam.

Finally, a method of beam control for exposing internal cylindrical surfaces is shown in Figure 12.

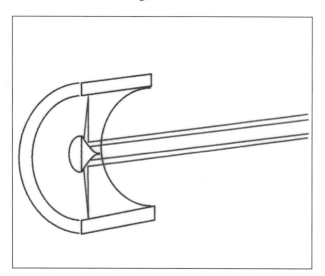

Figure 12. System for scanning interior cylindrical surfaces.

CHARLES E. ALBRIGHT

7.3 Results of Laser Heat Treatment

7.3.0 Introduction

The unique role of lasers and their virtually unlimited potential in surface engineering applications to selectively harden ferrous alloys will be illustrated (1–19, 22, 38–41). We will survey the laser heat treatment characteristics with a range of processing conditions for several ferrous alloys such as carbon steels, alloy steels, tool steels, and cast irons for various industrial applications such as camshafts, gear housing shafts, and gear teeth. Based on experimental findings, laser processing maps showing the ranges of required incident power density (0.8 to 40 kW/cm^2), specific energy (0.3 to 60 kJ/cm^2), and interaction time (0.03 to 9 s) regimes for the ferrous alloys using continuous-wave CO_2 lasers have been developed. However, the actual energy required to harden may vary depending on the surface absorptivity characteristics. The phases in the laser-heat-treated microstructures include one or a combination of lath martensite, ferrite, retained austenite, and proeutectoid ferrite-cementite together with highly dislocated substructures due to rapid quenching, depending on the ferrous alloy chemistry and laser processing parameters. The typical microhardness of the laser-heat-treated ferrous alloys were in the range of 450 to 975 kg/mm^2 (Fig. 11 of Section 7.3.5) and were better than or comparable to those obtained by conventional heat treatment methods.

For a proper treatment of this subject, we determined that some theoretical material was called for, and in that respect, this section differs from others in this *Handbook*.

7.3.1 Irradiance Versus Interaction Time

Laser heat treatment of steels and cast irons is usually done selectively to enhance the surface hardness and hence the resulting properties (e.g., improved wear resistance in applications such as tool steels, automotive crankshaft, camshaft, valves, cylinder liners, gear teeth, etc.) with minimal thermal distortion of the workpiece. This is usually accomplished by rapidly heating the surface to temperatures above the critical austenitization range in the solid state but well below that of the melting points of the particular alloy composition, then followed by rapid self-quenching by fast heat conduction to the bulk of the substrate at rates in excess of the critical cooling rates required for martensitic transformation.

Figure 1 shows the laser power density versus the interaction time together with specific energy regimes for various laser materials processing applications such as transformation hardening, melt-quenching, alloying, cladding, welding, cutting, drilling, and shock hardening. It also shows the differences between using continuous-wave high-power lasers and pulsed lasers. It is apparent that most of the laser hardening work on various materials has been performed using high-power CW lasers. The required laser power densities are usually lower than those required for surface melting such as alloying, welding, and cutting, but the duration of the laser beam interaction on the workpiece is relatively longer, as shown in the general laser processing regimes of Figure 1 (1, 4). The process advantages of the laser heat treatment process are as follows: high processing speeds (hence higher production rates), controlled input laser energy, reduced thermal distortion of the workpiece, selective hardening of the surface, self-quenching without the need for external quenchants, no vacuum requirement unlike electron beam hardening, time sharing of the laser beam by switching between workstations, hardening of difficult-to-access areas by suitable optics and/or fiber-optic beam delivery (e.g., Nd:YAG lasers), less/no post-heat treatment machining operations, amenability to computer process control, and environmentally clean processing (6, 12, 21).

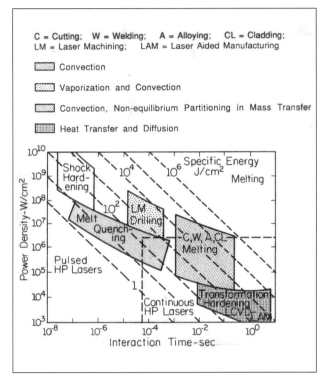

Figure 1. Schematic diagram of various laser processing regimes as a function of power density versus interaction time (1, 4).

7.3.2 Summary of Laser Heat Treatment Data
Some representative results including the processing parameters and microstructural and geometrical characteristics for laser-hardened ferrous alloys are presented in Table 1 (20, 23–37).

The experimentally obtained values of incident laser power density or irradiance (laser power/beam cross-sectional area), interaction time (laser beam size/process speed), and specific energy [laser power/(beam size × process speed)] are plotted in Figure 2 (12). This figure shows the typical range in which these materials have been successfully heat treated using continuous-wave CO_2 lasers. Such heat-treated materials include various types of low-, medium-, and high-carbon steels, low-alloy steels, tool steels, and cast irons. The hardening response and geometry (e.g., width and depth of hardening) depend on the initial microstructure, thermophysical properties such as conductivity/diffusivity, and photon absorptivity of the materials and the cooling rates as a function of the laser hardening parameters (e.g., at a given power density, higher process speeds give higher cooling rates). Figure 2 is limited to the range of data available in the literature.

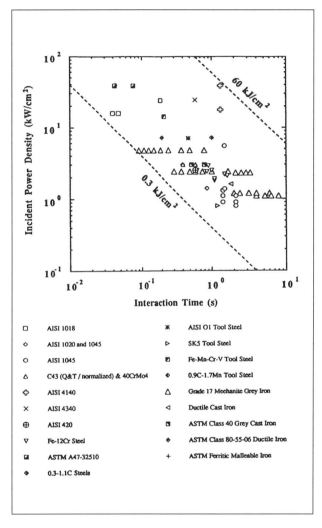

Figure 2. Laser heat treatment map for select engineering materials (12).

7.3.3 Effect of Process Variables
The major independent process variables for laser heat treatment include incident laser beam power, beam diameter, absorptivity of the coating and substrate, and traverse speed. Thermophysical properties of the substrate also play an important role. The dependent variables are considered to be case depth, microhardness, geometry of the heat-affected zone and its microstructure, and mechanical (e.g., strength, toughness, or fatigue) and wear resistance.

Laser Irradiance
Laser beam diameter and intensity distribution define the surface heat source. The laser beam power and diameter determine

Table 1. Laser Heat Treatment Data for Various Engineering Materials

Base Material (wt %)	Coating	Process Parameters: (a) Laser Type (b) Power (kW) (c) Beam Diam. (mm)	Process Parameters: (d) Transverse Mode (e) Process Speed (mm/s) (f) Interaction Time (s)	Process Parameters: (g) Power Density (kW/cm²) (h) Specific Energy (J/cm²) (i) Shielding Gas	Microstructural Characteristics and Properties	Geometrical Characteristics	Hardness (kgf/mm²)	Application	Ref(s)
AISI 1018 steel		(a) CO_2 (b) 9 (c) 12 × 12 (square)	(d) — (e) 63.5-169 (f) 0.071-0.20	(g) 6.25 (h) 444-1181 (i) air	Low-carbon martensite	HAZ = 254 μm	446		20, 23
AISI 1018 & 1045 steels		(a) CO_2 (b) 1.0 (c) 2.54	(d) — (e) 25.4 (f) 0.1-0.5	(g) 0.789-19.7 (h) 315-1600 (i) —	Ferrite + martensite; proportion of martensite in 1045 much higher than in 1018	depth = 254 μm width = 1.65 mm	AISI 1045 Base: 354 HAZ: 720		24
En 8 (0.36% C steel)	Graphite "Dag"	(a) CO_2 (b) 1.2-2.0 (c) 1.6-5.8	(d) Gaussian (e) 25-400 (f) 0.004-0.232	(g) 4.54-99.5 (h) 51.7-5000 (i) —	Martensite + proeutectoid ferrite	HAZ depth = 700 μm	500-680		25
AISI 1045	Black paint	(a) CO_2 (b) 2.5-4.15 (c) 18 × 18 (square)	(d) — (e) 8.5-12.7 (f) 1.42-2.12	(g) 0.772-1.28 (h) 1093-2712 (i) —	Martensite	HAZ = 520-1240 μm	446		26
AISI 1045	Black paint	(a) CO_2 (b) 8.8 (c) 12.5 × 25.4 (dual beam)	(d) — (e) 8.33 (f) —	(g) 1.38 (h) — (i) —	Martensite	HAZ = 1.2-1.3 mm	674-697	Gear teeth	26
Hypoeutectic, eutectic, hypereutectic, and ledeburitic steels	Specimens oxidized to improve absorptivity	(a) CO_2 (b) 1.25 (c) 9	(d) — (e) 5 (f) 1.8	(g) 1.96 (h) 2778 (i) —	Inhomogeneous structures for the hypereutectic, and ledeburitic steels; ferrite-cementite, austenite, & martensite in the HAZ		640-870		27
SK5 tool steel	Manganese phosphate	(a) CO_2 (b) 1.3 (c) 12 × 12 (square)	(d) TEM_{00} + TEM_{11} (e) 10 (f) 1.20	(g) 0.903 (h) 1083 (i) —	Martensite	HAZ Depth = 920 μm width = 6.8 mm	850		28
Tool steels A6-air hardened O1-oil hardened		(a) CO_2 (b) 1.0 (c) 2.54-12.7	(d) — (e) 38.1 (f) 0.0667-0.333	(g) 0.789-19.7 (h) 1462 (i) —	Martensite	HAZ = 305 μm	A6: 653-746 O1: 800-865		24
Tool steel (0.95C-1.7Mn-0.25Cr-0.25V)		(a) CO_2 (b) 2.8 (c) 5	(d) — (e) 23.3 (f) 0.215	(g) 14.3 (h) 2400 (i) —	Martensite		800		29
Fe/3.11 Cr/1.98 Mn/0.5 Mo/0.26 C (3 Cr) & Fe/9.85 Cr/1.0 Mn/0.5 Al/0.2 C (10Cr)		(a) CO_2 (b) 1.25 (c) narrow elliptical spot	(d) — (e) 4.23-8.47 (f) —	(g) — (h) — (i) He	Packet martensite (retained austenite films surrounding dislocated and fine twinned laths); martensitic laths oriented in re-solidified and unmelted parts of grains; in melted zone, grains large and fine cellular; just below melt zone, grains coarse and irregular; in HAZ, grains fine martensitic and irregular; presence of δ-ferrite		600-700		30
AISI 4140 steel	Black paint	(a) CO_2 (b) 3.5 at tip, 7.5 at cylindrical portion (c) 5	(d) annular (ring) (e) 1300 rpm 3.7 mm/s (f) —	(g) — (h) — (i) He	Martensite	HAZ Depth = 1.65-2 mm	653-674	Shaft	26
(a) AISI 4340 (b) AISI 8620 (c) ASI 52100		(a) CO_2 (b) 1.0 (c) 2.54-12.7	(d) — (e) 19-25.4 (f) 0.1-0.0667	(g) 0.789-19.7 (h) 310-2072 (i) —	In all cases very fine martensite; negligible distortion	HAZ depth/width μm (a) 406/2500 (b) 356/2300 (c) 178/1350	(a) 633-674 (b) 513 (c) 697-800		24

Chapter 7: Surface Treatment: Heat Treating

Table 1. Laser Heat Treatment Data for Various Engineering Materials (continued)

Base Material (wt %)	Coating	Process Parameters (a) Laser Type (b) Power (kW) (c) Beam Diam. (mm)	(d) Transverse Mode (e) Process Speed (mm/s) (f) Interaction Time (s)	(g) Power Density (kW/cm²) (h) Specific Energy (J/cm²) (i) Shielding Gas	Microstructural Characteristics and Properties	Geometrical Characteristics	Hardness (kgf/mm²)	Application	Ref(s)
AISI 4340 and 300-M		(a) CO_2 (b) 1.2 (c) 2.5	(d) — (e) 4.2 (f) 0.595	(g) 24.5 (h) 11429 (i) —	In 4340, a mixture of dislocated and twinned martensites with presence of twins in lath martensite; retained austenite; homogeneous dispersion of self-tempered cementite particles (both at the lath boundaries and along the internal twins) within the martensite; in both systems, substructure of grain boundary is blocky martensite (without twins or carbides) or massively transformed ferrite	HAZ depth = 1.1 mm width = 3.6 mm	AISI 4340 Base: 354 HAZ: 720		31, 32
12% Cr Steel (tempered martensitic)	Graphite	(a) CO_2 (b) — (c) —	(d) — (e) — (f) 0.63-1.62	(g) 1.8-2.9 (h) — (i) —	Very fine lamellar martensite with extremely high dislocation density	HAZ depth = 0.7-1.4 mm	HAZ: 500-600 Base: 300		34
Fe-6C-.09Si .99Mn-.24Cr & Fe-18W-4.25Cr-.75C-1.05V & Fe-11.5Cr-2.05C-.7W		(a) CO_2 (b) 1.3 (c) 19	(d) TEM_{00} (e) 10-400 (f) 0.0425-1.9	(g) 0.459 (h) 17.1-684 (i) —	δ-ferrite, austenite, & martensite	Fe.6C HAZ width = 550-800 μm softened tone = 200-500 μm	Fe-C: 800-1000 Fe-W: 800-1000 Fe-Cr: 460-530		35
ASTM class 40 grey iron & class 80-55-06 ductile cast iron	Manganese phosphate	(a) CO_2 (b) 0.4-1.2 (c) 6.35 (square)	(d) TEM^*_{01}, TEM_{00}, & square (e) 4.23-1.69 (f) 0.0375-1.50	(g) 0.992-2.98 (h) 37.3-4464 (i) —	Grey iron exhibits less distortion than ductile iron	Distortion less than 50 μm HAZ = 0-508 μm	800-1000		33
Grade 17 "Meehanite" grey cast iron	Colloidal graphite	(a) CO_2 (b) — (c) —	(d) — (e) — (f) 0.09-0.79	(g) 1.375-6.0 (h) 1000-4000 (i) —	Retained austenite + coarse martensite	HAZ depth = 0.05-1.62 mm			36
Ductile cast iron	Manganese phosphate	(a) CO_2 (b) 9 (c) 22 x 25 (oscillating)	(d) — (e) 12.7 & 3 (f) —	(g) 1.57 (h) — (i) —	Primarily a matrix of fine martensite containing flake graphite	Distortion less than 127 μm HAZ depth = 560 μm	550-630	Lobes of camshaft	26
ASTM A48 class 40 grey cast iron		(a) CO_2 (b) 1.0 (c) 2.54-12.7	(d) — (e) 25.4 (f) 0.1-0.5	(g) 0.789-19.7 (h) 315-1600 (i) —	Primarily a matrix of fine martensite containing flake graphite	HAZ depth = 0.5 mm width = 3.8 mm	735		24
Ferritic malleable cast iron		(a) CO_2 (b) 1.0 (c) 2.54-12.7	(d) — (e) 50.8 (f) 0.05-0.25	(g) 0.789-19.7 (h) 155-775 (i) —	Martensite surrounding tempered carbon	HAZ depth = 305 μm width = 2.03 mm	675		24
ASTM-A47-32510 ferritic malleable iron	Manganese phosphate	(a) CO_2 (b) 0.5 & 1.0 (c) 1.9	(d) TEM^*_{01} (e) 25.4 & 45.7 (f) 0.0748 & 0.0416	(g) 17.6 & 35.3 (h) 1036 & 1152 (i) —	Ferritic + martensitic regions surround temper carbon nodules	HAZ depth = 254-356 μm width = 2.5-15 mm	630-735	Power steering gear housing	37

the irradiance (or power density), and thus, coverage rate. The various methods of measuring the laser beam diameter include single isotherm contouring techniques, and photodiodes with various sampling techniques such as rotating needle and beam scan methods. Select beam diagnostic instruments and their characteristics have been described in Section 4.5. The recommended laser beam diameter as defined by $1/e^2$ of the peak intensity contains about 86% of the total laser power. In single isotherm contouring, the particular isotherm depends on the laser power and exposure time.

Unlike laser welding or cutting, which normally requires a tightly focused low-order-mode Gaussian beam (TEM_{00}), a laser beam with uniform energy intensity distribution (e.g., TEM_{01}^*) is preferred for laser heat treatment. Such uniform intensity distribution is desirable for producing uniform case depth. Courtney and Steen concluded when hardening En8 steel (0.36% C, 0.58% Mn, 0.22% Si, 0.25% Ni, 0.5% Cu, 0.08% Cr, 0.015% P, and 0.2% S) that the depth of hardening is closely correlated with the parameter $P/(D_b V)^{0.5}$, where P denotes laser power, D_b beam diameter, and V is the process speed. The relationship between this parameter and the depth of hardening is shown in Figure 3 (43).

The variation of case depth as a function of incident laser power for various coverage rates for plain carbon steels is shown in Figure 4 (44).

laser surface hardening. The interaction time for the CO_2 laser hardening of various steels and cast iron (Fig. 2) in the present view is in the range of 0.03–9 s.

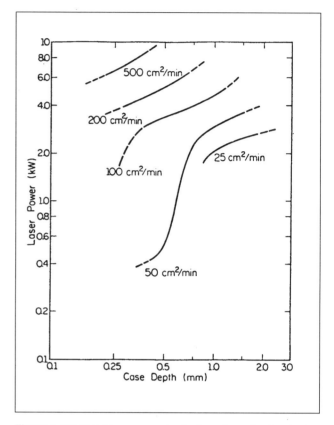

Figure 4. Idealized coverage rates for transformation hardening of typical plain carbon steels (44).

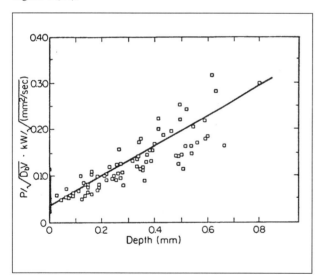

Figure 3. $P/(D_b V)^{0.5}$ versus depth of hardening (43).

Interaction Time

Both process speed and laser beam size determine the interaction time. It is inversely proportional to the depth of hardening, as shown in Figure 5 (58). It is apparent from Table 2 and Figure 5 that the alloy composition (e.g., carbon concentration) plays an important role in determining the extent of case depth for various traverse speeds. A minimum interaction time on the order of 10^{-2} s with a power density in excess of 10^3 W/cm^2 is needed for transformation hardening. A process speed of 0.5–5 cm/s is quoted by Gregson (44) as an approximate range for

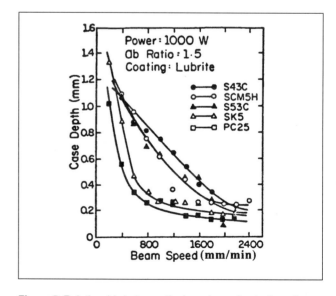

Figure 5. Relationship between the laser beam feed rate and case depth in various materials (58).

ISBN 0-912035-15-3

Chapter 7: Surface Treatment: Heat Treating

Table 2. Composition of Experimental Ferrous Alloys (58)

	C	Si	Mn	P	S	Ni	Cr	Mo	Cu
S43C	0.43	0.24	0.77	0.012	0.010	0.02	0.05	0.01	0.03
S53C	0.51	0.22	0.72	0.013	0.027	0.06	0.11	0.01	0.14
SCM5	0.47	0.31	0.79	0.23	0.022	0.10	1.18	0.20	0.18
PC25	3.38	1.83	0.49	0.031	0.058	0.08	0.04	< 0.01	< 0.01
SK5	0.83	0.17	0.45	0.18	0.017	0.02	0.19		0.03

Heat-Treatable Materials

The hardening response of various steels and cast irons can be classified as treatable or nontreatable. The treatable materials are low-, medium-, and high-carbon steels, low-alloy high-strength steels, especially ferrite-hardened and low-carbon martensitic tool steels, martensitic stainless steels, and pearlitic cast irons (gray, alloyed, malleable, and nodular). The nontreatable are work-hardenable austenitic stainless steels (Cr-Ni), ferritic stainless steels, and ferritic cast irons without pearlite (13).

The suitable microstructures in steels and cast iron for optimum laser hardening results are obtained with fine pearlitic structure and smaller grain size initially before heat treatment. Because of rapid heating rate, carbon may not have enough time for diffusion before being fully austenitized for complete transformation to martensite. Therefore, ferrous alloys with coarser grains and coarse graphite and/or carbide structures (e.g., nodular cast iron and spheroidized carbide microstructure) may not be conducive for laser hardening. However, a suitable combination of pearlitic and other carbide structure may promote hardening with relative ease. The quantity of residual austenite in the hardened microstructure plays a vital role in determining the final hardness. The processing parameters need to be optimized to avoid any spurious melting during hardening, which might lead to grain growth and retention of austenite and/or delta-ferrite phases with lower final hardness in the structure. Laser hardening of alloy steels result in greater depths than those of carbon steels, partly due to the lower thermal conductivity of alloy steels than carbon steels and change in hardening temperatures.

Because of the relatively higher quench rates possible using lasers than those obtained by conventional heat treatment techniques, some research findings indicate that there is a tendency for the formation of relatively more restrained martensite with a slight increase in the values of hardness in hardenable ferrous alloys. Also, laser hardening has been found to produce surface residual compressive stresses, which in turn are beneficial to minimize the crack growth tendency in the treated layers, thereby providing better fatigue and wear-resistant properties.

Surface Preparation

The efficiency of the laser heat treatment depends on the absorption of light energy by the workpiece. Any heat transfer calculation for laser processing is based on the absorbed energy. The infrared absorption of metals largely depends on conductive absorption by free electrons. Theoretical absorptivity of metals based on their electrical resistivity has been discussed in Reference (42). For ferrous alloys, it is estimated to be around 15%. Absorption increases when a keyhole is formed due to internal reflections. However, no melting or keyhole formation may be permitted during laser heat treatment. Therefore, some absorbent coatings are almost always used during laser heat treatment. Most commonly used absorbent coatings include colloidal graphite, manganese phosphate, zinc-phosphate, and black paint. A mixture of Na and K silicate is also known to produce high absorptivity. Nonetheless, exact absorptivity of any of these coatings is still a matter of debate.

Arata quoted 50–90% absorptivity for phosphate coatings without melting the substrate and dependency on interaction time (45), whereas Trafford et al. (46) quoted a value of around 70–80% for no-melt situations depending on the process speed as shown in Figure 6.

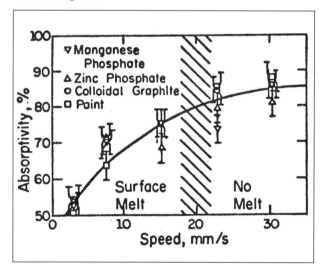

Figure 6. Absorptivity versus scan speed for four different absorbent coatings (46).

For colloidal graphite coating and paint coating, they reported an absorptivity in excess of 80%, whereas Courtney et al. (43) reported a value of around 60% for colloidal graphite coating. Data in Figure 6 were obtained by Trafford using calorimetric measurements for 0.4% C steel. The hatched region in Figure 6 corresponds to an intermediate region between "surface melt" and "no-melt" zones. Courtney et al. determined their absorptivity by comparing the experimental isotherms with the heat transfer model. It is in any case a general consensus that any of these coatings provides absorptivity around or in excess of 80%. The other variables that affect the absorptivity are surface roughness, surface microconstituents such as oxides, and absorbent coating thickness.

The suitability of fiber delivery for the Nd:YAG laser with a relatively shorter wavelength (1.06 µm) with better coupling characteristics than its CO_2 counterpart has been explored for heat treating in recent years successfully (47–49). One of the advantages of fiber-optic delivery is to harden difficult-to-access areas. The absorptivity characteristics as a function of angle of incidence, temperature and type of absorbent coatings or surface treatment such as graphite coat, preoxidizing, sandblasting, and milling for both CO_2 and Nd:YAG laser heat treatments are shown in Figures 7 to 9 (47, 48).

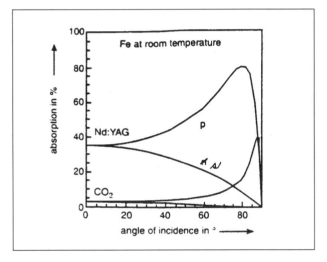

Figure 7. Absorption of iron at room temperature depending on angle of incidence, polarization, and wavelength (47), for the parallel (p) and perpendicular components of polarization.

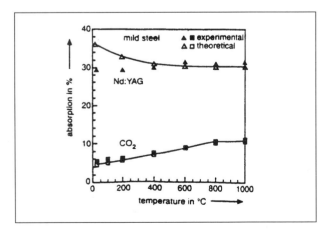

Figure 8. Temperature dependence of absorption in mild steel from the electrical conductivity calculations for CO_2 and Nd:YAG laser wavelengths (47).

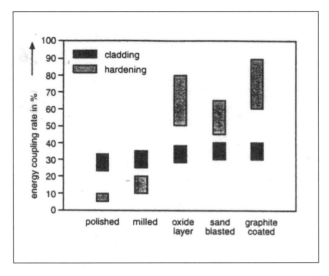

Figure 9. Effect of different surface conditions on the energy coupling rate for laser hardening (47).

7.3.4 Residual Stresses in Laser Heat Treatment

Residual stresses form in the laser-treated surfaces because of rapid thermal heating and constrained cooling due to clamping of the workpieces. The nature and magnitude of these stresses on the surfaces formed during laser processing depend on the type of processing, temperature gradients, and phase-change kinetics. This in turn may or may not give rise to cracking tendency after processing depending on the level of stress, the distribution and nature of the type of stress distribution, and the mechanical strength of the phases present in the laser-treated microstructures. Residual compressive stresses are beneficial to enhance the fatigue resistance because they will help to retard the crack growth. On the other hand, residual tensile stresses are deleterious for the fatigue resistance due to the enhancement of crack propagation rates. Hence it is generally recommended that a simple post-processing step such as annealing or a pretreatment step such as preheating of the base material before laser processing be carried out to minimize the chances of cracking tendency.

Measurement of Residual Stresses

Both destructive and nondestructive techniques are useful in the experimental measurement of residual stresses (50–53). In the former case, the procedure involves the movement or deflection of the specimens treated symmetrically on both sides as a result of the progressive removal of thin layers by electrochemical technique. Such a method results in stress relaxation due to elastic behavior, and therefore the values of pre-existing stresses can be determined after measuring the curvature of deflection. By recording the camber as a function of the removed layer thickness, the residual stress as a function of distance from the original specimen surface can be obtained by analytical techniques. The nondestructive measurement techniques include X-ray or neutron diffraction methods. In general, X-ray methods involve $\sin^2\chi$ technique (χ being the angle between the normal to the surface and the reflecting plane) and chemical etching rather than mechanical methods to avoid the problem of spurious stresses introduced into the surface (54).

Residual stress measurements of the CO_2 laser-hardened steels and cast iron using a destructive technique show that the important variables to assess the final residual stresses are the maximum temperatures reached during treatment, the depth of heating, and the boundary conditions (55, 56). For example, tensile stresses were present in steel samples as opposed to cast iron samples due to the relatively higher surface temperatures required for transformation in the former samples. It was possible to limit the onset of tensile stresses at the surface or to obtain compressive stresses by increasing the interaction time at a given power density. However, such long hold times resulted in less fine martensitic structure and therefore required several other optimum combinations of treatments. Gurkovsky investigated the difference in residual stresses induced by Nd:YAG pulsed laser hardening (PLH) and continuous-wave CO_2 laser hardening (CWLH) on 1045 steel plates (57). The substrate plates were hardened at 830°C and tempered at 520°C to obtain minimum residual stresses before laser-hardening treatment. Residual tensile stresses were found in the PLH samples, while tensile stresses in the CWLH samples for pulsed laser hardening without tempering resulted in reduction of yield, tensile strength, and ductility in comparison with unprocessed samples due to the formation of fragile martensitic structure of high hardness and residual tensile stresses. The hardened specimens fractured in these areas of brittle structure. Tempering at 230°C resulted in better mechanical properties than those in the initial condition. Mechanical properties of CWLH samples were better than those obtained by PLH and tempering. Further, the tempering treatment of CWLH samples at 230°C showed even better mechanical properties because of the presence of fine cubical martensitic structure and compressive residual stress. The distribution of residual stresses is shown in Figure 10 for comparison.

The discussion of selected experimental results as mentioned above illustrate the significance of residual stresses present in the as-processed layers due to laser hardening. It is important to know the residual stress states and their consequences in the component being processed with lasers before it can be used for real service conditions. This factor together with an appropriate choice of either preprocessing (e.g., preheating of the substrate) or postprocessing (e.g., thermal annealing) steps are essential and should not be overlooked in surface treatment and design. There are relatively few research publications on the residual stress estimation of the laser-surface-treated components. Nevertheless, these preliminary efforts provide some basic insights as to the needs for such residual stress measurements to ensure reliability of the processed parts with better mechanical properties.

7.3.5 Laser Heat Treatment Hardness Data

Relevant laser heat treatment data have already been presented in Table 1. Select microhardness data are shown in Figures 11, 12, and 13. Figure 11 shows the typical final hardness values of materials after laser hardening. The hardness values depend on the laser heat treatment parameters as well as the microstructural and alloy composition of the materials being treated. The published research data on hardness characteristics of the laser-hardened alloys include hardness variation along the depth and a single average value or range (see Table 1). Because of the unavailability of sufficient data of the processing parameters with specific hardness values as a function of laser heat treatment conditions (e.g., laser power, spot size, and process speed), the exact values of laser power density and process speed are not included in Figure 11. This figure and Table 1 serve as references for the readers to estimate average surface hardness available for various alloys. The general trend of the hardness data indicates that most of the high-carbon ferrous alloys such as bearing steel (e.g., 52100 steel), tool steels (#18, 19, 20 and 21), Fe-Cr-Mn-C, and Fe-W-Cr-V-C hardfacing alloy steels, have relatively higher hardnesses compared to the low- and medium-carbon and alloy steels. On the other hand, the cast iron materials show some overlap in the hardness values with the low- and medium-carbon alloy steels.

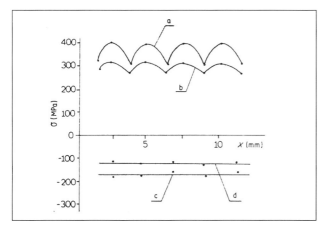

Figure 10. Residual stress distribution in a 1045 steel (initially hardened at 830°C and tempered at 520°C) (57) (a) pulsed laser hardening (1.06 μm wavelength; 30 J energy; 7 ms pulse, diam = 5 mm); (b) with tempering at 230°C after pulsed laser hardening; (c) CW CO_2 laser hardening (P = 1 kW; v = 42 mm/s; width and depth of hardening = 5 and 0.5 mm); (d) with tempering at 230°C after CW CO_2 laser hardening.

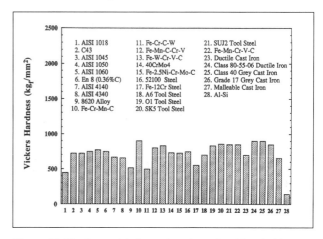

Figure 11. Hardness data for various laser-heat-treated ferrous and nonferrous alloys (12).

Figure 12 shows the distribution of hardness values obtained after laser hardening as compared to induction hardening. The higher values for laser hardening near the surface are due to the much finer and highly restrained martensites in the laser-hardened microstructures compared to the other case.

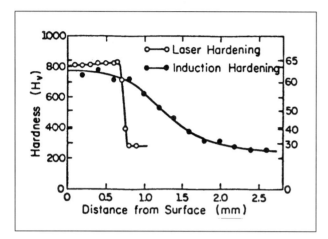

Figure 12. Hardness distribution comparison between laser hardening and induction hardening (58).

The hardness data shown in Figure 13 were obtained along the laser-hardened inclined tracks on a 0.45% C steel cylindrical specimen (quenched and tempered to initial hardness of 65.2 to 66.4 HRA) followed by high-frequency current (HFC) hardening to a hardnes of 76.5 to 81.5 HRA. The CW-CO_2 laser heat treatment conditions used were: power = 950 W; process speed = 10 mm/s; beam diameter = 3.4 mm; absorbent coating = ZnO.

The hardness scale is marked HRA on the y axis. The "HRA" stands for "Rockwell Hardness A." The Rockwell Hardness A is usually measured with a static indentation load of 60kg.

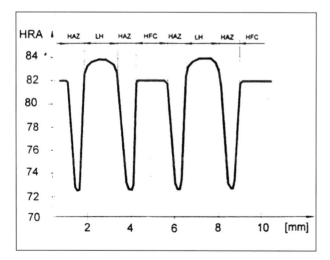

Figure 13. Variation of hardness for (a) HFC, high-frequency current hardening (b) HAZ, heat-affected zone, and (c) LH, laser hardening, along laser treatment direction (59).

References

1. M. Bass (Ed.), in *Laser Materials Processing,* North Holland-Publishing Company, Amsterdam, Chapters 1–5, 1983, Vol. 3, 1–296.
2. G. M. Eboo and A. E. Lindemains, *Proc. Conf. on Applications of High Power Lasers,* R. R. Jacobs (Ed.), SPIE, Bellingham, WA, Society of Photo-Optical Instrumentation Engineers, 1985, Vol. 527, 86–94.
3. B. H. Kear and P. R. Strutt, in *Design of New Materials,* D. L. Cocke and A. Clearfield (Eds.), Plenum Press, New York, NY, 1987, 229–56.
4. J. Mazumder, in *Interdisciplinary Issues in Materials Processing and Manufacturing,* S. K. Samanta et al., (Eds.), New York, NY, American Society of Mechanical Engineers, 1987, Vol. 2, 599–630.
5. R. J. Sanderson, in *Lasers in Metalworking - A Summary and Forecast,* Tech Trans Corporation, Naperville, IL, 1983.
6. J. Mazumder, *J. of Metals* **35** (5), 18–26 (1983).
7. P. A. Molian, in *Surface Modification Technologies - An Engineer's Guide,* T. S. Sudarshan (Ed.), Marcel Dekker, New York, NY, 1989, 421–92.
8. M. J. Pechersky, in *Surface Modification Engineering,* R. Kossowsky (Ed.), CRC Press, Boca Raton, FL, 1989, Chapter 6, Vol. II, 173–91.
9. W. M. Steen, in *Applied Laser Tooling,* O. D. D. Soares, and M. Perez-Amor (Eds.), Martinus Nijhoff Publishers, Dordrecht, The Netherlands, 1987, 131–211.
10. J. I. Nurminen and G. J. Bruck, in *Surface Modification Engineering,* R. Kossowsky (Ed.), CRC Press, Boca Raton, FL, 1989, Vol. II, 193–209.
11. D. M. Roessler, *Mater. Manuf. Proc.* **4,** 285–310 (1989).
12. K. Nagarathnam, in *Processing and Characterization of Laser-Synthesized Overcoats for Surface Engineering,* Ph.D. Thesis, Department of Mechanical & Industrial Eng., Univesity of Illinois at Urbana-Champaign, Published by UMI, Ann Arbor, MI, 1994, Order #9512495, 1–115.
13. R. Saunders, T. Conklin, G. Thomas, W. Shiner, and D. Bennett, in *Lasers-Operation, Equipment, Application, and Design,* J. Bellis (Ed.), McGraw-Hill, New York, NY, 1980, 123–35.
14. N. Rykalin, A. Uglov, I. Zuev, and A. Kokora, in *Laser and Electron Beam Material Processing - Handbook,* Moscow, Mir Publishers, 1988, 1–357.
15. G. A. Abil'siitov and E. P. Velikhov, *Opt. and Laser Technol.* **16,** 30–6 (1984).
16. A. G. Blake, A. A. Mangaly, M. A. Everett, and A. H. Hammeke, *Proc. Conf. on Laser Beam Surface Treating and Coating,* G. Sepold (Ed.), SPIE, Bellingham, WA, Society of Photo-Optical Instrumentation Engineers, 1988, Vol. 957, 56–65.
17. G. J. Bruck, in *Laser Beam Surface Treating and Coating,* G. Sepold (Ed.), SPIE, Bellingham, WA, Society of Photo-Optical Instrumentation Engineers, 1988, Vol. 957, 14–28.
18. R. B. Shingledecker, in *Metals Handbook,* H. E. Boyer and T. L. Gall (Eds.), American Society for Metals, Metals Park, OH, Chapter 28, 1989, 1–63.

19. W. Koechner (Ed.), in *Solid State Laser Engineering,* 1976, Springer-Verlag Publication, New York, NY.
20. D. Belforte and M. Levitt (Eds.), *The Industrial Laser Annual Handbook,* SPIE, Pennwell Publishing Company, 1986, Vol. 629.
21. C. Wick and R. F. Veilleux (Eds.), in *Tool and Manufacturing Engineers Handbook,* 4th edition, Dearborn, MI, SME, 1985, Chapter 13, Vol. 3, 17–22.
22. D. S. Gnanamuthu, *Opt. Eng.* **19**, 783–92 (1980).
23. D. S. Gnanamuthu, C. D. Shaw, Jr., W. E. Lawrence, and M. R. Mitchell, in *Proc. Conf. on Laser-Solid Interactions and Laser Processing,* S. D. Ferris (Ed.), New York, NY, American Institute of Physics, 1979, Vol. 50, 173–87.
24. M. Yes and R. P. Scherer, in *Source Book on Applications of the Laser in Metal Working,* E. A. Metzbower (Ed.), Metals Park, OH, American Society for Metals, 1981, 219–26.
25. C. Courtney and W. M. Steen, in *Source Book on Applications of the Laser in Metal Working,* E. A. Metzbower (Ed.), Metals Park, OH, American Society for Metals, 1978, 195–208.
26. O. Sandven, in *Metals Handbook,* 9th edition, Metals Park, OH, American Society for Metals, 1981, Vol. 4, 507–17.
27. L. S. Kremnev, E. V. Kholodnov, and O. V. Vladimirova, *Met. Sci. Heat Treat.* **29**, 695–98 (1987).
28. H. Kawasumi, in *Source Book on Applications of the Laser in Metal Working,* E. A. Metzbower (Ed.), Metals Park, OH, American Society for Metals, 1981, 185–94.
29. J. W. Hill, M. J. Lee, and I. J. Spalding, *Opt. and Laser Technol.* **6**, 276–78 (1974).
30. J. Kusinski and G. Thomas, in *Proc. Conf. on Laser Processing: Fundamentals, Applications and Systems Engineering,* SPIE, Bellingham, WA, Society of Photo-Optical Instrumentation Engineers, 1986, Vol. 668, 150–57.
31. P. A. Molian, *Mater. Sci. Eng.* **51**, 253–60 (1981).
32. P. A. Molian, *Mater. Sci. Eng.* **56**, 265–69 (1982).
33. P. A. Molian, *Surf. Eng.* **2**, 19–28 (1986).
34. M. Roth and M. Cantello, in *Proc. 2nd International Conference on Lasers in Manufacturing,* M. F. Kimmitt (Ed.), Birmingham, U. K., 1985, 119–28.
35. H. J. Hegge, H. De Beurs, J. Noordhuis, and J. Th. M. De Hosson, *Metall. Trans. A.* **21A**, 987–95 (1990).
36. D. N. H. Trafford, T. Bell, J. H. C. P. Megaw, and A. S. Bransden, *Met. Technol.* **10**, 69–77 (1983).
37. J. E. Miller and J. A. Wineman, *Met. Prog.* **3**, 38–43 (1977).
38. F. D. Seaman and D. S. Gnanamuthu, *Met. Prog.* **108**, 67–74 (1975).
39. G. H. Harth, W. C. Leslie, V. G. Gregson, and B. A. Sanders, *J. Met.* **28**, 5–11 (1976).
40. R. Menin, E. Ramous, and M. Magrini, in *Proc. 4th Int. Conf. on Rapidly Quenched Metals,* T. Masumoto and K. Suzuki (Eds.), Sendai, Japan, The Japan Institute of Metals, 1981, Vol. I, 193–96.
41. E. A. Metzbower (Ed.), in *Source Book on Applications of the Laser in Metal Working,* Metals Park, OH, American Society for Metals, 1981, 227–28.
42. J. Mazumder, *J. of Metals* **34** (7), 16–24 (1982).
43. C. Courtney and W. M. Steen, *Proc. of Int. Conf. on Advances in Surface Coatings Techology,* British Welding Institute, England, 1978, 219–32.
44. V. Gregson, *Proc. of 1st Joint US./Japan Int. Laser Proc. Conf.,* 1981, Laser Institute of America (LIA), Toledo, OH, Paper No. 15.
45. Y. Arata, *Proc. of 1st Joint US./Japan Int. Laser Proc. Conf.,* 1981, Laser Institute of American (LIA), Toledo, OH, Paper No. 2.
46. D. N. H. Trafford, T. Bell, J. H. P. C. Megaw, and A. S. Branden, *Heat Treatment '79,* The Metals Society, London, 1979, 33–8.
47. W. Bloehs, B. Grunenwald, F. Dausinger, and H. Hugel, *J. Laser Appl.* **8** (1), 15–23 (1996).
48. W. Bloehs, B. Grunenwald, F. Dausinger, and H. Hugel, *J. Laser Appl.* **8** (2), 65–77 (1996).
49. B. V. Hunter, K. H. Leong, C. B. Miller, J. F. Golden, R. D. Glesias, and P. J. Laverty, *J. Laser Appl.* **8** (6), 307–16 (1996).
50. A. J. Fletcher, in *Thermal Stress and Strain Generation in Heat Treatment,* Elsevier Applied Science Publishers, New York, NY, 1989, 1–203.
51. A. Solina, V. Bulckaen, and L. Paganini, *Rev. Sci. Instrum.* **54**, 346–52 (1983).
52. R. G. Treuting and W. T. Read, *J. Appl. Phys.* **22**, 130–4 (1951).
53. V. Bulckaen and N. Gucci, *Rev. Sci. Instrum.* **46**, 1402–9 (1975).
54. M. Kurita, in *Proc. of the Inter. Conf. on the Role of Fracture Mechanics in Modern Technology,* G. C. Sih et al. (Eds), Elsevier Science Publishers, North-Holland, 1987, 863–74.
55. A. Solina, M. De Sanctis, L. Paganini, A. Blarasin, and S. Quaranta, *J. Heat Treat.* **3**, 193–204 (1984).
56. A. Solina, M. De Sanctis, L. Paganini, and P. Coppa, *J. Heat Treating* **4**, 272–80 (1986).
57. S. S. Gurkovsky, *J. Mater. Sci. Lett,* **10**, 491–3 (1991).
58. M. Kikuchi, H. Hisada, Y. Kuroda, and K. Moritsu, *Proc. of 1st Joint US./Japan Int. Laser Proc. Conf.,* 1981, Laser Institute of America (LIA), Toledo, OH, Paper No. 12.
59. V. Munteanu, D. T. Levcovici, M. M. Paraschiv, and S. M. Levcovici, *Surf. Eng.* **13** (1), 75–8 (1997).

KARTHIK NAGARATHNAM
JYOTI MAZUMDER

7.3.6 Surface Hardening with Diode Lasers

Today's high-power diode lasers provide a wide range of output powers up to the multikilowatt level. Stacks with output power of up to 4 kW have been used for direct material processing applications. Higher power levels can be achieved by stacking more diode laser arrays. The beam quality and the intensity on the workpiece achieved with diode laser stacks is much lower than that of CO_2 and Nd:YAG lasers. Thus diode lasers are not used for cutting and deep penetration welding applications today. For surface heat treatment applications, however, diode lasers are an excellent tool.

The diode laser is superior to other lasers because of the following advantages. The short wavelength (typically in the range of 790 to 980 nm) exhibits good absorption on metal surfaces and makes the application of coatings dispensable. Since the use of these absorbing layers is critical and cost-intensive, the use of diode lasers improves the hardening process, which can be used more efficiently in industry. Furthermore, diode lasers exhibit a line-shaped focus geometry with a nearly rectangular top-hat distribution, which is favorable for scanning-surface applications. No special optical components, such as beam integrators, are necessary. In addition, a diode laser system requires significantly less space and energy to operate. With an efficiency of up to 30%, the requirements for the power supply and the chiller are decreased considerably.

High-power diode laser stacks are used for hardening of differently shaped parts. This is due to the ability to form the beam size and the aspect ratio by means of different optics. Here, the results of some applications are presented using different lasers equipped with several different optics.

Surface Hardening Using a 2-kW Stack

Samples of ¾-in. flat metal M1044 alloy have been hardened with a 2.0-kW diode laser stack. The carbon content of this steel is specified in the range between 0.4% and 0.5%.

The diode laser incorporates a zoom lens, which enables the user to vary the spot size in one direction, the slow axis, which coincides with the larger dimension of the focal spot. Tracks with different widths have been hardened to demonstrate the performance of the laser and the zoom lens and to determine the best parameters for the process.

The laser consists of single diode laser arrays that are stacked in an arrangement of 2 x 48 arrays. The focusing optic provides a working distance of 83 mm with a numerical aperture in the range of 0.42 x 0.18 to 0.42 x 0.09 depending on the setting of the zoom lens. The dimension of the focus spot varies in the range of 11 x 2.8 mm to 22 x 2.8 mm corresponding to the setting of the zoom lens.

Tracks have been hardened using different power levels and several speed settings. The experiments have been conducted with the 11- and the 22-mm line focus. Figure 14 shows a cross-section of a track processed with an 11-mm-wide line focus, a speed of 300 mm/min, and a laser power of 1.4 kW, corresponding to an irradiance of 4.5×10^3 W/cm^2 if averaged over the area of the focus spot. The actual width of the hardened track is less than 11 mm because of the larger heat transfer into the base material at the sides of the track. This leaves less energy at the limits of the track to heat the material sufficiently. The width of the hardened track is approximately 10.0 mm, depending on the definition of the depth of a hardened track. Furthermore, a slight drop in the depth of the hardened zone in the middle of the geometry can be seen. This is caused by the fact that the two diode laser stacks are mounted next to each other, leaving a small gap between them. Since the emitting surfaces of the diode lasers are imaged to the workpiece, the gap remains visible on the sample.

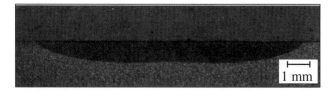

Figure 14. Cross-section of a 9-mm-wide hardened track.

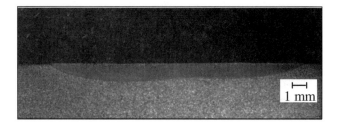

Figure 15. Cross-section of a 19-mm-wide hardened track.

The achieved depth of the hardened zone has to be measured where the gap is located, since only then is the required hardness guaranteed across the whole width of the track. The depth here is 0.65 mm, and the hardness amounts to a Vickers hardness (HV 0.05) of 750 for this sample.

Figure 15 shows a sample hardened with a wider focus line, a speed of 200 mm/min and a laser power of 1.8 kW, corresponding to a mean irradiance of 2.9×10^3 W/cm^2. Here, too, the gap in the middle of the track is imaged onto the workpiece. The width of the hardened track is approximately 19 mm, the depth of the track is 0.7 mm, and the hardness is 650 HV 0.5.

The results of a set of experiments have been monitored measuring the hardness and the width and depth of the tracks. The results obtained with a laser power level of 1.4 kW are shown in Table 3. The hardness of the tracks were measured as 650 HV 0.5 to 750 HV 0.5.

Table 3. Hardening Results Achieved with 1.4-kW Laser Power

Speed (mm/min)	Depth (mm)
300	0.65
350	0.55
400	0.50
500	0.35

Hardening of Cutting Edges

As an example, the hardening of the cutting edges of pliers was demonstrated. The pliers were fabricated from heat-treatable steel with a carbon content of 0.42% to 0.5%. A 1-kW diode laser stack was used for this application (60). The laser was operated with an output power of 600 W, and the feed rate was set to 1000 mm/min.

The focus of the diode laser was oriented in such a way that the elongated axis was parallel to the cutting edge. This way a fairly small area could be hardened. The depth of the hardened zone was 0.9 mm, and the a hardness was 900 HV 0.1. The geometry of the hardened zone can be seen in the cross-section of the pliers (Fig. 16).

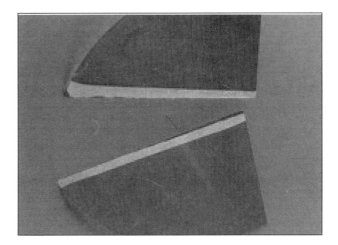

Figure 16. Cross-section of hardened cutting edges of pliers.

Hardening of Rim Geometries

The next example shows that specific tasks can often be accomplished with different lasers and different laser power levels. The example demonstrates the hardening of small rim-like geometries, such as piston rings. First, the hardening was completed with a high-power diode laser stack (61). The output power of the laser was 1.4 kW, and the dimension of the beam on the workpiece was 4.4 by 9.1 mm. A feed rate of 2.1 m/min was chosen, and the track was shielded with argon gas to avoid surface oxidization. The carbon content of the material was in the range of 0.5% to 0.6%. A cross-section of the hardened ring is shown in Figure 17.

The resulting hardness was measured as approximately 800 HV 0.05 with a depth of 0.4 mm. The detailed measurement can be seen in Figure 18.

A similar piston ring with a carbon content of approximately 0.8% was hardened with a fiber-coupled diode laser with an 800-μm fiber and a maximum output power of 70 W. The spot size was approximately 650 μm. The laser power was 60 W, and the selected feed rate was approximately 60 mm/min. No shielding gas was used. With this considerably lower energy input, a hardened depth of 0.1 mm was achieved. The hardness was 650 HV 0.1.

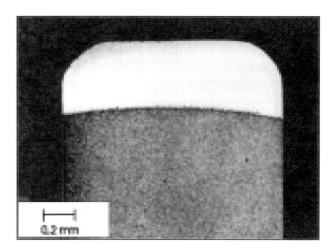

Figure 17. Cross-section of a hardened piston ring.

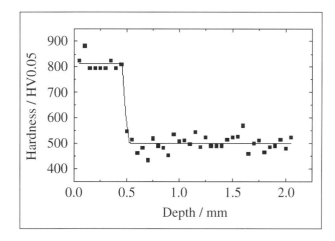

Figure 18. Vickers-hardness through the depth of a hardened piston ring.

References

60. Data and photos courtesy Fraunhofer ILT, Aachen, Germany
61. S. Bonz, B. Brenner, E. Beyer, and F. Bachmann, *Diode laser applications hardening and welding,* Proceedings of ICALEO'98, Orlando, FL, November 1998.

BODO EHLERS

7.4 Materials and Testing

7.4.1 Alloy Effects

Introduction

Laser surface heat treatment has developed into a multipurpose process for generating hard and wear-resistant layers on tools and components for toolmaking and mechanical engineering (1). Especially in the automotive industry, laser beam hardening is widely used for processing large dies for cutting and deep drawing of sheet material (Fig. 1).

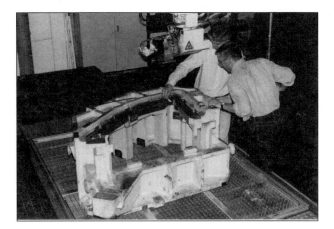

Figure 1. CO_2-laser beam hardening of large tools.

During the process the surface layer of the workpiece is heated to a temperature above the temperature for formation of austenite for a few seconds or less using a laser beam as the heat source. This is called short-time austenitization. The following cooling of the surface layer regularly takes place via heat flow into the substrate (self-quenching) without using any external quenchant. See Section 7.1 for further details.

The maximum temperatures are higher than those achieved using conventional (volume) heat treatments, resulting in the complete transformation and maximum homogenization of the austenite. In practice, however, melted areas or hot cracking occasionally occur. Therefore, further investigations were necessary to learn how to prevent these imperfections. In the following text some experimental investigations are presented concerning the suitability of steels for laser surface heat treatments.

Experimental Setup

Modified Jominy Test: According to the well-known Jominy test for measuring the hardenability of steels, a modified end quench fixture has been developed (Fig. 2). The specified cylindrical specimen (diameter: 30 mm; height: 10 mm) is water quenched on its lower surface, ensuring reproducible cooling conditions while the upper surface is laser beam hardened. The hardening is carried out using a suitable laser, for example, a 2-kW Nd:YAG laser with a spot size of 10 mm diameter with the surface temperature controlled by an optical pyrometer. This setup can be used to investigate the influence of the control temperature T_c and the exposure time on hardening depth, structure, and distortion of the specimen.

Gleeble Hot Tensile Tests: A servohydraulic tension testing machine with conductive heating system known as the Gleeble 1500 is used to determine the mechanical properties of the materials after rapid heating. The specimen is fixed by water-cooled specimen grips made of copper to promote electrical contact and heat transfer. The instantaneous temperature is measured and controlled by a Pt/PtRh thermocouple welded at the center of the specimen. Heating rates greater than 10^3 K/s and accurate temperature control are attainable during the tensile test (Fig. 3).

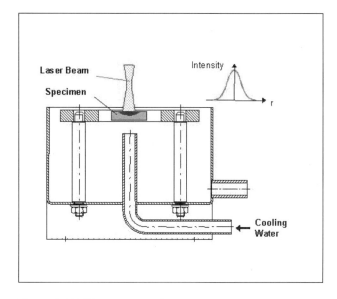

Figure 2. Modified Jominy end quench fixture.

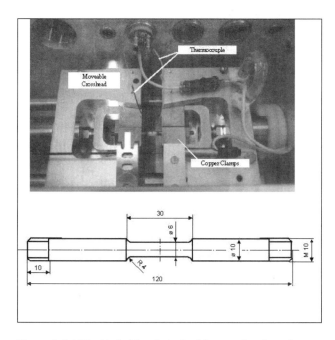

Figure 3. (a) Gleeble-hot tensile tests; (b) geometry of specimens.

Temperature Profile

The conductive heating and heat transfer via the water-cooled clamps result in a parabolic-shaped temperature profile along the x-axis of the specimen, which can be approximated by the equation

$$T(x, T_{max}) = T_{max} - a(T_{max})\, x^2$$

where T_{max} is the control temperature and the parameter $a(T_{max})$ is the axis intercept dependent on the control temperature and weakly dependent on the material. Figure 4 compares the experimentally determined temperatures (points) with the calculated approximation according to the above equation (traced lines).

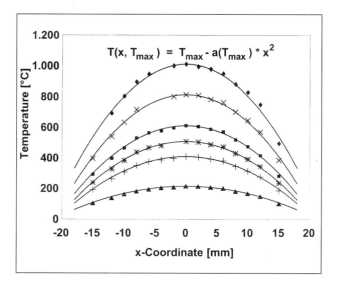

Figure 4. Resulting temperature field for a number of values of T_{max}.

Determination of the Reference Length

In contrast to conventional tensile tests with a constant temperature field, the local deformation is not homogeneously distributed along the measuring section of the specimen due to the temperature profile. Subsequently, the strain measurements cannot be obtained directly from the macroscopic elongation of the specimen (which is measured as the movement of the crosshead). Therefore, preliminary investigations are necessary to define a suitable reference length of the specimen gage length, thereby allowing for the calculation of stress-strain diagrams. Using an automatic microhardness tester, a number of specimens can be marked with a pattern of indentations and deformed with the Gleeble tester within the limit of proportionality. Measuring the deformation of the pattern allows for the determination the local deformation along the specimen for each control temperature (Fig. 5). The major part of the plastic deformation takes place within a narrow temperature range. Unfortunately the reference length depends on the material and changes irregularly with increasing temperature up to the alpha-gamma-transformation temperature.

Results and Discussion

Modified Jominy Test — Hardness Profiles: Based on the modified Jominy end quench test using temperature control, the resulting hardening depth depends on the control temperature and exposure time (Fig. 6). Exposure times of more than 10 s do not increase the hardening depth significantly due to the influence of the cooling water and the resulting stationary temperature field.

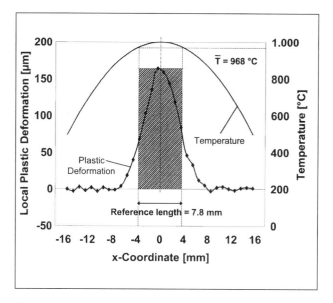

Figure 5. Determination of reference length via measurement of the local deformation.

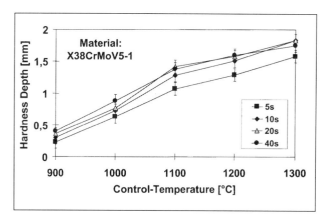

Figure 6. Surface hardening depth (X38CrMoV5-1).

Figure 7 displays the hardness curves for an exposure time of 10 s for four different materials. Plain carbon steels and low-alloyed steels show a marked transition from the high hardness level (even for laser beam hardening) to the hardness level of the substrate. In contrast to the low-alloyed steel 42CrMo4, the plain carbon steel C45W requires water cooling in order to reach sufficient cooling rates for the martensitic transformation and reasonable hardness. The hot working tool steel X38CrMoV5-1 shows a continously increasing hardness profile from the beginning of the hardening depth up to the surface of the specimen due to the increasing amount of dissolved carbon in the matrix. Hardening without external cooling results in lower cooling rates (especially at lower temperatures) and some kind of self-annealing of the martensite (loss of maximum hardness). In steels with higher carbon contents (e.g., the cold working tool steel X100CrMoV5-1) another phenomenon can be observed. If the control temperature exceeds 1000°C, a great amount of alloy carbides can be dissolved, increasing the amount of carbon in the matrix. Consequently the formation of retained austenite leads to a decreased hardness in the outer surface region.

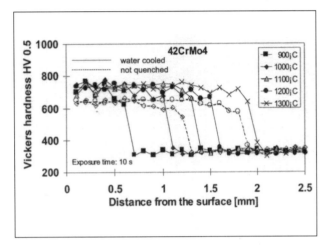

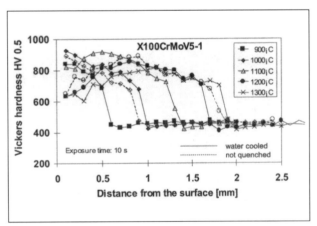

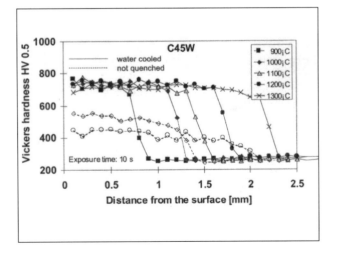

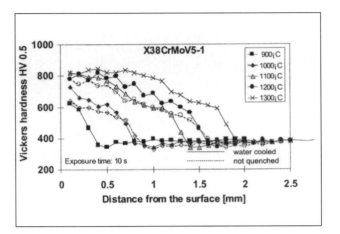

Figure 7. Hardness-depth profiles for different steels and control temperatures.

Grain Size: Figure 8 displays the grain size of the former austenite grains in the surface hardened region with 10 s exposure time for the X100CrMoV5-1. In comparison to the initial substrate grain structure determined prior to heat treatment, the grain size decreases by 1-3 ASTM units when the A_{c3}-isotherm is exceeded. Next to the surface the grain size of the former austenite grains increases due to grain growth at higher temperatures.

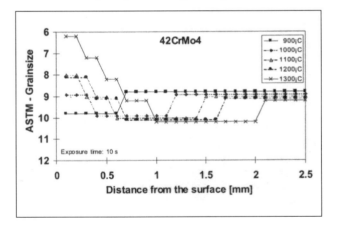

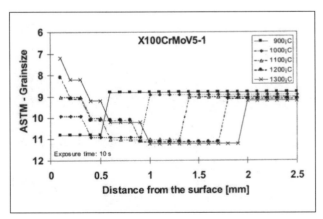

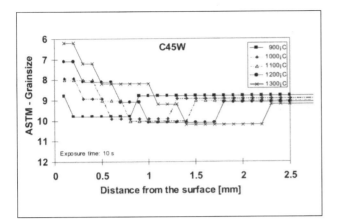

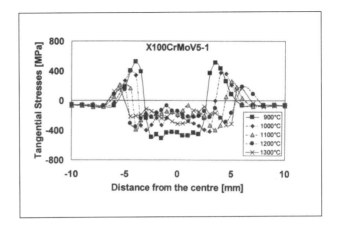

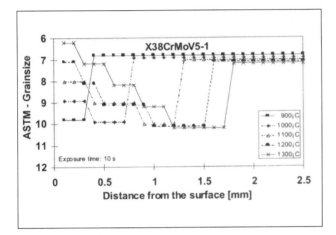

Figure 9. Residual stresses (X100CrMoV5-1, 10 s exposure time) for various control temperatures.

Gleeble Hot Tensile Tests — Mechanical Properties: With increasing temperature the deformation behavior of the material changes. While yield strength and tensile strength are decreasing, the elongation to fracture increases with temperature. At elevated temperatures the material starts losing its work hardening ability. At very high temperatures, the elongation to fracture breaks down from high values to a very low level within a range of 10 K. Instantaneously the mechanism of fracture changes from a ductile behavior to brittle fracture combined with creep effects at the grain boundaries and no visible reduction in cross-sectional area (see below). This tendency is common for all investigated steels after rapid heating and loading.

Figure 10 displays the temperature-dependent mechanical properties of X100CrMoV5-1 with three different structures. The cast structure is the weakest, followed by the annealed structure. The quenched and tempered material has the highest strength. Above the ferrite-austenite-transformation temperature the different initial structures show nearly the same strength with minimal difference between the yield strength and the tensile strength due to dynamic recrystallization effects.

Figure 8. Grain size-depth profiles for different steels and control temperatures.

Residual Stresses: The residual stresses at the surface of the specimen were measured with X-ray techniques. For the radial as well as the tangential stresses the well-known stress profiles can be observed with compressive stresses in the hardened region and tensile stresses in the heat-affected zone close to the substrate (2, 3). With increasing control temperature the hardened area becomes larger, resulting in reduced tensile stresses at the edge and decreased compressive stresses in the center (Fig. 9).

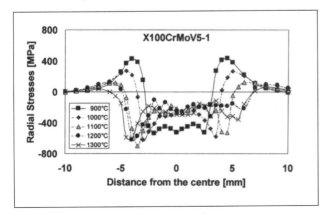

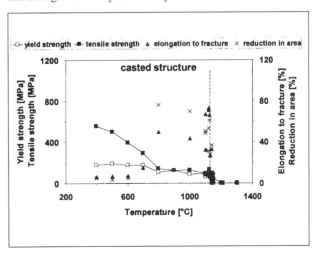

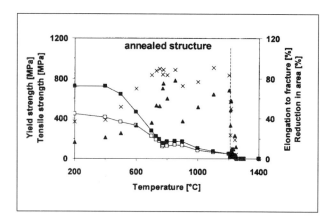

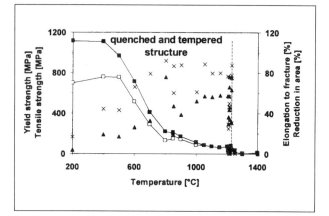

Figure 10. Temperature-dependent mechanical properties for different structures (X100CrMoV5-1).

The most important structural effect for the technical application of laser surface hardening is the difference in the transition temperature from the ductile to the brittle deformation behavior ("zero-strain area"). If this critical temperature t_{crit}, which can be locally different within the material, is exceeded even at one single point, the material may not be able to endure the tensile stresses developed during cooling. A damaged surface or even hot cracking is the consequence. In the practical application of laser beam surface hardening, it has to be guaranteed that the peak temperature does not reach the critical transition temperature t_{crit} of the material.

As Figure 10 shows, the annealed structure and the quenched and tempered structure have a remarkably higher critical temperature. Cast structures do not allow high austenitization temperatures (in short time processes). On the other hand, the diffusion distances are longer to attain sufficient homogeneity of the austenite (compared to quenched and tempered structures). This disadvantage can only be compensated with longer exposure times or repeated hardening. Quenched and tempered structures are most suitable for surface hardening because of their homogeneity (short diffusion distances) and small grain size. The major disadvantage is their hard workability.

Fractography and Structure: Figure 11 illustrates the tremendous changes in the fracture behavior. Testing at room temperature or insufficient elevated temperatures results in a cup and cone type of fracture with moderate reduction in area. The longitudinal section shows a slightly deformed ferritic-pearlitic structure. At higher temperatures the material deforms ductilely, reaching large elongation to fracture and small fracture cross-sections. This results in a dimple-like fracture surface, and a highly deformed structure can be observed. If very high temperatures are applied (close to the melting point of the material), an area is reached where the elongation to fracture decreases rapidly ("zero-strain area"). The specimen fails without any visible reduction in area, even at low stresses. In the SEM picture of the fracture surface single grains with molten grain boundary films can be observed, torn out of the polycrystalline aggregate.

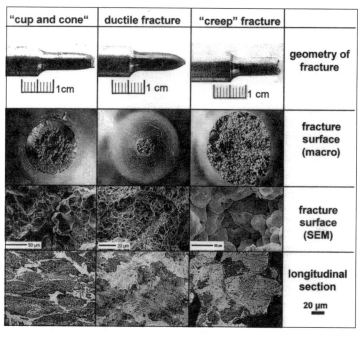

Figure 11. Changes in the fracture behavior (C45W normalized) at various temperature ranges defined in the text. In row 3, left to right, the scales represent 50, 20, and 50 µm respectively.

Conclusions
- Temperature-controlled laser beam hardening has been successfully used in production for many years.
- The modified Jominy end quench test is suitable for testing the qualification of the material for laser beam surface hardening.
- Although the modified Jominy test uses a fixed beam position, the results can be applied for hardening tracks (moving laser beam).
- For crack-free hardening the control temperature should not exceed the ductile/brittle transition for rapidly heated steels.

- Composition and microstructure of the steel must be considered in the choice of the control temperature.
- Inhomogeneous materials (e.g., cast structures) tend to melt at the grain boundaries and therefore are not suitable for laser surface hardening.
- Rolled, annealed, or quenched and tempered structures are preferred because of their homogeneity and grain size. Nevertheless the control temperature must be limited to prevent surface damage and hot cracking.

References
1. H. W. Bergmann and K. Messer, *Stand des Laserstrahlhärtens,* Proc. of the 6th European Conference on Laser Treatment of Materials ECLAT´96, Stuttgart, 16–18 September 1996, 265–76.
2. J. Domes, *Die Ausbildung von Makroeigenspannungen beim Laserstrahlrandschichthärten und anderen Verfahren der Lasermaterialbearbeitung,* Ph.D. Thesis, Erlangen 1995.
3. R. Lin, *On Residual Stresses and Fatigue of Laser Hardened Steels,* Ph. D. Thesis, Linköping, Sweden, 1992.

J. Bach, R. Damaschek, E. Geissler, and H. W. Bergmann, *Härtereitechnische Mitteilungen* **46,** 97–107 (1991).

H. W. Bergmann, H. Stiele, and F. Bohner, *Härtereitechnische Mitteilungen* **52,** 108–16 (1997).

7.4.2 Surface Condition

During laser beam surface hardening the total amount of energy put into the workpiece is very low compared to conventional (volume or surface) heat treatments because of the high power density of the laser beam. Therefore, the distortion that is to be expected is insignificant.

Subsequently laser-hardened tools and components can be finish shaped before the hardening process and afterwards often applied without final work. So the surface preparation regularly consists of cleaning. Depending on the laser system used, it may be necessary to provide coatings or oxide layers to improve the absorption of the radiation.

Coatings

When one uses CO_2-laser systems for surface heat treatment, the absorption of the laser radiation on the metallic surface of the workpiece (which depends on the wavelength, the incident angle of the beam, the temperature of the surface, etc.) is not such that much of the radiation will be reflected. Two different coatings are commonly used to improve the absorption of the radiation:

- Thin oxide layers can be generated by annealing at 300–400°C (for example in steam atmosphere).
- Graphite coatings are easy to handle, but carburizing of the outer surface layer (some micrometers depth) can occur.

The shorter wavelength of Nd:YAG lasers or diode-laser systems provide better absorption on the metallic surface at low temperatures. During the heating process, a thin layer of iron nitrides is developed on the surface, providing sufficient absorption for the laser radiation. Therefore, when one uses Nd:YAG lasers or diode-laser systems, coating of the surface is normally not necessary.

KLAUS MÜLLER
HANS WILHELM BERGMANN

7.5 Surface Properties

7.5.0 Introduction

Improvement in the performance of workpieces, so as to increase the safe life and efficiency of engines and mechanisms, is the main goal of laser surface heat treatment. In order to accomplish this, it is not only important to improve a particular performance characteristic, but to be able to achieve reproducible results with acceptable accuracy. In accordance with this, and also for the systematic accumulation of the information that is needed to create systems to control the laser surface treatment processes, it is best to examine the performance characteristics as the final section of a technological system (see Fig. 1, next page).

As can be seen, the performance characteristics of the workpieces are directly dependent upon the condition and properties of the workpieces's surface layer. These properties can be directly changed by organizing the corresponding physical-chemical processes (heat, thermodeformation, oxidizing, and others), determined by four main variables - temperature (T_h), time (t_h), heating time (V_h), chilling time (V_χ). The needed combination of these variables, resulting from the progress of the necessary physical-chemical process, can be received by registering and changing some of the factors connected with the laser beam, the irradiation conditions, and the treated workpiece. At the same time, there is a definite connection between the parameters of the process and the performance properties of the surface.

7.5.1 Chemical Composition

During the process of laser heat treatment, which can take place with or without the melting of surfaces, the quality of the chemical composition of the surface layer of the alloys does not change in quality. But the distribution of the alloy-forming elements and the mixtures changes in respect to the matrix. Particular interest lies in the redistribution taking place in a solid phase of the alloy elements and the mixtures in the laser heating zone (LHZ) of the alloys. During the pulse irradiation of the high-speed steel, the carbon from the lower layer of the LHZ, where the transformations were taking place in a solid state, migrates to the upper layer (Fig. 2). With a depth of the LHZ at 300 μm, the depth of the lower layer at 150 μm and the length of the pulse at 6 ms, the migration ratio of the carbon is 2.5×10^{-2} m/s (1).

A great redistribution of other alloy elements in this steel, both in the melting zone (MZ), as well as in the hardening zone from the solid state (HAZ), can be seen in Table 1.

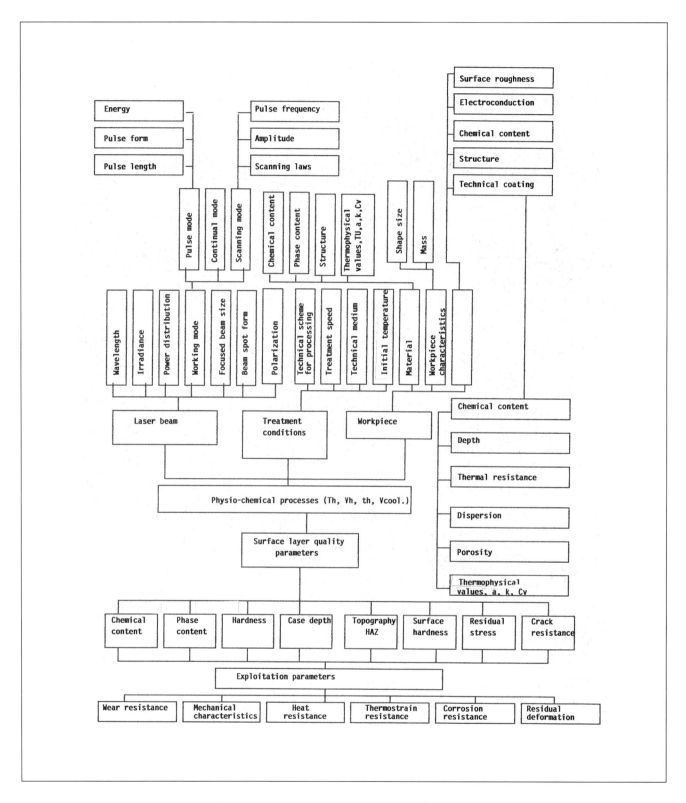

Figure 1. Laser surface treatment as a technological system.

Chapter 7: Surface Treatment: Heat Treating

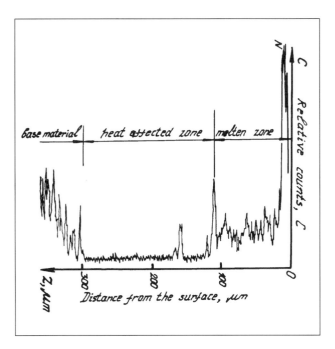

Figure 2. The distribution of carbon by depth in the LHZ in high-speed instrumental steel.

Table 1. The Changing of the Contents of Alloy Elements (in % of mass) in High-Speed Steel during Pulsed Laser Hardening Treatment. MZ: Melt Zone; HAZ: Hardened Zone.

Alloyed elements	Initial content	Treatment without melting	Treatment with melting	
			MZ	HAZ
W	3.8	6.0	5.8	5.4
Mo	6.9	10.2	9.3	8.6
Cr	4.0	3.9	4.7	4.0

The redistribution of the elements greatly depends upon the length of time of the laser heating, and, in particular, during pulse irradiation, from the pulse width τ (Table 2).

Table 2. The Effect of the Irradiation Conditions on the Redistribution of the Alloy Elements (in % of mass) in Mild Steel (0.2% C, 1% Mn, 6% Mo). MZ: Melt Zone; HAZ: Hardened Zone.

Alloyed element	Mn	Mo
Initial content	0.8–1.2	0.5–0.6
Pulse duration		
τ = 1.5 ms		
MZ	< 0.1	0.5–0.6
HAZ	0.4–0.6	0.6–0.7
τ = 4 ms		
MZ	2.6–8.0	< 0.1
HAZ	0.2–0.3	0.6–0.7
Continuous radiation		
MZ	6.4–8.0	0.2–0.4
HAZ	0.4–0.6	0.5–0.6

For most of the different types of steel, a large reduction of the amount of nonmetallic occlusions in the LHZ is characteristic (more than twice the amount).

An unusual mass transfer can be noticed during laser treatment (the power density $W_p = 3 \times 10^3$ W/cm^2; length of irradiation, $t = 0.1$ s) of Armco-iron, saturated with B, Ni, Cr by diffusion to depths of 150, 50, and 50 µm, respectively. After laser irradiation without surface melting, the depth of penetration for B was 1050 µm and for Ni and Cr was 400 µm, i.e., an increase of almost ten times. The migration rates of the elements would correspond to diffusion coefficients of $10^{-5} - 10^{-7}$ m^2/s, which is larger than those for the liquid phase. Because of this, this effect is of an anomalous nature, and cannot be explained by a diffusion mechanism.

On the basis of available information, we can propose that the nature of this feature lies in the stress-deformed state that occurs during laser irradiation. The elucidation of the mechanism of this witnessed mass transfer will make it possible to create new technologies for controlling the properties of the surface layers of the workpieces when applying laser treatment.

7.5.2 Hardness and Its Distribution Along the Surface

The hardness of the surface layer of alloys, and its distribution along the surface and depth has a great influence on the performance characteristics of materials. Under the conditions of laser irradiation, it is determined by the chemical composition and original structure-phase condition of the alloy and by the parameters of the thermal cycle, i.e., the "heating-cooling" cycle.

Information that has been accumulated allows us to formulate some propositions (1):

- Alloys, the hardness of which can be increased by traditional heating treatment, can be hardened by laser irradiation (Table 3–see page 253);
- The high cooling rates make it possible to apply this method for increasing the hardness of alloys that are not hardened by traditional methods of heat treatment;
- The treatment by pulse radiation in comparison to continuous radiation gives less opportunity to control the hardness and the depth of the hardened layer of the alloys (the hardened depth reached when treating with pulse and continuous radiation without melting the surface is 0.12–0.15 and 1–1.5 mm, with surface melting, 0.5–0.8 and 2–3 mm, respectively);
- The hardness of the hardened layer in alloys, which were subjected to bulk hardening treatment before laser treatment, does not differ from the hardness in alloys that were preannealed

- (hardened layers have a greater depth by 20–60% and a more uniform hardness structure);
- The greatest hardness, with uniform distribution, lowering the probability of having cracks and pores in most of the cast irons, is achieved during laser treatment with a low $W_p = (1-5) \times 10^3$ W/cm² and low treatment speed (0.8–1.5 m/min);
- The hardness of the hardened layer in cast irons with a pearlitic matrix is always greater than with a ferrite one;
- Laser hardening of cast irons without surface melting is distinguished by a non-uniform structure and greater spreading of hardness;
- During the same mode of laser treatment, the depth of the hardened layer in cast irons is 20–40% less than in steel;
- The hardness of cast aluminum alloys increases during laser treatment only with melting (eutectic composition by 1.5–2 times);
- The hardness of the hardened layer in aluminum alloys may be raised by 15–20% by doing a subsequent aging treatment at a temperature of 150°C for a period of 15 or more hours;
- Deformed dispersion-hardened aluminum alloys become weaker during laser treatment;
- The hardness of titanium alloys after laser treatment with melting is the greatest with air as a medium; in an inert medium it is 1.2–1.5 times less; without melting there is a greater spreading because of the non-uniform structure; the hardness of the hardened layer in titanium alloys decreases with the increase of the extent of its alloying;
- When hardening large-area surfaces, an uneven distribution of hardness takes place due to the fact that on the boundary of overlapping LHZs in steel and cast irons there are tempering zones with less hardness. In titanium alloys, there are zones of recrystallization with greater hardness. If this is undesirable then it is best to treat with a scanning beam (the width of the hardened zone with evenly distributed hardness can be increased to 16–20 mm);
- When hardening the external and internal surfaces of cylindrical details use toroidal focusing mirrors;
- For some types of steel and cast iron, laser treatment along with preheating the workpiece to the temperature of increased stability of supercooled austenite followed by cooling in water can be used.

7.5.3 Residual Stresses

The thermal processes taking place in the local bulk of the workpiece during laser hardening, and also the structural phase changes connected with them, determine the stress state of the workpiece's surface layers. Because the pure thermal processes (heating-cooling) determine the forming of stretched thermal structures, while structural phase transformations (martensitic) affect residual stress structures, the resulting stress state will be determined by their relationship. The size, sign, and distribution characteristics of the residual stresses depend upon the irradiation mode and the disposition of the hardened zones of the treated surface. During laser treatment of alloys by modes that do not produce hardening (the heating is less than the temperature of phase changes), stretched residual stresses are formed in the LHZ as a result of the pure thermal processes (1) (Table 4).

The zone in which the stress changes is larger than the size of the LHZ, and is symmetrical in relation to its center. The stress is greatest in the zone center, and minimum at the edge. In technically clean steel, during treatment with surface melting, different tensile stresses are formed in the center and on the perimeter of the LHZ (see Table 4). When the density of power increases, the effect of martensitic transformations increases. In the center of the LHZ, the tensile stress transforms into a compressive stress, and on the perimeter they increase as they move away from the center of the zone.

In middle-carbon steel, when a change in the structure and hardness of the surface layer can be noted, during pulse irradiation as well as during continuous irradiation, compressive stresses are formed in the zone's center, and at the edges tensile stresses. The greatest compressive residual stresses are characteristic of those structures with nonuniform martensite, the least for those with partial hardening or with tempered martensite. When the

Table 4. Distribution of Residual Stresses in the Heating Zone of Fe-C Alloys with Continuous Radiation by CO_2 Laser
T_{cr}: transformation temperature; T_m: melting temperature

Material	Beam power (kW)	Heating temperature, T_h	Stress (Mpa) Distance from the center LHZ (mm)						
			0	1	2	3	4	5	6
Carbon steel, 0.45% C	0.5	$T_h < T_{cr}$	380	380	330	150	200	—	—
Carbon steel, 0.8% C	0.5	$T_h < T_{cr}$	260	150	80	-150	-200	—	—
Chromium-tungsten manganese steel, 1% C.1, 1%Cr, 1.4% W	0.5	$T_h < T_{cr}$	450	380	230	-100	—	—	—
Low-carbon steel, 0.03% C	1.3	$T_{cr} < T_h < T_m$	80	0	170	250	170	-10	-100
Low-carbon steel, 0.03% C	2.0	$T_h > T_m$	-60	-40	0	190	210	10	-50
Low-carbon steel, 0.03% C	3.0	$T_h > T_m$	0	-25	25	180	280	220	10

Chapter 7: Surface Treatment: Heat Treating

Table 3. Hardness of Alloys Resulting from Laser Hardening from the Liquid State (MZ) and in Solid Phase (HAZ)

Material	Chemical content, %	Initial hardness Hv	Hardness, Hv MZ	HAZ
Low-carbon steel	C 0.03; Mn 0.05; Si 0.001	100	230–320	170–180
	C 0.2; Mn 0.5; Si 0.27	200	450–500	400–650
Carbon steels	C 0.45; Mn 0.65; Si 0.27	250	700–750	650–850
		440	700–850	700–850
	C 0.65; Mn 1.0; Si 0.27	180	900–1100	1000–1100
	C 0.8: Mn 0.25; Si 0.27	280	1000–1150	1050–1200
High-carbon steel	C 1.2; Mn 0.25; Si 0.25	280	1000–1200	1100–1300
Chromium steels	C 0.4; Cr 1.0; Mn 0.65; Si 0.27	280	800–900	800–850
	C 1.0; Cr 1.5; Mn 0.28; Si 0.25	300	1100–1200	950–1100
Nickel-chromium steels	C 0.4; Cr 0.6; Ni 1,2; Mn 0.7;	320	600–650	700–750
	C 0.12; Cr 0.8; Ni 3,0; Mn 0.5 ;	260	450–500	500–550
	C 0.14: Cr 1.0; Ni 3.0; Mn 1.0	280	700–800	800–900
Silicon-chromium steels	C 0.9; Cr 1.1; Si 1.4; Mn 0.5	700	700–900	950–1000
Manganese-wolfram chromium steel	C 1.0; Cr 1.1; W 1.4; Mn 0.9; Si 0.25	750	1000–1050	950–1100
High-alloyed tool steels	C 1.5; Cr 12.0; Mo 0.5; V 0.25;	780	500–600	1000–1100
	C 0.85; W 6.0; Mo 5.0; Cr 4.1; V1.9;	780	700–1100	980–1200
	C 0.75; W 18.0; Mo 1.0; Cr 4.2; V 1.2	800	700–900	950–1100
High-chromium steels	C 0.2; Cr 13.0; Mn <0.8;	230	660–720	600–700
	C 0.4; Cr 13.0; Mn <0.8	280	830–900	780–820
Grey cast irons	C 2.6; Si 1.2; Mn 0.4; S 0.12;	160	600–800	380–650
	C 2.9; Si 1.6; Mn 1.0; S 0.12	210	850–1000	850–890
	C 3.4; Si 2.0; Mn 0.8; S 0.02	250	900–1100	880–980
Grey cast iron with a higher concentration of:				
S	C 3.5; Si 1.8; Mn 0.5; S 0.2	250	930	250–930
P	C 3.5; Si 2.0; Mn 0.5; P 1.0	220	1180	220–1190
Si	C 3.4; Si 4.0; Mn 0.5; S 0.02	150	1100	150–1100
Alloy cast iron	C2.7; Si 0.3; Mn 1.0; Cr 27.5	—	600	450–600
	C 2.6; Si 2.3; Mn 1.0; Cr 2.0 Ni 21.0; S 0.02; P 0.02	200	450	200–450
	C 3.0; Si 0.7; Mn 0.8; Cr 1.8 Ni 4.2; S 0.06; P 0.06	—	300	400
	C 3.3; Si 2.1; Mn 6.0; Ni 12.0	180	700	180–700
Titanium alloys	Al 4.0; Mn 1.4	280	800–1600	350
	Al 1.5; Cr 2.5	180	780	200
	Al 5.1; Cr 2.0; Mo 1.9	340	750–890	360–500
	Al 5.0; Sn 2.5	300	800	340
	Al 6.0; V 4.6	340	860–890	490–510
	Al 6.5; Mo 3.3	280	600	400
	Al 2.7; V 4.5; Mo 5.0	380	486–510	300–430
Aluminum alloys	Cu 2.2; Mg 1.6; Si 0.8; Ni1.1	170	94–179	170
	Cu 4.2; Mg 1.5; Mn 0.8	152	103–165	152
	Cu 0.3; Si 9.5; Mg 0.3; Fe 0.64	55	86–96	55
	Si 7.0; Mg 0.3	85	95–122	85
	Si 5.0; Mg 0.4; Cu 7.0	84	122–257	84
	Si 12.0; Mg 1.0; Mn 0.5	117	235–265	117
	Si 13.0; Mg 0.9; Sn 0.01; Ni 1.0	109	179–203	109

ISBN 0-912035-15-3

content of carbon in alloys and the degree of its alloying increases, the retained austenite, the saturation of the solid solution and the disposition of the beginning and end point of martensitic transformations have an effect on the stress state. In eutectoid carbon steel in which there is 20–22% retained austentite in its hardened layer, tensile compressive stresses are formed, with values in the range 80 to 270 MPa. In steel with 0.45% of C during the same radiation mode, tensile stresses range up to - 400 MPa (Fig. 3). In chromo-tungsten manganese steel (1% C; 1.1 Cr; 1.4 W; 0.9 Mn), which contains up to 25–48% retained austenite in its hardened layer, the stresses become much larger (- 450 to -700 MPa) than in eutectoid steel. In this case, the dominating effect of the position of the beginning points of the martensitic transformation in relation to the content of retained austentite becomes apparent.

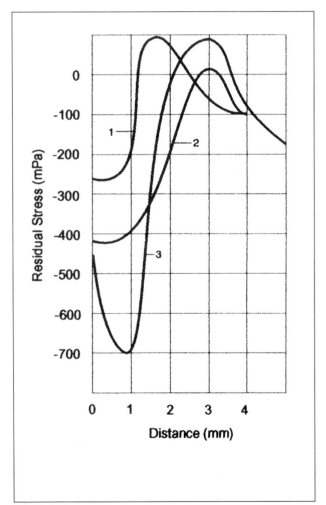

Figure 3. The distribution of residual stresses in the cross-section of the heating zones of steels by continuous irradiation with a CO_2 laser. 1. Eutectoid carbon steel; 2. Steel (0.45% C); and 3. Chromo-tungsten manganese steel.

In high-alloy steels, the effect of the above-mentioned factors is even greater. Because of this, in these steels, during laser hardening at modes different from optimal, tensile residual stresses are formed. Similar factors are characteristic of the changes of residual stresses during laser hardening of cast irons. In gray pearlitic cast iron during laser treatment without surface melting ($P = 0.9$ kW; $V = 0.6 - 1.2$ m/min; $d_o = 7$mm), compressive residual stresses are formed in the center of the LHZ, 1000 MPa, which evenly compresses to 520–550 MPa at the boundary of the zone and to 480–520 MPa beyond it. In high-chrome cast-iron (16% Cr), both with and without surface melting, tensile stresses, which lead to the formation of cracks, occur. In the melting case, along the boundary of the melted zone; in the case of no melting, in the zone itself. Laser treatment without surface melting, with preheating of the cast iron to 400°C, makes it possible to eliminate cracks from being formed, to lower the extent of residual stresses to 300 MPa and to receive an optimum structure with a hardness of 1070 HV.

There are different opinions about the effect on the residual stresses of the initial structure of alloys. There is information that the initial structure has an affect only on the position of the peak of the tensile strength in the tempering zone, and other data that not only does the size of the stress change, but sometimes the sign (1).

The nonuniform distribution of residual stresses within one LHZ (tracks or spots) changes the general stress state of the workpiece's surface layer, which is formed by a combination of such zones. During mutual overlapping of the LHZ, a partial relaxation of the stresses takes place as a result of the formation of tempered zones and the plastic deformation of the heated material of each following zone. The results of the measurements of integral residual stresses in steels and cast irons are shown in Figures 4 and 5 (1).

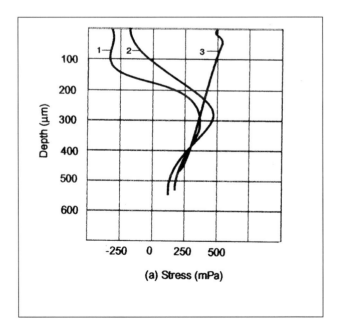

Chapter 7: Surface Treatment: Heat Treating

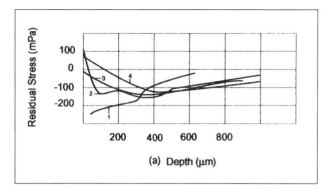

with an overlapping factor of 0.5, during both pulse and continuous irradiation, tensile stresses are formed in carbon steel and ferrite cast iron, mainly in the thin surface layer (Fig. 5).

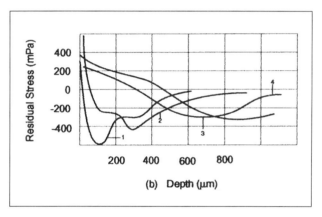

Figure 5. The distribution of residual stresses through the depth z of the surface layer of ferrite cast iron (a) and 0.4% C carbon steel after treatment with pulsed (1, 2) and continuous (3, 4) irradiation (1, 3 without melting, 2, 4 with surface melting).

7.5.4 Residual Deformation

During the laser strengthening of local sections of the surfaces of workpieces, particularly of those that have greater mass, plastic deformation, connected with the changes in their geometrical size and form, is not present. However, if workpieces are being treated that have low stiffness or hardening is being done on large area surfaces, then plastic deformation may be present and fairly large. The size and the sign of the deformation depends upon the length of the sample, the relationship between the thickness and depth of the strengthened layer. If the thickness of the sample is commensurate with the depth of the strengthened layer, then the sample will bulge toward the beam, but if it is much greater (the depth of the HAZ is less than 2–3%), then it will press in. During this, the deformation of samples of carbon steel (0.8% C), the thickness of which is 4 mm, hardened by pulse irradiation to a depth of 140 μm, is 0.8 mm and 0.65 mm for lengths of 25 and 110 mm (1), respectively.

During treatment with continuous radiation, which needs a longer heating period and consequently greater effective depths of the

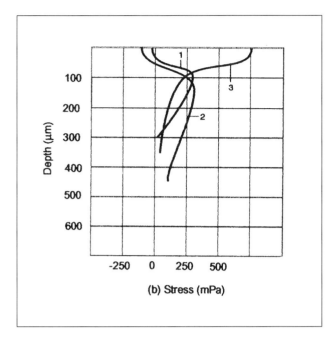

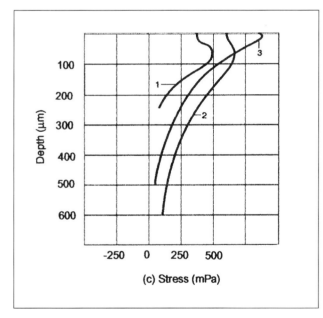

Figure 4. The distribution of integral residual stresses as a function of depth, z, in the hardened layer of different steels: 1-(1% C, 1.4% W, 0.9 Mn), 2–0.8% C, 3-(1.5% C, 12% Cr, 0.5% Mo), at W_p = 20, (a) 60, (b) 200, (c) kW/cm^2.

When arranging the zone of the pulse laser heating with an overlap factor $K_o = 0.7$ ($K_o = S/d_o$, where S is the distance between the centers of two zones, and d_o is the diameter of a single zone), compressive residual stresses are formed only in carbon and low-alloy steel when the treatment is done with melting. When the treatment is done without melting, tensile stress results. During all the different types of operation, in high-alloy steel tensile stresses are formed with different values. When arranging LHZ

HAZ (1-1.5 mm), the plastic deformation may become very large (Table 5).

Table 5. Residual Deformation in Steels and Cast Irons during Hardening with Continuous Laser Radiation

Characteristics of workpiece	Power (kW)	Treating speed (m/min)	Beam diameter (mm)	Deformation (mm)
Grey cast iron size, mm 50x120x1800	2.2	0.6	6.3	- 2.15
Carbon low-alloyed steels, 0.4% C, 1% Cr	2.7	0.3	4.5	- 0.6

The deflection of the sample is almost always toward the laser beam. Outside these above-mentioned factors, the size of the deformation is affected by the initial alloy structure. The harder it is, the more deformation there is. It is sometimes possible to lower the plastic deformation, and sometimes even to eliminate it, if the following approaches are used:

- On the side opposite the one that is being treated, bring in similar LHZs;
- When bringing in the next LHZ, allow a time interval between them;
- Before the laser treatment, introduce a forced bend bulged toward the beam;
- Place the LHZs uniformly and symmetrically on the treated surface.

7.5.5 Mechanical Characteristics

Laser hardening changes many of the major characteristics of the material's surface layer, including its disposition to form cracks, which is the main cause of the failure of workpieces. Pulsed laser hardening of carbon steel (0.45% C) and following tempering leads to, with static tension, a great increase in the limits of its strength and yielding, and to lowering the relative elongation. The raising of the level of the limit of strength and yielding increases with the portion of the hardened layer in the common cross-section of the sample.

The initiation of the failure of carbon and alloy steel samples, hardened by continuous irradiation, begins on the surface in the LHZ. In carbon steels this initiation takes place in accordance with the mechanism of intergranular cracking, and the end of the failure by the mechanism of intragranular transcrystallite chipping. In the hardened zone, in comparison with the initial material, the crack has a stable and relative slow growth.

The fatigue strength of the steel and cast iron samples, hardened with overlap of the LHZ decreases because of the presence of the tempering zones, which are metallurgical concentrators of stress. To eliminate such stress concentrators, it is best to do the laser treatment of the steel in the state of delivery without overlapping the LHZ, so that the treatment step will be wider that the width of the single zone. In this case the fatigue strength of the samples is greatly increased in comparison with standard thermal treatment. For samples of carbon low-alloy steel (0.4% C, 1.0% Cr), hardened in accordance with this scheme with surface melting (the roughness of the surface is 3–4 times less), the number of cycles before failure increases by 10–20 times. Another way to eliminate the tempering zone and to achieve uniform hardness is laser treatment of quick-rotating and forward-moving cylindrical samples (the scanning mode is realized) and also treatment using toroidal focusing mirrors (1).

The laser hardening of alloy steel in accordance with the first method without surface melting ($P = 2.5$ kW, $d_o = 3$ mm, the rate of linear transposition is 0.9 m/min, the rotation frequency is 285 rot/min) results in an increase of fatigue strength in comparison with the standard treatment by 70–80%. The treatment with melting and following fine polishing of the surface provides an increase in the fatigue strength only for low-carbon steel (0.3% C). Laser hardening of steels and cast irons by the second method gives an increase in the fatigue strength of 30%. This is connected with the formation of compressed residual stresses in the surface layer from 364 to 512 MPa (1).

Laser hardening, for low cyclic fatigue cycle modes (15–20 cycles/min), of workpieces of low-carbon steel (0.3% C), makes it possible to increase the durability with relatively small deformation levels (ε) (Fig. 6). At high deformation levels $\varepsilon > \varepsilon_{cr}$ the durability of nontoughened steel is higher than that of toughened. When toughened workpieces are cycled aggressively, the critical level of deformation lowers from $\varepsilon_{cr} = 0.9$ to 0.6. Along with this, the durability level decreases (Fig. 7), exceeding the corresponding figures for nontoughened workpieces. Because of this, laser hardening is best used to increase the resistance to corrosion-fatigue failure of steels, both for plastic and elastic stress.

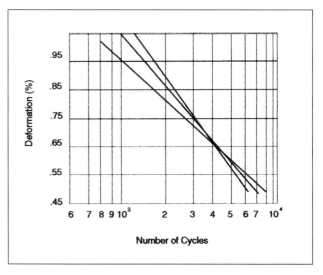

Figure 6. Low-cyclic fatigue of steel (0.3% C), treated with laser irradiation at different speeds in air. (1) 0.2 m/min; (2) 0.4 m/min; (3) 0.8 m/min.

Chapter 7: Surface Treatment: Heat Treating

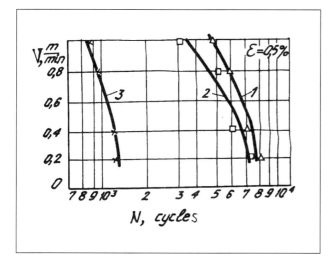

Figure 7. Dependence of steel (0.3% C) low-cyclic durability in air (1), in 3.5% aqueous solution of NaCl and in 25% aqueous solution of formic acid (3) as a function of the laser treatment speed (V).

7.5.6 Heat Resistance

The stability of the structure of the surface layers of alloys, hardened by laser irradiation with subsequent heating, is determined by the chemical composition of the alloys and the irradiation mode. In carbon steels, hardened by continuous radiation with a CO_2 laser at optimum modes with heating of up to 100°C and holding for 1 hour, there are no changes in the LHZ. The increase of the temperature to 200°C leads to a lowering of the microhardness of the hardened layer (Table 6) (1). This is connected with the decomposition of the martensitic hardening to martensitic tempering with the separation of ε-carbides.

Table 6. The Heat Resistance of Carbon Steel and Grey Cast Iron Hardened by Continuous Laser Radiation. MZ: melt zone; HAZ: hardened zone. Entries are Vickers hardness.

Heating temp. (°C)	Carbon steel			Grey cast iron (MZ)	Grey cast iron (HAZ)
	Low 0.2% C	0.45% C	0.8% C		
20	600	800	1200	950	900
100	500	780	1000	950	950
200	400	650	900	980	780
300	300	500	600	1000	700
400	220	320	480	900	500
500	200	240	350	750	380
600	200	240	280	500	320

In steel containing 0.45% C and 0.8% C, outside this temperature range the decomposition of retained austenite takes place. When the tempering temperature is raised to 300°C, in eutectoid steel further decrease of martensite and retained austenite takes place. Besides this, the ε-carbide transforms to cementite.

The hardness of the LHZ greatly decreases. The decomposition of martensite and the transformation of carbide is complete at the heating temperature of 400°C. From martensite, all the oversaturated carbon is separated in the form of cementite. The tetragonal feature of the lattice of the α-solid solution is eliminated and the martensite is completely transformed into ferrite. At tempering temperatures of 500 and 600°C in steels (0.22% C and 0.45% C), the structure of the ferrite changes, the density of the dislocation decreases, the grains become larger, and their form approaches equilibrium. With this the precipitation resulting from the laser hardening process is removed. Further coagulation of cementite takes place in the eutectoid steel.

The structure of the LHZ of high carbon steel is more sensitive to changes in the tempering temperature. The character of the change in the hardness of the LHZ of low-alloy chrome steels, heated at temperatures from 200°C to 300°C, is like the changes in the hardness of this steel after bulk hardening and the corresponding tempering. However, in the first case, the hardness level is always 150–250 HV less. It is noted that during the laser treatment of these steels without surface melting, the stability of the structure of the LHZ in relation to tempering depends upon the initial structure.

Heat resistance of high-alloy chrome steels, hardened by continuous laser irradiation, increases by 150–180°C. In high-speed steels the hardness of the LHZ after heating to 100–500°C and 600–650°C is, respectively, higher by 100–150HV and 250–300HV than the hardness of these steels treated by standard technology.

For cast irons a common mechanism can be seen. The hardness of the LHZ, received after treatment with melting, when heated to 300–450°C (depending upon the chemical composition of the cast iron and the form of the graphite) increases. This is connected with the decomposition of the retained austenite. When heated to a temperature of more than 400–500°C, the hardness of the LHZ greatly decreases because of the tempering processes of the products from the decomposition of retained austenite, the graphitization of cementite. The hardness of the hardened layer in cast irons treated by irradiation without melting lowers after being heated to 200°C (Table 6).

Heating of the casting aluminum alloys, hardened by laser melting, to a temperature of 150°C and subsequent holding for 17 hours, increases their hardness by 20–25%. When heated to 200–300°C, the hardness of these alloys decreases after the first hour of heating, but remains much greater than the hardness of nonhardened alloys after similar heating.

7.5.7 Corrosion Resistance

Corrosion resistance is a function of the properties of the material's surface layer. The main precondition for the improvement of corrosion resistance is to achieve the electro-chemical homogeneity of the surface or the formation of a corrosion-resistant structure.

Laser treatment of cast irons and aluminum alloys during melting makes it possible to greatly increase their corrosion resistance. In gray pearlitic cast iron, after treatment by continuous irradiation with a CO_2 laser and surface melting, a great slowing down can be noticed of cathode and anode processes during electro-chemical corrosion in a 5% mixture of H_2SO_4. This leads to a tenfold increase in the corrosion resistance. This is connected with the fact that in the melted zone, as a result of the dissolution of the graphite occlusions, a galvanic steam of iron-graphite is either absent or its quantity is less.

Laser treatment of austenic cast irons, alloyed with nickel (6–12%) and silicon (2–3%), treated with surface melting, raises the corrosion resistance from 40% to 100% in comparison with the initial state while testing during a period of 1024 hours in sea water. Such an increase is connected with the formation of a small crystal structure. The confirmation of this is an increase in the corrosion resistance of founding aluminum alloys, hardened by laser treatment and tested in neutral alkali and acid environments, and also pure clean iron and chrome steels.

In carbon steels where during laser treatment phase transformations occur, a decrease of the corrosion resistance of LHZ can be seen. The corrosion process intensifies with an increase in the content of carbon in steel. This is related to the formation of a complex heterogeneous martensitic-austenitic structure with a large quantity of small-dispersion carbide occlusions.

References
1. V. S. Kovalenko, A. D. Verhoturov, L. F. Golovko, and I. A. Podchernyaeva, "Laser Surface Hardening and Electric Spark Surface Hardening of Materials," *Journal of Soviet Laser Research,* Plenum Publishing Corporation, New York, NY, p. 276, 1988.

M. R. James, D. S. Gnanamuthu, and R. J. Moores, *Scripta Metallurgica* **18,** 357–61 (1984).

B. L. Mordike and H. W. Bergmann, "Surface Alloying of Iron Alloys by Laser Beam Melting," *Mat. Research Society Symposia Proc.,* Vol. 8, "Rapidly Solidified Amorphous and Crystalline Alloys," R. Kear, B. C. Giessen and M. Cohen (Eds.), North Holland, 463–83, 1982.

A. G. Grigoryants and A. N. Safonov, *Basic Laser Heat Hardening of Alloys,* Vischa Schola, Moscow, p. 159, 1988.

V. M. Andriyakhin, *Processes of Laser Welding and Heat Treatments,* Nauka, Moscow, p. 176, 1988.

LEONID F. GOLOVKO

7.5.8 Wear Resistance

Wear is one factor leading to component replacement, and enhanced wear resistance is often cited as justification for laser installations. Few concrete data are publicly available; for example, hardening of diesel engine cylinder liners was said to result in "greatly reduced" scuffing. Resistance to abrasive wear is generally associated with increased hardness, but other factors shown in Table 7 also have an effect (2). Laser treatment will affect all the factors except carbon content.

Table 7. Factors Influencing Wear Resistance of Steel

Hardness
Carbon content
Microstructure
Carbide volume
Nature of the carbides

To a first approximation, there is no reason to expect that steel of a given hardness produced by laser transformation hardening should be superior in wear resistance to that produced by other hardening processes. Secondary effects might occur; for example, the relative time-at-temperature during the hardening cycle may have minor effects on the microstructure and hence the wear resistance, but at the present time there are no data to support this.

Limited test data are available. A grey cast iron (2.9–3.2% C, 1.7–2.1% Si, 0.5–0.8% Mn) was subjected to two laser treatments; it was transformation hardened, producing a fully martensitic structure, and surface melted, producing a fine, filamentary lebeduritic structure (3). Wear rates of a specimen oscillated with a steady applied load against a silicon carbide pad are shown in Table 8. Both types of laser treatments produced a dramatic increase in wear resistance.

Table 8. Wear Rates of Untreated and Laser-Treated Cast Iron

Untreated material	1.1×10^{-11}
Hardened material	2.5×10^{-12}
Surface melted material	2.2×10^{-12}

Units: cm^3 of material removed per kg load per cm of distance moved

References
2. T. S. Eyre, "Wear Characteristics of Metals," in *Tribology International,* Vol. 9, Oct. 1976, reproduced in *Source Book on Wear Control Technology*, D. A. Rigney and W. A. Glaeser (Eds.), American Society of Metals, Metals Park, OH, 1978.
3. D. N. H. Trafford, T. Bell, H. H. P. C. Megaw, and A. S. Bransden, *Metals Technology* **10,** 69–77 (1983).

VIVIAN E. MERCHANT

7.6 Applications of Heat Treating

7.6.1 Steering Gear Assemblies

The first commercial production application of laser heat treating is an excellent example of the cost effectiveness of the laser's localized heating benefit.

Originally designed as a batch furnace heat treat process, the automobile power steering pumps shown in Figure 1 became a subject for process improvement as the cost of energy made a 24-hour furnace schedule expensive.

Chapter 7: Surface Treatment: Heat Treating

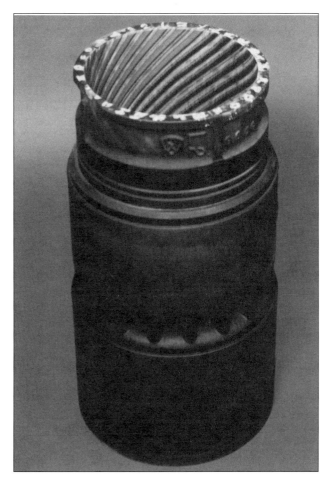

Figure 1. This auto steering pump has laser-hardened tracks to prevent piston scuffing.

Rather than through heating 5 kg of ferritic malleable cast iron, engineers at the steering gear division of a U.S. auto company decided to produce a localized wear-resistant surface on the inner bore of the pump housing, as protection against expected wear from the piston operating under heavier loads.

They could have changed to a tougher material, but this would have increased machining costs. Other hardening processes such as nitriding and tuftriding required an intermediate ancillary operation prior to final machining for concentricity.

Wear pattern analysis suggested that selective bore hardening would eliminate wear. Conventional induction hardening, which successfully produced a hardness pattern, caused excessive distortion of the bore diameter that would have necessitated a costly post-heat-treat honing operation.

Experiments with a defocused CO_2 laser beam indicated that a series of five hardened tracks, strategically placed, would produce sufficient wear resistance without part distortion. In practice, the beam from a kilowatt-level CO_2 laser is directed through a rotating optic device to the inside bore of the pump housing. A disposable, piston-mounted, mirror is sequenced up and down so the beam produces vertical stripes on the steering gear bore. A large-diameter, low-power-density spot of laser light produces the heat required to transformation harden a 2.5-mm-wide track to a depth of 0.35 mm. For an energy consumption analysis, approximately 2.5 g of cast iron need to be hardened, as opposed to the total 5 kg necessary in the furnace heat-treat method.

Low-power-density CO_2 laser beams are reflected by the smooth cast iron surface with reflectivity in excess of 92%. Thus an absorbent coating would normally be applied to couple laser energy long enough to cause the surface temperature to rise to a level where increased absorption occurs. For this application a preapplied manganese phosphate coating (required for rust prevention in downstream operations, and subsequently removed by machining) works for the purpose.

At one time 20 CO_2 lasers, powering dual workstations, were employed to harden 35,000 housings per day. Today, some 20 years later, this application, accomplished with 13 laser systems, is still in use at the auto component plant.

7.6.2 Diesel Engine Cylinder Liners

Fuel used to feed railroad diesel engines can vary in composition depending on the source of production. One trace element that can cause scuffing on the bore wall of malleable cast iron cylinder liners is vanadium, which abrades the smooth bore surface as the piston moves up and down the 68-cm bore length.

To compensate for wear scuffing from vanadium and other impurities, such as high sulfur content, a U.S. manufacturer of railroad diesel engine locomotives considered several ways to protect the bore from wear. The first, and most logical, choice was chrome plating, which provided a smooth, tough, chemically resistant, surface. Unfortunately, the chrome plating process produces severe environmental problems, specifically in treating the effluent from the process. Based on the engine volumes produced at the time of analysis, chrome plating liquid treatment and disposal would cost $250,000/year.

Other ways to produce a harder cylinder wall surface were explored. Among these were salt bath nitriding, induction heating, and laser transformation hardening.

The nitriding process did not produce the required hardened case depth, and the high process temperature of the salt bath distorted the bore and caused deterioration of the braze joints in the water jacket.

Induction heating did produce the required case depth, but the lack of control indexing the inductor along the walls of the 22-mm bore diameter caused an excessive bore distortion from overheating.

Based on the success of the steering pump hardening process, discussed above, engineers from the diesel engine plant, a sister to the auto division, conducted successful tests with their kilowatt CO_2 laser. As a result, an order was placed for 5-kW CO_2 lasers that could produce 500 cm² of 1-mm-deep hardened case in one min.

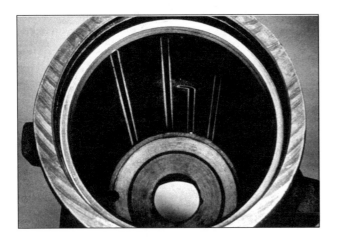

Figure 2. Laser hardening of this cylinder liner prevents wall scoring from abrasive fuels.

Because the cylinder liner shown in Figure 2 is too heavy for easy movement, a rotating beam delivery unit with a molybdenum mirror as the last optical element delivers an integrated rectangular beam onto the bore surface, producing a helical pattern. In this manner a hardened track of 0.7 mm case depth is presented, at all times, to the moving piston.

The machined cast iron surface is coated with a black enamel paint, sprayed on before laser treatment, which acts as an absorbing coating to couple the CO_2 energy into the surface. This paint is evaporated by the laser heat, leaving a clean surface that serves as a quality control check to validate the process.

Uniform case depth, even in areas where water cooling passages thin the cylinder wall, is obtained by the selective, localized heating effect of the laser beam. The increased hardness and small grain structure produced by the rapid heating and cooling effect of the laser process produces a superior wear resistance. This is proven by extended cylinder liner maintenance schedules.

DAVID A. BELFORTE

7.6.3 Turbine Blade Hardening

Another important application of laser heat treating involves hardening of blades for steam turbines. Turbine blades are eroded by water droplets during turbine operation. Other approaches to increase the hardness of the blades, like flame hardening or cladding with a hard metal-like stellite, have various disadvantages.

Laser heat treating has been used to harden turbine blades to reduce erosion and to increase their lifetime. This application has been in use for some time. In one typical investigation (1), turbine blades were hardened with a 6-kW CO_2 laser. The hardening track was 30 mm wide, and the speed was between 150 and 400 mm/min. The coverage rate could be as high as 120 cm²/min.

The hardened blades exhibited significantly reduced mass loss after 1.5 million revolutions, in comparison with the results of other hardening technologies. The laser-hardened blades had excellent wear properties and high fatigue strength. Extended life tests of the laser-hardened blades in steam turbines proved that the blades meet all requirements. Laser hardening of turbine blades have been used in several countries for a number of years.

Reference
1. E. Brenner and W. Reizenstein, *Industrial Laser Review*, p. 17, April 1996.

JOHN F. READY

7.7 Comparison with Other Technologies

7.7.1 Advantages/Disadvantages

Because of the directional nature of laser light, laser transformation hardening can be applied to specific areas of a workpiece. As a result, the heat input to the workpiece is minimal, resulting in low distortion.

Other technologies for case hardening are listed in Table 1. The chief disadvantage of laser hardening with respect to the other technologies is the high initial cost of the equipment. Also, it cannot cost effectively be applied to harden large areas. For small areas, it may be the method of choice.

Table 1. Other Technologies for Case Hardening

Flame hardening
Furnace hardening
Induction hardening
Gas carburizing

Flame Hardening

A torch such as oxy-acetylene is used to heat a nonlocalized area of the part to be hardened. The power density is low compared to laser hardening, and the heat is applied for a significant time period. Heat is conducted deep into material, and a liquid quench is usually required to produce the high cooling rates necessary to result in hardening. It is usually manually applied and leads to inconsistency in the hardness and depth of hardening due to poor control of flame and material temperature and positioning of the flame.

Furnace Hardening

The object to be hardened is heated in a furnace, and subsequently liquid quenched to produce hardening. Furnace hardening is slow and energy intensive, but has the advantage that very large objects can be hardened, and that the same equipment can be used for other operations, for example, annealing. Furnaces may be bulky, require considerable floor area, and make the whole work area uncomfortably warm. For irregularly shaped parts, the cooling rate as a function of depth, and the resulting hardness, is difficult to control and/or predict.

Induction Heaters

Induction heaters for case hardening have low capital and maintenance costs, and often require little floor space. The total energy input to the workpiece is higher than in laser heat treating, resulting in the possibility of workpiece distortion. The process is not easily adaptable to irregularly shaped workpieces, as the scanning coil must be located consistently close to the surface. Variations in the coil-to-work-surface air gap will adversely affect the resulting hardness and depth of hardness.

Gas Carburizing

Gas carburizing requires a long process time for the carbon to diffuse into the steel; as a consequence it is only cost effective with large batch lots. In carburizing selected regions of a workpiece, the regions not being carburized have to be masked off, with the masking subsequently removed in a secondary operation. Only certain grades of steels are amenable to gas carburizing. For these steels, however, a consistent hardening occurs, with no workpiece distortion.

7.7.2 Economic Considerations

Generally speaking, the economics of different hardening processes can only be compared on a case-by-case basis. Comparative costs of the hardening processes cannot be considered separately from the comparative costs of preparing the material for hardening and the cost of subsequent operations. A negative cost consideration for laser hardening is the need to pretreat the surface with paint to enhance the absorption of the beam, and the need subsequently to remove the remnants of the paint. A positive cost consideration is the absence of any post-hardening machining operation to correct for distortion.

The economics cannot be separated from the job requirements. If a high degree of consistency of hardening is not required, the less expensive flame hardening process can be used.

The high capital equipment cost for laser hardening is a disadvantage except when the equipment is fully utilized, for example, in a job shop environment where the equipment can be used for other functions, or in a high-production environment where the equipment cost prorated over the annual production results in a small value per part.

For hardening of gears, cost comparisons between laser hardening and gas carburizing are available. In an environment where the laser is busy two shifts per day, laser treatment was shown to be cost effective for large gears where a limited area was to be treated. One manufacturer that replaced gas carburizing with laser hardening cites the reasons given in Table 2 (1).

Table 2. Factors in Cost Effectiveness of Laser Hardening

1. Reduced hardening time
2. Reduced scrap rate
3. Elimination of complex quenching, plating, masking, stripping, and cleaning steps
4. Reduced work-in-progress inventory
5. Quicker turnaround, less material handling
6. Reduced floor space requirements
7. Reduced pollution by elimination of copper plating
8. Reduced energy use

References

1. M. A. Howes, "Lasers Can Replace Selective Carburization Economically," in *Laser Surface Modification,* Proceedings from the 1988 Conference, New Orleans, April 14–15, 1988, American Welding Society, Miami, FL, 43–60.

F. D. Seaman, "New Developments in Laser Surface Modification," *The Industrial Laser Annual Handbook*, D. Belforte and M. Levitt (Eds.), PennWell Publishing Company, Tulsa, OK, 1990.

VIVIAN E. MERCHANT

Notes

Chapter 8

Surface Treatment: Glazing, Remelting, Alloying, Cladding, and Cleaning

8.0 Introduction

Chapter 7 has described surface treatment involving phase transformation without melting of the surface. This has been the most widely used type of laser-based surface modification.

This chapter will discuss other methods of surface modification that do involve melting or vaporization. A number of these approaches involve melting only of the surface. These approaches include techniques like glazing and remelting, which use very rapid heating, melting, and cooling to modify the surface properties, and alloying and cladding, which involve melting of the surface plus material added to the surface to form a modified surface layer. Because of the importance of the rapid melting process, the chapter includes information on the basic physical processes, including convection in the melt pool and microstructures formed during rapid quenching of the melt.

The chapter also describes some methods that use lasers to clean surfaces. These methods generally involve vaporization or ablation of material.

JOHN F. READY

8.1 Rapid Melting

8.1.1 Melting Kinetics

Many of the applications described in this chapter depend on the process of rapid melting of a surface by laser irradiation. By rapid melting and subsequent rapid resolidification we mean that only a thin layer near the surface is melted. In contrast to welding applications, in which one desires penetration of heat into the volume of the workpiece, usually all the way through the workpiece, here one desires the heat to be confined near the surface. Also, one desires that the surface not begin to vaporize. Thus the time scale for these interactions is very short.

In this section, we discuss some of the physical phenomena that occur during this process. In the next section, we describe how the rapid resolidification affects the grain size near the surface.

When a laser beam with high irradiance is rapidly scanned over a metal surface, it produces a thin layer of molten material near the surface. The high energy density leads to localized surface melting with efficient use of the energy for melting. Thus almost all the energy is used for melting, and only a small amount is lost to subsurface heating. One maintains a cold subsurface while melting a thin surface layer. This leads to very rapid quenching of the molten material by conduction into the substrate after the end of the short irradiation.

For a Gaussian beam with radius d delivering an absorbed irradiance of F W/cm^2, beginning at time $t = 0$, to a surface initially at temperature T_0, the temperature at the surface and at the center of the beam is

$$T(t) = [Fd \tan^{-1}(4kt/d^2)^{1/2}]/\pi^{1/2}K$$

where k is the thermal diffusivity and K the thermal conductivity. Differentiating with respect to time, one obtains for the rate of change of temperature

$$dT(t)/dt = 2Fd^2k^{1/2}/\pi^{1/2}Kt^{1/2}(d^2 + 4kt)$$

With easily attainable conditions, one can obtain very rapid heating rates, around 10^8 K/s.

The time t_f to reach the melting temperature T_f is given, for a uniform absorbed irradiance F at the surface of a semi-infinite solid as

$$t_f = \pi K \rho c (T_f - T_0)^2 / 4F^2$$

where ρ is the density and c the heat capacity per unit mass. For many applications involving surface modification, one desires to treat relatively large areas at one time, so that the assumption of uniform irradiance is reasonable.

Table 1 presents calculated results for the time to reach the melting temperature for several metals at different values of irradiance. This time can be very short, often in the submicrosecond regime.

Table 1. Time t_f to Reach Melting Temperature

Metal	$F = 10^5$ W/cm^2 t_f (μs)	$F = 10^6$ W/cm^2 t_f (μs)	$F = 10^7$ W/cm^2 t_f (μs)
Aluminum	210	2.10	0.021
Copper	1350	13.5	0.135
Iron	649	6.49	0.0649
Nickel	565	5.65	0.0565
Titanium	90.9	0.909	0.00909
Tungsten	4190	41.9	0.419

It is possible to obtain a rough estimate for the depth melted by assuming that there are no losses of energy, that is, that all the incident energy goes toward heating and melting the given depth of material. This is in fact a reasonable assumption; in the rapid heating regime there is relatively little energy lost by thermal conduction out of the volume in which it is deposited. Also one does not desire vaporization of the surface to begin. Then the maximum depth melted will occur at the time t_v at which the surface just reaches its vaporization temperature.

ISBN 0-912035-15-3

The time t_v may may be calculated using an equation similar to that for t_f above, that is

$$t_v = \pi K \rho c (T_v - T_0)^2 / 4F^2$$

where T_v is the vaporization temperature. This equation neglects the latent heat of fusion. One may argue that the latent heat of fusion is small compared to the amount of heat required to raise the material to its vaporization temperature, that is, the integral of the heat capacity from T_0 to T_f plus the integral from T_f to T_v. For example, in aluminum, the latent heat of fusion is 2550 cal/mol and the heat content represented by the integrals of the heat capacity is 19,370 cal/mol. But the latent heat of fusion represents a nonlinearity in a moving boundary-value problem; so neglecting it, even though it is relatively small, could introduce an error. Thus this approach cannot be considered as giving more than a rough approximation.

For a better solution, one must solve the heat flow equation in both the solid and liquid regions, with the condition of conservation of energy at the moving boundary between solid and liquid. The general problem cannot be solved analytically. There have been solutions obtained by analog computer techniques and by finite-difference methods.

The maximum melted depth D may be estimated from an equation that essentially represents an energy balance, in which the energy input is equated to the total energy required to raise that depth to the vaporization temperature

$$F t_v = \rho D [c (T_v - T_0) + H_f]$$

where H_f is the latent heat of fusion. One first solves the equation for t_v and then this last equation for D. Table 2 presents some calculated values for t_v and D for several metals and for different values of the absorbed irradiance.

Table 2. Time t_v to Reach Vaporization Temperature and Maximum Depth D Melted

	$F = 10^5$ W/cm²		$F = 10^6$ W/cm²		$F = 10^7$ W/cm²	
Metal	t_v (µs)	D (cm)	t_v (µs)	D (cm)	t_v (µs)	D (cm)
Al	3670	0.045	36.7	0.0045	0.367	0.00045
Copper	8260	0.066	82.6	0.0066	0.826	0.00066
Iron	1860	0.0102	18.6	0.00102	0.186	0.000102
Nickel	1840	0.0106	18.4	0.00106	0.184	0.000106
Titanium	319	0.0027	3.19	0.00027	0.0319	0.000027
Tungsten	10,460	0.059	104.6	0.0059	1.046	0.00059

Table 2 indicates that the time to reach vaporization temperature may also be very short, less than a microsecond as the irradiance becomes high. The value of D decreases as the irradiance increases. This may seem paradoxical, but it results from the fact that the time available for heating without surface vaporization becomes very short as irradiance increases. The value of D is also very small, in the micrometer regime as the irradiance becomes high.

References
M. I. Cohen, *J. Franklin Inst.* **283**, 271 (1967).
J. F. Ready, *Effects of High Power Laser Radiation,* Academic Press, New York (1971).

JOHN F. READY

8.1.2 Absorption Mechanisms
In the solid state only a small part of the energy of the laser is absorbed, but upon melting, absorption increases significantly because of two important mechanisms: avalanche ionization and multiphoton absorption and ionization. Both mechanisms are capable of imparting large amounts of thermal energy into normally transparent liquids, much larger than that occurring through classical absorption. In both cases, neutral liquid molecules are ionized in the presence of the laser irradiation. The resulting free electrons form a nonthermal plasma that can result in extremely high absorption of the incident energy.

Avalanche ionization results when the initially free electrons in the liquid oscillate and gain energy in the electric field of the laser radiation. Collisions with neutral liquid molecules result in ionization and the generation of more free electrons, after which the process repeats. Avalanche ionization begins to become important once the threshold irradiance, I_t, is exceeded. If more than several percent of the liquid atoms are ionized, breakdown can occur, resulting in a spark and shock formation in the liquid. Breakdown irradiances vary widely, typically $10^7 - 10^{11}$ W/cm², depending on the wavelength and liquid. Multiphoton absorption and ionization occur at comparable irradiances, and result when a liquid molecule absorbs two or more photons, after which the molecule can ionize or dissociate. The resulting ionized electrons can absorb very strongly, in a fashion similar to avalanche ionization.

The threshold irradiance and dominating mechanism depend strongly on the wavelength, pulse duration, and liquid. In general, a given liquid must be characterized experimentally to determine I_t and the effective nonequilibrium absorption coefficient.

8.1.3 Effects of Convection
The portion of the liquid that the laser irradiation passes through is changed in two ways. First, the temperature of the liquid increases as a result of absorption of the laser irradiation, causing variations in the density and surface tension. Second, charged particles can be created in the liquid from ionization and dissociation processes, possibly altering the surface tension and initiating flow.

In the bath melted by a laser, a temperature gradient exists on the surface: The hottest region is that under the laser beam; the coldest, the region close to the liquid/solid contact area. In addition a temperature gradient extends into the depth of the bath. The surface temperature gradient is the cause of tension between the various areas of the surface, which in turn leads to a flow of liquid to the edges of the molten strip. The shear forces and the temperature gradient into the melt cause the liquid to advance toward the lower layers of the bath.

Chapter 8: Surface Treatment: Glazing, Remelting, Alloying, Cladding, and Cleaning

In addition to the effect of the temperature gradient on the flow, influence is also exerted by the pressure on the surface and by gravity. However, in laser treatment with no plasma present (laser irradiance up to 10^6 W/cm^2), the influence of the pressure is negligible, and the effective forces are:

Volume forces: temperature dependent/composition dependent
Surface forces: temperature-induced tension/composition induced

Mathematical models for analyzing the temperature field and the flow pattern (1–7) enable estimation of their effects on the geometry of the molten bath, on the distribution of the temperature therein, and the quality of the surface, as will be explained in the following. Convection has also been described in Section 5.4.4.

The Flow Profile

The nature of the flow (see Fig. 1) is determined by the temperature-effected changes in surface tension (γ) and by shifts (deformations) of the surface. If the latter are neglected (i.e., the surface is assumed to be flat), the flow profile takes the form illustrated in Figure 2.

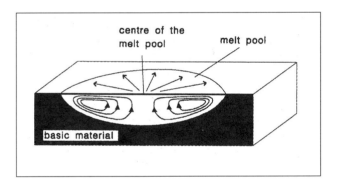

Figure 1. Melt pool convection for negative surface tension (3).

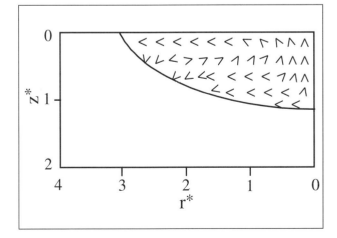

Figure 2. Convection flow profile in a laser-melted bath (1). Here Z^* is dimensionless depth, $Z^* = zr_0$, where r_0 is the radius of the laser beam and r^* is dimensionless radius, $r^* = r/r_0$.

That profile applies as long as $d\gamma/dT$ is negative (as it is, e.g., in metals), but if the surface tension increases as the temperature rises, the direction of flow is reversed.

The flow is directed radially outward from the center of the laser beam to the external field of the melt. At the edge of the molten bath the direction of the flow is downward, along the contact area, liquid/solid, to the bottom of the bath, and from there upward, closing the circle while preserving the mass (Fig. 1). Recently, this flow pattern has been proven experimentally (3).

The flow profile depends on the ratio between the diameter of the laser beam and the depth of the bath, as shown in Figure 3 (2).

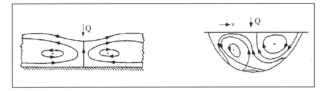

Figure 3. Flow profile: (left) in a shallow bath and (right) in a deep bath (2).

In a deep bath (Fig. 3b) intensive mixing of the melt takes place, although at its bottom a boundary zone exists, in which the flow is less effective. In Figure 4, which shows the microstructure for the two cases, flow lines are discernible that, qualitatively, correspond to those that are depicted in Figure 3.

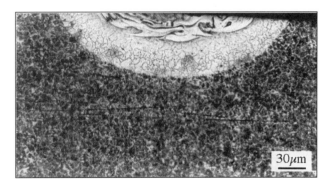

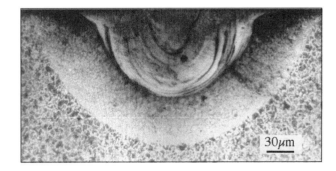

Figure 4. Flow profile in CW-CO$_2$ laser alloying. (top) Shallow bath and (bottom) deep bath.

The ratio between the depth of the bath and its width is also represented in the influence of the gravitational forces on the flow as compared with the contribution of the surface tension. In the case of a beam smaller than 1 mm (e.g., in welding) the forces of surface tension dominate, but in surface treatments with a wide beam, the model for calculating the flow must also take account of the gravitational forces and their effect on the flow profile. In cross section the flow profile is a function of the scan speed of the laser (7). Raising the scan velocity of the laser leads, on the one hand, to an increase in the flow velocity on the surface, on the other hand to a smaller bath depth, which slows the flow because of gravitational forces and the higher viscosity of the melt. Hence at the beginning of the scan velocity increase, the surface flow accelerates to a maximum of 2.7 m/s and then slows to values that equal the scan velocity. Since above the critical scan velocity the thermocapillary forces are insufficient to cause a recirculation flow on the surface, the mixing effect is suppressed (7).

Rippling

The liquid movement causes a depressed surface under the beam, that is, to a change in the focal distance and therefore in the energy absorbed by the surface. This, in turn, leads to a more uniform distribution of the surface temperature and thus reduces the force driving the flow. The surface deformation is diminished, the absorption again increases, and the flow is resumed. The interconnection between the surface deformation, the absorption, and the force driving the flow is the cause of the cyclic nature of the surface deformation, made manifest in the ripples characteristic of laser melting. Schematic representations of sections of the bath perpendicular to the direction of the laser movement are shown in Figure 5.

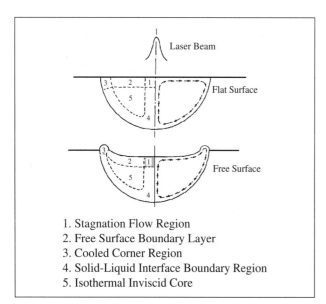

1. Stagnation Flow Region
2. Free Surface Boundary Layer
3. Cooled Corner Region
4. Solid-Liquid Interface Boundary Region
5. Isothermal Inviscid Core

Figure 5. Schematic representation of the laser-melted bath perpendicular to the direction of the laser beam movement for the assumption of a flat surface and for a free surface (4).

An approximate simulation of a free surface has been obtained by assuming the existence of small deformations (7). The asymmetry in the depression is connected with the asymmetry of the distribution of the surface tension in the direction of the laser movement. The simulation resembles the experimental results.

8.1.4 Temperature Distribution in the Melt

The temperature in the treated substrate directly under the laser beam during heating is given by:

$$T(z,t) = T_0 + \frac{AP}{2k\pi V_b \sqrt{t(t_i + t_0)}} \left[\exp\left\{-\frac{(z+z_o)^2}{4\alpha t}\right\} + \exp\left\{-\frac{(z-z_o)^2}{4\alpha t}\right\} \right] \mathrm{erfc}\left(\frac{z+z_o}{\sqrt{4\alpha t}}\right)$$

where A is the absorption coefficient, P the laser power (W), k the thermal conductivity (W/mm-K), V_b the scan speed (mm/s), t the time, t_1 the heating time, t_0 the time necessary for the heat to diffuse over a distance equal to the laser beam radius on the workpiece surface, $t_0 = R_b^2/4\alpha$, z the coordinate perpendicular to the treated surface, z_0 the distance over which heat can diffuse during the laser beam interaction time, for $t \gg t_0$,

$$z_0^2 = \frac{\sqrt{\pi}}{e}\left(\frac{\alpha R_b}{C V_b}\right)^{0.5} R_b$$

and for $t \ll t_0$

$$z_0^2 = \frac{\pi}{2e}\left(\frac{\alpha R_b}{C V_b}\right)$$

R_b the laser beam radius, C a constant = 0.5, and α the thermal diffusivity (m²/s).

This equation yields the surface temperature under the laser beam, which is maximal, but it drops toward the edge of the laser spot. However, the flow of melt over the surface, away from the center "smoothes" the surface temperature. Finally, when the melt flow changes direction following its encounter with the solid, further cooling takes place in the region of the edge, and the temperature gradient rises again (4).

The temperature distribution in the cross section of the bath perpendicular to the movement of the laser is shown in Figure 6 (1). The temperature gradient at the bottom of the bath and at its margins is not as steep as at the center of the upper part. This is due to turbulence, which transfers hot liquid to more distant areas, where it moderates the temperature gradient. The same state of things is observed in the surface temperature profile. The numbers on the curves are dimensionless temperatures T^*, defined as $T^* = k(T-T_0)/qr_0$, where k is the thermal conductivity, T_0 the ambient temperature and q the average absorbed irradiance in kW/mm².

Chapter 8: Surface Treatment: Glazing, Remelting, Alloying, Cladding, and Cleaning

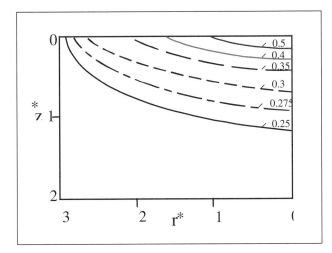

Figure 6. Temperature profile in the bath normal to the laser movement (1). The dimensionless parameters Z^* and r^* have been defined in the caption of Figure 2.

In laser alloying a situation may arise wherein the addition of alloying elements raises the surface tension together with a rise in temperature and a reversal of the flow profile (Fig. 7a), the latter causing a flow of very hot liquid from the region of irradiation toward the bottom of the bath, a deeper molten bath, and, surprisingly, steeper temperature gradients at the bottom (Fig. 7b).

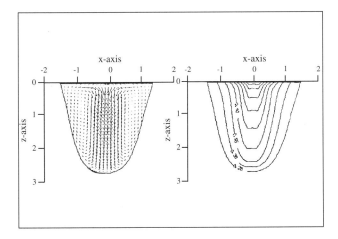

Figure 7. Flow profile (left) and temperature field (right) in the event of a rise in surface tension with rising temperature (4). The numbers on the curves in part b are the dimensionless temperature T^*, defined earlier. The x axis and z axis are the dimensionless parameters r^* and Z^*.

The flow profile of Figure 3b changes the temperature profile in the cross section, from a collection of isotherms concentrated round the point of contact with the laser beam (Fig. 6) to the profile shown in Figure 8.

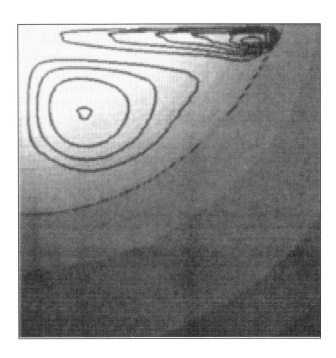

Figure 8. Temperature field in the bath, showing convection currents (5).

The difference between the temperature profile of Figure 6 and that of Figure 8 is due to the difference in flow profiles and to the different numerical conditions:
Pr - the Prandtl number: 0.15 (4), 0.01 (5);
Re - the Reynolds number: 10,000 (4), 1000 (5);
Ma - the Marangoni number: 1500 (4), 10 (5). (Ma = Re x Pr)

Convection distorts the circular profile of the isotherms in the bath, as can be concluded from a comparison of Figures 6 and 9.

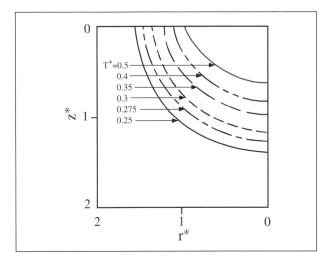

Figure 9. Isotherms without convection (1); T^*=0.25 is the liquid/solid front. The dimensionless parameters Z^*, r^*, and T^* have been defined earlier.

ISBN 0-912035-15-3

The Dimension of the Molten Bath

From Figure 9 one can conclude that the bath becomes wider and shallower when turbulence occurs (1, 4). The stronger the turbulence, the higher the Marangoni number, and thus the aspect ratio of the bath also rises, by up to 150% over that observed when there is no convection. In experiments the same behavior was found, but the calculated aspect ratios were 25% higher than the measured ones (1). The application of these rapid solidification concepts to melting of cast iron surfaces will be described in Section 8.5.2.

References

1. C. L. Chan, J. Mazumder, and M. M. Chen, *Materials Science and Technology* **3**, 306–11 (1987).
2. G. G. Gladush, L. S. Krasitskaya, E. B. Levchenko, and A. L. Chernyakov, *Sov. J. Quantum Electron.* **12**, 408–12 (1982).
3. H. Haferkamp, I. Burmester, and S. Czerner, in European Conference on Laser Treatment of Materials, ECLAT '98, B. L. Mordike (Ed), Werkstoff-Informationgesellschaft 1998, 111–16.
4. J. Mazumder, M. M. Chen, C. L. Chan, R. Zehr, and D. Voelkel in 3rd European Conference on Laser Treatment of Materials, ECLAT'90, H. W. Bergmann and R. Kupfer (Eds.), Sprecgsaal Publishing Group 1990, 37–53.
5. D. Morvan, Ph. Bournot, A. Garino, and D. Dufresne SPIE **1810**, 700–3 (1992).
6. D. Peidao, L. Jianglong, and S. Gongqi, *Lasers in Engineering* **2**, 75–9 (1993).
7. N. Pirch, E. W. Kreutz, L. Möller, A. Gasser, and K. Wissenbach, in 3rd European Conference on Laser Treatment of Materials, ECLAT'90, H. W. Bergmann and R. Kupfer (Eds.), Sprechsaal Publishing Group 1990, 65–80.

MENACHEM BAMBERGER

8.2 Rapid Solidification and Microstructure

8.2.1 Solidification

The prime condition for the solidification of a liquid is the reduction of Gibbs free energy of the system to the minimum. That process is attended by the redistribution of the system's elements among its various phases while at the same time preserving equal chemical potential of each component in these phases. Based on these principles, the phase diagram of the system can be calculated. In that diagram the phases constituting it are shown at equilibrium. For the diffusive redistribution of the elements among the phases, time is needed, so that in rapid solidification, in which the time available for diffusion or reaction is very short, a deviation from the state of equilibrium results, whereas the preservation laws and a pair of response functions at the liquid/solid front are maintained.

It is a common assumption that, despite the absence of equilibrium at the liquid/solid front, the free energy of each phase by itself is determined by its composition and its temperature. In this manner T_o, the temperature at which the free energy equilibrium of the solid and of the liquid exists, can be determined. The broken line in Figure 1 shows the temperatures at which, in principle, the transition from liquid to solid can take place while the composition remains unchanged. This is known as partitionless solidification.

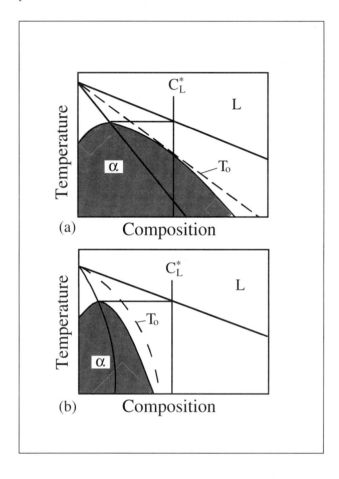

Figure 1. Dimensionless schematic diagram of the free energy equilibrium temperature of the liquid and the solid, T_o, for various compositions, as well as the range in which partitionless solidification takes place (8).

Cases (a) and (b) in the figure present different relationships between the T_o curve and the cooling of the alloy, which in turn will result in partitionless solidification in (a) and will not in (b). Also α is the solid phase (usually a solid solution of one element, e.g., B, in the other, A, and L is the liquid). The set of response functions exhibit the conditions at the solidification front, the temperature and the composition of the solid, as dependent on the conditions of the solidification. The conclusion to be drawn from these functions is that a liquid of composition C_L^* can undergo partitionless solidification within a range of compositions and temperatures that depends on the rate of solidification, rather than at one certain temperature T_o. This is shown by the dark areas in Figure 1. The line T_o represents the maximum temperature at which partitionless solidification can take place: in case (b) it cannot; in case (a) it can.

The curve, T_o, for phases having a limited solubility range has been found to apply to compositions close to that of the solubility limit of the phase because of the narrow range of the free-energy curve of that phase. This being so a number of characteristic curves of T_o are possible with eutectic alloys, as seen in Figure 2.

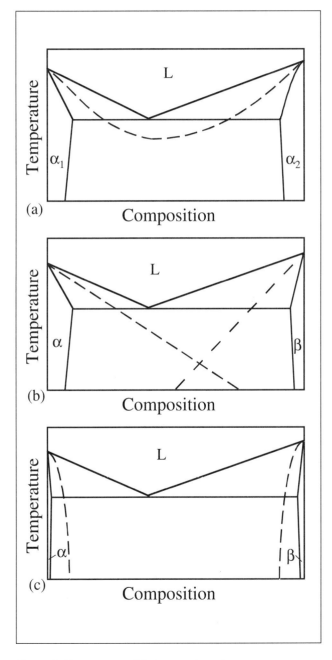

Figure 2. T_0 curves possible in eutectic systems.

In Figure 2a the two phases are the similar, so that T_o will be continuous over the entire range with a minimum close to the eutectic composition. In the system, Ag-Cu, T_o behaves in this manner and is situated only about 100°C below the eutectic temperature. This is why, after laser melting, columnar solidification of a supersaturated face-centered cubic phase occurs and no eutectic structure is obtained (9). The distance λ between the columns depends on the cooling rate (see Fig. 3). Different workers have obtained different expressions for this dependence.

$$\lambda = 50(\dot{T})^{-1/3} \text{ in } \mu m \quad (4)$$

$$\lambda = 21.4(\dot{T})^{-0.28} \text{ in } \mu m \quad (10)$$

with $\dot{T}$ the cooling rate in K/sec.

8.2.2 Temperature Distribution During Cooling

The temperature in the treated substrate during cooling is given by (12):

$$T(z,t) = T_0 + \frac{AP}{2\pi k V_b \sqrt{t(t_i + t_0)}}$$

$$\times \left[\exp\left\{-\frac{(z+z_0)^2}{4\alpha t}\right\} + \exp\left\{-\frac{(z-z_0)^2}{4\alpha t}\right\} - \exp\left\{-\frac{(z-z_0)^2}{4\cdot\alpha(t-t_i)}\right\} \right]$$

$$\times \text{erfc}\left(\frac{z+z_0}{\sqrt{4\alpha t}}\right)$$

This equation can be compared to the equation for $T(z,t)$ during heating presented in Section 8.1.4. The notation is the same as for that equation. Differentiation of this equation with respect to time yeilds the cooling rate.

8.2.3 Dendrite Spacing

Differentiation of this equation in Section 8.2.2 with time yields the cooling rate and hence the dendritic arm spacing λ can be correlated with the laser processing parameters using the equations at the end of 8.2.1. Results for dendritic arm spacing as a function of cooling rate are shown in Figure 3. The figure illustrates the very small dendritic spacings that may be obtained at high cooling rates.

Returning to Figure 2, Figure 2b is a eutectic diagram in which one phase is of limited solubility (β), which solidifies mostly faceted, and another, metallic, phase that solidifies nonfaceted and is of high solubility in the other element. In a case like this, remarkable undercooling of an off-eutectic composition may lead to eutectic solidification, provided that the alloy is in the "coupled zone" close to the eutectic composition (13). The distance d between the eutectic lamellae is connected with the cooling rate according to (14):

$$d = 1.04 \times 10^{-5} \dot{T}^{-0.5}$$

Higher undercooling leads either to partitionless solidification of one or the other phase or to the formation of a crystalline phase that is not one of the equilbrium phases in the system (10).

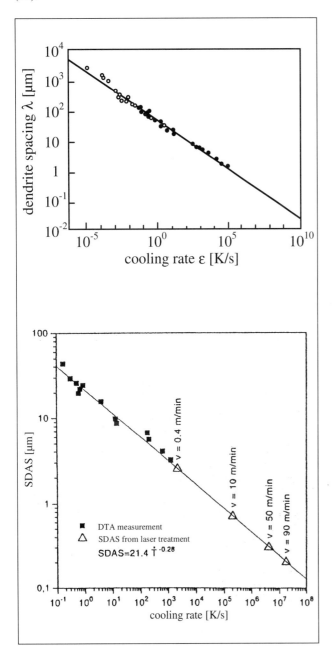

Figure 3. Dendritic arm spacing as a function of the cooling rate. DTA is differential thermal analysis and SDAS is secondary dentritic arm spacing. Bottom curve from Reference 10, top curve from Reference 11.

Figure 2c, on the other hand, is a diagram with two phases of limited solubility, and only a slight broadening of their solubility range is possible. A eutectic alloy in this system is a strong candidate for glass formation (10). The ratio between the temperature of the glass transition, T_g, at which the viscosity of the melt is 10^{13} poise, and the solidification temperature, T_f, determines the critical cooling rate R_c for obtaining the glass phase. The higher T_g/T_f is, the lower R_c becomes (10) (see Fig. 4).

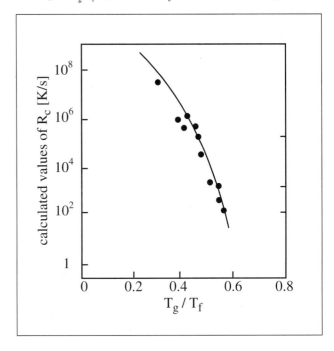

Figure 4. The critical cooling rate for obtaining the glassy phase as a function of the ratio between the temperature of the glass transition, T_g, and the solidification temperature, T_f.

An evaluation of the cooling rate that produces an amorphous structure can be obtained by calculating the time t required for the solidification of a small volume x at temperature T (15):

$$t = \frac{9.32\eta}{kT}\left[\frac{a_0^9 x}{f^3 N_v^0}\frac{\exp\left(\frac{1.024}{T_r^3 \Delta T_r^2}\right)}{\left\{1-\exp\left(\frac{-\Delta H_f \Delta T_r}{RT}\right)\right\}^3}\right]^{1/4}$$

where a_0 is the average atomic diameter, N_v^0 the average number of atoms per unit volume, T_r the normalized temperature = T/T_m, ΔT_r the normalized undercooling = $(T_m-T)/T_m$, ΔH_f the molar heat of fusion ($\Delta H_f/T_m$ = 10 J/kmol for most metals), η the viscosity at temperature T, f the fraction of sites on the interface at which atoms are preferentially added or removed (for metals, $f=1$), R the gas constant, k Boltzmann's constant. η as a function of the temperature with respect to metals and alloys is given in Reference 16. With that equation the time–temperature transformation (T-T-T) curve (see Chapter 7) of rapid solidification is calculated. The calculated cooling rate $R_c=(T_m-T_n)/t_n$, where

T_n and t_n are, respectively, the temperature and the time corresponding to the "nose" of the T-T-T curve for a small volume ($X=10^{-6}$) corresponds well with experimental results (15).

References

8. W. J. Boettinger, in *Rapidly Solidified Amorphous and Crystalline Alloys,* B. H. Kear, B. C. Giessen, and M. Cohen (Eds.), Elsevier Science Publishing, 15–31 (1982).
9. D. G. Beck, S. M. Copley, and M. Bass, *Metallurgical Transactions* **12A**, 1687–91 (1981).
10. R. W. Cahn, and P. Haasen (Eds.), 1996: *Physical Metallurgy,* North-Holland, Amsterdam.
11. K. Rabitsch, R. Sitte, R. Ebner, and F. Jeglitsch, *Prakt. Met. Sonderbd.* **26**, 545–56 (1995).
12. J. Grun and R. Sturm, in *Conf. Adv. Mater. Processes Appl.* 5th **3**, 3/155–3/159 (1997).
13. W. Kurz, and D. J. Fisher 1989: *Fundamentals of Solidification,* Trans Tech Publications, Switzerland.
14. B. L. Mordike, in R. W. Cahn, P. Haasen, and E. J. Kramer (Eds.), 1991: *Materials Science and Technology* **15**, VCH Weinheim.
15. H. A. Davis, J. Aucote, and J. B. Hull, *Scripta Metallurgica* **8**, 1179–90, (1974).
16. L. Battezzati, and A. L. Greer, *Acta. Metall.* **37**, 1791–802, (1989).

MENACHEM BAMBERGER

8.3 Appropriate Lasers and Optics

Nd:YAG and CO_2 lasers are the most widely used lasers for production alloying, cladding, and glazing because they are the only commercially available lasers currently producing multiple kilowatts of power for sustained periods of time.

8.3.1 Nd:YAG Lasers

The Nd:YAG laser, operating at 1.06 μm, is often used when very high irradiance levels are required, which can only be achieved by producing a very small focused spot size, when the processed materials have too high a reflectance for a CO_2 laser beam, and when power up to 3 kW CW is sufficient for the particular application.

The most common optical materials used for optics for Nd:YAG lasers are quartz (SiO_2) and borosilicate crown glass (BK-7), because they offer very high transmission at 1.06 μm, and they are compatible with in-line visible alignment and monitoring systems. Also, expendable/disposable cover glass slides, of these materials, can be used to protect the primary beam focusing optics. Silver-coated copper mirrors have also been used in Nd:YAG applications when the irradiance is too high for glass materials having low thermal conductivity. The copper mirrors are typically used only when the power levels are ≥2 kW and the life expectancy must be very high, or when irradiance levels are so high that direct water cooling of the optics is required.

One of the best features of Nd:YAG lasers is that fiber optics can be used to direct the beam to the workstation. This eliminates several beam-bending components that are typically required with CO_2 lasers.

8.3.2 CO_2 Lasers

The CO_2 laser, operating at 10.6 μm, is required when radiant power levels must be higher than 3 kW or when the processed materials have better radiant coupling efficiencies at 10.6 than at 1.06 μm.

The most popular and common optical transmitting material used for CO_2 lasers is zinc selenide, with gallium arsenide and germanium being the second and third choices, respectively. Zinc selenide is transparent to visible wavelengths and therefore compatible with in-line visible monitoring and alignment systems. When very high irradiance or power levels are used, or direct water cooling is required, then metal mirrors of copper or molybdenum are used. If the mirror must scan or dither at a high rate of speed, then aluminum, silicon carbide, or beryllium can be used. Each of these materials has trade-offs. Aluminum and molybdenum easily corrode when water cooled. Silicon carbide requires a reflective coating that can become contaminated by smoke from the processing application and thereby damages and burns off. Beryllium has a very high reflectance but is considered toxic, producing respiratory illnesses if inhaled.

Materials processing applications typically produce excessive amounts of smoke and debris that often contaminate the optical surfaces. This contamination causes additional absorption of the beam at the mirror surface, which leads to premature failure of the component, in addition to processing inefficiencies. Molybdenum is generally considered an easily cleaned optical surface, with little or no damage caused by the cleaning process. Copper is considered more difficult to clean than molybdenum. Its inherent soft surface is more easily scratched during cleaning, and it also corrodes faster. Copper is still the best choice, however, when water cooling is required, because the cost is significantly less than that of other candidate materials.

WALTER J. SPAWR

8.4 Laser Glazing

8.4.1 The Glazing Process

The term *glazing* means to make glassy, to make a solid with no crystalline structure. Laser glazing occurs when a beam of sufficient intensity to create a molten state is scanned rapidly across a solid. With the removal of the heat source as the beam moves away from a particular spot, the molten surface layer cools rapidly by conduction of heat into the bulk of the material. If the total heat input is low enough that the thermal gradients in the material are steep, the molten layer is shallow and very high cooling rates can occur. Calculated cooling rates exceed 500°C/μs. Cooling rates may be estimated using the equation in Section 8.2.2.

Laser glazing typically occurs with a partially focused beam incident on a sample spinning at high speed, for example, on a rotating turntable. Speeds of several meters per second are achieved. The depth of the melted and solidified regions is small, and can be only be increased at the expense of decreasing the cooling rate.

Metals

Cases in which a laser has produced glassy metallic structures were confirmed by broad circular steaks in an electron diffraction pattern. These include Fe-C-Si-B and Pd-Cu-Si alloys, usually of a eutectic composition. However, not all eutectic alloys will produce glassy structures. A pretreatment to homogenize the microstructure prior to the glazing pass of the laser beam has been used.

A more common result of irradiation with a scanning laser beam has been a single-phase microstructure that looks featureless through an optical microscope. The various constituents in the solid have dissolved, and rapid solidification has occurred with no time for segregation of the various alloying elements into regions of high and low concentration. In these cases, laser melting and rapid solidification would be a more suitable term than laser glazing. For example, laser glazing of Ti-6Al-4V produced a fine α martensite. Other alloys to which the laser rapid solidification process have been applied include copper-zinc alloys, nickel aluminum bronze, and a variety of cast irons and superalloys.

The single-phase microstructure produced during laser rapid solidification can also be produced when material is added during the laser melting process. This has been demonstrated with a powder feed for adding material and with a wire feeder for 0.25-mm-diameter wire. It is expected that the use of standard wire of the order of 1 mm diameter would require sufficient heat input that single-phase microstructure would not occur. In other cases, the added material has been in the form of a surface layer preapplied by plasma spraying; the laser serves to melt the surface layer with the substrate, producing a new single-phase alloy.

Ceramics

Scanning a focused laser beam across a ceramic surface produces a smooth glassy finish. Inevitably, surface cracks occur because of contraction during cooling of the melted surface. This process has been applied not only to solid ceramics but also to ceramic surfaces created by plasma spraying, which consists of a "splat" from the multiple impact of partly melted ceramic particles. Laser treatment improves adhesion of the surface layer.

In spite of the surface cracking, a laser-treated zirconia coating on an aerospace alloy was shown to have a superior lifetime when subjected to thermal cycling typical of turbine engine operation, and subjected to thermal cycling in an atmosphere of hot oxidizing gasses. Laser treatment of zeolite-based mortars produced a glassy surface, confirmed by X-ray diffraction, which reduced water absorption and damage during cyclic freezing and thawing.

Reference
E. M. Breinan and B. H. Kear, 1983: *Laser Materials Processing*, M. Bass (Ed.), North Holland Publishing Company, 235–95.

VIVIAN E. MERCHANT

8.4.2 Rapid Cooling

The laser glazing process depends on the very rapid cooling of a very thin melted layer in contact with a more massive substrate. Because of the rapidity of the process, the surface layer is melted while the substrate remains cool. Thus a very large temperature gradient is established and resolidification and solid-state cooling can occur very rapidly, freezing in nonequilibrium crystalline structures.

For a melt depth of 1 μm, which may be achieved with an irradiance around 10^7 W/cm², the cooling rate may be as high as 10^{10} K/sec. For lower values of irradiance, it will take longer to melt the material. The cooling rate will be lower, and the depth melted will be greater. Typical melt depths for laser glazing are usually in the range from 1 to 100 μm. For a melt depth of 100 μm, the cooling rate may be reduced to values around 10^6 K/sec. Estimates of maximum melt depth may be obtained using the methods described in Section 8.1.1.

There is a maximum melt depth that may be obtained with a given value of irradiance before surface vaporization begins. At the maximum melt depth, the cooling rate will be smaller than in the case of smaller melt depth.

Figure 1 shows how the cooling rate varies with absorbed irradiance for pure nickel (1). This is the maximum cooling rate, which occurs in the limiting case as the melt depth approaches zero. The pulse duration (or interaction time) is very short for this situation. The figure illustrates the very high quench rates that may be obtained.

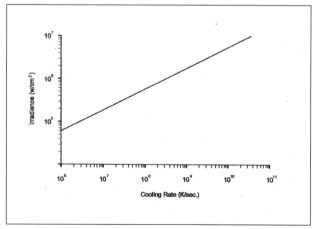

Figure 1. Maximum cooling rate as a function of absorbed irradiance for pure nickel.

One notes that the maximum cooling rate increases as the square of the irradiance.

One may use Figure 3 of Section 8.2.3 in conjunction with this figure to obtain the minimum dendrite spacing that may be obtained as a function of irradiance. At 10^7 W/cm^2 one may obtain dendrite spacings less than 0.1 μm.

Figure 2 compares the regimes of irradiance and interaction time for laser glazing and some related processes. Laser glazing is the most rapid of these processes. Laser remelting, to be described in Section 8.5, uses a longer time, resulting in a deeper melt and less rapid quenching. Transformation hardening, described in Chapter 7, uses lower irradiance and longer interaction times, and does not produce surface melting.

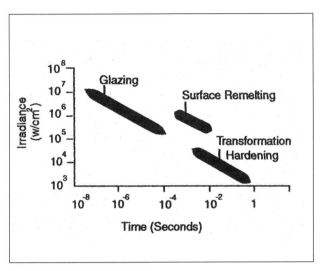

Figure 2. Regimes of irradiance and interaction time for laser glazing, remelting, and transformation hardening.

Laser glazing has been shown to yield a variety of interesting and potentially useful metallurgical microstructures. Despite the capability of laser glazing for producing unusual surface morphology, most of the work on laser glazing has been research oriented and there have been few production applications.

Reference
1. E. M. Breinan, B. H. Kear, and C. M. Banas, *Physics Today*, p. 44, November, 1976.

JOHN F. READY

8.5 Surface Remelting

This section describes the modification of surface properties through rapid melting and resolidification. The melt depth is somewhat greater and the cooling rates somewhat slower than for laser glazing (see Section 8.4.2). Surface remelting has been used to produce surfaces with very fine microstructures that extend the life of turbine engine bearings. This application is described in Section 8.5.1. The melting of cast iron surfaces and resultant hardening of the surfaces is described in Section 8.5.2.

8.5.1 Surface Remelting of Bearings

Surface remelting technology utilizes high-energy industrial CO_2 lasers and Nd:YAG lasers. A particularly effective method is based on a patented process of refining the carbide distributions in high-speed steels (HSS) by laser surface remelting (1). Similar processing can be performed on high carbon, high chromium steels, and nickel-based alloys.

Typically, a CO_2 laser is operated at approximately 3 kW with a beam diameter of 0.5 mm. The bearing races to be remelted pass through the beam at approximately 170 mm/s. To a first approximation, the interaction time is 0.003 s, and the irradiance is approximately 1.5×10^6 W/cm^2. The processing is very similar to laser glazing; however, the increased interaction time allows a deeper layer to be melted (2).

HSS alloys produced by conventional ingot metallurgical operations generally are used in a hardened condition. The steels have high tensile and compressive yield strengths, but are brittle. The major microstructural constituent in these alloys is tempered martensite, occasionally with amounts of retained austenite. Since these alloys contain molybdenum, vanadium, tungsten, chromium, and carbon ranging from 0.80% to 1.25% by weight, many large-alloy carbides exist in these steels. The solidification rates of these alloys are relatively slow. Thus the primary alloy carbides formed in these steels are quite large compared to carbides in conventional alloy steels. The local solidification time or interaction time for cast ingots may be as high as 100 s. After solidifying, the ingots are rolled into bars, plate, or wire. While some of the largest carbides fracture into smaller carbides during hot rolling, generally many large carbides are still present in the final wrought product. Since the carbides form in the liquid zone between dendrite arms, the carbides in the alloys are not uniformly distributed throughout the microstructure. The carbides become concentrated into bands that are parallel to the axis of deformation during rolling.

It is well known that in M50 HSS the large carbides are responsible for reduced bearing performance (3). To perform surface remelting, a rough machined cone is mounted on a fixture (see Fig. 1). The cone rotates about its x axis at an angular velocity of ω. The beam emerges from a CO_2 laser focusing head that is protected by a zinc selenide window. The beam, b, passes through a nozzle that has shielding gas coming in from the side, and exiting coaxially with the laser beam. The cone is positioned such that the laser beam illuminates its raceway, and the raceway of the cone is perpendicular to the beam. The focusing head is positioned so that the laser beam is in focus on or just below the raceway. Moreover, the design of the nozzle is such that the shielding gas completely floods the zone illuminated by the beam.

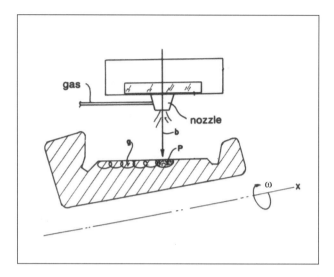

Figure 1. Schematic representation of a laser beam remelting the raceway of a bearing cone.

The laser beam melts the cone at its raceway and produces a liquid zone (Fig. 1). Since the cone revolves about its *x* axis, the point of impingement moves circumferentially along the raceway. Once the beam passes, this portion of the liquid zone immediately freezes at a very high rate of solidification due to the mass of the cone beneath it that is at room temperature. After approximately 1.3 to 1.5 revolutions, the cone is advanced axially. The path of illumination of the beam transforms from a circle to a spiral. The rate of advancement is such that the pitch of the path is less than the width of the puddle. In this manner, the entire raceway surface is remelted (Fig. 2). The remelted material has a very fine dendritic microstructure containing very small alloy carbides. In the unmelted steel large carbides and macroscopic banding are observed (Figs. 3a and b). (The remelted steel is in the upper portion of the micrographs.)

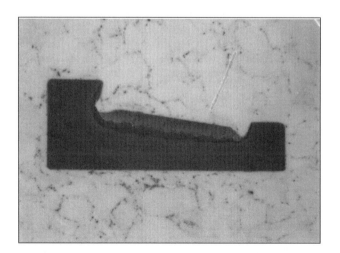

Figure 2. Longitudinal cross-sectional view of a surface remelted M50 tapered roller bearing cone.

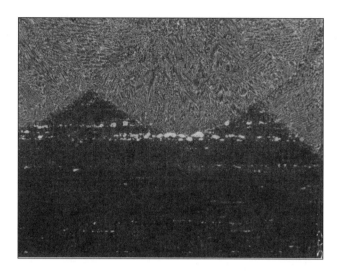

(a) 200 mm

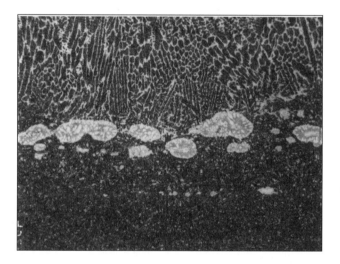

(b) 40 mm

Figure 3. Microstructure of M50 HSS laser glazed cone.

Laser surface remelting greatly enhances the fatigue life of bearing manufactured from M50 HSS (Fig. 4). As indicated, the point at which the cumulative failure probability, the so-called L10 life, of the cones that were laser surface remelted is almost an order of magnitude greater than similar cones manufactured from wrought bar product. There are two reasons for the enhanced performance. First, the steel has been remelted and then rapidly solidified. The rapid solidification rates greatly decrease the size of the alloy carbides. Second, since the direction of remelting and solidification is perpendicular to the longitudinal axis of the bearing cones, the macroscopic banding has been eliminated. Complete details of these microstructural features are described elsewhere (4). The patent pending heat treatments given to this class of steels is quite unique. While the composition of the alloys is uniform, compressive residual stresses similar to those developed in carburized components are created. In the figure, se and le refer to the small end and large end of the cones, respectively. The two conditions indicate the direction in which the remelting proceeded.

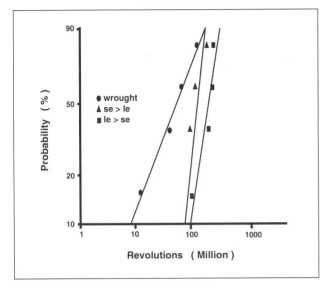

Figure 4. Weibull statistical analysis of M50 bearing cones. The values on the y-axis give the Cumulative Failure probability.

A similar type of processing has been developed for 440C stainless steel. Similar improvements in L10 fatigue life were realized for this material (Fig. 5).

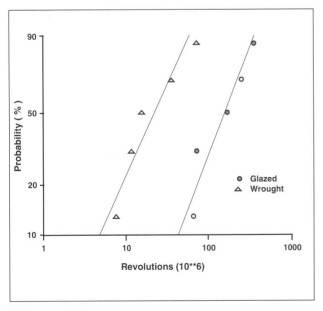

Figure 5. Weibull statistical analysis of 440C bearing cones. The values on the y-axis give the Cumulative Failure probability.

As a result of laser surface remelting, carbide refinement occurred and macroscopic banding was eliminated (Fig. 6).

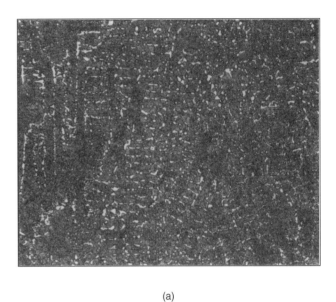

(a)

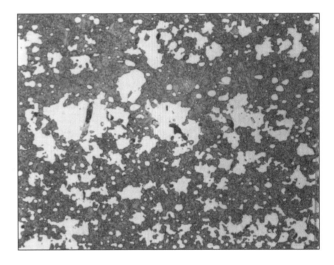

(b) 20 µm

Figure 6. 440C martensitic steel microstructures: (a) glazed, (b) wrought.

For these types of alloys, conventional heat treating was employed. As a result, the residual stress pattern in these cones was similar to that of any through hardened bearing; that is, the residual stress distribution was essentially zero from the surface to center of the cone.

This work was focused on a very specific application. Other work has been performed on HSS alloys. Successful laser surface remelting has been achieved with M1, M2, M4, and M7N high-speed steel alloys and several other ferrous-based materials. This processing should be beneficial to other types of alloys where large carbides or intermetallics develop by conventional slow solidification rate processing. For conventional alloy steels, laser surface remelting would not provide any enhanced performance because there are no large microstructural features in these alloys. Similarly, this processing would probably be impossible to use on nonmetallics such as ceramics because the high-energy inputs would probably lead to severe cracking. However, under the right conditions and for the proper alloys, laser surface remelting can offer extremely high performance levels when compared to alloys that are technologically considered the best by today's standards.

References
1. D. W. Hetzner, U.S. Patent No. 5,861,067, 1999, The Timken Company.
2. B. H. Kear, et al., "Laser glazing – a new process for production and control of rapidly chilled metallurgical microstructures," *Solidification and Casting of Metals*, The Metals Society, 1979, 501–9.
3. E. V. Zaretsky, et al., "Effect of Carbide Size, Area and Density on Rolling-Element Fatigue," NASA TN D-6835, 1972.
4. D. W. Hetzner, "Laser Glazed Bearings," Fifth International Symposium on Bearing Steels: Into the 21st Century, ASTM STP 1327, J. J. C. Hoo, Ed., American Society for Testing and Materials, 1997, 471–95.

DENNIS W. HETZNER

8.5.2 Melting Cast-Iron Surfaces

Cast iron – gray or nodular (spheroidal) – is a composite material consisting of a metal matrix, usually ferrite or pearlite, with a soft second phase, viz. graphite. The carbon and silicon contents as well as the shape of the graphite (lamellar or spherical, according to the type of cast iron) determine both the properties of the material and the structure of the surface after laser treatment, in addition, of course, to the contributions of the process parameters.

Phase Transformations as a Result of Laser Irradiation
Heating the surface with laser radiation at a relatively low energy density raises the temperature of the surface to the austenization range but short of the melting point. When the energy density is increased, the surface is melted, while the zone underneath the melted layer undergoes austenization processes similar to those to which the surface is subjected when it is heated but not melted. We shall accordingly focus our attention on two phase transformations that occur during laser irradiation, melting and austenization.

Melting the Surface
Melting the surface of cast iron to a depth of 500–1000 μm is achieved by CW-CO_2 laser irradiation at an energy density of 4000–5000 J/cm² (5, 6). At an energy density of 100 J/cm², the depth of the molten layer is only 100 μm (7). If one uses a pulsed Nd:YAG laser (pulse frequency 20 Hz, pulse duration 8 ms, scan speed 0.1 m/min, power 928 W, beam diameter 4 mm), a molten layer of about 1200 μm thickness is obtained (8). According to (9) the required energy densities are higher. The depth of the bath also depends on the microstructure of the substrate and its thermal conductivity, which in the case of gray cast iron is very high, so that the depth of the bath is maximal. For pearlitic spheroidal cast iron, its very low conductivity causes the bath to be shallower (7). The bath depth affects the dissolution of the graphite: The deeper the bath, the longer the graphite remains in contact with the melt, and the more complete is its dissolution. This is why graphite nodules are found on the surface of spheroidal cast iron that has undergone melting (7, 10, 11), whereas in melting the surface of lamellar cast iron under the same conditions, the graphite dissolves completely, and hence the composition of the surface after melting is very similar to that of the original material (5–8). The concentration of carbon in the liquid is given by

$$C(t) = C_s - (C_s - C_0) \exp(-At),$$

where C_s is the concentration of carbon in the specimen; C_0 the concentration of carbon in the liquid before the dissolution of the graphite (i.e., its concentration in pearlite = 0.8 wt.%), A a constant ($A=14$ for an alloy of 25 μm nodule size, $A=6$ for one of 75-μm nodule size), and t is the time of dissolution.

Surface Austenization
At an energy density of several hundreds of J/cm² a temperature above the austenization temperature (see Chapter 7) is obtained and austenization of the surface takes place in periods of 10^{-3}-10^{-2} s (5, 6, 12). In addition, it sometimes happens that the eutectic grain boundaries are melted, so that the region contains austenite, graphite, and liquid, an occurrence that is more frequent in the heat-affected zone underneath the molten bath (13).

Austenization begins on the grain boundaries and in the interface with pearlite colonies, because it is there that defects are present that serve as austenite nucleation sites. Because of the relatively high temperature needed for austenization and the very high heating rate, 5.64×10^4 K/s, the resulting austenite is equiaxial and not acicular (12). The austenite morphology also exerts its influence on the microstructure after cooling. The short austenization time does not enable the graphite to dissolve, especially if it is nodular. It can only cause the pearlitic matrix to transform to austenite. This is why nodular graphite is discerned in the specimen after heating with a laser (5, 14) and why ferritic cast iron cannot be hardened through austenization alone but only through surface melting (15).

Cooling and Solidification
At hypo-eutectic carbon concentrations, austenite is the first to solidify, while the residual liquid solidifies to fine ledeburite. At rapid solidification (10^4-10^6 K/s) (9, 12), the austenite transforms to martensite, and the microstructure then contains martensite, ledeburite, cementite, residual austenite, and nodules of undissolved graphite (5, 7, 8, 9). When melting the surface of lamellar cast iron, the carbon content is preserved close to the

eutectic because of its complete dissolution, and the martensitic transition temperature drops, producing a greater quantity of residual austenite than in the case of nodular cast iron (see Fig. 7) (16). The fact that in lamellar cast iron the melted bath is deeper also has an effect, viz. that the cooling rate is lower (7).

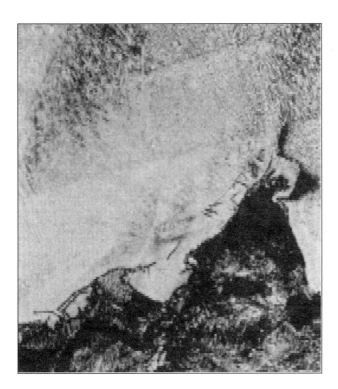

(a)

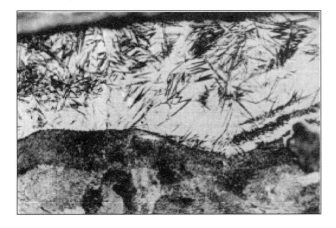

(b)

Figure 7. The metallographic structure of (a) lamellar and of (b) nodular pearlitic cast iron after laser melting of the surface (7).

The austenite in the heat-affected zone undergoes martensitic transformation because of rapid cooling, with only little retained austenite. In the heating stage the transformation to austenite was not complete, part of the graphite remained undissolved and stayed so after cooling. The heat-affected zone (HAZ) underneath the molten surface, or the surface that underwent austenization during laser surface heating, contains, after the rapid cooling, martensite, some residual austenite, and graphite (5, 10, 13). As was mentioned before, melting of the grain boundaries is possible, especially in the HAZ, and these regions solidify to a fine dendritic eutectic structure (13). The presence of martensite in the HAZ may lead to cracks in the relevant layer during heating or cooling in service and has therefore to be prevented if possible. It is accordingly common practice to heat the substrate to 350°C before the laser treatment in order to prevent the appearance of martensite (17).

Tempering and Graphitization

The microstructure of the surface after laser melting consists mainly of martensite and cementite, as was mentioned before. Accordingly a hardness of 700–900 Hv (5, 15), characteristic of fine martensite with cementite, is obtained. However, reheating of the martensite leads to local tempering followed by fluctuations in the hardness and a reduction in the overall hardness, as shown schematically in Figure 8.

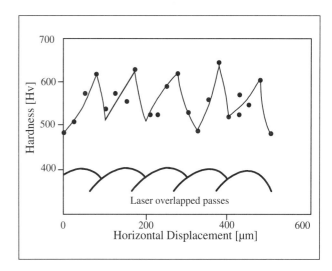

Figure 8. Hardness distribution parallel to the surface at a depth of 30 μm in ferritic nodular cast iron after laser melting (7).

The fluctuations in the hardness and the average hardness are a function of the conditions of laser melting, power, scan speed, and the percentage of overlap between adjacent passes. This is well known in all hardening processes based on metastable phases. In the case of laser surface treatment, however, an additional feature exerts an influence on the microstructure and the properties: local graphitization because of the renewed heating of the hardened region by the next pass of the laser. This is seen in Figure 9.

ures 9a and b. Figure 9c depicts the microstructure in the overlap zone, from which it is clear that in the underlying track, near the overlapping track, the cementite (the bright phase) has completely disappeared, and consequently the hardness has dropped to 200 Hv. This layer is 68–75 μm thick, regardless of the parameters of the laser treatment. The cementite has been transformed into graphite particles of about 1 μm diameter. Somewhat farther from the overlapping track there is a zone about 500 μm wide that has undergone partial graphitization; then comes a zone that has only been tempered, and yet farther away the following pass is without influence on the microstructure and the properties of the underlying track. The rate of graphitization is four orders of magnitude higher than what is common in the conventional technology, because of the following factors (8, 18):

1. The high content of graphitizers, mainly C and Si
2. The great number of nucleation sites in the interface, cementite/matrix, and the defects in the lattice typical in rapid cooling following laser surface melting
3. A heating process specific to pulsed-laser surface treatment, that is, a great number of brief heating cycles promoting precipitation from the supersaturated matrix and at the same time preventing the growth of precipitates

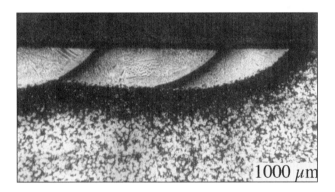

(a)

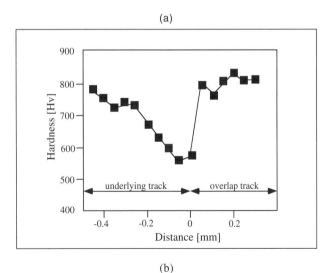

(b)

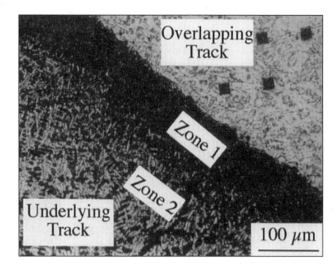

(c)

Figure 9. Section perpendicular to the direction of the laser beam's advance. (a) The tempered area; (b) hardness distribution; (c) the microstructure in the overlap zone.

Properties

The thickness of the laser-melted layer and its characteristic hardness depend on the processing conditions. Figure 10 shows the hardness distribution for the laser treatment of lamellar cast iron camshaft at a power of 4.5 kW, beam width 35 mm as a function of the distance from the surface, and different scan speeds (6). The higher the scan speed, the smaller the depth attained and the higher the hardness. The high hardness of the laser-remelted surface also improves the wear and abrasion resistance; the rate of abrasion is two orders of magnitude lower than that of the original material (Fig. 11).

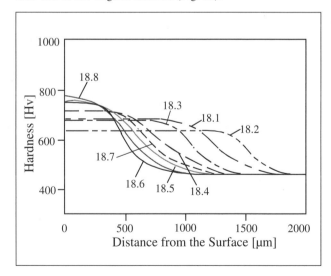

Figure 10. Hardness distribution on laser-remelted lamellar cast iron. The numbers on the curves indicate individual camshafts. The time for treatment was shortest for 18.8 and longest for 18.1.

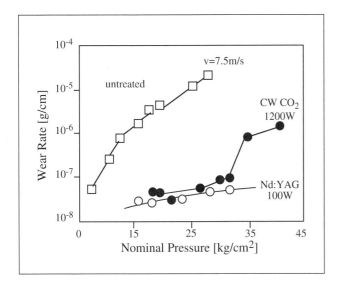

Figure 11. The abrasion rate of a laser-remelted surface compared with that of the untreated material.

Significant improvement was also noted in the resistance to erosion and to corrosion (9), but pores and cracks, typical of the rapid solidification of brittle materials, degrade the surface properties (7).

References
5. C. F. Magnusson, G. Wiklund, E. Vuorinen, Engström and T. F. Pedersen, *Materials Science Forum* **102–104**, 443–58 (1992).
6. S. Mordike, *Lasers in Engineering* **2**, 43–60 (1993).
7. M. Bamberger, M. Boas and O. Akin, *Z. Metallkunde* **79**, 806–12 (1988).
8. H. M. Wang and H. W. Bergmann, *Metallurgical and Materials Transactions* **26A**, 793–800 (1995).
9. S. P. Gadag, and M. N. Srinivasan, *Applied Physics A: Materials Science and Processing* **A63**, 409–14 (1996).
10. J. Adamka and J. Styk, in *Laser Treatment of Materials,* B. L. Mordike (Ed.), 1987, DFG, 235–42.
11. R. Dekumbis and P. Magnin, in *Laser Treatment of Materials,* B. L. Mordike (Ed.), 1987, DFG, 195–204.
12. L. Jianglong, S. Gongqing, D. Peidao, and O. Zhongxin, *Lasers in Engineering* **5**, 163–66 (1996).
13. L. Jianglong, *Lasers in Engineering* **1**, 185–91 (1992).
14. C. Papaphilippou and M. Jeandin, *J. Materials Science Letters* **15**, 1064–66 (1996).
15. B. L. Mordike, *Lasers in Engineering* **4**, 187–200 (1995).
16. P. Schaaf, V. Biehl, U. Gonser, M. Bamberger, and Ph. Bauer, *J. Materials Science* **26**, 5019–24 (1991).
17. B. L. Mordike in R. W. Cahn, P. Haasen, and E. J. Kramer (Eds.), 1991: *Materials Science and Technology* **15,** VCH Weinheim.
18. H. M. Wang and H. W. Bergmann, *Scripta Metallurgica et Materialia* **31**, 433–38 (1994).

MENACHEM BAMBERGER

8.6 Surface Alloying

8.6.1 Basics of Laser Alloying

Laser alloying of a surface involves melting the surface of a workpiece along with some material added to the surface. The added material is mixed in with the surface during the melting. The surface resolidifies rapidly. The composition of the surface layer is modified because of the additional material mixed into the surface. The result can be a thin hardened layer at the surface.

It is possible to add elements such as boron, chromium, silicon, nickel, and carbon to the surface of a workpiece.

The laser used for alloying is often a multikilowatt CO_2 laser. The high power is needed to provide reasonably high coverage rates. The rate of surface coverage is lower than that attained with transformation hardening, because melting of the surface is required.

The motivation for surface alloying is to provide a hardened layer on a relatively inexpensive substrate. One could produce a stainless steel layer on a low carbon steel workpiece by adding nickel and chromium.

In laser alloying, the mass of material melted on the workpiece surface is larger than the mass of the added material. In a related process, laser cladding, to be described in Section 8.7, the mass of the molten bath on the workpiece is less than that of the added material.

There has been a substantial amount of research work on the laser alloying process, but it has not yet reached widespread production application.

JOHN F. READY

8.6.2 Materials Deposition Techniques

Materials to be alloyed into a surface, referred to as a matrix surface, may be deposited before laser irradiation or may be introduced into the irradiated zone during laser treatment. In the first case the precoating may be performed using the following means.

Powder Distribution on the Surface

The technique is very simple. The powder of the alloying element (or elements) is distributed on the surface to be alloyed in a thin layer (0.2–0.5 mm) and then is subjected to laser radiation. Drawbacks include difficulties in controlling the layer thickness, high heat resistance between the layer and surface, usefulness only with horizontal surfaces, and problems with layer preservation on the surface; a high portion of the powder is wasted.

Painting with Alloying Materials

Alloying powder is mixed with glue or water glass and then brushed or sprayed onto the surface. The heat contact is better than in the previous technique, but alloying efficiency is not very high because of nonuniformity of the layer. The alloying depth does not exceed 200 μm. There is no limitation on surface location. The technique is widespread.

Powder Alloying in a Magnetic Field

This technique is an improved version of the first one. The magnetic or electromagnetic field confines the powder particles of ferromagnetic materials (ferroboron, ferrochrome, sormite, cermets, ferrosilicium) on the matrix surface and allows one to control the angle of the particles inclination to the matrix surface and thus to control to some extent the absorptivity of the surface to be laser treated. The absorptivity depends on the magnetic field intensity and affects other critical parameters of the process. Figure 1 shows how the surface absorptivity A, microhardness $H\mu$, and the HAZ depth h depend on the angle θ of particle inclination to the matrix surface. Because of the action of the magnetic field, the powder particles may be kept firmly in difficult-to-access areas of the component, and on vertical and ceiling surfaces. The magnetic field helps also to reduce the waste of alloying powder.

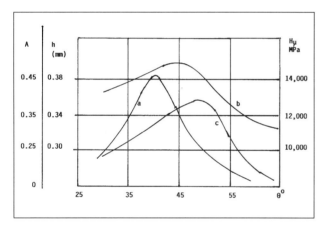

Figure 1. Microhardness $H\mu$ (a), absorptivity A (b), HAZ depth h (c) as function of the angle θ between powder particle axis and matrix material surface.

Foil Rolling

Foil made of material to be alloyed is rolled onto the surface of matrix material and then is subjected to laser irradiation. The thickness uniformity of the precoated layer makes the alloying efficiency higher and the alloyed depth larger (50–600 μm). By varying the foil thickness, one can control the amount of alloyed material. Drawbacks include problems with securing tightness of foil contact with the matrix. The technique is not applicable for matrix surfaces with a complex shape.

Electrodischarge Precoating

This technique is very efficient and rather simple, though it needs special equipment. The precoating of different refractory elements (Mo, W, Cr, Ti) and their carbides may produce layers 10–300 μm thick. There is negligible heat resistance at the layer border with the matrix because an intermediary zone 5–15 μm thick is formed. Drawbacks include the facts that the alloying elements have to be electrically conductive materials, and that for some combinations of metals there are limitations to reaching the needed layer thickness. The technique is widespread.

Plasma Precoating

This is a very efficient technique for material deposition that provides reliable heat contact of the coated layer with the matrix. It needs special equipment, but the technology is not complicated. Layers with a wide range of thicknesses from superhard alloys, carbides and nitrides of refractory metals, etc., may be deposited. The technique is rather widespread.

Detonation Precoating

This technique is based on the use of detonation in gases. The explosion of an acetylene-oxygen-powder mixture takes place in a special chamber where powder is supplied with nitrogen flow. During each explosion of duration 0.2 s, a coated layer 6–8 μm thick is formed. The multilayer coating thickness may reach 0.01–0.4 mm. The technique provides high-quality coating but is rather costly and needs quite complicated equipment.

Electrochemical Precoating

With electrochemical deposition it is possible to produce layers up to 150 μm thick with good heat contact with the matrix material. The high layer continuity allows one to control alloying element content in a wide range (up to 20–60%). A drawback is that because of a high amount of dissolved gas (hydrogen) in the coating, some pores may occur after matrix remelting. To improve coating quality, vacuum degassing is needed in some cases.

Vacuum Evaporation (Ion Implantation)

These techniques provide very uniform coatings, but the coating procedure is rather complicated and needs special expensive equipment. The size of the components to be laser alloyed are limited by the vacuum chamber dimensions. The thickness of the layer may be of the order of a few micrometers and is very even, which provides good control over alloying process quality. The technique is used for very precise alloying of small surfaces of delicate components.

The introduction of alloying material into the melted pool during laser irradiation may be performed using the following techniques.

Alloying in Gas Media

This technique may be realized in a closed chamber with a special window transparent to the laser beam and filled with a working gas – carbon containing propane-butane mixture, nitrogen, etc. The closed chamber reduces gas consumption and makes the process ecologically clean, but limits the dimensions of components to be laser treated. For large components a local gas zone is created by supplying gas through the nozzle. The gas flow increases in this case, and the process is not safe enough. Alloying in a closed chamber with gas at high pressure (2–10 MPa) under pulsed laser radiation causes nitride and carbide synthesis (so-called laser plasma alloying).

Alloying in Liquid Media

The component is located in a vessel with liquid alloying media. Water, glycerin, or other liquids may be used with the addition of alloying elements. In some cases, liquid nitrogen is used, providing not only alloying with nitrogen, but also increasing the temperature gradient at the matrix material leading to self-quenching. Drawbacks include the fact that the low concentration of alloying elements in the liquid does not allow an increase of the laser alloying efficiency, the need to clean the component after the end of the process, large waste of alloying elements, etc.

Powder Injection at Alloying

This technique is typical both for alloying and cladding. The powder supply is synchronized with laser irradiation of the matrix material. From the powder feeder via the transporting tube and nozzle, the alloying mixture is directed to the melted surface zone with flow of air or gas. As a feeder for powder injection, standard plasma cladding systems may be used.

Wire (Filler) Feed

The technique is widely used in welding and cladding. Filler-added laser welding is described in detail in Chapter 11. Alloying additions to the wire filler may improve resistance to crack formation and increase the strength of weld or cladded material.

Reference

V. S. Kovalenko, L. F. Golovko, and V. S. Chernenko, 1990, *Hardening and Alloying of Machine Components with Laser Beam,* Technica, Kiev, Ukraine, Chapter 4.

VOLODYMYR S. KOVALENKO

8.6.3. Mixing Characteristics

The final result of laser alloying, improvement of properties of the matrix material, depends on the type of material to be alloyed, the alloying elements (or their combinations), and the process conditions. Different thermochemical processes may be realized as will be described.

Laser Carburization

This process consists of steel surface layer saturation with carbon and unlike the conventional process does not necessarily need special thermal treatment, quenching, and low temperature tempering before carburization. Different types of carbon-containing media are used as well as pulsed and CW radiation (Table 1).

Depending on the amount of carbon introduced into the matrix of carbon steel, the microhardness may be increased from 4500 up to 14,000 MPa. For high-carbon steel in the martensite-austenite structure the carbides may appear.

Laser Nitriding and Cyaniding

The process is used to improve surface properties of steels, titanium, and other alloys. Alloying may be performed from media containing solid, gas, and liquid alloying elements (Table 2).

Laser Boronizing

For laser boronizing, a painting precoating is mainly used. The process is critically dependent on the level of laser irradiance, which must not cause boiling and evaporation of metal, because much energy is needed to melt the coating, which has low heat conductivity. Depending on the laser power, some critical thickness of precoated layers must not be exceeded. In comparison with conventional boronizing, this process is more versatile and provides good results in the wear resistance increase of the treated surfaces (Table 3). The painted coating is usually a mixture of boron, boron carbides, boron anhydride, borax, ferroboron powders, and glue.

Laser Diffusion Metallizing

For diffusion metallizing of iron and steels more than a dozen pure metals are used, such as Co, Cr, Sn, Mn, Nb, Ni, Mo, W, Ta, Ti, V, as well as alloys Cr-Mo-W, Ni-Nb, and others. The process may provide an abnormal concentration of alloying elements (36% Mo, 45% Ni, etc.), much exceeding the equilibrium concentration for corresponding systems. Depending on the matrix material, alloying with metal usually causes an increase of surface hardness (except for Ni), wear resistance, and other

Table 1. Laser Carburization

Matrix material	Alloying media	Deposition technique	Structure	Laser type (mode)	Comments
Stainless Steel	Propane-butane+argon Methane+argon	Alloying in gas media	Martensite Ledeburite	Nd:YAG, (pulsed) CO_2, CW	Hμ = 6380 MPa
Armco-iron	Graphite	Painting	Retained austenite (1.5% C)	Nd-glass (pulsed)	Hμ = 8680–10,650 MPa
Carbon steel	Graphite	Painting	Martensite-austenite	Nd-glass (pulsed)	Hμ = 7500–8000 MPa

characteristics. The introduction of Cr, for example, increases corrosion resistance of iron-based alloys. The depth of alloying and the alloying element concentration depend on laser power, working speed, and precoated layer thickness (Table 4).

Laser Alloying with Compositions

Unlike usual alloying, in this process it is possible to introduce into the matrix surface layer not only elements but different compositions – carbides, nitrides, oxides, etc. The commonly used materials are carbides (WC, TiC, B_4C), nitrides (TiN), diborides (CrB_2), disulfides (MoS_2), oxides (Al_2O_3), and others (pure or with binder).

Laser Alloying of Nonferrous Alloys

Among the most promising materials for laser alloying are titanium and titanium alloys. For these materials, a flow of nitrogen is used more frequently to increase surface wear resistance. Because of titanium nitride formation, increase of microhardness up to 10,000–20,000 MPa is observed, depending on the type of titanium alloy. For laser irradiation in methane or using graphite painting precoating, titanium carbide formation causes a microhardness increase up to 25,000 MPa. For complex alloying with carbon and boron, the microhardness increase may reach 38,950 MPa. To keep enough bulk matrix material plasticity, the optimal microhardness is considered to be in the range

Table 2. Laser Nitriding and Cyaniding

Matrix material	Alloying elements	Deposition technique	Structure	Laser type (mode)	Comments
Nitralloy	Ammonia	Gas media (chamber)	Nitrous martensite	Nd:YAG, (pulsed)	
Chromium steel, high-speed cutting steel	N_2 (flow under pressure)	Gas media		Nd:YAG, (pulsed)	$H\mu$ = 10,300 MPa
Carbon steel	Carbamide $CO(NH_2)_2$	Painting	Nitrous martensite+ $Fe_2N + Fe_2(C,N)$		$H\mu$ = 8400–9400 MPa
Carbon steel, chromium steel	$K_4Fe(CN)_6$	Painting	Nitrous martensite	CO_2, (CW)	2.5–3.0 times wear resistance increase
Carbon steel, stainless steel, high-speed cutting steel	Liquid nitrogen	Liquid media	Nitrous martensite	Nd-glass, (pulsed)	$H\mu$ = 10,700 MPa

Table 3. Laser Boronizing

Matrix material	Alloying elements	Precoating technique	Structure	Laser type (mode)	Comments
Armco iron	Boron	Painting	FeB, Fe_2B Fe_3B	Nd-glass, (pulsed)	Friction coefficient decrease from 0.045 down to 0.018
Chromium steel	Boron	Painting	Martensite + FeB, Fe_2B Fe_3B	Nd-glass, (pulsed)	$H\mu$ = 6000–16,800 MPa
Carbon steel	Boron	Painting	Martensite + FeB, Fe_2B	CO_2, (CW)	$H\mu$ = 25,000–30,000 MPa

Table 4. Cr Concentration and Alloying Depth Versus Laser Treatment Conditions

Power (kW) (CO_2, CW)	Working speed (m/min)	Precoated layer thickness (μm)	Alloyed depth (μm)	Cr concentration (wt %) experimental
4.5	0.5	100	1200	6
3.0	0.5	100	600	10
4.5	1.0	100	700	11
3.0	1.0	100	250	25
4.5	0.5	200	900	18
3.0	0.5	200	450	25
4.5	1.0	200	400	40
3.0	1.0	200	200	45
4.5	0.75	200	600	25
4.5	1.0	300	350-200	17–33
3.0	0.5	300	200-100	30–34
3.0	1.0	300	150-100	50–100

16,800–25,000 MPa. Combined laser carbonizing and siliconizing may give maximum microhardness up to 22,900 MPa, but the optimal level lies in the range 11,300–16,800 MPa.

Aluminum and aluminum-based alloys are another group of material suitable for laser alloying. For their alloying, silicon, iron, nickel, copper, zirconium, tungsten, manganese, boron, and other elements are used both separately and in different combinations. To alloy nickel-based alloys, working at high temperatures, cobalt, boron carbide (B_4C), titanium boride, and chromium boride are used.

References
A. G. Grigorynz and A. N. Safonov, 1987: Methods of surface laser treatment, "Vyshaya Schola," Moscow, Chapter 6.
V. S. Kovalenko, L. F. Golovko, and V. S. Chernenko, 1990: Hardening and alloying machine components with laser beam, "Technica," Kiev, Chapter 4.

VOLODYMYR S. KOVALENKO

8.6.4 Enhanced Surface Properties
For laser surface alloying, the most critical parameters are the depth of the alloyed zone, the concentration of the alloyed element in the matrix material, the mechanical properties of the alloyed zone (microhardness, friction coefficient, etc.), and surface geometry parameters (surface roughness, waviness). To evaluate these parameters, a variety of conventional and original methods are used. For example, to predict roughly the concentration C_2 of the alloying element in the alloyed zone of the matrix material, the following formula may be used:

$$C_2 = C_1 V_2 / (V_1 + V_2)$$

where C_1 is the alloying element concentration in the precoated layer, V_1 the volume of the precoated layer, and V_2 the volume of the alloyed zone. All these parameters are influenced both by the matrix material – alloying material combination and the working conditions (Table 5).

In addition to these improvements in surface properties, laser alloying may cause color changes (plastic metallization), changes of electric characteristics (in microelectronics), changes of magnetic characteristics (in magnetic systems for information recording), etc.

References
C. V. Draper, Laser Surface Alloying: The State of the Art, *Journal of Metal*, **34**, (4), 24–32 (1982).
V. S. Kovalenko, L. F. Golovko, and V. S. Chernenko, 1990: Hardening and Alloying of Machine Components with Laser Beam, "Technika," Kiev, Chapter 4.
N. N. Rykalin (Ed.), 1985: Laser and Electron Beam Material Machining, Machinostroenie, Moscow, Chapter 7.
W. M. Steen, 1991, Laser Material Processing, Springer-Verlag, London, Chapter 6.

VOLODYMYR S. KOVALENKO

Table 5. Influence of Different Factors on Surface Property Enhancement

Matrix material	Alloying element (composition)	Working conditions	Enhanced surface properties
Armco-iron	C	Painting with graphite	$H\mu$ = 8680–10,650 MPa
	B	Painting	$H\mu$ = 6000–16,000 MPa
	Mo	Foil rolling	Mo concentration: 28–36%
	WC, WC+Co, TiN	Powder injection	Hardness increase
Carbon steel	C	Painting	$H\mu$ = 7500–8000 MPa, heat resistance increase
	$K_4Fe(CN)_6$	Painting	Surface absorption increase, 2.5–3.0 times wear resistance increase
	B	Painting	$H\mu$ = 6000–16,000 MPa, friction coefficient decrease from 0.045 down to 0.018, heat resistance increase in the range 500–900°C
	Cr	Painting	Corrosion resistance increase
	$W + SiO_2 + B_4C$	Painting	$H\mu$ = 10,000–18,000 MPa
	TiC	Painting	6–8 times hardness increase
	WC	Painting	2.0–2.5 times alloyed zone thickness increase
	Al_2O_3	Painting	Hardness increase
	MoS_2	Painting	40% wear resistance increase
Stainless steel, high-speed cutting steel	C	Gas media	No heat treatment after
	N_2	Gas media	$H\mu$ = 8400–10,300 MPa
	B	Painting	$H\mu$ = 16,000–20,000 MPa
	Cr	Painting	Corrosion resistance increase
	Al_2O_3	Painting	Heat resistance and corrosion resistance increase
	TiC	Powder injection	Friction coefficient reduction from 0.45 down to 0.18
Titanium alloys	N_2	Gas media, Nd:YAG pulsed	$H\mu$ = 5000–5600 MPa
	C, TiC	CO_2, CW	$H\mu$ = 8000–16,000 MPa
	C, C+ B+ Si	CH_4, painting, Nd:YAG pulsed	$H\mu$ = 25,000 MPa $H\mu$ = 16,000–25,000 MPa, 1.5–50 times wear resistance increase, heat resistance increase at 500°C
Aluminum alloy	Ni+Mn	Powder injection, Nd:YAG, pulsed	2.8 times heat resistance increase
	Fe		4.5 times heat resistance increase
Nickel alloy	Co	Powder injection, CO_2, CW	Heat resistance increase
	B_4C	Plasma coating	Surface absorptivity increase and, hence, alloying depth increase up to 900 μm, $H\mu$ = 7000 MPa
Al_2O_3 ceramics	Ni+Ti	Powder coating 1 mm thick, CO_2, CW	Reliable ceramic/metal joint
	Ti	Foil coating 3 mm thick, CO_2, CW	Reliable ceramic/metal joint

8.7 Surface Cladding

8.7.0 Introduction

Laser cladding is characterized as welding of a filler material to the surface of a base material. The cladding mixes in a minimal manner with the base material. This is in contrast to the case of laser alloying, described in Section 8.6, in which the alloying material is thoroughly mixed with the surface matrix. The filler can be in the form of wire, strip, or powder. Generally, powder is preferred, as it is easier to control for lower feed rates. The process offers optimum bonding, great flexibility, low distortion, and low thermal load on the workpiece together with little need for after treatment.

8.7.1 Cladding Techniques

The process is simply described as having a laser beam melting the surface of the base material and then continuously injecting powder to the melt pool, thus forming a cladding. The powder is transported by an inert carrier gas or simply by gravity. Alternatively, the cladding material can be preplaced, but this technique is very rarely used. Shielding gas is always used to protect the molten material from the atmosphere. The cladding is performed as single or overlapping tracks, in one or several layers. Standard focusing optics are normally used with the laser beam pointing perpendicular to the surface. At higher power levels one can benefit from using an integrating mirror, as this provides a more uniform energy distribution and covers a larger area, for example, spot size 12 x 12 mm at 10 kW.

8.7.2 Feeding Principles

The powder can be supplied either from the side or coaxially with the laser beam. When feeding from the side, the powder is injected to the melt pool generated by the laser. The more advanced feeding nozzle consists of two concentric nozzles. The central nozzle feeds the powder and carrier gas if used. The outermost carries the shielding gas, which in addition collimates the powder stream so it is focused when entering the melt pool. The central nozzle has a diameter that corresponds to the diameter of the laser-generated melt pool. The powder is either supplied parallel with the cladded track or perpendicular to the track, with the unused powder spraying away from the cladded surface. Figure 1 illustrates powder feeding from the side.

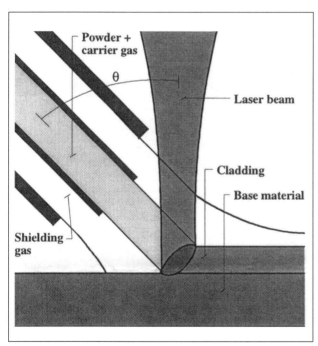

Figure 1. Powder feeding from the side. The powder is supplied parallel to the cladded track.

The coaxial principle is based on a nozzle that delivers the laser beam and the powder. The nozzle typically contains three concentric bores. The central bore guides the beam, the second feeds the powder suspended in an inert gas, and the outermost carries a gas supply for focusing the powder stream. The laser beam melts the powder to lay down tracks of molten material. Figure 2 shows coaxial feeding.

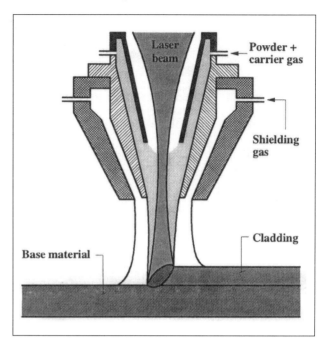

Figure 2. Coaxial feeding.

Generally, the advantage of using feeding from the side is the possibility of cladding very thin layers at lower power levels. This can be explained by the limited shadowing of the laser beam, caused by the powder stream. Furthermore, if the powder is supplied perpendicular to the track, the unused powder is spraying away from the cladded surface. Then the unused powder is not sticking to the cladded surface. This technique results in a cladding of very high quality with practically no inclusions. The advantage of using coaxial powder feeding is the simplicity when performing multidirectional processing, because of the symmetrical feeding.

8.7.3 Process Characteristics

For a certain laser power it is possible to perform the cladding in various ways. This is done by controlling the size of the melt pool on the substrate and the processing speed. It is most often an advantage to use a laser with a uniform energy distribution, like multimode beams. This type of energy profile is suitable for wide and shallow welding, which is very attractive for cladding. Using laser power ranging from 0.3 to 20 kW, one may clad a single track with a thickness of 0.1–2.0 mm and a width of 0.8–20 mm. The powder feed rates are typically in the range of 3.0–120 g/min. Table 1 gives some typical processing data for laser cladding using different lasers and power levels. When one uses overlapping tracks to clad a larger surface, an overlap in the range of 60% will be suitable for most applications. This figure is based on standard focusing optics. The high degree of overlap ensures a smooth and uniform surface with little dilution from the base material. If one uses special optics such as integrating mirrors, the overlap can be reduced significantly. Another important parameter is the utilization of the supplied powder. This process efficiency is very much dependent on the spot size and power level. For power levels in the range of 0.3 kW, the process efficiency is typically 10–20%. For power levels above 2 kW, the process efficiency is typically in range of 70–90%. In the low power range it is possible to increase the efficiency to approximately 50% by tilting the set-up by θ/2, where θ is the angle between the powder nozzle and the laser beam. In this set-up the reflected laser beam preheats the incoming powder stream, which improves the process efficiency effectively. However, the danger of using this set-up is the high risk of damaging the powder nozzle.

8.7.4 Cladding Characteristics

Laser cladding is characterized by very little mixing with the base material. For a cladding thickness of only 0.3 mm, it is possible to have a dilution of only 0–2% measured at the surface of the cladding. Furthermore, the heat-affected zone (HAZ) in the base material is extremely narrow. A varying transition zone will normally be observed from the base material to the cladding. This provides good bonding. The microstructure is much finer than that of arc welding. This forms the basis for the high wear and erosion resistance of the coatings. Imperfections in the surface layer like cracks are related to the chemical composition of the filler material and the base material. Often problems with cracking can be avoided by careful selection of processing parameters, which minimize the mixing with the base material. Figure 3 shows a micrograph of a two-layer cladding.

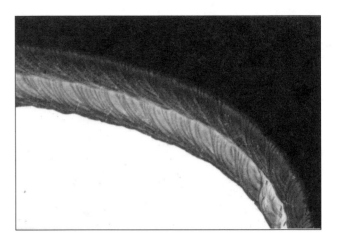

Figure 3. Two-layer cladding on elliptic surface. Magnification 20x.

8.7.5 Cladding Materials

As laser cladding is a welding process, the filler and base material must be weldable. This puts some limitations on material combinations and especially on the maximum obtainable hardness and wear resistance of the cladding. Typical materials for improved wear and corrosion resistance are the cobalt-based alloys, such as stellite, and the nickel-based alloys, such as hastelloy.

8.7.6 Process Benefits

It is possible to clad very thin layers in selected areas with a minimum of mixing with the base material. Compared to competitive processes like plasma spraying, the bonding to the base

Table 1. Typical Processing Data for Laser Cladding

Laser	Power (kW)	Mode Pulsed/cw	Feed (g/min)	Speed (m/min)	Spot Size (mm)	Thickness (mm/layer)	Width (mm)
Nd:YAG	0.3	Pulsed/150 Hz	3	0.75	Ø 1.0	0.1–0.2	0.8
Nd:YAG	2	CW	15	1.2	Ø 3.5	0.5	2.5
CO_2	0.7	CW	-[a]	-	-	0.3	1.5
CO_2	1	CW	8	0.5	-	0.5	1.5
CO_2	3	CW	-	-	-	1.5	-
CO_2	5	CW	35	0.6	-	1.5	5
CO_2	10	CW	30	0.6	12 x 12	0.8	11.5
CO_2	10	CW	80	0.6	-	1.5	10
CO_2	20	CW	120	1.2	-	1.5	10

[a]Data not available.

material is superior. Furthermore, there is practically no porosity and a much more homogeneous microstructure in the coating. Compared to plasma arc or gas tungston arc welding (GTAW), the mixing with the base material is very much lower. This means that the thickness of the cladding can be much reduced, resulting in less distortion of the cladded components. Because of the very low heat input, it is often possible to clad high-temperature-resistant steels without pre- or post-heating.

8.7.7 Process Drawbacks
Laser cladding is a rather costly process compared to the competitive processes mentioned previously.

8.7.8 Applications
Laser cladding has been used to provide:

- Improved wear resistance on valves, bearings, turbine blades, molds, etc.
- Repair of worn parts like engine cylinder blocks, molds, turbine blades, fins on labyrinth seals (e.g., in gas turbines), and valve seats and shafts (e.g., in power plants).

8.7.9 Special Applications
When multiple tracks are deposited on top of each other to build complex three-dimensional structures, it is called inverse machining or laser direct casting. Using this technique makes it possible to grow small metal parts, like 3D metal prototypes. Cladding of a preplaced polymer foil by scanning the laser beam is another special application that is used, for example, inside steel tubes.

THOMAS AABOE JENSEN

8.8 Cleaning

8.8.0 Introduction
This section presents three descriptions of laser cleaning applications. Each application targets a different industrial problem that can be approached using a more conventional, nonlaser, technology. In each instance, the author – a practitioner of laser cleaning – has found it advantageous to utilize lasers rather than competing technologies and discusses the arguments behind his or her positions.

The picture presented by these articles is intriguing; contaminants ranging from the unusually horrific (radioactive elements) to the seemingly benign (submicroscopic dust particles) can be effectively removed from surfaces using lasers; objects ranging in size from large commercial aircraft to microchips are potential targets for laser cleaning.

As industrial lasers become less expensive and more capable, the number of laser cleaning applications will surely increase. The applications cited in this section will compete even more favorably against traditional nonlaser cleaning methods that often pose environmental and safety hazards; expect new applications to emerge.

MARTIN C. EDELSON

8.8.1 Surface Cleaning
"Surface cleaning" can be used to refer to two distinctly different operations. The first, more properly referred to as "coating removal," generally refers to the removal of a layer on the surface of a substrate. In most cases the chemical and physical composition of the layer differs significantly from that of the substrate. The removal of paint from metals, an application with significant industrial potential, falls within this classification.

Another variant of surface cleaning, here called "laser surface decontamination," refers to the removal of impurities deeply embedded within the surface of a material by physically removing the upper layer of the substrate. In most cases the surface impurity concentration is small and there is little chemical or physical difference between the surface layer and the substrate. The decontamination of certain radioactive metals using laser ablation falls within this classification.

Laser surface decontamination differs from laser marking in that larger surface areas are targeted and the extent of material removed is dictated by the need to remove impurities rather than to prepare a careful surface pattern. Thus the optical systems used for focusing and process monitoring will differ significantly in the two operations.

To decontaminate surfaces, it may be necessary to remove significant amounts of material (e.g., steel primary coolant vessels used for long periods of time in a nuclear reactor can have radioactive metals ~100 µm below the physical surface of the vessel).

However, when one removes foreign particles from the surface of materials used in microelectronic applications (e.g., silicon wafers), cleaning must be done without affecting substrate properties. In this case surface cleaning is done without the removal (or heating) of substrate material. Microscopic (< 0.1 µm) impurities that cannot be removed using wet methods can be removed by laser surface cleaning methods.

All variants of laser surface cleaning require that contaminants removed from the surface be efficiently collected before they can redeposit on the surface. Fine particulates produced by short-pulse lasers can be efficiently collected using high-efficiency particulate air filters (HEPA). As the laser pulse width increases, the potential for surface melting and the ejection of droplets too heavy to be easily entrained in air flowing at moderate velocities also increases, making the collection of particles more difficult.

The atmosphere around the workpiece influences laser cleaning efficiency. Laser surface decontamination can be effected in air

ISBN 0-912035-15-3

at normal pressures, a convenient situation, but the presence of oxygen can lead to significant surface oxidation. Replacing air with a helium environment is known to improve surface cleaning efficiency even at atmospheric pressure. The efficiency of the laser ablation of metal surfaces is also known to increase with reduction of air pressure around the workpiece.

Advantages of Laser Surface Cleaning

Several advantages that laser surface cleaning offers relative to other surface cleaning technologies are presented in Table 1.

Table 1. Laser Surface Cleaning: Advantages

Advantages of laser surface cleaning over:
Chemical cleaning
Virtually no secondary waste produced
No worker exposure to corrosive chemicals
Little generation of toxic by-products
Little explosion or fire potential
CO_2 pellet blasting
Can remove deeply embedded contaminants
Can be applied to non- "line-of-sight" problems
Can be applied to small areas selectively
Cleaning progress can be monitored continuously
Easily automated with computer control
Shot blasting
Can be applied to delicate substrates
Can be applied to small areas selectively
Virtually no secondary waste produced
Can be applied to non- "line-of-sight" problems
Easily automated with computer control
Cleaning progress can be monitored continuously

The chief disadvantages of laser surface cleaning relative to nonlaser cleaning methods are the high initial capital cost and, in some cases, the increased processing time. However, both may be outweighed by the labor savings achieved through laser surface cleaning, which is a very highly automated process.

Lasers Used for Surface Cleaning

Several different laser systems have been successfully applied to surface cleaning. Some are listed in Table 2.

Table 2. Lasers Used for Surface Cleaning

Laser	Application
Excimer	Oxide layer removal (Al substrate)
	Removal of contaminants on silicon wafer surfaces
	Removal of radioactive surface contamination (metal substrates)
Nd:YAG	Removal of graffiti from metal surfaces
	Removal of paint from metal surfaces
	Removal of radioactive contaminants in metals
CO_2	Cleaning of the surface of F-16 radomes
	Cleaning of ship hulls
	Destruction of PCBs on metal surfaces

Laser Parameters

Technical parameters of three systems used for laser surface cleaning are collected in Table 3.

Table 3. Characteristics of Successful Laser Surface Cleaning Systems

Application	System Characteristics
Radioactive surface decontamination (1)	Nd:YAG laser
	Fiber-optic beam delivery
	5000 Hz
	~40 mJ/pulse
	~150-ns pulse width
	~1-mm spot diameter
Surface cleaning [fine particulate removal (2)]	Excimer laser (248 nm)
	Flowing inert gas tangential to surface
	30 Hz
	600 mJ/pulse
	34-ns pulse width
Laser-based paint removal system (3)	CO_2 laser
	< 150 Hz
	14–27 J/pulse
	1.5-µs pulse width
	~2-cm spot diameter

Process Monitoring

Laser-based processing technologies can often be monitored in real time. Laser surface decontamination is particularly amenable to real-time monitoring through the plasma emission signals that accompany the removal of surface material. An example of process monitoring using plasma emission spectroscopy is shown in Figure 1, where the removal of a cesium impurity from a hard surface coating on a metal was monitored by measuring the diminution of intensity of the cesium emission line at 852 nm as the surface cleaning continued. Note that by the fifth scan, no cesium signal could be observed. Subsequent analysis of the cleaned sample by x-ray fluorescence spectroscopy confirmed that over 99.5% of the cesium originally present had been removed.

Other phenomena can be used to control the laser cleaning process. For example, the acoustic signal generated when a focused laser beam strikes a metal surface can be monitored by a microphone and used to adjust the focus of the laser on the surface. Alternatively, position-sensitive detectors can be used to monitor the reflection of a small CW laser (e.g., He-Ne) for the same purpose.

As a surface is cleaned, its reflectivity changes, and as paint is removed from a surface, the "color" of that surface can be monitored to determine when, for example, an outer paint layer has been removed and the primer coat is exposed.

Beam Delivery

In many industrial laser applications it is advantageous to use fiber-optic delivery systems to port laser energy from a source to a point of application. Conventional fiber optics are very efficient close to the Nd:YAG wavelength (1064 nm), and radiation from such lasers can be transmitted efficiently using such fibers over relatively long distances. For short distances, even the fourth harmonic of Nd:YAG lasers (~266 nm) can be ported to a workpiece for light-duty surface cleaning applications (e.g., removal of auto clear coat imperfections).

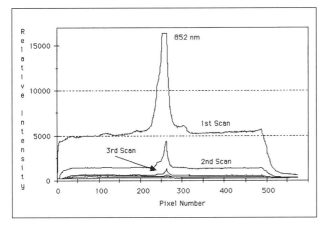

Figure 1. Real-time monitoring of the removal of Cs from a metal surface by laser surface cleaning. The plasma formed during cleaning using a Nd:YAG laser was monitored by a CCD attached to a small monochromator. The figure shows five consecutive scans over a surface originally contaminated with Cs. By the fifth scan, no Cs signal was observed.

Summary

Lasers have been used for the surface cleaning of priceless works of art, valuable microelectronic substrates, and radioactively contaminated metals. Given the availability of lasers with wavelengths from the deep ultraviolet to the far infrared, pulse lengths varying from infinity (i.e., continuous-wave lasers) to femtoseconds (i.e., 10^{-15} s), it is likely that many other laser cleaning jobs will be added to this list in the coming years.

References
1. M. C. Edelson, H-m. Pang, and R. L. Ferguson, A Laser-Based Solution to Industrial Decontamination Problems, in "Proceedings of the Laser Materials Processing Conference ICALEO '95," J. Mazumder, A. Matsunawa, and C. Magnusson (Eds.), 1995: Laser Inst. of America, Orlando, FL, 768–77.
2. A. A. Gruebl, J. A. Dehais, and A. C. Engelsberg, *SSA Journal* **10,** 39–44 (1996); B. R. Marx, *Laser Focus World* **32,** 33–35 (1996).
3. A. E. Hill, Physical Requirements and Methodology Necessary to Achieve Controllable Damage-Free Coating Removal Using a High Energy Pulsed Laser, in "Proceedings of the Laser Materials Processing Conference ICALEO '95," J. Mazumder, A. Matsunawa, and C. Magnusson (Eds.), 1995: Laser Inst. of America, Orlando, FL, 778–87.

MARTIN C. EDELSON

8.8.2 Contaminant Removal

The removal of surface contaminants or debris using high-energy photons has increased as the microelectronics industry has grown, producing surfaces that are more sophisticated and therefore more sensitive to particulates in the micrometer and submicrometer range. But lasers are also receiving considerable interest on the larger scale, even, for example, in paint removal from bridges, as current competing removal techniques become viewed as environmentally unfriendly. The contamination itself can consist of a variety of materials, some that were placed on the surfaces intentionally, such as paint, adhesives, dips, and protective coatings, and many that were unintentional, such as rust and scale, dust and residues, marine salts, and even bird droppings (1). The unintentional sources range from birds to air pollution, biological attack or natural weathering, and radioactive waste. The substrates are as varied as the sources and contaminants, including wood, metal, semiconductors, cloth, stone, ceramic, plastics, and even skin. This large multiplicity of source, contaminant, and substrate is reflected in Table 4, which is a compilation of much of the available information. It shows significant variation in laser parameters depending upon whether delicate semiconductor surfaces or more robust concretes are being decontaminated.

The need for removal of contaminants from surfaces has spurred the development of a large group of techniques such as (2) high-pressure jet spraying, mechanical wiping and scrubbing, wet chemical cleaning, etching, plasma cleaning, ultrasonic cleaning (2), megasonic cleaning, UV/ozone cleaning, CO_2 snow cleaning (3), thermal cleaning in high vacuum, chemical gas cleaning, ion cleaning, electrolytic cleaning, electrostatic cleaning, and cleaning by a synchrotron light source (2). Unfortunately for these techniques, they often have drawbacks in that they are prone to damage delicate parts, can add contaminants either to the surface itself or to the environment, or are simply not effective as the contaminant particle size decreases (3). Since lasers do not have these drawbacks, they are becoming a feasible alternative to many of these techniques. An additional advantage the laser has in cleaning is its lack of contact with the surface. It also does not rely on the use of chemicals or chemical reactions to complete its task, and can be highly localized if necessary to contain any by-products or effluence.

There appear to be two broad classes of adhesion mechanisms that enable a contaminant to adhere to the surface: mechanical and electrostatic (1). The physical mechanisms responsible for laser removal of contaminants can be classified into three categories: explosive vaporization, acoustic excitation due to rapid thermal expansion, and ablative photodecomposition (3).

Explosive vaporization is accomplished utilizing short-pulsed laser irradiation explosively to vaporize either the contaminant itself or other substances. In some cases, the other substance is a liquid film, which is deliberately introduced to assist the removal by generating the force to lift the contaminant from the surface.

Table 4. Contaminant Removal Results

Ref.	Surface	Laser	Species Removed	Fluence (mJ/cm²) or [Irradiance] (W/cm²)	Rep Rate (Hz) or [Pulses]	Pulse Width (ns)	Environment
4	Metals Cu, Al, SS	KrF	Organics and Inorganics	460	1	20	Air
		TEA – CO_2[a]				100	
5	304L SS	Q-Switched Nd:YAG	Metal oxides	366 [>120]	Single	10	Inert Helium
6	Aluminum 304 SS, 316 SS,	CW – CO_2[a]	Radioactive contamination	2 x 10³	150	25	Air
	Inconel 600 Copper	KrF			30	~8	
	Inconel 825 Hastelloy X	Nd:YAG			[~1000 pulses]	3 x 10⁴	
7	Metals Stainless steel Haynes 25 Lead brick	Q-Switched Nd:YAG	Radioactive contamination	2.4–7.4	4–5000	100	
8	Aluminum on Polyethylene Foil	Nd:YAG	Aluminum	[10¹³–10¹⁵]		0.7	3 x 10⁻⁵ Torr
9	Metals	Nd:YAG	Oxides: Al_2O_3 Cr_2O_3 ZrO_3	40–1 x 10³		14	Air
2	Ferrite Magnetic Head Slide	KrF	Epoxy resin	60		20	Air
	Glass Metals Copper SUS	TEA – CO_2[a]	Fingerprints Magic marker Oil and grease	500 500 62.5–450	[20 pulses]	100	
10	Glass Quartz	KrF	Fingerprints	450	10 [2 pulses]	20	Air
		CW CO_2[a] TEA – CO_2[a]				100	
11	Copper Stainless steel (304)	KrF	Oil and grease	460 830	1 [5 pulses] 1 [20 pulses]	20	Air Dry
	Aluminum	TEA – CO_2[a]				100	
12	Semiconductor - Silicon	KrF ArF	Covalently bonded methyl groups Environmental carbon	35	5		Inert (Flowing)
			Organics on metal Environmental carbon Si_p on Si Al flake on aluminum	9 x 10³	2		

Table 4. Contaminant Removal Results (continued)

Ref.	Surface	Laser	Species Removed	Fluence (mJ/cm^2) or [Irradiance] (W/cm^2)	Rep Rate (Hz) or [Pulses]	Pulse Width (ns)	Environment
13	Semiconductors Optical: Al/quartz Au/Ni/Al mirror	Excimer	Molecular films Chemical and metallic particulate	50–500	5	80	10^{-6} Torr Air
14	Silicon (Integrated circuits)	TEA – CO$_2$	9.5 μ Al$_2$O$_3$ 5 μ Al$_2$O$_3$ 1 μm polystyrene	2.6 x 10^3 - 13.15 x 10^3		100	Water vapor
15	Crystalline silicon, Chromium, TiC – Al$_2$O$_3$	KrF	Epoxy film 1 μm alumina particles	50–200	10	16	Dry 8% Isopropanol and Water
16	Silicon	KrF	0.1 μm alumina particles	120		16	20% methanol, ethanol or isopropanol and water
17	Silicon	TEA – CO$_2$	9.5 μm, 5 μm Al$_2$O$_3$ and 1 μm polystyrene	2.63 x 10^3 13.15 x 10^3		1 x 10^3	Water
18	Silicon	TEA – CO$_2$	1 μm alumina	Max 30 x 10^3		1 x 10^3	Water
19	Silicon lithography Masks	KrF or XeCl Q-Switched Er:YAG[a]	Latex and Alumina (0.35 μ) Silica Gold (0.2 μ)	350		16	Air Water
3	Crystalline silicon	KrF	1 μm alumina Epoxy/acetone	110–180	300	16	Isopropanol and water Dry air
20	Semiconductors Electronic components Optical components Magnetic components Optics, coated Automotive Aerospace	KrF	Paint particles, haze, rustoleum, rust Oxide, adhesive Fingerprints Oil	30 – 2.30x10^3	30		Flowing Inert
21	Art: marble, metal, terra cotta	Q-Switched Ruby Ruby	Black encrustations of dust, unburned Carbon residues Marine salts and Biological organisms	1 x 10^3 1 x 10^4		35 1 x 10^6	Air

Table 4 concludes on page 30.

Table 4. Contaminant Removal Results (continued)

Ref.	Surface	Laser	Species Removed	Fluence (mJ/cm²) or [Irradiance] (W/cm²)	Rep Rate (Hz) or [Pulses]	Pulse Width (ns)	Environment
22	Concrete	Pulsed - Nd:YAG CW – Nd:YAG	Radioactive contamination which soaked into walls Paint	[b]1.5–3.7 W 4.7–12 x 10³ Joules 620 W 18.6 x 10³ Joules		3.5 x 10⁶	Air Water
23	Stained glass	Ruby	Surface (flashing) encrustation	1 kW/cm²		1 x 10⁶	Air

[a]Not Effective [b]Inadequate information available to allow units to be changed where data was available. We noted processes that were to be ineffective.

Rapid thermal expansion of the surface can cause particles to be ejected at high speed when the substrate is rapidly laser heated with moderate energy density (<1 J/cm²).

If the surface and the contaminants have different absorptivities for laser irradiation and different ablation thresholds, the application of laser irradiation can either dissociate the contaminant or induce photothermal desorption. The energy density required for this is usually less than that for vaporization of the substrate.

The commonality of these three mechanisms lies in their use of short-wavelength lasers at short pulse durations. As can be seen in Table 4, when longer wavelengths were used, such as with TEA–CO_2 lasers, the cleaning process often was not effective. There also seems to be a critical fluence range to achieve effective cleaning without undesired damage to the substrate. This is determined largely by the particular adhesion mechanism and the morphology of the contaminant. Once above the critical value, a low fluence requires a large number of pulses to achieve cleaning. A higher fluence with fewer pulses can be used if the fluence remains below the damage threshold.

References

1. C. M. Young, William M. Moeny, R. D. Curry, Ken McDonald, and John T. Bosma, "Application of lasers and pulsed power to coating removal," *SPIE* Vol. 2374, 2–9 (1995).
2. Y. F. Lu, and Y. Aoyagi. "Laser cleaning - a new surface cleaning method without pollutions," *Mat. Res. Soc. Symp. Proc.* Vol. 344, 329–34 (1994).
3. Hee K. Park, Costas P. Grigoropoulos, and Andrew C. Tam, "Practical excimer laser-assisted cleaning of solid surfaces," *SPIE* Vol. 2498, 22–31 (1995).
4. Y. F. Lu, M. Takai, S. Komuro, T. Shiokawa, and Y. Aoyagi, *Appl Phys.* **A59**, 281–88 (1994).
5. H. C. Peebles, N. A. Creager, and D. E. Peebles, "Surface Cleaning by Laser Ablation," SAND–91-0505C, DE91 009189, Conf-910279-12.
6. Rick L. Demmer, and Russ L. Ferguson, "Testing and evaluation of light ablation decontamination," INEL-94/0134 UC-510, 1994: Prepared for the U.S. Department of Energy under DOE Idaho Operations Office Contract DE-AC07-941D13223.
7. M. C. Edelson, Ho-ming Pang, and Russell L. Ferguson, "A laser-based solution to industrial decontamination problems," DOE document IS-M–838 Conf-9511146-5.
8. Faiz Dahmani, and Tahar Ferdja, "Laser-intensity and wavelength dependence of mass-ablation rate, ablation pressure, and heat-flux inhibition in laser-produced plasmas," *Phys. Rev. A* **44**, 2649–56 (1991).
9. R. Oltra, O. Yavas, F. Cruz, J. P. Boquillon, and C. Sartori, "Modeling and diagnostic of pulsed laser cleaning of oxidized metallic surfaces," *Applied Surface Science* **96–98**, 484–90 (1996).
10. Yong-Feng Lu, Shuji Komuro and Yoshinobu Aoyagi, "Laser-induced removal of fingerprints from glass and quartz surfaces," *Jpn. J. Appl. Phys.*, **33**, 4691–96 (1994).
11. Y. F. Lu, M. Takai, S. Komuro, T. Shiokawa, and Y. Aoyagi, "Surface cleaning of metals by pulsed-laser irradiation in air," *Appl. Phys. A* **59**, 281–8 (1994).
12. Audrey C. Engelsberg, "Particle Removal from Semiconductor Surfaces Using a Photon-Assisted, Gas-Phase Cleaning Process," Mat. Res. Soc. Symp. Proc. Vol. 315, 1993: Materials Research Society, *Surface Chemical Cleaning and Passivation for Semiconductor Processing,* Gregg S. Higashi, Eugene A. Irene, and Tadahiro Ohmi (Eds.).
13. D. J. Flesher, "Lasers and High-energy light as a decontamination tool for nuclear applications," WHC-SA-2132-FP, 1993: Prepared for the U.S. Department of Energy Office of Environmental Restoration and Waste Management under Contract DE-AC06-87RL10930 (#7).
14. T. J. Magee, and C. S. Leung, "Scanning UV laser removal of contaminants from semiconductor and optical surfaces," *Particles on Surfaces 3*, K. L. Mittal (Ed.), 1991: Plenum Press, New York, 307–16.

15. H. K. Park, Costas P. Grigoropoulos, Wing P. Leung, and Andrew C. Tam, IEEE Transactions on Components, Packaging and Manufacturing Technology - Part A, Vol. 17, No. 4, December 1994, 139–42.
16. Andrew C. Tam, Wing P. Leung, Werner Zapka and Winfrid Ziemlich, *JAP 71* (7) 3515–23 (April 1992).
17. S. J. Lee, K. Imen, and S. D. Allen, "CO_2 laser assisted particle removal threshold measurements," *Appl. Phys. Lett.* **61** (19), 2314–16 (1992).
18. K. Imen, S. J. Lee and S. D. Allen, "Laser-assisted micron scale particle removal," *Appl. Phys. Lett.* **58** (2), 203–5 (1991).
19. W. Zapka, W. Ziemlich, and A. C. Tam. "Efficient pulsed laser removal of 0.2 micron sized particles from a solid surface," *Appl. Phys. Lett.* **58** (20), 2217–19 (1991).
20. E. C. Harvey, J. Fletcher, and A. C. Engelsberg, "A non-reactive excimer-based surface preparation and cleaning tool for broad-based industrial applications," Mat. Res. Soc. Symp. Vol. 397, 335–40 (1996).
21. J. F. Asmus, Carl G. Murphy, and Walter H. Munk, "Studies on the interaction of laser radiation with art artifacts," Proceedings of the Society of Photo-Optical Instrumentation Engineers, Vol. 41, 1974, for Meeting in San Diego, California, August 27–29, 1973, 19–27.
22. N. S. Cannon, and D. J. Flesher. "Lasers for the Radioactive Decontamination of Concrete," 1993: WHC-SA-2116-FP Prepared for the U.S. Department of Energy Office of Environmental Restoration and Waste Management.
23. J. F. Asmus, "Use of lasers in the conservation of stained glass," *Conservation in Archaeology and the Applied Arts,* London: International Institute for Conservation of Historic and Artistic Works, c1975.
24. Wayne Reitz, "Environmental aspects of coating removal technologies," *Advances in Coatings Technologies for Corrosion and Wear Resistant Coatings,* A. R. Srivatsa, C. R. Clayton, and J. K. Hirvonen (Eds.), *The Minerals, Metals and Materials Society* (1995) 329–52.
25. Audrey C. Engelsberg, "Removal of surface contaminants by irradiation from a high-energy source," U.S. Patent No. 5,024,968, Jun. 18, 1991.
26. "Environmentally Friendly Paint Removal," *Industrial Laser Review,* p. 4, September 1994.
27. Paul A. Lovoi, and A. M. Frank, "Method of and apparatus for the removal of paint and the like from a substrate," U.S. Patent No. 4,588,885.

MARY HELEN McCAY

8.8.3 Removal of Paint, Dielectric and Other Coatings

Laser ablation provides a method of selectively removing coatings with great precision from delicate substrates without causing damage, even when substrate and coating(s) are nearly indistinguishable from each other. Furthermore, the ejectant residue (sometimes hazardous) may be completely and safely captured. The recent development of special rep-pulsed CO_2 lasers, which combine high peak and average powers (1) (up to 50 MW peak and 10 kW average, respectively), makes it feasible to strip very large, arbitrarily shaped objects such as airplanes, ships, buildings, bridges, and oil derricks at speeds that are competitive with those characteristic of sand-blasting nozzles.

The capital equipment cost of laser-based paint (or other coatings) removal systems typically exceed that of more conventional systems, such as abrasive blasters, water blasters, or chemical-based systems. However, conventional systems nearly always damage sensitive substrates, cannot be carefully controlled, and create an enormous cleanup problem, usually resulting in serious environmental impact. Whenever one or more of those issues cannot be tolerated, the laser-based option should be explored.

The choice of CO_2 versus Nd:YAG lasers is driven primarily by the size of the job and secondarily by the need for flexibility of delivery. A specifically designed 10-kW average power CO_2 laser can remove 5-mil-thick paint at the rate of 600 ft^2/h. Nd:YAG lasers currently must operate in a multi-kilohertz, Q-switched mode to be effective for this application. Such lasers are not easily scaled to high average power levels, ~300 W average power the maximum as of the date of this submission. Small-scale parts cleaning or touch-up applications that fall within the power handling capability of available Nd:YAG lasers could well benefit from this laser's portability, low cost, and capability for fiber-optic beam delivery — at least up to the power handling capabilities of the fiber for Q-switched operation. Both CO_2 and Nd:YAG laser wavelengths are absorbed within a few micrometers in nearly all paints and most other dielectric coatings.

The required laser process is significantly different from more usual "thermal" processes, wherein a continuous laser beam is tightly focused in order to create a deep melt zone over a small area. Instead, this application requires that a very intense (~5 MW/cm^2) beam be distributed over a large area (a few cm^2 to tens of cm^2) and that its dwell time be limited to a specific, application-dependent pulse length — most typically a few microseconds (1), (2). A microscopically thin melt zone is created over the irradiated area, despite rapid heat loss into the cold substrate directly below. The coating temperature must be further elevated to the vaporization point, and energy deposition must continue long enough to evaporate a significant amount of material.

Figures 2a and 2b present the time history of thermal conduction with varying depths into acrylic and steel. Acrylic typifies the thermal properties of many paints and many delicate composite aircraft structures as well. The steel represents a classic alternative substrate having very large thermal conductivity, which tends to heat sink the removal process as the laser beam–material interface approaches the steel surface. Knowledge of the coatings' and substrates' thermal response data is useful in choosing the pulse period and repetition rate for a specific process.

Spatial resolution and control may be maximized by minimizing the depth of interaction. In turn, this is facilitated by maximizing the peak irradiance to the point of narrowly (but safely) escaping plasma formation. Thus peak irradiance, pulse shape, and energy density must be selected to control optimally the surface interaction depth and to avoid damage to the substrate.

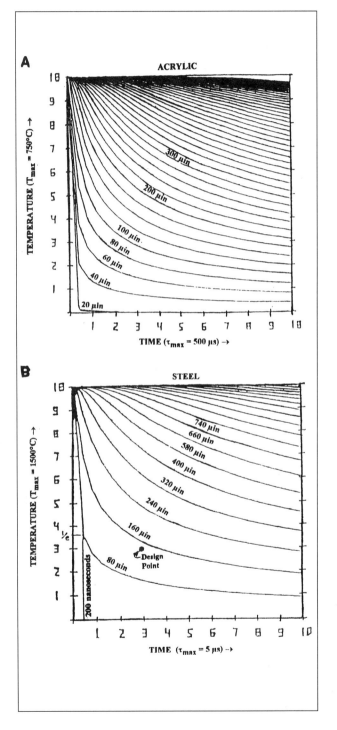

Figure 2. Time history of thermal conduction with varying depths into (a) acrylic and (b) steel. Depth contours are in microinches (μin.).

Plasma formation must be avoided for two reasons: (1) The shock wave it produces will severely damage any composite substrate and will also fatigue aluminum skin substrates, and (2) even if the substrate is indestructable, the plasma would block most of the laser beam from reaching the substrate. For the case of CO_2 laser radiation ($\lambda = 10.6$ μm), peak irradiance should be held to ~5 MW/cm² to avoid breakdown, allowing for the effects of aerosols and interference fringing. If metal reflections are to be encountered, further intensity reduction may prove necessary. For the case of Nd:YAG lasers, the plasma formation threshold is raised by a factor of 100 (i.e., 5×10^8 W/cm²). This is fortuitous since one *needs* to deliver 100-fold greater irradiance using a Nd:YAG laser compared to a CO_2 laser. This follows because a Nd:YAG laser's pulse energy is down by a factor of ~1000 and its pulse period is down by a factor of ~10 compared to an electrically pulsed CO_2 laser.

If the pulse length is too great, much energy will be lost to heating the substrate, and nonmetallic substrates will be damaged, as is evident from Figure 2.

If the pulse length is too short, then an insufficient amount of energy is deposited into the substrate and the ablation process becomes inefficient. Only that fraction of energy applied *after* the surface has reached the ablating point causes physical removal; the energy that is applied from turn on up to the ablating point is simply heat sunk into the substrate which, except for thermal build-up, is lost. Figure 3 illustrates this effect for the case of a 1.5-μs CO_2 laser pulse applied to Phantom F-4 radome paint. Note that 5 J/cm² couples ~90% of the absorbed laser energy into material ablation. Had the fluence been 0.5 J/cm², 90% of the energy would have been lost rather than absorbed. On the other hand, raising the fluence to level toward 10 J/cm² pushes the laser's electric field strength dangerously close to creating air breakdown.

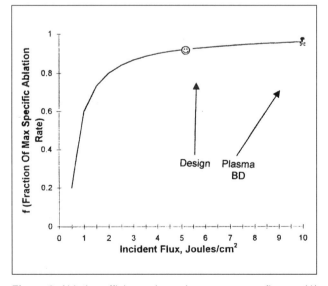

Figure 3. Ablation efficiency dependence on energy fluence (J/cm²-pulse) for the case of 1.5-μs flat-top CO_2 laser pulses.

Because of the necessity to avoid air breakdown, a CO_2 laser's pulse shape significantly affects its ability to do useful work as a paint stripper. For example, conventional CO_2 TEA lasers deliver ~50% of their pulse energy in a ~100-ns spike, followed by a long tail. It is evident from Figure 3 that this pulse shape restricts the peak irradiance to less than ~1.5 J/cm^2, since the first three-quarters of a joule produces ~7.5 MW/cm^2, a peak irradiance that borders on creating air breakdown. Figure 3 shows that, depending on the actual plasma formation point, at least 30%, and perhaps up to 50%, of the available energy is lost. By comparison, if 1–2-μs-wide flat-top pulses are applied, less than 10% of the energy is lost to substrate heating.

Moving from laser architectural specifications to the mechanics of beam delivery, the foremost consideration is to avoid thermal build-up. Figure 4 depicts the temporal history of the surface temperature in response to a sequence of 1 μs laser pulses spaced 10 ms apart and applied to a fixed position. The actual temperature coordinate depends on the specific material. The lower dashed line denotes the coating boiling temperature, while the upper dashed line denotes a temperature at which the underlying substrate will be damaged when the floor of the ablated area reaches the substrate. When the pulses overlap at high repetition rates, the surface temperature does not have time to decay fully between pulse applications. Therefore, both upper and lower temperature envelopes increase with succeeding pulses until an asymptotic limit is reached at steady state.

Prior to reaching steady state, the maximum temperature may exceed the damage threshold for the substrate, and, as the "floor" of the ablated area approaches the substrate, damage will begin. In cases where the substrate is not subject to damage, a certain level of thermal build-up can be used to enhance the process efficiency. It is desired to control the repetition rate and the scan rate such that the ablation efficiency is enhanced, but damage to the substrate is circumvented. In the example of Figure 4, where the laser rests 10,000 times longer than its pulse length, no more than 6 pulses should successively overlap at any given point.

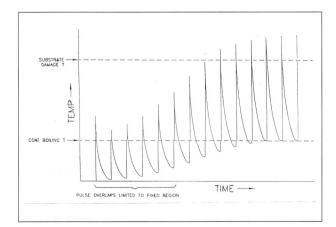

Figure 4. Thermal build-up in response to 1-μs flat-top laser pulses at 100 pps for acrylic paint.

If the pulse length were more than 10 μs long (instead of 1 or 2 μs long), pulse overlap should be avoided. The beam must instead be rastered such that many positions, widely separated from each other, are targeted prior to repeating the pattern.

A scan methodology is exemplified in Figure 5. This illustrates that if the coat is initially irregular, a linear, overlapping scan trajectory will preserve the spatial irregularities as we approach the substrate with each succeeding pass. As the substrate comes into view, "islands" of residual coat remain that correspond to places where the initial coat was thickest.

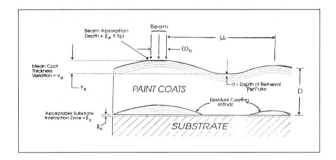

Figure 5. Matching laser scan parameters with surface topology. Requirements: d << D if substrate has high thermal conductivity or high reflectivity (i.e., metal); ω_b<<μ for efficient "island" cleanup; d is chosen to voice substrate damage, such as, (1) τ_{pulse} is sufficiently short to restrict thermal penetration beyond δ_d, (2) power density is high enough that ablation velocity >> thermal velocity, and (3) scan speed and overlap are chosen to avoid thermal build-up.

If the substrate is delicate (i.e., fiberglass), a vision system may become necessary that blocks out individual laser pulses wherever the substrate has been reached. Neither computer storage nor processing is needed because the gate status is determined immediately prior to triggering each laser pulse. In order spatially to resolve "island" clean-up, the irradiation area should be small compared to the coatings' spatial undulation period. Furthermore, the total thickness of material removed over a single full area scan (including x and y overlap) should normally be much smaller than the total coat thickness. Increasing the number of total passes reduces the amount of energy coupled to the substrate and increases the efficiency of "island" clean-up.

Sensitive substrates may require a large number of passes to avoid damage, while insensitive, thermally conductive substrates such as metals can tolerate a reduced number of passes. However, reducing the number of passes may, because of heat loss, significantly reduce the efficiency and thus increase the process time.

There is no limit to the depth of removal that can be achieved by overlapping pulses, followed by overlapping scans. In general, the footprints should overlap in both scan and scan-step directions (x and y). For example, if two-tenths mil is removed for each pulse (typical for application of parameters presented) and, if the footprint is overlapped 5 times in both x and y coordinates, then 5 mils depth will be removed for each raster scan over the full area being processed.

A large fraction of all applications will fall into one of two distinctly different categories:

Case 1: Coat and substrate are vastly differentiated by reflectivity, thermal conductivity, and boiling temperatures (e.g., paint on steel or aluminum)

Case 2: Coat and substrate have similar properties, although the substrate may be a composite (e.g., paint on fiberglass)

For Case 1, the beam is easily absorbed by the coat and nearly reflected by this substrate, and there is no need to control the process. It is highly efficient and fully discriminatory. The beam may be manually scoured over the surface as though it were blasted sand. For the case of deeply textured metals, the paint can be removed from the deepest crevices given sufficient time and without affecting the metal. Also, the peak power requirement for this case can be relaxed.

For Case 2, there is no significant discrimination by virtue of the physical process, *and* the substrates are generally delicate. This case generally requires monitored control of the scan, repetition rate, and pulse gate in accordance with all the considerations presented in this section. For the simplest cases, visual monitoring may suffice.

Tables 5–8 are offered as a guide to set up processing scenarios for Cases 1 and 2. Many dielectric coats, paints, grease layers, or even biological tissue are similar in their physical properties and can be approximated by the generic "paint" properties offered.

Table 5. Physical Properties of Coats and Substrates

Material	Reflectivity	Thermal conductivity K (W/cm-deg)	Melting temperature (°C)
Coat			
Paint	~5%	0.002	~400°C
Primer	similar	similar	similar
Substrate			
Resin	similar	similar	similar
Fiberglass	similar	0.0076	~800°C
Steel	~95%	1.13	1535°C
Aluminum	~95%	2.04	660°C

Table 6. Coating Removal Rates

Paint on smooth composite substrate	250–300 ft^2·mil/kW-h
Paint on smooth metal substrate	Similar
Paint below surface of textured metal substrate	<125 ft^2·mil/kW-h

Table 7. Suggested Range of Pulsed CO_2 Laser Parameters

Case 1: Paint on Metal	
Pulse length	1–100 μs
Peak irradiance	50 kW/cm^2 – 7.5 MW/cm^2
Energy density/pulse	5–750 J/cm^2
Repetition rate	50–1000 pps
Case 2: Paint on Composite	
Pulse length	1–10 μs, 1–3 μs, typically optimal
Peak irradiance	4–7.5 MW/cm^2
Energy density/pulse	4–7.5 J/cm^2
Repetition rate	50–200 pps

Table 8. Suggested Range of *Q*-switched Nd:YAG Laser Parameters

Case 1: Paint on Metal	
Pulse length	30–500 ns
Peak irradiance	≥ 500 MW/cm^2
Energy density/pulse	5–50(?) J/cm^2
Repetition rate	3000–15000 pps

Notes: (1) Cases 1 and 2 become indistinguishable; (2) limited energy necessitates a small spot requiring high-speed mechanical scan in one dimension.

The laser cavity should be designed to generate a uniform spatial beam distribution, consisting of the maximum possible number of modes that can be transmitted through the beam delivery system, recalling that the beam divergence scales proportionally to the square root of the mode number. Long-distance delivery systems, particularly those subject to large variations in optical path length during a scan scenario, may *require* use of a single-mode beam in order to accommodate beam delivery. In this case a mode scrambler should be incorporated near the point of delivery.

Fortunately for the case of CO_2 lasers, large-mode-number beams may be focused from several meters distant to produce footprints of appropriate size (5–10 cm^2) on the target, and the depth of field can well exceed ± 30 cm. So the focal distance (z) is not critical, and neither are the x-y coordinates. Therefore, a manually controlled articulated arm could be used even if the substrate is fragile, as long as simple safety backup systems (which probably incorporate feedback) are provided to ensure against overstrip. Alternatively, the process may be fully automated, but without a requirement for precision positioning control.

Since the ablating process produces shock waves, some means of acoustic abatement may be necessary. In addition, a vacuum cleaner-like debris suction and filter capture system will typically be needed. Following the laser strip procedure, slight carbon soot deposits may remain that can easily be wiped away with a damp cloth. In most cases, the final result can be a surface that is virtually indistinguishable from its condition prior to having been painted. Alternatively, the primer coat may be left intact.

ISBN 0-912035-15-3

References

1. A. E. Hill, The physics and methodology of laser surface ablation: DOD Industry Advanced Coatings Removal Conference, Phoenix, Arizona (1995).
2. A. E. Hill, Physical requirements and methodology necessary to achieve controllable damage-free coating removal using a high energy pulsed laser: Proc. ICALEO '95, Laser Institute of America, Vol. 80, Laser Materials Processing. 778–87 (1995).

ALAN E. HILL

8.9 Disk Texturing

Zone texturing is a laser-based manufacturing process that improves the performance of computer hard-disk drives. The laser creates microscopic "bumps" in a specific region on the disk surface. These bumps optimize the interaction of the disk surface and the drive head by creating a rough zone where the slider can land on the otherwise extremely smooth surface of the disk. Because of higher storage densities, lower fly heights for the sliders are necessary, translating into smoother surfaces in the data storage areas. The problem of stiction on landing associated with the extremely smooth surfaces is thus minimized and disk magnetics can be decoupled from mechanical issues in manufacturing.

A typical process is to place a dedicated "landing zone" on the inner portion of the disk and outside the magnetic area, where the slider can be parked. The width of the zone is only about 2 to 3 mm – comparable to the slider width. There is little or no material removal in an optimized process. Process conditions are optimized so that ablation is avoided, but a melt and reflow produces the desired microstructure. These bumps can take several different shapes, depending on set-up conditions, including "sombrero" and new-Gaussian. Feature sizes thus attained vary from a few up to about 30 μm in diameter and up to 100 nm in height.

The laser typically used is a high-repetition-rate, diode-pumped solid-state laser, usually Nd:YLF in the fundamental frequency. This wavelength interacts well with the NiP-plated aluminum substrate to create the bumps rapidly by a melting process. The laser must be highly reliable and have excellent pulse-to-pulse stability in order to achieve the necessary uniformity. Pulse repetition rates of 10 to 100 kHz are usually employed with single pulse energies of 10 to 20 μJ and stability of 1–2% rms (s <1–2%). The spatial output is TEM_{00}.

In a typical set up, the laser output is adjusted to a power level appropriate to achieve the desired bump shape and height. This output is then focused onto the surface of the substrate, which is mounted on a rotating spindle. In addition to rotary motion, it is also necessary to move either the beam or the part laterally during processing. A shutter is placed in the beam and, after loading when the spindle has reached the desired relative speed and position, the shutter opens and the laser begins firing, creating a spiral of distinct bumps on the NiP surface. The separation between bumps is less than 100 μm and provides excellent support for the contacting slider. Employing this technique, a textured landing zone 2 to 3 mm wide can be made in a few seconds of lasing time.

References

P. Baumgart, D. Krajnovich, T. Nguyen, and A. Tam, *Safe landings: Laser texturing of high-density magnetic disks*; Data Storage (March 1996).

P. Baumgart, D. Krajnovich, T. Nguyenand, and A. Tam, *A new laser texturing technique for high performance magnetic disk drives*; IEEE Proceedings, 2946–51 (1995).

R. Ranjan, D. N. Lambeth, M. Tromel, P. Goglia, and Y. Li, *Laser Texturing for Low-flying-height Media*; *J. Appl. Phys.*, **69**, 5745–47 (1991).

RONALD D. SCHAEFFER

Notes

Chapter 9

Brazing/Soldering

9.1 Process Definition

Brazing is defined as a process where the base material remains in the solid state and a solder material reaches the liquid state, thus wetting the base material. Brazing is divided into soft brazing (temperature below 450°C) and hard brazing (temperature above 450°C).

There is a variety of heat sources available for this process. If one uses a furnace, induction-heating equipment, or a flame in combination with small components, the joint can be formed over the total length at one time. This is an effective technique with through-heating of the base material or at least a large heat-affected zone. Another possibility is to heat the joint only locally and to move the heat along the seam. This can be done by a flame, an arc, and also by a laser. The technique is very similar to welding; so the advantages and disadvantages are comparable.

Brazing is done generally with a base metal, a braze metal, and in many cases a flux, which will destroy and remove the oxides from the base metal and protect the base metal and the solder from oxidation during the process. The fluxes can cause corrosion and then have to be removed carefully from the brazed components. Fluxes and braze metals are often unhealthy for workers, and safety must be considered.

The most important requirements for achieving high-quality joints are clean surfaces, normally inside a small gap, and a guaranteed working temperature over the whole brazing area. Under these conditions the solder material can flow into the gap because of capillary forces and wet the surfaces. It is clear that the absorbed laser energy that is conducted from the irradiated area to the surrounding material can produce the correct working temperature only in thin sheets and for short conduction distances. If longer distances between the area of laser absorption and the gap where the solder has to be melted are necessary, a higher temperature difference between these two areas results. In this case, even for hard brazing, an undesired melting of the laser-irradiated area occurs. Therefore, for laser brazing the laser should be positioned directly above the gap to heat both base materials.

Typical geometries for brazing are the overlap seam and the flanged seam. In both cases the necessary gap can be maintained by clamping both sheets together. An adjustment of the width of the gap is not necessary. Laser brazing can be carried out at all orientations. The braze metal can be supplied as filler wire, as a braze metal sheet, or sometimes in combination with the flux as a powder or a paste. For special applications the use of gas mixtures, mostly containing hydrogen, can destroy oxides and substitute for the flux.

The advantage of laser brazing compared to other brazing techniques with a moving brazing area is the low heat input, resulting in a low distortion. Brazing cannot be done with a keyhole and a focused laser beam. Defocusing of the laser beam is common and is accompanied by a decrease in energy density.

The distortion can be minimized with a small overlap of the sheet ($\approx$ 2 mm), leading to a sufficient tension or shear strength, and an optimized heat input achievable by maximum feed rate with the highest possible energy density. The limitation for an optimized heat input is that an appropriate temperature level over the whole gap has to be maintained. With decreasing velocity both the maximum value of the temperature field and the distance between the isotherms increase. Higher energy density leads to higher maximum temperature at the place of absorption. The maximum temperature of the temperature field should be below the melting temperature of the base metal. The minimum width of the isotherms of the working temperature must be equal to the width of the overlap area. Normally this adjustment leads to sufficient brazing processes.

Using this technology, many types of steels, titanium alloys, and other alloys can be brazed. For aluminum alloys a limitation is the available braze metals, which have a melting temperature near the melting point of aluminum and make brazing difficult. Braze metals containing Ge and In are under development for aerospace applications and will work at approximately 570°C but further research is necessary to make braze metals affordable. Another limitation is the available fluxes, which can work sufficiently well with Mg contents below 3%.

Because of the high temperature gradient resulting in laser brazing, joining of dissimilar metals and alloys is possible. A growth of critical intermetallic phases can be controlled, and combinations of aluminum, steel, or titanium can be joined.

9.2 Appropriate Lasers

Brazing with lasers does not use a keyhole, which means the energy must be absorbed directly at the surface of the base material. Generally the absorption of a metal decreases with increasing wavelength of the laser beam. Therefore, if other technical requirements allow it, lasers close to the visible wavelength range are recommended.

For materials processing two types of lasers have been used most often: CO_2 lasers (wavelength 10.6 μm) and Nd:YAG lasers (wavelength 1.06 μm). The wavelength of these lasers differs by a factor of 10; so the absorption of Nd:YAG lasers is generally higher. The beam quality of both laser types is more than sufficient for brazing, because the beam is normally defocused. Better beam quality could be used if a greater distance between the process area and the working head of the laser system is used to prevent contamination of the optics by dust and dirt.

CO_2 laser systems have a few disadvantages for brazing. The comparably long wavelength leads to a low process efficiency because of the high reflected laser power. The reflected power can damage surrounding objects, but also the process itself is influenced. The reflection normally varies, depending on the surface quality of the material; so absorption along a seam is not totally constant. In combination with the low absorption (steel: 2-10%) very high laser powers are necessary (> 4 kW). The difference of absorption along the seam can lead to local overheating in areas of a high absorption (e.g., with flux on the surface) and lead to insufficient wetting in areas of low absorption. Therefore, CO_2 lasers cannot be recommended for brazing technologies.

Nd:YAG laser systems offer some advantages for brazing compared to CO_2 lasers but also one disadvantage. The disadvantage is the high operating cost. The use of Nd:YAG systems at high power levels leads to a short lifetime of the lamps (500-600 h, depending on the laser system and the maximum beam power), which has to be recognized for cost calculations. The advantage of brazing for this kind of laser system is the short wavelength, which leads to a stable process (absorption of steel ≈ 40%) and no problems with reflected energy of the laser beam.

Since 1997 a third laser system has been available over the range of 1-3 kW. These are semiconductor lasers or high-power diode lasers. The advantage of this laser is the high efficiency of up to 30% compared with 2-4% for Nd:YAG systems and 10-15% for CO_2 lasers. High-power diode lasers are serious competitors for established lasers. The wavelengths of diode laser systems are in the range 800 to 1000 nm at power levels up to 3 kW. The relatively poor beam quality is sufficient for laser brazing but can cause trouble for protecting the optics when critical metals like zinc-coated steels or metals with lubricants on the surface are to be brazed. Because of its very compact design, the complete diode laser can be installed in a robot with a capacity of at least 20 kg. The power and cooling supplies can be connected via cable and are very small compared to other laser systems. No systems with mirrors or fibers are necessary for beam delivery. The beam is delivered directly from the laser source to the process. The use of diode lasers for soldering is described in Section 9.4.4.

9.3 Beam Manipulation Techniques

As mentioned previously, Nd:YAG lasers are used with a defocused beam. For brazing the dimension of the working spot is more important than the dimension of the focus or the beam quality.

Different geometries of the working spot can be chosen. Normally a circular spot is used following beam delivery through an optical fiber. The main advantage is that the process result is independent of the orientation between the laser spot and the seam. Additionally, curved seams can be generated with a 2D-CNC system. A circular spot is obtained by defocusing the beam, using a normal working head for laser welding and greater distances along the z axis. But there are some disadvantages. If one uses a filler wire instead of pastes or brazing sheets, the orientation between the filler wire and the seam has to be constant. With the filler wire mounted on the working head of the laser, a rotation of the head above the curve is necessary. This can be done only by a three-axis CNC system, and normally a four-axis system is used to adjust the z axis too. A rectangular beam can be obtained by special optics.

The spot of a high-power diode laser, normally used without a fiber, is rectangular. The beam of a diode laser is described by the divergence in two directions, which are called the fast and slow axes. For joining curved seams the laser has to be rotated to achieve stable results.

A rectangular working spot offers some advantages for brazing, especially for coated material. The problem with coated materials is that they often have relatively high reflectivity. This can be overcome by a higher energy density, leading to a local evaporation of the coating at the process area. A defocused circular working spot after a fiber, with an energy density distribution similar to a Gaussian distribution, offers a high energy density only in the center of the beam. This nonuniform distribution leads to an increased reflection outside the beam center compared to a uniform rectangular spot, so that the sublimation can start only in the central area. Of course with a uniform energy density over the whole beam, the total energy is higher than with a Gaussian distribution at the same maximum energy density. Practically, higher feed rates are achievable with a rectangular beam distribution.

Theoretically, an optimized distribution of energy density looks like a chair, with a maximum peak at the front resulting in high temperature gradients, a flat part behind it causing a constant temperature, and finally a sudden fall resulting in high temperature gradients with a rapidly decreasing temperature. Up to now experimental studies on the effect of energy distributions have been done only for hardening.

A third type of beam manipulation with a normal working head is a setup with an angle between the z axis and the axis of the laser beam. The resulting geometry of the spot is elliptical, so that results comparable to rectangular spots can be achieved, but with lower efficiency. Joining of curved seams is more complicated because of the angle between the beam and the z axis. Because of this a second axis has to be considered with possible problems during the adjustment of a tool center point (TCP) in three- and four-axis systems. The motivation behind the similarity to a rectangular spot was the possibility of overcoming problems with reflected laser light. If this problem does not occur, the use of an elliptic spot cannot be recommended.

Figure 1 illustrates the dependence between a movement of the laser head in the z direction and the resulting movement of the beam in a second direction (here in the x direction). If the movement is done by the handling system, a movement of the TCP results. To follow a curved seam requires special handling systems.

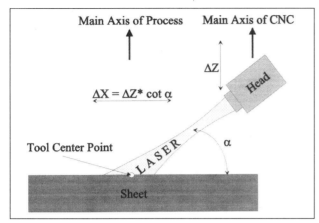

Figure 1. Dependence between the movement in the z direction and the movement of the TCP using an angular beam.

A special type of beam manipulation is the simultaneous use of two lasers. The advantage is the possibility of working with two working spots, which can be formed separately, as described. This offers the opportunity of controlling the temperature of the lower and upper sheet separately. The disadvantage is the additional cost for the second laser. Overlap joints with an overlap up to 10 mm can be brazed with such systems.

9.4 Applications and Results

Laser brazing, except for the joining of electronic components, is a young technology. The first industrial applications are under development. A potential is seen for applications in the automotive industry, where thin sheets of steel have to be joined with low distortion and high surface quality.

The main target of development is hybrid joints of dissimilar materials (e.g., steel and aluminum), which became possible using the resulting high temperature gradients.

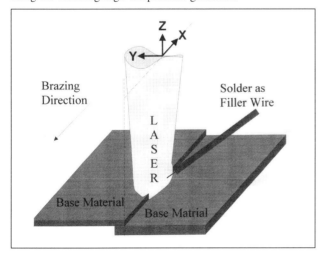

Figure 1. Setup for brazing or joining with filler wire.

Figure 1 shows a setup for brazing and joining with filler wire. The adjustment of the filler wire depends on the solder used, the feed rate, and the diameter of the wire. For an easy adjustment, an adjusting element for movement of the target point at the end of the filler wire along the x axis is recommended. The filler wire should meet the sheets at the edge of the sheets between the center and the end of the working spot.

9.4.1 Brazing of Steel

For brazing of steel many different solders with different properties are available. Depending on the solder and the base material, an appropriate flux has to be chosen. An optimal choice of brazes and fluxes is dependent on many factors, such as the necessary strength, the corrosion behavior, the color after coating, etc., and especially the cost. For example, the price of silver-based solders is up to ten times higher than other braze materials.

Figure 2 shows a cross section of brazed steel sheets. The width of the overlap is 5 mm. This is possible with a low brazing speed and an appropriate heat input. Because of the great width of the overlap and the high temperature gradients, defects like pores and insufficient wetting can occur. Smaller overlap joints are more common for laser brazing. Above a critical width of the overlap, the tensile strength of a brazed specimen cannot be increased. The critical width for the overlap for mild steel (1.0 mm) and braze metals like L-Ag55Sn or L-CuNi10Zn42+Ag is 1 mm. Further details are given in References 1 and 2.

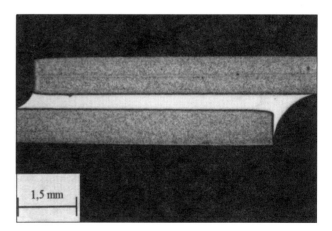

Figure 2. Brazing of steel St12O3 1.0 mm with L-Ag55Sn, F-SH 1. Nd:YAG-laser power $P = 300$ W, speed $v_b = 1.5$ mm/s, feed rate of filler wire $v_w = 5$ mm/s, imaging ratio 2:1, defocusing $z_f = 15$ mm, overlap width $w = 5$ mm, done in vertical position.

Another example is given in Figure 3, where a cross section of an X5CrNi18 9 brazing is shown. The solder formed a concave fillet at each edge. This form is favorable in case of dynamic loads and is a result of the good wetting behavior between the solder, the braze metal, and the flux.

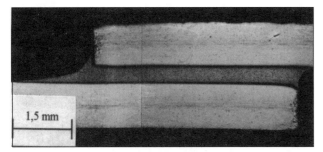

Figure 3. Brazing of steel X5CrNi18 9 1.0 mm with L-Ag55Sn, F-SH1. Nd:YAG-laser power $P = 350$ W, speed $v_b = 2$ mm/s, feed rate of filler wire $v_w = 7.5$ mm/s, imaging ratio 2:1, defocusing $z_f = 15$ mm, overlap width $w = 5$ mm, done in a vertical position.

An example of a joint between zinc-coated and uncoated steel is given in Figure 4. This is also an example of joining materials of different thickness. The width of the overlap is 2 mm, which is a good compromise between a small overlap for highest speed and a larger overlap for an easy adjustment with higher tolerances.

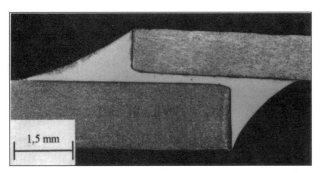

Figure 4. Brazing of steel St1203 1.0 mm uncoated with steel and St1203 coated with zinc, solder L-Ag55Sn, flux F-SH1. Nd:YAG-laser power $P = 345$ W, speed $v_b = 1$ mm/s, feed rate of filler wire $v_w = 3.3$ mm/s, imaging ratio 2:1, defocusing $z_f = 15$ mm, overlap width $w = 2$ mm, done in vertical position.

The above examples were generated with argon gas shielding from both sides of the sheet. This is necessary only to reduce the quantity of flux, and is not necessary for the brazing process itself because the flux can remove all oxides. The use of an exact quantity of flux is not recommended if a layer of flux wets the sheets inside the gap. This parameter can be optimized sufficiently for a given application.

Using laser powers up to 1.5 kW, the possible joining speeds in a horizontal position are between 350 and 750 mm/s, depending on the surface quality of the materials.

The tensile strength of a brazed specimen reaches the values of the base material, if the width of the overlap is higher than the critical distance. In case of a brazed butt joint (not typical for brazing) of mild steel brazed with the high-strength solder L-CuNi10Zn42+Ag, the tensile strength is 335 N/mm², the value of the base material.

9.4.2 Brazing of Titanium

Titanium is a highly reactive metal that can react with oxygen or nitrogen from the atmosphere at temperatures above 200°C, resulting in an embrittlement of the material. Therefore, gas shielding is recommended to prevent negative reactions between the atmosphere and the material. The advantage of titanium for brazing is the possibility of the material to dissolve its own surface oxides at higher temperatures. Therefore, fluxes are not always needed. Figure 5 gives an example with a special gas mixture (5% N_2H_2, 95% Ar) and an aluminum wire. T-joints are also possible with argon as the shielding gas.

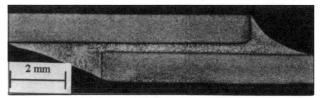

Figure 5. Brazing of titanium 1.0 mm SG-AlSi12, Nd:YAG-laser power $P = 225$ W, speed $v_b = 1$ mm/s, feed rate of filler wire $v_w = 3.1$ mm/s, imaging ratio 2:1, defocusing $z_f = 15$ mm, overlap width $w = 2$ mm, done in a horizontal position. Shielding gas: 5% N_2H_2 95% Ar.

The critical distance for the overlap in this case is 2 mm, which is double the sheet thickness. The tensile strength is 343 N/mm². This value is below the strength of the titanium base material (470 N/mm²) because the heat effects the base metal.

9.4.3 Joining of Dissimilar Materials

One interesting aspect of laser brazing is the possibility of joining dissimilar materials (3). This can be done in two ways.

One possibility is to braze materials with a solder that can wet both base materials. An example is shown in Figure 3, where steel is brazed with zinc-coated steel. The combination of steel and austenitic steel is another example, because both metals can be brazed with L-Ag55Sn. In this way many other material combinations can be brazed.

A second possibility is a mixture between welding and brazing. If one base material has a lower melting temperature than the other, the material with the higher melting temperature can be heated by the laser beam and conduct the heat to the other material. If the other base metal starts melting, it can wet the second base metal. The problem in that case is that often intermetallic phases are formed in reaction between the materials. These materials are mostly highly brittle and can lead to an insufficient joint. The first example of this type of joining is the use of aluminum filler wire for brazing titanium. In the same way titanium can be brazed with aluminum. But a more interesting joint with a high potential for industrial applications is joining aluminum to steel. For this application, high-power laser systems with an output of at least 1.5 kW are recommended. Figure 6 shows a cross-section of such a joint.

ISBN 0-912035-15-3

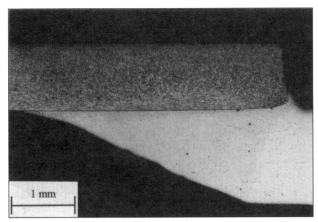

Figure 6. Joining of St12O3 0.9 mm to aluminum AA 6016, 1.2 mm. Nd:YAG-laser power P = 1.75 kW, speed v_b = 900 mm/s, imaging ratio 1:1, defocusing z_t = 30 mm, overlap width w = 2 mm, done in a horizontal position, flux F-LH2.

The joint between these materials is acceptable for industrial applications, if the thickness of the intermetallic layer between the base metals is below 10 µm. Figure 7 shows a cross-section of the joining area. The thickness of the intermetallic phase layer is below 5 µm. The tensile strength of the joint is up to 200 N/mm² (calculated from the thickness of the aluminum, which is the fractured base material). The fracture after a tensile test occurred in the heat-affected zone of the aluminum sheet or in the base metals. The dynamic stress resistance is independent of the number of load cycles at a level of 50 N/mm².

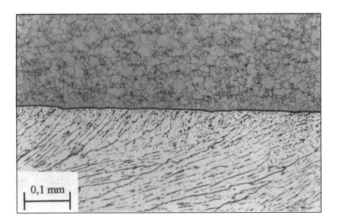

Figure 7. Cross-section of the contact area between aluminum and steel.

Figure 8 shows an example of a curved joint between aluminum and steel, done with a 1.5-kW high-power diode laser. The laser was mounted to a six-axis robot. The rectangular spot of the laser and the filler wire demand a rotation of the laser along the direction of the seam. Other component joints with a total length up to 4 m were manufactured with a Nd:YAG laser at a beam power of 2 kW.

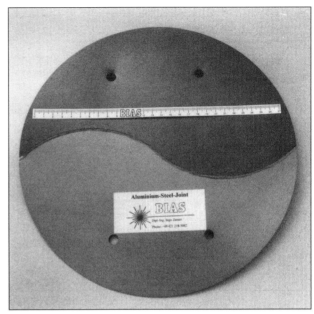

Figure 8. Nonlinear tailored blank with steel (dark gray) and aluminum joined with a high-power diode laser 1.5 kW.

References

1. Schubert, E., Kohn, H., Radscheit, C., and Sepold, G., 1996: Grundlagenuntersuchungen zum flußmittelarmen Hartlöten mit kontinuierlichen Festkörperlasern. Abschlußbericht zum BMBF-Vorhaben "Präzisionsbearbeitung mit Festkörperlasern (Fügen), Teilvorhaben: 13N 6047," Düsseldorf, VDI-Verlag, pp. 1-70.
2. Radscheit, C., Schubert, E., and Sepold, G., 1995: Laserstrahlhart-löten – ein geeignetes Fügeerfahren für metallische Werk-stoffe im Feinblechbe-reich. In: Geiger, M., *Vortragsband zur Veranstaltung: "Schlüsseltechnologie Laser: Herausfordung an die Fabrik 2000,"* Bamberg: Meisenbach-Verlag, pp. 334-335.
3. Schubert, E., and Zerner, I., 1997: Neue Verbindungsmöglichkeiten mit dem Laser. Strahltechnik, Band 10; Bremen: Verlag BIAS.

E. SCHUBERT, I. ZERNER, G. SEPOLD

9.4.4 Soldering Applications with Diode Lasers

This section will focus on soldering with diode lasers. Diode lasers can be used for soft soldering in two different ways. The diode laser beam can be transported to the solder joint either by means of an optical fiber, or it can be focused on the work piece directly, without any optical guidance.

The first approach has the advantage of very flexible beam delivery (1). Only small masses and volumes have to be handled directly at the work piece, since the laser itself is located in a rack or on a table. Fiber-coupled diode lasers are used if a circular spot geometry is mandatory for the application. Depending on the application, the user can choose from a wide range of power levels and fiber diameters.

The second method of using high-power diode lasers for soldering does not employ a fiber optical device. The laser beam is focused directly on the solder joints by means of an imaging optic. Since the laser beam typically exits a rectangular aperture at the emitting facet of the diode laser array, the intensity distribution on the work piece also exhibits a rectangular shape. The rectangular shape enables the soldering of a line-shaped solder joint or a line of circular solder joints.

There are several advantages in using a high-power diode laser over an Nd:YAG laser (both fiber coupled), such as higher efficiency, smaller size, lower maintenance costs and lower investment costs. For the soldering process, an irradiance typically below 10^4 W/cm^2 is required. This irradiance can be achieved with a diode laser at much lower costs than with an Nd:YAG laser.

When using a fiber-coupled diode laser, the out-coupling end of the optical fiber is typically re-imaged to the joint with an imaging ratio of 1:1. However, the ratio can be varied to decrease the spot size by a factor of two, when using high quality optics comprised of aspherical lenses. In order to magnify the spot size, a larger focal length of the focusing lens has to be chosen (see Fig. 1). Depending on the required power, the fiber core diameter ranges between 150 μm and approximately 1.5 mm. The power level of such devices ranges between 10 W to approximately 100 W.

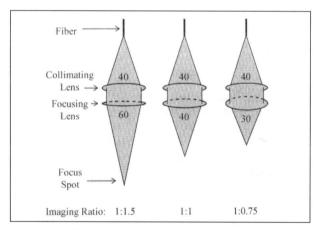

Figure 1. Different re-imaging heads for fiber-coupled laser beams.

Since the heat input into the solder joint is very localized and the intensity on the work piece is higher when using a diode laser compared to conventional techniques, the parameter window of the process is narrower. This means only small fluctuations in the irradiance of the laser beam on the workpiece can be tolerated. The variation of the absorption among the solder joints and a displacement of the laser spot are predominantly respon-

sible for such a variation in irradiance. In order to eliminate this effect, a pyrometer can be integrated in the process to enable closeloop control. The pyrometer measures the surface temperature of the workpiece and adjusts the laser power accordingly, to maintain the preset reflow temperature. A temperature ramp can also be directly preset. The laser power then follows the required temperature time dependence.

The final data used for a soldering application can vary considerably from case to case. The main influence on the process is caused by the heat conduction of the parts forming the joint and their absorption coefficient. In order to give some typical parameters for the diode laser soldering process, some soldering applications are demonstrated and the process data are listed.

Bead-on Plate Experiments
As a first example of soldering with a fiber-coupled diode laser, results of a bead-on-plate experiment are shown. A lead-free, water-soluble solder paste is reflowed on a thin film evaporated gold coated ceramic board. This experiment serves as a preliminary study for a micro-electronic application. Such a bond is commonly achieved with a silver epoxy. Soldering of such bonds is difficult with conventional soldering techniques because of the small dimensions and the sensitivity of the parts. Laser soldering can produce small submillimeter bonds with very little heat input on the surrounding material. The data for this set up are shown in Table 1.

Table 1. Parameters of the Bead-on Plate Experiment

Parameter	Value
Film thickness	0.3– 0.5 μm
Size of solder joint	150 μm
Spot size	200 μm
Laser power	4.5 W
Reflow time	1.5 sec.

When using this solder paste, the best results are achieved with relatively long reflow times. Usually much smaller process cycles are applied, as demonstrated in the following examples. The tolerable deviations from the optimum process parameters are fairly small. One example is the thin gold layer of approximately one micrometer. Thus, the heat conduction effect is very small. The values for the power and the reflow time can vary considerably, depending on the solder paste, the size of the solder and the thickness of the base material.

Soldering of a Ni-ribbon to a Ni-pad
In this application, a nickel ribbon has been soldered to a nickel pad using a fiber coupled diode laser (2). The process data for this application are summarized in Table 2.

Chapter 9: Brazing/Soldering

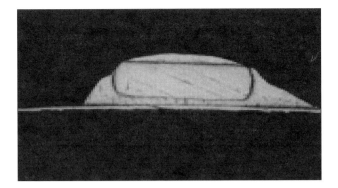

Figure 11. Cross-section of the Ni-Ni joint.

Table 2. Process Parameters of the Ni-pad Soldering

Parameter	Value
Pad thickness	5 µm
Ribbon thickness	50 µm
Size of solder joint	~350 µm
Laser spot size	600 µm
Laser power	~10 W
Reflow time	0.5 to 1.0 sec.

The results are visualized using a cross section of the joint. Figure 11 shows the 50 µm ribbon soldered to the 5 µm Ni-pad. Here, the process cycle time is much shorter and the power level has been set higher than in the previous application. The larger geometry of the joint configuration accounts for better heat conduction. A high-quality bond with a high repeatability can be achieved.

Soldering of Leads with a Fiber-coupled Diode Laser
The next example illustrates the soldering of leads of an integrated circuit to solder pads. The IC consists of 12 pins which have been soldered sequentially with a laser spot size of approximately 0.8 mm. The data are given in Table 3.

Table 3. Lead Soldering with a Fiber-coupled Diode Laser

Parameter	Value
Solder material	AgPbAg
Spot size	0.8 mm
Laser power	10 W
Reflow time	100 msec.

The quality of the solder joint is visualized using a cross section that has been prepared along a lead perpendicular to the surface of the board. It is shown in Figure 12. The photo shows a homogenous joint with no inclusions and no cracks.

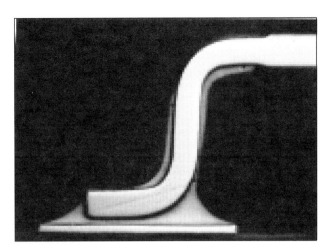

Figure 12. Cross-section of an individually soldered lead.

A comparison of the process data for this application to those of the previous one shows that the reflow times vary considerably, with the output power of the laser remaining the same. This is due to the larger dimensions of the ribbon compared to the size of the lead that was soldered in this application. Hence, the overall heat input into the joint is lower in this application.

Lead Soldering with a Diode Laser Stack
In the next application, leads and pads similar to the former example are soldered simultaneously. Here, a stack of non-fiber-coupled diode laser arrays is used to create a line-shaped focus on the work piece, which has the same width as the row of pins. Diode laser stacks with an output power of up to 400 W have been used for this application. Typically, the reflow time is in the range of 150 ms. The parameters are given in Table 4.

Table 4. Parameters of the Soldering of a Row of Pins

Parameter	Value
Plating thickness	~5 mm
Plating material	80% Sn
Lead material	Cu
Lead width	0.17 mm
Lead pitch	0.4 mm
Width of pin row	25 mm
Laser power	~200 W
Reflow time	200 ms

Because of the considerably thicker base material, which has about a 5 µm thickness, the overlap of the laser beam over the actual solder joints causes no overheating, a consequence of sufficient heat conduction through the base material.

References

1. Beckett, P. M., Fleming, A. R., Foster, R. J., Gilbert, J. M., and Whitehead, D. G., 1995: "The application of semiconductor diode lasers to the soldering of electronic components," *Optical and Quantum Electronics* **27**. pp. 1303–11.

2. Legewie, F., Bosse, L., Gillner, A., and Poprawe, R., "Laser beam joining for the micro technology," Proceedings of ICALEO'98, Laser Institute of America, Orlando, FL.

BODO EHLERS

Chapter 10

Conduction Welding

10.0 Introduction

At relatively low values of laser power, less than approximately one kilowatt, the irradiance at the surface of a workpiece to be welded is limited. The laser energy is absorbed at the surface and is conducted into the interior of the workpiece by thermal conduction. This is a relatively slow process which limits the depth which can be melted effectively and hence limits the welding depth. This regime is often called conduction welding, the process which is the subject of this chapter. Conduction welding with laser sources is widely used for welding of relatively thin materials.

At higher values of laser power, other physical phenomena come into play. This often occurs when the power is in the 1–1.5 kW region, but, depending on materials, wavelength and focusing, may occur at powers as low as a few hundred watts. In this regime, especially at multikilowatt levels, the laser energy may be deposited deeper in the workpiece. This allows production of welds having greater depth. This regime, often called penetration welding, is the focus of Chapter 11.

This chapter presents welding results in terms of penetration depth and weld rate and the like for specified conditions of irradiation. These data have been obtained from a number of sources. In later chapters, similar tabulations and figures will present results for drilling and cutting. However, the exact results obtained for a welding operation, or for cutting and drilling, depend on a wide variety of parameters, which may vary from one laser installation to another. These factors include focusing conditions, beam quality and surface finish. These parameters are usually not specified well enough to allow one to duplicate exactly the conditions for a particular laser materials processing operation. Thus the tabulated and graphed data must be regarded as indicating an approximate range of results that may be obtained. The user must optimize the parameters for a particular processing operation experimentally in order to obtain the best results.

JOHN F. READY

10.1 Basic Description of Laser Welding

10.1.1 Use of Laser Welding

Laser welding is used when it is essential to limit the size of the heat-affected zone (HAZ), to reduce the roughness of the welded surface and to eliminate mechanical effects. Solid-state lasers operating in the continuous or pulsed mode can function as welding sources. Present-day lasers can provide very high levels of power per unit area, while the beam spot is comparable in area to the square of the wavelength (1–4). For comparison, Figure 1 presents the power densities, in W/cm^2, for various energy sources. Pulsed lasers provide higher power density than any other available source.

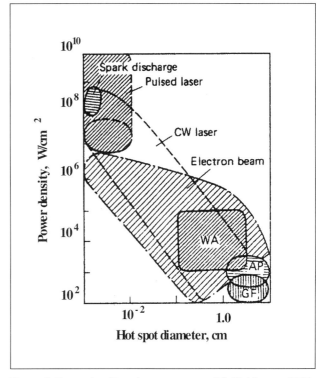

Figure 1. Power densities of energy sources (5). Welding arc (WA); arc plasma (AP); gas flame (GF) (1).

Figure 2 illustrates possible applications of lasers operating either in the continuous or in the pulsed mode for various heat treatment processes used in industry.

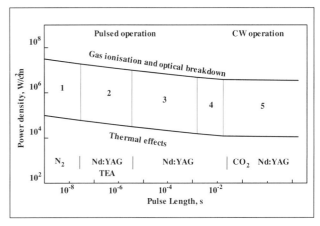

Figure 2. Use of lasers for heat treatment processes: 1) thin-film vaporization; 2) scribing and film vaporization; 3) hole drilling and punching; 4) spot welding and surface heat treatment; 5) deep melting, gas-assisted cutting, surface hardening, and splitting. TEA, transversely excited atmospheric pressure CO_2 laser (5).

References

1. N. G. Basov and V. A. Danilychev, 1985: *Industrial High-Power Lasers. Science and Mankind*, Znanie, Moscow, 261–78.
2. G. Chryssolouris, 1991: *Laser Machining: Theory and Practice*, Springer-Verlag, Mechanical Engineering Series, New York.
3. A. M. Prokhorov (Ed.), 1978: *Laser Handbook*, Vol. 1, Sov. Radio, Moscow, 504.
4. A. M. Prokhorov (Ed.), 1978: *Laser Handbook*, Vol. 1, Sov. Radio, Moscow, 400.
5. A. G. Grigoryants, 1994: *Basics of Laser Material Processing*, Mir Publishers, Moscow.

GEORGE CHRYSSOLOURIS
STEFANOS KARAGIANNIS

10.1.2 Metal Reflectivity

For laser welding to take place, the laser energy must be absorbed into the parts to be welded in order to create sufficient heating to develop a melt puddle. The reflectivity of a metal increases with its conductivity and also increases with the increasing wavelength of laser light impinging on the surface.

Reflectivity values of solid metals in the 0.4 to 11 µm wavelength range are high. The values for absorption are rather low, often less than 10%. The reflectivity of metallic surfaces, and its variation with wavelength and temperature, are described in detail in Section 5.3.

The initial high value of reflectivity and its associated loss of laser energy can be overcome if a melt puddle is created on the surface of the metal to increase absorption. A liquid metal has a much lower conductivity than a solid because of its higher temperature. This phenomenon of overcoming the base metal reflectivity and creating a substantial melt puddle is termed *coupling* into the material.

There is another advantage to creating a melt puddle. It is found in the geometry the melt puddle takes as the beam impinges upon it; the melt puddle forms into a crater. It is lower at the center and rises at the edges. This is due to the surface tension of the melt puddle and the variation of the surface tension with temperature. At the center, the melt puddle is lowest and the surface tension is at a minimum as compared to the cooler edges next to the solid material. Metal vapor is boiling off the melt puddle and heated by the beam. The recoil force of this vapor depresses the melt puddle downward forming the crater shape (see Fig. 3).

Any laser light that is not absorbed by the liquid metal is reflected down toward the center of the melt puddle with multiple opportunities for absorption at each reflection. This increases the heating of the center of the melt puddle and will increase the depth of the crater. Absorption can be increased from less than 5% as a solid metal to more than 95% once coupling occurs (see Fig. 4).

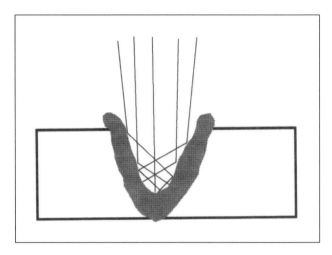

Figure 3. Formation of weld puddle crater resulting in increased absorption at the center.

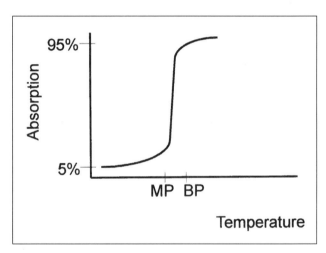

Figure 4. Coupling of laser energy into the melt once the melting point (MP) and boiling point (BP) are reached.

Other physical characteristics of the surface also determine reflectivity. These include surface roughness, the physical joint shape, and any surface contamination. The first, roughness, is a simple concept. If the surface of a metal is polished, it is much more like a mirror than a metal with a brushed finish, a surface with machining marks, or a rough as-cast finish. These small imperfections channel laser light into the bottom of the pits and valleys, increasing the amount of absorbed light on the bottom and sides of the imperfections. This also occurs on a macroscopic scale. For example, if two machined tube sections are to be butt welded together, they might have slight shoulder bevels on each end where the sharp edges have been removed. These form a v-notch at the joint that guides the laser energy into the weld seam. The same is true for the seam created between the two edges of tube as it is rolled into a circle in a tube mill. These surfaces will meet in a V-shaped joint that will trap laser energy at the bottom of the joint improving absorption of laser light substantially (see Fig. 5).

Chapter 10: Conduction Welding

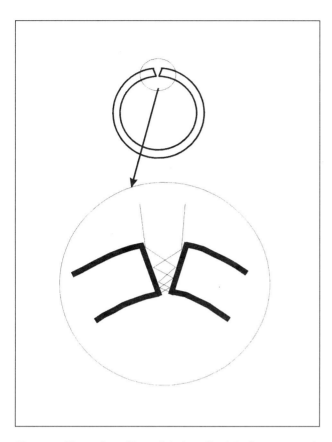

Figure 5. Channeling of laser light by reflectivity from a v-notch seam (6).

Surface Contamination Effects
Surface contamination can also increase absorption of laser light by providing a local surface material with much higher absorption than the base metal. This is the case with tarnish on silver, a nickel plating on copper components, or surface oxides on materials such as copper and aluminum. Oxides are not good conductors like the parent material, and their absorption may be quite high. For example, aluminum with an oxidized surface has an absorption coefficient of 28 to 50% because of the layer of oxides. Laser energy absorbed by contaminants will conduct into the parent material. Oxides can also be created by the laser welding process itself, especially if oxygen is present in the alloys or weld joint or when inert gas shielding around the parts is nonexistent or poor.

These surface variables and their effect on reflectivity can often determine the viability of a laser welding project. For example, copper components are often nickel plated to reduce reflectivity so that a low-power pulsed Nd:YAG laser can produce welds of sufficient penetration. Surface finish and surface oxides can cause problems in laser processing if these attributes vary the reflectivity substantially along the weld joint. If the oxides on copper create much better absorption in some areas, the laser interaction can be much stronger in those areas than on the rest of the component. This can cause localized metal loss because of a vigorous absorption, resulting in areas of excessive penetration or excessive heating of the part. Another detriment of surface oxidation is that these oxides can be porous enough to trap water, cutting fluids, finger oils,etc. which will explosively expand during rapid laser heating cycles.

Alloys with Reflectivity Challenges
Reflectivity constraints are not a problem with most metal alloys where laser welding is employed. All ferrous metals, nickel alloys, titanium alloys, zirconium alloys, and refractory alloys can be laser welded with lasers with average powers well below 500 W CW and with pulsed lasers with very low average power and modest peak powers.

Typically only the most reflective alloys, such as copper, silver, gold, and aluminum, add a tighter constraint on laser choice for successful welding at these power levels. Carbon dioxide lasers are not capable of breaking down the reflectivity of these metals at this low power level even when high peak power pulsing is used. Pulsed Nd:YAG lasers are the correct choice for welding these very reflective metals. Nd:YAG lasers produce high peak power pulses at the shorter wavelength of 1.06 μm that will overcome the reflectivity of the part and create very high quality welds. See Section 10.2.1 for more information on laser characteristics.

References
6. L. Tapper, K. Nilsson, A. Bengtsson, Final report of ICA Project No. 389, International Copper Association, May 1991.
T. R. Kugler and H. N. Bransch, *Photonics Spectra*, Laurin Publishing Co., May 1992.
J. Mazumder, *Laser Beam Welding,* ASM Handbook Vol. 6.

THOMAS R. KUGLER

10.1.3 Thermal Properties of Metals
Once laser energy is absorbed by the material creating a temperature rise, the resulting heat input and weld characteristics are a function of the thermal properties of the metal(s) involved. Attributes of interest to laser processing are the melting point, boiling point, latent heat of fusion, heat capacity, density, and thermal conductivity. Thermal properties are described in Section 5.1, but they will be reviewed here as they apply to welding.

Melting Point and Boiling Point
Of course, higher temperatures must be reached to weld a metal with a higher melting point; however, the amount of energy needed to raise the temperature to this point is related to the density of the metal and its heat capacity. This topic will be discussed below. Since lasers have no source temperature such as a flame or oven, the temperature achieved by the laser interaction is determined by the amount of energy absorbed by the target material. Lasers can easily input enough energy into any metal to raise it to its melting point and even well above the boiling point. What is most important to consider is the melting and boiling points of each metal when welding dissimilar metals, metals with a coating, or metal alloys.

Zinc is the most common example of melting point and boiling point mismatches in laser welding. When one attempts to weld brass, the result is explosive metal loss and only a very shallow weld on the surface of a crater or trench that was the weld area. The reason is that the zinc boils at 907°C and copper melts at 1085°C. As the temperature of the melt puddle rises, the zinc explosively vaporizes just as the copper becomes molten, ejecting metal from the puddle. The same is true for zinc-coated steels, such as hot-dipped galvanized steels. Platinum alloys welded to dissimilar metals also create some complications. Platinum melts at 1772°C while stainless steel melts about 1425°C. There is no problem here with explosive vaporization of the stainless; however, there is minimal mixing of the metals in the melt puddle because of the short time in the molten state. What does occur is the very fast solidification of the platinum alloy while the stainless is still molten. This causes weld porosity because the puddle solidifies before any gasses from the bottom of the melt pool depression can rise out of the melt puddle. Only through the use of long weld times with ramp down of power can porosity free spot welds be produced.

Thermal Diffusivity

When one considers heat capacity, density, and thermal conductivity, one realizes what the most important parameter is in determining how much energy will be lost through thermal conduction instead of the energy being used to efficiently create a very localized melt puddle. This parameter is termed *thermal diffusivity* and is determined by all three properties.

Thermal conductivity, κ (W/m K), describes the property of a metal to conduct heat away from the melt. The laser must introduce more heat into a melt puddle than is lost to the base metal if the weld nugget is to grow and increase weld penetration and or width. Thermal conductivity is proportional to the electrical conductivity in metals, so a good conductor of electricity will have a high thermal conductivity. For example, copper and iron have thermal conductivities of 3.94 and 0.75 W/cm K, respectively.

Heat capacity, c_p, (J/g K), is another value of importance. This term is related to the amount of heat energy required to raise the temperature of a known mass of the metal one degree in temperature. For example copper requires 0.9 J of energy to raise one gram by one degree Kelvin and iron requires 0.46 J. Density, ρ (g/cm^3), is the measure of the amount of mass per unit area of a material. Copper has a density of 8.98 g/cm^3, and that of iron is 7.87 g/cm^3.

The product of the density and heat capacity (ρc_p=J/cm^3 K) determines the amount of energy required to raise a specific volume by one degree. For copper and iron this value is 3.45 and 3.62J/cm^3 K, respectively. The lower this number, the larger the volume of metal that will be heated by a given amount of energy. If the thermal conductivity is divided by this product, one has a measure of the way in which heat energy is lost to temperature rise and to conductivity into the rest of the metal during the transient laser heating. This measure is called the thermal diffusivity, α ($\kappa/\rho c_p$). So any metal with a high thermal conductivity and low values for density and heat capacity will require more laser energy per unit time to create and sustain a melt puddle. For example, the values of thermal diffusivity for copper and iron are 1.14 and 0.208 (cm^2/sec), respectively, so copper will remove heat from the weld area at a rate approximately 5.5× that of iron. Therefore welding copper will require approximately 5.5× the laser power density for similar results with iron alloys. See Table 1 for more information on the thermal properties of some metals.

Table 1. Thermal Properties of Some Metals

Element	Density ρ (g/cm^3)	Heat capacity C_p (j/g K)	Heat conductivity κ (W/cm K)	Thermal diffusity α (cm^2/sec)
Al	2.699	0.9	2.21	0.91
Cu	8.96	0.385	3.94	1.14
Au	19.32	0.131	2.97	1.178
Fe	7.87	0.46	0.75	0.208
Ni	8.902	0.44	0.92	0.235
Pt	21.45	0.131	0.69	0.245
Ag	10.49	0.234	4.18	1.705
Ta	16.6	0.142	0.54	0.23
Sn	7.2984	0.226	0.63	0.38
Ti	4.507	0.519	0.22	0.092
W	19.3	0.138	1.66	0.62
Zr	6.489	0.28	0.21	0.12

Reference

J. Eagar, Energy Sources Used for Fusion Welding, ASM Handbook Vol. 6.

THOMAS R. KUGLER

10.1.4 Fusion Front Penetration

Modes of Laser Welding

Weld penetration is determined, of course, by the fusion front penetration into the material to be welded. The depth and shape of the weld cross section is determined by many factors including the joint geometry, thermal characteristics of the metals, and the laser parameters. For this discussion we will focus on the basic beam–material interaction as a primer in laser welding modes of penetration. Three distinct modes of laser welding apply to welding with less than 1 kW beams. These are conduction mode, penetration mode, and keyhole mode welding. Each is possible with lasers in this power range.

Keyhole Mode Welding

Consider a CW or pulsed laser focused onto the surface of the part to be welded. The laser beam is sufficiently focused to couple with the metal and the laser beam is absorbed at the surface. Solid metal turns to liquid and this liquid melt puddle grows as heat is conducted in a hemispherical geometry around the impingement point. If the laser beam has sufficient irradiance (power density), the liquid surface will deform because of the surface tension gradients and the vapor and recoil pressure of the metal vapor above the pool. This traps the laser energy in the depression and the laser beam is concentrated at the center further forcing the depression down into the puddle.

For CW or peak powers of approximately 500 W or more focused to a spot size of 0.2 mm or less in diameter, this interaction results in a keyhole of hot ionized metal vapor surrounded by liquid metal. The vapor pressure of the ionized gas holds the liquid metal against the edges of the liquid/solid interface and the laser beam nearly reaches the bottom of the melt zone, as shown in Figure 6. A pulsed laser will reform the keyhole during each pulse with reflow and solidification of the melt puddle at the end of each pulse.

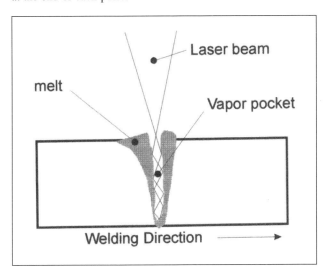

Figure 6. Keyhole formation with deep vapor pocket.

Keyhole mode welding is possible only with small focal spot sizes at less than 1 kW of average power. Sufficient average power and power density at the focus are needed to form a keyhole, maintain enough vapor pressure to preserve the keyhole cavity, and overcome the energy losses to conduction. The depth of the keyhole is determined by the CW power or peak power of the laser for pulsed units. The lower the average power, the shallower the keyhole before conduction losses equal laser power and the keyhole depth limit is reached. When one moves the keyhole across the part during a seam weld, the fusion front penetration is determined by the keyhole depth. As the processing speed is increased, the keyhole depth will decrease but the weld cross section will retain a keyhole or "nailhead" geometry. At slower speeds, the weld penetration will increase to a virtual maximum determined by the keyhole depth of near zero travel speed. At this point, the weld width will increase as more melt is created by conduction of heat from the keyhole but keyhole depth is not appreciably increased with the longer localized interaction time of slower speeds. This effect is characterized by the weld cross section losing its high aspect ratio keyhole shape and becoming a weld with an aspect ratio less than 3:1 as shown in Figure 7 (next page). If a deep narrow weld is required, the laser power must be sufficient to produce a keyhole to the required depth of penetration. The very efficient coupling of keyhole mode welding and the funneling of the laser energy to the bottom of the keyhole results in a very high aspect of ratio weld nuggets with ratios (weld penetration to the width at half penetration) exceeding 6:1.

Conduction Mode Welding

At low power density, the melt puddle depression does not occur and the laser energy input creates a smooth shallow liquid pool. This pool will grow in size until the laser energy delivered into the puddle equals the energy lost to conduction into the rest of the solid metal. Upon solidification of the puddle, a cross section of the parts will show a weld that has a penetration no greater than half the width of the weld. The surface of the weld is very smooth and cosmetic because the melt puddle is not recoiling during solidification. For lasers less than 1 kW and typical ferrous alloys the penetration of these types of welds does not exceed about 0.3 mm (see Fig. 8).

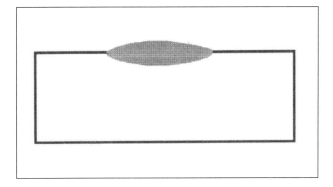

Figure 8. Typical cross section of a conduction-mode weld.

Penetration Mode Welding

Low-power lasers with focal spot sizes larger than about 0.3 mm in diameter cannot form a stable small keyhole. Laser energy density at focus is too low to produce a large volume of metal vapor with sufficient pressure to hold the liquid layer against the edges of the keyhole. These lasers do, however, have a welding regime somewhere between conduction mode welding and keyhole welding termed *penetration-mode welding*. Lasers such as pulsed Nd:YAG lasers weld in this regime. Their larger focal spot size and high peak power will create a large weld puddle depression but no stable keyhole. The depression traps laser energy at its center and efficiently absorbs and channels the laser energy creating a weld that has an aspect ratio of up to 3:1 (see Fig. 9, next page). Pulsed lasers of this type can produce penetrations up to 2.5 mm at average powers below 50 W but peak power of > 3 kW. This welding regime is less efficient than keyhole welding but creates a weld nugget with significantly less heat input than that from conventional processes and can weld to penetrations not possible with CW lasers with power less than 1 kW.

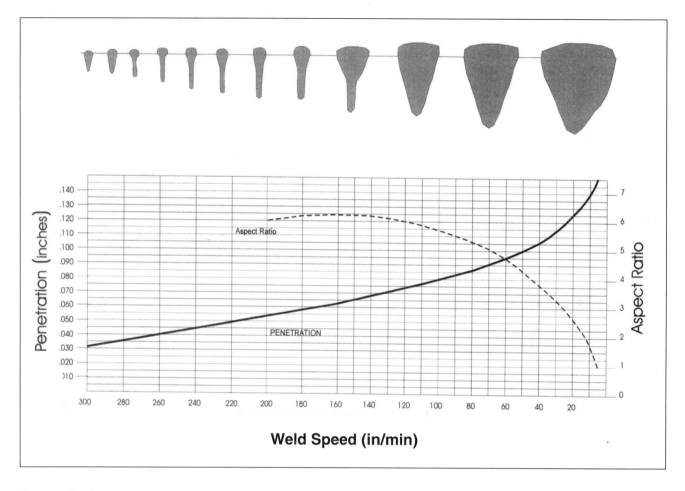

Figure 7. Varying penetration and aspect ratio of welds with a 1200 W CO_2 laser. Note the lower aspect ratio cross sections at lower speeds with little increase in weld penetration.

Also, these lasers can produce spot welds with much larger interface diameters than the narrow keyhole spot welds. Seam welds are simply a series of overlapping spot welds.

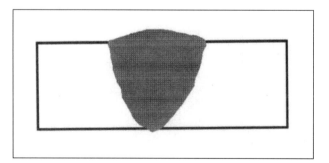

Figure 9. Typical cross section of penetration-mode weld.

In conclusion, there are three basic modes of laser welding that are determined by the laser power and focal spot size. At 300 W of average or peak power with a focal spot size of less than 0.2 mm diameter, the laser power density is sufficient to create and maintain keyhole mode welding. The depth and aspect ratio of the weld is determined by the average power and weld speed with aspect ratios up to 6:1. Penetration mode welding is achieved with high-peak-power pulsed lasers with focal spot sizes larger than approximately 0.2 mm. A rather large puddle depression is created with resulting weld cross sections that are wider and have a lower aspect ratio than true keyhole welding. Conduction mode welding occurs with lower power density at the surface of the workpiece than the other welding modes. Focusing to a larger focal spot size or operating the laser at lower average or peak power will result in this regime. The aspect ratio of this type of weld never exceeds 0.5:1 with a characteristic smooth surface.

References

T. R. Kugler and H. N. Bransch, *Photonics Spectra*, Laurin Publishing Co, May 1992.

T. R. Kugler and H. N. Bransch, ICALEO 1993 Proceedings LIA Volume 77.

J. Eagar, Energy Sources Used for Fusion Welding, ASM Handbook Vol. 6.

THOMAS R. KUGLER

10.1.5 Thermal Conduction Limitations

Keyhole and penetration mode welding modes improve efficiency in laser welding but the weld size and geometry are determined by the conduction of heat from the laser interaction surface into the bulk metal. As discussed in Section 10.1.3, the thermal properties of the material determine the melt size, shape, and volume once the laser energy is absorbed.

Heat Energy Flow

Thermal conductivity and, more truly, the thermal diffusivity of the metal determines the limitations in laser welding, especially at low average power. To understand the principles it is best to investigate the energy flow within the laser weld.

Energy input is provided by the laser alone. In welding there typically are no exothermal reactions or phase changes from solid to liquid that release energy. Energy losses are due to thermal conduction, black-body radiation from the melt surface, and energy lost through the convection of metal vapor leaving the weld area; the rest of the energy is used for melting metal. All of the energy losses except for conduction losses are minimal and can be neglected in the discussions here.

Limits to Heat Conduction

During laser welding the generation of a melt puddle will continue and the melt volume will increase until the energy lost equals the laser energy absorbed. As the melt volume increases, the surface area of the melt puddle grows in interface area with the solid metal. Doubling the diameter of the melt puddle increases the surface area by a factor of 4. Because of this fast increase in conducting surface area, the laser weld pool is quickly limited in size. For this reason welding rates are not a linear function of penetration.

Benefits of Keyhole and Penetration Mode

Only with the creation of a keyhole or penetration-mode welding depression does weld penetration increase with the minimum increase in conduction surface area. Thus the keyhole welding mode will result in the deepest penetration possible. The only way to increase weld penetration is to increase laser power or pre-heat the part to reduce the energy flow from the hot melt puddle to the base metal.

Bulk Heating Effects

Preheating is usually not done in practice to increase welding penetration, but the laser energy itself can heat the part during laser seam welding. This effect, which is usually seen in small parts or parts with a substantial weld volume, will result in laser welding penetration that increases during the welding as the components are pre-heated by the laser energy (see Fig. 10). Usually this preheat effect is seen in the first centimeter of the weld for large parts because the temperature rise reaches a local equilibrium rather quickly. In small parts the weld penetration increase can occur throughout the weld. Methods to compensate for this vary. Many users will simply ensure that the weld penetration is sufficient at the very start and allow the penetration to increase later in the weld. For higher tolerance applications, the laser weld is initiated while the part is stationary for up to a second and then motion begins. The initial stationary phase preheats the local area, and weld penetration is then constant. Most users deal with this effect in circular welds by overlapping the weld start area so that the penetration is increased during the overlap.

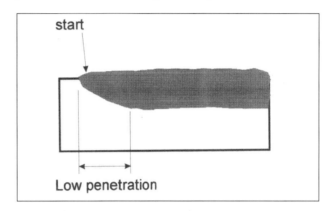

Figure 10. Effect of bulk heating on weld penetration during initial phases of the weld cycle.

Alloys with Dissimilar Thermal Properties

Welding of dissimilar metals with varying conductivity or thermal diffusivity is another area where laser penetration is greatly affected by thermal properties. Considering a butt weld of pure copper to another compatible alloy such as nickel is the best way to illustrate this phenomenon. Absorption is best in nickel and the thermal diffusivity is 4.8 times lower in nickel as compared to copper. Inspection of the weld nugget will show a very asymmetric cross section with much more penetration into the nickel and very little fusion of the copper, as shown in Figure 11. Weld cross section is improved in several ways. First, since the nickel side of the joint has much better absorption, it is often best to favor the nickel side with the laser beam relying on the conduction of heat into the edge of the copper from the nickel. Second, it is very beneficial to provide a small gap between the components so that the laser energy channeled into the interface in a quasi-artificial keyhole of the gap. This technique will greatly improve the weld penetration.

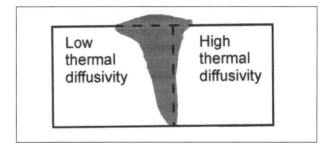

Figure 11. Typical weld cross section between two parts with very different thermal diffusivity values.

The conductivity differential between components is most drastic with lap joints. If the higher conductivity component is on the surface, it will require a great deal of laser energy to create a melt nugget at the interface that will produce fusion between the two parts. Conversely, if the high conductivity component position is reversed, penetration is improved but the weld interface might be much smaller than the fusion width in the low conductivity component (see Fig. 12).

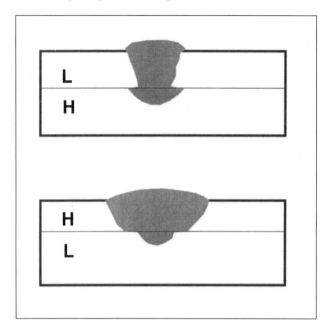

Figure 12. Lap joint interface variation with materials with very different thermal diffusivities. H = high thermal diffusivity, L = low thermal diffusivity.

Barriers to Thermal Energy Flow

Another effect of conductivity is one related to the insulative properties of the actual joint gap especially in lap welding configurations. Heat must be transferred from the top component into the bottom one by conduction if the laser keyhole does not reach into the bottom component. The gap between the parts can be a substantial barrier to this conduction even when the gap is rather small. A very small weld width at the interface or lack of fusion is usually the result of such an effect. Welding rates are often much slower in lap welded components as compared to bead-on-plate welding rates or butt-welding rates. A keyhole welding regime usually minimizes this gap effect as long as the gap is not so large that the two melt puddles cannot bridge the gap. By definition of a keyhole weld, the laser beam reaches to the bottom of the keyhole and the beam will strike the bottom component if the keyhole penetration is greater than the component thickness. For all of these reasons it is best if lap welding is performed by thin-onto-thick so that gap effects are minimized and the efficiency of the laser weld is optimized.

Although the subject of this chapter is conduction welding, comparisons to penetration welding and other welding matters are touched on. Penetration welding is covered in detail in Chapter 11.

Reference
J. Eagar, Energy Sources Used for Fusion Welding, ASM Handbook Vol. 6.

THOMAS R. KUGLER

10.2 Welding Procedures

10.2.1 Laser Characteristics

Laser Types

Lasers are usually differentiated by their different lasing mediums and their associated wavelengths. For the discussions here we will describe carbon dioxide lasers (CO_2), Nd:YAG lasers, and Nd:glass lasers. While there are other types, they are not used for laser welding tasks. (Chapter 2 provides an overview of different laser types.)

Laser Output Characteristics

The application of one particular laser over another is often determined by the laser output characteristics and not the wavelength of a particular laser type. Most lasers are characterized by their power output over time. These fall into several categories. Figure 1 illustrates their output characteristics.

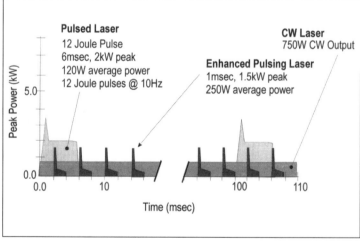

Figure 1. Typical output characteristics of CW, Pulsed, and Enhanced Pulsing Lasers. Note the time base and peak power level for each type.

CW Lasers

Lasers operating in a continuous wave output (CW) mode produce a beam continuously with no pulsing action. These lasers have a power supply that can continuously send excitation energy to the lasing medium. Usually CW lasers can operate in ranges from 0 to 20% of their maximum rated power up to 120% of their CW power rating. Gating the laser energy on and off is a typical feature of these units and many of these units can gate the beam on and off at repetition rates up to 500 Hz or more. This can be considered pulsing, but true CW lasers do not produce gated pulses with peak powers higher than their CW ratings. Both CO_2 and Nd:YAG lasers are available as CW lasers. CW Nd:YAG and CO_2 lasers are available with ratings of a few milliwatts to several thousand watts.

Enhanced Pulsing Lasers

There are typically lasers that will operate in the CW mode but can pulse or modulate the laser output with peak powers from 1.5 to 5X their CW rating. This is usually accomplished by storing some energy in the power supply during the beam off time. Extra energy sent to the lasing medium during turn-on of the laser results in a short duration of high peak power. If the laser were to remain on in the CW mode, the output would fall to the CW level after a few hundred msec. These lasers are often very practical in the < 1 kW power range because they provide high peak power to overcome thermal diffusivity yet they have high average powers for fast processing. CO_2 and Nd:YAG lasers are available with this type of output.

Pulsed Lasers

Pulsed lasers employ a power supply designed for delivering high peak powers during the laser pulse and do not have CW capability. Lasers with high peak power pulses are capable of much more material processing than their average power rating might indicate. High peak power overcomes the thermal diffusivity and reflectivity of precious metals, copper, and aluminum. They can also weld large volumes with a single pulse. It is common for Nd:YAG and Nd:glass lasers to produce peak powers of 3 to 10 kW or more from a laser with an average power rating of less than 50 W. Solid state lasers like the Nd:YAG and Nd:glass lasers develop these peak powers from the very energetic pumping of the lasing medium during pulses that are from 0.1 msec to over 20 msec long. Since this high peak power enhancement applies to the entire pulse duration, the pulse energies produced are quite high with typical lasers being able to produce 0.1 to 50 J of energy per pulse.

Pulsed Laser Output Terminology

Most lasers are rated by their CW output, but pulsed lasers have pulse energy and peak power terminology that must be understood when discussing pulsed laser applications. When discussing spot welding, the laser average power is not a factor for each weld. What is important is the energy of the laser pulse, measured in Joules.

A laser operating at 5 J/pulse and 10 pulses/second has an average power of 50 W (5 J x 10 Hz = 50 J/sec = 50 W). To weld at twice that speed, a repetition rate of 20 Hz is required or a 100 W laser. The other important factor to consider is the peak pulse power of the laser. If the 5 J laser pulse has a pulse duration of 2 msec, the peak power is 2.5 kW (5 J/2 msec = 2,500 J/sec = 2.5 kW). The pulsed energy can be changed in different ways. First, the power supply can be programmed to deliver less energy in the same 2 msec pulse duration so that the laser's energy and peak power are both reduced. In this example, if the output is reduced to 4 J in 2 msec, the peak power is reduced to 2 kW. Second, the laser pulse width can be reduced with the same peak power so in the same example the pulse duration can be reduced to 1.5 msec with the same 2.5 kW peak power to produce a 3.75 J pulse with 1.5 msec duration. Pulse energy and peak power increases can be made in much the same way. Both the laser pulse energy and the peak power have a substantial effect on weld penetration and weld cross-section geometry.

Beam Quality of the Laser

For small weld features and for high power densities at focus with low power lasers, good beam quality is important. Also, for very good repeatability the consistency of the focus spot size and the energy distribution are also very important. Chapter 3 explores the theory and practice of laser beam quality and the focus of laser beams and should be referenced by readers with questions in this area. It is sufficient at this stage of our discussion to note that most suppliers of lasers < 1 kW can offer units that will produce focal spot sizes of 100 µm and larger but that good beam quality lasers are usually lower power lasers.

Laser Choices

The choice of which laser is required for a task will depend upon many factors but the most important are: average power, pulse energy, and peak power. Other factors such as cost and size are not relevant here.

Average Power

Processing speed and average power are synonymous. If a CW laser has the capability to weld to the required depth in the CW mode, a laser with the same focal spot size and higher average power will process at a faster rate. Higher CW powers also produce a deeper keyhole for more efficient welding and less heat input into the workpiece. For pulsed lasers, higher average powers will result in faster processing speeds also, but the efficiency will usually not be increased because keyhole welding is not possible with pulsed lasers of this power range and beam quality. With pulsed lasers, the speed increase is simply an increase in the pulsing rate for the same pulse energy.

Pulse Energy

The energy per pulse in pulsed lasers determines the volume of the melt puddle for each pulse. There is a minimum pulse energy required for weld penetration to a certain depth in a given material. If this energy is not available from the laser, the process cannot be improved by using more pulses, especially with low power lasers. Also, if optics are used to produce more than one focal spot from a single laser, the laser energy at each focal spot must be sufficient to perform the welding task. For example, many pulsed Nd:YAG laser systems employ fiber optics in an energyshare configuration to divide the laser output into multiple fibers. If 10 J pulses are required for a single focal spot, then 30 J pulses would be required for a three-way energyshare system.

Peak Power

Peak power from pulsed lasers breaks down reflectivity and

overcomes thermal diffusivity. Higher peak power lasers are required for precious metal welding and aluminum welding. For both pulsed lasers and lasers with only enhanced pulsing, the peak power will improve welding efficiency and consistency in the more reflective materials or where low average power is necessary to minimize heat input. For pulsed lasers, peak power is vital in producing large spot welds with minimum heat input. Once again, if energyshare systems are required, the laser peak power must be increased when compared to single focal spot scenarios. Using the same example as above, a laser producing 10 J of energy in 10 msec for one focal spot must produce 30 J in 10 msec if a three-way energyshare is employed to perform the same task at three focal spots. As illustrated here, a three-way energyshare system triples the peak power requirements, greatly changing the laser specification.

10.2.2 Optics

Almost all applications of lasers in the category of 1 kW or below employ transmissive optics to focus the laser beam for welding. Delivering the laser beam from the laser to the focus optic can be accomplished by conventional mirror delivery, fiber optic delivery, and, sometimes, a combination of both. Beam delivery is treated in Chapter 3. Here beam delivery systems are described with relevance to welding systems.

Up Collimators

Focal spot size is determined by the divergence of the laser beam and the focus lens choice for a laser system. The simplest way to reduce beam divergence is to increase the diameter of the collimated laser beam. Up collimators, also called beam expanders, are often used at the laser source to increase the beam diameter. Doubling the diameter of the beam reduces the beam divergence by a factor of two and can, with the proper focus lens system, produce a focal spot that is half the size that one would have had without the collimator. For CO_2 lasers with powers above 500 W this is usually not necessary. The raw beam diameter from these lasers and their low divergence eliminates any need for an up-collimator. However, for low-power CO_2 lasers and most Nd:YAG lasers, an up collimator is used to increase beam diameter from approximately 6 to 10 mm in diameter to 12 to 25 mm in diameter.

Focusing Optics

Transmissive focus lenses are the norm for low-power welding applications. Parabolic mirrors can focus laser beams but are generally used for laser powers of > 1.5 kW from CO_2 lasers. Focus lenses are typically plano-convex lenses because of their low cost and minimal spherical aberration characteristics for f-numbers above 5. The f-number is defined as the focal length of the lens divided by the beam diameter. For example, a 25-mm beam diameter being focused by a 150-mm lens has an f-number of 6. For f-numbers smaller than 4, more complex optical systems than a simple plano-convex lens are required to provide good focusing. As the f-number decreases, problems with spherical aberration become more severe.

With CO_2 lasers at small f-numbers, there are two typical optics employed. The lowest cost option is to use meniscus shaped singlet lenses. A meniscus lens has a convex top (first) surface and a concave bottom surface. At the high index of refraction that ZnSe and GaAs have at 10.6 μm, the meniscus shape produces minimum spherical aberration from a singlet lens. Meniscus optics are a good choice for focus lenses with f-numbers as low as approximately 3. For f-numbers from 3 to 2, diffractive optics can be used or more complex optical systems involving air-spaced doublets. f-numbers below two will require triplets or more.

Plano-convex lenses are the best optical shape for the index of refraction of glass at the 1.06 μm Nd:YAG laser wavelength. Optical systems with f-numbers as low as 4 can employ plano-convex lenses. Nd:YAG laser systems with f-numbers smaller than 4 usually employ doublet lenses, which are two types of glass, ground at their interface to mate together. These are standard optics used in photographic and projection systems in industry; they are low cost and are readily available in many different sizes. These optics are often referred to as *achromatic doublets* or *achromats* since they are also designed to focus the visible spectrum with color correction. Achromatic doublets focus Nd:YAG lasers with near zero aberrations down to f-numbers of 2. For smaller f-numbers, triplets or other, more complex, focus lens systems must be employed. Table 1 outlines the best lens choices.

Table 1. Best Lens Shape Choices for Nd:YAG and CO_2 Lasers at Various f-numbers

f-number range	CO_2 optic	Nd:YAG optic
4+	plano-convex	plano-convex
3 to 4	meniscus	plano-convex
2 to 3	diffractive-convex	doublet
< 2	triplet	triplet

Focus Lens Choices

When one welds with low-power lasers, the choice of a focus lens is determined by the optical information given above and the capabilities of the laser itself. With CW lasers a small focal spot size is required for keyhole welding. The focus lens system should have a sufficiently small f-number to produce and maintain the keyhole. For CO_2 lasers in the 500 to 1000 W range, this is an 80 to 125 mm focal length lens. Longer focal length lenses will produce spot sizes that are too large to create a keyhole in the metal. For lower average powers, at the 300 to 500 W level, a focal length of 63 mm might be required. Lasers with enhanced pulsing can use a longer focal length lens because the peak power of the pulsing will create a momentary keyhole. Enhanced pulsing CO_2 lasers in the 100 to 300 W range can weld with lenses of 63 to 80 mm while lasers at the 300 to 1000 W range can employ up to 200 mm focal length lenses for keyhole welding. If conduction mode welding is required, focus lenses of 125 to 250 mm focal length are the usual choices for lasers in the 500 to 1000 W level.

Pulsed laser systems can use much longer focal length lenses because of their very high peak powers. For small weld sizes, a short focal length is used to produce the minimum diameter melt puddle. However, for typical pulsed laser welding tasks, lenses with focal lengths from 100 to 200 mm are common. Highly reflective materials might require shorter focal lengths but the vast majority of applications are covered with 100 to 200 mm focal length lenses. Conduction mode welds are possible with these same lenses by simply reducing the laser peak pulse power.

Conventional Mirror Delivery
All CO_2 systems and many Nd:YAG laser systems use turning mirror systems to deliver the laser beam to the workpiece. These systems can be simple one-mirror systems to complex systems employing up to 10 mirrors. All systems generally use mirror mounts that have fine steering adjustments and easy access to the mirrors themselves for inspection, cleaning, and replacement. At 1 kW power levels and below there is little need to provide any cooling to the mirror mounts. CO_2 laser systems at these power levels use silicon substrates with metallic and dielectric coatings to produce mirrors with greater than 99.5% reflectivity. Nd:YAG laser systems will typically use glass substrates with dielectric coatings.

There are some limitations to mirror delivery systems. The mechanical mounting of the mirror holders must be rigid and the mirrors cannot move relative to each other or the system will momentarily or permanently lose alignment. As the laser beam travels it diverges. If the length of the beam path is long or the divergence is high, the beam might expand to a diameter larger than the optics in the beam path. If this is the case, the beam must be conditioned with lenses in the beam path. This is called a *relay system*, where the beam is imaged by lenses to the focus lens position.

Fiber Optic Beam Delivery
Only Nd:YAG lasers can employ this type of beam delivery because the 1.06-mm wavelength can be transmitted by glass fibers. This type of beam delivery minimizes the complications of mirror delivery, especially with long distances, and is used on most Nd:YAG welding systems. Focal spot size is extremely consistent with fiber delivery, which in not the case when using Nd:YAG lasers with mirror delivery. Fiber delivery also makes energyshare and timeshare systems inexpensive and viable. Limitations to fiber delivery include the minimum bend radius of the fibers of 100 to 200 mm. Fibers can degrade the beam quality producing larger focal spot sizes than mirror delivered systems. In general, fiber delivery is used on most welding systems, except those where focal spot sizes smaller than 100 μm are required. See Chapter 3 for further information on fiber optic beam delivery.

Lens Protection
Some welding processes produce weld soot and spatter that can attach to the focus optic. Any debris on the focus optic will reduce the transmission and cause a localized absorption source on the optic that will damage the optic's surface and any coatings. This is especially true when welding with short focal length lenses or when welding volatile or contaminated metals. If lens life is severely reduced by this type of debris, a lens protection window or *cover slide* is placed just after the lens as a low cost, sacrificial optic that is replaced as needed. Nd:YAG and Nd:glass lasers almost always employ cover slides because the glass slides are inexpensive. With CO_2 lasers of low average power, the use of protection slides is much less common because of the cost and life limitations of the slide material. CO_2 cover slides are usually KCl or NaCl windows that are polished on both sides. These windows will absorb water from the atmosphere so will change their transmission during their life.

References
T. R. Kugler and H. N. Bransch, *Photonics Spectra*, Laurin Publishing Co., May 1992.
F. A. Jenkins and H. E. White, 1976: *Fundamentals of Optics* McGraw-Hill, New York, NY.

THOMAS R. KUGLER

10.2.3 Focus Position
Generally all laser processes with low-power lasers are carried out "in focus," where the waist of the beam focus is at the surface of the parts being welded. There is some tolerance to focus position in laser processes, and the amount of tolerance is based on two factors. The first is the *f*-number of the focus lens system. Small *f*-numbers, meaning short focal length lenses and/or large beam diameters, have less depth of focus and vice-versa (see Section 3.3). Another factor is the tolerance of the process to focal spot size that encompasses variables such as reflectivity, the power density at focus, and the surface condition and joint condition of the parts. Most welding applications should be performed with a focus lens just short enough to provide consistent coupling with the materials being used. A 125-mm focal length lens or longer is considered a long focal length lens in this power range. Lenses from 80 to 125 mm are intermediate focal lengths and any lens shorter than 80 mm is considered a short lens.

It is often debated whether focus position other than at the surface produces a better result. Typically this is a topic most appropriate to lasers with over 1 kW of average power; however, some applications can benefit from pushing the focus into the components to be welded. Provided that the power density at the surface of the part is sufficient to create a keyhole, a beam focal point below the surface will increase the power density in the keyhole and will slightly increase the keyhole depth into the part. The amount that the focus varies from the surface is small, usually no more than 1% of the len's focal length. If there is too much of a defocus from the surface, the weld penetration will become variable because the keyhole will become unstable when insufficient power density exists at the surface. For conduction mode welds, the laser should be focused on the surface. If the power density at focus is too high, keyhole welding can occur but the best practice is not to defocus to achieve conduction mode welding but to change the laser parameters or use a longer focal length lens. A longer focal length lens will result in a larger focal spot size that will not produce keyhole welding. If one works at the actual focal point, the maximum depth of focus is available for the task.

Reference
T. R. Kugler and H. N. Bransch, *Photonics Spectra*, Laurin Publishing Co., May 1992.

THOMAS R. KUGLER

10.2.4 Surface Conditions
Laser coupling, weld integrity, and weld cosmetics are affected by the surface conditions of the weld joint much more so than for traditional welding techniques. Laser welding creates a very fast melting rate in the weld and contaminants can create local areas of poor metallurgy, or if the contaminants are volatile, will create explosive metal loss in the weld. The very low heat input and autogenous nature of laser welding results in very little molten metal volume to reflow and very little time for that small molten volume to flow into any flaws.

Surface Oxides and Contaminants

Section 10.1.2 discusses the effects of surface finish on reflectivity. An oxidized surface has the greatest effect in this regard. Surface oxides also affect the localized weld metallurgy. Most metal oxides have a very high melting point and act as a brittle ceramic constituent during solidification. Therefore oxides in the weld will cause cracking and loss of ductility. These oxides are also rather porous, trapping volatile constituents such as water, oils, and other debris. These volatile constituents will produce porous welds and undercutting because of the explosive vaporization of the contaminants and the molten metal that is expelled.

Contaminants can be introduced in other ways, usually by abrasion of tools that form or machine the parts. Diamonds from diamond tooling can be transferred into the surface of parts during machining. Weld flaws from diamond contamination usually are small voids that occur when the diamonds are vaporized explosively, flying away as small sparks and leaving voids and craters. Components that are drawn though dies will often have some kind of low viscosity lubricant on their surface that can be imbedded into the surface of the metal as it is deformed by the die. These lubricants can contain lead, sulfur and other volatile and nonvolatile constituents. The volatile components cause the usual problems but the nonvolatile elements can create metallurgy defects from intermetallics formed by combining with sulfur or other constituents.

Surface coatings

Many engineering alloys will be plated or coated for various reasons, most often for the prevention of oxidation, hardness, or for future brazing or soldering applications. Zinc coatings cause problems discussed in Section 10.1.3. In general, zinc coatings are easiest to cope with when they are thin, as when used as an electrogalvanized coating instead of thick hot-dipped coatings. Zinc boiling problems are also minimized by having a gap in the joint where the vapors can escape with minimum metal loss. Other coatings such as electroless nickel platings can be a problem with ferrous alloys because of the phosphorus trapped in the plating. Phosphorus causes intermetallic formation in the grain boundaries of ferrous alloys so phosphorus-free electrolytic nickel should be used. Gold platings can also be a problem because of intermetallic formation in many alloys except copper alloys. Since gold plating must be underplated with nickel on ferrous alloys, the nickel plating must be electrolytic to eliminate intermetallics from phosphorus also.

Reference
S. Gorscak, H. N. Bransch, and T. R. Kugler, *Hybrid Circuit Technology*, August 1991, IHS Publishing Group.

THOMAS R. KUGLER

10.2.5 Joint Design: Configurations and Tolerances
The laser beam welding process utilizes joint designs much like those of the arc welding processes, but the narrow deep penetration characteristics of the laser weld permit some added capabilities while at the same time enforcing greater restrictions in some aspects of joint design. In this section, we illustrate common joint configurations for laser welding and provide guidelines for joint tolerances, weld geometry and location and part orientation.

Autogenous Laser Welding Joint Configurations

Table 2 illustrates some commonly used laser weld joint configurations. These joints are primarily intended for use in autogenous laser welding (i.e., welding without filler addition). Although the illustrations show sheet/plate material, these joints may be used equally well on pipe, tubing or more complex shapes.

Filler Wire Addition

Laser welding is usually performed autogenously (i.e., without the addition of filler wire). However, filler wire addition can prevent undercut if the joint gap cannot be maintained within the tolerances required for autogenous welding. It can also provide alloying additions necessary to improve weld metal strength and to prevent weld metal cracking (a problem with autogenous welding of 6000-series aluminum alloys, for example). Filler wire additions in relatively moderate amounts may be used with all of the joint designs shown in Table 2.

Although some job shops have used filler-added welding procedures in production applications, the practice is known to be very demanding in terms of setup precision because of the small dimensions of the focused laser beam. In general, fillet joints require less-accurate wire positioning than most other joint configurations because the base metal serves to constrain the filler wire, guiding it toward the weld centerline.

Thickness of Materials

The maximum thickness of the parts that can be joined by laser welding is usually limited by the laser power that is available. Data showing depth of penetration for a variety of materials and

Chapter 10: Conduction Welding

Table 2. Joint Designs and Considerations for Use

Joint Type	Applicability	Considerations For Use
Butt	Very commonly used in ferrous, other alloys having medium to high viscosity when molten.	• Maximum allowable gap = 0.05 x thickness. • Beam/seam alignment requirement approx. 0.5x focus spot diameter • Joint strength dependent on degree of penetration and weld metal strength.
Butt With Backing	Commonly used with aluminum-bronze alloys and others with low viscosity when molten.	• Consumable backings of same composition as base material most common. • Root porosity found in partial penetration laser welds may be removed by machining backing strip in some applications. • Ceramic and non-consumable (e.g. copper) backings not usually applicable.
Lap Welding	Commonly-used in all materials.	• Maximum allowable gap = 0.05 x thickness of thinner member. • Tolerant of beam/seam misalignment. • Thin-on-top/thick-on-bottom joints easily accommodated. • Thick-on-top/thin-on-bottom joints less desirable • Joint strength determined by weld metal strength, weld width (multiple passes can increase joint strength).
Stake Weld	Can produce "blind welds" that are difficult or expensive to accomplish using arc processes.	• Laser beam/web plate alignment tolerance dependent on web thickness, beam diameter. • Maximum gap = 0.05 x flange thickness. • Joint strength dependent on degree of penetration and weld width (multiple passes can increase join strength).
Edge Weld	Usually applied in thinner gauges where the laser weld bead consumes all or most of the thickness of both members.	• Wide range of included angles possible with appropriate forming of edges (as illustrated). • Maximum gap = 0.05 x thickness of thinner member. • Joint strength dependent on degree of penetration and weld metal strength. • Delamination of metal an important design strength consideration.
"Skid" Fillet Weld	Full penetration possible with sufficient power.	• Small beam centerline/flange angle (approx. 10 degrees or less). • Maximum gap = 0.05 x thickness of web plate. • Beam/seam alignment approx. 0.5 x focus spot diameter. • Joint strength dependent on degree of penetration and weld metal strength.
Corner Weld	Full penetration possible with sufficient power.	• Beam/seam alignment (approx. 0.5 x focus spot diameter). • Joint strength dependent on degree of penetration and weld metal strength. • Maximum gap = 0.05 x thickness of web plate.

laser powers are found throughout Chapters 10 and 11. Using a 25 kW CO_2 laser, butt welds in 7/8-in. steel have been made on a production basis and larger thickness is possible. The lower limit on thickness is often determined by distortion. For a given laser, the beam quality determines the smallest focal spot that can be achieved. This, in turn, largely determines the smallest weld size that can be produced. Weld widths that are substantially larger than the sheet thickness often result in unacceptable levels of distortion. Materials 0.001-in. and less have been welded using sub-hundred watt lasers with high beam quality.

Fitup Tolerance

Laser welding demands tighter fitup than most arc welding processes because of the small size of the heat source as well as the fact that most welds are autogenous. The effect of excessive gap is usually lack of fusion (in the worse cases) or undercut (for smaller gaps). The amount of undercut that will be experienced in, for example, a butt weld is directly related to both gap size and weld size, with narrow welds being more sensitive to gap-induced undercut. Most practitioners use a rule of thumb that the maximum fitup gap should be less than 5% of the thickness of the thinner material being welded. This rule applies to both butt welds and lap welds. Table 2 (previous page) includes information on the maximum gap for various configurations.

DAVE F. FARSON

10.2.6 Joint Design: Choice

A given joint design may be chosen for a number of reasons, such as ease of assembly, allowance for fabrication tolerances, reduced material costs, and/or simpler fixturing methods. Some joints must allow for motion of the part just before welding so that the position can be set for alignment or calibration. A joint design is sometimes selected simply because "that is the way it has always been done." Laser welding is most successful when the joint design is chosen for optimum results.

Joint Types

Butt, lap, and fillet joints are the common types. All other joint designs can be considered variations on these three basic types. Because of the autogenous welding methods employed by lasers, the fitup requirements of joints are much more stringent than those for more conventional welding techniques. In most cases, the joint gap between components should not exceed 10% of the thickness of the thinnest component in the weld. The requirement can be relaxed for materials thicker than approximately 0.6 mm and might require even tighter tolerance for components thinner than 0.1 mm.

Butt Joint

The butt joint allows for the minimum heat input weld and all of the weld penetration achieved directly results in a stronger joint as compared to other joint designs. Butt joints are the best joint geometries for hermetic welds because all of the weld nugget is in the sealing volume and voids or cracks must continue to the top surface of the weld for leaks to occur. Low tolerances exist, however, for the alignment of the focal spot to the weld seam. This can require a high tolerance stack-up of complex assemblies. Butt joints are easy to inspect for weld quality, especially if the weld penetration required is 100% and the bottom of the weld joint is visible. Butt joints also allow favoring one side of the weld joint or the other if one alloy has better metallurgy or beam absorption characteristics over another.

Lap Joint

Lap joints allow for the largest tolerance of beam position but there are several limitations. Lap welds require the maximum heat input from a laser because the top component is melted without creating any weld joint until the bottom component begins to melt. For this reason the laser lap weld should always be "thin onto thick" to minimize heat input and maximize welding speed. The weld nugget at the interface is also smaller than the top of the weld nugget and this can be difficult to inspect. A thinner weld interface also makes hermetic sealing less tolerant because a smaller nugget is present and porosity deep in the weld is closer to the joint area. Weld penetration in lap welds determines the metallurgical mixing of two dissimilar components but this can be a positive attribute, especially if the bottom material has poorer metallurgy. Minimum penetration into the bottom layer can improve the metallurgy of the weld nugget. In most cases it is the weld beam width at the interface that determines the weld strength so if the weld nugget interface is larger than the thinner component weld strength is maximized.

Fillet Joint

Fillet joints are often used in small components or where machining is difficult. These are considered high heat input welds if the top layer is rather thick. The welds are easy to inspect, however, and hermeticity is easy to achieve with good fitup and good metallurgy. Surface tension forces pulling at the solidifying melt puddle and the concave bead result in very high stresses in the weld. Cracking is a very common problem in fillet welds with marginal metallurgy. Also, the fillet weld makes favoring one material over another difficult because a good melt puddle is required on both sides to get good melt flow and fusion. These welds might require a laser beam orientation of about 45 degrees to the joint for thick materials, but welding normal to the materials is possible with a thin top component such that the edge will flow over onto the bottom material.

References
S. Gorscak, H. N. Bransch, and T. R. Kugler, *Hybrid Circuit Technology*, August 1991, IHS Publishing Group.
T. R. Kugler and H. N. Bransch, *Photonics Spectra*, Laurin Publishing Co., May 1992.

THOMAS R. KUGLER

10.2.7 Elements of Quality

Weld Penetration

The most common determination of weld quality is the penetration. This is often easy to judge from cross sections of test parts or by inspecting the backside of a through-penetration weld. In most cases the penetration requirement is set by the mechanics of the alloys, strength tests during process development, and accepted safety margins. Various measurement techniques are used that allow for welds at angles to the surface, undercutting at the top or bottom of a weld, or to specify penetration by the depth of penetration into the bottom component of a lap weld.

Weld Strength

Strength of a weld is determined by all of the physical properties of the weld, its metallurgy, the components that are welded and even the type of forces and their cycling. Weld strength is usually determined by pull tests, burst tests, torque tests, and/or fatigue tests and many of these can include corrosive atmospheres. Weld strength can be improved if weld placement is also considered. For most weldments the ultimate strengths can be determined by the geometry of the weld joint and the strengths determined from simple coupon and tensile tests. Penetration and weld integrity determine the majority of weld strength attributes. Butt joints are strongest with higher penetrations, and lap and fillet welds are strongest with wider weld widths at the interface. Lack of porosity and undercutting in the weld bead also improve the integrity of the nugget increasing weld strength.

The basic metallurgy of the joint is another important factor. Many alloys can be laser welded with weld nugget properties that are better than the parent metal. Ferrous alloys typically have this characteristic. Welds in ferrous alloys and stainless steels are often stronger than the surrounding area. Other alloy systems, however, have reduced strength or hardness because of the annealing or grain refinement characteristics in the nugget or in the heat-affected zone (HAZ). Aluminum and titanium alloys exhibit this characteristic. Heat treatments can restore weld strength in some systems and this technique should be investigated if deemed necessary as a result of weld testing.

Hardness and Ductility

Weld metallurgy and post weld heat treatments usually determine the hardness and ductility of a weld joint. In ferrous alloys it is the carbon content and cooling rate of the weld that determine the ultimate hardness of the weld. In many cases with ferrous alloys, the HAZ is the hardest region because of the high rate of heat conduction into the parent metal and out from the weld nugget. The relative size of the weldment as compared to the weld nugget volume will also determine the heat input and resulting metallurgical changes. Preheating to reduce postweld cooling and postweld heat treatments are often used to achieve the required weld ductility while maintaining the required hardness in the parent metal.

Laser welding is usually chosen for its speed, lack of part deformation, and minimum weld volume. Welding tasks that require high heat inputs for proper weld metallurgy can negate many of the advantages that lasers can provide.

Cracking

Weld cracking is not desired in welded assemblies but sometimes occurs to a limited degree that can be considered acceptable, especially with some alloys that have a difficult metallurgy. If cracking is not allowed, crack presence is determined by visual inspection, ultrasonic inspection, dye penetrant inspection, metallurgical sections, and even radiography. Cracks are usually caused by metallurgical problems from poor base metals or contaminants from coatings, platings, or unclean parts.

Weld cracks, if allowed, are usually classified by their length, width, and location in the weld. If a weld is simply used to hold a component in place until further assembly tasks or is used to stake a part to eliminate movement, then weld cracking might not be a problem. Strength tests, torque tests, and other tests will determine if cracking or the extent of cracking will produce any failures.

Undercutting

Metal flow into a weld joint can create an undercut in the weld bead so that there is a localized reduction in weld cross section. This can occur at the top and bottom of a butt joint or between plates in a lap weld. Undercutting can also result from metal loss due to contaminant expulsion in the melt. Undercutting always results in loss of strength and potential stress risers in a structure.

Porosity

Voids of any kind within a weld are usually termed porosity, but their causes can vary a great deal. The most common is from volatile constituents in the joint or parent metal. Oxidized surfaces can trap volatile materials such as cutting oils, lint, air, and water vapor in their porous structure. When these come into contact with the melt, their rapid expansion will create small pores in the nugget that might not reach the surface by convection before the melt freezes. Powdered metals, castings, metals with surface oxidation such as aluminum alloys, or any metals that are not well cleaned before welding can cause this problem. Metals that have been extruded can have extrusion lubricants embedded in their surfaces or metals that have been machined with diamond tools can have small volatile diamond grit lodged in their surfaces.

Another cause of weld porosity is the trapped gasses from the bottom of the weld keyhole. In deep narrow welds the keyhole is a vapor pocket in the melt. If the position of the keyhole quickly shifts in the melt, the vapor in the previous keyhole cavity root can be trapped by melt that flows over the bottom of the pocket. The trapped gas often cannot rise to the surface before solidification, so it will become a pore in the nugget, forming what is called root porosity. These are usually seen in fast keyhole welding tasks or in pulsed laser welds where the peak power of the pulses is high to improve the weld nugget penetration. Slowing the welding rate and moderating the peak power improves root porosity. Full penetration welds rarely have root porosity because the keyhole extends through the metal and does not quickly shift position but is very stable.

Porosity can also form from gases trapped in a closed volume being sealed by the laser weld. These gases are warmed and expand from the heat input of the weld. Any trapped gases will be under a higher pressure and will push into the nugget creating porosity. In sealing small devices, it is often necessary to delay the final sealing length of weld and wait for the gas temperature in the part to reach equilibrium and stop flowing out.

Hermeticity

A hermetic weld is one that encloses a volume and seals that volume to a maximum leak specification. Most medical devices and military devices specify their leak rate to meet various specifications. Typically the leak rate is measured in small volumes of helium per second because helium is a small atom and will leak through the smallest of openings. Measuring these small leak rates requires special equipment with vacuum pumps and a mass spectrometer to measure the amount of helium that leaks out into the vacuum around the part. Helium is usually present in the atmosphere during welding or is forced into the package under high pressure after the sealing weld by a practice called "bombing". Most specifications form hermeticity require a leak rate no higher than 5×10^{-7} cc of helium/sec. Hermetic welds with this specification require clean surfaces, good weld metallurgy, and proper part design and fixturing; however, hermetic welding is very common and can be done with consistent results with the proper methodology. Weld cracks, plating contaminants, porosity, and poor fitup are the major problems in hermetic sealing.

Other hermeticity requirements can be much less stringent, with leak rates specified as less than 1×10^{-3} cc of air/sec. This is common with automotive parts that require a seal designed more to prevent dust and water ingress than to be completely gas-tight.

Weld Cosmetics

A rather difficult quantity to specify but one that is very important to many manufacturers is weld aesthetics. Many consumer devices have welds that are visible and good weld cosmetics improve the appearance and perceived quality of the devices. In these cases the welds must be as smooth as possible and have a very consistent quality to the width, surface roughness, and bead height. Although all of these factors can be measured, samples of acceptable or unacceptable characteristics can be used by quality control.

Often the cosmetics will improve functionality. Implanted medical devices must be smooth so they will not cause damage to organs or other devices. Welds must often have a consistent bead height so that the proper wall strengths are achieved or they will be machined down to form a consistent surface for other assemblies in a later operation. The existence of oxides on the surface greatly influence weld cosmetics and can result in weld integrity problems especially when oxides or nitrides reduce strength or toughness.

References
S. Gorscak, H. N. Bransch, and T. R. Kugler, *Hybrid Circuit Technology*, August 1991, IHS Publishing Group.
W. A. Baeslack, J. R. Daves, and C. E. Cross, Selection and Weldability of Conventional Titanium Alloys, ASM Handbook Volume 6.

R. P. Martukanitz, Selection and Weldability of Heat-Treatable Aluminum Alloys, ASM Handbook Volume 6.

THOMAS R. KUGLER

10.2.8 Processing Gases

Welding with laser power below 1 kW may be performed in the continues wave mode (CW) or pulsed mode. Although the laser power is relatively low, a short-focal-length lens can create high irradiance during CW operations. During pulsed operations, the peak power may be considerably higher than the average power of 1 kW. Consequently, deep penetration welding is possible as well as conduction welding.

During conduction welding, the material is molten, but it is not vaporized. The task of the process gas is mainly to shield the molten pool.

During deep penetration welding, the material is partly vaporized and ionized. The ionized vapor is called a *plasma*, and it can absorb laser light, especially if the wavelength of the laser light is long. Therefore, in CO_2 laser welding, the assist gas is used for plasma control and shielding of the molten pool. In Nd:YAG laser welding, its main task is shielding of the molten pool. Because of the shorter wavelength of the Nd:YAG laser, a strong plasma is not likely to occur.

Assist Gas for Plasma Control

Effective means of avoiding a strong plasma during CO_2 laser welding are:

- Using an assist gas with a high ionization energy
- Using an assist gas with high heat conductivity
- Using an assist gas with small specific weight

Consequently, helium is a suitable assist gas because it combines a high ionization potential and a high thermal conductivity with low specific weight (see Table 3). In addition, it is an inert gas and does not react with the molten pool. However, many low-power CO_2 laser welding applications do not require helium as an expensive plasma control gas because the intensities employed are not high. It has been found that up to 2 kW, argon, and up to 8 kW argon-helium or other gas mixtures can be applied successfully.

In Nd:YAG laser welding, argon is preferred as a shielding gas because it is less expensive, gives an excellent coverage because it is heavier than air, and will not create a plasma because the wavelength of the Nd:YAG laser is 10 times shorter than the CO_2 wavelength. Its inert character provides also excellent shielding.

Nozzle Position and Gas Consumption

Plasma control is also possible if one uses different assist gas nozzle designs. As shown in Figure 2, the coaxial nozzle and the off axis jet nozzle are the two principle choices and are sometimes offered as options by the machine manufacturer. The off-axis nozzle allows higher-gas-flow rates without blowing the melt out of the molten pool. It thereby cools the plasma, keeps it small and decreases the plasma absorption.

Table 3. Properties of Gases Used in Laser Welding

Gas	Density (kg/m^3)	Ionization potential (eV)	Thermal conductivity (10^{-4} W/m K)
Argon	1.650	15.7	161.0
Carbon Dioxide[b]	1.1833	14.4	157.0
Helium	0.165	24.5	1482.0
Hydrogen[b]	0.0834		174
Nitrogen[b]	1.153	15.5	250.0
Oxygen[b]	1.326	13.2	2.39

[a]The values for density are valid at 70°F (21.1°C) and 1 atm.
[b]Dissociation energy has to be considered in polyatomic gases.

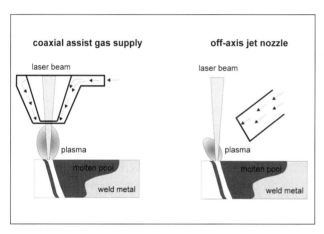

Figure 2. Plasma formation using different nozzle designs.

In some cases, i.e., welding of stainless steel or titanium, a second nozzle is required for root protection. In case of a hollow structure it may also be possible to purge the structure with an inert gas such as helium, argon or nitrogen.

The flow rate of the gas depends on the type of gas and the nozzle arrangement. The flow rates in Table 4 are for an off-axis jet nozzle with 4–6 mm inner diameter or a coaxial nozzle that has one or more orifices in a similar total cross section.

The gas purity of helium and argon that can be used for laser welding of mild steel and stainless steel is:

- helium: 99.996%
- argon: 99.99%

For titanium, higher purity levels and low moisture contents are recommended.

Table 4. Gas Consumption in Laser Welding Used in Industry

Gas type	Coaxial nozzle		Off-axis jet[a]	
	CO_2	Nd:YAG	CO_2	Nd:YAG
Helium or mixtures with high helium content	10–30 liter/min	10–30 liter/min	10–40 liter/min	10–30 liter/min
Argon or mixtures with high argon content	not suitable	5–20 liter/min[b]	20–40 liter/min	5–20 liter/min[b]

[a]Recommended for welding with more than 8 kW laser power
[b]Flow rate reduced due to specific weight of argon

Assist Gas for Melt Pool Coverage

Helium and argon are the predominant gases in laser welding. They form the basis for a number of gas mixtures where components are added to meet special goals.

Which gases are added is mainly dependent on the material to be welded. The right assist gas can affect the joint appearance and its mechanical properties by:

- Creating a pore-free weld metal
- Avoiding embrittlement of the weld metal
- Creating a smooth surface without undercut

Pores in the weld metal can be a typical phenomenon of laser welding. Pores may appear because the molten pool is very deep and the time for gases to escape is too short because of high welding speeds. The number of pores is strongly dependent on the metal purity and weld joint configuration. A joint configuration where gases cannot escape at the root side of the weld and the penetration depth is more than 1/4 in. should be avoided.

Pores can also be created by out-gassing during solidification of the molten metal. This can occur when the solubility of the gas in the molten metal is higher than in the solid metal. In this case, outgassing during solidification leads to high porosity. Examples are given in the Figures 3 and 4 for hydrogen and nitrogen in iron and aluminum.

Gas (nitrogen, carbon dioxide and oxygen) can be soluble in the molten metal. The fact that the gas can react with alloying elements of the material increases the possibility of mechanical defects in the welded metal. Gas mixtures that contain hydrogen, nitrogen, carbon dioxide or oxygen can be beneficial in many applications but a substantial knowledge about their effects on process performance and weld quality is necessary.

Welding under atmosphere (without any assist gas) may be seen as the most inexpensive solution but can be justified only for lower quality joints and after comprehensive investigations of the static and dynamic mechanical properties of the weld.

A modified stretch-draw test to assess the formability of butt joints showed a significant reduction of the formability of welds made with nitrogen and carbon dioxide compared to welds made with helium and argon because of a large number of pores.

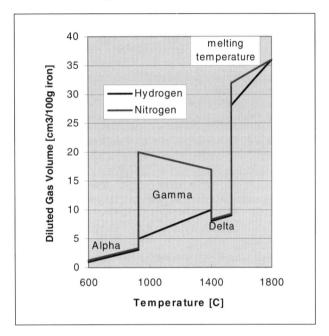

Figure 3. Solubility of hydrogen and nitrogen in iron.

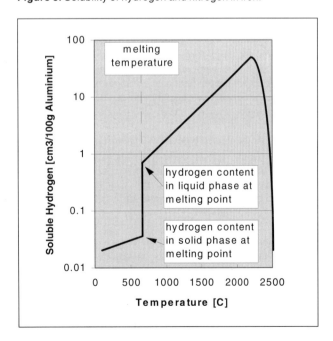

Figure 4. Solubility of hydrogen in aluminum.

Because in most cases the gas-related costs are below 1% of the total welding cost, it is recommended that one use a gas cover and avoid performance problems and defects in the weld.

Gas Mixtures for Different Materials

Materials that can be laser welded include mild steel, stainless steel, titanium and aluminum. Aluminum, however is more difficult to weld than steel because of the low-laser-light absorption and the lower viscosity of the molten pool.

Mild steel is weldable if the carbon content is lower than 0.22% and no other alloying elements are significantly diluted.

Alloying elements such as zinc or zinc coatings for corrosion protection may cause problems because of the relatively low boiling point of the zinc. This is in particular true in the case of lap joints with zinc coatings between the material.

Stainless steel is welded quite often in industry. Helium is used most of the time for the CO_2 welding of stainless steel; argon is the right choice for Nd:YAG welding operations.

A general point of concern is corrosion resistance after welding. In particular intercrystalline corrosion may occur in ferritic stainless steel but also in austenitic stainless steels because of the formation of chromium carbides. The formation of chromium carbides lowers the amount of chromium along the boundaries of the grain and can start corrosion. Because carbon is needed to generate those carbides, CO_2 as an assist gas is not appropriate.

In addition to argon, helium and argon-helium mixtures, argon-hydrogen mixtures are beneficial for welding of austenitic steel. Small amounts of hydrogen are very effective in controlling plasma formation; they reduce the surface oxides and positively affect the viscosity of the melt.

- Hydrogen should not be used with ferritic steels because of the possibility of hydrogen embrittlement.

Nitrogen and mixtures with nitrogen may be used for those austenitic steels that are alloyed with nitrogen. Thereby the losses of nitrogen in the weld metal can be reduced.

- Nitrogen is not appropriate for austenitic steels that are alloyed with titanium and niobium. The corrosion resistance of these materials would be impaired because of the formations of titanium and niobium nitrides.

Aluminum has a molten pool with very low viscosity. It is therefore characterized by highly dynamic motion of the molten pool. The dynamics of the molten pool lead to different evaporation rates at the keyhole front, and the different evaporation rates then create an unstable vapor and plasma formation. In the case of Nd:YAG welding, the vapor does not interfere with the laser beam so that this laser may be preferred for welding of aluminum. However, because of the limited power of Nd:YAG lasers, CO_2 lasers may be considered for some applications. In this case the unstable vapor formation reacts with the CO_2 laser beam, which can cause unstable energy coupling and inhomogeneous welding depth. Argon used in an argon-helium mixture can stabilize the process by increasing the plasma plume slightly and creating an V-shaped keyhole, which is less sensitive for changing evaporation rates and vapor pressures inside the keyhole.

Titanium's weldability and that of its alloys in general are good. However, for temperatures above 300ºC, titanium and its alloys show a high affinity to oxygen, nitrogen, and hydrogen. Higher content of these gases in the weld metal influences the ductility of the weld metal in a negative way and makes the joint brittle.

To minimize the negative effects on the mechanical properties, the gas content should be lower than 0.20% of oxygen, 0.07% of nitrogen and 0.125% of hydrogen. To achieve this it is necessary to cover the top and the back of the molten pool as well as the top and backside of the solidified weld metal behind the pool with a good inert gas cover. Depending on the laser power and the weld position, higher flow rates of helium and argon are appropriate.

Reference
Facts about: Laser welding gases, Information AGA Gas Inc.

JOACHIM BERKMANNS

10.2.9 Guidelines

Edge Preparation

Machining, shearing, slitting, and thermal (e.g., flame, plasma or laser) cutting, and other similar processes may all be used to prepare materials for laser welding. Where the cut surfaces are to be consumed by the weld (such as with butt welds), the maximum roughness of the cut edges should be about 5% or less of the thinner joint member. This can be a demanding requirement for thermal cutting processes, so mechanical methods are often preferred. Also, it is recommended that dross and oxides resulting from thermal cutting be removed by grinding or particle-blasting prior to laser welding.

Weld Geometry and Location

Several general guidelines regarding weld geometry and location can be stated.

> Straight or circular weld geometries should be used whenever possible to minimize the cost of machining the joint and the cost and complexity of the tooling needed to manipulate the beam and/or the part during welding.

> Welds should be full penetration rather than partial. Partial-penetration laser welds almost always contain some root porosity caused by gas. In many cases, this root porosity is acceptable, but it is avoided in full penetration welds. This is one reason that lap welds are usually made so that the weld fully penetrates the bottom sheet even when penetration through the interface between the two sheets would suffice.

Another advantage of full penetration welds is that they are easily visually inspectable for adequate penetration.

Weld widths in thin materials should be approximately equal to the sheet thickness. This rule of thumb is based on a trade-off between weld strength (for lap welds) and distortion considerations. In lap welds, the joint strength is directly affected by the weld width at the interface. Although design calculations should be performed to ensure an adequate weld size, a weld width of 1–2 times the sheet thickness is usually adequate. In the butt weld configuration, the weld need only be wide enough to consume the weld interface. In thin sheet materials, weld distortion dictates that the weld size be no larger than is necessary for adequate strength.

Line-of-sight access from the last turning mirror (or off-axis focusing mirror) to the joint is necessary. The length of this line of sight depends upon the focusing optics and beam power that are being used. For example, in the specialized focusing head for welding 38-mm-diameter tubes from the inside diameter, the line of sight is only 19 mm, this distance being measured from the center of the last turning mirror to the inner diameter of the tube.

The laser beam should be normal to the part in both the planes perpendicular to and parallel to the travel direction. In some cases this is not possible and some angle must be accepted. However, increased angles inevitably cause the weld width to grow (due to focal spot spreading) and require higher heat input than would be the case for normal impingement. Increased reflection can also be a problem as beam angle is increased. Some process developers use 30 degrees from perpendicular as a rule of thumb for the maximum allowable angle. However, if focal spot size is minimized, angles in the range of 45 degrees can be feasible.

A flat (or downhand) weld position is most common, but horizontal, vertical, and overhead positions can also be used for welding of many materials. In fact, some advantages are realized in the vertical-up position. The root porosity commonly associated with partial penetration laser welds is minimized, and slightly deeper weld penetration can be achieved. It should be noted that welding in the overhead position is very rare and very little data or experience exist concerning this configuration.

DAVE F. FARSON

10.3 Laser Welding Results

10.3.1 Nd:YAG Laser Welding

The widespread application of solid-state Nd-doped lasers — such as neodymium-doped yttrium-aluminium-garnet (Nd:YAG) lasers — in industry testifies to the fact that they are reliable, safe to operate, and simple to control. They can emit power in a pulse as high as 10^7 W or more and can process materials at an extremely high rate. A typical repetition rate varies from 0.05 to 50.0 kHz, and the average power reaches 20 to 50 W with an efficiency of 4–7%. At low frequencies, 0.1–1.0 Hz, these lasers can yield up to 10 J in a 100-μs pulse and can emit 10^5 W peak power. Increasing lasing efficiency and power is a prerequisite for increased quality and capacity in laser material processing.

There are a number of problems, though, associated with solid-state lasers, such as:

- Large beam divergence, because of the inhomogeneous structure of the synthetic crystals or the irregular doping of the host material;
- Synthetic crystal's low thermal conductivity that causes difficulties in cooling lasing elements; and,
- Their comparatively low lasing efficiency and power generated, owing to the limited size of the linear dimensions of the synthetic crystals used.

Having the balance of properties required to produce an efficient welding source, the Nd:YAG laser is the most acceptable solid-state laser used for this purpose.

Nd:YAG laser welding covers a large variety of techniques capable of producing welds in various metals, ranging from a few micrometers to tens of millimeters in thickness. Figure 1 illustrates laser welding methods classified by the *beam energy characteristics*, *performance parameters*, and *process characteristics*.

Beam Energy Characteristics

These are the laser power density (irradiance), I, and the action time or dwell time, t. The latter depends on the welding speed in continuous wave (CW) laser welding, and on the pulse duration (pulse length) in pulsed welding.

Laser welding presupposes an upper limit to the irradiance defined as the threshold irradiance, I_{th}, above which the metal vaporises vigorously, while the material ejection impairs the weld joint. In practice, the welds are made at an irradiance in the range 10^5–10^7 W/cm^2. Irradiance below 10^5 W/cm^2 is insufficient to provide quality welds. In this case, a traditional welding technique with melting can be considered a better choice.

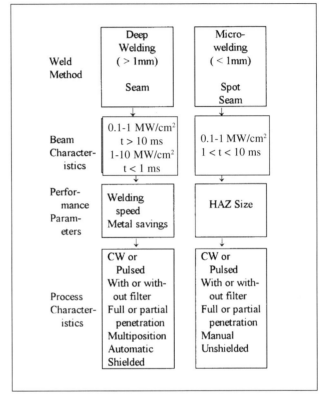

Figure 1. Classification of laser welding methods (1).

A feature specific to laser welding is that it requires a definite

Table 1. CW Nd:YAG Laser-Beam Irradiances for Melting and Welding of Metals

Material	Welding speed (cm/s) v_w	Beam diameter (μm) d	Penetration depth (mm) h	Irradiance for melting (10^6 W/cm^2) I_m	Irradiance for welding (10^6 W/cm^2) I_w
Al-6000 (2)	13.330	450	1.0	0.910	1.60
Al-6082 (3)	18.330	300	1.0	1.380	2.00
Al-5754 (4)	6.350	600	2.0	0.280	0.82
Vanadium (5)	3.390	500	1.6	0.110	0.71
	1.020	500	2.2	0.100	0.71
	0.677	500	2.4	0.098	0.71

Notes: v_w, welding speed in cm·s^{-1}; d, beam diameter in mm; h, penetration depth in mm; I_m, irradiance for melting in 10^6·W·cm^{-2}; I_w, irradiance for welding in 10^6·W·cm^{-2}.

combination of the irradiance and dwell time. Three combinations of I and t are possible for application purposes in laser welding.

First combination: 10^5 W/cm^2 ≤ I ≤ 10^6 W/cm^2 and $t > 10^{-2}$ s. This combination is typical of CW laser welding. Table 1 summarizes irradiances required for melting and welding of metals. The variation of I and t in the specified limits allows the fusion welding of various materials to be carried out, covering a wide range in thickness.

As can be seen from Table 1, the laser irradiance required for welding is affected by the welding speed, beam diameter, and penetration depth. The dwell time, in this case, can be defined as the ratio of the diameter of the focal spot, d, to the welding speed, v_w: $t = d / v_w$. Usually, CW Nd:YAG lasers are rated by their average power, which constitutes a suitable measure of performance. CW Nd:YAG lasers are often equipped with an acousto-optic Q-switch that makes them useful for integration into resistor trimming and laser marking systems. With CW Nd:YAG lasers, the average power rating has a virtually linear relation to the processing speed and production capability.

Second combination: 10^6 W/cm^2 ≤ I ≤ 10^7 W/cm^2 and $t < 10^{-3}$ s. This combination is used for pulsed welding with recurrent pulses, whose rate reaches tens and hundreds of Hz. The pulse duration (pulse length), t_p, is much shorter than the dwell time defined in the first combination, but the total action time of a few overlapping pulses is sufficient to ensure deep penetration. Pulsed welding under these conditions can yield welds in a wide range of depths and requires a much lower heat input than continuous laser welding does. Peak power, pulse energy, and pulse repetition rate are useful indicators for determining the processing speed and capability of pulsed Nd:YAG lasers. Furthermore, low to average power pulsed Nd:YAG lasers that produce a short pulse duration can be focused on a small spot to achieve very high irradiance needed to make deep spot and seam weld joints. These features permit low average power pulsed Nd:YAG lasers to be a cost effective solution for a broad range of precision metal joining applications.

Third combination: 10^5 W/cm^2 ≤ I ≤ 10^6 W/cm^2 and $10^{-3} < t < 10^{-2}$ s. Here the dwell time is approximately the same as it is in the second combination, but the pulse duration (pulse length) is longer. A train of pulses can yield a spot weld of a requisite depth that is comparatively small.

The optimum pulse duration range and the depth of the molten zone can be determined for each material, and within this range a weld is obtained without excessive removal of the material from the HAZ. The optimum pulse duration ranges are different for different materials. For the higher pulse energies, the optimum pulse duration is longer. For a shorter pulse duration, there is not enough time for melting, while for a longer duration, the pulsed irradiance is not sufficient.

Figures 2 and 3 present estimates of the temperature at the center of the focused spot on the surface of the irradiated material, and of the depth of the molten pool, respectively, for copper, aluminium, tungsten, and steel at $\alpha = 0.74 \times 10^6$ cm^{-2} and $r = 25$ μm; where α is the concentration factor determining the focusing property of the radiation source, and r is the heated spot radius.

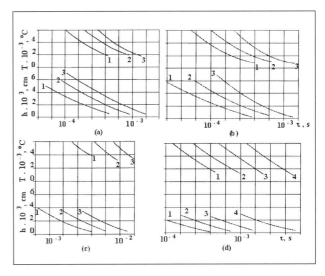

Figure 2. Temperature at the center of the focused spot on the surface of the irradiated material, and depth of the molten pool as functions of the pulse duration t at various pulse energies (6): (a) Copper; 1: 10^{-2} J; 2: 2.0×10^{-2} J; 3: 3.0×10^{-2} J; (b) Aluminium; 1: 2.5×10^{-3} J; 2: 5.0×10^{-3} J; 3: 10^{-2} J; (c) Tungsten; 1: 5.0×10^{-2} J; 2: 10^{-1} J; 3: 0.3 J; (d) Stainless Steel; 1: 10^{-3} J; 2: 2.0×10^{-3} J; 3: 4.0×10^{-3} J; 4: 10^{-2} J.

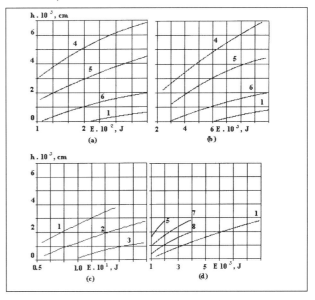

Figure 3. Molten pool depth as a function of pulse energy E at various lengths of pulse duration (6): (a) Copper; (b) Aluminium; (c) Tungsten; (d) Stainless Steel; 1: 10^{-3} s; 2: 2.0×10^{-3} s; 3: 4.0×10^{-3} s; 4: 10^{-4} s; 5: 2.0×10^{-4} s; 6: 5.0×10^{-4} s; 7: 4.0×10^{-4} s; 8: 6.5×10^{-4} s.

For a given pulse energy there is a pulse duration in which the depth of the molten pool becomes the largest (Fig. 4).

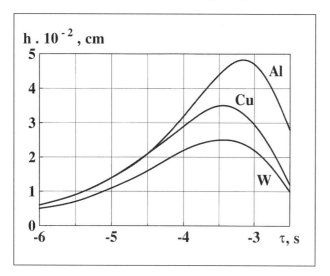

Figure 4. Maximum welding depth as a function of the logarithm of pulse duration (6) for constant pulse energy (1.5 J).

Table 2 summarizes optimum pulse duration ranges for some common materials.

Table 2. Optimum Pulse Duration (6)

Material	Optimum pulse duration range (s)
Copper	1.0×10^{-4} to 5.0×10^{-4}
Aluminium	5.0×10^{-4} to 2.0×10^{-3}
Steel	5.0×10^{-3} to 8.0×10^{-3}

Performance Parameters

These figures of merit determine the effectiveness of a welding process and include the welding speed, the factor used to account for metal saving, and the spot size or HAZ size.

Continuous laser welding can be carried out at speeds several times exceeding those of conventional welding processes. A high welding speed raises the process capacity at a reduced heat input, i.e., the power needed per unit weld length. The speed of pulsed welding, though, is much lower than that of continuous welding and, generally, comparable to that of the conventional welding processes. The welding speed affects both the weld depth and the weld width (Fig. 5), and has certain effects on the hardness profiles of the weld — namely, they increase with decreasing welding speed. Regarding weld quality, it can happen in many practical applications that the width of the HAZ may not be a critical factor, so it is likely that the process speed (welding speed) will need to be maximized in order for the desired hardness properties to be acquired.

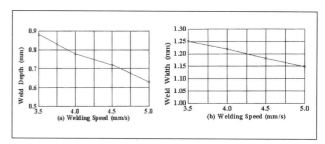

Figure 5. Weld depth (a) and weld width (b) as functions of welding speed (7). Source: pulsed Nd:YAG laser at a wavelength of 1.06 μm, power 200 W, pulse repetition frequency of 10 Hz, and pulse duration of 10 ms. Material: high carbon steel gage plate 0.88 mm thick.

The process of continuous laser welding of plates, 15 to 20 mm thick, affects savings in metal since, unlike arc butt welding, it dispenses with a bevelled plate and filler wire and can form a weld in a single pass. In laser welding of thin sheets, savings in metal are insignificant.

A laser beam focused on a spot of 0.1 mm or less in diameter provides a narrow heat-affected zone, which rapidly cools without inducing large plastic strains. So, laser welding can serve as an effective tool for the fabrication of precision weldments (8). In materials with high heat conduction and comparatively low boiling point at normal pressure (i.e., copper, aluminium, and other metals) the heat transfer from the laser-heated surface does not, practically speaking, affect the temperature of the specimen, while for metals such as W, Mo, Ti, and steel heat transfer can have a certain effect on the specimen temperature if the laser pulse duration is sufficiently long. For titanium the critical spot radius is 140 μm, for tungsten 200 μm, for molybdenum 400 μm, and for steel 500 μm in the case of vacuum heating (6).

Depending on the welding application, the HAZ can be subjected to the following restrictions:

- Limited size of the HAZ (for instance, in welding of metal foil and semiconductor, welding in the vicinity of a heat-sensitive component, etc.);
- Restriction of the material removal from the HAZ (this restriction is typically needed to obtain strong welds);
- Limited temperature gradient;
- Limited time of contact between solid and liquid phases to prevent the formation of intermetallic layers and embrittlement of the HAZ;
- Sufficient depth of the molten pool without any material removal in order to obtain strong welds;
- Prevention of surface oxidation of the materials, by using protective atmosphere or vacuum.

It is difficult to satisfy simultaneously all (or most) of the conditions enumerated above.

Process Characteristics

Regarding penetration depths, the laser welding process can be,

Chapter 10: Conduction Welding

roughly, categorized into two types: one that provides penetration depths above 1 mm, and one that provides penetration depths below 1 mm. Both CW lasers and repetitively pulsed lasers are suitable for penetration welding, and micro-welding (micro-joining) at small heating depths. In the latter case, the laser operates under less rigid conditions, in which the heat source only melts the base metal without raising the temperature to the vaporization point. In cases either of reduced requirement — regarding the assembly accuracy or alloying the weld metal in the process of welding — one can use filler materials in the form of a powder or a thin wire (1.5–1.0 mm in diameter or even less) that must be precisely fed into the interaction region.

Welding under small-penetration conditions relies on the thermal effect produced by the laser beam, as the latter interacts with an opaque material. For efficient melting of the metal to take place, the pulse duration must correspond to the thermal time constant for the given metal, approximately defined as $t \approx \delta^2/4k$, where δ is the thickness of the processed part; $k = K/c\rho$, the thermal diffusivity; c, the specific heat; ρ, the density; and K, the thermal conductivity. The values of the thermal time constant for thin parts, 0.1–0.2 mm thick, are comparable to the free-running laser pulse duration (pulse length) in the order of a few milliseconds. On the other hand, for parts, thicker than 1.0 mm, the thermal time constant appreciably exceeds the longest pulse duration (highest pulse length) and presents difficulties in implementing the process of pulse welding.

Full-penetration welding mostly applies to the processing of critical load-bearing units, while partial penetration welding serves either to form an air-tight joint between thin parts or to join them to thicker parts. It should be noted that the optical system can direct the beam to any location in order to produce the weld at any position in space.

Penetration welding commonly calls for protection of the molten metal against oxidation and contamination by shielding gases, while the welding of thin low-carbon steel parts can proceed without protection by any shielding gas. The latter case includes also thin parts produced from some other materials.

A deep-penetration weld involves the phenomenon of keyholing, which is the rapid vaporization of the metal at the focused spot, allowing the laser beam unimpededly to penetrate into the part and form a deep cavity. At an appropriate welding speed, the cavity profile acquires a dynamic stability. Since laser energy penetrates deep into the target and efficiently couples with the cavity walls, the beam forms a narrow weld with a large aspect ratio. This is discussed in more detail in Chapter 11.

Weld quality is appreciably affected by the process of molten metal transfer in the pool, under the action of the reacting forces of vapours. Experiments reveal that the speed of the molten metal transfer reaches 1000–2000 mm/s at a welding speed of 2–5 mm/s. The recurrence rate of mass transfer varies in proportion to the welding speed and ranges from 10 to 50 Hz.

Overlapping pulsed welding relies on the use of pulses of 10^{-3}–10^{-6} s long at an irradiance of 10^6–10^7 W/cm^2 and a repetition rate of 100 to 1000 Hz. As with CW laser welding, spot welding under deep-penetration conditions depends on the keyholing process, during which the hole does not clog as the pulse decays.

The power in a pulse may reach 100 kW at a mean power of 1 kW. The metal rapidly heats to its boiling point over a short time. The reacting forces of vapors displace, periodically, the molten metal from the front wall of the cavity to the back one at a certain pulse repetition rate (9). As there is no time for the cavity wall to cool down at a high pulse repetition rate, the penetration depth can be even deeper than that when welding with a CW laser.

A periodic generation and relaxation of the plasma above the target surface is the result of repetitively pulsed laser welding. The plasma plume builds up after some time delay, t_1, from the instant the pulse arrives at the target surface, and then abates for a time interval, t_2, after the pulse ceases, affecting considerably the melting efficiency of the material. Table 3 presents information on the effect of various shielding gases.

Table 3. Parameters of Laser Melting in Shielding Gases (1)

Shielding gas	h (mm)	h/b	h/h$_{He}$	ρ_0 (kg/m^3)	$\theta \times 10^4$ (m^3/s)
He	6.1	2.8	1.00	0.178	5.00
CO$_2$	5.1	1.8	0.84	1.980	2.83
Air	4.9	2.1	0.77	1.290	–
N$_2$	4.2	1.9	0.72	1.250	2.83
Ar	1.0	0.6	0.14	1.780	2.83

Notes: where h, depth; b, average width of the melt zone; ρ_0, gas density at 0°C and 0.1 MPa; h/h$_{He}$, ratio between the depths of melting in a given gas and in helium, with h$_{He}$ taken equal to unity; θ, gas flow rate.

The basic parameters of a repetitive wave form are the pulse duration (pulse length), $t_p = 1/gf_p$, and the time, $t_{sp} = (1/f_p) - t_p$, between the successive pulses; where g is the pulse-period to pulse-duration ratio and f_p, the pulse repetition rate. The plasma effect on the melting efficiency can be minimized, by selecting a wave form for which $t_p < t_1$ and $t_{sp} > t_2$. On the other hand, a proper choice of a shielding gas at atmospheric pressure for laser welding can improve the melting parameters as Table 3 shows.

Spot Welding

Advances in manufacturing technology and the trend for smaller part geometry have opened the door for new metal-joining applications where traditional TIG and resistance welding methods no longer meet precision, quality, or productivity requirements. Pulsed Nd:YAG laser spot welding technology is now being used to replace these processes, often with increased productivity and lower overall cost. Moreover, the demand for greater precision in high-performance assemblies has favored the use of these lasers as a more cost-effective alternative to the resistance welding that has been used for decades. Nd:YAG laser spot welding eliminates problems associated with resistance welding, including electrode sticking, and cleaning or replacement. Also, since laser welding is a noncontact process, there is no metal deformation of the component parts.

Spot welding is the simplest form of laser welding. There are two types of spot welding modes: conduction and penetration. The conduction welding mode is employed for micro-joining purposes (refer back to Fig. 1). Penetration welding permits aspect ratios (ratio of depth to width) much higher than unity. Related to the process are parameters such as the welding speed, the focal length of the beam focusing lens, the workpiece position relative to the beam focal point and the shield gas type and flow characteristics (see Table 3).

There are some conditions, though, which must be satisfied in laser spot-welding (6):

- Highly accurate positioning of the components to be welded.
- Accurate positioning of the component in the focus of the laser to prevent large variations in the irradiance.
- Creation of a protective atmosphere. If the materials to be welded are easily oxidized in air, welding must be done in a protective — for instance, argon — atmosphere. It has been found that argon protection of the welding zone increases the plasticity of the weld in laser welding.
- Symmetrical laser heating.

Before selecting a pulsed Nd:YAG laser system for spot welding purposes, several factors have to be considered. Users should be certain that the laser performance specifications exceed their basic requirements, and meet weld quality and repeatability expectations. The most significant feature is pulse energy as it permits deeper weld penetration, higher throughput and more energy available for multiple fiber outputs. Maximum pulse energy usually lies in the range of 10–15 J for an air-cooled laser, and in the range of 25–50 J for a water-cooled laser. Peak power (in kW) is also a significant feature as it represents the highest power value achievable during a single pulse, and is associated with faster welding speed, deeper weld penetration, and more options for multiple fiber outputs. Pulsed Nd:YAG laser systems, typically, offer peak powers of 3–5 kW, and are available with multiple fiber outputs. Another factor to be taken into account is that the first laser pulse must deliver the same power as all subsequent pulses in order to maximize welding speed and flash-lamp life. Lasers that require *dummy* shots in order to warm up, will exhibit shorter flash-lamp life.

The use of graded index (GI) and stepped index (SI) fibers allows the user to tailor the beam delivery system to its specific tasks, optimizing the laser welding process. Flexible, silica core fibers transmit high peak power laser pulses over several dozen meters to the laser workstation without any meaningful transmission losses. Many pulsed Nd:YAG laser devices offer multiple fiber-optic outputs from a single supply, a feature that permits a number of welds to be performed, simultaneously, with a single pulse of laser power. GI fibers produce a more intense beam profile and a smaller spot diameter than SI fibers. GI fibers provide up to three times greater weld penetration compared to SI fibers, which makes them ideal for laser welding thicker materials. SI fibers are more suitable for thinner metals where the top-hat energy distribution profile produces a larger, more uniform weld nugget.

Fiber-optic beam delivery also enables the user to take advantage of time and energy sharing features available with most pulsed Nd:YAG laser devices. Time sharing allows the use of several, independently, controlled fibers from one laser source. Each time-sharing output may be programmed to deliver up to 100% of the available energy either in series or in a random program. With an energy-sharing configuration, the user pre-determines the percentage of energy needed to be delivered through each fiber.

Pulsed Nd:YAG laser devices are easily integrated into high-speed factory automation equipment to produce four or more spot welds every second. Most advanced manufacturing applications for pulsed Nd:YAG lasers require some operational control via a PC or a PLC (programmable logic control) for selecting the proper laser welding schedule and setting laser process parameters, fire commands, data feedback and motion control functions. The laser power supply and the beam delivery system should be capable of working with standard factory automation and computer systems.

The majority of laser spot welding applications use parts made of galvanized low carbon 1010 and 1100 cold-rolled steel along with 304, 306, and 400 series low-carbon stainless steel, ranging in thickness from 0.41 to 1.57 mm. The effects of spot welding on these common materials are well known and documented. Welding associations as well as laser welding device suppliers, publish spot welding parameter tables for the most common materials.

Some battery manufacturers are using nickel tabs for spot welding of the interior and exterior of the battery in order to provide electrical contact and mechanical strength without thermal damage or deformation of the components. Many manufacturers of automotive components are introducing pulsed Nd:YAG lasers for precision spot welding applications.

Lab tests with a 50 W pulsed Nd:YAG laser welder show that a 6 J laser pulse is required for consistent battery tab spot welds. Four AA-size lithium ion batteries can be laser spot welded 30% faster with a pulsed Nd:YAG laser than with resistance welding, saving 15 to 30 minutes required for periodical cleaning in the latter case. Each laser weld nugget increases the tab pull strength by about 8.89–13.35 N. A laser beam spot diameter between 0.076 and 0.089 mm is required in order to achieve sufficient irradiance to fuse the nickel tab to the steel case and produce an intimate contact between them. In production, about 50% of the cycle time is allotted to laser welding with the remaining time needed for battery pack moving and tab fixturing.

Multiple laser outputs are usually specified to meet high-volume production requirements.

Seam Welding

Seam welding is one of the simplest forms of laser welding. There are two seam welding modes: conduction and penetration. The conduction welding mode is employed for micro-joining purposes (refer to Fig. 1). Penetration welding, discussed in detail in Chapter 11, permits aspect ratios (ratio of depth to width) much higher than unity. A hole is drilled in the material and this hole is then propagated through the material to form the fusion zone.

Some of the parameters that determine important characteristics of the seam welding process are related to material properties (i.e., surface optical properties at the wavelength of the laser beam), to thermal properties (i.e., conductivity, diffusivity, heat capacity), and to the melting and vaporization temperatures and to weldability. Related to the laser beam are power, power distribution in time, power distribution across the beam, and wavelength. Finally, the welding speed, the focal length of the beam focusing lens, the workpiece position relative to the beam focal point, and the shield gas type and flow characteristics are related to the process characteristics. Refer to Figure 1 and Table 3.

Laser seam welding, using pulsed radiation with a high pulse rate, is, in practice, spot welding with the spots overlapping each other, by their radius. In pulsed laser welding the thickness of the metal parts to be welded is limited by the energy and the duration of the pulse; if one increases the power and the duration of the laser pulse, the permissible thickness of the parts to be welded increases (10). Spot welds, overlapping each other to a large extent, ensure a complete-penetration weld. In this case the distance between the centers of the spot welds does not exceed the diameter of the molten zone from the backside of the welded part. Figure 6 illustrates butt welding of two plates.

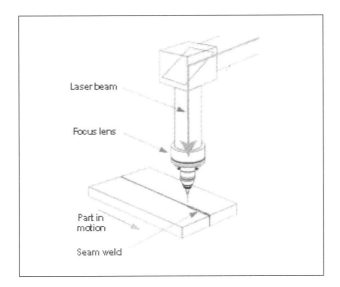

Figure 6. Schematic of laser seam welding (butt welding).

Steels, like other materials, obey the general regularities related to changes in the weld geometry with welding conditions. Table 4 lists the values of some parameters of CW welding of certain steel grades. The process of welding with the values of the parameters presented in Table 5 ensures the best geometry of the weld and high strength of the weld metal. The optimal conditions of welding cover the range of welding speeds from 80 to 120 m/h, at which the laser power required to weld 1-mm steel reaches 1.0–1.3 kW. The depth of the focal point below the target surface varies with the design of the welded structure and the focal length. These parameters relate to butt welding but lend themselves to adjustment so as to produce slot, corner, tee, and other welds.

In laser seam welding the reflection and absorption losses amount to 10–12%. Measurements of the reflectivity conducted on steel surfaces of varying roughness, and irradiated by a laser beam have shown (11) that the reflectivity decreases with decreasing angle of incidence. Intense mirror reflection occurs when the surface roughness is less than or comparable to the wavelength of the laser beam; thereafter, it decreases steadily with increasing roughness of the surface. With the surface roughness about 0.694 μm, the diffuse reflection is slight (about 5.5%); it increases to a maximum at a roughness of 2.4 μm (6).

Table 4. Parameters for CW Welding of Various Steel Grades (1)

Steel grade	h (mm)	P (kW)	v_w (m/h)	f (mm)	h_{fp} (mm)
Low-carbon, low-alloy	3.0	3.1	110	120	1.5
Medium-carbon	2.0	2.8	100	120	1.5
Medium-carbon, alloyed	3.0	3.2	100	120	1.5
High-alloy	3.0	3.3	100	160	1.0
High-alloy, austenitic	5.0	5.0	75	150	1.0
High-alloy	2.0	2.5	100	160	1.0
High-alloy, maraging	3.0	3.5	80	500	1.5

Notes: where h, steel thickness; P, laser power; v_w, welding speed; f, focal length; h_{fp}, focal point depth.

The irradiance on the surface of the material can be controlled by defocusing the beam, that is, by placing the workpiece nearer or farther from the objective of the optical system. The irradiance in the heated spot decreases with defocusing, and the size of the molten zone is changed (Fig. 7).

Among the advantages of Nd:YAG lasers for seam welding are their very high precision, their very low thermal damage, their capability for welding difficult-to-weld metals, their high welding efficiency, their high process rates, and the spatial compactness of the system. The automotive industry has been at the forefront of laser-beam-welding development and implementation. Laser beam welding has replaced numerous processes in the manufacturing of power trains and other components, and has enabled manufacturers to design products that are smaller and lighter. The most revolutionary application of laser beam welding is *tailored blanks* that increase material utilization and improve product performance, while reducing manufacturing and capital costs. Tailored blank welding is described further in Chapter 11. Other industries, such as the aerospace, have used the unique properties of laser beam welding to incorporate difficult-to-weld materials, for example, high temperature alloys, in their product designs, resulting in improved overall efficiency. More recent developments in laser beam welding include welding of heavier section steels for fabrication and construction purposes.

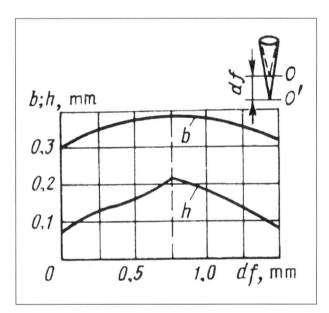

Figure 7. Variation in width, b, and depth, h, of the molten pool produced by a laser pulse with duration of 2.2 ms in a steel plate (2.6-mm thick, initially) as a function of position of the focal spot (focal distance 20 mm). O - focal plane of the focusing system; O' - focused spot of the laser beam (6).

Seam welding with pulsed Nd:YAG lasers normally requires a programmable CNC Cartesian motion system and/or a rotary stage. However, because of the energy requirements of typical weld joints and the limitations of CNC motion systems, most pulsed Nd:YAG laser welding is completed at a pulse repetition rate between 10 and 30 Hz. A 0.50 spot overlap ratio ensures good mechanical strength, while a 0.70 spot overlap ratio is needed to ensure hermetic joining. For X- and Y-motion, the CNC and the laser systems must communicate with each other, electronically, in order to synchronize the laser start and stop commands with the motion system. Complex seam welds may require a multi-axis motion system to move either the part or the laser beam focusing head in the XY, YZ and ZX planes. Perimeter welds are less complex and, usually, require a slow turning rotary stage. The operator programs the exact number of laser weld pulses in order to complete the full 360° seam weld, plus a few extra pulses for overlap, then inserts and removes parts while the rotary stage is in motion, and fires the laser at any time during part rotation.

Welding speed, considered as a function of pulse energy and pulse repetition rate, may not exceed the rated average power of the laser source. The use of multiple fibers will greatly increase production, provided the total output does not exceed the average power capacity of the laser source.

In selecting a pulsed Nd:YAG laser system for seam welding purposes, users should make certain that the laser performance specifications exceed their basic requirements, by at least 20%, and meet weld quality and repeatability expectations. Laser system characteristics presented in the discussion of spot welding are also applicable to the case of seam welding. Laser systems may be equipped with CCTV focusing heads to allow the user direct viewing of the work in progress.

Micro-joining

Micro-joining is another form of laser welding used in many applications in the electronic, aerospace, and medical product industries. Micro-joining involves both seam and spot welding (refer to Fig. 1). The difference from the other laser welding techniques lies in the small size of the parts to be welded, since it is necessary to make everything smaller. Micro-joining can be performed both with CW and repetitively pulsed Nd:YAG lasers at powers up to 1 kW. The thickness range for *small scale* micro-joining is from 0.125 to 0.51 mm, and from 0.0125 to 0.125 mm for *micro scale* micro-joining.

Highly accurate, narrow, and precisely located welds do not require subsequent dressing or machining and allow for a compact layout of the components of devices and assemblies. The use of micro-joining, for example, in the fabrication of electronic circuits leads to a considerable increase in the packing density of components on the board, which reduces the overall dimensions and mass of the devices. The precise locality of welds manifests itself most vividly in pulsed micro-joining.

The main parameters of the process of pulsed micro-joining are the pulse energy, the pulse duration, the pulse repetition rate, the focused spot radius r, and the position of the focal point relative to the target surface. The pulse duration determines the time of melting of a metal, depending on its properties and thickness. Approximate values of pulse duration needed to melt some typical metals were given in Table 2. More accurate values for the required pulse duration can be derived from experiments.

The trapezoidal or triangular wave-form with a steep leading edge and a gently sloping trailing edge is the best pulse shape for micro-joining. The size of the irradiated area and the laser power density, I, are determined by the focal spot diameter, d. The focal spot diameter must be chosen in the range from 0.05

to 1.0 mm to ensure an irradiance in the range from 10^5 to 10^6 W/cm^2. The simplest way to adjust the spot diameter and, thus, the irradiance is to defocus the beam, by placing the focal spot of the least diameter above or below the target surface.

The possibility of achieving successful laser micro-joining is affected by the part geometry, the heat balance between the parts, and the HAZ created by the laser beam. The primary goal of part design for weldability is to use geometry to affect a heat balance among disparate parts. As the size of the parts to be welded decreases, the region of HAZ and the surface finish quality of each part become of greater importance.

Seam welding applied in the conduction mode can serve micro-joining purposes. In conduction mode welding, the beam impinges on the material at an irradiance at which fusion is achieved, but no substantial vaporization takes place, and beam energy is transferred to the base material by conduction. Weld fusion zone aspect ratios (ratio of depth to width) are typically limited to about 1.0. Welds are made by overlapping weld spots at a definite overlap ratio, recommended range from 0.3 to 0.9, that varies with the type of the weld, its strength, and the required air-tightness. The speed of seam spot welding depends on the weld spot diameter (approximately equal to the diameter d of the focused beam), the overlap ratio a, and the pulse repetition rate f_p. Solid-state Nd:YAG laser welding set-ups can produce a weld seam at a speed up to 5 mm/s and f_p up to 20 Hz. An increase in f_p can lead to a higher value of the welding speed, v_w.

In cross section, there is a small fusion zone associated with a spot weld. A short dwell time results in a high cooling rate of 10^5 to 10^6 K/s inside this zone that displays a fine-grained dendrite structure with inter-dendrite inhomogeneity. The size of the HAZ that has an inhomogeneous structure is, generally, small and ranges from 100 to 150 µm in cross section. A filler material introduced into the weld pool in the form of a powder, wire, or strip serves:

- To change the chemical composition of the weld metal,
- To adjust its structure, and
- To increase the cross-sectional area of the weld to eliminate the weld concavity.

The filler can either be sprayed or smeared on the part edges to be welded.

The broadest use of spot welding is in electronic engineering for assembling components with butt, lap, and corner joints, and, especially, for joining small pieces to large parts.

Figure 8 illustrates joint designs for welding small parts to massive components, with arrows showing the laser beam direction. In the joint design of Figure 8a, a thicker body of revolution is cut to provide a ledge for a thinner part. If the two parts differ considerably in thickness, the beam falls on a thicker part to equalize the temperature field and, uniformly, melt both parts. In the tee joint design of Figure 8b, the joint preparation is more complex and calls for grooving the thicker part so as to form flanges raised on both sides of the thinner part. The groove cut in the massive part of Figure 8c accommodates a thin part to be seam welded along the edges of the groove or spot welded at individual points to a penetration depth below the thin part. In the joint design of Figure 8d, a thin part has a hole to allow the beam to melt over the hole edges and the surface of the thick part along the circumference.

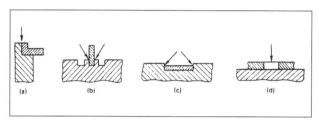

Figure 8. Designs of weld joints between thin and thick parts. Arrows show the laser beam direction (1).

An optimal joint design is one that ensures the most efficient melting and solidification of the metal. In preparing a butt joint it is essential that the gap and the edge skewing should be held as small as possible (1).

Seam welding lid assemblies with glass-to-metal feed-through for medical implants and electronic packages are ideal applications of pulsed Nd:YAG laser small scale micro-joining. Titanium, kovar or stainless steel constitute both the lid and case materials, ranging typically from 0.254 to 0.504 mm in thickness. If one uses TIG or resistance welding techniques, the glass-to-metal feed-through often cracks because of thermal stresses. The use of pulsed Nd:YAG laser welding techniques, instead, results in a significant reduction of the size of the thermal stresses because of less heat input, not damaging the glass-to-metal feed-through and producing a hermetic seam weld, as well.

As an example, consider a typical rectangular lid (31.75×6.35 mm) with a glass feed-through that has a total linear welding length of 76.20 mm. By using a 50% spot overlap ratio, a 1 J pulse, and a 30 Hz pulse repetition rate, this seam may be completed in about 6 sec. The same seam-weld could be completed in about 14 sec, with a 80% spot overlap ratio. The time cycles could effectively be reduced to half by using two laser beams.

References
1. A. G. Grigoryants, 1994: *Basics of Laser Material Processing*, Mir Publishers, Moscow.
2. J. Berkmann, R. Imhoff, K. Behler, and E. Beyer, Proc. Automotive Laser Applications Workshop, March 6–7, Dearborn, MI (1995).
3. F. Dausinger, F. Faisst, R. Hack, J. Rapp, H. Hugel, and M. Beck, Proceedings of Laser Materials Processing Symposium, ICALEO 95, J. Mazumder, A. Matsunawa, and C. Magnusson (Eds.), November 13–17, San Diego, CA (1995).
4. R. P. Martukanitz and B. Altshuller, Proceedings of Laser and Electro-Optics for Automotive Manufacturing ICALEO

5. K. H. Leong, H. K. Geyer, K. R. Sabo, and P. G. Sanders, *Journal of Laser Applications*, **9** (5), 227–31 (1997).
6. N. Rykalin, A. Uglov, and A. Kokora, 1978: *Laser Machining and Welding*, Mir Publishers, Moscow.
7. S. NG. Eng and I. A. Waston, *Journal of Laser Applications* **9** (5), 243–52 (1997).
8. G. A. Nikolaev and A. G. Grigoryants, *Izv. Akad. Nauk* **47** (8), 1458–67 (1983).
9. A. A. Vedenov and G. G. Gladush, 1985: *Physics of Laser Material Processing*, Energoatomizdat, Moscow, p. 207.
10. R. H. Fairbanks and C. M. Adams, *Welding Journal* **43** (3), 97-S, 102-S (1964).
11. M. S. Baranov, M. L. Voshchinsky, and I. N. Geinrikhs, 1971: *Lazernaya svarka metallov* (*Laser Welding of Metals*), Mashinostroenie, Moscow.

GEORGE CHRYSSOLOURIS
STEFANOS KARAGIANNIS

10.3.2 Nd:YAG Laser Welding Guidelines

When considering Nd:YAG laser welding applications under 1 kW, two primary subcategories are immediately evident, namely pulsed and continuous wave (CW) applications. A pulsed laser produces a beam with a very short, intense burst of energy, while a CW laser produces a beam of constant, steady state power. The primary considerations between pulsed and CW have to do with either product limits (i.e., pulsed versus CW capability on a given laser) or process limits (focused spot irradiance requirements for a given application), or both. While there is some overlapping of applications, there are specific areas where either a pulsed laser or a continuous-wave (CW) laser is more suitable.

Pulsed Welding Applications

Pulsing implies that the laser's active medium is excited by a very quick response stimulus. This allows the laser to transmit a burst of energy for a brief length of time (generally milliseconds). Peak pulse powers can reach values over 30 times greater than the maximum average or CW power levels. This allows low-to-medium power lasers to provide enough power to reach vaporization temperatures for most materials.

The short duration pulse produced by a pulsable laser guarantees minimum heat input, which is particularly important for parts sensitive to distortion. However, pulsing action slows down welding speeds since duty cycles (the percentage of time that the laser is emitting energy during a weld) are less than 100%. Most welding applications require that the pulses overlap to produce a pseudo continuous, and sometimes hermetic, weld. Pulse shaping is available on some lasers, and can be used to create unique pulse shapes that either enhance coupling efficiency or reduce weld bead roughness, or both.

Frequency and Overlap

If a pulsed laser is utilized, then pulse rate in Hz (f), average weld spot diameter (d_w), and weld speed (V – distance per second) have to be matched to produce the required percent overlap (%OL). The typical %OL values for both hermetic and non-hermetic welds are indicated below. For nonhermetic welding, the lower %OL allows for faster weld speeds, but weld beads can have a rough surface. In general, the larger the %OL, the smoother the weld, but the slower the weld speed. The following relationships may be helpful, especially for Nd:YAG applications where frequency is a limiting factor (about 1000 Hz maximum compared to about 10 kHz for CO_2 lasers):

Overlap = $d_w - V/f$ (ignoring oblong effect due to travel)

%OL = $100[(d_w - V/f)/d_w]$, and rearranging yields

$f = 100V/(d_w)(100-\%OL)$

For hermetic welds: $75 < \%OL < 80$
For typical nonhermetic: $50 < \%OL < 70$

Then: $f = 5V/d_w$ (for %OL= *80*)

The average weld spot diameter is not a trivial issue, because no weld profile is perfectly parallel. Therefore, the appropriate weld spot diameter must be carefully considered. Table 5 gives some recommendations that should be considered when determining the appropriate value of d_w.

Table 5. Recommended Values for Weld Spot Diameter, d_w

Weld joint configuration	Recommendations	
	d_w *standard*	d_w *conservative*
Overlap weld	0.9 x average weld width @ interface	Focused spot size
Butt weld (*full penetration*)	Focused spot size	0.9 x average weld width @ root
Butt weld (*partial penetration*)	Focused spot size	0.9 x average weld width @ 90% weld depth

Example: Calculate the pulse frequency required to produce a hermetic pulsed weld on an overlap weld joint configuration, using a weld speed of 30 mm/sec and an average weld width at an interface of 1.0 mm. First, calculate $d_w = 0.9 (1.0) = 0.9$ mm. Next, substituting into $f = 5V/d_w$ yields: $f = (5)(30)/(0.9) = 167$ Hz.

Pulse Energy

In pulsable Nd:YAG laser welding, energy per pulse (average power multiplied by the pulse length, or the ratio of average power to pulse frequency), peak power per pulse (the ratio of energy per pulse to pulse width) and pulse width (laser pulse "on" time) are key weld parameters.

For a given energy per pulse, short pulse width times yield high peak powers. When peak power gets too high, the resultant weld can have either undercutting or voids (or both). This occurs because the high peak power results in a high irradiance per pulse, which can vaporize material constituents out of the molten weld pool that at lower power densities would remain molten (refer to the *General Guidelines for Normal Pulse Welding Applications* below). In general, high peak powers produce welds via keyholing, resulting in deeper weld penetration and less overall heat input into the component being welded. Keyholing for deep-penetration welding is covered in Chapter 11. On the other hand, the deep and narrow keyhole welds require better part fit-up. If hermetic welds are required, the weld speed may suffer because of the smaller molten spot diameter and because high peak powers occur at lower frequencies (especially for Nd:YAG lasers).

Pulse Width

Long pulse width times yield low peak powers and produce welds via conduction, which geometrically tend to be wide and shallow. This geometry is more tolerant to part fitup, and is also beneficial when overlap welding a thin component onto a thicker component (e.g., diaphragm welding). However, low peak irradiance results in greater overall heat input into the welded component, and can yield severe back reflections off the weld joint.

Example: Calculate the peak power per pulse of a weld utilizing 5 J and a 2 ms pulse width. Since peak power is defined as the ratio of energy per pulse to pulse width, then peak power = 5/.002 = 2500 W. To calculate peak irradiance per pulse, simply divide this value by the area of the focused spot.

General Guidelines for Normal Pulse Welding Applications

General guidelines for pulsed welding are difficult to compose because of the interaction between many parameters (e.g., power, focused spot size, weld speed, weld joint geometry, weld joint fit-up, material characteristics, and so on). However, two general situations are worthy of comment, namely adjustment of parameters for increasing or decreasing weld penetration, while minimizing weld spatter. The guidelines below, in combination with Table 6 and Figure 9 (next page), will aid in process parameter determination for Nd:YAG pulsed welding applications.

I. Inadequate Weld Penetration:

   a. With weld spatter expulsion caused by peak power:
   Guideline: Increase pulse width.

   b. Without weld spatter expulsion:
   Guideline: Increase peak power by decreasing pulse width and keeping energy per pulse constant.

II. Excessive Weld Penetration:

   a. With weld spatter expulsion caused by peak power:
   Guideline: Increase speed (and pulse frequency to keep overlap constant), and/or reduce pulse energy by reducing peak power.

   b. Without weld spatter expulsion:
   Guideline: Increase speed (and pulse frequency to keep overlap constant), and/or reduce pulse energy by reducing pulse width.

Table 6. Typical Process Parameters for Pulse Welding
Range of values goes from thin (th) to thick (tk) material as noted.

	Pulse energy E_p (J)	Pulse width (ms)	Average power P_{ave} (W)	Peak power P_p (kW)	Frequency (Hz)
	th–tk	th–tk	th–tk	th–tk	tk–th
Steel	1–20	1–3	10–2000	1–4	10–1000
Al	10–20	1–10[a]	500–2000	2–10	10–75

[a]Typically 6–15 ms if pulse shaping is used.

CW Welding Applications

Continuous-wave lasers maintain their output over the entire span of processing (100% duty cycle). The main advantage of CW operation is that there is a greater amount of power per unit time. This generally leads to faster welding speeds than for the pulsed mode. In some lasers, pulse or (superpulse) schedules can be used in combination with CW power (with perhaps some reduction in pulse peak power, depending on CW power level). The combination of the two can be used for weld seam smoothing (especially on aluminum).

Keyhole Welding

Keyhole welding, covered in Chapter 11, is dependent on focal spot power density (i.e., laser power and focused spot size), welding speed, material melting temperature, material reflectivity, material conductivity, and the like. In general, keyhole welding of steels and stainless steels is possible above 600 W. For materials such as aluminum and copper, keyhole welding is generally not possible in the CW range below 1000 W.

Conduction Welding

Conduction welding is possible when the absorbed energy is sufficient to melt the weld zone, but insufficient for vaporization and plasma formation. Conduction welding of steels and stainless steels at low power typically requires a relatively small focused spot (in the range of 250–300 μm) in order to obtain efficient coupling of the energy into the weld joint. In general, conduction welding of steels and stainless steels is possible down to about 100 or 200 W, while conduction welding of materials such as aluminum and copper is only possible above 500 W. In general, conduction welds require higher heat input, which results in a wider weld and makes oxide free welding more difficult to obtain.

Weld Troubleshooting

Determining the appropriate weld parameters when all is well is one thing; determining what went wrong when all is not well is quite another. The *Checklist* (following Fig.9 on next page) presents a few of the primary causes of weld degradation, and it arranges them in the form of a diagnostic checklist. While not

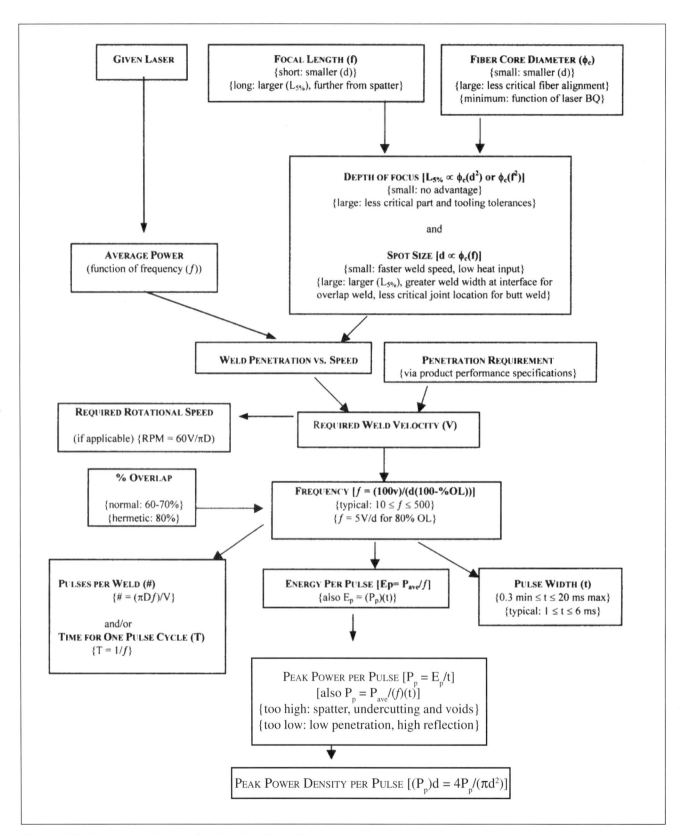

Figure 9. Weld process development flowchart for pulse welding.

Chapter 10: Conduction Welding

intended to be ultimately comprehensive and complete, it yields a methodology which is fundamentally sound and gives the welding engineer or technician an excellent start at diagnosing weld problems in the field.

Sample weld trouble-shooting checklist for Nd:YAG laser welding applications

Preliminary Data:

a. Date? _____ mo/dy/yr
b. Shift? _____ shift
c. Person performing maintenance? _____ name
d. Laser model? _____ RS model #
e. Laser serial number? _____ SN
f. Number of shots on flash lamps? _____ shots, lamps 1–4
g. Expected weld power at laser control? _____ W
h. Present weld power at laser control? _____ W
i. Expected weld normal speed? _____ m/min (in./min)
j. Present weld speed? _____ m/min (in./min)
k. Expected weld penetration at normal speed?
   _____ mm(in.)(or full/partial)
l. Present weld penetration at normal speed?
   _____ mm(in.)(or full/partial)

1. *Focus Unit*: Inspect cover slide and focus unit optic(s). Are they clean and in good condition?
   (   ) Yes (go to 2)
   (   ) No (clean, go to 9)
   Note: check focus optic protection device if applicable.

2. *Beam Delivery Power Loss*: Measure power at focus unit with nozzle cone (if used) and cover slide in place, and record. Measure power in front of incoupler, and record. Subtract the first reading from the second, and record. Is the difference greater than 10% (100 W for 1000 W weld)?
   _____ W @ focus unit
   _____ W @ incoupler
   _____ W difference
   (   ) Yes (align in coupler, replace fiber optics if required, go to 9)
   (   ) No (go to 3)

3. Measure power at focus unit with nozzle cone (if used) and cover slide removed, and record. Compare with that measured at focus unit in step 2. Record. Is the difference greater than 1–2%?
   (   ) Yes (Inspect nozzle cone integrity and alignment, correct and go to 9)
   (   ) No (go to 4)

4. *Out of Focus*: Check focus. Is focus at optimal position?
   (   ) Yes (go to 5) *Note: A gage calibrated to best focus position can be used to confirm this.*
   (   ) No (correct, go to 9)

5. *Shield Gas Nozzle:* Is shield gas nozzle clean and located properly (unobstructed, stand-off, aiming, angle)?
   (   ) Yes (go to 6)
   (   ) No (correct, go to 9)

6. *Shielding and Plasma Suppression:* Measure shield gas flow rate. Does actual shield gas flow rate match expected?
   _____ Expected: liter/h (scfh)
   _____ Actual: liter/h (scfh)
   (   ) Yes (go to 7)
   (   ) No (correct, go to 9)

7. *Poor Part Cleanliness:* Is the weld zone free of oil, water, dust, rust, or other residue or contamination? *Check that the parts are clean and dry at the exit of the parts washer.*
   (   ) Yes (go to 8)
   (   ) No (correct, go to 9)

8. *Poor Part Fitup or Poor Weld Joint Location:* Is the weld joint location and fitup consistent? *Check for conditions such as poor part fitup, part or tolling run-out, inconsistent chamfer on weld edges, damaged tooling, weld spatter on tooling, etc.*
   (   ) Yes (go to 9)
   (   ) No (correct, go to 9)

9. *Post Correction Data:* Indicate step(s) where correction was necessary, and postcorrection weld penetration. If expected weld penetration is not achieved by correction, continue with the step following where the correction was made.

Step 1 (   ) _____ mm (in.) / or full/partial
Step 2 (   ) _____ mm (in.) / or full/partial
Step 3 (   ) _____ mm (in.) / or full/partial
Step 4 (   ) _____ mm (in.) / or full/partial
Step 5 (   ) _____ mm (in.) / or full/partial
Step 6 (   ) _____ mm (in.) / or full/partial
Step 7 (   ) _____ mm (in.) / or full/partial
Step 8 (   ) _____ mm (in.) / or full/partial

10. Indicate any comments that may be necessary for detailed explanation of root cause problems.

DAVID HAVRILLA

ISBN 0-912035-15-3

10.3.3 Nd:YAG Laser CW Seam Welding of Common Materials

Low-power (less than 1 kW) CW (continuous wave) Nd:YAG lasers are used for precision shallow penetration welding of common engineering materials. In contrast to the deep penetration welding mechanism of *keyholing*, the melting is done in the conduction mode. The weld cross section is commonly in a semicircular shape with aspect ratio less than 1.0. Highly reflective materials such as copper and aluminum are difficult to weld with low power CW Nd:YAG lasers because of their low irradiance unless special optics are used to concentrate the beam to a very small spot.

A continuous wave laser must be several times higher in power to be equal to a pulsed laser for the equivalent weld penetration, since the pulsed laser has several times higher peak power. Figure 10 shows the comparison of CW Nd:YAG, pulsed Nd:YAG, and CW CO_2 laser welding performance (12, 13). As shown, the weld penetration is limited since the melting is conduction limited when low power CW Nd:YAG lasers are used.

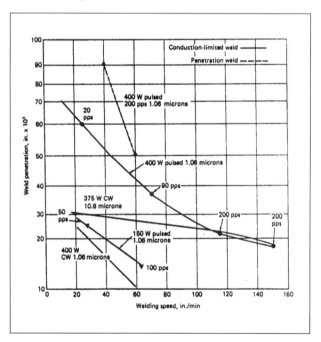

Figure 10. Comparison of CW Nd:YAG, pulsed Nd:YAG, and CW CO_2 laser welding performance (12, 13).

For single-spot welding, it is rarely necessary to provide inert gas shielding to prevent excessive oxidation of welds for many common engineering materials. The metal is at an elevated temperature for a short period of time so that significant oxidation does not occur. In case of overlapping-spot welding and CW seam welding, shielding gas is necessary to prevent excessive oxidation of welds.

Most low-power Nd:YAG laser welding has been done successfully in pulsed operation. Low-power CW Nd:YAG laser welding is not as prevalent as pulsed laser welding, but new applications are emerging in the areas of medical components, electronics, and automotive applications.

The advantage of Nd:YAG laser welding over CO_2 laser welding is the ability to transport the laser beam through fiber optics, better coupling of the beam to metals and the lower maintenance because of the simplicity of the solid-state laser. The disadvantages include low beam quality (larger spot size, low power density, less penetration) and low-energy-conversion efficiency.

The main advantages of CW Nd:YAG laser welding over pulsed Nd:YAG welding is the smoothness of resulting welds. Pulsed welding, however, is beneficial for deeper penetration welds because of better beam quality and high peak power. The weld experiences less heat accumulation for the same penetration.

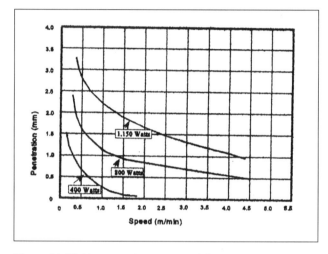

Figure 11. Weld penetration versus welding speed with an 1200 W CW Nd:YAG laser (14).

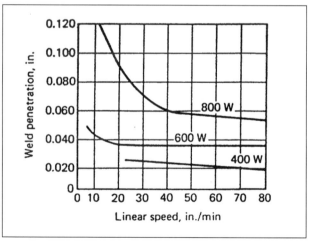

Figure 12. Weld rates obtained with a continuous-wave Nd:YAG laser on type 304 stainless steel (12).

Chapter 10: Conduction Welding

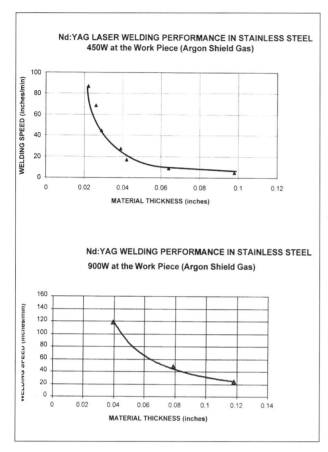

Figure 13. Upper and lower: Nd:YAG welding performance in stainless steel (16).

Typical welding performance curves are shown in Figures 11 and 12. Figure 11 shows weld penetration as a function of welding speed with a 400 W, 800 W, and 1,150 W CW Nd:YAG laser (14). Figure 12 shows weld rates obtained with a CW Nd:YAG laser on type 304 stainless steel (12). Figure 13 illustrates the Nd:YAG laser welding performance in stainless steel at 450 W and 900 W (16).

Low-power laser welding applications are typically for delicate and precision components, which require precision positioning of the beam to the workpiece. Precision tooling or seam tracking often is necessary with a low-power Nd:YAG laser welding.

Thin guage (0.002 to 0.008 in. thick) diaphragms of stainless steels are edge welded to form metal bellows. Low-power Nd:YAG became a powerful heat source to weld metal bellows 5 to 10 times faster than conventional arc welding such as gas-tungsten-arc welding (TIG welding) (15).

The conventional bellows arc welding systems have inherent limitations in terms of productivity and quality. The welding speed is slow and the weld quality degrades as the electrode tip wears. An operator watches the welding arc through a stereo microscope for alignment before and during welding. Constant adjustments and finesse are needed to track the weld seam and to maintain the weld quality, which depends largely on the skill, experience, acuity, and attentiveness of the operator. The process is labor intensive and is not well suited for automation.

An Nd:YAG laser welding system with a precision seam tracking device made automatic metal bellows welding possible. The productivity increase, quality improvement, and cost savings are reported to be substantial (6 months' payback period). Moreover, the repeatability of the weld quality is the primary advantages of precision automatic laser welding.

Other applications examples include precision medical devices and electronic components welding.

References
12. Metals Handbook, 9th Ed., Vol. 6, Welding, Brazing, and Soldering, American Society for Metals, 1983.
13. M. L. Marshall, *High-power, High-pulse-rate YAG Laser Seam Welding, Lasers in Modern Industry*, p. 184, First Edition, 1979, SME.
14. H. N. Bransch, "Welding with High-Power CW and Pulsed Nd:YAG Lasers," *Photonics Spectra*, September 1991.
15. D. U. Chang, Automatic Laser Welding of Metal Bellows with Precision Seam Tracker, ICALEO'96 Proceedings, Vol. 82, Lasers and Electro-Optics for Automotive Manufacturing, LIA.
16. Lumonics, Laser Welding Rate Charts.

DALE CHANG

10.3.4 Nd:YAG Pulsed-Seam Welding

Peak Irradiance
For each pulsed Nd:YAG welding task there are two possible welding modes: conduction-mode welding or penetration-mode welding. The factor that determines which type is created is the peak irradiance. Refer to Section 10.1.4 for more information on this subject and to Chapter 11 for details on penetration welding. Peak irradiance is the peak power of the laser divided by the focal spot area. Peak irradiance values up to approximately 400 kW/cm^2 will produce a conduction-mode weld in a common material such as stainless steel. Penetration-mode welds are best performed in the range of 400 kW to 1 MW/cm^2. These values correspond to 1–2 kW peak power pulses focused to 0.5 mm diameter spots on the workpiece. For highly reflective alloys such as copper and aluminum, higher values are needed, perhaps up to 2.5 MW/cm^2.

Focal Spot Size
Weld width is typically larger than the focal spot diameter, especially with high penetration welds, so the focal spot size should not be larger than the required weld width. If small diameter welds are required, a correspondingly small focal spot size is necessary.

Sufficiently small focal spot sizes are required to produce the peak irradiance needed for welding tasks. For low-peak-power lasers, a small focal spot might be required for penetration-mode welding since the peak irradiance constraint is the limit. Consistent focal spot size is key to consistent welding. The size of the focused spot can change with conventionally delivered Nd:YAG lasers because of thermal lensing of the laser, so weld parameter development should take this into account. Operating the laser at a constant average power during parameter development should eliminate thermal lensing effects on focal spot size. With fiber-delivered lasers, the focal spot size will be constant. This is therefore the most common form of beam delivery for Nd:YAG laser welding. Once an optical system is selected (laser power, up-collimation ratio, and focus lens) the laser's peak power is adjusted in a series of test welds to determine the values that produce the desired welding mode.

In some instances, the optical system may produce spot sizes that require peak powers higher than the laser can produce. This typically occurs when long focal length lenses are used. In such a case, the optical system must be modified by either using a shorter focal length lens or increasing the up-collimation ratio.

Pulse Energy

The energy per pulse determines the melt volume produced with a laser pulse. Changing the pulse energy is typically the way in which weld penetration is adjusted. If increased penetration is required, the energy per pulse should be increased at the same peak power. In this way the weld cross section shape will not change but simply be a scaled-up version of the lower energy parameters. Once proper weld penetration is achieved, some changes in the peak power can be attempted to improve the aspect ratio of the weld without introducing excessive voids or undercutting.

Pulse Repetition Rate

Pulsed Nd:YAG lasers produce seam welds by overlapping a series of spot welds. Only at average powers about 1 kW or greater does the melt puddle remain molten between pulses. At low average powers, the pulsing rate of the laser results in faster or slower seam welding as the rate is increased or decreased. The welding rate limit is reached when the laser cannot pulse at higher rates with the same energy per pulse or the speed of the motion system used cannot be increased. Higher average powers can result in changing optical spot sizes with mirror delivered systems so this effect must be kept in mind.

Overlap

Pulse to pulse overlap is required to perform a seam weld as compared to a series of spot welds separated by unwelded metal. Overlap is increased with increasing spot diameter, increasing repetition rate or decreasing speed.

The weld speed V and the weld overlap percentage OL are related to the repetition rate R and the weld diameter D by the equation:

$$V = D(1 - OL/100)R \qquad (1)$$

This equation is represented in Figure 14. Minimum weld overlap for seam welding is typically 50–60% and this allows for maximum speed. Since the individual pulse weld nuggets resemble a cone with the tip at the root of the weld, the overlap can also determine the average weld penetration. When welding components with a hermeticity specification, higher overlap values of 85–90% are common. High values for overlap mean that the same weld area is melted and resolidified many times which fills voids and undercuts along with more consistent penetration and smoother surfaces.

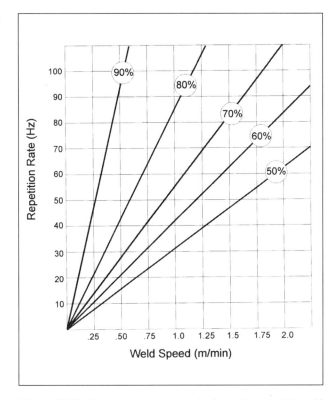

Figure 14. Welding speed versus overlap for a 1.0-mm-wide weld based on Equation 1, for the indicated values of overlap percentage.

Penetration

As discussed above and in Section 10.1.4, the average power of a pulsed laser has a much smaller effect on weld penetration than keyhole welding lasers. For conduction-mode welding, the penetration is limited to about 0.5 mm in penetration with weld widths of at least twice the weld depth. Increasing penetration over this value requires penetration-mode welding.

Changing pulse energy is the most direct method of varying penetration in the penetration-mode welding regime. Doubling pulse energy will increase weld volume by approximately 60–90% and increase weld penetration by 30–70%. The incremental gains in penetration with pulse energy are most efficient in penetrations of less than 0.75 mm and become less and less efficient for deeper penetrations. Figure 15 shows how penetration increases with pulse energy for both welding modes.

Chapter 10: Conduction Welding

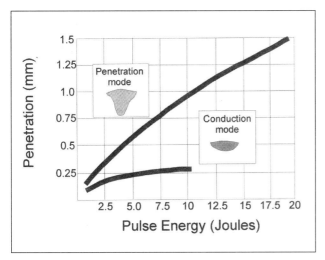

Figure 15. Penetration versus pulse energy for spot welds produced in conduction and penetration modes in 304 stainless steel.

Increases in penetration are also possible with increases in the laser average power. This is mostly because of the bulk heating of the parts to be welded, especially small parts and parts with poor conductivity. The temperature rise of the surrounding area will result in more molten metal per pulse. This is especially true after the start of the weld so the first few millimeters of a weld will show steadily increasing penetration and then one usually reaches a consistent penetration because of a quasi-equilibrium temperature reached at the surroundings of the melt puddle (see Section 10.1.5).

Repeatability

For the laser welding process to be repeatable, several parameters must be held constant in addition to the tolerances on the material and fitup. These are the laser parameters (energy, peak power, pulse duration), velocity, focus position at the joint, and focal spot size on the surface of the material. When these factors are controlled, the laser penetration can be held to better than 5% or about 12.5 μm, whichever is larger.

Heat Input

Pulsed Nd:YAG lasers have a very distinct advantage over CW and enhanced pulsing lasers. The penetration of the pulsed Nd:YAG laser is independent of the average power. For example a pulsed laser can produce a seam weld that is 1 mm in penetration at over 30 pulses/sec or slower than 1 pulse/min. Adjusting the laser's pulsing and welding rate to minimize the heat flow into the part allows welding of extremely heat sensitive assemblies. Laser welds can be made within 0.5 mm of glass-to-metal seals or polymer components. Detonation initiators for automotive air bags or explosive bolts can be welded live in cans that are less than 0.5 mm in thickness.

In developing a weld schedule on this type of component the laser welding parameters are tested with thermocouples attached to the sensitive areas or hermeticity and visual checks of seals are performed as the average power is increased. Once thermal limits or damage develops, the laser power cannot be increased without increasing the thermal capacity of the part via quench blocks, heat sinks, external cooling, etc.

Optimization with Pulsed Nd:YAG Lasers

Weld parameter development should have a specification requirement as a target, if possible. Easily measurable attributes such as weld penetration, strength, hermeticity, etc., work best. Below is a quick synopsis of the parameter development process.

1. Determine the required focal spot size needed to produce the weld. Longer lenses for large weld widths and/or shallow welds; short lenses for narrow welds or welds that require a higher aspect ratio for the weld nugget.

2. Adjust the peak power of the laser pulses to produce the required welding mode, that is, penetration-mode or conduction-mode welding. Several trials of spot or seam welds with varying peak powers are used to determine the correct value. Welds that have only shallow surface melting will require higher peak powers for increased penetration-mode effects. Welds that suffer from porosity, metal loss through expulsion, or undercutting will require less peak power. Some lasers can produce pulses with variations in the peak power throughout the pulse. This is called pulse shaping and can be used to optimize metallurgical results and cosmetic results.

3. Optimize the pulse energy at a constant peak power to produce the correct weld penetration. Energy changes will change the volume of weld metal and, therefore, the penetration. If pulse energy limits are reached, a shorter focus lens might be required or a laser with more energy employed.

4. Vary the laser repetition rate and/or part travel speed to achieve the required weld overlap.

5. Determine if average power effects are present and change the laser parameters or weld schedule to eliminate any problems. These will usually be increasing weld penetration during the weld or overheating of the assembly during the weld because of the part's small relative volume or the presence of temperature sensitive components.

6. Optimize other factors such as inert shield gas delivery, weld position, metallurgical constraints, etc., as needed.

Trade-Offs with Pulsed-Seam Welding

Pulsed Nd:YAG lasers have excellent spot welding characteristics and the low-heat-input welding capability outlined above. Any welding task that requires spot and seam welding with penetrations of 1.5 mm and lower are excellent candidates for this type of laser system (see Fig. 16). Many times seam-welding speeds can be increased by using CW lasers but these lasers are not good choices for spot welding. Also, the heat input with CW lasers might be too high for the devices being welded. In this case the trade-off is between speed and flexibility. The pulsed laser provides all of the spot and seam welding capability but lower seam welding speeds. The CW laser is the faster seam welder but a marginal spot welding system at best.

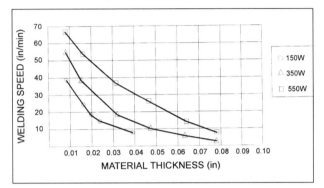

Figure 16. Welding speeds for a: 150 W, b: 350 W, and c: 550 W pulsed Nd:YAG lasers in stainless steel.

Welding materials such as copper alloys, aluminum, or silver will require a laser with very high peak power, and the pulsed Nd:YAG laser is the best choice. In this example there is no trade-off. The pulsed YAG is the only choice for these alloys.

Most often the trade-off will be between several different pulsed Nd:YAG lasers with varying specifications of average power, pulse energy, and peak power. It is usually best to have sufficient average power to easily meet throughput requirements and sufficient pulse energy to weld the required components. High peak powers are not usually necessary for welding but are usually available for systems that also drill. Units with small focal spot sizes might be necessary for extremely small welding tasks.

Reference
S. Gorscak, H. N. Bransch, and T. R. Kugler, *Hybrid Circuit Technology*, August 1991, IHS Publishing Group.

THOMAS R. KUGLER

10.3.5 Spot Welding with Pulsed Nd:YAG Lasers

On the basis of the unique process characteristics relative to other processes, laser micro spot welding enables new production technologies and design of parts. The significant advantages are:

- Contactless and forceless joining process; the position of the parts does not change during the welding process.
- Low specific heat input creates only a small heat-affected zone.
- Extremely rapid cooling rates.
- No filler wire necessary; only the base material determines the weldability.
- No tool wear and therefore a good repeatability of the welding process exists.
- Welding of dissimilar metals is possible in most cases (17).

Most often, optical fibers are used as a beam delivery system. This makes it possible to integrate the laser into an existing production machine very easily. Furthermore, it is possible to weld a metal piece both with one weld spot and with several simultaneously welded spots. For this, the laser energy is divided into equal portions by means of beam splitters and guided with an optical fiber to the workpiece. This welding strategy is called *energy sharing*.

A direct beam with a processing head can also be used. If it is necessary, a shielding gas is used for the welding process. The gas protects the objective lens and prevents the oxidation of the weld bead. Moreover, the gas influences the plasma ignition threshold because of different ionization potentials (18).

Theoretical studies of the spot welding process are found for example in (19) and (20).

Table 7 compares practicable results for the spot welding process with a pulsed Nd:YAG laser for different types of material.

In this table, s is the material thickness, E the pulse energy, τ_H the

Table 7. Typical Spot Welding Applications for Different Beam Delivery Systems and Materials

Material	s (mm)	E (J)	τ_H (ms)	f_P (Hz)	Fiber (μm)	f_L (mm)	Gas	d_E (mm)
Titanium	1.40	1.30	2.00	10	no	100	Ar	0.60
Copper/copper	0.20	1.80	3.00	2	no	100		0.65
Inox	0.12	0.23	0.80	50	no	100	Ar	0.25
Inox	0.12	0.28	1.00	5	200	50		0.25
Iron/nickel	0.07	0.30	1.00	5	200	100	N_2	0.40
Tin/lead	0.30	8.30	6.00	5	400	100		0.65
Zinc/steel	1.30	3.55	5.00	10	400	100		0.65
Cobalt/iron	0.20	3.50	4.00	2	600	100		0.80
Copper/zinc	0.50	6.00	6.00	5	600	100		0.80

Chapter 10: Conduction Welding

pulse duration, f_p the pulse repetition rate, f_L the lens focal length, and d_E the weld nugget diameter.

We next present some examples of spot welds. Three pieces of a relay are welded with four weld spots by means of a beam scanning system in the *x*- and *y*-direction, which is shown in Figure 17. The material is copper with a thickness of 0.3 and 0.9 mm. With this system, spot welds are achieved with a diameter of 0.6 mm. The necessary time to weld this relay is shorter than 1 second.

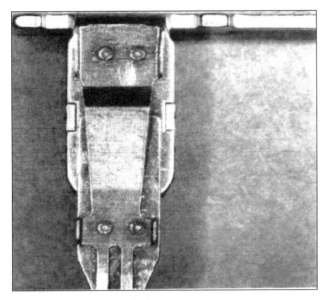

Figure 17. Part of relay (21).

Another microelectonic part is the connector in Figure 18. In this case the base material is again copper, but the left part is tinned and the right part is gold-plated. A pulse energy of 6.6 J with a pulse duration of 1.2 ms is used to weld these parts with two spots. A weld spot diameter of 0.4 mm is obtained by means of an objective with a focal length of 100 mm, together with a beam expansion of 2.

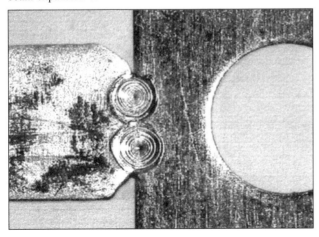

Figure 18. Connector with a material thickness of 0.2 mm (21).

Figure 19 illustrates a metallographic section of a micro-weld bead. Tin-coated copper was welded using a single laser pulse at a pulse energy of 5 J and a pulse duration of 2.5 ms. The thickness of each part is 0.3 mm. Only a very small heat-affected zone around the weld bead can be observed.

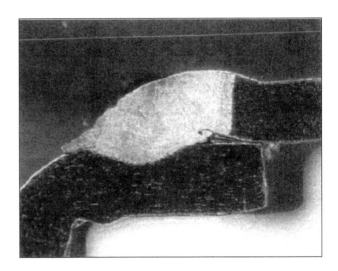

Figure 19. Laser weld in a tin-coated copper (21).

Figure 20 shows a photograph of a ball race welded by eight weld spots. The material is austenitic steel and the thickness of each ring is 0.5 mm. The diameter of the ball race ranges from 10 to 25 mm. A pulse energy of 15 J at a pulse frequency of 10 Hz is used to weld through both rings with one laser pulse.

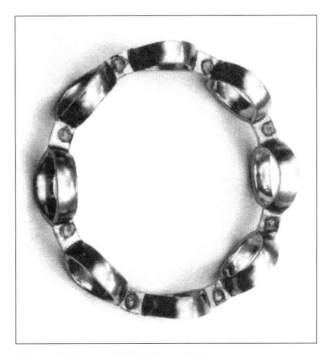

Figure 20. Laser-welded ball race (21).

ISBN 0-912035-15-3

A typical welding application in the watch industry is the microwelding of the balance spring with the axis, which is shown in Figure 21. The diameter of the weld spot is 0.15 mm and the dimensions of the spring are 0.1 × 0.025 mm. It is possible to weld the balance spring in a way that the spring does not bend. The advantage of this process is the exact positioning of the spring, which replaces an expensive process.

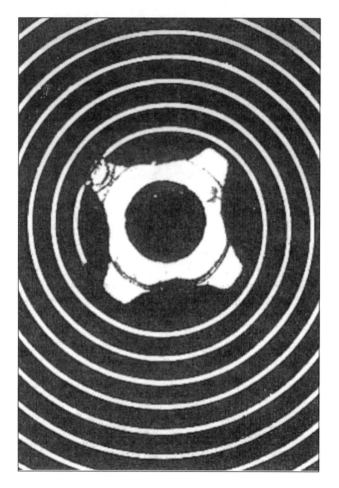

Figure 21. Balance spring of a mechanical watch (21).

References
17. C. Banas, *High Power Laser Welding*, in: The Industrial Laser Annual Handbook, D. Belforte and M. Levitt (Eds.), 69–86 (1986).
18. J. T. Luxon and D. E. Parker, *Industrial Lasers and their Applications*, Prentice-Hall Inc., Englewood Cliffs, Chapter 12-2 (1985).
19. M. R. Frewin and D. A. Scott, *Numerical and Experimental Investigation of Pulsed Nd:YAG Laser Welding*, in: Proc. Laser Materials Processing ICALEO '95, Vol. 80, LIA, 904–13 (1995).
20. C. J. Nonhof and R. Schimmel, *Physics of Laser Spot Welding with Pulsed Nd-Lasers*, in: Proc. 8th Int. Congress LASER '87, W. Waidelich (Ed.), Springer Verlag, 512–6 (1987).
21. Photographs: Lasag AG Industrial Lasers, Thun, Switzerland.

HANSJOERG ROHDE

10.3.6 Microjoining with Nd:YAG Lasers

Fabrication of welds with the Nd:YAG laser can be accomplished in both the continuous and pulsed beam mode. For low-power welding, the process is typically used in the pulsed mode at frequencies up to 200 Hz because of the extremely high irradiance available. The calculation in the example below shows the irradiance available with a continuous versus a pulsed beam at 250 W average power for typical laser parameters.

I = Irradiance = average power/area = W/cm^2
area = πr^2, where r is the radius of the focal spot

Continuous Beam: Assume 250 W and 0.0254 cm focal spot.

$$I_{continuous} = 250 \text{ W}/\pi (0.0254/2)^2 = 493,381 \text{ W/cm}^2$$

Pulsed Beam: Assume 250 W (average power), 20 pulses/sec 2 millisec pulse length, 0.0254 cm focal spot.

Average power/pulse = 250 W/(20 pps x 0.002 sec) = 6250 W/pulse

$$I_{pulsed} = 6250 \text{ W}/\pi (0.0254 \text{ cm}/2)^2 = 12,334,533 \text{ W/cm}^2$$

This characteristic high irradiance yields the lowest heat input fusion welding process available to industry. This is because very low average power can be used with the pulsed process, yielding threshold values easily exceeding those required for melting of most metals. This resulting low heat input required for most welds makes Nd:YAG welding the process of choice in the fabrication of very intricate, precision, and very often heat sensitive devices. It should be noted that when discussing pulsed laser welding, it is typical to reference energy per pulse rather than power levels. The energy per pulse is determined by dividing the average power by the pulse repetition frequency being used.

The process advantages are as follows:

1. Low heat input allowing for welding extremely close to heat sensitive materials (i.e., explosives, glass-metal seals).
2. Minimal heat induced distortion of the welded assembly. The dimensional stability of the assembly is maintained after welding.
3. Ability to weld very thin sheet materials and small diameter wires without burning back of the materials.
4. The beam can be focused to a small area allowing for welding of very small components, which are often closely spaced.

The process disadvantages are as follows:

1. Close fitup of the materials to be welded is required. Precision fixturing is often necessary to ensure intimate contact between the pieces to be welded depending on the power level used.

2. The low heat input used yields extremely rapid weld metal solidification, which can result in weld cracking in materials not typically sensitive to cracking and weld porosity.
3. Beam to joint alignment is very critical because of the small diameter of the weld.
4. Special techniques are required for high reflectivity materials (i.e., copper, aluminum, gold, silver).

Low-power Nd:YAG welding is typically accomplished in the conduction energy transfer mode versus the keyhole mode which is typically used for high power laser welding, discussed in Chapter 11. Very often, laser power must be reduced or laser spot size increased to prevent vaporization/drilling of the substrate material, which can result in excessive spatter adjacent to the weld bead.

Frequently, low-power Nd:YAG laser welding is used for hermetic sealing applications resulting in welds with leak rates less than 1×10^{-6} atm-cc/sec. In the pulsed mode, a pulse overlap of 60–75% is recommended for effective sealing. The part travel speed required for a 70% pulse overlap condition is calculated as shown below:

Assume: 0.76 mm laser weld diameter
20 pulses/s
70% overlap
Total weld length of 25.4 mm

a. Distance between pulses = 0.76 mm/pulse x 30% = 0.228 mm/pulse
b. # of pulses required = 25.4 mm/(0.228 mm/pulse) = 111 pulses
c. Weld time required = 111 pulses/(20 pulses/s) = 5.55 s
d. Part travel speed required = 2.5.4 mm/5.55 s = 4.58 mm/s

For welding of high reflectivity materials, it is often necessary to use a laser pulse that incorporates a "leading edge" spike. The use of the leading edge spike allows for extremely high peak powers, which initiate a small amount of melting in the substrate. This drastically increases the absorption by the substrate when the metal is molten, allowing for increased coupling of the laser beam to the workpiece.

Joint Design
The majority of low-power laser welds are designed to be autogenous welds (i.e., welding without filler material addition). Because of the increased crack sensitivity of low-power Nd:YAG laser welding, it is sometimes necessary to incorporate filler materials into the weld metal for increased control of weld metal chemistry. Filler material can be added in the form of foils placed between the joint or added as filler wire supplied from an independent wire feed system. The problem with adding filler wire is that the size of the wire must be small (0.005–0.020 in.) because of the small weld pool diameter. This necessitates a precision wire feed system that accurately locates and places the wire during the welding process. If at all possible, it is best (and in the long run often least expensive) to incorporate materials at the joint that have excellent weldability. Very often, these filler materials are the standard filler materials used for arc welding processes, which include 308L steel for austenitic stainless steels, 4043 Al for aluminum alloys, and hastalloy W for nickel-based alloys. Careful control of the weld joint material chemistry must often be dictated to the part manufacturer. Weldability testing before part fabrication is also commonly done to ensure fitness for service. When considering weld joint design, any gaps between the mating parts to be welded must be minimized with intimate contact between the mating parts preferred and often required depending on part thickness. Refer to Section 10.2.5 for additional discussion on typical weld joint designs.

Weld Evaluation
Because of the small size of low-power Nd:YAG laser welds, it is very difficult to nondestructively test the resultant welds using standard NDT techniques. For hermetic sealing applications, helium leak testing can be utilized on a 100% basis. For applications requiring a minimum weld throat dimension for a strength application, it is often necessary to use weld process control samples. These weld process control samples can be metallographically sectioned, tensile pull tested, or hydrostatically burst tested to ensure that adequate weld penetration has been obtained. An alternate method would be to monitor all critical weld parameters (power, pulse shape, travel speed, focus dimension, etc.) with a data acquisition system to ensure process repeatability.

Microjoining Applications
The low heat input associated with the pulsed Nd:YAG process results in superheating of the materials to be welded to above the melting point, yet yields a temperature near ambient extremely close to the weld pool. This is shown graphically in Figure 22 in a thermocouple study conducted on a component containing explosive materials. The weld was made between a 0.005-in.-thick disc and a 0.030-in.-thick sleeve. Explosive powder is located directly against the sleeve. The requirement was to keep the temperature at the sleeve-to-explosive interface below 100°C. Thermocouples were laser welded directly onto the inside diameter of the sleeve to monitor temperature rise.

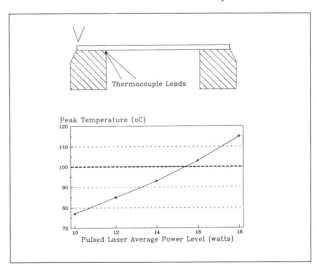

Figure 22. Graph of pulsed laser average power versus temperature rise at sleeve-to-explosive material interface.

The Nd:YAG process can be readily used to attach thin material to thicker substrates without melt/burn back of the thin material. A metallographic section of a thin sheet material (0.005-in.-thick 304L stainless steel) to 304L stainless steel is shown below in Figure 23. The weld consists of a series of overlapping pulses yielding a hermetically sealed component.

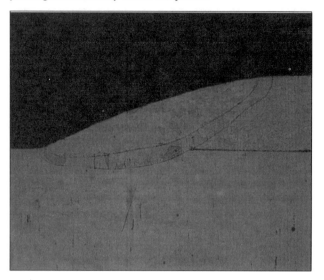

Figure 23. Metallographic section of 0.005-in.-thick 304L stainless steel disc welded to 304L stainless steel substrate. Laser parameters: 2 millisec pulse length, 40 W, 30 PPS, 4.08 mm/s travel speed.

The process is also readily used for circumferential welding of small cylinders. Figure 24 shows a metallographic cross-section of two inconel 718 shells laser welded using a thin foil of hastalloy to provide filler material. Although not shown in the figure, the weld has been made in close proximity to glass-to-metal seals on both inconel pieces. The hastalloy foil is used to enhance the weldability of the material combination.

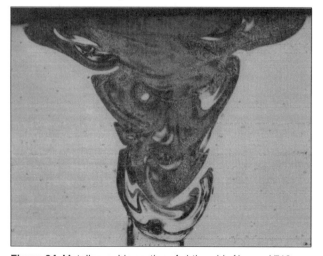

Figure 24. Metallographic section of girth weld of inconel 718 materials using hastalloy filler material. Laser parameters: 5 millisec pulse length, 90 W, 20 PPS, 5.22 mm/s.

Figure 25 below shows another girth weld between kovar and hastalloy showing a depth of penetration of 0.56 mm extending past the root of the joint.

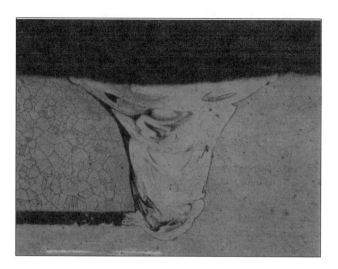

Figure 25. Metallographic section of girth weld between kovar and hastalloy materials.

The metallographic sections shown in Figures 26 and 27 illustrate one of the unique capabilities of the Nd:YAG pulsed welding process in joining a very thin material to another. A 0.15-mm-thick 308L stainless steel sleeve has been girth welded to a 0.165-mm-thick hydodermic needle material and is shown in Figure 26. The resultant weld is 0.36 mm in width.

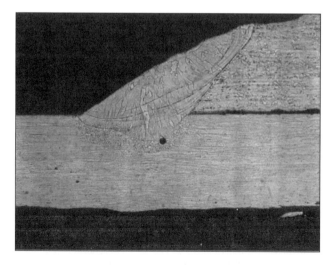

Figure 26. Metallographic section of girth weld between 0.15-mm-thick 308L SS sleeve and 0.165-mm-thick hypodermic needle.

Figure 27 shows a transverse cross section of a weld in 0.10-mm-thick Haynes Alloy 25 material. The weld is a longitudinal seam weld used to form a cylinder. A butt weld joint configuration was used.

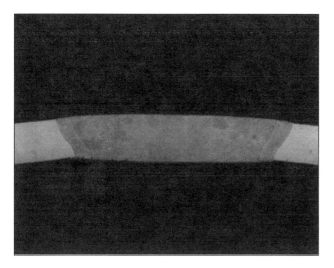

Figure 27. Metallographic section of a longitudinal seam weld using 0.10-mm-thick Haynes Alloy 25 material.

The above applications illustrate welds made using a multipulse laser system. Figure 28 illustrates one of the many single pulse applications for Nd:YAG lasers. A 0.005-in.-thick pure nickel foil has been laser welded to the end of a 0.040 in. hastelloy pin. The hastalloy pin has been sealed in a glass-ceramic material. The seal is not perturbed by the heat of welding. Note the presence of the small pore which can be typical of pulsed laser welds. The indications along the sides of the weld in the nickel foil are etching artifacts due to alloying of the materials.

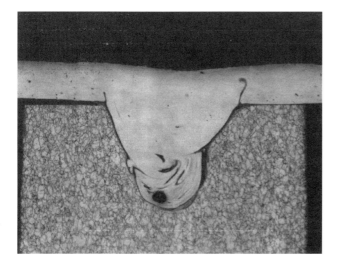

Figure 28. Metallographic section of a single-pulse laser weld between nickel foil and hastalloy pin.

Other single-pulse applications include welding of thermocouple junctions, attachment of small diameter wires to electrical leads and, in particular, tacking of assemblies to temporarily hold pieces together prior to final welding.

JOSEPH J. KWIATKOWSKI

10.3.7 Conduction Welding with CO_2 Lasers

In conduction welding, the laser energy is absorbed in a thin layer near the surface of the metallic workpiece. It is transported into the interior of the workpiece by thermal conduction. The surface begins to melt when the latent heat of fusion of the material has been supplied at the surface and a fusion front begins to propagate into the material. For many welding applications, the fusion front should propagate all the way through the thickness of the material. This is a relatively slow process, so that the welding speed is limited when one is operating in the conduction welding regime. Still, for thin materials, the welding rate may be adequate for a cost-effective production application.

Figure 29 shows some results for welding of steels with CO_2 laser radiation at different power levels. The top curve is for a conduction-mode weld, not for a penetration-mode weld, despite the fact that the power was 1500 W.

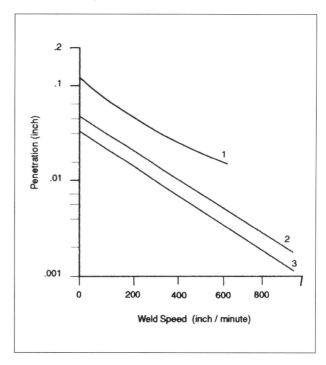

Figure 29. Penetration depth versus weld speed for steels welded by continuous CO_2 lasers. Curve 1. Welding of 302 stainless steel at 1500 W. Curve 2. Welding of carbon steel at 375 W. Curve 3. Welding of 300 series stainless steel at 375 W. Curve 1 based on S. L Engel, *Laser Focus*, p.44, February 1976. Curves 2 and 3 based on data from Photon Sources, Inc.

The figure shows several things. For relatively thin material, 0.01 in. or less, the welding rate can be reasonably high, high enough to be attractive for production applications, even with a few hundred watts of laser power. But for thicker material, greater than 0.1 in., the welding rate is unacceptably low. If the power is increased to 1500 W, the penetration is deeper, but the weld rate is still near zero for material with thickness greater than 0.1 in.

The effect of material parameters is also apparent. For stainless steels, with very low values of thermal conductivity, the penetration depth is less than for carbon steel, which has higher thermal conductivity. This illustrates the limitations imposed by thermal conduction in this welding regime.

JOHN F. READY

10.3.8 Welding with Low-Power CO_2 Lasers

A CO_2 laser emitting only a few hundred watts of power can be an effective welding tool, at least for thin materials. Table 8 (next page) presents some results for welding with CO_2 lasers in this range of power, both for continuous and pulsed devices. The higher peak power of short pulse lasers allows the surface to be broken down more easily and its reflectivity at the 10.6-μm wavelength is thus reduced. More energy can be coupled into the surface by pulsed lasers, so that at the same level of average power, pulsed lasers will have greater welding capability than continuous devices.

The results in the table are from a variety of sources, which used different measurement conditions. The results will vary depending on beam quality, focusing conditions, surface preparation, etc. Thus the results cannot give an exact prediction of what will occur in the user's facility, even for the same power and material. Still the table does give an indication of the range of welding capabilities that can be achieved with CO_2 lasers at power levels up to a few hundred watts.

References
22. J. M. Webster, *Metals Progr.* **98,** 59 (1970).
23. M. J. Yessik, *Opt. Eng.* **17,** 202 (1978).
24. The Engineering Staff of Coherent, Inc., *Lasers, Operation, Equipment, Applications and Design,* McGraw-Hill Book Co., New York (1980).
25. R. J. Conti, *Welding J.* **48,** 800 (1969).

JOHN F. READY

10.3.9 Welding with Diode Lasers

Laser welding processes are separated into two categories, distinguished by the occurrence of a plasma during the process. One category is plasma welding or deep penetration welding process that has high efficiency because of the occurrence of a keyhole. This accounts for the high absorption of the laser radiation during the process. The absorption is considerably higher than the absorption through the surface of flat sheet metal. The second category is the heat conduction welding process. Here the absorption of the laser radiation takes place solely through the surface of the workpiece. For the wavelength of high-power diode lasers, the absorption is generally in the range of 25–70% depending on the material and angle of the laser with respect to the workpiece.

To create plasma on the workpiece, a certain irradiance threshold has to be breached. As a rule of thumb, this threshold is around 10^6 W/cm^2 for high power lasers used for steel welding. Commercially available high-power diode laser stacks in the multi-kilowatt range provide a maximum irradiance of 10^5 W/cm^2 on the workpiece. This level is adequate to melt the steel, however, not sufficient to ignite a plasma on the workpiece. Thus, heat conduction welding is the only welding process a high-power diode laser is capable of today.

With heat conduction welding, the heat input into the workpiece is kept below the critical threshold. This threshold is marked by the vapor pressure of the evaporated metal. There is no significant vapor pressure during the heat conduction welding process, hence, no capillary (keyhole) forms. The geometry of the melt pool and the penetration depth is determined predominantly by the heat conduction of the workpiece, the irradiance of the laser beam, and the overall heat input.

Because of the absence of a capillary, the penetration depth is comparatively low. Hence, this process is primarily used to weld thin materials such as wires, thin sheet metal plates, and tubes.

According to Fresnel's equations (see Section 5.3), the absorption coefficient varies with the wavelength, angle and polarization of the laser beam. By making use of the polarization of a laser beam, the absorption can be increased. Since diode lasers exhibit a high degree of polarization, which is typically around 95%, this technique is applicable here. However, the welding speed that can be achieved is still considerably slower than that achieved with high-power CO_2 or Nd:YAG lasers.

Butt Joint Welding of Stainless Steel Sheets
A 2-kW diode laser stack has been used for heat conduction welding. The focus exhibits a line shape having the dimensions of 2.8 by 11.0 mm. The numerical aperture is 0.38 by 0.20. The samples to be welded were austenitic, chrome-nickel stainless steel sheets, type 304, with thickness of 0.90 and 0.45 mm. The chemical data and the melting temperature of this material are given in Table 9.

Table 9. Properties of Stainless Steel Type 304

Chromium (%)	18–20
Nickel (%)	8–11
Carbon (%)	0.08 max
Manganese (%)	2.0 max
Silicon (%)	1.0 max
Melting temperature (°C)	1400

The sample pieces had dimensions of 30 by 100 mm. They were

Table 8. Laser Welding Results for Low-Power CO_2 Lasers

Continuous lasers					
Material	Weld type	Power (W)	Penetration (mm)	Weld rate (cm/sec)	Source
321 Stainless steel	Butt	250	0.125	3.8	Ref. (22)
321 Stainless steel	Butt	250	0.250	1.48	Ref. (22)
321 Stainless steel	Butt	250	0.417	0.47	Ref. (22)
302 Stainless steel	Butt	250	0.125	2.11	Ref. (22)
302 Stainless steel	Butt	250	0.203	1.27	Ref. (22)
302 Stainless steel	Butt	250	0.250	0.42	Ref. (22)
Inconel	Butt	250	0.100	6.35	Ref. (22)
Inconel	Butt	250	0.250	1.69	Ref. (22)
Nickel	Butt	250	0.125	1.48	Ref. (22)
Monel	Butt	250	0.250	0.64	Ref. (22)
Titanium	Butt	250	0.125	5.90	Ref. (22)
Titanium	Butt	250	0.250	2.11	Ref. (22)
Low-carbon steel	Unspecified	375	0.5	4.8	Ref. (23)
Low-carbon steel	Unspecified	375	0.25	10.5	Ref. (23)
304 Stainless steel	Bead on plate	200	0.51	1.27	Ref. (24)
304 Stainless steel	Bead on plate	300	1.02	1.27	Ref. (24)
304 Stainless steel	Bead on plate	400	5.1	1.27	Ref. (24)

Pulsed lasers							
Material	Weld type	Pulse length (sec)	Rep rate (Hz)	Average power (W)	Penetration (mm)	Weld rate (cm/sec)	Source
Phosphor bronze	Edge lap	0.3	3.9	95	0.11	0.21	Ref. (25)
304 Stainless steel	Edge lap	0.0002	1000	95	0.10	0.13	Ref. (25)
304 Stainless steel	Edge lap	0.22	3.6	95	0.10	0.28	Ref. (25)
Monel	Edge lap	0.07	500	95	0.10	0.13	Ref. (25)
Cupronickel	Edge lap	0.33	2.9	95	0.10	0.13	Ref. (25)
320 Stainless steel	Butt	0.00004	75	100	0.076	2.4	Honeywell, Inc.
304 Stainless steel	Bead on plate	Unspecified	Unspecified	200	0.64	1.27	Ref. (24)
304 Stainless steel	Bead on plate	Unspecified	Unspecified	300	1.09	1.27	Ref. (24)
304 Stainless steel	Bead on plate	Unspecified	Unspecified	400	1.55	1.27	Ref. (24)

put into the fixture shown in Figure 30 and welded. Argon was used as a shielding gas to prevent oxidation of the weld seam. The gas was applied from both sides.

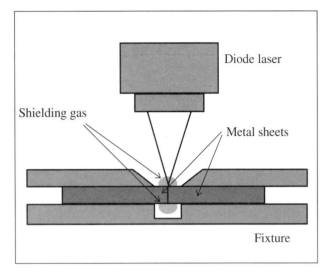

Figure 30. Set-up for the conduction welding process.

The appropriate welding speeds for two thicknesses were found experimentally. They are given in Table 10.

Table 10. Process Parameters for Conduction Welding

Power (kW)	1.7
Irradiance (kW/cm^2)	6.2
Focus dimension (mm^2)	2.5 x 11.0
Speed for 0.45 mm thickness	2.0 m/min
Speed for 0.90 mm thickness	1.0 m/min

The weld seam exhibits a smooth surface after the welding process. However, the color of the surface neighboring the weld seam changes. Usually, a multi-colored zone that is referred to as the heat-affected zone (HAZ) arises (see Fig. 31). Optimization of the shielding gas flow and the fixture can further decrease this effect.

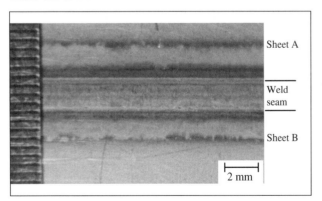

Figure 31. Weld seam of heat-conduction welded sheets.

For this set-up, the width of this zone is dependent on both the width of the laser beam on the workpiece and the welding speed. Figure 32 shows the cross section of the weld seam of the two stainless steel sheets, thickness 0.45 mm, welded together with the parameters given in Table 10.

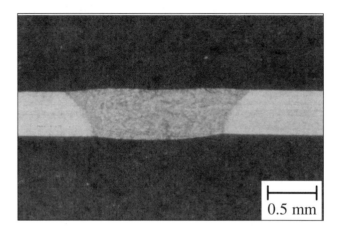

Figure 32. Cross section of the diode laser welded sheets.

Overlap Welding of Stainless Steel Sheets
This application also involves stainless steel, however an overlap joint was used. The arrangement of the sheets is shown in Figure 33. The two sheet metal parts are shown before the welding process.

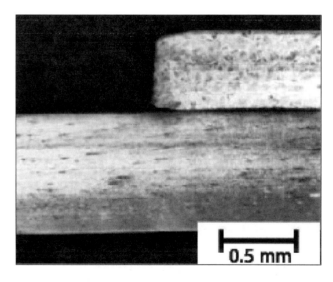

Figure 33. Overlap joint configuration before welding.

The weld was performed with a laser power of 1450 W at a feed rate of 2000 mm/min. The spot size of the laser was measured to be 1.8 by 3.8 mm, where the longer extension of the beam was oriented along the weld seam. The cross section of the weld seam is shown in Figure 34.

Chapter 10: Conduction Welding

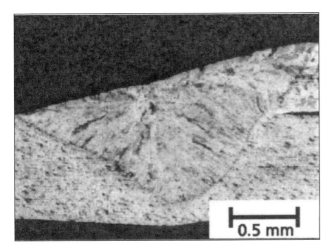

Figure 34. Cross section of overlap joint.

Butt Joint Welding of Aluminum Sheets

The process is not limited to steel but can also be applied to aluminum. As a demonstration two aluminum flats with a thickness of 0.8 mm were welded together in a butt-joint configuration. The same laser as in the last application was used with a spot size of 1.8 by 3.8 mm. Again the longer dimension of the beam was oriented along the direction of motion. The result is shown in Figure 35.

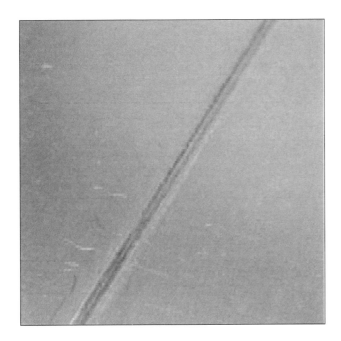

Figure 35. Heat-conduction-welded aluminum sheets.

The laser power was chosen to be 2.0 kW with a feed rate of 1100 mm/min. The weld seam quality is shown in cross section in Figure 36.

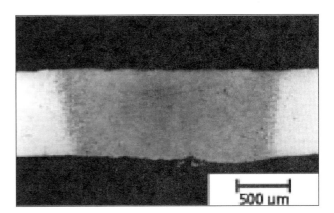

Figure 36. Cross section of butt-joined aluminum sheets.

Reference
S. Bonss, B. Brenner, E. Beyer, and F. Bachmann, "Diode laser applications hardening and welding", Proceedings of ICALEO'98, Orlando, FL, November 1998.

BODO EHLERS

10.3.10 Welding with Photolytic Iodine Lasers (PILS)
The photolytic iodine laser is described in Section 2.5.5. A photolytic iodine laser has been used for welding stainless steels.

Thin 0.004-in.-thick 302 stainless steel sheets were lap welded using a 20-µm PILS beam. The best results produced 40-µm-wide welds on the top and bottom using Ar as the assist gas. The heat-affected zones (HAZ) were small compared to those of Nd:YAG and CO_2 lasers, given the same parameters. The use of helium in any percentage mixture resulted in no metal processing because the helium appeared to absorb the beam. The use of oxygen in any percentage mixture resulted in odd welds because of the intense beams. A thin weld between the sheets was made, but both tops and bottoms of the sheets were essentially vaporized. Welds with argon as the assist gas resulted in welds with strength of 75–80 % of the base material as shown in Figure 37. Figure 38 illustrates the welds with small HAZ.

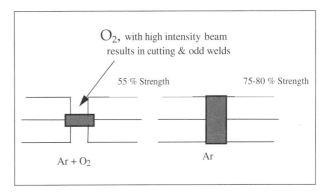

Figure 37. Welds with and without O_2 assist gas.

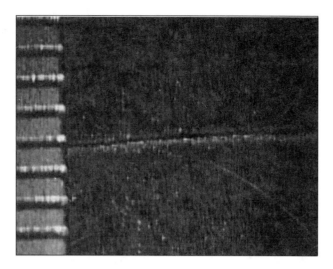

Figure 38. Photograph of 40 micrometer lap weld of 0.004 in. stainless steel using argon as assist gas and standard 5 in. focus lens (power 17 W, feed rate 0.02–0.11 in./s and Ar assist gas 13 psig).

PHILIP R. CUNNINGHAM
L. A. (VERN) SCHLIE

10.4 Materials Issues

10.4.1 Tabulation of Materials and Weldability

Weldability is defined as: "The capacity of a material to be welded under the imposed fabrication conditions into a specific, suitably designed structure and to perform satisfactorily in the intended service" (1). Some factors, which must be considered when evaluating the weldability of materials, include:

- homogeneity of chemical composition
- uniformity of mechanical properties
- level of fracture toughness
- degree of freedom from surface defects
- maximum size and number of metallic inclusions
- internal soundness
- nature and uniformity of microstructure (2)
- constraints in joint geometry

In addition, weldability may have application-specific implications. For example, a material which may be considered to have good weldability for an appliance application may be unsuited for an aerospace application where the weld cannot reliably endure the rigorous aerospace environment, and failure could result in loss of life.

Table 1 lists candidate materials that may be laser welded. Since it is not practical to list all such available materials, the materials listed in Table 1 are categorized as various types with similar weldable properties. Each of these materials have particular laser weldability characteristics, and some of these will be discussed in subsequent paragraphs.

Table 1. Candidate Materials for Laser Welding

Carbon and Alloy Steels
  low-carbon steel < 0.2% carbon
  moderate-carbon steel > 0.2% < 0.5% carbon
  high-carbon steel > 0.5% carbon
  alloy steels

Stainless Steels and Superalloys
  austenetic stainless steel
  martenistic stainless steel
  ferritic stainless steel
  nickel-base superalloy
  nickel-iron base superalloy
  cobalt base superalloy

Aluminum and Aluminum Alloys
  1100 series
  2000 series
  5000 series
  6000 series
  7000 series

Reactive Metals
  titanium
  zirconium
  tungsten
  tantalum

Other Metallic Materials
  lead
  copper

Nonmetallics

The first and foremost consideration for all materials is chemical composition, including impurities and inclusions. Material structure, which is strongly influenced by the basic metallurgical background, or history, is another important consideration. Good weldability begins on the foundry floor where the metal is cast. In general, for good weldability, contaminants must be kept to a minimum. For almost all materials, high oxygen content results in poor weldability, so it is important that material for laser welding be procured with low oxygen content. In general, it has been found that metals produced by powder metal techniques do not respond well to laser welding. This is because powder metals usually contain more volatile constituents than wrought metals. These volatile constituents vaporize violently in the molten pool during welding resulting in severe porosity and unacceptable weld surface quality.

Valuable insight into the weldability of various materials may be obtained from the references cited at the end of this section.

Filler Material
The weldability of many materials may be enhanced by the addition of filler material in the form of wire, powder or foil. Wire may be added at room temperature, or heated by resistance heating. Filler material addition may result in the following desirable features:

- provide additional material to compensate for poor fitup
- change chemical composition, resulting in enhanced fusion zone properties, such as strength and durability
- refine fusion zone structures

Carbon and Alloy Steels

The first and most extensive group of laser weldable materials is *carbon steel,* which includes both low- and high-carbon steels and many alloy steels. Common features of these steels, required for good weldability, include low oxygen content and minimal nonmetallic inclusions. Best welding occurs in low-carbon steels, (< 0.2% carbon), that are aluminum or silicon killed. Laser welds in these materials are usually uniform and contain little or no porosity. Laser welds in rimmed, capped, or semi-killed steels may exhibit varying amounts of porosity depending on oxygen and impurity content, weld parameters and material thickness. Filler metal that can deoxidize the weld metal may be used to produce sound welds in these materials. Also, surface coatings containing high aluminum content may promote smooth continuous welds in thin rimmed, capped, or semi-killed low-carbon steel.

Steels that are manufactured for *free machining* are usually poor candidates for laser welding. These materials normally contain high percentages of sulfur or lead, which are not soluble in the base metal matrix, and which vaporize at temperatures significantly lower than the base material. Laser welds in these materials may be nonuniform and contain significant amounts of porosity.

High sulfur and/or phosphorous content also effect laser weldability. In general, the ratio of manganese to sulfur plus phosphorous should be maintained below 40 to 1 for acceptable weldability. Other contaminants, such as the rare earths, also may have a deleterious effect on weldability of low carbon steels.

Steels containing moderate carbon content (between 0.2 and 0.5%) are usually weldable by laser processing techniques, but are subject to higher hardness in the fusion and heat-affected zones. This is because minimum heat inherent in the laser welding process results in very high quench rates, such that the fusion and heat-affected zones remain in the untempered martensitic state upon cooling to room temperature. Preheating and/or post-heating may be necessary when welding carbon steel with a carbon content of 0.2% or higher to reduce the cooling rate and reduce the propensity for fusion zone and heat-affected zone cracking.

Steels containing greater than 0.5% carbon may be laser welded under special conditions. However, welds in these steels usually exhibit high hardness in the "as welded" state, and may be susceptible to cracking, especially when weld joints are constrained. Preheat and post-heat treatments are normally required when welding these steels.

High-strength, low-alloy steels, chrome alloy steels and other alloy steels may be laser welded with acceptable results following procedures that are usually successful for the more conventional processes, such as gas tungsten arc welding, or gas metal arc welding.

Stainless Steels and Superalloys

The basic metallurgy used in the manufacture of these materials usually results in materials of high quality with insignificant amounts of contamination. The more common austenitic stainless steels, such as AISI 302 or AISI 304, usually have good laser weldability. However, austenitic stainless steel with higher alloy content, such as AISI 316 and AISI 347, may be a bit crack sensitive. Weldability depends on material thickness, and parameter selection. Free machining stainless steel, such as AISI 303, is not usually weldable.

Feritic and martensitic stainless steel are usually weldable by lasers, except those containing moderate amounts of carbon are subject to the same precautions necessary for welding carbon steels with moderate to high carbon content.

Superalloys are classified as heat resisting alloys with nickel, nickel-iron, or cobalt as their base. These alloys exhibit a unique combination of mechanical strength and resistance to surface degradation when exposed to elevated temperatures. Four groups of these materials include; solid-solution-strengthened alloys, precipitation-hardened alloys, dispersion-strengthened-alloys, and cast alloys.

Many of the superalloys respond well to laser welding. Their response to laser welding is similar to conventional welding and reference should be made to AWS Welding Handbook, Eighth Edition, Volume 3, "Materials and Applications" Part I for unique weldability characteristics of specific alloys.

Aluminum and Aluminum Alloys

While not laser welded as extensively as steel and the other alloys mentioned above, aluminum and some aluminum alloys are welded in production using laser techniques. Most aluminum materials welded to date have been relatively thin, up to one or two millimeters thick. Aluminum is highly reflective, and this feature makes it difficult to laser weld because laser irradiance high enough to overcome reflectivity tends to be excessive and overheats the material. Also, the surface of aluminum usually has an oxide skin, which forms at room temperature and continues to thicken with time. This aluminum oxide layer interacts with the molten aluminum, and may cause porosity and other weld defects. In addition, because molten aluminum reacts readily with oxygen, the face and root of the molten pool must be protected by inert gas coverage, such as helium or argon, while welding.

Even with the above limitations, many aluminum alloys are being welded in production. Recent work has indicated that Nd:YAG laser welding of aluminum is sometimes more effective than CO_2 laser welding, because reflectivity of the shorter Nd:YAG wavelength is less than for the CO_2 laser, and the laser beam more readily couples into the material.

Pure aluminum (1100 series), and some of the 2000 and 5000 series are good candidates for laser welding. Other alloys, such as 6000 and 7000 series, can sometimes be welded, but are more susceptible to cracking.

The primary defects in aluminum laser welds are porosity and cracking. Suppression of these defects is accomplished by careful cleaning techniques, complete inert shielding, and proper selection of laser processing parameters. Filler material may also be used when laser welding aluminum, to compensate for joint fitup, or to change chemical composition.

Aluminum alloys up to 12 millimeters thick and greater have been welded using high power CO_2 laser welding techniques with reasonable results, but few applications if any are in production.

Other aluminum alloys in wrought, forged or cast condition may be laser welded, depending upon their response to the laser beam. Weldability would have to be determined for each specific application.

In general, all laser welds formed in aluminum and aluminum alloys exhibit mechanical properties poorer than those of the base metal. Therefore, applications where laser welding of aluminum are applied must be carefully evaluated to assure that the component will perform its service function.

Reactive Metals

Most of the reactive metals listed in Table 1 can be laser welded by applying compatible processing techniques and laser parameters. Cleanliness procedures are important when welding reactive metals, and inert shielding must be provided not only in the vicinity of the interaction point, but also beyond to the point that the material has cooled below its oxidation temperature. Indeed, it is quite common to laser weld these materials in a "dry box" using sufficient purge to create an oxygen free environment for laser processing.

Titanium and zirconium and their alloys, which can be welded by conventional techniques, are especially receptive to laser welding. Reactive metals, such as tungsten and tantalum, may be laser welded, but fusion zones in these materials usually contain large grains, causing them to be brittle. Post-heat treatment may be used after welding to regain acceptable properties.

Other Metallic Materials

Lead has been successfully joined by laser beam welding, but thickness is limited and weld parameters require stringent control. Thin copper is weldable using pulsed Nd:YAG laser beams, and limited success has been attained in material up to 0.25 in. (6-mm) thick using high power CO_2 lasers. Weldability of metals not mentioned above would have to be determined by test.

Nonmetallics

Some ceramics and plastics may be laser welded. Because these materials differ dramatically, the best way to determine weldability for a specific material is to evaluate its response to the laser beam.

References
1. American Welding Society, *Welding Handbook,* Eighth Edition, Vol. 1 Appendix A.
2. G. E. Linnert, *Welding Metallurgy,* 4th Edition, Vol. I, Fundamentals, Chapter 5, Pg. 431.

American Society of Metals International Handbook, Vol. 6, "Welding, Brazing, and Soldering."
American Welding Society, *Welding Handbook,* Eighth Edition, Vols. 1, 2, and 3.

R. F. DUHAMEL

10.4.2 Welding of Dissimilar Materials

Material Weldability

Low power laser welding often involves the joining of dissimilar materials. Applications include the welding of automotive fuel injectors, heat exchangers, medical devices, and electronic components. Figure 1 shows some examples.

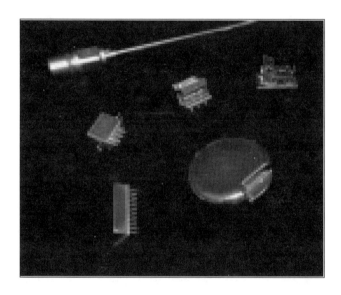

Figure 1. Typical applications of low-power laser welds using dissimilar materials. Examples pictured include medical devices, electronic interconnects, and hermetic enclosures for various devices.

These types of components use a variety of materials, usually selected for electrical performance, strength in thin sections, non-magnetic properties, or corrosion resistance. Weldability should not be neglected during the selection process. Table 2 lists many commonly found materials in current use of medical and electronic applications. Table 3 (3) is a matrix of materials, some which are included in Table 2, stating their ability to be joined as dissimilar weldments.

ISBN 0-912035-15-3

Chapter 10: Conduction Welding

Table 2. Common Materials Found in Medical and Electronic Devices

Material	Electrical and medical applications
Gold	Wires, electrodes, contacts
Platinum	Wire, electrodes, contacts
Tungsten	Wire, electrodes, contacts
Titanium	Wires, orthopedic implants, sensor contacts
Stainless steels	Endoscopy instruments, housings, clips, clamps
Nickel alloys	Wires and orthopedic devices
Copper	Wires, heatsinks, contacts
Silver	Wires, conductors, contacts
Aluminum	Housings, enclosures, conductors, wire

General Considerations

Many low-power welds are low power because of the thin materials being joined. Thin materials can have extremely efficient thermal conductivity because the portion away from the weld zone can act as a heat fin, promoting rapid cooling of the weld zone. When welding dissimilar metal joints, it is good practice to aim the laser spot at the material with the higher thermal conductivity. The intent is to use the direct energy of the laser to heat up the metal quickly and not allow the high conductivity to pull heat away from the weld zone. Often, the addition of a filler material can help, such as using silicon-bearing alloys when welding combinations of aluminum. The high cooling rate of thin materials will extend the normal solid solubility of alloys and can avoid the development of brittle intermetallics. In pulsed welding, use high-energy short-duration pulses at a minimum repetition rate. This will allow for good penetration, low total heat input, and rapid cooling. In continuous-wave (CW) welding, use the power and speed combination that yields the fastest speed (feed rate) and lowest power weld. This again will allow for rapid cooling and minimum heat input.

The downside of this approach is stress. The use of high-intensity pulses or fast travel speeds and rapid cooling can give rise to stresses in the weld zone. The most robust process will be a balance between the energy and cooling rate needed to reduce formation of intermetallics and at the same time keep stresses from causing cracks.

Be aware as well of fixturing, and its contribution to the heat balance. Many microjoining low-power applications can be successful with a minimum of tooling.

The materials to be welded will define the irradiance required to melt and fuse the joint. Weldibility is improved when materials are chosen that have similar melting points and vapor pressures. Welds between materials with wide differences in melting point will be difficult to achieve. Most ferrous metals such as stainless steel, CRS, kovar, Inconel, and hastalloy will require similar irradiance. Gold, copper, beryllium, and alloys with high reflectivity and thermal conductivity will require significantly higher power density to achieve fusion (4).

Table 3. Weldability Matrix for Common Materials Used in Medical and Electronic Devices

	W	Ta	Mo	Cr	Co	Ti	Be	Fe	Pt	Ni	Pd	Cu	Au	Ag	Mg	Al	Zn	Cd	Pb
Ta	E																		
Mo	E	E																	
Cr	E	P	E																
Co	F	P	F	G															
Ti	F	E	E	G	F														
Be	P	P	P	P	F	P													
Fe	F	F	G	E	E	F	F												
Pt	G	F	G	G	E	F	P	G											
Ni	F	G	F	G	E	F	F	G	E										
Pd	F	G	G	G	E	F	F	G	E	E									
Cu	P	P	P	P	F	F	F	F	E	E	E								
Au	*	*	P	F	P	F	F	F	E	E	E	E							
Ag	P	P	P	P	F	P	P	F	P	E	F	E							
Mg	P	*	P	P	P	P	P	P	P	P	F	F	F						
Al	P	P	P	P	F	F	P	F	P	F	P	F	F	F					
Zn	P	*	P	P	F	P	P	F	P	F	F	G	F	G	P	F			
Cd	*	*	*	P	P	P	*	P	F	F	F	P	F	G	E	P	P		
Pb	P	*	P	P	P	P	*	P	P	P	P	P	P	P	P	P	P	P	
Sn	P	P	P	P	P	P	P	P	F	P	F	P	F	F	P	P	P	P	F

E = Excellent, G = Good, F = Fair, P = Poor

Effects of Fusion

Laser welds typically require full fusion of the parent materials. This is in contrast to solid-state welding where no bulk melting of the parent materials occurs. In dissimilar welds, this fusion causes mixing of the alloy constituents originally present in the parent materials, yielding a weld zone that has some of each parent material represented in it. The degree of mixing can have a drastic effect on the weld quality. The intensity of the laser beam with its high energy density, even in lower power welding, is sufficient to vaporize low boiling or high vapor pressure constituents such as zinc and sulfur. Laser welds of brass, bronze, and free machining grades (sulfur or lead added) of steels have shown reduced quantities of these elements in the weld zone. Elements can also be simply redistributed across the weld zone or even within the smaller areas near grain boundaries. Stainless steels can have altered corrosion resistance because of nickel and chrome redistribution near grain boundaries after welding. These effects are often exacerbated in dissimilar welds because of the formation of precipitates and intermetallics in addition to the normal elemental redistribution that occurs.

Development of Microstructure

Microstructure will be defined by the extent of heating and cooling of the weld metal during processing. The rate of cooling can help or hinder the growth of intermetallics, precipitates, and cracks across the weld zone. One of the key issues in dissimilar welds is to determine the susceptibility of the weld metal to cracking. Several of the key issues in weldability will be briefly discussed below. Detailed information is available from several sources (5–7).

The chemistry of the weld zone will be dictated by the solubility of the various elements in the molten weld pool and the redistribution of elements in the heat-affected zone (HAZ). If intermetallic compounds form, they will be deleterious only if they reach a certain threshold value of thickness. If the intermetallic layer is less than the critical value, the weld will be stable, and will be unstable above this value. Soluble elements will be absorbed into the weld zone, while insoluble elements will float away from the liquid solid interface. The formation of eutectic alloys is very important to note, because these will be the lowest melting point constituent in the weld zone. This low melting alloy can segregate to grain boundaries and cause cracking during cooling, because the liquid material between the grains will be insufficient to support any stress. The extent of the melt zone, HAZ, and parent material zone can be predicted (8).

The best place to begin when welding dissimilar materials are with listings of phase diagrams. These can be used to assess the major constituents of the alloy and their propensity to form intermetallics or eutectics. The phase diagram shown in Figure 2 is for an alloy of nickel and lead. These materials form a solid solution over a wide range of alloy additions. The point at 11.5 atomic percent lead is characteristic of a eutectic point. The wide clear area below the liquidus-solidus curve represents a large, solid-solution region of stable nickel-lead alloy.

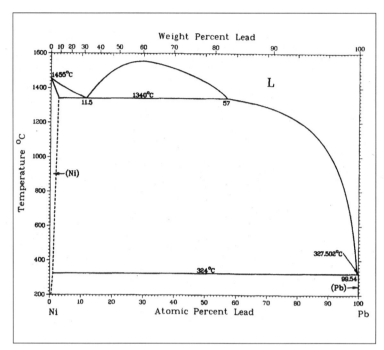

Figure 2. Phase diagram of nickel lead. Note that the solid phase zone is free of lines and zones. This is an indication that intermetallics will not form between these elements if they are present in the weld zone.

Note that the solid solution zone is free of any lines indicating a lack of immiscible or intermetallic alloys. Compare this to Figure 3, the phase diagram of iron and thorium.

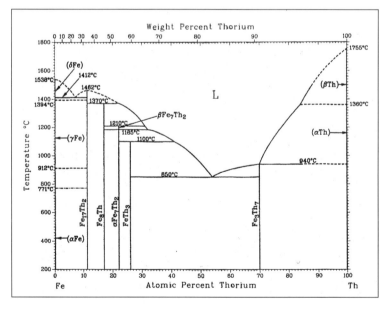

Figure 3. Phase diagram for iron thorium. Note the many lines and zones in the solid phase region. These are indicators of intermetallics. The narrower the zone, the more likely the alloy will be a brittle intermetallic, detrimental to weldability.

This diagram contains many intermetallics as indicated by the narrow vertical regions in the solid-phase zone. These narrow bands in a phase diagram typically indicate intermetallic compounds, which can be assumed to be brittle. These brittle intermetallic layers will usually define the stress limit of the weld, if it can be welded at all. Often the presence of the intermetallics or eutectics will lead to the formation of cracking in the weld zone.

Other helpful data can be discerned from the phase diagram. These include the difference in melting points of certain alloys, and temperature differences between the solid-liquid interface and the bulk liquid in the weld zone. The greater the difference between the solid-liquid interface and the bulk liquid in the melt zone, the greater the tendency for a hot crack to occur (9).

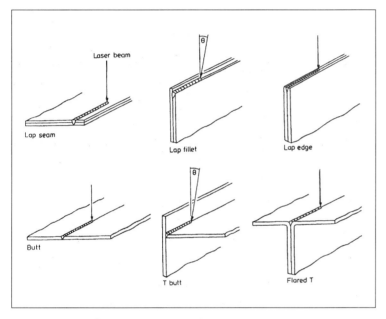

Figure 4. Common laser weld joint designs. Joint gap can be no more than 10% of the thinner material thickness. Contact of the mating surfaces is generally preferred.

Joint Design

Joint design can directly effect the weldability of a component because of the resultant stress in the joint after cooling. Heat flow during the weld process and especially during the cooling cycle can define the extent of the HAZ and the degree of grain size change seen across the weld zone. In many microjoining applications requiring low-power welds, stresses in the weld area can be an issue. Thin materials used in full-hard or half-hard condition will be fully annealed in the weld zone. This change in grain size across the weld zone can cause cracking in the HAZ, or have insufficient strength for the service environment. If the rapid solidification is causing warping or cracking, the addition of more heat can help. The general idea is to slow down the cooling rate. This can be achieved by extending the pulse width, increasing the repetition rate, or slowing down on feed rate. In CW welds, increasing average power or slowing down can often help. Joint gaps should be minimum, with nominal press fits or tight clamping preferred. This will prevent weld material from having to cross the gap in addition to suffering from cooling stresses. Joints that allow for a free-standing edge, such as a flange weld are also recommended. The weld stress can be taken up by simple deflection of the thin section of the flange, avoiding a weld crack. Examples of common laser weld joint designs are given in Figure 4. Tolerances on the fitup of the parts have been discussed in Section 10.2.5.

References
3. Z. Sun and J. C. Ion, *J. Materials Science* **30,** 4205–14 (1995).
4. C. Morley, *YAG Laser Welding Guide,* Unitek-Miyachi Corporation, Monrovia, CA.
5. K. McEwain and D. R. Milner, Pressure Welding of Dissimilar Metals, Welding Technology (1962).
6. J. Lippold, Solidification Behavior and Cracking Susceptibility of Pulsed Laser Welds in Austenitic Stainless Steels, Welding Research Supplement, June 1994, 129–39.
7. A. L. Schaeffler, *Metals Progress* **56,** (1949) 680.
8. ASM Handbook, Welding Brazing Soldering, Vol. 6, p. 12 (Equation 48).
9. ASM Handbook, Welding Brazing Soldering, Vol. 6, 45–55.

KEVIN J. ELY

10.5 Comparison of Laser Welding with Other Technologies

10.5.1 Advantages/Limitations

Joint Preparation for Laser Welding

There are a number of methods for joining metals; Table 1 gives a partial list of welding processes. Several welding processes, such as shielded-metal-arc welding, gas-metal-arc welding, and submerged-arc welding cannot be used without adding filler metal, whereas most often laser welding is used without a filler metal, for butt joints between two pieces of material. A different joint preparation, such as a V groove or a double V groove, is used with these welding processes. Because filler metal is added, these welding processes are more tolerant of a gap between the two pieces being welded than is laser welding. Laser welding usually requires a machined joint, prepared to minimize the gap between the parts being welded. Fitup tolerances are covered in Section 10.2.5.

Table 1. Welding Processes

Shielded Metal Arc Welding (SMAW)
Gas Metal Arc Welding (GMAW)
Gas Tungsten Arc Welding (GTAW)
Submerged Arc Welding (SAW)
Plasma Arc Welding (PAW)
Laser Welding (LBW)
Electron Beam Welding (EBW)
Resistance Welding (ERW)
Oxyacetylene Welding

Aspect Ratio of Welds

Laser welding and electron-beam welding are commonly considered deep penetration or keyhole welding processes, in which welds are created with a high aspect ratio (depth to width). By contrast, in the arc welding processes, heat is absorbed at the metal surface and conducted sideways as well as into the depth of the material, resulting in a lower-aspect-ratio weld. Because of the high aspect ratio, a weld is made with lower heat input, reducing the possibility of distortion. Plasma arc welding is sometimes considered a keyhole process, but is not capable of welds of the same aspect ratio as EBW and LBW.

Although electron-beam welding produces a weld with similar characteristics to laser beam welding, this process usually takes place inside a vacuum system. This limits the throughput of the process. Laser beam welding does not have this limitation.

Comparative Welding Heat Input

Table 2 presents a comparison of laser welding of 6 mm plate with other methods. The table shows that although a greater power is absorbed by the workpiece in laser welding, because of the higher welding speed, there is a lower heat input per unit length, and less total heat into the part. Both the GTAW and the PAW had a V-shaped weld, which resulted in considerable distortion of the plate. Less distortion resulted from the EBW and the LBW in which the welds were of relatively uniform cross section through the thickness of the material.

Ramifications of Lower Heat Input

Because of the lower heat input and because of the ability to precisely deposit the heat, laser welding is often employed when it is required to make a joint close to a glass-to-metal seal, rubber seal, or on other heat-sensitive material. There may be no practical alternative welding process that can perform this function.

Limitations of laser welding are summarized in Table 3.

Table 2. Comparison of Processes for Welding 6 mm Plate

LBW	GTAW	PAW	EBW
Power absorbed by workpiece			
4 kW	2 kW	4 kW	5 kW
Total power used			
50 kW	3 kW	6 kW	6 kW
Traverse speed			
16 mm/s	2 mm/s	5.7 mm/s	40 mm/s
Energy per unit length absorbed by the workpiece			
250 J/mm	1000 J/mm	600 J/mm	125 J/mm
Alignment accuracy required			
± 0.5 mm	± 1.0 mm	± 1.0 mm	± 0.3 mm

Table 3. Limitations of Laser Welding

High capital and operating cost of equipment
Machined joint required to ensure good fitup
Accurate seam tracking required

10.5.2 Economic Considerations

Laser welders have a high capital and operating cost. However, laser welding is characterized by a high welding speed. The high throughput results yield a cost per welded part that can be competitive with other welding processes. The competitiveness depends on keeping the machine busy, either through application in a mass production environment or in a job shop processing large numbers of small jobs.

Cost Factors

Factors that should be taken into account in evaluating the relative cost associated with laser welding and other technologies are listed in Table 4. Installation may include the cost of providing electrical power at the location, of the laser and chiller and perhaps special transformers. The capital expense is amortized over the expected life of equipment, taking into account the expected usage (one, two, or three shifts a day), to arrive at an hourly cost. Estimates of the maintenance costs should be available from laser vendors, and can be converted to an hourly cost.

Table 4. Cost Factors in Evaluating Welding Processes

System cost, including chiller
Installation cost
Amortization of capital expense
Electrical power
Water cooling (if chiller not used)
Laser gas (for CO_2 laser welders)
Shielding gas
Cost of maintenance time
Replacement flashlamps (Nd:YAG laser welders)
Replacement cover glasses (Nd:YAG laser welders)
Replacement laser and focusing optics
Replacement water and gas filters

Floor Space Requirements

Floor space and location can be a major factor in laser installations. In some instances, for example, as when putting a new welder into an existing production line, or where the welding must take place inside clean rooms or dry rooms, the laser generator can be located some distance away from the welding location and only the welding system needs to be installed in the space critical area. The beam can be delivered from the generator to the welder via beam tubes or fiber optics.

Reduction in Scrap and Rework

Laser welding is a precise process, with a high degree of control over the welding energy and the deposition of the energy into the material. This has led in some installations to substantial reductions in the amount of scrap or rework necessary to produce a satisfactory product. The savings in cost of rework may be sufficient to justify laser welding.

Throughput Considerations

In some instances, welding is the time limiting step in the overall factory output. In these cases, installation of a more expensive but faster welding process may be justified because it increases the throughput of the whole factory. Examples (although systems have not been engineered to utilize laser technology in these applications) are laser welding in ship yards and in pipeline construction.

VIVIAN E. MERCHANT

10.5.3 Comparison of Welding Results

The ability of the laser to deliver high power to a small area makes the laser a source far superior to any conventional welding sources. Electron-beam devices, competing with lasers in critical parts welding, require a high vacuum in the welding chamber for the process to proceed steadily. Laser welding, in contrast, can take place in a shielding gas atmosphere, preferably, argon, helium, or carbon dioxide. The lens-mirror system can easily direct the laser beam in space in order to process elements of any dimensions and difficult-to-reach locations, allowing for simple automation of the material treatment process. By adjusting the beam energy parameters, the laser welding process is easily controlled. Unlike the electron beam and arc, the laser beam is not affected by the magnetic field of a workpiece, thus yielding a quality weld throughout its length. A comparison of laser to other competitive welding processes is given in Table 5.

Table 5. Comparison to Competitive Welding Processes (1)

Characteristics	Laser	Electron beam	Resistance spot	Gas-tungsten arc
Heat generation	Low	Moderate	Moderate	Very high
Weld quality	Excellent	Excellent	Good	Excellent
Weld speed	Moderate	High	Low	Low
Initial cost	Moderate	High	Low	Low
Operating/maintenance costs	Low	Moderate	Low	Low
Tooling costs	Low	High	High	Moderate
Controllability	Very good	Good	Low	Fair
Range of dissimilar materials	Very wide	Wide	Narrow	Narrow

Reference

1. M. M. Schwartz, Laser Welding, Metals Joining Manual, McGraw-Hill, New York, 1979.

GEORGE CHRYSSOLOURIS
STEFANOS KARAGIANNIS

Notes

ISBN 0-912035-15-3

Chapter 11

Penetration Welding

11.0 Introduction

Chapter 10 has emphasized conduction welding, in which laser energy is absorbed at the surface and is conducted into the interior of the workpiece by thermal conduction. This relatively slow process limits the depth that can be melted effectively and hence limits the welding depth.

At higher values of laser power, a keyhole may be formed in the material and the laser energy may be deposited deeper in the workpiece. This allows production of welds having greater depth. This regime, often called *penetration welding,* will be emphasized in this chapter.

The chapter presents welding results like penetration depth and weld rate for specified conditions of irradiation. The exact results obtained for a penetration welding operation depend on a wide variety of parameters that may vary from one laser installation to another. These parameters are usually not specified well enough to allow one to duplicate exactly the conditions for a particular operation. Thus the tabulated and graphed data must be interpreted as indicating an approximate range of results that may be obtained. The user must optimize the parameters for a particular processing operation experimentally in order to obtain the best results.

JOHN F. READY

11.1 Description of Penetration Welding

11.1.1 The Deep-Penetration Process

Precisely focused laser beams are used for the welding of metals. Depending on the laser irradiance, either a conduction-limited or a deep-penetration mode is possible. Conduction-limited welds are obtained in metals at an irradiance less than 10^6 W/cm^2. At these irradiance levels, the focused laser beam is absorbed by the metal workpiece, generating heat that is rapidly conducted into the metal, thus melting the laser-irradiated surface and the subsurface layers. This process goes on without vaporization of molten surface layers. Conduction-limited welds are obtained at weld speeds less than 20 in./min. Metallographic cross sections of such welds reveal an aspect ratio of weld depth to weld width less than 4 to 1. Conduction-limited welds are applicable to metal thickness up to 2 mm. Details and examples of conduction-limited laser welds can be found in Chapter 10.

Deep-penetration laser welding of metals requires a laser irradiance in excess of 10^6 W/cm^2. Such irradiance levels can be obtained with a continuous CO_2 laser beam.

During this process, the laser beam melts through the metal workpiece thickness and produces a narrow cylinder of liquid metal. Furthermore, vaporization of the liquid through a finite thickness occurs, producing a column of metal vapor. The vapor column, commonly referred to as a vapor cavity or keyhole, is surrounded by liquid metal. Because of temperature gradients existing along surface and subsurface liquid layers, the surface tension varies dramatically along these liquid layers, promoting localized convection. When the workpiece is translated past the laser beam, the metal along the leading edge of the keyhole is melted through its entire thickness. The liquid metal flows around and along the base of the keyhole, eventually resolidifying at the trailing edge. The stability of the keyhole is based on laser irradiance and welding speed. At high enough irradiance, excessive vaporization leads to keyhole formation through the thickness of the metal, leading to liquid metal drop-through, as in laser cutting; at low irradiance, vaporization of the liquid metal is not sufficient to form a keyhole, and therefore there is incomplete weld penetration. At low weld speed, the weld fusion zone is large and wide, resulting in liquid metal drop-through; at high enough weld speeds, weld penetration is incomplete, not penetrating through the metal thickness. Metallographic cross sections of deep penetration laser welds reveal an aspect ratio of weld depth to weld width greater than 4 to 1.

Figure 1 shows an example of typical shapes of the weld beads obtained with conduction welding and with deep-penetration welding.

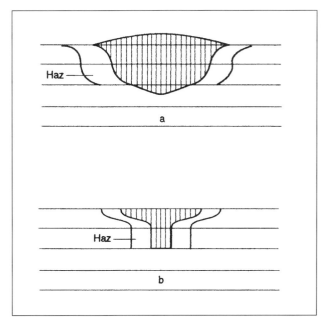

Figure 1. Typical shapes for weld beads for conduction-limited welds (a) and deep-penetration welds (b). HAZ is the heat-affected zone.

When metal vapor that is formed is further irradiated by a laser beam with an irradiance normally used for deep-penetration welding, the metal vapor breaks down into a plasma consisting of ions and electrons. This plasma over the metal surface is opaque to the laser beam and effectively minimizes beam coupling to the metal surface. To weld with a laser beam, plasma formation should be minimized. This is accomplished by directing a high-velocity jet of inert gas into the weld region and removing the plasma to one side.

Thermal conduction does not limit penetration; laser beam energy is delivered to the metal through the depth of the weld, not just to the top surface. Once the energy of the laser beam begins to be absorbed by the metal, the amount of energy that is required to melt the metal locally where it is irradiated by the laser beam is a function of the thermophysical properties of the metal, such as density, heat capacity, melting temperature, and latent heat of fusion. The total energy q required to bring a mass of metal from room temperature to a temperature above the melting temperature is:

$$q = \rho V(C_{ps}\Delta T_s + H_f + C_{pl}\Delta T_l)$$

where ρ is the density, V the volume of metal, $C_{ps}\Delta T_s$ the heat required to raise the solid metal to its melting point, H_f the latent heat of fusion, and $C_{pl}\Delta T_l$ the heat required to raise the liquid metal from the melting temperature to a temperature below the boiling temperature.

From the thermophysical properties of the metal, a first-order approximation of the amount of energy required to melt the metal can be calculated.

Laser light reflected from the surface of a metal constitutes a loss for the process. At low laser irradiance, the reflectivity of metals increases from about 50% at visible wavelengths (argon ion, ruby) to as much as 95–98% for the longer-wavelength infrared (CO_2, Nd:YAG) lasers (see Table 1). The reflectivity of metals decreases at high temperature and with surface condition (presence of surface oxides, chemical treatment and coatings). When applied laser irradiance for metals is sufficient to ensure that the absorbed intensity exceeds a threshold of the order of 10^4 W/cm^2, surface melting and enhanced laser absorption occur. This has been discussed in more detail in Chapter 5. Additionally the absorbed power must be sufficiently high to overcome energy losses due to thermal conduction. The minimum energy needed to melt most metals ranges from 2 to 12 kJ/cm^3.

Table 1. Reflectance at Normal Incidence (Room Temperature)

Wavelength (μm)	Nickel	Chromium	Gold	Silver
0.4880 (Ar II)	0.597	0.437	0.415	0.952
0.6943 (Cr^{3+})	0.676	0.831	0.930	0.961
1.06 (Nd^{3+})	0.741	0.901	0.981	0.964
10.6 (CO_2)	0.941	0.984	0.975	0.989

Time-dependent solutions of the heat diffusion equation indicate that at an applied irradiance of the order of 10^6 W/cm^2, vaporization at the surface of metals becomes very rapid so that the interaction of the laser beam with metal becomes highly complex. Deep penetration welds in which the absorbed energy is efficiently convected by capillary and gravitational forces are then possible. At even higher irradiance around 10^8 W/cm^2, explosive boiling beneath the surface of the liquid can occur. At laser irradiance in the range 10^5–10^9 W/cm^2, the associated electric fields are often sufficiently strong to ionize the atmosphere immediately over a metal work surface. The resulting plasma shields the workpiece from the laser and so precautions are necessary to inhibit the ionization process (see Section 11.2.8).

Laser welds made at approximately 1 kW continuous wave on a slab or with pulsed low-repetition-rate lasers yield conduction-limited welds.

Laser welds made at continuous multikilowatt power levels yield deep-penetration welds. As the laser beam traverses the workpiece, metal melts ahead of a deep void (or keyhole) sustained by the pressure of the metal vapor and the liquid behind the void, leaving a characteristically narrow weld. The benefits of deep-penetration welding are the high energy efficiency of the process, so that thermal distortion is minimized, and the possibility of making single-pass welds. The plasma formed above the workpiece in multikilowatt laser welding can often be eliminated by using a suitable transverse gas jet just above the surface. The metal vapor within the keyhole maintains the liquid cavity, but may ionize and so attenuate and dissipate the focused laser beam.

The high irradiance of the laser source enables deep penetration welding to be achieved. Thus square-edged sections may be butt welded in a single pass with minimal thermal distortion. Similarly to the electron beam, the laser is able to penetrate because of the formation of a keyhole, which acts as a black body absorber. The hole is maintained open by the metal vapor pressure. The keyhole translates with the laser beam, metal being melted ahead of it and flowing around to solidify behind, leaving a deep narrow weld. While one of the significant advantages of a laser over electron beam welding is the ability to operate at atmospheric pressure, such operation has the potential difficulty that the electrons from the metal workpiece can initiate a laser-sustained plasma in the gas above it. The plasma absorbs the incident beam. In general, helium shield gas directed across the laser beam near the workpiece surface is sufficient to reduce plasma formation and its effects to an acceptable level. When argon is used as a shield gas, the melt depth is reduced by approximately 70% compared to helium as a shield gas. The weld penetration is limited by the laser beam absorption process within the keyhole and not in the plasma above the surface.

It has been shown by Swift-Hook and Gick (1) that in a simplified model of a deep penetration melt, the power input to the melt volume corresponds to approximately one-half of the total power input, the rest being lost by conduction. Thus it is estimated that the efficiency with which laser power is coupled into the metal is about 75%.

Most metals can be melted with an absorbed irradiance of 10^4 W/cm^2, and surface vaporization occurs at irradiance around 10^6 W/cm^2. The minimum energy density to melt metals ranges from approximately 2.5 (Al) to 12.5 kJ/cm^2 (W), and the energy density to vaporize ranges approximately from 30 to 80 kJ/cm^2. The high room-temperature reflectivity and thermal conductivity of most metals implies that much higher irradiance is required for the processing of metals. However, once a threshold irradiance is exceeded, the surface absorption and the energy efficiency of the process can be enhanced by the strong temperature dependence of the reflectivity. At higher irradiance, local heating becomes so rapid that conduction can be neglected. Incident laser radiation is absorbed in a surface layer as thin as 1 μm (compared to nearly 100 μm for electron beams), and considerable energy is transported by metal vapor and molten metal.

For many applications, the high electrical efficiency of the CO_2 laser (greater than 10%) is an advantage.

Welding lasers are usually designed to operate with an optical cavity producing the lowest-order transverse mode so that the output beam divergence is diffraction limited. That is, the beam can be focused using a large aperture and low aberration focusing optics to a minimum spot size with a diameter of the order of the wavelength of the laser beam. Focal spot sizes from about 1 μm for an argon laser to about 15 or 20 μm for the CO_2 laser can be obtained. This means that high positional accuracy and narrow weld zones are possible. Deep penetration welds in which the absorbed energy is efficiently convected by capillary and gravitational forces are then possible.

References
1. D. T. Swift-Hook and A. E. F. Gick, Penetration Welding with Lasers, Welding Research Supplement, *The Welding Journal* **52,** 492-s (1973).
E. V. Locke, E. D. Hoag, and R. A. Hella, *IEEE J. Quantum Electronics* **QE-8,** 132 (1972).

DAN GNANAMUTHU

11.1.2 Motion of the Keyhole
The level of laser power is not so important for defining the deep-penetration mode of laser welding as are the physical processes. The penetration welding process is illustrated in Figure 2. The figure shows the formation of the keyhole. The laser beam moves across the surface, and the keyhole is translated through the material. The keyhole is stable as the beam traverses the surface. The keyhole moves through the material surrounded by molten metal. This weld pool characteristically has a teardrop shape. Molten metal flows around the hole and fills in behind it. The molten metal then rapidly resolidifies, producing a seam weld as the beam moves across the surface.

An irradiance around 10^6 W/cm^2 is required for the keyhole to form. For values of irradiance above 10^7 W/cm^2, there is excessive vaporization. Thus penetration welding is usually performed in the range of irradiance between 10^6 and 10^7 W/cm^2.

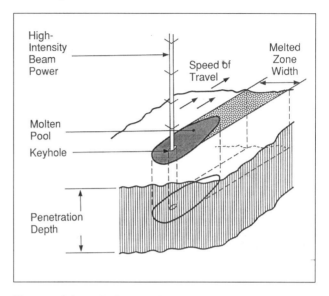

Figure 2. Schematic diagram of the process of keyhole formation and deep-penetration welding. (From D. T. Swift-Hook and A. E. F. Gick, Welding Research Supplement, *Weld. J.,* 492-S, November 1973.)

JOHN F. READY

11.1.3 Penetration
The penetration depth increases with laser power at constant beam traverse speed. Figure 3 shows how weld penetration depth increases as a function of laser power. The figure is based on data relevant to welding of steel with a CO_2 laser, but does not show exact data for any specific case. Such data are presented in the sections to follow in this chapter. The purpose of this figure is to show the general shape of the functional relation between penetration depth and laser power.

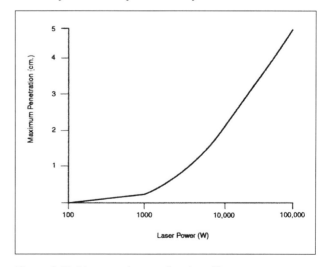

Figure 3. Weld penetration as a function of laser output power.

ISBN 0-912035-15-3

At levels below 1000 W, the process is conduction welding. Penetration increases slowly with power, and the penetration is limited. Around 1000 W, one reaches the threshold for penetration welding and the curve bends upward. The exact value of this threshold depends on many factors. The threshold is often in the 1–1.5 kW region, but depending on materials, wavelength, beam quality, and focusing, it may occur at powers as low as a few hundred watts.

Well above the threshold, the penetration increases as the 0.7 or 0.8 power of the laser power, reaching about 5 cm for steel near the 100-kW level.

The results obtained in a particular welding application will depend on the specific circumstances, including focusing, the beam traverse velocity, type and angle of the gas jet used to dissipate the plasma, etc. For fixed laser power, the penetration is inversely proportional to the weld speed. There does exist a minimum welding speed below which the keyhole is no longer stable. The maximum penetration for the given conditions is achieved at speeds just above this minimum.

JOHN F. READY

11.1.4 Lasers for Penetration Welding

Deep-penetration laser welding has been performed mostly with multikilowatt CO_2 lasers. Until fairly recently there had been no well-developed multikilowatt Nd:YAG lasers. This situation has changed, and reliable stable multikilowatt Nd:YAG lasers are now available. The following sections will present results for both CO_2 and Nd:YAG lasers in detail. Here we simply indicate that a suitable Nd:YAG laser can perform penetration welding at lower levels of power than a CO_2 laser, largely because of its shorter wavelength, which allows a higher value of irradiance to be delivered to the surface of the workpiece.

Most of the applications for multikilowatt laser welding have so far used CO_2 lasers, because they developed first, but because the Nd:YAG laser has greater welding capability at a given power, we may expect to see applications for that laser develop.

In addition, recent work with high-radiance lasers, such as experimental copper vapor lasers and dye lasers, has indicated that laser welding can be performed with high weld velocity. These were high-radiance experimental lasers developed at Lawrence Livermore National Laboratory, and they are not available commercially. But the work indicates that as high-power lasers with high radiance become more common, we may expect laser penetration welding to be performed with other types of lasers.

JOHN F. READY

11.1.5 Melting Efficiency

Deep-penetration welding may be performed with efficient use of the laser energy. Figure 4 shows results obtained with a 5-kW CO_2 laser. The parameters in the figure are given in terms of a dimensionless weld speed parameter, Vb/k, where V is the seam welding rate, b the width of the fusion zone, and k the thermal diffusivity averaged over temperature, and a dimensionless power parameter, P/hKd, with P the laser power, h the weld penetration, K the thermal conductivity averaged over temperature, and

$$d = T_m - T_0 + H/c$$

with T_m the melting temperature, T_0 the ambient temperature, H the latent heat of fusion, and c the heat capacity. The diagonal lines in the figure represent constant melting efficiency, which is defined as the ratio of the minimum energy required to melt the specified volume of material divided by the laser energy. Because V_{bh} is the volume of material welded per unit time and

$$\rho[c(T_m - T_0) + H]$$

is the energy per unit volume to melt the material, then at 100% melting efficiency (i.e., all the laser energy is utilized in supplying the sensible heat and latent heat required to melt the material), one has

$$P = (Vbh)\rho[c(T_m - T_0) + H]$$
$$= (Vb\rho c/K)hK(T_m - T_0 + H/c)$$
$$= (Vb/k)hK(T_m - T_0 + H/c) = (Vb/k)hKd$$

which means that for 100% melting efficiency

$$Vb/k = P/hKd$$

This situation is represented by the line marked 100% melting efficiency in the figure. Other diagonal lines define other lower values of melting efficiency.

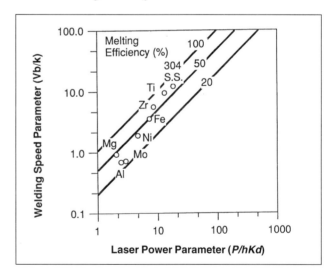

Figure 4. Normalized weld speed as a function of normalized laser power. The symbols are defined in the text. The diagonal lines indicate specified values of the melting efficiency. (From E. M. Breinan, C. M. Banas, and M. A. Greenfield, United Technologies Research Center Report R75-111087-3, 1975.)

For metals with low thermal conductivity like stainless steel, high values of melting efficiency are attainable, up to 70%. This means that 70% of the incident laser energy is utilized in melting metal and only 30% is lost. Some energy loss is inevitable because of thermal conduction out of the weld zone, but this can be relatively small. The melting efficiency for metals with higher thermal conductivity, like aluminum and molybdenum, is lower, because of thermal conduction of heat out of the weld zone. We note that the high values of melting efficiency are attainable only if the initial surface reflectivity is reduced during the welding process, as has been described in Chapter 5.

Because melting efficiency can be so high, the input energy per unit volume required to make a weld is lower than for most conventional welding processes. It is about a factor of ten lower than for processes like resistance welding. This fact contributes to the smallness of the heat-affected zone in laser welding and is one of the attractive aspects of laser welding.

JOHN F. READY

11.2 Welding Procedures

11.2.1 Laser Choice

Of the hundreds of laser types that have been developed during the past thirty plus years, only two are currently suitable for multikilowatt industrial applications. These are the neodymium-YAG (available in units with power to 6 kW) and the carbon dioxide (with continuous power to 50 kW) systems. The fundamental technology for these industrial laser workhorses dates back to the 1960s; principal developments since then have been in making the units more suitable and reliable for production use. It is anticipated that solid-state diode lasers, which are currently experiencing intense development, will challenge Nd:YAG and carbon dioxide for some multikilowatt applications within the next several years.

Neodymium-YAG Lasers

Industrially suited, neodymium-YAG lasers are available with continuous power ratings to 6 kW. The lasing medium is neodymium, which was originally used in a glass host in some of the earliest laser systems. YAG (yttrium aluminum garnet) was substituted to provide a host material with more favor- able thermal properties than glass. Lasing output is at 1.06 µm in the near-infrared portion of the electromagnetic spectrum. Although this wavelength is beyond the visible range, which extends from approximately 0.38 to 0.77 µm, it is readily transmitted by common optical materials as well as the human eye. For this reason, even a few milliwatts of Nd:YAG radiation can cause eye damage. Accordingly, appropriate safety provisions should be taken and are seriously addressed in current industrial systems. For a discussion of safety considerations, refer to Chapter 6.

Stable resonator cavity optics are customarily used in multikilowatt, CW, Nd:YAG laser systems. Because of imperfections and thermal effects within the lasing solid, attainable focus spot size usually exceeds the diffraction limit, but the resultant irradiance that can be attained is more than adequate for effective welding applications. Initial beam coupling to metals is higher than it is for carbon dioxide lasers, as noted in Section 5.3. In view of the higher initial absorption, the Nd:YAG system may offer significant advantages over carbon dioxide lasers in welding of highly reflective materials such as aluminum and copper alloys. It should be noted, however, that net beam absorption for welding is strongly influenced by radiation trapping in keyhole welding, as discussed in Section 11.1.

Excitation energy for Nd:YAG systems is commonly provided by high-intensity, electric-discharge lamps. Electrical conversion efficiency, defined as the ratio of output laser power to lamp power, is, typically, in the range 3–5% depending on the required optical quality of the output beam. Somewhat higher efficiency and improved optical quality may be achieved by diode excitation (1). This technique is currently under development for applications requiring improved optical quality such as precision drilling of small holes. The increased cost of such systems may be justified for such applications, but may not be for routine production welding.

The cost of lamp-pumped Nd:YAG systems is generally higher than that of carbon dioxide systems of equivalent power. A selection of Nd:YAG is, therefore, dependent upon the establishment of superior process characteristics as well as upon other factors that can influence overall production system cost. A prime factor relating to the latter is that fiber optic delivery, as described in Section 3.2.2, may be used for the Nd:YAG beam, thereby offering the potential for significant system simplification and cost reduction. Another factor to be considered is that plasma formation problems (discussed in Sections 5.7 and 11.2.8) are less severe with Nd:YAG than with carbon dioxide. This characteristic may reduce plasma suppression gas flow requirements with a corresponding decrease in system operational costs.

Carbon Dioxide Lasers

Multikilowatt carbon dioxide lasers are available from several suppliers in the power range 5–20 kW. Higher-power systems are currently available only from a single supplier.

Carbon dioxide systems utilize a circulating gas mixture of helium, nitrogen, and carbon dioxide; the latter is the lasing medium, while helium and nitrogen serve to improve conversion efficiency and cooling. Excitation of the lasing medium is by rf, dc, or high-frequency ac electric power. The output beam wavelength is 10.6 µm, which is well into the infrared. The 10:1 relationship between the wavelengths of Nd:YAG and carbon dioxide may, perhaps, be surprising, but is apparently coincidental. Electrical-to-optical beam conversion efficiencies for carbon dioxide are typically in the range of 12–14%. Values of 18–20% are attained with rf-driven systems, but these values should be adjusted for conversion losses associated with generation of rf power.

Single or multimode stable cavity optics are typical for units to 5 kW. In the intermediate high-power range, either multimode stable or unstable oscillator optics are used. At power levels above 20 kW, unstable oscillator optics are customary. As shown in Figure 1, "unstable" oscillator optics yield an annular output beam characterized by a ratio M of the outer to inner beam diameter. The term *unstable* stems from the fact that a photon generated within the laser cavity tends to move outward toward the cavity walls rather than inward as in a stable oscillator. This, perhaps confusing, terminology relates to optical details and does not imply unstable system operation. When focused, the annular, unstable oscillator beam inverts to provide a sharp central power peak with a prominent circular outer ring. Beyond focus, the beam reverts to its initial annular form.

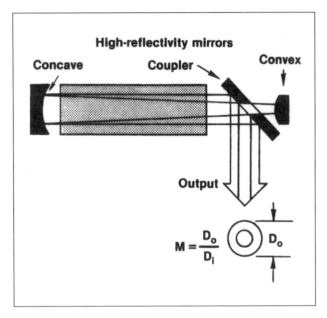

Figure 1. Unstable resonator optical arrangement. D_i is the diameter of the inner ring.

At multikilowatt power levels, carbon dioxide lasers currently offer the lowest cost per unit power. Typical cost is of the order of $50/W at the 5-kW level and drops to $30–35 in the intermediate range. The specific price increases at the high-power end of available units because of increased technological requirements as well as the low production volume.

Common optically transparent materials (glass, quartz, clear acrylics, etc.) are totally opaque to the 10.6 μm lasing wavelength. A disadvantage of this characteristic is that special, and more expensive, infrared transmitting materials such as zinc selenide and single crystal alkali halides must be used. On the other hand, the long wavelength facilitates eye protection from the carbon dioxide laser beam while providing convenient visual access to the welding process.

11.2.2 Optics

Transmitting Optics

At the lower end of the multikilowatt power spectrum, transmitting optics, usually of zinc selenide composition, are used effectively. Care must be exercised to keep the optical elements clean and cool. The former is often accomplished by shrouding the optical element in a focus head and providing a protective flow of inert gas. The latter is accomplished by edge cooling of the element at lower power levels and by more elaborate surface convection at higher power.

Reflective Optics

At highest powers, reflective metal optics are used. These are typically formed with copper substrates provided with "thin skin" cooling provisions designed to minimize temperature gradients and potential thermal distortion of the element. The temperature of the cooling medium for industrial systems is normally set slightly above the highest anticipated dew point in the installation so that condensation does not occur on the optical surfaces. It is not essential that reflective optical elements be cold, only that they have uniform temperature. The copper substrate is often hard coated with a material such as electroless nickel into which the final optical figure is generated. The mirrors are then coated with gold or a multilayer coating designed to yield maximum durability and reflectivity at the lasing wavelength. Reflectivity values exceeding 99% are readily available.

For focusing, corrected spherical and/or aspheric elements may be used, depending on process convenience. For example, off-axis parabolic optics may be used to both redirect, as well as focus, the beam. This can eliminate requirements for an additional directing mirror within the focus head and can provide a convenient means for rotational motion capability around the beam path centerline. Advantages, however, should be weighed against requirements for increased beam alignment precision as the off-axis angle of the parabolic element increases.

In high-volume production applications involving materials subject to spatter, molybdenum focus optics may be employed. Although the reflectivity of such optics is lower than for gold or multilayer coatings, the loss in efficiency is offset by production durability. In fact, solid molybdenum mirrors can sustain liquid steel spatter without damage; regular cleaning is, of course, required. Some two-element molybdenum focus heads have yielded more than 100,000 h of reliable operation in 9-kW welding applications.

Focusing Factors

The diameter of the focused spot on the workpiece is one of the most important process variables because, together with power, it defines the incident beam irradiance. As noted previously, irradiance determines the nature of the beam-material interaction. For example, as shown in Figure 2, incident irradiance governs the transition from thermal-diffusion-dominated to keyhole welding behavior.

The spot size D_s is dependent upon the focal length F and is inversely proportional to unfocused beam diameter d (Section 3.3)

$$D_s = K\lambda F/d \qquad (1)$$

Chapter 11: Penetration Welding

in which K is a constant dependent upon beam quality and λ is the laser wavelength. The ratio of focal length to beam diameter, F/d, is commonly referred to in photography as the f/number and is chosen for specific applications on the basis of process requirements. Nominal values of $f/6$ to $f/10$ are representative for multikilowatt welding with appropriate values increasing as power level and required weld penetration increase. For reference, it is noted that the predicted minimum spot diameter for a plane wave ($K = 2.44$) at 10.6 μm and an f/number of unity, is of the order of 0.025 mm.

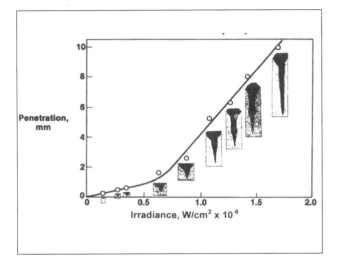

Figure 2. Effect of irradiance on welding response.

11.2.3 Focus Position

The exact location of focus relative to the surface of the workpiece for most effective welding is somewhat of a matter of individual process development. Usually, the most useful starting point for process development is with the focal point located at the material surface. This condition, together with an f/number appropriate to the material thickness, will usually produce the narrowest weld at the highest speed for the penetration required. It may well be, however, that the bead profile under these conditions is not ideal for the application under development. Small variations of focal spot location, above and below the material surface, will usually identify the most suitable conditions. It should be noted that the off-focus characteristics of different focusing elements (spherical, parabolic, elliptical, etc.) may differ for elements yielding identical spot size at principal focus.

In electron beam welding of thick materials, it has been found that improved bead characteristics are obtained if the focal point is located near the center of the required penetration. Since most industrial laser welding applications to date involve material thickness less than 12 mm, this is not, generally, an option for laser welds. At 50 kW, however, the available single-pass penetration is of the order of 40 mm, so that some benefit may accrue from positioning of the focal spot within the material.

Another electron beam practice, oscillation of the focal spot, is more difficult to implement with lasers. In contrast to electro-

magnetic beam deflection, laser spot oscillation at high power must rely on oscillation of one the optical elements. Since high-power optical elements are relatively heavy, attainment of required high frequency is difficult but not impossible. A guideline for the oscillation frequency required is that the characteristic thermal response time for many engineering materials is of the order of 1 ms. At frequencies above 1 kHz, therefore, the material will respond to the integrated energy input rather than the instantaneous input. A further constraint on frequency occurs in high-speed welding. It is essential that part motion not exceed focused spot diameter in one cycle. At a speed of 30 m/min, for example, surface motion is 0.5 mm in 1 ms. If a spot diameter of 0.5 mm is being used, then a minimum oscillation frequency of 1 kHz is required to obviate a zig-zag weld track. Oscillation can significantly influence bead shape and width as well as reduce defects, particularly in aluminum alloys. One of the other means for modifying the weld bead profile is to distribute the beam energy at focus by using dual focus spots. As shown in Figure 3, transverse separation of beam spots is a very effective means for increasing weld width, particularly in thin materials.

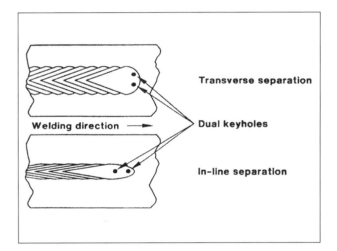

Figure 3. Effect of twin spot focus separation on weld profiles.

With a single spot, increased weld width entails decreasing weld speed, positioning the material surface away from the plane of principal focus, or a combination of these two procedures. In very thin materials, the former is often marginally effective because the fraction of beam energy that passes through the material increases as speed decreases and weld width remains roughly equivalent to focal spot size. The latter is limited by the fact that incident irradiance decreases as spot size increases so that welding performance may suffer. On the other hand, twin spots yield significant capability for broadening a fusion zone and also have the benefit of moving the high-intensity central portion of the focused beam off the weld seam; this can reduce loss of beam energy through the joint, can reduce the tendency for "blow through" of weld metal, and thus can have a major positive influence on production of sound welds in thin materials that do not have perfect fitup.

A second benefit of spot separation is attained if the spots are separated in line with the weld direction. This stems from the fact that keyhole welds experience a fluid dynamic instability leading to "humping" at high speeds. It has been shown that the wave instability can be delayed to higher speeds if the length of the laser melt pool is increase. Conditions for the humping instability may be inferred from the nondimensional hydrodynamic Froude number, V^2/lg, in which V is velocity, g is the acceleration of gravity, and l is a characteristic length, which is appropriately taken as the length of the melt pool. The Froude number represents the ratio of dynamic forces to the forces of gravity and is used to scale surface wave effects on ships. As may be noted in Figure 4, stable surface conditions occur at low values of Froude number and instabilities grow with increased values.

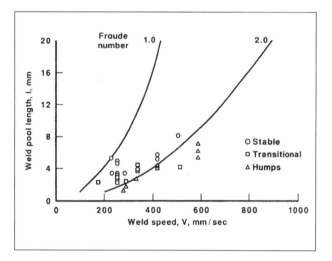

Figure 4. Effect of Froude number on high-speed weld stability.

11.2.4. Surface Conditions

The effect of surface impurities on weld characteristics can be severe or essentially nonexistent depending upon the nature of the material and the process parameters. As a general rule, materials such as paint and/or oil that have vaporization temperatures below the melting point of the material being welded will be vaporized by the high-intensity laser beam with little influence on the weld characteristics of common steels. Evaporation of such materials, however, can lead to formation of a high-density plasma above the workpiece surface, as discussed in Section 11.2.8 and in Chapter 5, which can lead to a marked reduction in welding performance. These comments refer only to the surfaces of the material that are only peripherally involved in the weld. On the other hand, weld faying surfaces (i.e., the surfaces being joined) must be free of contaminants or severe weld defects may occur.

Surface contaminants that have comparable or higher melting points than the weldment must be removed prior to laser welding if the highest weld quality is to be obtained. Examples are mill scale on as-received material, carburized steel surfaces, and surface oxides. In carbon dioxide laser welding, the high absorptance of aluminum oxide (up to 98% at 10.6 μm) as compared to that of freshly scraped aluminum, which exhibits 98% reflectance, has spawned some tests designed to take advantage of the oxide absorption to increase welding performance. If the oxide, which has a much higher melting point than the metal, is not removed from the surface of the workpiece, however, it will be thoroughly mixed with the fused material during the welding process with resultant detrimental effects on weld quality.

In highly reactive metals such as titanium alloys, zircaloys, etc., it is essential that all material that will undergo fusion be appropriately cleaned. Preweld cleaning procedures used in conventional welding practice are usually suitable for laser welding. Degreasing should be employed unless this introduces other production difficulties and process development has shown that required weld integrity can be obtained without it. Other procedures include mechanical scraping for such materials as aluminum alloys as well as various machining and chemical procedures. Rinsing of the faying and adjacent surfaces with ethyl alcohol is an effective final preparation for materials sensitive to residue and moisture.

11.2.5 Joint Design

The laser beam welding process effectively utilizes joint designs similar to those of more conventional welding processes and, in particular, those used for electron beam welding. The narrow, deep-penetration capabilities of the laser permit some latitude in joint configuration, but also introduce restrictions on the tolerances and nature of some of the designs.

Autogenous Welds

Commonly used joint configurations for autogenous welds have been illustrated in Section 10.2.5, which has also discussed fit-up tolerances.

Although these joints are primarily intended for use without filler addition, small quantities of filler may be added to influence chemistry and/or reduce thermal distortion. The maximum effective gap in a butt joint is about 3% of the material thickness. For gaps beyond this approximate value, an underfilled fusion zone will be obtained unless filler material is added. For a gap that exceeds 3% of the material thickness, but is less than 5%, some underfill may be experienced that may not only be acceptable but desirable for certain applications. For example, a positive bead reinforcement is often detrimental for welds in sheet metal components (tailored blanks) that are to be subsequently formed. Since the strength of the fusion zone in such materials is usually higher than that of the parent metal, the slight reduction in material cross section at the joint does not compromise weldment integrity. Finally, it is noted that the 3% rule of thumb does not apply to thick materials when its use would predict a gap larger than the focused beam diameter. Under these conditions, it is possible that the beam will pass through the joint without interaction with the material.

In deep-penetration (keyhole) laser welds, the width of the fusion zone in very thin materials being welded at high speed is typically of the order of the focused spot diameter. As noted previously, attempts to increase weld width by reducing welding speed usually result in excess beam energy being transmitted through the material. In thicker materials, fusion zone depth-to-width ratio is influenced by incident beam power intensity, power, depth of focus, and welding speed; a depth-to-width ratio about 5:1 is common, but values greater than 10:1 are possible. The highest depth-to-width ratios are obtained near the upper limit of irradiance for effective welding with a depth of focus comparable to the material thickness. With reference to Equation 1, it is noted that the depth of focus D_f is given by the product of the spot diameter and the f/number:

$$D_f = D_s f = K\lambda f^2 \qquad (2)$$

This equation predicts that an f/number of 8.0 will produce a depth of focus comparable to a material thickness of 6.4 mm if the value of K yields a spot diameter of 0.8 mm. This should provide a good starting choice for process development. If beam optical quality is not sufficiently high to yield the 0.8-mm-diameter spot which has been selected to yield the desired incident power intensity, a smaller f/number is required. Primary emphasis in such circumstances must be on spot diameter and irradiance; depth-of-focus provisions should be considered of second order.

In lap welds, joint strength depends upon the cross-sectional area of the fused zone at the interface. For this reason, a wide weld at the interface is to be preferred; extensive penetration into the lower segment is not a basic requirement, although full penetration may be chosen to eliminate potential "blind penetration" root bead imperfections and/or to facilitate a qualitative means for weld quality monitoring. A somewhat broader weld can be achieved by locating the focal point slightly above or below the material surface and welding at lower power and speed. In some multikilowatt systems, the focal spot may be slightly elliptical, and a wider fusion zone may be simply achieved by orienting the weld direction at 90 degrees to the major axis of the focus ellipse. Another means for broadening the fusion zone is to reduce plasma suppression provisions so that a small, controlled plasma is established in close contact with the material surface. Although effective, this latter technique requires close process control. Finally, pronounced bead broadening can be achieved by utilization of a twin-focus or spot oscillation means, as noted earlier.

Fitup

Permissible gap width for a laser keyhole weld should be identified in terms of the fraction of the thickness of the material rather than on an absolute basis. Typically, the maximum gap that will still permit generation of a completely filled weld joint is of the order of 3% of the material thickness. Thus an 0.8-mm-thick material could sustain a 0.024-mm gap before underfill occurs, while a 25-mm-thick material could endure a 0.75-mm gap. In some applications, such as tailored blank welding, a slightly underfilled weld is desirable to avoid difficulties in postweld forming. Generally, total lack of fusion may occur if the gap width between faying surfaces significantly exceeds 5% of the material thickness. This limit may be extended somewhat if the beam is inclined slightly with respect to the weld seam, and/or fusion zone width is increased by transverse beam oscillation, dual-spot techniques, or other procedures.

11.2.6 Edge Preparation

Acceptable edge preparation for laser welding is subject to the requirements of the application. For high-quality, autogenous welds, a square, machined edge is preferred. Other edge preparation can, however, be utilized successfully for laser welding providing that certain basic criteria are met. Suitable means include shearing, flame cutting, and plasma cutting. With respect to the latter two, it is essential that the HAZ from the thermal cutting process be either so small that it is refused during laser welding, or that the characteristics of a residual HAZ are acceptable for the final weldment.

In addition to the requirements for faying surface cleanliness, as discussed in Section 11.2.4, it is also necessary that the effective gap width of the irregular surface not exceed previously noted limits. Filler metal addition can, to a degree, offset the imperfect fitup, as can the utilization of beam weaving transverse to the weld seam to involve more of the parent material in the weldment.

11.2.7 Fixturing

In general, the overall fixturing requirements for laser welding involve maintaining the relative position of the weldment components while providing beam access to the weld seam. Although these requirements are relatively straightforward, it is worth noting that forces induced during laser welding may well exceed the elastic limit of the material. Even though specific energy delivery to the workpiece is low, gradients are high and significant thermal distortion may occur. If fixturing is adequately robust, distortion may be prevented, but high residual stresses may be generated.

In many welding applications, it may be desirable to tack weld the assembly prior to the final weld pass. This may be done with a conventional welding process, or with the laser, depending upon process convenience. In a linear weld, for example, a short tack at the end of the weld will prevent separation of the faying surfaces as the weld progresses. Similarly, pretacking of an axisymmetric weldment can significantly reduce the clamping forces required to keep the units properly aligned. This may take the form of a 360-degree, high-speed, partial-penetration pass or several short tacks at selected angular locations. Care should be taken to minimize oxide formation during the tack pass, which could adversely influence final weld quality as discussed in Section 11.2.4. In a lap weld configuration, care should be exercised to ensure proper fitup along the entire weld length.

In a butt joint configuration, "wing up" of the mating elements may occur during welding. This behavior stems from the fact that lateral shrinkage occurs in a keyhole laser weld, and the degree of shrinkage is directly proportional to the width of the fusion zone. A tapered fusion zone, therefore, exhibits greater shrinkage at the bead face than at the root, thereby causing distortion. Such distortion may be restrained by robust fixturing, but significant residual stress may result in the weld component. The best means to deal with this behavior is to develop process parameters yielding a parallel-sided fusion zone. This requires adequate irradiance and a suitable depth of focus. It is generally obtained in what might be termed an overpenetration condition; that is, significant power loss may occur through the root of the weld. Such energy loss can be justified if the tolerances on the weldment can be met with this technique.

In various laser welding applications involving overlapping of materials, there is difficulty in providing adequate, local clamping pressure while still providing unobstructed beam access to the weld point. Dynamic clamping utilizing pressure rollers before and after the weld point may be effective in such instances. Pressure rollers can also be used in conjunction with appropriate guides to establish a controlled gap between faying surfaces in a butt joint configuration. This arrangement can be used to prevent generation of a positive overbead or underbead.

11.2.8 Shielding and Plasma Control

One of the negative characteristics of the multikilowatt laser welding process is that intense laser beams have the capability to ionize the atmosphere adjacent to the beam-material interaction point, thereby creating a high-optical-density plasma. In some surface treating applications this may enhance beam-material coupling and, in special circumstances, as noted in Section 11.2.5, establishment of a controlled plasma may facilitate attainment of desirable weld characteristics. In general, however, plasma formation inhibits effective beam energy delivery to the workpiece and is detrimental to deep-penetration laser welding performance.

Plasma Formation Factors

Classical electromagnetic theory relates the optical breakdown threshold (point at which a high-optical-density plasma is formed) to the strength of the electric field within the focused beam (note that the laser beam is an electromagnetic wave). The breakdown threshold is inversely proportional to the square of the wavelength. Theory yields a breakdown potential of 3×10^9 W/cm^2 for carbon dioxide lasers; an exponent of 11 is appropriate for Nd:YAG (note the implications relative to the comparative plasma sensitivity of carbon dioxide and Nd:YAG). Short-pulse laser output at this irradiance will produce a spark in free air at the beam focal point. It is to be noted that the level predicted for carbon dioxide is three orders of magnitude higher than that which is used in effective laser keyhole welding. In the keyhole process, however, metal vapors are generated that have much lower ionization potentials than atmospheric gases. Such metal vapor provides free electrons, which can directly absorb beam photons by the process of inverse Bremsstrahlung, and eventually, atmospheric breakdown occurs. The reduction in breakdown threshold is similar to the behavior of a spark gap in dry air when a small quantity of moisture is introduced. More extensive discussion of plasma formation factors is given in Chapter 5 and in (2). A comparison of ionization potentials is shown in Table 1. A plasma is kindled more easily in materials with lower ionization potentials.

Table 1. Typical Ionization Potentials

Medium	First ionization potential, (eV)
Argon	15.7
Carbon dioxide	14.4
Helium	24.5
Nitrogen	14.5
Aluminum	6.0
Chromium	6.7
Iron	7.8

Since the number of species at any energy level, N_i, is exponentially dependent upon the energy level, E_i,

$$N_i = \text{const}\, (Ne^{-E/kT}) \qquad (3)$$

the impact of the presence of metal vapor on the number of free electrons available for photon absorption is quite evident.

Suppression Techniques

Based on the above-noted considerations, effective laser welding obviously requires effective plasma suppression. This is accomplished by providing a flow of high-ionization-potential gas (helium is best) over the beam-material interaction point such that seed ionization is swept from the region. The specific flow means to this end are almost as numerous as the number of multikilowatt installations. Regardless of the suppression geometry, however, suppression effectiveness increases with suppression jet velocity. Helium has an advantage in this respect because of its low density, which results in much lower dynamic pressure compared to other gases flowing at the same velocity. This factor is illustrated in Table 2, which compares the dynamic pressure of different shielding gases for a suppression flow rate of 40 L/min through a rectangular 2.5 x 5.0 mm jet. To provide an indication of the potential influence of the suppression jet on the liquid metal in the melt pool, the dynamic pressure is represented in terms of an equivalent column of liquid steel. This is similar to representing barometric pressure in mm Hg.

Table 2. Comparison of Suppression Flow Dynamic Pressure (2.5 x 5.0 mm jet; 40 L/min)

Gas	Dynamic pressure, (mm of steel)
Argon	13.8
Carbon dioxide	15.2
Helium	1.4
Nitrogen	10.0

If the dynamic pressure of the suppression gas approaches the thickness of the material being welded, the potential for significant disruption of the melt pool exists.

In contrast to suppression requirements, protection of the fusion zone from atmospheric contamination is generally facilitated by relatively quiescent atmospheres of inert gases more dense than air. Argon is a common choice for conventional welding but is, unfortunately, highly prone to plasma breakdown, particularly with carbon dioxide lasers. Argon may, however, be used at lower powers, and mixtures of argon and helium (with the fraction of helium increasing with power) are quite effective. From the above considerations it is obvious that requirements for plasma suppression and atmospheric shielding are at odds, and compromise established by process development is usually required.

Shielding Provisions

In many steels, and in high-thermal-diffusivity materials such as the aluminum alloys, local shielding may be adequate to yield desired weld properties. In other materials, local shielding is inadequate, and extended shielding with advance and/or trailer segments may be required, as shown in Figure 5.

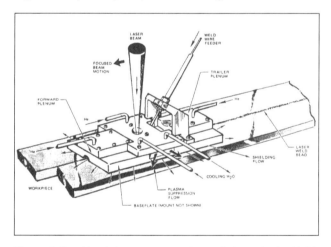

Figure 5. Combined plasma suppression and atmospheric shield.

In shields of this form, gas used in the advance and trailer sections may be chosen solely on the basis of atmospheric contamination protection; suppression gas need only be used at the beam-material interaction point. It should be noted, however, that a shield of the type shown in Figure 5 is sensitive to the geometry of the weldment. In a short, flat specimen, for example, shielding effectiveness is compromised when the advance or trailing sections pass beyond the edge of the weldment because gas containment by the workpiece is lost. Run-on and run-off tabs, which maintain the plane of the weld surface, are, therefore, essential. Such tabs are also essential to the formation of a uniform weld over the entire joint without start and end defects and, therefore, serve a dual function. Further, underbead shielding is also highly important to the generation of high-quality welds. Effective underbead shielding can be obtained with relatively small gas flow rates provided that uniform dispersion is assured as with a porous, extended delivery tube. In addition, it is beneficial to maintain a slight (of the order of 5 mm of water) positive pressure on the underbead, which can be monitored by a draft gage. Overall attainment of effective shielding is often attested by formation of carbon-like deposits parallel to the weld. These represent a layer of small (of the order of 400 μm diameter), shiny metal particles, which appear jet black because of geometric light trapping. In some instances with reactive metals, these particles flash and burn if they are at elevated temperature as they emerge from the inert gas cover.

For materials that are extremely sensitive to atmospheric contamination (e.g., the zircalloys) effective shielding may require that the workpiece be placed in an enclosed, inert-gas chamber (similar to a glove box used in conventional welding). The laser welding chamber should be provided with a controlled through flow of inert gas to prevent buildup of weld fumes, which can adversely influence welding performance. A small plasma suppression jet can be provided above the beam-material interaction point to prevent atmospheric breakdown, and a small opening can be used to permit beam delivery to the workpiece. The suppression jet gas choice may be helium; argon, or a mixture of argon and helium, can be used in the chamber.

Reducing Shielding Gas Cost

It is worth noting that the highest gas costs associated with production laser welding may be for the requirements of plasma suppression and shielding and not from the consumption of laser gases. At the lower end of the multikilowatt power spectrum, gases other than helium can effectively be used for laser welding of some materials. Carbon dioxide, for example, is commonly used in gas metal arc (GMAW) welding of low-carbon steel. Carbon dioxide can also be used for both plasma suppression and shielding in keyhole laser welding of low-carbon and alloy steels, particularly at the lower-power end of the multikilowatt spectrum. Required flow rates may be higher than those for helium and maximum weld penetrations may not be attained. For modest penetrations, however, carbon dioxide can sometimes yield a more desirable bead profile, as shown in Figure 6, particularly if a small quantity of helium is added.

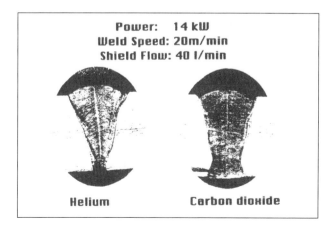

Figure 6. Shield gas effects on bead characteristics.

The cost implications of reducing helium requirements can be significant. For example, substituting a mixture of 95% carbon dioxide and 5% helium for 100% helium in a production application involving a 5-day, 3-shift operation at 80% duty cycle can yield an estimated annual cost savings of the order of $25,000 in the United States; higher values pertain in other industrial nations. Such savings can scale to the order of $1 million for plants utilizing tens of multikilowatt systems in six- or seven-day-a-week production.

Other Suppression Means

Other than the removal of seed ionization by flow of an appropriate inert, or minimally reactive, gas over the beam-material interaction point, plasma suppression may also be attained by reducing ambient pressure in the weld region to approximately 1/3 of an atmosphere. This procedure is not generally cost effective, but may be in welding of highly atmospheric-sensitive materials, which require processing in an enclosed chamber in order to prevent atmospheric contamination.

Another means for plasma suppression is use of a controlled, high-frequency interrupted output from the laser (3). This is possible because plasma breakdown does not occur instantly, but may require an onset time of the order of 100 ms under laser welding conditions. (Note that this is a consequence of the fact that welding irradiance is below the spontaneous breakdown level and breakdown occurs only when a sufficient density of free electrons is generated to initiate breakdown.) Decay of ionized species, on the other hand, takes place on a much more rapid time scale. Therefore, if the beam is turned off briefly before breakdown occurs, seed ionization essentially disappears and levels for plasma ignition are not attained.

11.2.9 Preheating

Preheating is commonly used in conventional welding of transformation-hardenable materials such as high-equivalent-carbon steels, or other materials subject to cracking during solidification and cooling. In view of the high cooling rates characteristic of keyhole laser welding, preheating is equally important for attainment of sound laser welds in thermally sensitive materials. A guideline for the preheat level required for beam welding may be obtained from that used in conventional welding. In general, the required preheat level increases with equivalent carbon content of the workpiece, as shown in Table 3.

Table 3. Representative Preheat Temperatures
(To ½ in. section thickness)

Material	Preheat temperature (°C)
1330 steel	180–230
4140 steel	200–260
5145 steel	200–260
8640 steel	180–230
D2 steel	370–480
M2 steel	510–590
Gray iron	320 min

Preheat may be achieved by flame, infrared heating with quartz lamps, electric resistance heating, or induction. The latter has the advantage of rapid local heating in depth. If preheat is used in thicker materials, care must be taken to provide sufficient thermal soaking time to ensure attainment of uniform temperature. Preheat temperature may be monitored with a pyrometer, thermocouple, temperature-indicating paint, or other means convenient to the application.

11.2.10 Spatter Control

Weld spatter is influenced by the characteristics of the material being welded as well as by the laser processing parameters being used. Rimmed steel, for example, is highly subject to spatter because of the presence of entrapped gas within the "rim." In this material, a thin coating of aluminum (which may be applied as an aluminum spray paint) serves to "kill" the fused material during the welding process. The positive influence of this simple procedure on the quality of beam welds in rimmed steel is very marked.

Effect of Irradiance

A sharply focused beam with good penetration characteristics has the tendency to expel material from the root of the fusion zone. This is particularly true if weld conditions are in an over-penetration mode in order to satisfy bead profile requirements. Under such conditions, an increase in weld speed, a slight defocusing of the beam spot, and/or a reduction in laser power will all tend to reduce the degree of spatter.

Dynamic Factors

In general, the higher the irradiance, the greater the probability that spatter will occur. This is influenced not only by the dc characteristics of the laser beam but by possible temporal variations. Many multikilowatt industrial laser systems exhibit an ac ripple in their power output that exceeds the dc variation but does not affect, and in some cases may enhance, typical laser welding performance. The effects of temporal power variations diminish at high frequencies, but can be significant at frequencies below 400 Hz, particularly if high welding speeds are involved. Consider, for example, a nominal 10-kW welding application for which a 20% peak-to-peak ripple exists in the output at a frequency of less than 1 kHz. Instantaneous power under these conditions fluctuates from 9 to 11 kW. At the upper power level, the higher power intensity can be instrumental in a significant increase in spatter because of overpenetration even though the general fusion zone characteristics are not affected. It is important in critical applications, therefore, to examine the temporal as well as the dc output characteristics of the beam. Minor modifications to the system, e.g., added power supply filtering, may be sufficient to mitigate such effects.

In some cases, the characteristics of the material and the required production rates do not permit total elimination of spatter during the welding process. In such instances, means may be taken to shield sensitive areas from spatter. Coating of adjacent material with conventional weld spatter spray will inhibit spatter adhesion; convective cooling of spattered material prior to its impingement on adjacent surfaces may also be beneficial in some circumstances.

11.2.11 Process Monitoring Systems

Optical Monitors

Various techniques are available for monitoring of the laser welding process (see Chapter 4). By far the most common are optical systems that measure the radiation from the beam-material interaction point. Typically such units measure both the infrared and the ultraviolet emission from the weld region.

The infrared emission from the weld zone is characterized by the melt zone temperature as well as its extent. If a standard acceptable emission band is established for the process, the system will respond to a signal outside the acceptable band and call attention to a potential defect. For example, if laser energy delivery to the workpiece is reduced as the result of any of various causes, the infrared signal from the resultant melt pool will decrease and a potentially unacceptable weld will be indicated.

The ultraviolet emission from the weld region is a measure of the intensity of the optical plasma adjacent to the workpiece surface. Note that, based on the general definition of a plasma as an electrically conducting gas, a "plasma" is normally present at the beam-material interaction point. Unacceptable conditions occur only when breakdown of the atmosphere occurs such that a high-optical-density plasma is formed that has the capability totally to block laser energy delivery to the workpiece. Acceptable weld conditions dictate that plasma emission be steady and within a bandwidth that has been established by processing experience. If atmospheric breakdown occurs, ultraviolet emission from the region will increase dramatically. Similarly, if emission is reduced, this may signal that plasma suppression means have failed, that laser energy delivery to the workpiece has been reduced, that an unacceptable joint gap has been encountered, and/or that other factors have changed that render weld quality suspect.

Optical monitoring systems designed for production laser weld use are available from several manufacturers. All offer associated computer capabilities that not only store but provide automatic information processing to yield statistically based limits.

Acoustic Monitors

Extensive evaluation of acoustic signals from laser welds has been conducted. Such tests have involved direct mounting of an acoustic sensor on the weldment, sensor mounting on system tooling, laser beam pickup from the material, and other indirect coupling means. Ultrasonic frequencies have typically been explored. The acoustic signals from laser welds are often complex and require innovative processing in order to simplify identification of potential defects. The potential for acoustic monitoring is attested by experience with audible emission from some welds. A steady, uniform hiss is generally indicative of uniform conditions and a "sound" weld. As with optical systems, a standard signal identifying an acceptable weld is first established on the basis of process experience. The standard acoustic signal, as processed, is then used to monitor the welds being generated.

Vision Systems

Direct viewing of the weld interaction point, or the completed weld, is also a means for monitoring weld uniformity. In such applications, the use of laser illumination of the weld region, in combination with appropriate wavelength filters, permits viewing of the weld without the obscuring interference of the laser-induced plasma above the workpiece surface. With such systems the width and other general features of the weld may provide an acceptable means for process monitoring. Further, a vision system can be used in advance of the weld to identify gaps between the faying surfaces. Gap information can then be utilized to modify weld parameters as a function of measured gap such that acceptable weld conditions are maintained. Such a modification may involve a change in the amplitude of beam weaving, a change in weld speed, and/or a change in filler metal delivery rate. Finally, if visual access to the root bead is available, this means can be used to verify attainment of adequate penetration as well as the existence of potential root bead defects.

11.2.12 Post Treatment

Although the laser provides unique welding capabilities, it does not result in obviating basic metallurgical requirements for attainment of desired fusion zone properties. As with other welding processes, the result of fusion is a recast structure that may, or may not, have the required properties. If fully hardened and aged aluminum alloys are welded, for example, the resultant fusion zone will not exhibit the same mechanical properties as those of the parent material even if appropriate filler material is used. For this reason it may be desirable to weld such material in a non-fully-aged condition so that the entire assembly can be postweld heat treated and aged to final conditions. Such a procedure can also eliminate potential weld cracking in fully strengthened materials.

Other examples of materials requiring postweld thermal treatment include inconel alloys, titanium alloys, and maraging steels. For these materials, final mechanical properties of the weldment are critically dependent upon the postweld heat treating process. Such is the case also for alloy steels that have restrictions on maximum-allowable fusion zone hardness (because of possible stress corrosion problems, etc.) even though as-welded mechanical properties are within acceptable limits.

The primary guideline for post-treatment of laser-welded materials is critically dependent on the characteristics of the material and its intended use. In some instances, as is the case with some titanium alloys, a simple elevated temperature stress relief may be adequate. Maraging steel must be aged following welding with the degree of aging dependent on the required service properties. In some materials slated for use in critical applications, e.g., inconel 718 in aerospace applications, complex high-temperature solution heat treatment and aging are required to develop the weldment's potential. Conventional welding practice and sound metallurgical guidelines (4) are the laser welder's allies in attainment of desired weldment characteristics.

11.2.13 Filler Material Considerations

Although laser welding is more generally suited to autogenous welding, filler material addition is feasible and sometimes desirable and/or essential in specific laser welding applications. The primary reasons for filler addition to laser welds are: (1) to compensate for imperfect fitup, (2) to modify fusion zone chemistry in order to attain desired weld properties, (3) to minimize part distortion and shrinkage during welding, and (4) a combination of these factors.

Laser welding with filler is most effective if keyhole welding characteristics are maintained. For this reason, applications that involve use of the laser as an alternative energy source for filler-added, thermal-diffusion-controlled welds are seldom cost effective. Within the keyhole welding restriction, filler materials established for conventional welding may be used as a starting point for laser welding applications. Filler material compositions recommended for specific classes of materials and applications are available from manufacturers as well as from welding handbooks, Mil specs, etc. As stated later, however, the relatively small dilution attainable in laser filler welds suggests that much higher alloying content may be appropriate for laser welding. Very little work has been done in this area and it represents a fruitful avenue for further research and development. Table 4 presents some suggested filler materials for aluminum alloys.

Table 4. Suggested Filler Material for Various Aluminum Alloys[a] (Note that selection is influenced by results desired.)

Base metal	Filler alloys[a]	
	Preferred for maximum as-welded tensile strength	Alternate filler alloys for maximum elongation
EC	1100	EC/1260
1100	1100/4043	1100/4043
2014	4145	4043/2319
2024	4145	4043/2319
2219	2319	–
3003	5183	1100/4043
3004	5554	5183/4043
5005	5183/4043	5183/4043
5050	5356	5183/4043
5052	5356/5183	5183/4043
5083	5183	5183
5086	5183	5183
5154	5356	5183/5356
5357	5554	5356
5454	5554	5356
5456	5556	5183
6061	4043/5183	5356
6063	4043/5183	5183
7039	5039	5183
7075	5183	–
7079	5183	–
7178	5183	–

[a]Source: From Kaiser Aluminum and Chemical, Inc., Welding Kaiser Aluminum (1967).

Fundamental to the filler addition process is that the extent of the fusion zone generated is primarily dependent upon power, irradiance, and welding process speed. Stated colloquially, the laser does not care whether the material being fused is parent or filler; the welding process energy balance determines the quantity of material melted. For this reason, a bead-on-plate penetration is an excellent starting point for developing a filler-added weld. Provided that the gap between weld and faying surfaces does not extend beyond the limits of the bead-on-plate weld, a laser weld with appropriate filler addition should proceed at essentially the same power and speed as that of the bead-on-plate penetration.

In traditional welding with filler addition it is customary to add filler material at the leading edge of the melt pool. This arrangement enhances mixing and is facilitated by the slow speeds and large extent of a conventional welding pool. In laser or electron beam welding, however, melt pool dimensions ahead of the beam impingement point are extremely small and require precise placement, control, and uniformity of welding conditions for successful implementation. In many high-power laser welding applications, therefore, it has been found advantageous to introduce filler wire into the trailing side of the melt pool. This approach relaxes positioning tolerances and permits convenient addition of significant amounts of filler material. Filler addition capability can be further enhanced by utilization of hot wire techniques.

A further consideration in the use of filler in laser welding is that the level of dilution attainable is relatively small. In contrast, the fusion zone composition of a conventional weld is quite often that of the filler. Mechanical test results for the "weld" therefore reflect the properties of the recast filler material and not those of the parent metal. Since filler dilution of a keyhole laser weld may only be of the order of 20%, the composition of a standard filler material may be totally inappropriate for laser welding. One approach to this dichotomy is to assume that the desirable composition of the material in the fusion zone should match that of the conventional filler material. Based on this assumption, the composition of an appropriate filler material can be calculated by a simple ratio of the known composition of the parent material and the assumed filler dilution rate. Development of appropriate filler material can be facilitated by the use of powder fill or hollow core wire. Figure 7 shows the joint geometry used with filler for a butt weld. Figure 8 shows the geometry used with filler for a tee weld. More information on the use of filler material is presented in Section 11.3.8.

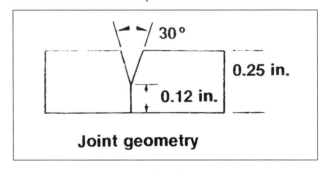

Figure 7. Joint geometry with filler for a butt weld.

Chapter 11: Penetration Welding

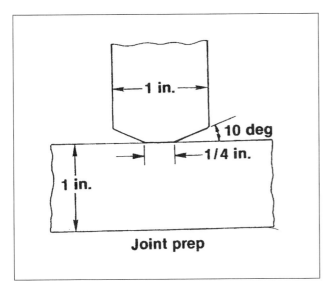

Figure 8. Joint geometry with filler for a tee weld.

References
1. J. Machon, et al., *Journal of Laser Applications* **8**, 225–32 (1996).
2. D. C. Smith, and M. C. Fowler, *Journal of Applied Physics* **46** (1), 138–50 (1975).
3. D. Belforte, and M. Levitt, (Eds.), 1986: *Industrial Laser Handbook,* 69–86, Pennwell Publishing, Tulsa, OK.
4. G. E. Linnert, *Welding Metallurgy,* Vol. 1, 4th Edition, AWS, 1994.

CONRAD M. BANAS

11.3 Welding Data Summary

11.3.1 High-Power Laser Welding of Common Materials

Process Requirements

The high-power (keyhole) laser beam welding of a metal (depicted in Fig. 1) is controlled by parameters that affect the absorption of the beam, the conduction of heat within the metal, and the stability of the weldpool. The first two effects determine the minimum irradiance and the beam power necessary to weld. Since the formation of plasma above the metal surface tends to absorb or defocus the beam energy, the beam focus position is normally placed inside the metal surface. In some instances, particularly with reflective metals, insufficient beam power or irradiance may necessitate the placement of the focus at the surface. The plasma caused by inverse Bremstrahlung is a function of the wavelength of the beam and the ionization potential of the metal vapor and the shielding gas used. The plasma tends to decrease penetration for CO_2 welding and is usually insignificant for the Nd:YAG case. Although the metal vapor tends to have a major effect on the plasma, the use of gases (e.g., argon, helium, carbon dioxide, nitrogen) with high ionization potential helps to decrease plasma formation. Helium with its high thermal conductivity that aids in thermal coupling is often preferred for the CO_2 case. Consequently, the use of cross-jet gas shielding to blow away the plasma usually increases penetration or weld speed for CO_2 laser welding. The cross-jet shielding works best when the plasma is blown away from the part to be welded.

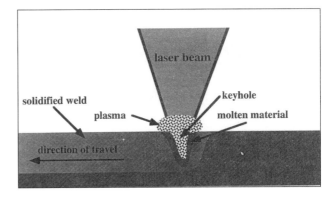

Figure 1. Schematic of laser beam keyhole welding process.

Before a keyhole is formed, the laser beam interacts with the metal and delivers the energy that is not reflected by the metal surface or absorbed by a plasma that may be present to the substrate metal. The reflectivity of metals tends to be high and decreases with wavelength and temperature. Table 1 lists absorptivities for some common metals at the melting point. The substantially higher absorptivities for the 1.06 μm wavelength of the Nd:YAG beam results in a lower beam irradiance requirement for welding than for CO_2 lasers. The minimum laser beam irradiance needed to initiate melting is obtained from the solution of the conservation of heat equation, giving the simple equation

$$I_m = k(T_{melt} - T_o)/Ad\, J_{max} \qquad (1)$$

where k is the thermal conductivity of the metal, T_{melt} is the melting point, T_0 is the initial temperature, A is the absorptivity of the surface, d is the diameter of the beam at the surface, and J_{max} is a nondimensional parameter obtained in the solution of the conservation of heat equation and is a function of the ratio of the thermal diffusivity to the product of the beam velocity and diameter (1). J_{max} increases somewhat linearly from 0.1 to 0.46 for α/vd of 0.01 to 1.0 (here α is the thermal diffusivity and v the weld speed) and has a limiting value of 0.52 for $\alpha/vd > 10$. Equation 1 predicts that higher irradiance is required when the absorptivity, beam diameter, or J_{max} is lower and the thermal conductivity or the melting point is higher. This trend is consistent with the physical phenomenon of heat transfer. Equation 1 accounts for the thermal conductivity of the substrate and the thermal diffusivity in relation to the welding speed and beam diameter. The behavior with beam diameter may not be immediately obvious and well known but helps to explain the differing requirements for welding aluminum with different laser systems, producing different focused beam diameters (2).

The threshold laser beam irradiance required for welding is greater than I_m with a value generally less than $10 I_m$ but $>10^5$ W/

Table 1. Thermophysical Properties at the Melting Point of Laser-Beam Welded[a] Metals

	α (cm^{2}s^{-1})	k (Wm^{-1}K^{-1})	T_{melt}(K)	A-10.6 μm(%)	A-1.06 μm (%)	η (kg m^{-1}s^{-1})	σ (Nm^{-1})
Al	0.68	210	933	5	-11	0.45	0.86
Cu	0.79	330	1357	5	25	0.34	1.3
Fe	0.063	30	1811	10	45	0.67	1.7

[a]Data from (3–8). α is the Thermal Diffusivity, k is the Thermal Conductivity, T_{melt} is the Melting Point, A is the Absorptivity, η is the viscosity, and σ is the surface tension.

cm^{-2} for CO_2 and Nd:YAG lasers to maintain the plasma and keyhole (3). The simple predictive equation provides a practical guide for the high-power laser welding of a variety of metals (1).

Welding Performance

The bulk of welding data and experience are for steel, an alloy that is well suited to laser beam welding. The relevant thermophysical properties of some common metals are listed in Table 1. The high reflectivity, thermal diffusivity, and thermal conductivity of aluminum necessitate the use of a substantially higher beam irradiance for welding. The surface tension and viscosity of molten steel are relatively high so that a stable keyhole can be obtained for a range of welding parameters. The low surface tension and viscosity of molten aluminum produces an unstable keyhole during welding, resulting in high spatter and low surface weld quality with undercut (2). In addition, dropout occurs for some alloys, particularly for wider welds. An optimal weld can be obtained with aluminum but with a much narrower range of parameters than steel. The higher absorptivity of aluminum for the 1.06-μm-wavelength beam of the Nd:YAG laser results in a lower threshold beam irradiance requirement for welding. Consequently, a more stable keyhole and better surface weld quality can be obtained using continuous wave Nd:YAG lasers compared to CO_2 lasers.

Use of an adequate value of the beam irradiance does not necessarily produce a good weld. The stability and condition of the molten weld pool will govern the surface quality, and the thermophysical properties of the constituents will determine the properties of the weld. For a given laser beam irradiance (i.e., power and spot size used) a higher weld speed will result in lower weld penetration and narrower weld widths. For a full penetration weld, low weld speeds may produce dropout. To maintain the weld penetration, the laser beam irradiance has to be increased for higher weld speeds. In practice, for a given laser system, the power is increased. However, as power and speed are steadily increased, the weld surface transitions from being relatively smooth to ropey to humping with undercut. These different regimes are shown in Figures 2a and b for full penetration welds on stainless steel and carbon steel (9). Innovative techniques can be used to extend the regime of smooth welds. One is the use of the dual-beam technique with the beams aligned in the direction of welding. Good welds at a higher speed regime can be obtained compared to using a conventional single beam at the same power. An alternative to this technique is the use of an oblong or high-aspect-ratio beam with the long axis aligned in the direction of welding. This technique is easier to implement using two mirrors than two laser beams.

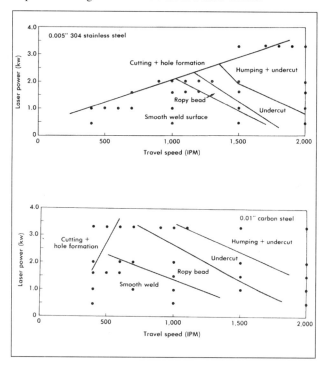

Figure 2. Map of weld bead profiles as functions of weld speed and laser power. (a) 0.12-mm-thick 304 stainless steel; (b) 0.12- and 0.25-mm-thick carbon steel (9).

It should be noted that the tendency of metals to have a higher absorptivity for shorter laser beam wavelengths does not imply more efficient welding with Nd:YAG lasers compared to CO_2 lasers when keyhole stability is not a problem. When threshold irradiance is exceeded, the beam couples efficiently with the plasma and keyhole and the weld is determined by the beam power available. This situation is demonstrated in Figure 3, which compares the welding speed at full penetration on stainless steel at different beam powers (10). Although the beam quality of the CO_2 beam was significantly better and the spot size was smaller than the Nd:YAG case, the weld widths obtained were similar, resulting in similar weld speeds for the same beam power applied. The data include CW and pulsed beams and show the energy-limited nature of the process when beam power is efficiently coupled into the metal.

Chapter 11: Penetration Welding

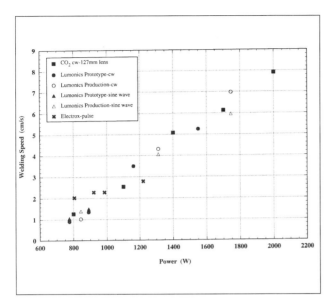

Figure 3. Welding speeds obtained for full penetration lap welds on two layers of 0.8-mm-thick aluminum-bearing stainless steel (12 SR). A Rofin-Sinar RS 6000 laser produced the TEM_{20} CO_2 beam with a focused spot of 0.3 mm. The Nd:YAG lasers used 1 mm fibers for beam delivery with M^2 of approximately 150 and a focused spot of 0.5 mm.

Welding with Pulsed Beams

Pulsed laser beam welding generally is slower than cw laser welding. The need to overlap pulses and the cooling or dissipation of heat between pulses limits the efficiency of the process. However, note that the pulsed Nd:YAG results in Figure 3 exhibit a different trend. At low average power (< 1000 W), the weld speeds achieved using the pulsed Electrox laser are significantly higher than those obtained using cw laser beams. For low average power, the peak power of the Electrox pulses was 4 kW with a substantially higher penetration capability than the lower power of the cw lasers. This high peak power more than compensates the low-welding-speed limitation of relatively low-repetition-rate pulsed welding. At power levels > 1000 W, the irradiance available is adequate to penetrate the material without resorting to significant weld speed reduction. Consequently, the weld speeds achieved with CW lasers are higher than in the pulsed case. The high-peak-power capability of low-average-power Nd:YAG lasers is cost efficient when relatively deep penetration is required but weld speed is not important.

The high peak power produced by pulsed laser beams may be a disadvantage when welding metals that have low viscosity or surface tension in the molten state. For the case of most industrial pulsed Nd:YAG lasers, the maximum average beam power output is produced with high-peak-power pulses and low repetition rate or low-peak-power pulses with high repetition rate. Frequently, the maximum pulse repetition rate is limited to several hundred per second and the maximum average power is obtained with higher-peak-power pulses and lower repetition rates. Welding of aluminum requires low peak irradiance above the threshold value to obtain optimal weld bead quality (smoothness). This situation compromises the maximum average power and consequently welding speed that can be used to produce good welds on aluminum or other metal with low viscosity or surface tension in the molten state.

Weld Metallurgy

Compared to conventional arc welding techniques, laser beam keyhole welding typically produces narrower joints with smaller heat-affected zones. Since the incident energy is focused on the region to be welded, very little energy is wasted on microstructural changes in the surrounding material. This allows more of the material to retain its original structure, and minimizes the volume of material in which weld defects may occur and distortion of the workpiece. Figures 4 and 5 show partial and full penetration laser beam keyhole welds on steel that are used to illustrate typical characteristics and defects. Figure 4 is a bead-on-plate (BOP) weld on 1045 steel, and Figure 5 is a full-penetration BOP weld on 1020 steel. The weld sections were etched to delineate the fusion heat-affected zones and the base metal.

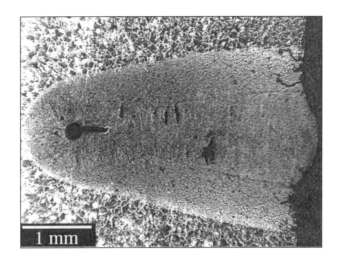

Figure 4. Micrograph of a CO_2 laser beam weld on 1045 steel showing root porosity and solidification cracking. The partial penetration bead-on-plate weld was made at 3.9 kW and 100 ipm with focus at the surface using a 6 in. off-axis parabola producing a 400-μm spot size.

The nugget geometry of a laser beam keyhole weld is quite different from that obtained with arc welding techniques. Because of the high energy density, the fusion zone is generally small with a large depth-to-width ratio (see Figs. 4 and 5). The small size and large surface area to volume ratio of the fusion zone allow more rapid cooling and solidification, which produces small grain sizes and a fine dendritic microstructure. The high strength and uniform phase distribution of this rapidly solidified structure produces high-quality welds.

In addition to the small fusion zone, laser welds also have narrow heat-affected zones. This is particularly important in steels, since the formation of martensite can be a significant problem. The hard and brittle martensite phase is not very tough, and cracks or a sudden jolt can lead to failure in this region. Minimizing the volume of material in the heat-affected zone greatly reduces the chances that this region will fail. Steels with higher carbon contents form martensite, which is harder and more brittle, which makes it particularly difficult to produce crack-free welds in these materials.

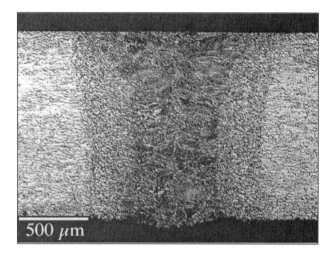

Figure 5. Micrograph of a CO_2 laser beam weld on cold-rolled 1020 steel. The full penetration bead-on-plate weld was made at 4.1 kW and 170 ipm with focus at the surface using a 6 in. parabola and a 400-μm spot size.

Porosity in laser beam welds is no more common than in other types of welding, but there are several instances when it may become a problem (11). When relatively deep, blind welds are made and vapors from outgassing or bubbles cannot escape, the narrow keyhole closes and the material solidifies, leaving pores at the root of the weld. Figure 4 shows a weld with root porosity. Hydrogen porosity is common in aluminum welding, since the solubility of hydrogen in molten aluminum is much higher than in the solid. Hydrogen from water vapor or solvents is dissolved in the molten metal during welding, and when the material solidifies, the hydrogen comes out of solution and forms pores. It is common for aluminum welds to have several small (<0.1 mm) voids in the fusion zone, which typically do not degrade the weld integrity or strength.

There are several types of cracks observed in laser beam welds (11). Solidification or hot cracking occurs at temperatures between the liquidus and the solidus when the material is not completely solidified and under contraction stresses. The liquid film between dendrites may pull apart due to solidification contraction stresses, leaving behind cracks. These cracks are typically near the centerline of the weld, which is the last place to solidify. The smaller the solidification temperature range, the less likely that these types of crack will occur. This is one reason why lower-carbon steels exhibit less cracking than higher-carbon steels. Crack-free welds are obtained in 1020 steel (Fig. 5), as opposed to the poor welds in 1045 material (Fig. 4). High sulfur levels in steel can also promote cracking by the formation of a low-melting-point iron sulfide.

Cold cracking in steel is typically aided by the presence of hydrogen, a brittle martinsitic microstructure, and residual stresses from weld solidification. The cracks usually form in the heat-affected zone, where their growth is aided by the hydrogen released and the contraction stresses from the solidification process. Another type of crack in the heat-affected zone is a liquation crack, which forms when a low-melting-point compound is melted and pulls apart due to weld solidification contraction stresses. Liquation cracks are common in aluminum alloys containing low-melting-point eutectics.

Mechanical Properties

When a sound weld is produced with little porosity and no cracks, weld strength is usually not an issue. The fine microstructure resulting from the rapid solidification of steel welds usually has higher hardnesses and tensile strengths than the base metal. However, a material's ductility usually decreases as its strength increases. For this reason, steel welds usually do not exhibit the same ductility and formability of the base metal. Sound welds and designs that limit stress concentrations are necessary to achieve acceptable fatigue properties.

As the hardness of the metal increases, so does the tensile strength. Approximate equivalent hardness numbers and tensile strengths are available for carbon and alloy steels in the annealed, normalized, and quench and tempered conditions (12). This allows comparisons of hardness values measured on different scales, as well as an estimate of the tensile strength. The weld microstructure is in the as-solidified condition; so this table should be used cautiously.

A hardness profile of a weld in a low-carbon steel (Fig. 5) is shown in Figure 6. The highest hardness was measured in the weld region, in which rapid solidification produced a fine microstructure of martensite, bainite, and ferrite. The heat-affected zone had an intermediate hardness, and the base metal was the softest. Similar measurements in a steel with a carbon level of 0.45% reveal that the hardness of the heat-affected zone is actually higher than the fusion zone, since the heating and rapid cooling of the heat-affected zone leads to formation of a very hard martensitic structure.

The strength of welds in aluminum alloys may be higher or lower than the base material. Evaporation and dissolving of alloying elements generally leads to lower strengths. The strength of the weld may be higher because of a finer weld microstructure and oxide inclusions. The greater thermal conductivity of aluminum alloys helps to produce a finer microstructure, while a greater affinity for oxygen increases the chance of oxide inclusions in the weld. Improved gas shielding above the requirements for welding steel may then be necessary to prevent significant oxide formation. Heat-affected zones in aluminum can be softer because of dissolving of precipitates and annealing of cold worked structures.

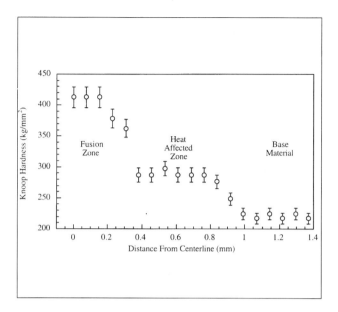

Figure 6. Hardness profile of the weld region in Figure 5 showing variation across the fusion and heat-affected zones and base metal.

The tensile strength of welds is measured using tensile specimens with the weld either perpendicular or parallel to the stress axis (2). Since the weld is usually stronger than the base material for steel, failure usually occurs near the weld interface. Incompatibility stresses result between the deformed base material and the undeformed weld. Welds in some aluminum alloys may be softer than the base material; so failure can occur within the weld. In addition, the presence of undercut would tend to decrease weld strength with the decrease in material thickness. Fracture may also occur in the weld if undercut is significant, since stress concentrations may result from the decreased cross-sectional area in the weld.

Ductility and formability are measures of the deformation of a material before failure. Ductility is typically the elongation or strain to failure in a tensile test. Formability is a more strenuous test, in which the material is deformed biaxially until separation. Typical formability tests involve deforming a square sheet of metal into a dome, with the formability specified as the dome height when cracking occurs. The results of a formability test are particularly important in the case of tailor blank welding, in which the welded sheet stock is subsequently stamped or formed. Since the weld is usually stronger than the base metal (steel), it is more resistant to deformation. Once again, this incompatibility between the weld and base material alters deformation patterns, and cracking usually initiates at the weld interface.

Fatigue failure of welds is caused by the cyclic loading and unloading of the joint. Fatigue is the most common failure mechanism in welded joints, since the stresses needed to produce fatigue failure are usually lower than those necessary for plastic deformation. The fatigue process generally consists of nucleation and growth of cracks. The nucleation of cracks within the weld is aided by residual solidification stresses, stress concentration from sharp edges and undercut, and the presence of hydrogen. Existing weld defects such as cracks and porosity enable the fatigue process to proceed directly to the crack growth phase. Laser welds typically have higher fatigue resistance because of smaller weld and heat-affected-zone volumes.

References

1. K. H. Leong, H. K. Geyer, K. R. Sabo, and P. G. Sanders, *Threshold Laser Beam Irradiances for Melting and Welding*, J. Laser Applications **9**, 227 (1997).
2. K. H. Leong, K. R. Sabo, P. G. Sanders, and W. J. Spawr, *Laser Beam Welding of Aluminum Alloys*, SPIE Proceedings Lasers as Tools for Manufacturing II **2993**, (1997).
3. C. J. Nonhof, 1988: *Material Processing with Nd-Lasers*. Electrochemical Publications, Ayr, Scotland
4. Y. S. Touloukian, R. W. Powell, C. Y. Ho, and M. C. Nicolaou, 1973: *Thermophysical Properties of Matter, Thermal Diffusivity* **10**, IFI/Plenum, New York.
5. Y. S. Touloukian, R. W. Powell, C. Y. Ho, and M. C. Nicolaou, 1970: *Thermal Conductivity Metallic Elements and Alloys, Thermophysical Properties of Matter* **1**, IFI/Plenum, New York.
6. A. M. Prokhorov, V. Konov, I. Ursu, and I. N. Mihailescu, 1990: *Laser Heating of Metals*, Adam Hilger, New York.
7. B. Hüttner, *Optical Properties of Polyvalent Metals in the Solid and Liquid State*: Aluminum, J. Phys. Condensed Matter **6**, 2459–74 (1994).
8. J. Elliott, and M. Gleiser, *Thermochemistry for Steelmaking*, Addison-Wesley Publishing Company, Inc., Reading, **1**, 296 (1960).
9. C. E. Albright, and S. Chiang, *High Speed Laser Welding Discontinuities*. Proceedings of the 7th International Conference on Applications of Lasers and Electro Optics ICALEO, Santa Clara, CA, 207–13 (1988).
10. K. H. Leong, L. A. Carol, and H. N. Bransch, *Welding with High Power CO_2 and Nd:YAG Lasers,* Industrial Laser Review (June 1994).
11. C. Dawes, 1992: *Laser Welding*, McGraw-Hill, New York.
12. H. E. Boyer, and T. L. Gall (Eds.), 1985: *Metals Handbook*, ASM International, Metals Park, OH.

KENG H. LEONG
PAUL G. SANDERS

11.3.2 CO_2 Laser CW Seam Welding of Common Materials; Conditions for Penetration Welding

Low-power CO_2 CW seam welding encompasses two distinct modes of laser welding: conduction welding and deep-penetration (keyhole) welding. Irradiance (power density) at the work surface will determine which of the two modes will dominate the process. Because of the high surface reflectivity and thermal conductivity of aluminum and copper alloys, low-power CW CO_2 welding has virtually no application for them. Data presented in this section will deal mainly with iron-based alloys.

Conduction Mode

Characterized by surface melting only, conduction welding is relatively inefficient and limited to shallow penetration. For iron-based alloys, irradiance in the 10^5 W/cm^2 range will couple to the material surface without creating a keyhole. The melt volume is created by conduction heating. Welds made in the conduction mode are roughly hemispherical, with an aspect ration of 1:1 or less. For CO_2 laser radiation, a large percentage of the laser energy will be reflected from the material surface. Maintaining sufficient irradiance to cause surface melting yet not causing vaporization limits the practical applications for conduction welding.

Deep-Penetration Mode

The deep-penetration mode is desirable for most applications. Irradiance greater than 10^5 W/cm^2 is necessary to generate the keyhole for deep-penetration welds. At power levels below 1000 W, relatively short focusing lenses are required to achieve this irradiance. Table 2 shows examples of typical lens and power combinations required to achieve deep-penetration mode at low power.

Table 2. Examples of Power and Lens Combinations for Deep-Penetration Welding

Power (W)	Focal length (mm)	Lens type	Spot diameter (mm)	Irradiance (MW/cm²)
200	63.5	Aspheric	0.120	1.8
1000				8.8
400	95.3	Meniscus	0.170	1.7
1000				4.4
700	127	Plano-convex	0.220	1.8
1000				2.6

Input beam diameter, 15 mm. $M^2 = 1.7$

According to the table, deep-penetration welding can occur with total power as low as 200 W if the conditions are right.

Depth of Focus

A difficulty with using a short-focal-length lens is the reduced depth of focus. For example, the depth of focus for a 63.5-mm-focal-length lens with a spot diameter of 0.120 mm is approximately 0.5 mm. This can create significant difficulty in maintaining optimum focus conditions in production welding. Alternatively, a 127-mm-focal-length lens, with a spot diameter of 0.240 mm, has a depth of focus of approximately 1.7 mm. This allows for more variation in focus-lens-to-work distance while maintaining optimum focus.

Shielding Gas

Weld-penetration plasma effects from shielding gas are not generally of concern with low-power welding up to 1 kW. With its higher ionization potential and higher thermal conductivity, helium will provide an improvement in penetration over argon up to 20% above 1 kW.

Penetration

For a given material, weld penetration is controlled by the combination of power, focused spot size, and travel speed. Different combinations of these parameters can yield the same penetration results but will produce different weld width. For example, high irradiance at fast travel speed will produce a weld with narrow width. Lowering the travel speed, while maintaining the same irradiance, will increase both penetration and width.

Increasing travel speed and power will increase melting efficiency and therefore provide lower heat input. Melting efficiency is the ratio of heat necessary to melt the fusion zone to the heat absorbed by the workpiece (13). High melting efficiency will reduce distortion and allow welding near heat-sensitive components.

Developing a set of operating parameters to meet a specific weld requirement is frequently done on a trial basis. Graphs of penetration and travel speed are often consulted to establish initial parameters for weld trials. Figures 7 to 10 show several examples of penetration and travel speed comparisons at specific operating conditions for relatively low-power CW CO_2 welding. Caution should be used when consulting such graphs to verify similar operating conditions. Comparable graphs can be user generated for particular laser and operating characteristics and can be consulted for future weld development to ensure accurate results.

According to Table 2, these figures represent conditions at or above the threshold for penetration welding to occur.

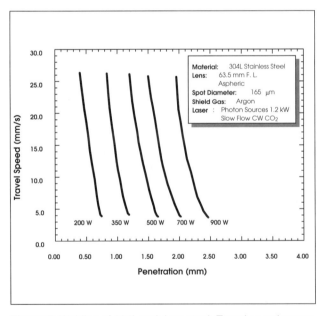

Figure 7. Welding of 304L stainless steel. Travel speed versus penetration at several power levels for a 63.5-mm-focal-length-focus lens.

ISBN 0-912035-15-3

Chapter 11: Penetration Welding

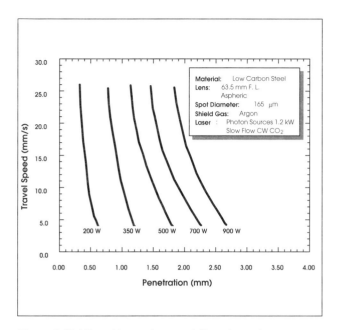

Figure 8. Welding of low carbon steel. Travel speed versus penetration at several power levels for a 63.5-mm-focal-length-focus lens.

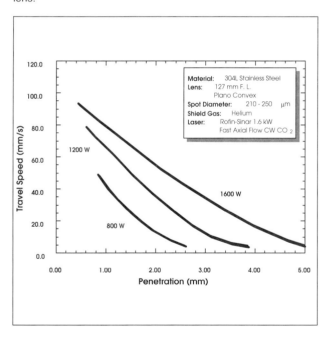

Figure 9. Welding of 304L stainless steel. Travel speed versus penetration at several power levels for a 127-mm-focal-length-focus lens.

Repeatability

The repeatability for the CW CO_2 welding process is highly dependent on process control. Inconsistencies can arise from any of various process parameters. Table 3 lists the primary parameters for which particular attention is required to ensure repeatability.

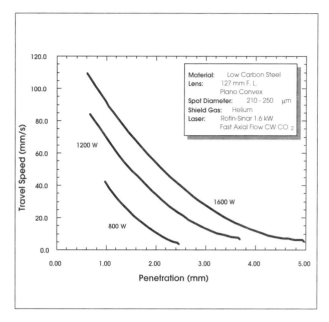

Figure 10. Welding of low carbon steel. Travel speed versus penetration at several power levels for a 127-mm-focal-length-focus lens.

Table 3. Welding Parameters and Related Causes for Weld Inconsistencies

Parameter	Possible causes
Irradiance	Power variation.
	Inconsistent focus spot size.
Power	Laser resonator problems.
	Contaminated or damaged mirrors.
	Contamination or damage to focus lens.
Focus spot size	Lens damage. Incorrect focus position.
	Inadequate depth of focus.
Travel speed	Machine control error. Drive system faults.

References

13. P. W. Fuerschbach, *Welding Journal* **75** (1), 24s–34s (1996).
L. Migliore, (Ed.), 1996: *Laser Materials Processing*, Marcel Dekker, Inc., New York, NY, Chapter 7.

ROBERT J. STEELE

11.3.3 CW CO_2 Laser Welding of Common Materials

CO_2 laser beam welding of common materials can be conveniently divided into thin and thick section welding. Thin section welding usually refers to a depth of penetration less than 6 mm.

Thin-Section Welding

Common engineering alloys that can normally be fusion welded can normally be autogenously laser beam welded in thin sections with a CO_2 laser. Figure 11 shows the welding speeds as a function of thickness for two laser powers and for both carbon and stainless steel. These welds were fabricated with a 150-mm focusing optic and argon shielding.

ISBN 0-912035-15-3

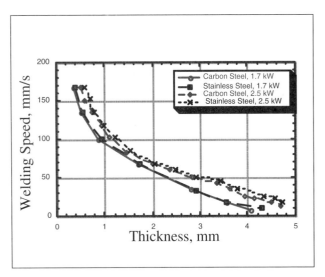

Figure 11. Welding speed as a function of thickness for two laser powers and carbon and stainless steel.

Most aluminum alloys are difficult to weld with the CO_2 laser. This is a result of the depletion of alloying elements during the welding process, both in conduction and keyhole welding. Some aluminum alloys are also prone to solidification cracking.

Titanium and its alloys have been successfully welded with the CO_2 laser. Some of these welds are hermetic seals.

Thick-Section Welding

Thick-section laser beam welding has only recently been embraced by the auto industry. Most of these applications are aptly described as "little round parts." However, a significant effort has established that laser beam welding of thick-section steel fabricates welds that have the required properties. The chemistry of the steel and especially the carbon content should be used as a guide as to the autogenous weldability of the steel. The more stringent the requirements for conventional welding, the less likely that laser beam welding will be successful.

The laser beam welding of steels depends on the irradiance, the focal point relative to the top surface of the plate, the welding speed, and the composition of the steel. Figure 12 shows the range of thickness of A36 steel that can be welded with satisfactory properties at different laser powers measured at the top surface of the steel and different welding speeds. For each thickness of steel, there is an envelope formed by the upper and lower limits of successful welds fabricated at the laser power and travel speed. All these welds were made with the steel horizontal and the laser beam vertical (down hand position) and with the focal point of the laser beam inside the steel and an f number of about 8. Although the diagram is for A36 steel, the data can be used as an approximation for most other steels.

The hardness of A36 steel laser beam welds in the as-welded and stress relief condition is shown in Figure 13. The hardness of the fusion zone is almost twice the value of the base plate. This is a result of the very fast cooling rate of laser beam welding and the carbon content of A36 steel. This figure also indicates the narrowness of both the fusion and HAZ in a 13-mm-thick plate.

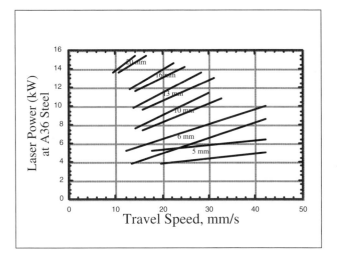

Figure 12. Laser power as a function of welding speed for different thickness A36 steel.

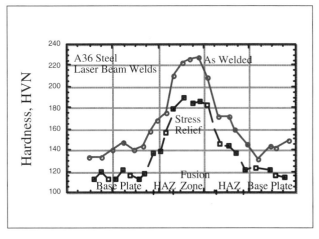

Figure 13. Hardness traverse across a laser beam weld of A36 steel.

The Charpy V-notch values as a function of temperature for the A36 steel base plate (two orientations, T-L and L-T), the as-welded and stress relief condition are shown in Figure 14. Charpy specimens were taken from 13-mm-thick laser beam weldment. The laser beam welds denoted as LB-SR were stress relieved at 900°C for 1 h. Above 20°C, the Charpy V-notch values of the LB-SR specimens were very near the limit of the testing machine. At least three specimens were tested at each temperature, and the average is plotted.

Thick-section aluminum alloys are welded only with difficulty and often require the addition of filler metal to retain adequate properties.

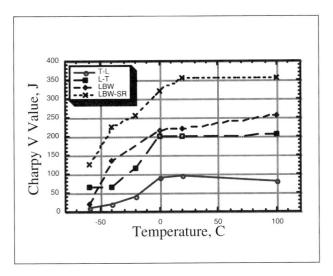

Figure 14. Charpy V-notch values as a function of temperature for A36 base plate and laser beam welds (LBW).

Titanium and its alloys have been successfully laser beam welded. Alpha titanium alloys do not require a postweld heat treatment, whereas alpha and beta titanium and beta alloys usually require annealing. Care must be taken to avoid the pick up of oxygen when laser beam welding titanium and its alloys.

Reference
E. A. Metzbower, R. A. Hella, and G. Theodorski, *Applications of Lasers in Materials Processing,* ASM International, Materials Park, OH, 1983.

E. A. METZBOWER

11.3.4 Pulsed CO_2 Laser Welding of Common Metals
Pulsed CO_2 laser welding may also be performed with average power in the multi-kilowatt regime with deep penetration. Table 4 (next two pages) presents results obtained for pulsed CO_2 laser welding of a variety of metals, for average powers up to 5.4 kW.

CHRIS RICKERT

11.3.5 Nd:YAG CW Welding of Common Materials
Since the early industrial application of Nd:YAG lasers, they have been widely used in the pulsed mode for welding, either for spot welding or by overlapped spots for seam welding. Typical average powers have been 100 W, with pulsed operation necessary to give sufficient irradiance to achieve the melt depth (typically < 2 mm) to affect the weld. Historically, the major use has been in electronics and other industries for precision-type applications.

Although a 1.1-kW CW Nd:YAG laser was first built in 1972, the technology for industrial kilowatt lasers was not developed until the end of the 1980s, and only in the past 2–3 years have applications begun to emerge. Although the current installed base is small (probably only 100–200 CW Nd:YAG lasers of 1 kW power and above in industrial applications by the middle of 1997), the number is rising rapidly. In comparison, market studies (14) show that the total number of industrial Nd:YAG lasers currently sold each year is 4,000. The great majority of kilowatt Nd:YAG laser installations are for welding tasks.

During the 1980s, a number of initiatives were undertaken to raise Nd:YAG laser power. A major stimulus for this was the realization that fiber-optic beam delivery, available with Nd:YAG lasers, provided an opportunity to increase the application of the technology in manufacturing, particularly if the laser power could be significantly increased to raise welding speed and penetration. Work centered on higher-average-power pulsed systems (e.g., by adding laser amplifier stages) and quasi-CW systems formed by interleaving pulsed beams. The results showed that, not only was fiber-optic beam delivery usable at these powers, but that at greater than 500 W, the welding transitioned from surface conduction to a penetration process. This effect seems to have been first noted in 1976 (15). Since beam irradiance is important to the welding process, major effort was made by laser suppliers not only to develop products with high power, but also to ensure that the beam could be focused to a small spot on the work at an acceptable working distance; typically 75–200 mm. In practice, this has meant developing kilowatt Nd:YAG lasers with fiber-optic beam delivery using fibers of core size in the 400–1000 μm diameter range.

The state of the art for CW Nd:YAG products today is 4 kW available on the work delivered via a 600-μm core silica fiber, focused to a spot in the range 300–1000 μm diameter. There appears to be no physical reasons why laser powers to 10 kW cannot be delivered by a single fiber of this size, and industry forecasters expect to see products to this power developed as kilowatt welding with the current products becomes more widely established.

The welding procedures developed with kilowatt Nd:YAG lasers have shown that pulsed or modulated operation is probably only advantageous with products to 1–2 kW average power, e.g., to achieve improved coupling in high-conductivity materials such as aluminum alloys, or to maximize penetration in thick-section materials. Figures 15 and 16 are examples showing the improvement in penetration achievable with a 2-kW laser operated modulated at 100 Hz to 3.5-kW peak power in low-speed welding of carbon steel and stainless steel or nickel-based alloys, respectively (16). In these cases Ar cover gas was used; other welding parameters were unchanged, and the average power at the work was constant at 1.7 kW. For welding at laser powers above this range, experiments show that the results are usually superior with CW beams. Recently CW Nd:YAG products with fiber-optic beam delivery to 2–4 kW power at the work have become commercially available. A major stimulus for the development of these products has been automotive applications.

The availability of Nd:YAG lasers of 2–4 kW power has been so recent that the welding performance is still the subject of major study. The effect of some key parameters (e.g., beam power, spot size, gas cover, etc.) on welding performance is becoming clear, and the following data are taken from the recent literature.

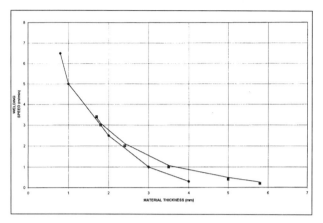

Figure 15. Welding performance in carbon steel. Diamonds: CW operation at 2000 W. Squares: Modulated to 3500 W peak power.

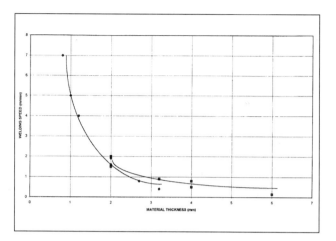

Figure 16. Welding performance in stainless steel and Ni-based alloys. Diamonds: CW operation at 2000 W. Squares: Modulated operation at 3500 W peak power.

Table 4. Pulsed CO_2 Laser Welding of Common Metals

Material	Pulse width (ms)	Average power (kW)	Frequency (Hz)	Travel speed (mm/s)
Aluminum 5005	76	3.0	10	17
Aluminum 5005	15.3	3.0	50	50
Aluminum 5251	76	3.0	10	17
Aluminum 5251	15.3	3.0	50	50
Aluminum 5754	76	3.0	10	17
Aluminum 5754	15.3	3.0	50	67
Aluminum 6061	76	3.0	10	17
Aluminum 6061	7.6	3.0	100	67
1008	5	2.5	100	16.67
1008	5	2.5	100	33.34
1008	5	2.5	100	50
1008	3.33	2.5	300	16.67
1008	3.33	2.5	300	33.34
1008	3.33	2.5	300	50
1008	6	2.5	100	33.34
1008	7	2.5	100	33.34
1008	8	2.5	100	33.34
1010	Gated	1.5	40,000	63
1010	Gated	3	40,000	63
1010	Gated	3.6	40,000	63
1010	Gated	4.2	40,000	63
1010	Gated	4.8	40,000	63
1010	Gated	5.4	40,000	63
Hastelloy X	0.2	0.45	250	22
Inconel 718	0.2	0.45	250	22
Inconel 718	17	3.2	50	25
Nitronic 30	Gated	4.2	50,000	42
Nitronic 30	Gated	3.6	40,000	63.5
Nitronic 30	Gated	5	50,000	74
316 S.S.	2.25	0.16	125	10.6
316 S.S.	2.25	0.07	125	10.6
304 S.S.	Gated	1.5	40,000	63.5
304 S.S.	Gated	1.5	40,000	63.5
304 S.S.	0.9	0.4	200	25

Chapter 11: Penetration Welding

Steel welding speed versus penetration data published for the Hobart HLP3000 (now Lumonics MW3000) laser, which operates to 2.5 kW on the work, is presented in Table 5.

Table 5. Hobart HLP3000 Welding Data: 600-μm Fiber, 2.5 kW at Work

Thickness (mm)	Description	Speed (m/min)
2 x 0.8	Uncoated steel, butt joint	10.2
2 x 0.8	Zn-coated steel, butt joint	10.2
2 x 0.8	Uncoated steel, lap joint	5.1
2 x 0.8	Zn-coated steel, lap joint	4.6
1	1020 Steel, bead on plate	12
2	As above	4
4	As above	1.2
6.8	As above	0.6
8	As above	0.2

Maximum speeds in the 5–10 m/min range are possible for welding thin automotive-type low-carbon steel body shell materials. There is also an interest in 2D and 3D laser welding of Al-alloy sheet (typically in the 1–2.5 mm range) for the automotive industry, and this has been studied. Table 6 is a comparison using the Haas HL3006D laser, of the welding speeds for low-carbon steel and 6000 series Al alloy with 3 kW at the work. Despite the significant difference in material conductivity, the table shows similar speeds are achievable under these conditions of welding with the laser focused to a small spot, corresponding to an irradiance of 5 MW/cm^{-2}.

In many practical situations, jigging and fit-up issues preclude use of a tightly focused laser beam for welding. Welding results have been obtained with different combinations of focusing optics to give a range of spot sizes. The results for welds in two types of Al alloys, with a beam of 3.3 kW focused to 0.3–0.8 mm on the work, are given in Table 7. The results show that, once sufficient irradiance is achieved to couple power into the work, the speed is not too sensitive to the focused spot size.

Focus position (mm)	Shielding gas	Weld type	Penetration (mm)	Comments
0	He	Butt weld	2.0	8.7% elongation
0	He	Butt weld	2.0	6.3% elongation
0	He	Butt weld	2.0	14% elongation
0	He	Butt weld	2.0	13% elongation
0	He	Butt weld	2.0	12 % elongation
0	He	Butt weld	2.0	17.2% elongation
0	He	Butt weld	1.6	5.0% elongation
0	He	Butt weld	1.6	4.5% elongation
0	He	Bead on plate	7.5	
0	He	Bead on plate	6	
0	He	Bead on plate	5	
0	He	Bead on plate	6	
0	He	Bead on plate	4.75	
0	He	Bead on plate	3.75	
0	He	Bead on plate	4.5	
0	He	Bead on plate	3.5	
0	He	Bead on plate	4	
0	He	Bead on plate	2	Undercut
0	Hc	Bead on plate	2.5	Undercut
0	He	Bead on plate	6.25	
0	He	Bead on plate	6.5	
0	He	Bead on plate	7.5	
0	He	Bead on plate	8	
0	He	Bead on plate		
0	He	Bead on plate		
0	He	Bead on plate	3.0	
0	He	Flare	4.3	
0	He	Flare	3.8	
0	He	Flare	5.6	
0	He	Edge	0.762	
0	He	Edge	0.381	
0	He	Fillet	0.5	
0	He	Fillet	0.5	
0	He	Bead on plate		

Table 6. Haas HL3006D Welding Data: 600-μm Fiber, 3.0 kW at Work

Low-carbon (mild) steel, bead on plate		Aluminum alloy (6000), bead on plate	
Thickness (mm)	Speed (m/min)	Thickness (mm)	Speed (m/min)
1.5	12.5	1.6	11
2	8	2	9
2.5	4.5	2.5	6.2
3	3.5	3	3.9
3.5	2.8	4	2
5	1		

Table 7. Lumonics Nd:YAG Welding Data: Effect of Spot Size at Constant Power[a]

Material type	Thickness (mm)	Spot size (mm)	Power at work (kW)	Speed (m/min)
6082 Al alloy	1.6	0.3	3.3	11
		0.5		11
		0.6		7.5
		0.8		0
	3	0.3	3.3	3.8
		0.5		3.5
		0.6		3
		0.8		0
5083 Al alloy	1.6	0.3	3.3	13
		0.5		12
		0.6		9.6
		0.8		7
	3	0.3	3.3	5
		0.5		5
		0.6		4
		0.8		3

[a]All results are bead on plate.

The foregoing discussion has emphasized welding speed. In terms of weld quality, the results with kilowatt Nd:YAG lasers are often compared with those achieved with CO_2 lasers, because the latter have been used at kilowatt power for ~ 20 years in welding applications and a wide database of information has been acquired. The welding results with Nd:YAG and CO_2 laser beams are reported to be quite similar when the penetration is over 2–3 mm (17). In this case, it seems that the keyhole is sufficiently deep that the beam power couples very efficiently into the material at both wavelengths. With thinner-section higher-speed welding, the lower reflectivity of materials at the Nd:YAG 1-μm wavelength provides better coupling than that of 10-μm radiation from CO_2 lasers, and achievable speeds (watt for watt at the same spot size) are faster at the Nd:YAG wavelength.

In overlap and butt welds made in automotive-type steels by kilowatt Nd:YAG laser beams, it is found that the weld bead is narrow and can be of high quality with negligible porosity, cracking, or undercut. In the case of Zn-coated material, it is important to leave a gap (typically ~ 0.05–0.1 mm) between welded sheets to avoid the excessive occurrence of blowholes. These occur with CO_2 laser welding as well, and are thought to be caused by the low-boiling-point Zn at the interface surfaces escaping from the weld. In all cases where the weld integrity is good, tensile strength tests show that failure occurs in the parent material rather than the weld.

A difference between kilowatt CO_2 and Nd:YAG laser welding concerns the effect of the plume on the process. In the case of CO_2 laser welding, He is predominantly used as the cover gas to mitigate plasma blocking effects. With kilowatt Nd:YAG beams, early work suggests that (cheaper) Ar can be used in the majority of cases. However, in the welding of Al alloys this might not be possible. Here, the molten weld material is of low viscosity, making control of "drop through" a key problem, and the rapid thermal cycling makes welds in many alloys subject to cracking and porosity. Preliminary results suggest that He cover gas mitigates these effects in kilowatt Nd:YAG welding of Al alloys. Early tensile test results with kilowatt Nd:YAG welded Al alloys, show that failure is invariably through the weld and that this occurs typically at 60–80% of the tensile strength of the parent material. In addition, for equivalent thicknesses and spot sizes, it has been found that welds in some 5000 series Al alloys can be made faster than in some 6000 Al alloys. This effect has also been noted in the CO_2 laser welding of Al alloys and with lower-power Nd:YAG beams.

The welding of stainless steels, titanium alloys, and nickel alloys up to 6-mm thickness with 1–2 kW Nd:YAG laser beams has been described in the literature (18–20). The results show high-quality welds, generally comparable to the best achieved with kilowatt CO_2 lasers. However, in more recent thicker-section welding (~ 6–12 mm) at higher Nd:YAG laser power, results show some plasma plume effects. At slow welding speeds, the plume can be a problem with Ar cover gas, sometimes leading to "nailhead"-type weld sections and unacceptable porosity in the weld. The situation is worst at the slowest speeds (down to ~ 0.2 m/min), but it is reported that use of He cover gas significantly mitigates the effects.

References

14. "Annual Market Survey," *Laser Report* **33** (1), 1 Jan 1997, PennWell Publications, Nashua, NH.
15. H. L. Marshall, High-Power, High-Pulse-Rate YAG Laser Seam Welding, SPIE Vol. **86,** Conference on Industrial Applications of High Power Laser Technology, 1976.
16. I. M. Norris, C. N. D. Peters, and K. Withnall, Supra-Kilowatt Nd:YAG Lasers - Their Development and Processing Performance, Proceedings of ISATA 1993, Aachen Germany, Automotive Automation Ltd, UK.
17. H. Hugal, Laser Welding of Aluminium Materials; Problems, Solutions, Readiness for Applications, Proceedings of the

European Laser Marketplace Meeting, Hannover, Oct. 1994.
18. B. Wedel, R. Dommaschk, J. Migl, D. Pathe, P. Zopf, and U. Bethke, Welding with a 2.8 kW CW Nd:YAG Laser in Oscillator Amplifier Configuration with a 600 μm FOBD System, p. 405, Proceedings of ISATA 1994, Aachen, Germany, Automotive Automation Ltd, UK.
19. A. P. Hoult, Current and Future Prospects for High Power Lasers in the Aerospace Industry, *Aircraft Engineering,* Sept 1989, p. 14.
20. I Norris, T. Hoult, C. Peters, and P. Wileman, Materials Processing with a 3 kW Nd:YAG Laser, Proceedings of LAMP 1992, Nagaoka Japan, June 1992, p. 489.

C. L. M. IRELAND

11.3.6 Nd:YAG Laser-Pulsed Welding of Common Materials

List of Symbols

A_b	Absorptivity
C_p	Specific heat (J/kg K)
d	Weld pool depth (m)
E	Energy per pulse (J)
f	Pulse frequency (Hz)
F_0	Fourier number
ΔH_f	Latent heat of fusion (J/m^3)
I	Irradiance of laser beam on the workpiece (W/m^2)
I_0	Irradiance at $r = 0$
k	Thermal conductivity (W/m K)
M^2	Beam quality
O_v	Percent overlap of individual spot welds in a seam weld
P_d	Average irradiance of the incident laser beam (W/m^2)
P_m	Mean laser power (W)
P_p	Peak pulse power (W)
q_0	Irradiance of the absorbed incident beam at $r = 0$ (W/m^2)
t_p	Pulse time (s)
T	Temperature (K)
T_{mp}	Melting temperature (K)
T_0	Room or preheat temperature (K)
v	Welding speed (mm/s)
V	Volume of weld metal (m^3)
w	Weld width (m)
Y	Distance between individual spot welds in a seam weld (m)
α	Thermal diffusivity (m^2/s)
σ	Distribution coefficient of a Gaussian distribution (m)
η	Nondimensional axial coordinate $\eta = z/\sigma$
η_{mr}	Melting ratio
ρ	Density (kg/m^3)
ξ	Nondimensional absorbed heat flux

Pulsed Nd:YAG lasers are used to make either individual spot welds or seam welds in a wide range of alloys between about 0.1 to 2 mm thickness. Seam welds are made by making a series of partially overlapping spot welds along the weld joint. In most cases, these welds are autogenous. Some typical applications of pulsed Nd:YAG laser welds are shown in Table 8.

Table 8. Typical Applications of Pulsed Nd:YAG Laser Welding

Application	Material
Brake sensors	400 Stainless steel
Circuitry enclosures	Aluminum alloys
Hermetic seals on pacemakers	304 Stainless steel
Heat exchanger tubing	Nickel-based alloys
Razor blades	Martensitic stainless steel
Hermetic seals on optoelectronic devices	Kovar
Air bag caps	Stainless steel
Reading/writing heads	Carbon/spring steel
Fuel injectors	409 Stainless steel

There are two basic Nd:YAG laser welder configurations, which differ in their method of beam delivery. As shown in Figure 17a, a binocular viewing head can be fixed to the laser head and a mirror used to direct the laser beam down through the final process lens to the weld specimen. This configuration allows the operator a coaxial view of the welding operation, either directly (using the appropriate laser safety glasses) or indirectly using a CCD camera. This can be advantageous for precise positioning of the laser weld. To make a weld using this configuration, the laser beam is fixed in space and the weldment is moved either manually or automatically using CNC positioning tables. A silica cover glass slide is normally placed between the process lens and the specimen to protect the process lens from weld spatter and vaporization. In addition, coaxial inert gas shielding is used to prevent excessive oxidation of the weld metal or gas porosity in the weld. The best type of shielding gas to use (e.g., argon, helium, etc.) will depend on the alloy being welded (21).

As shown in Figure 17b, fiber-optic cables can also be used to deliver the beam to the weld specimen. Here, the beam is directed down a fiber-optic cable of the desired length and then passed through a final process lens head. This lens head may contain just a recollimator lens and a process lens. If coaxial viewing of the weld is desired for focusing and beam positioning purposes, a mirror and CCD camera can be incorporated into the final lens assembly. While welds can be made using this configuration by fixing the final lens head and laser beam in space and, as before, moving the weldment either manually or automatically with CNC positioning tables, welds can also be made by fixing the weldment in space and moving the final lens head and laser beam along the weld joint. By fixing the final lens assembly to a robot, it is also possible to weld three-dimensional parts using this beam delivery configuration. As before, a glass cover slide is normally placed between the process lens and the specimen, and coaxial shielding gas is used.

ISBN 0-912035-15-3

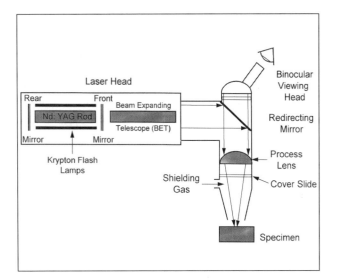

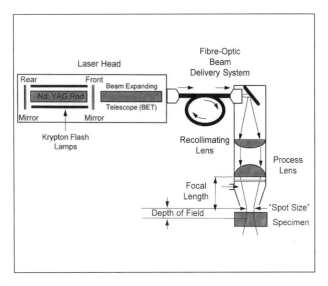

Figure 17. Beam delivery systems used for pulsed Nd:YAG laser welding: (a) binocular viewing head and (b) fiber-optic cable.

Input Characteristics

The simplest form of laser pulse has a "square" temporal pulse shape as illustrated in Figure 18. The laser pulse is created by discharge of the krypton flash lamps, giving a nominally constant peak laser power, P_p, for a predetermined pulse time, t_p. Characteristically, there will be a short power spike at the beginning of the pulse, but this does not significantly affect the final weld dimensions or weld quality of welds made in common alloys such as steels, stainless steels, and nickel-based alloys. The total pulse energy, E, contained in this pulse is given by the product of peak laser power times the pulse time, i.e., $E = P_p t_p$. Note that the pulse conditions are fully defined by P_p and t_p; however, they are not fully defined by E, since there is an infinite number of combinations of P_p and t_p that will give the same pulse energy.

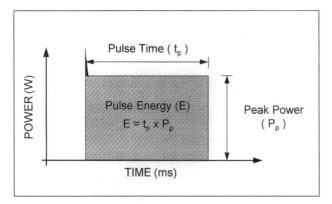

Figure 18. Parameters for a temporally "square" laser pulse with constant peak power, P_p, pulse time t_p, and pulse energy E.

When the pulsed laser welder is first turned on, a series of laser pulses are generated at a predetermined frequency or repetition rate, f, as shown in Figure 19, and these pulses are deflected by a shutter to a beam dump located within the laser head. In this case, the mean laser power P_m is given by the product of $E\cdot f$. It is important to realize that P_p and P_m are quite different. Individual spot welds are made by opening the shutter to allow out a single laser pulse. Alternatively, a series of spot welds or seam welds are made by moving the part relative to the laser beam at a welding speed, v, while leaving the shutter open to allow a continuous series of pulses to leave the laser welder.

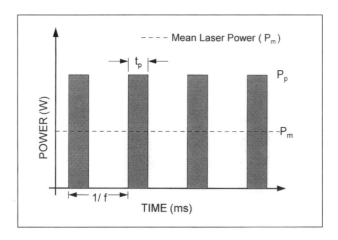

Figure 19. Power versus time for a series of laser pulses showing peak power, P_p, and mean laser power, P_m.

During the laser pulse, the peak power is distributed over a certain area. The spatial distribution of power depends on the laser, the optical components used, and the mean laser power. The output of Nd:YAG lasers is generally multimode with M^2 values as high as 50, but frequently the intensity distribution is well described by a Gaussian distribution, as shown in Figure 20. In this case, the intensity distribution is given by the relation

$$I_o(r,t) = I_o \exp(-2r^2/\sigma^2)$$

where I_o is the maximum beam intensity at $r = 0$, r is the radial distance from the beam center, and σ is the distribution coefficient, defined in this case as the radius at which the intensity has fallen to $1/e^2$ of I_o. The beam intensity distribution shown in Figure 20 has a distribution coefficient of $\sigma = 205$ μm.

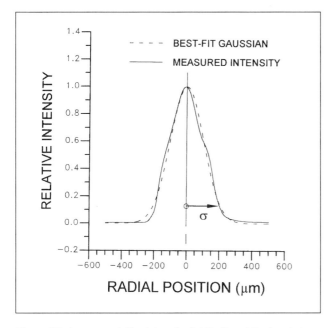

Figure 20. A representative intensity distribution at the focal plane of a pulsed Nd:YAG laser beam.

The average irradiance of the incident laser beam, P_d, is frequently used as a characterizing welding process parameter. This is calculated by dividing P_p by the area over which the beam acts. This area is calculated using some measure of the beam "spot size." The spot size of multimode beams can be defined in a number of ways, including the diameter of a circle that encloses 86% of the beam power, or four times the square root of the second moment of area of the intensity distribution. For the Gaussian-distributed beam shown in Figure 20, the spot size can be defined as the width at which the intensity has dropped to $1/e^2$ of I_o, that is, 2σ. In this case, $P_d = P_p/\pi \sigma^2$. Because the spot size of a multimode beam will depend on the method used to define it, the definition of the beam spot size should always be reported for a calculated average power density. Also, it should be noted that P_d depends strongly on the beam "spot size." For example, while a 10% increase in P_p will increase P_d by 10%, a 10% increase of σ will decrease P_d by about 20%. When using a binocular viewing head such as illustrated in Figure 17a, the focused beam "spot size" will increase with mean laser power and the laser beam mode will change because of "thermal lensing" effects caused by heating of the Nd:YAG rod (22). This "thermal lensing" effect necessitates adjustment of the lenses in the beam expanding telescope (BET) for each mean laser power used in order to minimize beam divergence and to bring the optical focal plane of the viewing head in coincidence with the focal plane of the 1.06-μm wavelength laser beam. Also, because thermal lensing effects cause the "spot size" to increase with increased P_m,

with a set P_p and t_p, P_d will decrease as P_m is increased. As will be shown later, this change in P_m will cause the weld dimensions to change even though the same pulse conditions are used.

When using a fiber-optic cable beam delivery (Fig. 17b), the BET does not have to be adjusted with each new mean laser power, rather the fiber-optic cable tends to "homogenize" the laser beam and produce a multimode beam at the focus with a Gaussian distribution. Also, the distribution coefficients of beams that have traveled through fiber-optic cables do not change significantly with P_m. Hence, when using the same pulse conditions, P_d, and therefore the weld dimensions, should not change significantly with changes of P_m.

In addition to the simple temporally square pulse shape illustrated in Figures 18 and 19, various temporally shaped pulses may be employed to improve weld quality, as discussed later. A schematic of a temporally shaped pulse is shown in Figure 21. Here, the pulse has been constructed using a series of pulse sectors, each with different peak powers and pulse times. For example, a series of ramp-up sectors may be used at the beginning of the pulse to eliminate the characteristic leading edge spike (see Fig. 18) or to control the rate of heating and melting. The main weld sector will be of sufficient peak power and duration to generate a weld of the desired dimensions. Finally, the series of ramp-down sectors at the end of the pulse can control the rate of solidification and cooling of the weld.

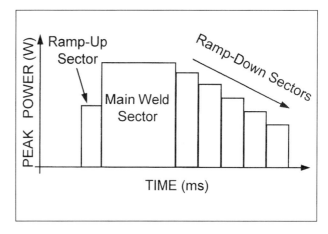

Figure 21. A temporally modified laser pulse with a ramp-up sector, a main welding sector, and a series of ramp-down sectors.

Welding Performance

When the laser beam hits the surface of a metal part, only a fraction of the light energy is absorbed at the surface and converted to heat while the balance is reflected off the surface. The fraction absorbed is defined by the absorptivity, A_b, which depends on the material and its surface finish (22). Reflective metals such as gold, copper, and aluminum alloys have low absorptivities (< 0.1), while alloys such as steels and stainless steels have higher absorptivities (~0.3). At low irradiance, the absorbed beam energy will heat and melt the material to produce a conduction-mode weld as illustrated in Figure 22a. In conduction-mode welds, heat is conducted from the incident surface into the bulk of the metal primarily by thermal conduction and convection in the liquid weld pool. The depth-to-width ratio of conduction-mode welds rarely exceeds 0.5. A heat-affected zone (HAZ) will be created in the base metal immediately adjacent to the fusion boundary. At higher power densities, the metal surface is heated well above the vaporization temperature of the metal and a keyhole-mode weld is produced as illustrated in Figure 22b. In this case, a plasma-filled keyhole is created that acts as a beam trap, thereby increasing the effective absorptivity to values greater than 0.9. Much greater depth of penetration is possible with keyhole-mode welding. The depth-to-width ratio of these welds is always greater than 0.5.

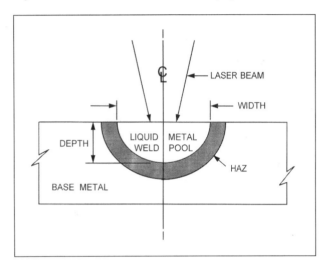

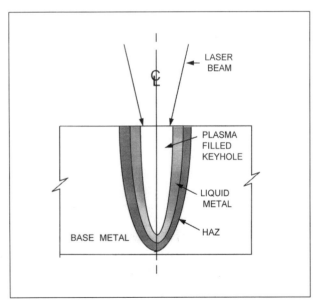

Figure 22. Schematic diagrams of (a) conduction-mode and (b) keyhole-mode laser spot welds.

The final width and depth of a laser spot weld depends on a combination of the irradiance and pulse time, as illustrated by the weld pool profiles in AISI 409 ferritic stainless steel in Figure 23 (23). Only conduction-mode welds are produced at the lowest irradiance, while keyhole-mode welds are produced at the higher irradiances. The depth of penetration of these welds increases with both irradiance and pulse time, while the width of the welds increases at a much lower rate.

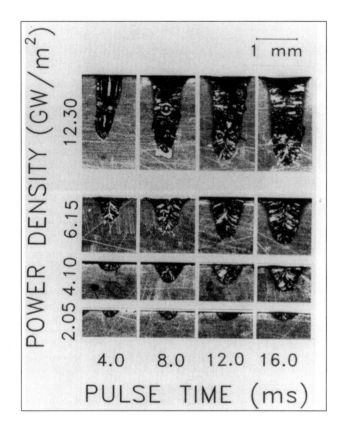

Figure 23. Cross sections of pulsed Nd:YAG welds in AISI 409 ferritic stainless steel as a function of power density and pulse time ($\sigma \approx 205\ \mu m$) (23).

Measurements of the weld pool width and depth in the same AISI 409 stainless steel welds as a function of irradiance and pulse time are summarized in the surface plots shown in Figures 24a and b (23). At irradiance less than about 4 GW/m^2 conduction-mode welds are produced. The dimensions of these welds increase rapidly during the first 2 ms, after which steady-state conditions are approached. The transition from conduction- to keyhole-mode welding, about 4 GW/m^2, is indicated in the plots by the sudden increase in the weld pool dimensions with increasing power density. As before, there is a rapid increase in keyhole-mode weld dimensions during the first 2 ms. After this, the weld dimensions continue to increase with time but at a slower rate. Note that the weld dimensions depend strongly on irradiance and are, therefore, very sensitive to changes of peak power and beam "spot size."

Chapter 11: Penetration Welding

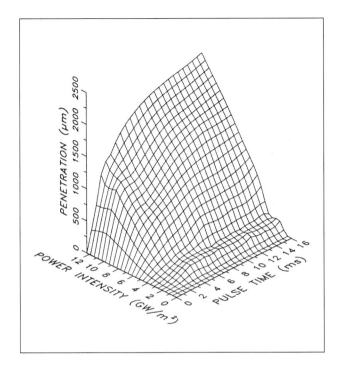

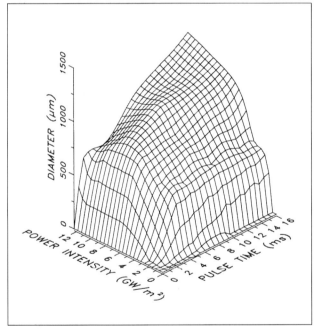

Figure 24. Average weld pool dimensions for Nd:YAG laser spot welds in AISI 409 stainless steel versus pulse time and irradiance (a) weld penetration and (b) weld width (23).

A map of the combined effects of power density and pulse time on the welding modes and weld quality of the AISI 409 stainless steel welds is shown in Figure 25 (23). Pulse energy isopleths have also been included on this graph, because the energy per pulse is measured and reported by most laser welders. The threshold for melting occurs at about 0.7 GW/m². Conduction-mode welds are produced between irradiances of 0.7 to 4 GW/m² while keyhole-mode welds are produced at irradiances greater than 4 GW/m². Finally, drilling occurs in this alloy at irradiances greater than 10 GW/m². Note that the laser-material interaction mode, i.e., surface heating, conduction-mode welding, keyhole-mode welding or drilling, and the dimensions of the spot welds are not uniquely defined by the energy per pulse but rather by the combination of the irradiance and the pulse time.

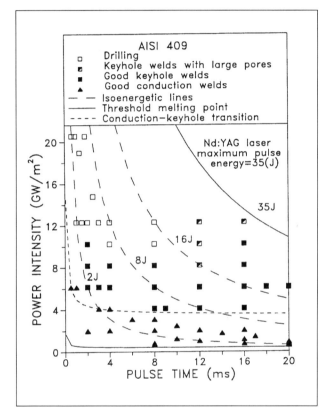

Figure 25. Summary of the effects of power density and pulse time on melting, transition conditions, and weld quality in AISI 409 stainless steel (23).

Maps similar to those shown in Figures 24 and 25 can be produced for other materials such as plain carbon steels and aluminum alloys, and these can be expected to exhibit the same general characteristics, that is, transitions from surface heating to conduction-mode welding to keyhole-mode welding and finally to drilling as the irradiance is increased. However, the threshold and transition irradiances will be different because of differences in absorptivity and thermophysical material properties. For example, using the same pulsed Nd:YAG laser, the threshold irradiance for 1100 aluminum is about 3.2 GW/m² and the transition from conduction- to keyhole-mode welding occurs about 10 GW/m² (24). Much greater irradiances are required when welding aluminum alloys, because their absorptivity is much lower than stainless steels and because they have higher thermal conductivities.

ISBN 0-912035-15-3

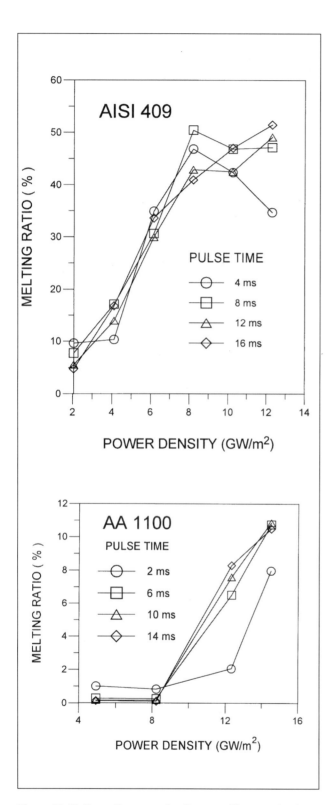

Figure 26. Melting ratios versus irradiance at different pulse times for (top) AISI 409 stainless steel (23) and (bottom) 1100 aluminum (24).

Melting Ratios

For most pulsed Nd:YAG lasers, the conversion efficiency of electrical energy to optical energy is relatively low, typically less than 5%. However, when considering the overall welding efficiency, it is usual to consider only the effectiveness of this output optical energy in forming a fused joint. This can be characterized by the melting ratio, η_{mr}, which is defined as the ratio of energy required to melt the weld metal to the energy incident on the workpiece, or

$$\eta_{mr} = \frac{V\,[\rho C_p(T_{mp} - T_o) + \Delta H_f\,]}{E}$$

Measured values of η_{mr} versus t_p and P_d for AISI 409 stainless steel and 1100 aluminum are shown in Figures 26a and b, respectively (23, 24). The melting ratio of conduction-mode welds in the stainless steel is about 10% and there is a rapid increase to about 50% as the power density is increased and keyhole-mode welds are produced. On the other hand, the melting ratio of conduction-mode welds in 1100 aluminum is only about 1%, and this increases to a maximum of only 10% as the power density is increased beyond 8 GW/m² and keyhole-mode welds are produced.

The melting ratios of the 1100 aluminum are much lower than that of the 409 stainless steel for two main reasons; more of the incident energy is reflected because of aluminum's lower absorptivity, and more of the absorbed energy is conducted away without causing melting because of its higher thermal conductivity. Similar low values of melting ratios can be expected for other high-conductivity, low-absorptivity alloys such as copper and gold alloys. For a given material, the melting ratio is greater for keyhole-mode welds than for conduction-mode welds, since the effective absorptivity is greater with keyhole-mode welds. Moreover, η_{mr} increases with increased P_d, since as the keyhole becomes deeper, more of the incident beam is trapped.

Optimum Lens Combinations

Different types of lenses and different focal length lens combinations can be used in the binocular head or collimator lens head of the fiber-optic beam delivery system (see Fig. 17). The optimum lens combination depends on the application. The lens combination affects the sensitivity of the welding process to positioning of the workpiece and to welding process variables, and also determines the final weld dimensions for a given set of pulse parameters.

With an increased focal length of the process lens, the workpiece is farther away from the process lens. This can be an advantage for robotic applications with complex workpiece shapes. Moreover, the depth of focus increases with increased focal length, allowing more flexibility of the workpiece position with respect to the process lens. Also, the laser beam "spot size" increases with increased focal length, so that for a given P_p, P_d decreases, which will result in a significant decrease of weld penetration (see Fig. 24a). Therefore, when a longer-focal-length lens is used, either t_p or P_p must be increased to maintain a given weld penetration. Finally, the larger laser spot size produced by longer-focal-length lenses will result in increased weld widths and increasing tolerance to lateral beam positioning with respect to the weld joint.

Seam Welds

Seam welds are made by opening the shutter for a longer predetermined period, while moving the workpiece laterally relative to the laser beam (or vice versa), at a welding speed v. This results in a series of overlapping laser spot welds being produced along the weld joint. The distance Y between weld centers is given by $Y = v/f$. If the spot weld width is w, then the percent overlap, O_v, of each weld on its predecessor is given by

$$O_v = (1 - Y/w)100$$

Typically, 70 to 95% overlap is used to make seam welds. Because of the geometries and aspect ratios of conduction versus keyhole-mode welds, consistent depth of penetration in a seam weld can be obtained with lower values of O_v when making conduction-mode welds, but higher values are required when making keyhole-mode welds. Note that for a fixed pulse peak power and pulse time, increased mean laser power permits use of a higher pulse frequency. Therefore, use of increased mean laser power permits higher welding speeds for a fixed overlap of pulses.

The same principles apply for seam welds as for individual spot welds, since seam welds are a series of partially overlapping spot welds. However, after an initial transient, the actual conditions that are suitable for seam welds are generally different from those for spot welds, because of the preheating effects of prior pulses. For a given power density and pulse time, the steady-state penetration and weld width in a seam weld will be greater than those of individual welds. Therefore, the irradiance usually must be reduced when making partial- or full-penetration seam welds.

In some applications such as hermetic sealing of pacemaker or optoelectronic packages, it is desirable to maximize the melting ratio and therefore minimize the amount of energy conducted into the part and subsequent heating of the parts. This can be accomplished through optimization of the lens combinations and process parameters used to make the seam weld. The smaller beam size and higher power density produced with a shorter focal length permits a lower value of P_p, which in turn results in a lower energy per pulse. For a given available mean laser power, this permits use of a higher pulse frequency, thus permitting a faster welding speed. Hence, less time is available for conduction into the workpiece, the process efficiency is increased, and the overall temperature of the weldment is decreased.

Weld Procedure Development Tools

There are a number of challenges that must be addressed when developing welding procedures for laser spot welding applications. These are related specifically to reliable and accurate measurement of the spot weld dimensions and to measurement and control of all weld process parameters. As shown in Figure 27, these welds are typically less than 1 mm in width, and this, in combination with the narrow, pointed geometry of keyhole-mode welds, makes it difficult to use standard metallographic techniques to section along the center line of individual spot welds for the purpose of measuring weld width and depth. In Figure 27, welds are shown that were produced in 304 stainless steel using a binocular head beam delivery system (see Fig. 17a), three different pulse parameters, 4, 12, and 16 J/pulse and three different mean laser powers, 60, 140, and 220 W. Note that thermal lensing causes a change in mode structure of the focused beam and an increase in the "spot size" of the beam with increasing P_m. Even though the same pulse conditions were used, the changes in the intensity distribution caused dramatic changes in the weld penetration that are not apparent from viewing the top surface of the final spot weld. Thus control over the weld dimensions requires effective techniques for measurement and control of the intensity distributions of the high-power, pulsed laser beams. There are a number of techniques that have been developed that address these specific challenges to weld procedure development and quality control.

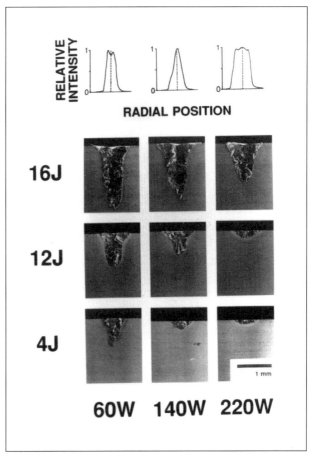

Figure 27. Thermal lensing effects on beam mode, "spot size," and resultant weld shapes and dimensions in 304 stainless steel.

The burn-pattern technique, in which a single laser pulse is used to burn a hole in a thin film of KAPTON™ is commonly used as a rapid method of measuring the "spot size" of pulsed Nd:YAG laser beams (25). As shown in Figure 28, however, the diameter of the hole produced varies depending on the energy of the pulse used to produce the hole. Therefore, while this is a very rapid and inexpensive way to check the "spot size" of the beam, the pulse energy used to make the hole must be kept constant. Note that this technique cannot be used reliably to measure the intensity distribution of the laser beam.

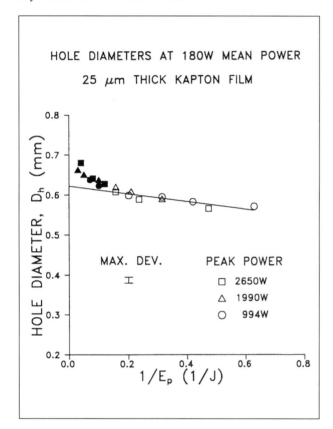

Figure 28. Measured hole diameters in Kapton film versus energy per pulse (25).

There are a number of techniques that may be used to measure the intensity distribution at the focus of the pulsed, high-power laser beams. Figure 29a is a schematic diagram of a rotating-wire-type laser beam analyzer in which a 1-mm-diameter, polished Mo wire is rotated through the focus of the laser beam and reflections of the beam are detected and recorded. Note that the analyzer and laser must be synchronized so that the wire sweeps through the focus during the laser pulse. This technique was used to measure the intensity distributions shown in Figures 20 and 27. A second technique is shown schematically in Figure 29b. This rotating pinhole technique requires that a hollow needle with a 10–30 μm diameter hole be swept through the focus during the laser pulse. The small portion of the sampled beam that passes through the hole is reflected down the hollow needle and is recorded by a detector to give a measure of the beam intensity as a function of position at the beam focus. A third technique involves insertion of a beam splitter at the focus of the beam which reflects only a small fraction of the beam into a CCD camera. All these techniques can be used to measure line scans of the intensity distribution at the focus of these beams or to produce three-dimensional surface maps of the beam intensity as a function of position. These can then be used to determine the effective "spot size" and irradiance, P_d, at the focus of the high-power, pulsed laser beam.

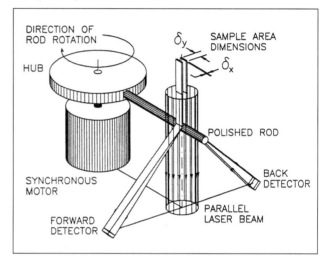

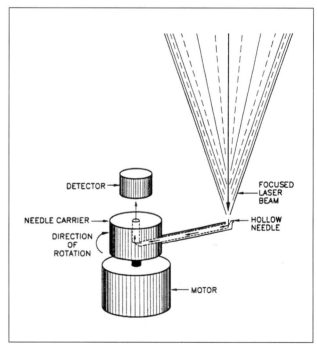

Figure 29. Schematic diagrams of (a) rotating-wire-type and (b) rotating hollow-needle-type laser beam analyzers.

While the width and depth of penetration of laser seam welds can be measured using standard metallographic sectioning techniques, it is extremely difficult to section precisely down the

Chapter 11: Penetration Welding

center line of individual laser spot welds in order to measure the depth of penetration or to measure and characterize weld defects. Instead, the "split-specimen" technique as shown schematically in Figure 30 may be used effectively (26). As indicated, the incident and joint surfaces of two individual specimens are carefully machined and polished and then firmly clamped together in a butt-joint configuration. Individual laser spot welds are then made centered over the joint using the desired welding parameters. After cooling the specimen (sometimes in liquid nitrogen to promote brittle fracture), one end is held in a vice and the other end given a sharp blow, as shown in Figure 30. This causes the welds to fracture, thus revealing their shape, dimensions, and defects, which then can easily be measured using standard metallographic microscopes and image analysis techniques. All the welds shown in Figures 23 and 27 have been produced and sectioned using this technique.

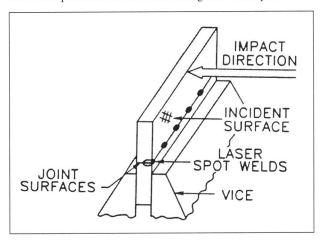

Figure 30. Schematic diagram of the split specimen technique.

Mathematical models and similarity relationships can be used effectively during weld procedure development to predict the welding conditions required to produce welds of desired size and shape prior to performing experiments, or to predict the expected effect of a change of a weld process parameter on an existing welding procedure. For example, assuming a Gaussian-distributed intensity distribution, the temperature at any position in a conduction-mode laser spot weld as a function time can be predicted using the following equation

$$T(r,z,t) = T_0 + \frac{A b\, q_o\, \sigma^2}{8k} \int_0^\infty J_0(\lambda r)\, e^{\sigma^2 \lambda^2/8}$$

$$\left\{ e^{-\lambda z}\, erfc\left[\frac{z}{2\sqrt{\alpha t}} - \lambda(\alpha t)^{1/2}\right] \right.$$

$$\left. - e^{\lambda z}\, erfc\left[\frac{z}{2\sqrt{\alpha t}} - \lambda(\alpha t)^{1/2}\right] \right\} d\lambda$$

in which $erfc$ is the complementary error function and J_o is a zeroeth order Bessel function. Solution of this equation can easily be implemented into an interactive, PC-microcomputer-based code and used to solve for (1) the hot-spot temperature $T(0,0,t)$ as a function of time; (2) the weld pool width, depth and aspect ratio as a function of time; and (3) the temperature field in the base metal at the end of the laser pulse (24). An example of predicted and measured weld pool width and depth as a function of time during melting and solidifying of a conduction-mode weld in inconel 600 is shown in Figure 31. Note that there is good correlation between predicted and observed weld pool dimensions. The weld pool grows quickly in the first 5 ms, but then approaches a steady-state size where the heat loss into the material by conduction is equal to the heat entering from the laser beam.

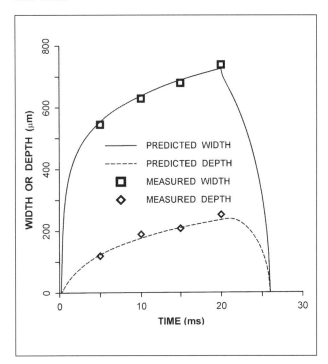

Figure 31. Predicted and measured weld pool dimensions versus time in inconel 600 (P_p = 422 W, t_p = 20 ms, σ = 320 µm, A_b = 0.32).

Similarity Relationships

Similarity parameters for the laser spot welding process may be derived by nondimensionalizing the governing energy equation and thermal boundary conditions. Using σ as the characteristic length scale, the nondimensional radial and axial coordinates can be defined as $\delta = r/\sigma$ and $\eta = z/\sigma$, respectively. Similarly, time can be nondimensionalized by the Fourier number, F_o.

$$F_o = \alpha t/\sigma$$

Substituting these into the governing equation and incident surface boundary condition, it can be shown (24) that geometrically similar welds will be produced, provided that both the nondimensional Fourier number, F_0, and the nondimensional absorbed heat flux, ξ, are kept the same. Here, ξ is defined by

$$\xi = 2A_b P_p / \pi \kappa \sigma (T_{mp} - T_0)$$

By holding F_0 and ξ constant, different welding conditions can be defined that will produce welds with geometric similarity (similar depth-to-width ratios), differing only in the absolute size of the weld. Alternatively, the welding parameters required to produce weld pools with exactly the same size and shape in different materials can be identified, provided that both F_0 and ξ are kept the same. Assuming that the absorptivity of each material is known, the required pulse time can be determined from the equation for F_0 and the pulse peak power from the equation for ξ.

In Figure 32, the nondimensional weld pool width, δ, and depth, η, are plotted versus F_0, for values of ξ up to 15. These plots were generated using the analytical model for pulsed laser welding [the equation for $T(r,z,t)$] and can be used for any material, provided the thermophysical properties and the absorptivity of the material are known. Note that melting is not predicted to occur unless $\xi > 1.67$. Figures 32a and b can be used effectively during the initial stages of weld procedure development for prediction of the process parameters required to obtain desired weld pool dimensions. They can also be useful for predicting the effects on weld pool dimensions of changes in various weld process parameters such as laser beam "spot size." For example, the inconel 600 welds in Figure 31 were produced with $\sigma = 320$ μm and $P_p = 422$ W. If a different laser was used with a smaller distribution coefficient of $\sigma = 250$ μm, but the same weld depth was required, that is, $d = 235$ μm (see Fig. 31) then the nondimensional depth, $\eta = d/\sigma = 235/250 = 0.94$. Assuming a pulse time of 20 ms and $\alpha = 5.2 \times 10^{-6}$ m²/s, from the equation for F_0, $F_0 = 5.2 \times 10^{-6} \times 20 \times 10^{-3} / (250 \times 10^{-6})^2 = 1.66$. From Figure 32b, with $\eta = 0.94$ and $F_0 = 1.66$, ξ must be ~ 8.5. Therefore, assuming $k = 26.2$ W/mK and $T_{mp} = 1656$ K, the peak pulse power required would be

$$P_p = \xi \pi k \sigma (T_{mp} - T_0) / 2 A_b$$

$$= (8.5\pi) 26.2 (250 \times 10^{-6})(1656-293)/2 \times 0.32$$

$$= 370 W$$

Finally, from Figure 32a with $F_0 = 1.28$ and $\xi = 8.5$, $\delta \sim 2.40$, or the expected weld pool width would be $w = \delta \times \sigma = 2.40 \times 250$ μm $= 600$ μm.

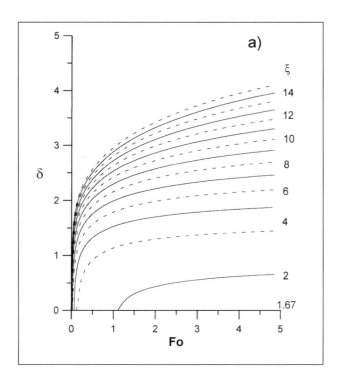

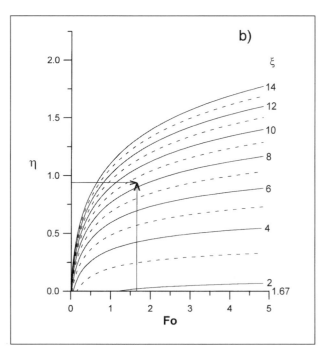

Figure 32. (a) The nondimensional weld pool width, δ, and (b) depth, η, versus the Fourier number, F_0, for values of ξ up to 15 (24).

Weld Metallurgy and Weld Defects
While many of the metallurgical and process issues frequently faced during pulsed Nd:YAG laser welding are not unlike those

commonly encountered with other fusion welding processes (21), there are some process specific problems as well. These include spatter and cratering, occluded vapor porosity, gas porosity, and solidification cracking in laser spot welds. Figure 33 shows an example of a keyhole-mode weld made in 409 stainless steel that has two types of defects, cratering and occluded gas porosity. Cratering is an indication that a significant fraction of the weld metal has been lost to spatter or vaporization and is most often seen at the beginning of the pulse when making keyhole-mode welds (23). In some cases, temporal pulse shaping can be used to reduce or eliminate spatter and cratering. The effects of temporal pulse shaping on cratering in 304 stainless steel is illustrated in the plots in Figure 34. Here, there is little metal loss and cratering in all conduction-mode welds produced at 1.5 GW/m². However, most keyhole-mode welds produced at the higher power densities exhibit cratering. The most severe cratering occurred when a ramp-down pulse shape (C) was used, while it was significantly reduced when using either a square (A) or ramp-up (D) pulse shape. This suggests that cratering and spatter can be minimized by using ramp-up sectors at the beginning of a pulse and keeping the maximum irradiance in the pulse as low as possible.

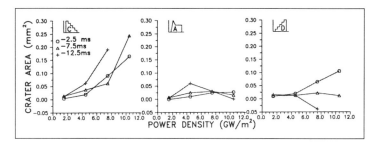

Figure 34. The effects of square, ramp-up, and ramp-down temporal pulse shapes on crater area in 304 stainless steel spot welds.

Occluded vapor porosity, also evident in the 409 stainless steel spot weld shown in Figure 33, is only observed in keyhole-mode welds and is thought to be created during the collapse of the keyhole at the end of the laser pulse (23). In some cases, temporal pulse shaping can be used to reduce or eliminate occluded vapor porosity. As shown in Figure 35, occluded vapor porosity in 304 stainless steel spot welds is also affected by temporal pulse shaping. Keyhole-mode welds made with a ramp-up (D) pulse shape have the greatest occluded vapor porosity, while those made with the ramp-down (C) pulse shape have the least porosity. This suggests that ramping down the power at the end of the pulse helps to control the collapse of the keyhole at the end of the pulse, thereby minimizing occluded vapor porosity.

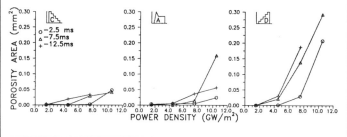

Figure 35. The effects of square, ramp-up, and ramp-down temporal pulse shapes on occluded vapor porosity in 304 stainless steel spot welds.

It is evident from Figures 34 and 35 that a ramp-up pulse shape will reduce spatter and cratering, but will also increase the amount of occluded vapor porosity. Alternatively, occluded vapor porosity can be reduced using a ramp-down pulse shape, but this will increase spatter and cratering. These opposing effects can be combined with a normal square pulse shape as shown in Figure 21 effectively to reduce both types of defects. That is, a ramp-up at the beginning of the pulse will reduce spatter, the square or main weld sector creates the weld of desired dimensions, and ramp-down sectors at the end of the pulse can control the collapse of the keyhole, thereby reducing the amount of occluded vapor porosity in the weld. The optimum rates of ramp-up and ramp-down as well as peak power and pulse time of the main weld sector must be determined experimentally for each new application and material.

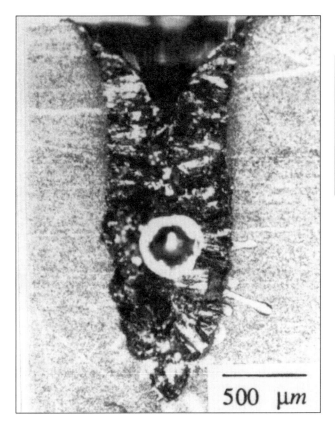

Figure 33. Cratering and occluded vapor porosity defects in a 409 stainless steel laser spot weld (23).

Another type of porosity commonly seen in laser spot welds is gas porosity. An example of spherical and worm-hole shaped gas porosity in an aluminum weld is shown in Figure 36 (24). Gas porosity is typically located close to the fusion boundary and can be caused by a number of different mechanisms, including insufficient shielding gas, welding parts with surfaces that are wet or contaminated with paints, oils, or grease (21, 27). The source and type of gas responsible for gas porosity and the appropriate precautions to use to avoid gas porosity including the best shielding gas to use will depend on the alloy being welded (24, 27). For example, in plain carbon steels, CO boil is most often the cause of gas porosity, while in aluminum alloys such as shown in Figure 36, gas porosity is most often caused by evolution of hydrogen during solidification (21, 24, 27). In many cases, this porosity in aluminum alloys can be minimized by mechanically removing the aluminum oxide or anodized surface layer prior to welding and by using inert gas shielding during welding (21, 24). In all cases, all surface contaminants should be removed from the weld specimens prior to welding.

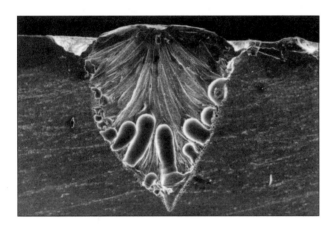

Figure 36. Spherical and worm-hole-shaped hydrogen gas porosity located near the fusion boundary of an aluminum alloy laser spot weld (24).

Solidification cracking is frequently observed in laser spot welds in crack-sensitive alloys such as 316 stainless steel, inconel 600, and various aluminum alloys. An example of severe solidification cracking in an Al-3.73 wt % Cu alloy, which was seam welded using a square temporal pulse shape, is shown in Figure 37. Typically, these cracks occur during solidification of the weld and run parallel to the solidification microstructure. As shown in Figure 37, these cracks can propagate through a number of overlapping welds.

Solidification cracking in pulsed laser welds is a result of complex interactions between the alloy composition, the welding process conditions and the resulting solidification process, and the thermomechanical strains that are generated during welding. Temporal pulse shaping has been shown to be effective in reducing or eliminating solidification cracking in various stainless steel and aluminum alloys; however, fundamental understanding of the influence of the temporal pulse shape on the cracking event has yet to be established. Figure 38 shows an example of a crack-free seam weld produced in the same Al-3.73 wt % Cu aluminum alloy using an optimized ramp-down temporal pulse shape. Depending on the alloy, however, temporal pulse shaping is not always effective in eliminating solidification cracking. For example, solidification cracking has also been reduced in austenitic stainless steel by increasing specimen preheat, by increasing pulse frequency, and by increasing percentage overlap between pulses. The best approach to elimination of solidification cracking will depend on the alloy and application and must be determined experimentally.

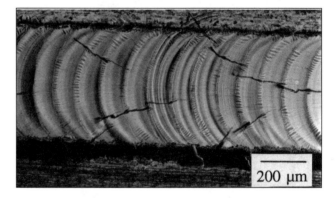

Figure 37. Severe solidification cracking in seam-welded Al-3.73 wt % Cu alloy welded using a square temporal pulse shape.

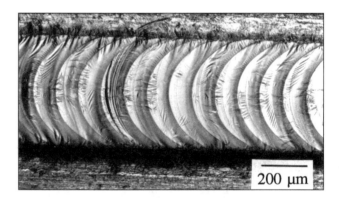

Figure 38. A crack-free seam weld produced in Al-3.73 wt % Cu aluminum alloy using an optimized ramp-down temporal pulse shape.

Laser Welding of Coated Metals

There are many applications where laser welding of coated sheet metals in the lap joint configuration is required such as welding of zinc-coated sheet steel, as illustrated in Figure 39a. The well-known problem with welding these materials in this joint configuration is related to the low boiling point of the zinc (906°C) compared with the melting temperature of steel (» 1550°C). During seam welding, the two zinc coatings at the interface vaporize and expand rapidly when the molten weld pool approaches the interface between the two sheet steels. With no gap between the sheets, this vapor can only escape through the weld pool, and this typically results in excessive weld porosity or complete expulsion of the weld metal.

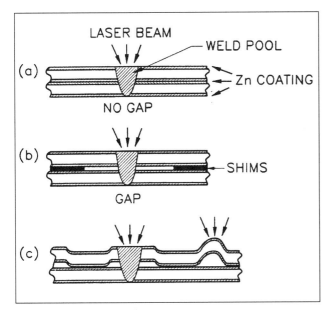

Figure 39. Schematic diagrams of lap-joint geometries for laser seam welding of zinc-coated sheet steels: (a) no gap between the sheets, (b) a defined gap between the sheets using preplaced shims, and (c) a defined gap using prestamped projections in the top sheet.

There are a number of different techniques that can be used to produce laser seam welds between sheet metal parts that have been plated with metals with boiling points below the melting point of the sheet. All these techniques involve modification of the lap-joint geometry to allow venting of the vapor generated during welding between the two sheets. For example, preplacement of shims of known thickness between the two sheets prior to welding as shown in Figure 39b has been shown to be sufficient to allow laser seam welding of galvanized sheet steels. Similarly, prestamping various groove geometries on one of the sheets to produce a gap between the sheets as shown in Figure 39c has also been used. A variation of this approach is seen in Figure 40, where a groove is prestamped in the top sheet, the parts clamped together and a laser seam weld made down the line of contact between the sheets. This geometry allows the zinc to vaporize and escape sideways in both directions between the sheets, permitting production of sound welds when using either pulsed or continuous-wave laser welders.

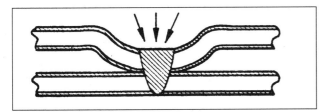

Figure 40. Schematic diagram of the groove-projection joint geometry used to laser seam weld coated sheet steels.

References

21. ASM Handbook, Vol. 6, *Welding, Brazing, and Soldering*, ASM International, Materials Park, OH, 1993.
22. C. J. Nonhof, 1988: *Material Processing with Nd-Lasers*, Electrochemical Publications Ltd., Ayr, Scotland.
23. J. T. Liu, D. C. Weckman, and H. W. Kerr, *Metall. Trans.* **24B**, 1065–76 (1993).
24. D. C. Weckman, H. W. Kerr, and J. T. Liu, *Metall. Mater. Trans.*, B **28B**, 687–700 (1997).
25. Z. Y. Wang, J. T. Liu, D. M. Hirak, D. C. Weckman, and H. W. Kerr, *J. Laser Appl.* **5** (1), 5–12, (1993).
26. H. N. Bransch, Z. Y. Wang, J. T. Liu, D. C. Weckman, and H. W. Kerr, *J. Laser Appl.* **3** (3), 25–34, (1991).
27. *Welding Handbook, Vol. 3, Materials and Applications, Part I,* American Welding Soc., Miami, FL, 25–8 (1996).

DAVID C. WECKMAN
HUGH W. KERR

11.3.7 Comparison of Penetration Welding with Nd:YAG and CO_2 Lasers

For otherwise comparable conditions, Nd:YAG lasers can provide greater welding capabilities (higher speed, greater penetration) than CO_2 lasers because of their shorter wavelength. Figure 41 shows data on the penetration welding of mild steel with Nd:YAG lasers and CO_2 lasers at various power levels.

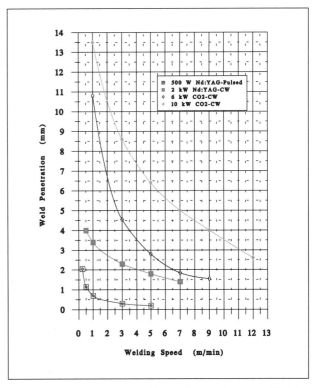

Figure 41. Representative weld speeds for CO_2 and Nd:YAG lasers on mild steel.

DAVID HAVRILLA

11.3.8 Laser Welding with Filler Wire

As with conventional welding, the use of filler wire provides new fields of application for laser welding. The special characteristics of laser beam welding require certain facts to be taken into consideration: The small laser spot diameter, the narrow distance between the welding gas nozzle and the metal surface, the small joint, and the small melt pool with its high speed dynamics are altogether limiting the field of parameters for laser beam welding with filler wire compared to conventional welding. Therefore, all parameters have to be adjusted carefully. The following subsections cover the applications of filler wire.

Gap Bridging

The small spot size of the laser beam requires a high-precision joint geometry. Even a gap of tenths of millimeters can lead to poor welds (see Fig. 42).

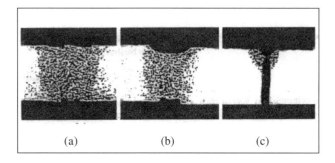

Figure 42. Butt welds with different gaps: (a) 0.1mm; (b) 0.2 mm; (c) 0.3 mm. Parameters are: beam power 1.9 kW; welding speed 2.0 m/min; mild steel; thickness 1.5 mm; wire SG2, ⌀ 0.8 mm.

When one uses filler wires, larger gaps are allowed. The filler wire not only helps to bridge gaps, but also provides additional absorption of laser power, which would be transmitted through the gap and therefore be lost without wire.

A basic condition for determining the maximum gap can be derived from the fact that the beam diameter has to be larger than the welding gap width:

$$a \leq 0.7\, d_s$$

where d_s is the laser beam diameter and a the gap size. Using this condition and the obligation to provide the necessary laser intensities, the allowable misalignment is as shown in Figure 43.

The permissible gap has been shown to increase by a factor of 3 to 6 when using filler wire (Fig. 44) in material with thickness up to 6 mm.

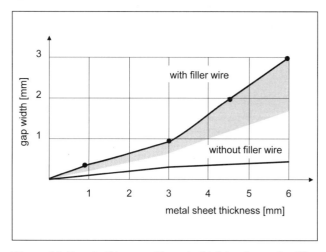

Figure 44. Permissible gap of laser butt joints when using filler wire [• – realized gap sizes].

Designing the Weld Geometry

Use of filler wire can avoid weld arching, underfilling, and undercutting. A refined and even scaled top weld seam can be achieved. Mechanical postprocessing is reduced or unnecessary (see Fig. 45).

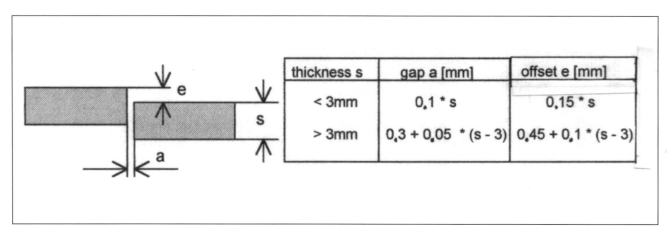

thickness s	gap a [mm]	offset e [mm]
< 3mm	0.1 * s	0.15 * s
> 3mm	0.3 + 0.05 * (s - 3)	0.45 + 0.1 * (s - 3)

Figure 43. Permissible misalignment of laser welded butt joints without filler wire.

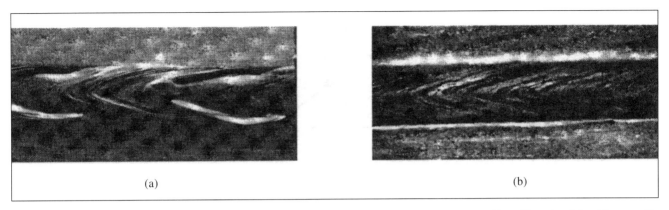

Figure 45. Top view of a laser welded seam (wire and base material: aluminum) (28). (a) Weld seam without filler wire; (b) weld seam with filler wire.

Joining of Difficult-to-Weld Materials

Difficult-to-weld material combinations, such as low-alloy steel with stainless steel, can be welded using laser beam welding with additional wire. The alloy of the wire has to be selected carefully to fit both welding partners. Because of the narrow fusion zone, only small quantities of molten metal will be mixed, thus allowing intermediate and weldable metal mixtures with both of the joint partners.

Multilayer Laser Beam Welding of Large Gaps

Because of the facts mentioned above, laser beam welding is limited to small joint cross sections and welding depths. Welding depths of more than about 10 mm require both a specially adapted joint geometry and a multilayer welding process. Therefore, a root bead (mostly without wire) is used to enable the melt pool of the following layers. Additional wire is used to fill the gap by multilayer laser welding.

The reduced heat input, per pass, leads to some advantages: It provides less distortion and fewer corrosion effects and allows welding even if there are heat-sensitive areas close to the joint. On the other hand, the repeated melting and cooling down of the weld and the heat-affected zone might cause problems with the metallurgical system.

Improvement of Mechanical and Technological Properties

As a result of the high temperatures during laser beam welding, significant vaporization of some low-melting-point alloys occurs. This especially affects laser beam welds of aluminum or other lightweight alloys, where the loss of magnesium, manganese, and lithium leads to a decreased corrosion resistance and less mechanical strength.

With the help of filler wire with selected alloy distribution, replacement of the lost amounts of alloys can be attained and good weld properties can be achieved. Increase of tensile strength, reduction of the hardness of the seam (see Fig. 46), improvement of the fatigue strength, reduction of hot cracking, and improved resistance against wear and corrosion can be attained with filler addition.

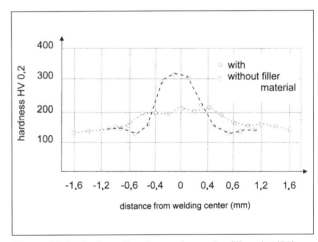

Figure 46. Reduction of hardness when using filler wire (29).

Improvement of the Weldability of Aluminum

The use of filler wire improves the weldability of aluminum by increasing the absorption and thus supporting both, the start of the welding and the deep penetration process (keyhole welding).

Improvement is especially apparent at relatively low irradiance in the range of 1.2×10^5 to 1×10^6 W/cm^2. Weld seam cross sections can be enlarged by 30–95% (application of CO_2 lasers). Attenuation of the otherwise highly turbulent dynamics of the melt pool occurs, thus stabilizing the pool and therefore getting a better weld with a refined scale and reduced roughness (28). Dropthrough, high porosity, and undercutting are reduced or disappear. If one uses appropriate alloy filler wire, hot cracking is reduced significantly (see Fig. 47 on next page).

Set-Up of Filler Wire Equipment

The equipment used for setting up a filler wire welding system with lasers is similar to conventional cold wire systems. A roll of filler wire provides the material, which is fed to the melt pool by a motor-driven unit. Because of the small diameter of the wire, a straightener may not be required. The wire is fed at an angle of 30 to 60 degrees (see Fig. 48 on next page).

Both dragging and lancing wire systems are used. If a sensing unit is needed, a lanced feeding is preferable because of the better visibility of the joint in front of the beam. A lanced feeding system involves the risk of sticking the wire to the solidified material, if the alignment is not perfect.

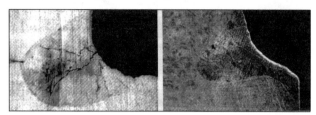

Figure 47. Reduction of hot cracking (left) using filler wire (right). Material: aluminum.

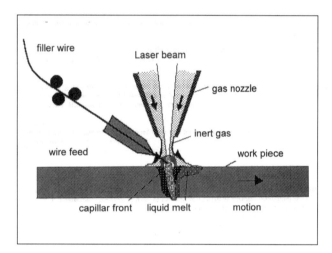

Figure 48. Principle for set-up for laser welding with filler wire (dragged wire feeding).

The shielding gas is fed either concentric with the wire, with the laser beam, or by a separate nozzle, depending on the design of the other components. The wire has to be fed directly to the melt pool. To avoid misalignment, a high-precision adjustment (± 0.2 mm in all directions) and a short free wire tip (< 5 mm) are required. Limits may vary with the size of the weldment, power, and weld speed. To prevent the nozzle tip from melting, it is made of tungsten and sometimes cooled additionally. A Teflon-coated spiral wire may be used to prevent adhesion and to reduce the slide resistance.

Typical filler wire units provide wire speed to 15 m/min. To avoid droplets at the end of the welding process, a defined retraction of the wire is required. As the gap may not be constant along the joint, sensors are needed to detect the joint position and gap width in order to adapt the wire speed using a control unit.

Melting Characteristics

Depending on the wire speed, three characteristic phases can be defined (see Fig. 49).

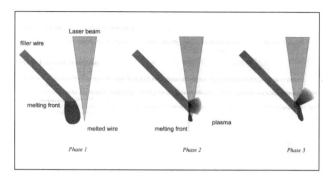

Figure 49. Melting characteristics of free-ending wires.

Phase 1. At low wire speed the wire is melted by the heat emission of the laser beam before entering the entire beam. The melting front is parallel to the workpiece surface. The molten material tends to form droplets.

Phase 2. With increasing wire speed the wire enters the entire beam and is melted by the laser radiation. The melting front swings to a position almost parallel to the beam. The molten material continuously bridges the gap between the wire and the workpiece. A plasma is produced. The solid part of the wire partly shades the beam.

Phase 3. Continued increase of the wire speed leads to a complete penetration of the entire beam by the wire. The wire will be melted only at its top side, shading the workpiece.

To maintain keyhole welding, it is advantageous to feed the wire at the trailing edge of the melt pool so as to avoid direct interaction of the wire with the beam.

Positioning

Accurate welds require phase 2 conditions, characterized by a stable bridge of molten wire material. To achieve this, precise positioning is essential. The crossing point of the wire (or its enlarged centerline) and the surface of the workpiece should be between 1 mm before the beam center and the beam center. A distance of more than 1 mm leads to beam shadowing (phase 3) and to the adhesion of the wire; values less than zero cause droplets (phase 1).

Control can be established in order to keep the height of the wire nozzle and the bridge of the molten wire material constant by varying the wire speed. Small wire diameter is required to realize the desired wide range of control. The diameter is limited by the availability of the wire and by handling problems, such as the risk of buckling. Typical diameters are in the range between 0.8 and 1.2 mm. Wires are available from 0.5 to 3 mm.

Calculating the Wire Speed

The wire speed can be calculated based on the fact that the wire has to fill the gap. The equation is:

$$v_{Dr} = F\,(v_s\,4\,s\,a) / (\pi\,d_{Dr}^{\,2})$$

Chapter 11: Penetration Welding

where v_{Dr} is the wire speed (m/min), v_S the welding speed (m/min), F the superelevation (e.g., 20% = 1.2), s the thickness of the workpiece (mm), a the gap width (mm), and d_{Dr} the wire diameter (mm).

A simple approximation results if the diameter of the wire is 0.8 mm and $F = 1$. Setting $\pi d_{Dr}^2 \approx 2$:

$$v_{Dr} = v_S \, 2 \, s \, a$$

As a result, welding of 3 mm material with gaps in the range of 0.2 to 0.5 mm leads to a wire speed – welding speed ratio of 1.2 to 3 and wire speeds of 3.0 to 9.0 m/min accordingly.

Required Power

The power for melting the wire must be taken from the laser beam. The beam will melt the same quantity of material at the same power and speed. If use of filler material yields a wider weld, more material is fused and laser power must increase.

The use of steel wires for gap bridging reduces the welding speed to about 60% compared to autogenous welding with the same weld width and perfect joint fitup.

Because of its low heat capacity, aluminum wires need less power. Especially if no gap bridging is desired, the wire speed is very low and the power needed is accordingly low.

Figure 50 (next page) shows the power needed for welding with steel and aluminum wire as a function of wire velocity.

Wire Materials; Filler Wire for Steel Welding

When welding high-alloy stainless steel, an even higher-alloyed filler wire is required to prevent the loss of low-vaporization-temperature melting alloys within the melting zone. Additional alloying with nickel improves the ductility.

Table 9 presents chemical compositions of wire suitable for mild and stainless steel welding.

Table 9. Filler Wire for Mild and Stainless Steel Welding

Wire material		Chemical analysis mass fraction %					
Short sign	Internat. reg. no.	C	Si	Mn	P	S	Cu
SG 1		0.06 to 0.12	0.5 to 0.7	1.0 to 1.3	≤ 0.025	≤ 0.025	≤ 0.30
SG 2, G421CG3Si1	ER70S-6	0.06 to 0.13	> 0.7 to 1.0	> 1.3 to 1.6	≤ 0.025	≤ 0.025	≤ 0.30
SG 3, G462CG4Si1	ER70S-6	0.06 to 0.12	0.8 to 1.2	> 1.6 to 1.9	≤ 0.025	≤ 0.025	≤ 0.30

Table 10. Filler Wire for Aluminum Welding (Al Mg Si Types)

Wire material		Chemical analysis (maximum values) mass fraction %								
Short name	Internat. reg. no.	Si	Fe	Cu	Mn	Mg	Cr	Zn	Ti[a]	Rest
S-AlSi5	4043	4.5 to 5.5	0.40	0.05	0.1	0.1	—	0.20	0.25	0.15
S-AlMg4,5Mn	5087	0.5 to 0.9	0.40	0.05	0.6 to 1.0	4.3 to 5.2	0.05 to 0.25	0.25	0.1 to 0.25	0.15
S-AlSi12	4047	11.0 to 13.5	0.6	0.05	0 to 0.5	0.05	—	0.20	0.10	0.15

[a] Titanium can be substituted with any refining alloy.

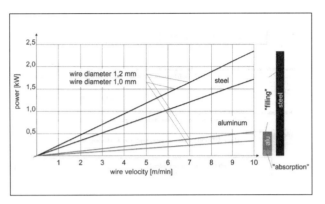

Figure 50. Required melting power for steel and aluminum wire versus wire velocity (28).

Mild and low-carbon steels should be welded using a low-equivalent-carbon wire to reduce the martensitic fraction in the weld, thus reducing the hardness due to the laser-induced heat treatment (see Fig. 46).

Filler Wire for Aluminum Welding

Manganese increases the strength, magnesium and zirconium increase the resistance against corrosion, and tin improves the mechanical properties. The tendency for hot cracking is reduced by silicon, copper, and manganese. Table 10 (previous page) presents chemical compositions of wire suitable for aluminum welding.

References

28. Chr. Binroth, Beitrag zur Prozeßstabilität beim CO_2-Schweißen von Aluminium mit Zusatzwerkstoff, Dissertation Universität Bremen, 1995.

29. M. Panten, J. Schneegans, M. Hendricks, A. Huwer, and L. Jacobskötter, Laser beam welding with filler wire, IIW COC.IV-545–90, ISF Aachen, 1990.

ANDREAS GEBHARDT

11.3.9 Welding with Other Lasers

High-Power Lasers Other than CO_2 and Nd:YAG

As important high-power (> 1 kW) laser sources other than CO_2 and Nd:YAG, the 5-μm-band CO laser and the 1.3-μm chemical oxygen-iodine laser (hereafter referred to as COIL) should be cited. Although both are still under development, they have many attractive features when their applications to welding are considered. In Table 11 the characteristics of these two new industrial lasers are compared with those of the present CO_2 and Nd:YAG lasers. See Chapter 2 for more information.

In laser welding, the process efficiency and sometimes even process quality are influenced by the laser wavelength, because the coupling of the laser energy to the workpiece is dominated by the surface absorption and/or the plasma absorption, both of which strongly depend on the laser wavelength. In general, the penetration depth increases with decreasing wavelength when other conditions remain unchanged.

The CO lasers can produce scalable outputs with as high efficiencies as achieved by CO_2 lasers with an output wavelength (5-μm band) shorter than that of the CO_2 laser (10.6 μm). For the reasons mentioned, therefore, higher-performance welding is expected with CO lasers than with the CO_2 lasers, especially at very high power levels, where the plasma absorption plays an important role for energy coupling.

Table 11. Characteristics of High-Power Lasers

Laser type (wavelength)		Nd:YAG laser (1.06 μm)	COIL (1.3 μm)	CO laser (5-μm band)	CO_2 laser (10.6 μm)
Maximum available output	Commercial	~ 4 kW	—	2 kW	45 kW
	R & D	5 ~ 6 kW	~ 1 kW (CW) > 5 kW (quasi-CW)	~ 20 kW	> 100 kW
Operating efficiency		Generally low	High (chemical pump)	High	High
Beam quality		Generally low	High	High	High
Pulsing characteristics		Excellent	Limited	Fair	Fair
Fiber-based beam delivery		Possible (> 1 kW)	Possible (> 1 kW)	Under R & D (~ 200 W)	Difficult
Interaction with metals	Surface absorption	High ⇐	⇐	⇐	⇐ Low
	Plasma absorption loss	Low ⇒	⇒	⇒	⇒ High

Chapter 11: Penetration Welding

Because the output wavelength of the COIL (1.3 μm) is close to that of the Nd:YAG laser (1.06 μm), the COIL laser beam can be delivered through quartz fibers. In addition, because of the nature of the gaseous lasers, the beam quality of the COIL is generally higher than that of the Nd:YAG lasers, which enables one to use narrower fibers for beam delivery. Although welding experiments with CO lasers and COILs started fairly recently, some important data have been reported.

Data on CO Laser Welding

In the past few years, welding experiments with multikilowatt (1-4 kW) CO-laser beams have been performed for aluminum alloys and steel. Most data are based on bead-on-plate welding.

Figure 51 shows the dependence of the penetration depth on the laser power with CO and CO_2 lasers around 1 kW for various aluminum alloys (30). For all such alloys, deeper penetration is obtained with the CO laser and the threshold laser powers for a deep-penetration fusion zone being formed are lower for the CO laser than for the CO_2 laser. Because this experiment is performed with CO and CO_2 lasers of similar beam quality, the different welding characteristics can be attributed to the difference in the wavelengths of the two lasers. It is known that for the non-transition metals including aluminum, the surface absorption depends less on the wavelength than for the transition metals. But the deeper penetrations obtained with the CO laser might be mainly due to the higher surface absorption at the shorter wavelength of the CO laser, because the energy coupling does not seem to be influenced by the laser-induced plasma at the laser power levels tested.

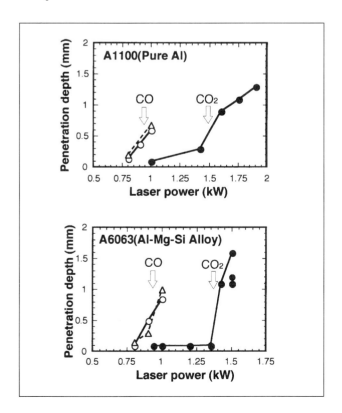

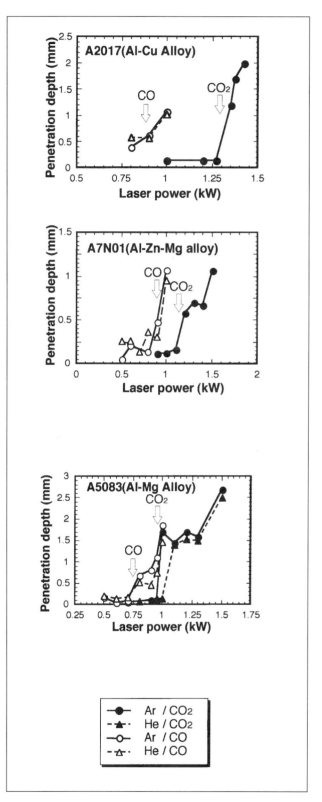

Figure 51. Dependence of the penetration depth on the laser power with CO and CO_2 lasers for various aluminum alloys (30). The arrows show the threshold powers for keyhole formation.

In Figure 52 the penetration depth obtained with the CO laser is compared with that obtained with the CO_2 and the Nd:YAG lasers for the AlMgSi1 alloy at a welding power of 2.2 kW, but the beam quality of these three lasers is evidently different. The penetration obtained with the CO laser is deeper not only than that of the CO_2 laser but also than that of the Nd:YAG laser. This can be explained by the fact that the beam quality of the Nd:YAG laser (fiber delivered) is lower than that of the CO laser, in spite of the Nd:YAG laser's shorter wavelength. More important, it is observed in this experiment that the bead surface quality for the CO laser is higher than that of the CO_2 laser, presumably because of the smaller plasma interruption of the laser beam for the CO laser than for the CO_2 laser.

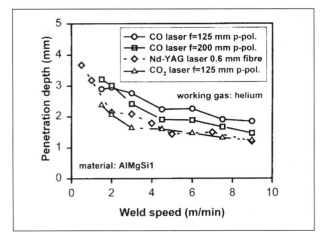

Figure 52. Dependence of the penetration depth on the laser power with CO, CO_2, Nd:YAG lasers for AlMgSi1 alloy (31).

Figure 53 also demonstrates that the CO laser gives deeper penetration than the Nd:YAG laser around 4 kW for the A5083 alloy. This may again be interpreted as being due to the difference of beam quality of the lasers used. Figure 54 shows the cross section of the CO-laser-welded bead at a welding speed of 0.75 m/min under Ar gas shielding. A penetration depth of more than 4 mm is obtained.

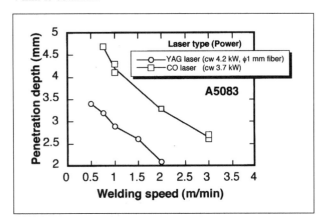

Figure 53. Dependence of the penetration depth on the laser power with CO and Nd:YAG lasers for the A5083 alloy.

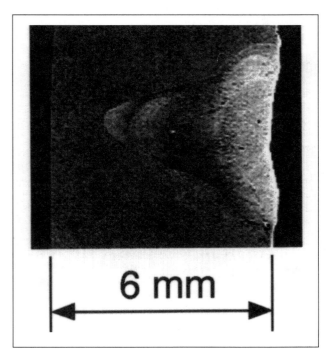

Figure 54. Transverse cross section of the weld bead with a 3.7-kW CO laser beam in the 6-mm-thick A5083 plates.

There are fewer data on the CO laser welding of steel. But for the C/Mn steel, penetration depths of 3.5–4.8 mm are obtained with a 1.8-kW CO laser beam at a welding speed of 0.6 m/min under both Ar and He shielding conditions. In another experiment using a wedge-shaped mild steel of 1–10 mm thickness, a maximum penetration around 6 mm was obtained at 4 kW under He shielding, while a maximum penetration of around 7 mm was obtained at 4.3 kW under Ar shielding (33).

These CO laser welding data are summarized in Table 12 (next page). Because much more intense laser-induced plasma is formed under Ar shielding than under He shielding, a higher-energy coupling and hence a deeper penetration is expected for the He shielding. But in many cases shown in Table 12, the influence of the type of shielding gas is not clear. The reason for this may be related to the fact that the heavier Ar gas can sometimes suppress the plasma more efficiently than He gas can, especially when the gas is supplied from a tube not from a coaxial nozzle.

Data on COIL Welding

Data on COIL welding are very scarce, but it is reported that very thick (40-mm) stainless steel plates (type 316L) can be successfully joined based on a multipass welding with a filler wire (34). For a narrow groove, a 15-pass welding procedure was performed at 3.4 kW under N_2 gas shielding. Figure 55 shows the cross section of the COIL-welded bead. The welding speed and the wire feeding speed were 0.3 and 1.7 m/min, respectively. The transverse shrinkage of the joint was as small as 2.3 mm.

Chapter 11: Penetration Welding

Table 12. Summary of CO Laser Welding Data

Material	Thickness (mm)	Shielding gas		Laser power (kW)	Spot diam. (μm)	Welding speed (m/min)	Penetration depth (mm)	Remarks	Ref.
		Type	Flow rate (L/min)						
A1100	6	He Ar	40	1	~300	1	0.7 0.6	A coaxial nozzle with a 6-mm-diam. hole is used for shield gas supply.	30
A2017	6	He Ar	40	1	~300	1	1.0 1.1		
A5083	6	He Ar	40	1	~300	1	1.5 1.9		
A6063	6	He Ar	40	1	~300	1	1.0 0.85		
A7N01	6	He Ar	40	1	~300	1	0.95 1.2		
AlMgSi (A6082)	6	He	30	2.2	150 240	2 9 2 9	3 1.9 3 1.5	A 4-mm-diam. tube is used for shield gas supply.	31
A5083	6	Ar	40	3.7	~600	0.75 3	4.7 2.7	A coaxial nozzle with a 6-mm-diam. hole is used for shield gas supply.	
C/Mn steel	6	He Ar	30 30	1.8 1.8	400 400	0.6 0.6	3.5–4.8 3.7–4.6	A 4-mm-diam. tube is used at 45° for shield gas supply.	32
Wedge-shaped mild steel	1–10	He Ar	60 15	4 4.3	~360 ~360	1	6.3 7.3	The spot diam. is measured at the focal point.	33

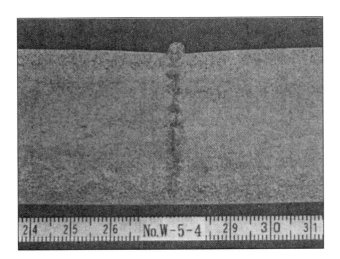

Figure 55. Cross section of the 15-pass weld bead with a 3.4-kW COIL beam in 40-mm-thick 316L stainless steel (34).

Outlook for the Future

Along with the development of practical high-power CO lasers and COILs, much more data on welding will be collected and reported. In the next few years, the usefulness of these two lasers for welding will be more clearly determined.

References
30. B. A. Mehmetli, K. Takahashi, and S. Sato, *J. Laser Applications* **8,** 25–31 (1996).
31. M. Schellhorn, and A. Eichhorn, *Optics & Laser Technology* **28,** 405–7 (1996).
32. R. J. Ducharme, P. D. Kapadia, J. M. Dowden, P. A. Hilton, S. T. Riches, and I. A. Jones, *Proc. ICALEO'96,* D/10–19 (1996).
33. M. Schellhorn, and H. v. Bülow, *SPIE* **2502,** 664–9 (1995).
34. T. Sakurai, K. Yasuda, T. Osaki, E. Tada, K. Koizumi, and M. Nakahira, *Proc. ICALEO'96,* E/28–37 (1996).

SUNICHI SATO

11.3.10 Operating Costs for Penetration Welding
This section estimates operating costs for some penetration welding applications. The approach is to calculate a per hour cost for expendables while amortizing some of the maintenance costs on an hourly basis.

ISBN 0-912035-15-3

Table 13 presents costs for CO_2 laser welding, and Table 14 presents costs for Nd:YAG laser welding. For the Nd:YAG laser, the lamp life is strongly dependent on laser power and duty cycle.

These estimates may be altered to cover other laser applications.

DAVID HAVRILLA

Table 13. Operating Costs for CO_2 Laser Penetration Welding

A 6000-W transverse flow laser, welding carbon steel with a 200-mm-focal-length focusing optic, and requiring a 5-mm (0.2 in.) weld penetration, with helium shield gas @ 40 scfh.

Welding speed	2.4 m/min (95 in./min)	
Laser electrical power	(70 kVA) (0.8 pf) ($0.08/kW h)	[1] 4.48
Laser gas, carbon dioxide	(0.07 scf/h) ($0.12/scf) =	0.01
Laser gas, helium	(1.00 scf/h) ($0.14/scf) =	0.14
Laser gas, nitrogen	(0.53 scf/h) ($0.08/scf) =	0.04
Chiller electrical power	(30 kW) ($0.08/kW h) =	2.40
Chiller additive	(0.10) (200 gal) ($20/gal)/(6000 h) =	0.07
Laser optics (2000 h)	($3720)/(2000 h) =	1.86
Laser optics (4000 h)	($3120)/(4000 h) =	0.78
Shield gas, helium	(40 scf/h) ($0.14/scf) =	[1] 5.60
Exhaust system power	(5 kW) ($0.08/kW h) =	0.40
Exhaust system filters	($50)/(100 h) =	0.50
Maintenance labor	(12 h/2000 h) ($45) =	0.27
Total approximate operating cost per hour (full power continuous weld)		$16.55/h
[1] Cost per hour (assuming 75% duty cycle)		$14.03/h

Table 14. Operating Costs for Nd:YAG Laser Penetration Welding

A 2000-W CW laser, welding carbon steel with a 120-mm-focal-length focusing optic, and requiring a 3-mm (0.12 in.) weld penetration, with helium shield gas @ 40 scfh.

Welding speed	1.3 m/min (50 in./min)	
Laser electrical power	(75 kW) ($0.08/kW h) =	[1] 6.00
Chiller electrical power	(40 kW) ($0.08/kW h) =	3.20
Chiller additive	(0.35) (75 gal) ($10/gal)/(4000 h) =	0.07
Laser arc lamps	($250) (8)/(1000 h) =	2.00
Shield gas	(40 scf/h) ($0.14/scf) =	[1] 5.60
Cover slide	($50)/(1000 h) =	0.05
Exhaust system power	(5 kW) ($0.08/kW h) =	0.40
Exhaust system filters	($50)/(100 h) =	0.50
Maintenance labor	(5 h/2000 h) ($45) =	0.11
Total approximate operating cost per hour		$17.93/h
[1] Cost per hour (assuming 75% duty cycle)		$15.03/h

11.4 Industrial Applications of High-Power Laser Welding

11.4.1 Introduction

The success of laser cutting in the industrial marketplace has led to the natural emergence of laser welding. Laser welding presents a fundamentally more challenging integration difficulty into industry as compared to laser cutting, because a weld must be load bearing. In this section we will examine the key aspects of laser welding for industrial applications, covering carbon and stainless steel, aluminum alloys, and selected plastics.

This section details important laser welding parameters and the advised considerations for welding particular material types and thickness. Sections dedicated to material thickness follow, with general observations, and detailed successfully implemented welding operations. A number of specific areas are then addressed, including weld tolerances and innovative hybrid welding techniques combining the arc and the laser.

11.4.2 Key Aspects

Laser Power and Processing Speed

The first decision to be made is the required welding speed based on penetration and production throughput. Once this starting point is made, the other parameters can be selected and optimized for the particular process. As a simple rule of thumb, the speed, power, and penetration relationship is given by $P = vd$, where P is power (kW), v is welding speed (m/min), and d is thickness (mm). The approximate figure for the necessary laser power is now known, though this is only a part of the story. How the optical energy is delivered to the workpiece, material heat cycling limitations, gas delivery, joint preparation, and weld analysis are other aspects.

Selection of Focusing Optics

The choice of focal length directly affects the focused spot and depth of focus, which impacts welding efficiency, alignment tolerances (vertical, seam tracking, gap width), and optic-to-workpiece distance.

Unfortunately, to attain high welding efficiency, by which is meant using the exact optical depth of focus that matches the depth of the material, the user immediately minimizes all tolerances and ultimately the processing window. For example, consider welding 1-mm mild steel. The speed requirement is as fast as possible with a 5-kW laser. To maximize the use of optical energy, match 1 mm with the depth of focus for that laser. Assuming a raw beam size of 20 mm ($1/e^2$), and using the definition of depth of focus as an increase in beam diameter by 5%, we have

$$\text{depth of focus} = 2\lambda/\pi \, (2F/D)^2$$

(approximately 2% of focal length), where λ is the laser wavelength, F the focal length, and D the beam diameter at the optic ($1/e^2$).

This gives a focal length of 120 mm, with a corresponding spot size diameter ($d_f = 4\lambda FM^2/\pi D$) of 0.12 mm. In real life both these will be slightly larger, but the approximate tolerances are very demanding: vertical misalignment around 0.35 mm (@ 40% material thickness), seam tracking around 0.05 mm (50% beam size), and gap width around 0.05 mm (50% beam size). Therefore, the choice of optics is a compromise between speed, tolerances, and available space. Metal optics are recommended over plano-convex ZnSe lenses when the power is over 2 kW, and/or the material thickness is over 2 mm (back-spatter problem). The reflective optics are oriented such that the mirror immediately above the weld and in line of the back spatter is an inexpensive flat or spherical mirror. As a matter of course, a lateral or downward protective gas jet should be used. Care must be taken in the orientation, positioning, and pressure setting of the jet to ensure no interference/contamination of the weld area. The flow area should be below the smallest opening possible and should be at least twice the cross section of this area. The pressure of the jet must be set so that it does not actually suck in contaminants.

The position of focus for welding material less than 3 mm thick is generally at the surface of the workpiece; this may be varied above and below to optimize the process for penetration, tolerances, wire feed, or weld bead smoothness. For thickness 3 mm and greater, the position of focus may be on or below the surface. With increasing thickness the keyhole acts as a waveguide for the radiation; thus it is not always best to be below the surface. The position of focus can be established for a CO_2 laser by moving the beam quickly over a Perspex sheet angled slightly from the vertical. For a Nd:YAG laser, Kapton film or exposed photographic paper can be used.

Thermal Cycling

The optical energy density that gives laser welding its characteristic advantages results in the weld metal and heat-affected zone experiencing an intense thermal cycling, with solidification rates around 1000 C/s. For steels the carbon equivalent (CE) equation is a useful guide.

$$CE = C\% + Mn\%/6 + (V\% + Cr\% + Mo\%)/5 + (Ni\% + Cu\%)/15$$

A steel with CE less than 0.4 is weldable; above this value further investigation is necessary to control heat input by welding more slowly than usual, using filler material, or using pre- or postweld heat treatment. For aluminum alloys the levels of volatile elements and heat treatment are important. Thus the 5xxx series is more weldable than the 6xxx series.

Gas Delivery

A nonreactive or inert welding assist gas serves several functions, such as suppressing the welding plume, protecting optics from weld spatter, preventing weld oxidation, and improving weld penetration/width.

The formation of a welding plume is unavoidable, though it can be minimized. The predominant loss effect of the plume is to enlarge the focus spot size by refracting the radiation as it passes through, plus absorbing some percentage of the beam energy directly. For sheet welding and/or using a Nd:YAG laser up to 2 kW, the type of gas and method of delivery can be argon, helium, and sometimes air (clean) with a 2–5 mm diameter coaxial delivery nozzle, at flows around 10–20 L/min. The higher power required for thicker material causes significant plume effects and must be seriously addressed by the gas shield type or mixture and mode of delivery. For steel two approaches can be adopted. The approaches are summarized in Table 1.

The direction of the gas jet can be either following or perpendicular to the direction of welding. The jet should not be ahead of the weld directed back along the completed weld. The use of a carbon dioxide assist, or oxygen additions up to 10% to the main shielding gas, has the effect to narrow and increase weld penetration. When welding up to 6-mm-thick material the use of argon/helium combinations should be considered, with exact percentages found for specific cases. Beyond this thickness, 100% helium is recommended. Galvanized steel is optimally shielded using a cross-flow jet, positioned either horizontal with the workpiece or at an angle less than 30 degrees pointing across or along the line to be welded.

For aluminum alloys, a diffused helium jet is required, typically at 20-mm distance from the keyhole, with a 5–10 mm bore at a flow of 20 L/min. In addition, an underbead flow is required, and in order to fill the underside region some choking of the flow at the exit is required. Underbead flow can also be used with steels for reasons of oxidation; usually argon is used, though some stainless steels require nitrogen.

Joint Preparation

The preparation of the weld faces, specifically for butt welding, is very significant. The edge squareness and uniformity over a cut length are crucial. For sheet parts the three major techniques of guillotine, stamp, and laser cut offer different edge qualities. The industry norm is precision shearing using double-guillotine-blade technology, typically offering ± 0.05 mm tolerance. Laser cutting is similar but as a thermal process causes an oxide and heat-affected zone area. The edges should be free from dirt, with degreasing preferred but not essential. For aluminum alloys the edges must be extremely clean. Degreasing is essential, and for critical welding operations pickling is also used. This also applies to titanium.

Table 1. Approaches for Shielding Gas Delivery for Laser Welding

Gas	Flow rate (L/min)	Pipe/nozzle bore diameter (mm)	Distance from keyhole (mm)	Pointing tolerance (mm)	Interaction point of pipe
Unoptimized 100% helium	Coaxial – 30 45° jet – 30	5	10	± 1–2	At laser spot, around 45 degrees
Optimized Ar/He/CO_2/O_2 combinations	Jet – 15	2	5	± 0.5	Around 1 mm ahead From 15 to 45 degrees

Table 2. Thin Sheet Welding Examples – Miscellaneous Applications

Material	Laser	Power (W)	Speed (m/min)	Weld type	Additional information
Stainless steel/nickel plated steel 0.2 mm	CO_2	270	NA	Spot	63.5-mm lens Nitrogen shroud Pulse duration 48 ms
Aluminum 0.35 mm		1.5 kW CW	40 m/min	Tack butt	150-mm lens Nitrogen assist gas
Stainless steel 0.03 mm thick		125 W CW	7.5 m/min	Hermetic lap	68.5-mm lens Nitrogen assist gas
Stainless steel 304 0.15 mm		700 W CW	25 m/min	Butt	125-mm lens defocused to 1-mm beam diameter Argon assist gas
Stainless steel	Nd:YAG	400 W av	NA	Spot	68.5-mm lens 1-ms pulse width
	CO_2	235 W av	NA	Spot	68.5-mm lens No assist gas 1.4-ms pulse width

For thicker sections, plasma and flame cutting can also be used with filler material.

11.4.3 Welding Thin Sheet Material (< 0.5 mm)

The welding of such material has been industrially implemented for the welding of razor blades. A number of systems manufacturers offer battery case welding. When the welding material is this thin, the lap configuration is firmly recommended over abutting, because butt welding tends to produce blow holes unless conduction welding is used. Also the lap weld avoids the significant difficulty of ensuring a close-fitting vertical-aligned butt joint with metal that is easily deformable.

The original market leader for this operation was the Nd:YAG laser, though this is now being challenged by RF-excited CO_2 lasers, which have high pulsing controllability and flexibility. Table 2 (previous page) presents some samples.

11.4.4 Sheet Material (1–3 mm)

The welding of this thickness of material largely relates to the automotive industry and more recently the ship building industry. The laser has the capability to join material of different thickness and grades in both the butt and lap/stake weld configurations. Table 3 shows a selection of the wide range of welding combinations. When welding this thickness of material, the position of focus is typically at the surface of the material. When one makes a step butt weld, the laser may be angled into the step by up to 15 degrees according to the weld surface profile requirements.

The use of filler material for the 6xxx series of aluminum alloys is required for the CO_2 laser, but not with the Nd:YAG laser. This largely relates to the larger spot size, around 0.6 mm compared to 0.4 mm with the CO_2 laser, and to the flat-top mode that stabilizes out-gassing and melt pool flow. The cross-section weld geometry for sheet materials of different thicknesses is dependent on the positioning of the beam with respect to the joint line centerline. A faster weld with low fatigue requirements can be welded on the joint line; however, when a smooth curvature is required, some offset of the beam to the thicker material is necessary – anywhere between 0 and 0.3 mm.

In the shipbuilding industry, the use of a new type of panel construction is offering large weight savings and a versatile design. The construction is two panels that sandwich a corrugated centerpiece. The exact dimensions of the corrugation and sheet thickness are tailored to meet strength requirements. The fabrication requires a stake weld between the flat and corrugated materials.

Table 3. Sheet Welding Examples – All Automotive Applications

Material	Laser	Power (kW)	Speed (m/min)	Weld type	Additional information
Cold-rolled mild steel 1.8–1.4 mm	CO_2	6	5	Butt	250-mm lens He gas assist
Cold-rolled or galvanized 2.0–0.8 mm		6	6	Butt	250-mm lens He gas assist
Stainless steel 409 1 mm		6	6	Butt	
Aluminum 5182 1.5–3 mm		5.1	4.5	Step butt	SG-AlMg4.5Mn (DE63) 1-mm filler wire used at 6.8 m/min (1)
Aluminum 6016 1.2 mm thick		3.5	2.5	Butt	SG-AlSi5 f 1 mm Helium at 20 L/min top and root (1)
Aluminum 6082 1 mm thick	Nd:YAG	2.8 CW	4	Butt	Helium shielding gas

Table 4. Examples of Sheet Stake Welding – Shipbuilding Industry

Material	Laser	Power (kW)	Speed (m/min)	Weld type	Additional information
Stainless steel 3xx 1.5–1.0 mm	CO_2	1.5	1.35	Thru stake	87-mm focal length Nitrogen shielding gas (2)
2.0–1.0 mm			0.8	Thru stake	
1.0–2.0 mm			1.85	Partial stake	

Excellent contact between the layers is essential for providing the fitup for a sound weld. Table 4 (previous page) presents some examples.

11.4.5 Welding Plate Material (4–12 mm)

For this thickness of material, at least 5 kW is required to achieve a reasonable welding speed and the required weld depth. The primary applications at this thickness are pipe welding and primary panels for the shipbuilding industry. One of the major considerations is a fitup that can be realistically maintained over long weld lengths. This has led to the use of filler material. An additional consideration with these structural steels are the post-weld mechanical properties in relation to material composition, with current limits being 0.12% C, 0.01% S, and 0.015% P. Examples are presented in Table 5.

11.4.6 Weld Tolerances

The weld tolerances that can be accommodated are largely re-

Table 5. Examples of Thick Section Welding for Shipbuilding and Pipe Manufacture Applications

Material	Laser	Power (kW)	Speed (m/min)	Weld type	Additional information
Carbon steel 12 mm	CO_2	9	0.8	Butt	Helium or He/10% O_2 shielding gas, at 30 L/min. Autogenous welds up to 0.4-mm gap width.
			0.4	Butt	1-mm Gap width Filler metal cored 1.2 ϕ mm
Carbon steel 9 mm	Nd:YAG	4	0.3	Butt	Argon shielding gas
Carbon steel 6 mm	CO_2	9	1.6	Butt	
		25	10	Butt	381 Focal length 870° C Preheat 50 L/min He through 10 mm ϕ pipe (3)
Carbon steel 5 mm		4	0.6	Butt	190-mm lens Helium coaxial assist at 40 L/min

Table 6. Summary of Welding Tolerances for Sheet and Plate Laser Welding

	General welding tolerances	
	0.5–2 mm thickness	5–12 mm thickness
Lens	200 mm Spot size of 0.2 mm	200–700 mm with beam diameter of 35–80 mm; Spot sizes between 0.4 and 0.8 mm
Gas assist	He, coaxial, or jet	He or He/10% O_2, using 1.8–10 mm diameter pipe with flow rate of 10–60 L/min
Gap width	Autogenous 0.1 mm See hybrid welding	Autogenous gap width of 0.4 mm, with ability to weld to 1.5 mm using filler and adaptive control
Joint preparation	Precision sheared	Thermal cut, thermal cut and sand blast, thermal cut and ground, milled
Vertical mismatch	Up to 50% material thickness	Up to 2 mm
Angular mismatch		5 degree from both directions. An 8 degree prep can be used if required
Primer/oxidation	Paint should be removed, oxide coating can be tolerated, but weld width is reduced by 30%	Can be tolerated
Filler addition	If attempted, must be precision feed, requiring a tolerance of ± 0.1 mm	The composition is typically similar to the parent material For steels – low C, Mn, S (0.07); For aluminum – high Mg, Si Wire diameter around 1.2 mm, positioned around 1–2 mm ahead of the beam, angled at 60 degrees. Wire feed speed around 6 m/min, with flame cut edges requiring adaptive control

lated to the optical setup and welding speed chosen. Intuitively a wider beam and slower welding speed are most tolerant. Table 6 (previous page) summarizes some general tolerances for both sheet and plate materials.

The major consideration in the thick section welds is the requirement of filler material, which is totally dependent on the likely fitup and cut quality of the joint edges. The amount of filler material logically relates to the gap width:

wire speed = (welding speed x gap cross section) wire cross section

It is advisable to minimize the wire diameter to the size of the gap width, and to ensure that gas shielding is adequate, typically using a coaxial, side and trailing jet each delivering helium at flows around 20 L/min. When one uses filler material, the speed of wire input and amount of defocus need to be optimized.

The filler technology for laser welding has largely used metal wire; recently the use of powders has been considered (4). These can be introduced ahead of the keyhole into the front of the melt pool, or in annuli around the keyhole. The particulate nature of the powder offers some unique benefits, including excellent mixing, multidirectional welding, and the ability to customize weld and powder compositions.

11.4.7 Hybrid Welding

The combination of the arc/preheat and the laser in certain applications offers a unique welding technique. The development of hybrid welding has been pursued for a number of reasons. Laser energy is expensive; arc energy is inexpensive. The advantages of both processes can be utilized to produce a host of welding solutions. The use of the equivalent arc energy allows the welding speed to be increased by up to 50%; in addition, the enlarged melt pool width can increase the fitup tolerances by around 200%. The hybrid technique of induction preheat effectively smoothes the thermal cycling of the weld; therefore, steels with carbon contents in excess of 0.25% become weldable. Table 7 presents some examples of hybrid welding.

The arc torch is positioned at the incident point of the laser beam, with gas mixtures of helium and argon usually used.

11.4.8 Weld Testing

The evaluation of sheet welding is more straightforward than plate welds, and simple visual inspection of the surface offers more reliable information than for the thicker sections. Quick sight checks include:

- Uniform weld width, showing regular chevron pattern top and underside
- Moving the fingernail over the weld reveals no distinct undercuts
- No obvious blue/gold coloration of the weld, indicating oxidation
- In-hand bend test (if possible)
- No obvious surface/underside bulging, or excessive weld spatter

Once these criteria have been satisfied, the formal mechanical testing (tensile, formability, sectioning, bend, hardness, radiography, fatigue, corrosion) can be completed as required. Problems arise when impact and fracture testing may be necessary; the laser welds are tough and undersized, and the usual procedures are no longer valid. According to one's resources, a fitness for purpose or customized test can be carried out. For example, for the Charpy impact test, overlapping welds can be made to increase the weld area to a standard size. A welding standard for laser and electron beam welding exists for structural steel. The standard is BS EN ISO 13919-1:1997 – *Welding: Electron and Laser Beam Welded Joints. Guidance for Quality Levels and Imperfections*. This is also a good guide for other materials.

11.4.9 Plastic Welding

The extremely high or low absorptivity of plastics, and the complication of multilayered sheets, means the weldability of plastics is limited to a few thermoplastics. The laser tends to ablate plastic, or is not absorbed by the plastic. In addition, the heating and cooling cycles of plastics must be adhered to, usually with

Table 7. Examples of Hybrid Laser Plus Arc Welding – Automotive and Pipe Applications

Material	Laser	Power (kW)	Speed (m/min)	Weld type	Additional information
Galavanized steel 1.2–1.8 mm	CO_2 + plasma	5 + 1.5	4.5	Step butt	Gap widths up to 0.5 mm Seam misalignment 0.4 mm (5)
Galvanized steel 1.0 mm	Nd:YAG + Plasma	2 + 1	0.9–2.0	Lap	Inter gap spacing up to 0.5 mm Helium shielding gas (5)
Mild steel 1–2 mm	CO_2 + TIG	4 + 4	10	Step butt	(6)
Aluminum AlMgSi05 4 mm	Nd:YAG + TIG	1.9 + 4	2.4	Butt	Filler wire S-AlSi5 1.6 mm diam. used (6)
Tempered steel 5 mm	CO_2	6	2	Butt	Preheat between 600 and 800°C, induction heating at 13 kHz (6)

the use of some compressive force on the joint. A few cases of welding operations involve lap welding of up to 0.3-mm-thick polypropylene with a CO_2 laser. This material has been welded by cutting and fusing the top layer to the bottom. Butt welds can be made in cut and weld operations, thin-sheet polyurethane being a good example. Plastics require extremely low irradiance, typically as low as 25 W/cm² for lap welding. Therefore a subkilowatt laser is usually more than sufficient.

11.4.10 Material Welding Summary

Table 8 summarizes some of the materials welded with lasers in industry.

References

1. T. Pohl and M. Schultz, *Laser beam welding of aluminum alloys for lightweight structures using CO_2 and Nd:YAG laser systems.* Laser Assisted Net Shape Engineering 2, Proceedings of LANE 97, Meisenbach Bamberg, 181–92, 1997.
2. A. Furio and J. Bird, Laser welding in ship construction. 6th International Conference on Welding and Melting by Electron and Laser Beams, 299–306, 1998.
3. T. Hayashi, Y. Inaba, Y. Matuhiro, T. Yamada, and T. Kudo, *Development of high power laser welding process for pipe.* International Congress on Laser and Electro-Optics (ICALEO) – Section D, Detroit, 132–40, 1996.
4. G. J. Shannon and W. M. Steen, *Thick section laser butt welding of structural steel using a coaxial filler nozzle.* International Congress on Laser and Electro-Optics (ICALEO), San Diego, Section G, 282–99, 1997.
5. J. Biffin, *Plasma augmented lasers shine ahead in auto body application,* Weld & Metal Fabrication, April, 19–21, 1997.
6. E. Beyer, B. Brenner, and R. Propawe, *Hybrid laser welding techniques for enhanced welding efficiency,* International Congress on Laser and Electro-Optics (ICALEO) – Section D, Detroit, 157–66, 1996.

Dawes, C. *Laser welding – A practical guide.* Abington Publishing, 1992. ISBN 1 85573 034 0.

GEOFF J. SHANNON

11.4.11 Laser-Welded Tailored Blanks

Tailor-welded blanks are flat sheet metal blanks produced from two or more individual sheets that have different properties. The property variations include gauge, material strength, and coating type. Most tailored blanks are steel, but aluminum blanks are being developed. The benefits of tailored blanks for the auto industry include lower weight, fewer assembly operations, improved crash energy management, and lower overall manufacturing cost. Tailored blanks are produced from rectangular, trapezoidal, or configured sheets to form the flat blank shape required by the metal forming (usually stamping) operation. After forming and trimming, the blanks proceed to assembly operations. This manufacturing approach gives designers the flexibility to build in or "tailor" performance characteristics at the locations on the automobile body where they are needed. For example, galvanized sheet material components can be used in locations that are most subject to corrosion, and thicker material can be used in areas where high stress demands it. Alter-

Table 8. Summary of Materials Currently Welded with a Laser

Material	Comments
Aluminum alloys	5000, 6000 series up to 3 mm depth – both require filler material; Nd:YAG lasers offer benefits over CO_2 lasers in terms of requiring filler material
Copper	High laser beam quality allows welding up to 3-mm sheet
Cast iron	Nodular cast iron can be welded with nickel filler wire
Nickel alloys (Hastelloy, Inconel, Waspaloy)	Some are highly weldable, subject to specific alloying elements
Steels - low carbon (<0.2%)	Highly weldable
- medium and high carbon (>0.2%)	Weldable, requiring filler and/or heat treatment
Alloy steels (BS4360 50D)	Structural and pipeline steels are weldable. Levels of Mn, S, Si elements are important considerations
Stainless steels: Austenitic (AISI 304-321)	Highly weldable (exception of 303 and 303e)
Ferritic (AISI 403-446)	Grades with low carbon and chromium weld best
Martensitic (AISI 410-440)	Problems with HAZ embrittlement – filler and past welding heat treatment are required
Titanium alloy (6Al-4V-Ti)	Highly weldable provided all usual precautions and weld prep are made
Plastics (thermoplastics – polyethylene, polypropylene)	Thin sheets weldable up to 300 µm. Absorption tuning of sheets/laser and the use of interface dies can enhance weldability. Penetration to 3 mm has been attempted; however, this is more a cut and press technique.

nately, thinner material can be incorporated in areas where controlled, crash energy absorption is critical. Figure 1 shows an example.

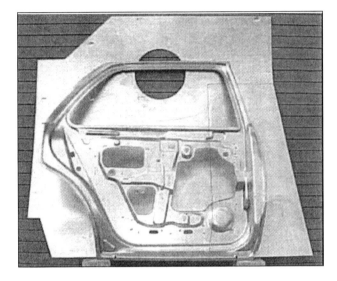

Figure 1. Door-inner panel formed from a tailored blank, illustrating nonlinear laser weld.

From a welding standpoint, there are several key factors to be considered in tailored blank manufacturing. High integrity is needed in the joints, since subsequent forming processes are likely to fracture welds, which have lack of fusion, concavity, porosity, or other discontinuities. The demand for consistent weld quality is such that on-line weld quality monitoring systems are often desired. Consistent blank dimensions are needed to ensure that parts are repeatably positioned in the subsequent forming dies. This concern is particularly an issue with large blanks or those consisting of many components. Dimensional accuracy also demands a low-distortion welding process. Finally, process cost is always an issue in high-production, mass-market products such as automobiles. Of the many possible welding processes that could potentially be used in this application, mash seam welding and laser beam welding have proven to be the most viable, and account for practically all automotive tailored blank production.

Laser welding of tailored blanks is a conceptually simple but practically demanding process. The joint configuration is an autogeneous straight-butt, usually with two different material thicknesses. The weld path is usually a straight line, requiring only one primary axis of motion to complete the weld, but nonlinear laser welds in tailored blanks are also used in large-scale automotive platforms. These two-dimensional blanks are more difficult to produce because of the precision edge preparation requirement and the need for unique, custom fixtures for each blank design.

Blank Component Preparation

Most tailored blank welding applications use steel sheet materials. The most common applications use uncoated, galvanized, and galvannealed material in thicknesses ranging from 0.6 to 2.3 mm. While the blank welding process tolerates many combinations of coating types, most tailor-welded blanks are produced from similarly coated sheets to aid in the consistency of subsequent forming, welding, and painting operations.

Precise preparation of blank components is an essential prerequisite to achieving consistently high weld quality and productivity. The ideal weld joint is one with perfectly flat mating edges, butted with no measurable gap at any point along the seam. Under these conditions and all other equipment factors remaining constant, the minimum laser focus spot size and, consequently, the maximum welding travel speed can be attained. Generally speaking, joint edge imperfections and gaps require a larger weld cross section and hence, larger focus spot size (or perhaps two focus spots) to avoid defects. Lack of fusion and weld bead concavity are the two defects most often resulting from excessive gap or poorly shaped edges. The consequence of larger focus spot size is reduced productivity since the travel speed must be reduced as focus spot size increases (power remaining the same). Regardless of focal spot size and travel speed, it is recommended that fitup gap should be no greater than 0.1–0.15 mm, depending on material thicknesses.

When the blank is designed with straight weld seams, precision shearing of the weld edges is a common way of achieving the required level of edge quality. A cross section of a typical sheared edge is illustrated in Figure 2 (next page). It consists of two regions, one that has been parted by shearing (the shear region) and another that has been parted by fracture (the break region). The nature of stresses during the cutting process are such that the break region forms a slight angle with the sheet surface, whereas the sheared region generally is much closer to perpendicular. When two sheared edges are abutted, a smaller gap is obtained if the edges are predominantly sheared, rather than broken. As a general rule, it is desirable that the ratio of the thickness of the shear region to that of the break region (shear-to-break ratio) be greater than one. Precision shearing also reduces the corner radius above the sheared region and the camber (nonstraightness along the length) of the sheared edges. Component edges are sometimes sheared or resheared immediately before welding to eliminate the risk of weld defects due to edge damage incurred during shipping and handling. This practice also improves the edge quality and dimensional accuracy of components fabricated by less accurate methods.

Cost-effective edge preparation techniques for two-dimensional blanks (having nonlinear weld seams) are not nearly as well developed as those for linear weld seams. Shearing is not feasible in this case, but press blanking still is, although at a premium cost and perhaps somewhat lower edge quality. Laser cutting offers an alternative, nonlinear edge preparation technique but certainly raises the cost hurdle for the overall blank welding application justification.

Part Fixturing

The main points regarding fixturing are similar to those appearing under the heading of blank preparation. To maintain maximum productivity, the gap between the abutting edges must be minimized. This is accomplished with part-positioning mechanisms, which ensure tight fitup prior to clamping and robust clamps, which are strong enough to minimize motion due to thermal distortion. Figure 3 shows an example of a clamping system.

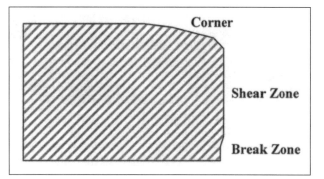

Figure 2. Sketch showing three zones of sheared edge.

In addition to eliminating fitup gaps, the second role of fixturing is to position the parts at a precisely known location. Because of the small focus spot size generally found in an optimized laser blank welding process, beam-seam alignment is critical to prevent lack of fusion defects. For a variety of possible welding system reasons, the use of a seam tracking system may be required to follow the joint.

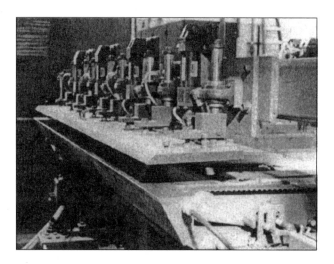

Figure 3. Clamping system for straight-line laser welding.

For the most common steel sheet thicknesses (0.8 to 1.8 mm) and straight weld lengths of about 1 m, maximum gaps of 0.05 to 0.1 mm can be achieved using precision shearing as well as carefully maintained blanking tools. Edge preparation on very long parts or those produced from steel strip with poor shape or high residual stress can yield gapping in excess of 0.2 to 0.3 mm. Gaps at the upper end of this range are generally not weldable by conventional, single-spot laser welding to normal weld quality standards.

Motion Systems

Typical tailored blank production rates are high enough that welding is invariably performed on systems designed specifically for this task. The most common motion system design approach for welding blanks with linear seams is a moving part system, using a single linear travel axis. Since blank welding is always done on flat components, only a small range of vertical motion is needed for focus adjustment and to accommodate varying sheet thicknesses. A small amount of controlled linear cross seam motion is also usually provided for beam-seam alignment. In applications where two-dimensional seams are to be welded, moving beam systems can offer the advantage of less moving mass. This simplifies seam following and process control around sharp contours and corners. However, the moving beam systems present concerns with laser focus height and focus spot size variation caused by changes in distance between the laser generator and the focusing optic. These can be compensated at the expense of a more complicated beam delivery system.

Laser Type and Process

CO_2 lasers in the 6–8 kW range and Nd:YAG lasers in the 4–5 kW range are usually selected for tailored blank welding. The debate about laser choice is ongoing. There is a much larger installed base of high-power CO_2 lasers and consequently more industrial experience with this source. It is available in higher powers at comparable cost to lower-power Nd:YAG units. However, Nd:YAG lasers offer the convenience of fiber-optic delivery, which reduces system complexity and facilitates beam sharing. Also, there is a growing consensus that YAG laser welding can tolerate larger fitup gap.

Table 9. CO_2 Laser Welding Parameters

Parameter	Value (units)
Part thickness	0.8 to 1.8 (mm)
Power on part	5.5 (kW)
Focus spot size	0.6 (mm)
Travel speed	7 (m/min)
Suppression gas	He

A sample weld parameter set for production CO_2 laser blank welding is shown in Table 9. These should be regarded as "typical" rather than optimized parameters for this process. The most notable characteristic of the process is the relatively high travel speed. A major factor in CO_2 laser beam welding is the requirement for a helium plume suppression gas. The detrimental effect of the plasma plume in CO_2 laser welding and the plume-suppressing effects of helium shielding gas are addressed in Section 11.2.8.

Some typical Nd:YAG process parameters are shown in Table 10. Note that the specified Nd:YAG process uses argon for shielding. In some cases, Nd:YAG welding with no shielding gas also produces satisfactory results.

Table 10. Nd:YAG Welding Parameters

Parameter	Value (units)
Part thickness	0.8 to 1.8 (mm)
Power on part	3.5 (kW)
Focus spot size	0.6 (mm)
Travel speed	8 (m/min)
Suppression gas	Ar

The dual-spot method of laser welding has utility in accommodating wider than optimum joint gaps. In this process variant, a special optic inserted in the beam path results in the laser energy being focused into two focus spots. By varying the spot spacing and their orientation relative to the travel direction, different effects can be obtained. Aligning the two spots in the travel direction increases the upper travel speed if it is limited by bead humping (a weld bead shape defect). Aligning the two spots transverse to the travel direction increases the weld width, and hence the amount of joint gap that can be accommodated. Of course, this benefit comes at the expense of travel speed, which must be reduced from single-spot levels.

Weld Quality Monitoring

As mentioned at the outset, the laser tailored blank welding application is fairly demanding in terms of weld quality, and there is often an interest in sensor-based systems for on-line weld quality monitoring. All aspects of this technology are not fully mature, and no technique has emerged as a clear favorite for blank weld monitoring. Real-time laser beam analyzers have been employed to provide continuous measurements of laser beam power, power distribution, pointing, and the like. Optical and computer vision-based measuring systems have been used to check the part fitup ahead of the weld and to inspect for visible defects in the completed weld. Other systems (described in some detail in Section 4.9) measure optical, acoustic, and plasma charge emissions during welding to detect and warn of process irregularities.

Process Economics

The consumable material costs of blank welding differ somewhat depending on the type of laser. For the CO_2 laser welding process, major consumables are electricity, laser gas, and helium process gas. The Nd:YAG laser welding process consumes considerably more electricity, arc lamps, and (perhaps) argon process gas. It happens that differences in the detailed operating costs for the two laser types tend to offset each other to some degree; so the operating costs of each are similar. The CO_2 laser uses less electrical power, but the saving is decreased by the increased cost of helium process gas as compared to a smaller volume of less expensive argon process gas needed for the Nd:YAG laser process.

While the consumable costs are significant, the system depreciation and labor costs for laser blank welding operations are substantially greater. In these welding systems the laser itself often a small part (10–30%) of the overall system cost, which can be dominated by automation equipment, fixturing, controls, etc. With automated handling equipment, the welding time is typically a large, sometimes the largest, component of the total cycle time. As a result, the process economics are sensitive to welding speed. This cost driver is one factor that can justify considerable attention and expense to obtain good weld joint preparation and fitup so that welding speed can be maximized. Additionally, large, automated systems can often benefit from laser power upgrades if overall system performance can be improved.

DAVE F. FARSON

11.4.12 Automotive Applications

Car-Body Cutting and Welding

A combined laser cutting and welding process was used by a German car manufacturer to achieve a nonvisible seam (see Fig. 4). In preparation for the filler wire supported welding, laser cutting of the edges of the joint was carried out in the same clamping device using interchangeable cutting and welding lenses. Because of the defined seam geometry, the post-treatment was reduced to only a grinding process. Smoothing the seam with a surfacer could be avoided as well as distortion that was caused by the former TIG-welding.

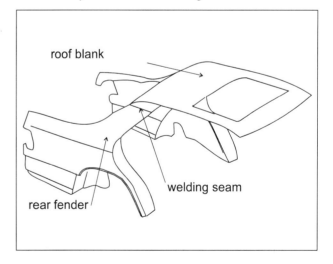

Figure 4. Car body joint geometry.

Clutch Housing Welding

A clutch housing was required to be sealed against oil loss. The gap was large (1.5 × 1.5 mm) and post-treatment had to be avoided (see Fig. 5 next page). To succeed in one-step welding, the beam was enlarged by defocusing. Consequently, only fusion welding was applicable, thus making travel speed poor. Filler wire was applied, "lancing" into the last third of the melt pool to achieve a stable process (see Fig. 6 next page).

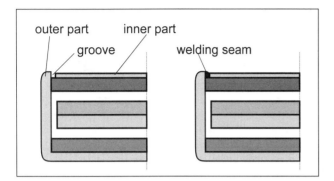

Figure 5. Joint geometry of a clutch housing.

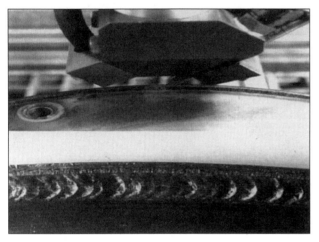

Figure 6. Welding process (above) and seam (below).

Flange Welding

Laser filler wire welding was used to avoid the disadvantages of conventional TIG-welding: distortion and post-treatment. A rather big (250 mm diameter) and thin-walled (2.5 mm) flange (Fig. 7) was welded using two seams. Both seams were welded using the same clamping device.

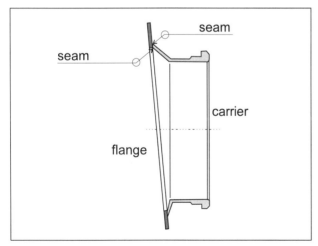

Figure 7. Flange cross section.

Steering Shaft Pinion

Welding of high carbon steel is difficult because of micro cracks. Special heat treatment is used as well as welding additives. A pinion made of high carbon steel (CK45) had to be joined to a high carbon steel steering shaft (CK50) without cracks. Using a 450 W Nd:YAG laser, an overlap geometry with a 6-mm fillet-joint was realized using a Ni-alloyed low-carbon filler wire (Fig. 8). This allowed the carbon to be absorbed in the melting pool and cracks were avoided.

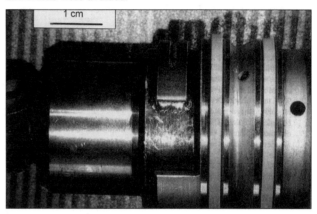

Figure 8. Filler wire fillet-joint of low-carbon materials (steering shaft and pinion).

ANDREAS GEBHARDT

11.5 Comparison of Laser Welding to Other Welding Technologies

11.5.1 Alternate Welding Technologies

Each welding technique has a particular set of characteristics, both technical and economical, that make one technique preferred over another in a specific welding application. This choice should be made with all the relevant information on all practical alternatives. In comparison to arc techniques, laser welding is still in the early stages of worldwide industrial usage, although it has been well established in automotive and niche industries for many years. The expansion of laser welding is expected to be significant, as the awareness of the process and its capabilities are discovered. This section offers a brief description of competing techniques followed by a comparison of welding capabilities to laser welding. No cost information has been covered, as the cost benefit of introducing laser welding, or in fact any welding operation, is usually complex and totally application specific encompassing any up- or down-stream benefits, product design enhancement, or a new innovative welding operation.

Welding techniques fall into two basic categories, high- and low-energy density processes. High-density processes include the laser, electron beam, and plasma arc sources. Low-density processes cover other generic arc, electrical, and friction sources that individually encompass a wide range of subgroups. These key differences in the welding characteristics of the two categories are presented in Table 1.

Chapter 11: Penetration Welding

Table 1. Fundamental Weld Characteristics of High- and Low-Density Techniques

High density	Low density
High welding speeds	Wide, shallow weld beads
Narrow deep welds	Large fitup tolerances
Low thermal input	Low–moderate welding speeds
Flexible heating source	Massive range of weldable materials
Precise heat input control	Very robust process
Single-side noncontact access	1–6 degree welding capability
Ease of automation	
In-process control capability	

Table 2. Characteristics of Submerged Arc Welding

Material	Voltage/current	Weld geometry	Speed (mm/s)
Carbon steel 6.4 mm thick	28 V 650 A	Flat square butt	20 (1 pass)
Carbon steel 16 mm thick	37 V 500A		7 (2 pass)

Submerged Arc Welding (SAW)

The SAW process is an electric arc welding process in which joining of metals is achieved by heating via an arc produced between a bare consumable electrode and the workpiece. The arc is blanketed in a granular flux and metal powder that are preplaced over the weld line ahead of the process. With up to 60% heat losses, a large-diameter electrode is required to provide sufficient input energy; this confines the process to sections of around 6 mm and above, though sheet welding is possible.

This easily automated robust process is predominantly used in joining carbon steel, low-alloy, and alloy steels in flat butt or fillet configuration. A number of welding examples are given in Table 2.

Gas Metal Arc Welding (GMAW)

The GMAW process is an electric arc welding process that produces the joining of metals by heating with an arc established between a continuous filler metal electrode and the workpiece. A number of metal transfer methods exist: spray, globular, short circuit, and pulsed. The spray and globular transfer of metal allows high deposition rates suitable for sections of 6 mm thickness, but the need for oxidizing gases to stabilize the arc limits suitable materials. Short-circuit and pulsed welding offer low and pulsed currents that enable thin sections to be welded. The shielding gas composition can be varied with the inclusion of carbon dioxide to increase penetration. GMAW is suited to welding all types of materials, with thickness from 1.6 to 30 mm. The deep-section welding can be accomplished by narrow-gap GMAW, using electrode positioning such that side-wall fusion occurs, the weld gap varies from 6.4–12 mm, according to access (see Table 3).

Flux Cored Arc Welding (FCAW)

The FCAW is an electric arc process that produces an arc be-

Table 3. Characteristics of Gas Metal Arc Welding

Material	Voltage/current	Weld geometry	Speed (mm/s)	Additional comments
Carbon steel 1.6 mm thick	18 V 95 A	Flat vee butt	6.8 (1 pass)	Short circuit. CO_2 or 75% Ar + 25% CO_2
Carbon steel 19 mm thick	29 V 450 A	Double vee butt	5.1 (4 pass)	Spray. Ar + 5% O_2
Austenitic ss 3.2 mm thick	24 V 125 A	Butt	7 (1 pass)	Short circuit. 90% He, 7.5% Ar + 2.5% CO_2

Table 4. Characteristics of Flux-Cored Arc Welding

Material	Voltage/current	Weld geometry	Speed (mm/s)	Additional comments
Carbon steel 3.2 mm thick	28 V 325 A	Flat square butt	17 (1 pass)	CO_2 shielding gas. Root opening 1.6 mm
Carbon steel 25.4 mm thick	32 V 525 A	Single vee butt	4.7 (6 pass)	CO_2 shielding gas. No root opening

tween a continuous metal filler electrode and the workpiece. This process combines facets of GMAW, SAW, and shielded welding, with a shielding gas protecting the weld during formation, and the flux contained in the fed consumable, protecting the weld during solidification with a covering slag. The process combines high deposition with quality, being ideally suited for carbon and low-alloy steels, stainless steels, and cast iron. Table 4 (previous page) presents some examples.

Gas Tungsten Arc Welding (GTAW)

The GTAW is an electric arc process that produces joining by heating with an arc established between a nonconsumable tungsten electrode and the workpiece. The use of pulsed sine and square-wave power supplies offers good control over heat input, and thus allows the technique to produce high-quality welds. The relatively slow welding rate limits GTAW to sections under 10 mm thick, though it is ideally suited to thin-section welding. Depending on the type of welding operation, either a pure argon gas shield is used or helium or hydrogen is added. Recently the development of preplaced fluxes and narrow-gap welding technology are overcoming the speed limitations of the process.

Similarly to GMAW, GTAW has developed a thick-section narrow-gap welding technique that allows a 50-mm-thick plate to be welded with only 2 deg of wall angle. The use of hot wire feed and localized heating enables competitive welding times. Table 5 presents some examples.

Plasma Arc Welding (PAW)

The PAW process is a modification of the GTAW process, where the arc is formed in an inner chamber, then discharged under the action of gases through an orifice concentrating and collimating the plasma. An outer part provides shielding gas to the weld. The increased energy concentration provides deeper narrower welds, which when operating at higher current levels begin to enter the high energy-density levels of laser and electron beams. The combination of plasma control through nozzle design with the inherent control of the power supply, offers a range of plasma welding modes; micro (0.1–15 A) for thin sheets below 0.1 mm thick, medium (15–100 A) for mid-thickness welding, and keyhole (100+ A) for single-pass penetration of plates. Table 6 presents some examples.

Friction Stir Welding

The basics of friction welding and friction surfacing have been combined to produce friction stir welding. The weld is initiated by inserting a rotating shoulder element into the metal, slightly above the depth required. By moving either the friction stud or the sample along the joint line, plasticized material is transported from the front of the rotating element to the rear forming the weld. Only metals with low melting points, such as aluminum (658°C) and copper (1083°C) can be welded, subject to the tool durability. Sound clamping of all parts is crucial to success, with backing a requirement and also the removal or filling in of the hole left at the end of the weld. Welding is currently limited

Table 5. Characteristics of Gas Tungsten Arc Welding

Material	Voltage/ current	Weld geometry	Speed (mm/s)	Additional comments
Carbon steel 1.6 mm thick	18 V 95 A	Flat vee butt	6.8 (1 pass)	Short circuit. CO_2 or 75% Ar + 25% CO_2
Carbon steel 19 mm thick	29 V 450 A	Double vee butt	5.1 (4 pass)	Spray. Ar + 5% O_2
Austenitic ss 3.2 mm thick	24 V 125 A	Butt	7 (1 pass)	Short circuit. 90% He, 7.5% Ar + 2.5% CO_2

Table 6. Characteristics of Plasma Arc Welding

Material	Voltage/ current	Weld geometry	Speed (mm/s)	Additional comments
Carbon steel 3.2 mm thick	28 V 185 A	Flat square butt	5 (1 pass)	Ar shield
Titanium 9.9 mm thick	38 V 225 A		4.2 (1 pass)	
Austenitic ss 0.76 mm thick	11 A		2 (1 pass)	95% Ar, 5% H shield

Chapter 11: Penetration Welding

to flat workpieces or those where backing can be provided. The tool design and speed must be established for each individual material alloy. Table 7 presents some examples.

Table 7. Characteristics of Friction Stir Welding

Material	Weld geometry	Speed (mm/s)
Aluminum 6082-T6 5 mm thick	Flat square butt	12.5
Aluminum 4212-6 25 mm		2.17
Copper 5010 0.76 mm		8.8
Copper 5010 7.4 mm		6.33

Electron Beam Welding

The EBW uses a stream of high-velocity electrons to produce a high-energy-density process, capable of deep single-pass welds, with extremely high quality. The process can be operated in several decreasingly effective environments; high vacuum (0.13–133 mPa), medium vacuum (133–3200 mPa), and at atmospheric pressure. An additional factor is the need to shield the surrounding area from x-rays produced during welding.

High-vacuum welding offers phenomenal welding capabilities in terms of penetration depth or welding speeds. Creating vacuum conditions requires substantial tooling costs; thus it is applied only to low-volume, high-value fabrication. However, more recently applications have used no-vacuum conditions. EB welding is ideally suited to high-quality welds in titanium, aluminum alloys, and copper as well as carbon steels.

The use of nonvacuum electron beam welding requires the final aperture of the gun to be less than 13 mm from the workpiece; otherwise the electrons become scattered and diffuse. This can be partially alleviated by employing a helium downblow jet that effectively clears a path for the electrons. Table 8 presents some characteristic results.

Electrical Resistance Welding

The welding is achieved between two electrodes that impart an electrical current and force to melt and fuse the weld metal. The shape and size of the electrode force and applied current offer a variety of welding methods, including: spot, projection, seam, upset, flash, and high frequency. The heating cycle is generally higher than the arc processes, and is controlled by the thermal sink of the electrode and the contact time with the weld. In terms of laser welding, spot, seam, and high frequency are worth considering. The requirement and effect of good electrical contact, pressure, and double-sided access have somewhat limited the application of this technique; however, it is extremely effective when the requirements can be met. Material thickness is usually limited to 3 mm. Table 9 presents an example.

11.5.2 Key Aspects of Comparison

Weld Bead Geometry and Fitup Tolerance

The laser with an irradiance around 10^6 W/cm^2 produces welds that are typically 0.2–2 mm wide, with penetration depths of 1–20 mm. The arc sources with power densities around 10^4 W/cm^2 produce welds typically 3 mm wide and 2–3 mm deep. The diameter of the focused laser can range from 0.1 to 0.8 mm, as

Table 8. Characteristics of Electron Beam Welding

Material	Voltage/current	Weld geometry	Speed (mm/s)	Additional comments
Carbon steel AISI 4340 7.5 mm thick	175 kV 6.4 kW	Flat square butt	15	Gun-to-work distance 6 mm
Aluminum alloy 6082 20 mm thick	150 kV		33.3	Vacuum
Carbon steel 101.6 mm thick	33 kW		2	

Table 9. Example of Electrical Resistance Welding

Material	Voltage/current	Weld geometry	Speed (mm/s)	Additional comments
Mild steel 1.6 mm	130 kVA	Overlapping	100	High frequency

compared with an arc source that is typically 2–3 times larger. This is reflected in the joining efficiencies, given in Table 10 for each process. Arc welding suffers from significant conductive losses and sideways melting. This can be particularly important when thermal distortion is an issue.

Table 10. Comparison of Welding Efficiency Based on Joint Line Penetration

Process	Approximate joining efficiency (power/speed x thickness) (J/mm^2)
Gas tungsten arc (GMAW)	0.8–2
Submerged arc (SAW)	4–10
Flux cored arc (FCAW)	3–4
High-frequency resistance	65–100
Electron beam (EB)	20–30
Laser	15–25

On the opposite side of reduced welding efficiency, the larger diffuse heating source of the arc techniques has the capability of welding under poor fitup conditions and materials sensitive to severe thermal cycling. Laser welding becomes increasingly difficult when tolerances, specifically gap width, increase above the nominal values of fractions of millimeters. The arc sources weld comfortably between 1- and 3-mm tolerance sizes, where the application of a laser becomes increasingly untenable. The diffuse nature of the arc source provides a less severe thermal cycle with lower solidification rates avoiding weld material overhardening or embrittlement.

Equipment Aspects

The final delivery component of the energy source for arc techniques is the torch or gun. This has physical size limitations and inflexible working distances, though power and gases are supplied through flexible cables. Electrical resistance welding requires double-sided access (usually) plus force, as does friction welding. The delivery of laser energy from the "laser head" to the workpiece is either by reflective mirrors (Nd:YAG and CO_2) or flexible fiber delivery (Nd:YAG only – peak power limitations exist). The final component of the laser system is a transmissive/reflective optic, with flexible working distances that focus the beam with divergence only a few degrees, offering good accessibility.

Conclusion

Many welding techniques exist, the selection between them must be made with a knowledge and awareness of all competing processes.

Table 11. Comparison of Laser Welding to Conventional Welding Processes

Characteristics	Laser beam	Electron beam	Resistance	Gas tungsten arc	Friction	Capacitive discharge
Weld quality	Excellent	Excellent	Fair	Good	Good	Excellent
Weld speed	High	High	Moderate	Moderate	Moderate	Very high
Heat input into welded part	Low	Low	Moderate	Very high	Moderate	Low
Weld joint fitup requirements	High	High	Low	Low	Moderate	High
Weld penetration	High	High	Low	Moderate	High	Low
Range of dissimilar materials	Wide	Wide	Narrow	Narrow	Wide	Wide
Range of part geometries/sizes	Wide	Moderate	Wide	Wide	Narrow	Narrow
Controllability	Very good	Good	Fair	Fair	Moderate	Moderate
Ease of automation	Excellent	Moderate	Excellent	Fair	Good	Good
Initial costs	High	High	Low	Low	Moderate	High
Operating/maintenance costs	Moderate	High	Moderate	Low	Low	Moderate
Tooling costs	High	Very high	Moderate	Moderate	Low	Very high

ISBN 0-912035-15-3

References
Welding Handbook, Eighth Edition, Volume 1 – Welding Technology. Volume 2 – Welding Processes. Volume 3 – Materials and Applications I. Volume 4 - Materials and Applications II. Published by the American Welding Institute.

GEOFF J. SHANNON

11.5.3 Laser Welding Comparisons
Attractive features of deep-penetration laser welding are the high energy efficiency so that thermal distortion is minimized and the possibility of making single-pass welds. Conventional arc, submerged arc, MIG, and TIG welding, on the other hand require the abutting edges to be chamferred to facilitate access, so that several overlapping passes using filler metals are necessary to complete the weld.

The metal vapor within the keyhole of a laser weld constitutes a less tractable problem, since it helps to maintain the molten cavity but may ionize and so attenuate the laser beam. Electron beam welders exhibit less attenuation from plasma that may form above the workpiece, so that the weld penetration depth per incident kilowatt of power is less for the laser than for a vacuum electron-beam welder. Under optimum welding conditions, the difference may be no more than 20% for 9-mm-thick stainless steel coupons. As the welding speed is decreased, laser penetration asymptotically approaches a maximum, while electron beam penetration continues to rise.

As a welding source the laser has potential performance comparable to electron beams and constricted plasma arcs. Laser welding does not present the problems of instability sometimes experienced with arc techniques and does not require vacuum as is the case for electron beam welders. Laser welding also offers advantages over electron beam welding because laser beams can be transported over large distances and into inaccessible joints.

DAN GNANAMUTHU

11.5.4 Comparison of Welding Technology Results
Table 11 (previous page) presents a comparison of the results (such as weld quality and speed) obtained with laser welding and several competing technologies.

DAVID HAVRILLA

Notes

ISBN 0-912035-15-3

Chapter 12

Laser Cutting

12.1 Basic Description of Laser Cutting

12.1.1 Cutting Processes

Laser Cutting

Laser cutting, the most established laser materials processing technology, is a method for shaping and separating a workpiece into segments of desired geometry. The cutting process is executed by moving a focused laser beam along the surface of the workpiece with constant distance, thereby generating a narrow (typically some tenths of a millimeter) cut kerf. This kerf fully penetrates the material along the desired cut contour.

Laser cutting is a thermal cutting process. During the process, part of the laser radiation is absorbed at the end of the kerf, called the *cutting front* (see Fig. 1).

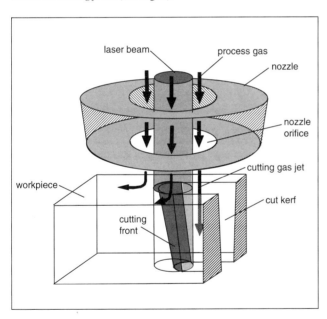

Figure 1. Cutting front with shaded projection of the laser beam and coaxial nozzle orifice with gas flow indicated by arrows.

The absorbed energy heats and transforms the prospective kerf volume into a state (molten, vaporized, or chemically changed) which is volatile or which can be removed easily. Normally, the material removal is supported by a gas jet, impinging coaxially to the laser beam. This cutting gas accelerates the transformed material and ejects it from the kerf.

Three standard laser cutting processes are defined according to their dominant transformation process, fusion cutting, oxidation cutting, and vaporization cutting. These are described in turn in the following.

Laser Fusion Cutting

In laser fusion cutting the kerf volume is transformed dominantly into the molten state and blown out of the kerf by a high-pressure (up to 2 MPa) inert gas jet. Therefore, this process is also called *high-pressure* or *inert gas cutting* (see Fig. 2).

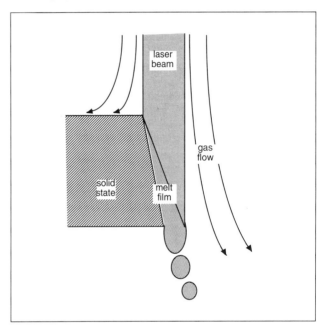

Figure 2. Sketch of laser fusion cutting.

Fusion cutting is applicable to all metals, especially stainless and other highly alloyed steels and aluminum and titanium alloys, to many thermoplastic polymers and some ceramics. During laser fusion cutting, the laser beam is the only heat source. The inert gas jet (mainly nitrogen or argon) is responsible for melt ejection and for shielding the heated material from the surrounding air. The resulting cut edges are free of oxides. The main technical demand is to avoid adherent melt (dross attachment) at the bottom edges of the kerf.

Laser Oxidation Cutting

Laser oxidation cutting, sometimes also called *laser oxygen cutting* or simply *laser gas cutting*, uses oxygen as the cutting gas. The laser beam is mainly responsible for igniting and stabilizing a burning process within the kerf (see Fig. 3).

This exothermic reaction of the oxygen with the material (mainly steel, especially mild and low alloyed steel) supports the laser cutting process by providing additional heat input. In some cases, this heat may be the dominant heat source. The result is higher cutting speeds compared to laser cutting with inert gases.

The formation of an oxide layer on the cutting front increases the absorption of the laser radiation (at angles of incidence below 80°) compared to the absorption of a pure metallic melt. Especially with mild and low alloyed steel, the oxides reduce the viscosity (at temperatures above 1900 K) and surface tension of the melt and thereby simplify melt ejection. The resulting cut edges are oxidized.

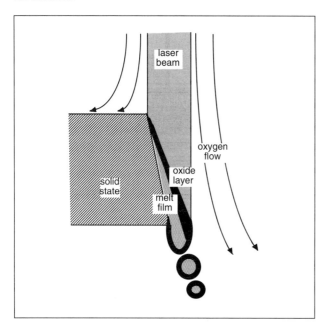

Figure 3. Sketch of laser oxidation cutting.

It is important to balance the laser power and other process parameters to avoid burning of sharp corners, small circles, or narrow bridges.

Laser Vaporization Cutting
In laser vaporization cutting, the kerf formation is mainly realized by vaporization of the material (see Fig. 4).

Typical materials that are cut by this kind of processes are acrylic, thermoset polymers, rubber, some thermoplastic polymers, wood, paper, leather, and some ceramics. To avoid precipitation of the hot, gaseous emissions on the workpiece and to prevent them from condensation within the developing kerf, a process gas jet is used for blowing the material out of the kerf. Vaporization cutting of metals is possible only if the relative contribution of the molten state is minimized by using repetitive, short laser pulses in conjunction with high power densities. If different processes can be applied for cutting of metals, vaporization cutting is the method with the lowest speed, but it is suitable for very precise, complex cut geometries in thin workpieces.

Mixed Processes
In practice, the cutting process is often not based on one individual transformation process but rather on two or more simultaneous transformations. For example, for reducing costs sometimes compressed air is used instead of oxygen or nitrogen as the cutting gas (e.g., during cutting aluminum and plastics). The oxygen content within the air leads to partial burning of the kerf material or the emitted by-products. On the other hand, this oxidation does not dominate the power and mass balance of the whole cutting process but only contributes to a mixed process.

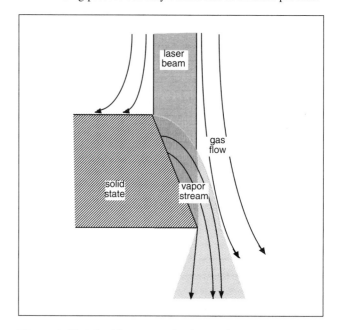

Figure 4. Sketch of laser vaporization cutting.

Another example of a mixed process is the laser inert gas cutting of thin sheet metal with high irradiance, resulting in partial evaporation of the superheated melt film of the cutting front.

Special and New Processes
There are a number of special or modified variants of laser cutting. Particular specialities include:

- Extreme process ranges (e.g., high-speed cutting by creating a vapor capillary instead of a simple cutting front [1])
- Additional media (e.g., water sprayed onto the workpiece for cooling and preventing burnoffs [2])
- Additional heat sources (e.g., burning-stabilized laser oxygen cutting [3])
- Modified system technology (e.g., high-power laser cutting with rugged mirror optics instead of a lens for beam focusing [4])
- A mixture of the above types (e.g., microjet cutting with a high-pressure water jet guiding the laser beam to the workpiece, cooling the workpiece and removing the kerf material [5])

Single- and Multidimensional Cutting
Laser cutting is suitable for one-, two- and three-dimensional applications. One-dimensional industrial applications are slitting of sheet metal coils into stripes and cutting or perforating

sheets, plates, or coils of various materials to length and width. Most typical for laser cutting is the two-dimensional cutting of complex shapes out of flat material, but also cutting of three-dimensional components, such as car body parts or tubes and profiles, is state of the art.

Process Parameters

The parameters for laser beam cutting include:

- Workpiece parameters: material thermophysical and optical properties, thickness.
- Laser beam parameters: wavelength (type of laser), irradiance, spatial distribution or mode structure, beam quality, type and degree of polarization, raw beam diameter at focusing system, laser beam power below cutting head, pulse duration, and repetition rate (if applicable)
- Cutting gas parameters: type of gas, gas pressure, type of nozzle, geometry of nozzle orifice, nozzle distance
- Focusing parameters: type of focusing optics, focal length, focal position
- Machine parameters: cutting speed

This list constitutes a complete set of typically relevant parameters. But other values can also become important, for instance, the cutting head inclination for bevel cuts and for cuts out of three-dimensional parts with special kerf angles. Other technically relevant parameters include piercing parameters, families of characteristics to define speed-adapted power control algorithms, and dynamical features of the machine axes (e.g., acceleration).

Advantages

The main advantageous features of laser cutting technology include flexibility regarding geometry, material and number of parts, speed, which affects productivity and availability of parts, quality, which affects precision, and accuracy and the lack of necessity for post-treatment.

Setting and Optimization of Parameters

The generalization of certain parameter settings as rules of thumb is subject to uncertainty. Nevertheless, some more or less clearly identified rules (and some specifications or exceptions) for laser cutting can be mentioned.

- Cutting speed: Sound and safe cutting results are practicable at feed rates of about 80 to 90% of the maximum possible cutting speed. For certain quality demands, the speed may have to be reduced. If the speed is too low, during fusion cutting dross formation and during oxidation cutting burnouts can occur. These two defects can be avoided by pulsing the laser.
- Focal position: In laser fusion cutting, the focal position should be near the bottom plane of the workpiece to simplify dross prevention and near or above the middle to maximize speed. In laser oxidation cutting, the focal point should be positioned in the upper half of the material. In the thick section range of 10 mm or more the optimum focal positon is often some millimeters above the surface of the workpiece.
- Gas pressure: In fusion cutting, the pressure has to be high (up to 2 MPa), increasing with workpiece thickness. On the other hand, a certain upper limit must not be exceeded to avoid a shielding plasma resulting in a kerf collapse. In oxidation cutting, typical pressure values are in the range of 0.1 to 0.5 MPa. In the case of thick (10 mm or more) mild steel, the oxygen pressure should be below 0.08 MPa to avoid burn-outs.
- Coaxial rotational symmetry: This is the most important rule for laser cutting of two- or three-dimensional contours. The cutting tool components and the spatial distribution of their properties have to be rotationally symmetrical and coaxially adjusted to each other as carefully as possible. An asymmetric tool would cause differing cutting and cut properties depending on the direction of travel. This means that the power distribution and the nozzle orifice have to be circular, or otherwise their orientation has to be adapted to the cutting direction by rotating devices. In any case the position and orientation of laser beam, nozzle, and moving machine have to be aligned properly and checked regularly. In addition, the alignment has to correspond with the programmed tool center point coordinates.

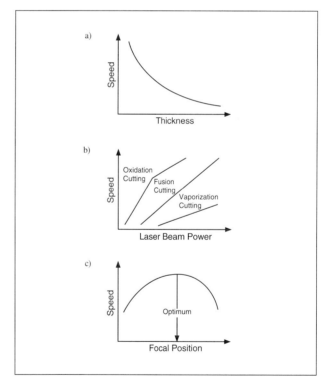

Figure 5. Typical course of functions in laser cutting. (a) Speed versus thickness, (b) speed versus laser beam power for different processes, (c) speed versus focal position.

Important Functions

Important functions to be considered in laser cutting are cutting speed versus thickness, power, and focal position for different materials and processes. The quality of the cut, including average roughness, dross attachment, and kerf width, depends on these parameters also. Some typical functional relationships are illustrated in Figure 5 (previous page) in schematic form.

Cutting Head

The cutting head combines the focusing optics and the gas nozzle (see Fig. 6). The device includes the mountings, adjustments, and cooling as well as the inlet connections for gas and sometimes also the water supply.

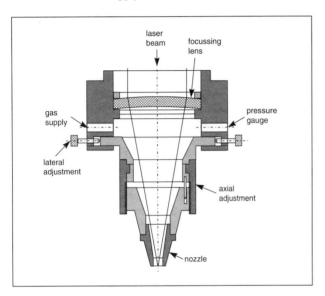

Figure 6. Laser beam cutting head.

Additionally a capacitive or mechanical distance sensor for closed-loop control of the height of the cutting head along the z axis can be integrated within or around the nozzle.

Cutting System

Besides the cutting head, the cutting system contains the laser source, including power and gas supply, chiller and control unit, and the handling machine, including motor drives for the different axes, optical beam guiding system, systems for material support and transport, exhausting unit, and a computer numerical control (CNC) system.

References
1. K. U. Preissig, D. Petring, and G. Herziger, SPIE Vol. 2207, 96–110 (1994).
2. C. Banchi, *Industrial Laser Review,* March 1996, 11–13.
3. J. W. Franke, W. Schulz, D. Petring, and E. Beyer, Proc. 11th Int. Congress Laser '93, Munich, 62–7 (1993).
4. D. Petring, K. U. Preissig, H. Zefferer, and E. Beyer, Proc. 3rd Int. "Beam Technology" Conf., Karlsruhe, DVS-Berichte Bd. **135,** 12–15 (1991).
5. B. Richerzhagen, *Industrial Laser Review,* Nov. 1997, 8–10.

DIRK PETRING

12.1.2 Power Balance

Important Parameters

Sophisticated computer simulations allow development and production engineers effective and efficient calculations of the laser cutting process for off-line parameter analysis, optimization, and prediction. These software tools give insight into the control of the laser cutting process (see Fig. 7).

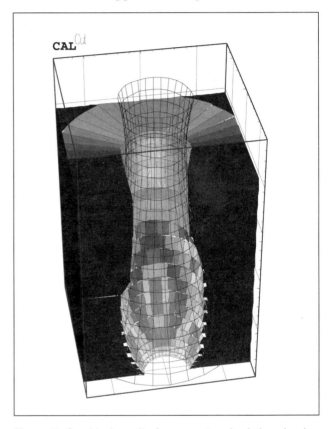

Figure 7. Graphical result of a computer simulation showing the laser focus caustic, the self-adjusting cutting front and cut kerf geometry, and the distribution of the absorbed power density. The example has been calculated for a CO_2 laser at 8 kW beam power cutting a 40-mm-thick stainless steel plate.

Nevertheless, some simple approximations are available that allow illustrative process understanding and formulation of acceptable estimates. The most significant input parameters of the laser cutting process, besides the relevant material properties of the workpiece, are:

- The laser beam power
- The laser beam diameter at the surface plane of the workpiece
- The thickness of the workpiece
- The cutting speed

It is helpful to have an overall scheme connecting these parameters within a simple formula to be able to estimate any of these parameters, if the others are given. This can be achieved most easily by calculating the power balance.

Chapter 12: Laser Cutting

Power Balance Calculation

A stable, steady-state cutting process requires a proper balance of the incoming and outgoing power contributions. The laser beam power absorbed and, in the case of oxidation cutting, additionally the exothermal reaction power have to be identical with the power necessary for heating and transforming the material along the cutting track.

The overall power balance for laser cutting can be written as

$$AP_L + P_r = P_{Tp} + P_m + P_v + P_l \quad (1)$$

with the absorptivity A, the laser beam power P_L, the reaction power P_r arising from possible exothermic reactions, the power P_{Tp} for heating the kerf volume up to the process temperature T_p, the power P_m for melting the kerf volume, the power P_v for evaporating (part) of the kerf volume, and the power P_l for compensating heat conduction losses into the material near the kerf. The different terms on the right-hand side of Equation 1 are calculated by the following formulas:

$$P_{Tp} = b_m\, s\, v_c\, \rho\, c\, [(1-\delta_v)(T_p - T_0) + \delta_v(T_s - T_0)] \quad (2)$$

$$P_m = b_m\, s\, v_c\, \rho\, \varepsilon_m \quad (3)$$

$$P_v = \delta_v\, b_m\, s\, v_c\, \rho\, \varepsilon_v \quad (4)$$

$$P_l = b_m\, s\, v_c\, \rho\, c\, (T_m - T_0) \left[\frac{\sqrt{2\pi/Pe}}{\varepsilon^{Pe^2/4} \kappa_o(Pe^2/4)} + 1 \right] \quad (5)$$

In Equation 5, κ_o is the modified Bessel function of the second kind and zeroth order.

Within Equations 2–5, b_m is the kerf width, s is the material thickness, v_c is the cutting speed, ρ is the mass density, c is the heat capacity, δ_v is the proportion of vaporized kerf volume, T_s is the surface temperature of the cutting front, T_0 is the room temperature, ε_m and ε_v are latent heat of fusion and evaporation, T_m is the melting temperature, Pe is the Peclet number (defined by $Pe = b_m v_c / 2\kappa$), and κ is the average thermal diffusivity in the solid state. The different terms within the power balance are illustrated in Figure 8.

Some of the above parameters are well known, such as from material data handbooks. Others have to be calculated from additional equations within a self-consistent approach or approximated by plausible or experimental values.

In pure laser fusion cutting, δ_v is equal to 0; in pure laser vaporization cutting, δ_v is equal to 1. In both cases $P_r = 0$. The kerf width b_m can be approximated by the diameter of the laser beam at the surface plane of the workpiece or measured from kerf cross sections. The process temperature T_p is nearly identical with the melting temperature T_m for metals with high heat conductivity like copper and aluminum and is approximately the average value of melting and evaporation temperatures for other materials like steel and titanium. In the case of vaporization cutting, T_p is identical with T_s and amounts to the vaporization or degradation temperature T_v.

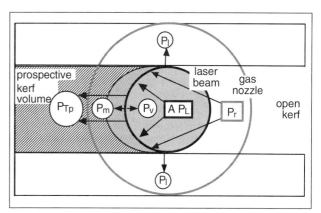

Figure 8. Illustration of the power balance contributions.

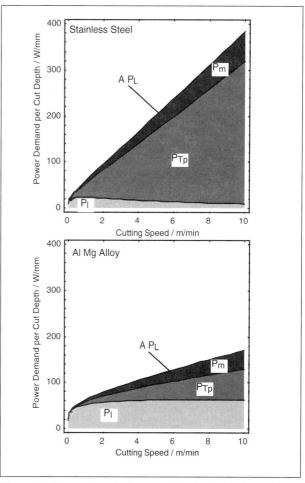

Figure 9. Power absorbed per cut depth during laser beam fusion cutting (b_m = 250 µm), calculated with Equations 1–5. Compared to the steel, the aluminum alloy has a higher power demand at low speeds because of its higher thermal diffusivity and a lower demand than steel at higher speeds because of its low melting temperature.

Figure 9 (previous page) shows the result of power balance calculations for laser beam fusion cutting of stainless steel and for an aluminum–mangnesium alloy.

Laser Beam Absorption

For metals the absorptivity during fusion cutting is typically in the range between 0.15 and 0.3. During oxidation cutting, higher values can be assumed, if the angle of incidence in below 80°, which is only true for correspondingly flat cutting fronts or divergent beams. For infrared laser radiation, the absorption behavior of oxides is similar to that of many plastics and other nonmentals. Total absorption of all the laser radiation during cutting is not usual. The laser beam is propagating along a steep cutting front, and generally part of it is reflected or transmitted through the open kerf.

Exothermic Reaction Power

The reaction power P_r can be estimated from the power P_{O_2} made available by the oxygen flow to the burning cutting front

$$P_{O_2} = (\pi/4)\, b_m^2\, v_{O_2}\, \rho_{O_2}\, E_{Ox} / m_{O_2} \quad (6)$$

and the power P_{Fe} made available by the workpiece material flow into the interaction zone

$$P_{Fe} = b_m\, s\, v_c\, \rho\, E_{Ox} / m_{Fe} \quad (7)$$

Within the above equations v_{O_2} is the oxygen velocity (depending on gas pressure), ρ_{O_2} is the oxygen density, E_{Ox} is the energy per single reaction, m_{O_2} is the mass per oxygen molecule, and m_{Fe} is the mass per iron atom. The minimum value of the two powers from Equations 6 and 7 is a good approximation to the maximum available reaction power $P_{r\,max}$, because the reaction is limited by the flow rate of the rarer type of reactant.

$$P_{r\,max} = min(P_{O_2}, P_{Fe}) \quad (8)$$

The laser power to be absorbed can now be calculated from the total power demand of the cut reduced by the maximum reaction power and from the obligatory power $P_l(T_i)+P_{Ti}$ indispensable for heating the cutting front to ignition temperature T_i. The final laser power demand for oxidation cutting is the maximum value of both cases:

$$AP_L = max[P_{Tp}+ P_m + P_v + P_l - P_{r\,max},\, P_l(T_i)+P_{Ti}] \quad (9)$$

In reality it is not that simple because the oxidation process is diffusion limited and shows strong dynamical behavior. In any case a stable laser oxidation cutting process requires at least an absorbed laser beam power high enough to heat the kerf volume to the ignition temperature and to compensate the corresponding heat conduction losses. Above a certain cutting speed, an additional increase P_Δ in laser power demand with speed is observed because of the limited reaction power P_r. In that case P_r cannot provide all the additional power necessary for heating to the ignition temperature. On the other hand, at low speeds the exothermal reaction can lead to an excess reaction power P_{ex},

which can be avoided by reducing the gas pressure and pulsing the laser beam. The reaction power P_r leading to a stable steady-state process can be deduced from Equations 1 and 9 as

$$P_r = P_{Tp}+P_m+P_v+P_l - AP_L = P_{r\,max} - P_{ex} \quad (10)$$

A comparison of the power balance for fusion and oxidation cutting of mild steel is shown in Figure 10.

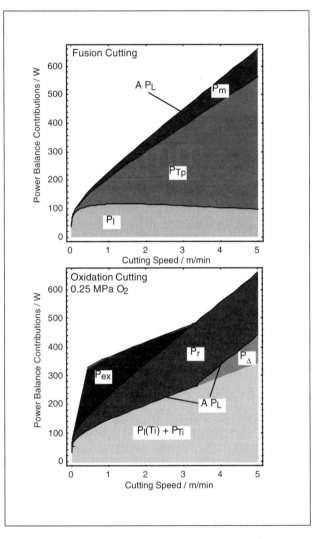

Figure 10. Power balance calculations for fusion and oxidation cutting of mild steel ($s = 3$ mm, $b_m = 250$ μm), calculated with Equations 1–10.

Reference

D. Petring, 1995: *Anwendungsorientierte Modellierung des Laserstrahlschneidens zur rechnergestuetzten Prozessoptimierung,* Verlag Shaker, Aachen.

DIRK PETRING

12.1.3 Appropriate Lasers

CO_2 Lasers

The most established laser cutting application is flat sheet metal cutting with CO_2 laser systems in the power range between 0.5 and 4 kW. The excellent beam quality ($M^2 < 2$) and the acceptable efficiency (10–20%) of these laser sources have continuously improved. Also, available output power has increased. Moreover, the CO_2 laser can be well controlled both in continuous operation and in the pulsed mode, with pulse durations below 100 μs and repetition rates up to 10 kHz. For certain cutting applications (e.g., highly reflective metals, filigree contours, or thermally sensitive ceramics) some suppliers have developed special pulse modes, such as the superpulsed mode with about five-fold increased peak power at the start of each pulse and the hyperpulse mode with superpulses and an additional lower CW-power contribution.

Sealed-off CO_2 lasers at power levels of 500 W and below are very compact, low-maintenance sources, mainly used for thin metal and nonmetal cutting. In the power range below 100 W, desktop systems for cutting and engraving are controlled via a simple PC interface.

At very high powers, above 3 kW, thick plate cutting CO_2 laser systems are increasingly equipped with rugged cutting heads using exclusively reflective optics and special nozzle design (see Section 12.1.4).

Nd:YAG Lasers

Pulsed or *Q*-switched Nd:YAG laser radiation in the power range below 100 W can be focused to 20 μm. Nd:YAG lasers have been used for many years for high-precision or microprocessing applications. Also fiber-coupled CW systems of 1 kW output power (fiber diameter, e.g., 300 μm) are installed for two-dimensional flat sheet metal cutting width thin sections and for three-dimensional cutting of car body and hydroformed parts with robots.

Other Lasers

Carbon monoxide lasers and chemical oxygen-iodine lasers have been used for cutting applications. Excimer and copper-vapor lasers are still more or less exceptions in industrial cutting applications. Nevertheless, their special features with respect to focusability, material absorption, and (in the case of the excimer laser) nonthermal material removal are valuable for certain micromachining applications.

12.1.4 Gas Assist Techniques

Besides the focused laser beam the cutting tool has a second component, the cutting gas jet. The tasks of the cutting gas are:

- Acceleration and ejection of transformed kerf material by momentum transfer via shear forces (friction) and pressure gradients
- Protection of focusing optics against vapor or spatter emitted from the interaction zone
- Protection of the interaction zone against oxidation from ambient air, or in contrast to this
- Providing the interaction zone with reactive gas (oxygen) to burn the kerf material (oxidation cutting)

Most cutting machines are now equipped with proportional valves and electronic sensors to allow the numerical controller to control the gas pressure. Generally the effect of the cutting gas jet can be enhanced by increasing the gas pressure or the nozzle orifice cross-section and by decreasing the clearance. In addition the process gas efficiency can be improved by a wider top kerf width. The kerf width is mainly dependent on the dimensions and the position of the laser focus. Section 4.8 has already presented information about gas nozzles. Here we consider nozzles specifically for cutting applications.

Standard Configuration Nozzles

Normally, the laser beam is focused through the cutting gas nozzle in a coaxial arrangement, which means the laser beam and the gas jet coincide. Laser cutting nozzles are made from copper, which is resistant to laser light and process heat because of its low absorptivity and high thermal conductivity.

The gas pressure is built up in a stagnation chamber below the focusing lens. This is also where the pressure gauge is installed to measure the stagnation pressure.

In standard cutting nozzles, the gas expands through a circular, narrowing channel leading into a cylindrical exit aperture (see Fig. 11). The height of the cylindrical bore, its diameter, and the clearance between nozzle tip and workpiece surface is typically of the order of 1–3 mm.

The cutting gas pressure is defined by the overpressure within the stagnation chamber relative to the ambient pressure. It is often higher than 0.09 MPa, which is the critical value for oxygen, nitrogen, and air. Above this pressure an underexpanded gas jet leaves the nozzle at sonic speed, expanding outside the nozzle and within the kerf to supersonic flow. At cutting gas pressures about 2 MPa, the gas flow can reach a velocity of more than twice the speed of sound, that is, Mach numbers of 2 or more. The underexpansion at the nozzle tip and the subsequent supersonic flow result in a complicated flow pattern with alternating expansion and compression, shock formation, and boundary-layer separation within the kerf (6). These effects are responsible for a nonlinear pressure and standoff dependence for the cutting process. They have been visualized by Schlieren-optical methods.

Laval Nozzle

With a Laval-type (convergent-divergent) nozzle a supersonic, parallel gas jet expanded to ambient pressure can be created (see Fig. 11). For that, the stagnation pressure has to be set near a specific operation value, depending on the ratio of the cross sections at the narrowest passage (nozzle throat) and the nozzle orifice. Accordingly, a homogeneous flow pattern between nozzle and workpiece and big distance tolerance are achievable. Nevertheless, within the cut kerf the gas flow pattern is very similarly structured to that of a standard nozzle. The Laval-type nozzle is seldom used because of its limited operating range regarding pressure and the interference of its inner nozzle throat with parts of the focused laser beam.

High-Power Nozzles

At laser beam powers of 3 kW and more one may use reflective optics for focusing to avoid thermal drift and strain within a transmissive lens or window. This calls for a special nozzle design to build up the stagnation pressure without a sealing window for the laser beam transition. There are mainly two solutions:

- Arranging two or more off-axis Laval nozzles symmetrically around the laser beam axis so that the individual jets are inclined toward the center, before they are redirected downward by an oblique shock into a common jet (7).
- Using a double-wall conical design with a converging annular flow passage in between, which leads into a central (e.g., cylindrical) orifice. This type of nozzle is called an "autonomous nozzle" because it governs the same gas jet conditions as a standard nozzle but independently of any transmissive window for the laser beam (6) (see Fig. 11).

Additional Nozzles

In some cases additional nozzles support the central cutting gas jet. These can be shaped as an annulus or can be single or multiple off-axis nozzles. Normally they have an individual gas supply. Additional nozzles are used, for example, to prevent or at least reduce precipitation of vapor on the workpiece surface near the cut edge by inducing a pressure gradient directed at the laser axis. The same arrangement, but with a lower pressure in the shielding ring jet, can be used to preserve the purity of the cutting gas on its way from the nozzle tip into the kerf. In a dragging configuration an additional nozzle supports melt ejection and avoids dross formation or post-burning behind the laser beam.

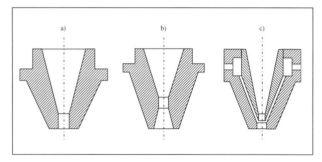

Figure 11. Different nozzle designs: (a) standard nozzle, (b) Laval nozzle, (c) autonomous nozzle.

Capacitive Distance Sensor

In modern laser cutting machines the nozzle tip operates simultaneously as a capacitive distance sensor. The second part of the capacitor is the metallic workpiece. If the distance between workpiece surface and nozzle tip is changed, the capacitance varies and an electronic oscillating circuit is detuned. This results in a signal that depends linearly on the distance and can be utilized in a closed-loop distance control. For proper operation the nozzle tip is electrically isolated from ground. If nonmetals are to be cut, then specially adapted capacitive and tactile distance sensors are used to control the cutting head clearance.

References

6. H. Zefferer, D. Petring, and E. Beyer, Proc. 3rd Int. "Beam Technology" Conf., Karlsruhe, DVS-Berichte Bd. 135, 210–4 (1991).
7. R. Edler and P. Berger, Proc. ICALEO '91, San Jose, 253–62 (1991).

12.1.5 Cutting of Complex Shapes

Starting a Cut

How one starts the cutting process depends on the special demands of the cut contour. In general there are two possibilities.

One is to start from an existing inner or outer edge of the workpiece. This is an appropriate method for cutting plates or coils to length or for trimming existing contours of a workpiece.

The second, more frequently applied method, which is called *piercing*, is necessary if inner contours, like complex-shaped holes, have to be produced. Piercing involves drilling a start hole, which can be continued as a cut. Laser drilling is described in detail in Chapter 13. The fastest piercing procedure is executed with one long laser pulse at full power, resulting in a big, low-quality drill hole. This is suitable only if the piercing hole is positioned on a scrap part of the workpiece. For high-quality piercing (e.g., on the cut contour itself or within small parts to be cut out) certain pulse sequences are applied. For optimum results the duty cycle, pulse frequency, and average power are gradually increased during the progress of piercing. The duration of high-quality piercing varies from a fraction of a second for thin sheet material in the range of 1 mm to more than 10 s for heavy section steel plates of more than 10 mm thickness.

A special method to start a cut is piercing on the fly. In this case the laser is switched on during movement of the cutting head above scrap material shortly before arriving at the start of the next cut part. This method is mainly utilized during fast cutting of thin sheets to minimize time loss.

Special Aspects of Contour Cutting

In principle a contour cut is nearly the same as a straight line cut, especially if the cutting tool is rotationally symmetric, as it should be in laser cutting (see Section 12.1.1). Nevertheless, experience shows that the parameters for straight line cutting or cutting of big radii often are not appropriate for the cutting of complex shapes, small holes, and narrow geometries. There are three main reasons for this:

- Heat conduction is obstructed in small workpiece geometries that are isolated by the kerf formation. This results in buildup of heat, subsequent overheating of critical parts, and their burn-off.

- In small radii cutting and during acceleration and slowing down, each machine has kinematic limits depending on the dynamical properties of the drives for the participating axes. This leads to periods when the travel speed is below its programmed value and thus to changed process conditions, particularly in small contours. This may lead to dross formation.
- A sudden or continuous change of cutting direction can disturb the formation of a steady cutting front. In consequence, a nonstationary process occurs with unsymmetrical and unstable heating and material removal.

Also, the polarization of the beam must be controlled as one changes directions in a complex cutting operation. This will be discussed in Sections 12.1.7 and 12.1.8.

Methods for Critical Geometries

It is obvious that under these circumstances the adaptation of parameters is necessary. If the dimensions of a contour are in the range of twice the workpiece thickness or smaller, the geometry has to be considered critical. The following methods are applied to stabilize the cutting process in these critical regions:

- Switching the laser beam into the pulsed mode with reduced average power, adapted to the actual cutting speed by varying pulse duty cycle and/or pulse frequency.
- Cutting loops with "corner overshooting" instead of driving directly around sharp corners. This is applicable only if an outer contour has to be cut.
- Short stop at corners, to give the process time for the new orientation and to cool the workpiece with the cutting gas.
- Rounding sharp corners with at least a small radius.
- Significantly reducing cutting speed and using the pulsed mode.
- Using water in addition to the cutting gas to cool the workpiece effectively.

Also the thermal load, stress, and distortion within the workpiece can be significantly reduced by controlling the order in which different parts of a cutting job are executed.

Minimizing Scrap

Another economical aspect during cutting complex shapes is to minimize scrap by nesting the parts to be cut out of one plate. The parts are positioned and oriented as closely as possible to each other, but a minimum distance in the range of one workpiece thickness should be maintained between different outer contours. Smaller parts are cut first out of the larger cutouts of big parts that would be wasted otherwise. This procedure is supported effectively via computer by CAD/CAM tools. Also the programming of partly common cutting kerfs for adjacent components is desirable.

12.1.6 Post-Cutting Operations

After the cut of a part is finished, it has to be separated from the scrap material and transported to the next work stage. This is done either manually or automatically.

Quality Aspects

The quality of a cut is usually specified by geometrical parameters:

- The size and form tolerances of the part
- The extent of dross or burr attachments
- Burnouts
- The average roughness
- The rectangularity of the cut edge

Other important properties of the cut edge and its heat affected zone (HAZ) are

- Chemical (oxidation, segregation, corrosion resistance)
- Metallurgical (depth of recast layer and HAZ, hardness)
- Mechanical (crack formation, bending and tensile strength)

Post Treatment

If the quality of the part does not meet the demands, it is waste or it has to be post machined, such as by deburring or grinding, again either manually or automatically. Normally this is not necessary with laser cuts because of their high quality. Other possible processes are partly independent of the cut quality but result from the raw material quality. These include cleaning, rust removal, and post-heat treatment of the material.

Further Processing Steps

Depending on the final product, additional post-cutting operations can be necessary. These include forming operations like bending, deep drawing, or hydroforming, refining operations like coating or painting, and completing or assembling operations like joining of cut parts, such as by laser welding.

DIRK PETRING

12.1.7 Polarization Effects in Laser Cutting: Basics

In laser cutting, the laser light is coupled into the material in the cut front as shown in Figure 12.

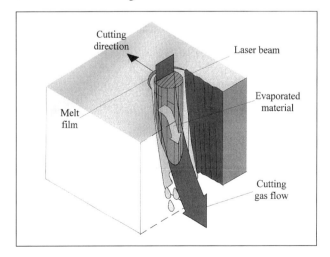

Figure 12. Coupling of laser light into the cut front.

ISBN 0-912035-15-3

Usually in laser cutting, the light is strongly absorbed by the material. The light absorption takes place in a thin surface layer, normally a thin molten layer.

In laser cutting, relatively high irradiance is used. Plasma formation can occur, especially with CO_2 lasers. However, the plasma absorption in laser cutting is normally relatively small compared to laser keyhole welding, because the strong gas flow reduces the ion density in the interaction zone. Therefore, plasma absorption can normally be neglected when describing the light coupling in laser cutting.

The reflectivity of the laser light impinging on the melt surface is dependent on:

- Angle of incidence of the laser beam
- Plane of polarization of the laser light
- Optical properties of the molten material

Normally the cut front has a semicircular shape and the angle of incidence of the laser beam, ϕ, is close to 90° (see Fig. 13).

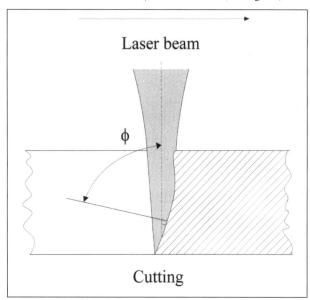

Figure 13. Orientation of beam in laser cutting.

The reflectivity of opaque surfaces has already been described in Section 5.3. Here we extend the description to derive the effects of polarization of the beam on laser cutting.

The reflectivity on the cut front can be calculated from the Fresnel formulas:

$$R_p = \left| \frac{\tan^2(\phi_t - \phi_i)}{\tan^2(\phi_t + \phi_i)} \right| \quad (11)$$

$$R_s = \left| \frac{\sin^2(\phi_t - \phi_i)}{\sin^2(\phi_t + \phi_i)} \right|$$

where R_p and R_s are the reflectivity of light polarized parallel and perpendicular, respectively, to the plane of incidence of the light. ϕ_i and ϕ_t are the angles of incidence and transmittance, respectively, of the beam.

The Snell theorem relates the ϕ_i, ϕ_t and index of refraction of the material $\tilde{n}$:

$$\sin \phi_t = \tilde{n} \sin \phi_i \quad (12)$$

The optical properties of the material and thus the index of refraction are dependent on the wavelength of the laser light and the material to be cut.

The index of refraction is a complex number:

$$\tilde{n} = n - i\kappa \quad (13)$$

where n is the refractive index and κ the extinction coefficient.

The refractive index n is the ratio of the velocity of light in vacuum to the velocity of light in the material. The extinction coefficient κ expresses the damping of the light in the material. The intensity $I(z)$ of light propagating through a material can be described by:

$$I(z) = I_0 \, e^{-\alpha z} \quad (14)$$

where I_0 is the intensity at the surface and z is the distance from the surface and

$$\alpha = \frac{4\pi\kappa}{\lambda} \quad (15)$$

The polarization of a laser beam can be linear, elliptic, circular, or random.

In the case of circular polarization, the coefficient of reflectivity R_c can be expressed by:

$$R_c = \frac{R_p + R_s}{2} \quad (16)$$

The efficiency of laser cutting depends on efficient energy coupling into the material, which in practice means a sufficiently high value of α and thus of κ. The material properties and thus the reflectivity are in general temperature dependent.

Both CO_2 and Nd:YAG lasers emit infrared light. For most metals, both n and κ are high for infrared radiation. This results in typical coefficients of reflectivity as shown in Figures 14 and 15 (next page).

Chapter 12: Laser Cutting

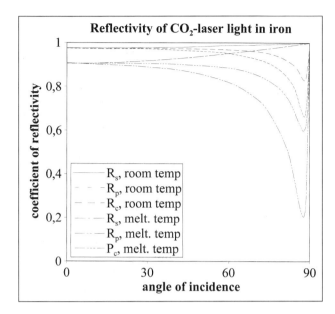

Figure 14. Reflectivity of CO_2 laser light versus angle of incidence for iron.

Figure 14 shows calculated coefficients of reflectivity R_p, R_s, and R_c for CO_2 laser radiation for Fe at room temperature and at the melting temperature. This shows a strong dependence of the reflectivity on the angle of incidence and the plane of polarization. It further shows that the light coupling improves when the material is heated to the melting temperature.

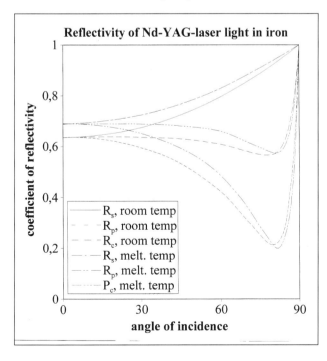

Figure 15. Reflectivity of Nd:YAG laser light as a function of angle of incidence for iron.

Figure 15 shows similar calculations for Nd:YAG laser light in iron. At this wavelength there is a strong dependence on polarization, although it is smaller than for CO_2 laser light.

Figure 16 shows the ratio A_p/A_s for iron at room and melting temperatures for the wavelengths of CO_2 and Nd:YAG lasers, where A_p and A_s are the absorption coefficients for the two different planes of polarization.

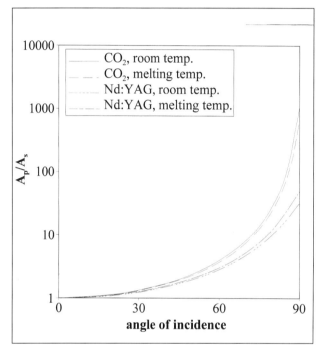

Figure 16. Ratio of absorption coefficients for the parallel and perpendicular components of polarization as a function of the angle of incidence for iron and for the conditions indicated.

These curves show the influence of the polarization of the laser beam on laser cutting. The reflectivity has a minimum around the Brewster angle, which is typically around 80°. In general the laser beam will form the cut front so that the angle of incidence will be close to the Brewster angle, where the most efficient energy coupling is obtained. See Section 5.3 for a discussion of Brewster's angle.

At this angle of incidence Figure 16 shows a strong dependence of energy coupling on polarization.

In the case of cutting materials with low reflectivity at normal incidence, the ratio A_p/A_s will be smaller. The influence of the polarization normally can be neglected.

In cases of laser cutting with linear polarization in metals, the differences in absorption in the cut kerf will cause different cutting results in different cutting directions.

Figure 17 shows a linearly polarized laser beam cutting metals. The figure shows where in the cut kerf on the workpiece the strongest absorption of the laser beam will take place, depending on the orientation of the plane of polarization relative to the cutting direction.

In cases of cutting in the direction of the plane of polarization, the strongest absorption will take place in the central part of the cut front, whereas in case of cutting in a direction perpendicular to the plane of polarization, the strongest absorption will take place at the sides of the cut front. This means, that the highest cutting rate and smallest cut kerf width can be obtained when cutting in the direction of polarization rather than when cutting in the perpendicular direction.

When cutting in other directions relative to the plane of polarization, the absorption will be asymmetric, and the kerf will bend to the side of the strongest absorption as shown.

These effects of polarization are strongest in case of metal cutting with CO_2 lasers. Methods for minimizing these effects will be presented in the next section.

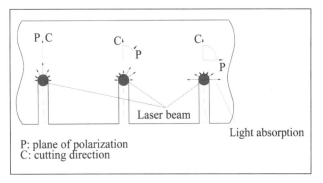

Figure 17. Schematic representation of relative strength of absorption for different orientations of the direction of cutting and the direction of polarization.

To overcome these problems, CO_2 laser cutting is normally performed with circularly polarized beams. The circular polarization is obtained by ensuring that the laser emits a linearly polarized beam with a well-defined plane of polarization and thereafter inserting a phase-shift mirror in the external beam path. For CO_2 lasers it is easy to control the plane of polarization, because any folding mirror inside the laser resonator will favor amplification in the plane perpendicular to the plane of incidence on the mirror.

In most practical applications, cutting rates obtained with circularly polarized laser beams are almost as high as those obtained using linearly polarized laser beams, parallel to the cutting direction.

Uniform cutting performance in contour cutting requires good polarization control. Degradation of mirrors or just multiple mirror beam paths can result in elliptical polarization on the workpiece, which can cause differences in cutting rates in different cutting direcations. Errors in polarization can be found by careful examination of cut kerfs. Even a sligthly elliptical polarization can cause differences in cutting performance in different directions.

FLEMMING O. OLSEN

12.1.8 Control of Beam Polarization Effects in Cutting

The beam emitted from a high-power CO_2 laser is usually polarized. Because of the problems described in the preceding section, this needs to be corrected before metals can be cut successfully. Correction is usually achieved by reflecting the beam off one or two coated mirrors to produce a depolarized or circularly polarized beam. These special mirrors have a number of names including phase-retarding mirrors, phase-change mirrors, depolarizing mirrors, and circularly polarizing mirrors.

If the coating on these mirrors becomes damaged by dirt, scratches, or overheating, they will not perform well, and the laser beam will return to its original polarized state. The use of a polarized beam when cutting metals means that a cut disc or hole will be circular only on its top face (see Fig. 18a). The bottom face of such a disc or hole will be noticeably oval, and the degree of ovality will increase if thicker sheets are cut. For example, in 10-mm-thick mild steel, a 15-mm hole will be 15 mm in diameter if measured on the top face and an ellipse with axes having lengths of ~14 and ~16 mm if measured on the bottom face. Similarly in 10-mm-thick material, a 100-mm square cut with a polarized beam will measure 100 x 100 mm on its top face and ~99 x ~101 mm on its bottom face, as shown in Figure 18b. Polarization problems of this sort are relevant to metal cutting, but do not occur when cutting low-conductivity materials such as plastics. Most nonmetals can be cut accurately with polarized or depolarized beams.

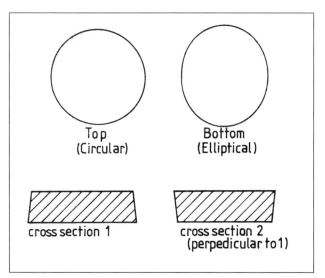

Figure 18. (a) A schematic top and bottom view of a "circle" cut with a polarized beam. (b) The inclination of the cut edge when cutting a square with a polarized beam. (In certain cases, when the cutting direction and the polarity are aligned, a perpendicular cut edge will be achieved for one of these cross sections) (8).

Chapter 12: Laser Cutting

It is worth noting that the directional properties of linearly polarized light also apply to the speed at which the beam will cut steels. A polarized beam is capable of cutting at higher speeds than an unpolarized beam but only in one direction. Fortunately, this is the same direction as the one in which it produces a perpendicular cut rather than a cut that slopes away from the vertical. This means that if a laser is used for a single-direction slitting operation, the maximum speed can be achieved with a linearly polarized beam, but the laser machine will need to be positioned at the correct angle to the oncoming material in order to produce a vertical cut. Some lasers change their polarization direction every few seconds and cannot be used in this way. Also, for contour cutting, it would be difficult to change the direction of polarization of a linearly polarized beam continuously to match the contour.

The physics behind polarization phenomena is briefly outlined in Figures 19 and 20. Each photon has an electrical and a magnetic vector associated with it, as shown in Figure 19a. In a polarized beam all these vectors point in the same two directions, as shown in Figure 19b. This type of beam can be tilted by metal as it passes through it to produce a cut. The resulting cut edges therefore slope toward or away from each other, depending on the cutting direction, as shown in Figure 18. After being reflected from a specially coated mirror, the photon vectors all point in different directions, as shown in Figure 20. In this case there is no overall tilt direction when the light passes through the cut zone and objects are cut accurately with perpendicular edges.

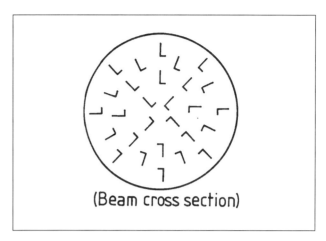

Figure 20. The alignment of the electrical and magnetic vectors of a depolarized or circularly polarized beam. Compare this with Figure 19b (8).

Thus most operations involving cutting of metals use laser beams that have been circularly polarized by the use of mirrors or phase-retarding elements.

Reference

8. J. Powell, 1993: CO_2 *Laser Cutting*, ISBN 3-540-19786-9, Springer Verlag.

JOHN POWELL

12.2 Laser Cutting of Metals

12.2.1 The Metal Cutting Process

Most laser metal cutting is performed with a gas assist. The beam from a laser is focused on the workpiece with a lens or, rarely, by a mirror. The irradiance must be high enough to melt the metal. The assist gas, introduced through a nozzle, mechanically removes the molten metal. Figure 1 schematically shows the process.

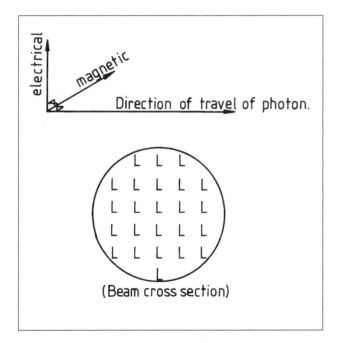

Figure 19. (a) A schematic of the electrical and magnetic vectors associated with a photon. (b) The alignment of the vectors in a polarized laser beam. A beam of this type will have directional properties (8).

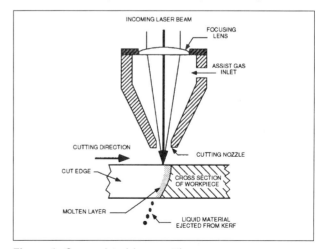

Figure 1. Gas-assisted laser cutting.

This process is successful only if the melt zone completely penetrates the workpiece. Laser metal cutting, then, is generally restricted to thin sections. While cutting has been reported through 100-mm sections of steel (1), the process is more typically used on metal sheets 6 mm or less in thickness.

Assist Gas

The assist gas may be reactive or inert. For most metals, oxygen and air are reactive, whereas nitrogen and argon are inert. The use of a reactive gas increases the energy available for cutting, but generally leaves reaction products on the cut edges. Cutting with inert gases produces cleaner edges at the cost of process speed.

The assist gas is critical for laser metal cutting, because it performs the actual removal of material. Table 1 outlines typical gas choices for several common metals.

Table 1. Gases for Metal Cutting With CO_2 Lasers

Metal	Gas	Comments
Carbon steel	Oxygen	Good finish, high speed; oxide layer on cut surface
Carbon steel	Nitrogen	Requires high power; cutting limited to material < 3 mm thick
Stainless steel	Oxygen	Heavy oxide slag on cut edges
Stainless steel	Nitrogen	Good edge quality; high gas pressure required
Aluminum	Air	Moderate quality
Aluminum	Oxygen	Highest cutting speeds, poor edge quality
Aluminum	Nitrogen	Slightly better edge quality than air
Titanium	Argon	Good edge quality
Titanium	Argon/helium	Best metallurgical quality

Gas pressure has a great effect on cut quality. For oxygen-assisted cutting of steel, a pressure of 300 kPa produces smooth edges on sheet below 2 mm in thickness. In thicker steel, such pressures cause burning and roughness on the cut edge; so the pressure must be dropped. Plates up to 8 mm thick may be cut with 200 kPa, whereas pressures as low as 50 kPa are necessary for plates above 12 mm.

Laser Duty Cycle

The highest cutting speed, and often the highest quality, is achieved using a beam that is on all the time. There are, however, many situations that require that the laser beam be pulsed.

The first condition mandating pulsing is that many lasers do not operate in a continuous-wave (CW) mode. Most lamp-pumped Nd:YAG lasers, and some RF-excited CO_2 lasers, fall into this category. All cutting with such equipment, then, is pulsed mode cutting.

A less trivial situation results from the ability of laser/CNC equipment to cut complex patterns. It is impossible, for reasons of mechanical inertia, to follow an intricate path at high speed. As an example, 16-gauge (1.5-mm) carbon steel may be cut at a speed of 4 m/min using 500 W CW. This speed cannot be maintained along small radii or in corners. If the laser power level is maintained at 500 W when negotiating such features, the material will burn away from the cut path. Reducing the CW power level does not alleviate this problem because the cutting mechanism is nonlinear.

The solution to this problem is to pulse the laser, maintaining a high irradiance while reducing the thermal input. A duty cycle of 10%, for example, will allow the cutting speed to be reduced to 0.2 m/min on 16-gauge steel while retaining high edge quality.

12.2.2 Characteristics of Laser-Cut Edges

Kerf Width

Kerf widths produced by laser cutting range from 0.05 to 1 mm. The widths vary with material thickness. In general, the goal is to generate the narrowest kerf possible, because that minimizes the amount of material removed. Narrow kerfs in thick material make it difficult for the cut material to be ejected; so in that case better results are achieved with wider kerfs.

Inert gas cutting of stainless steel requires high gas velocities to prevent the attachment of recast material to the bottom of the cut. Wide kerfs, on the order of 0.4 mm, are needed to allow complete ejection of molten material.

Surface Roughness

Thin carbon steel cut with an oxygen assist has relatively smooth edges. A surface roughness of 1 µm or better can be produced on 20-gauge (0.8-mm) carbon steel. As the steel gets thicker, the edge roughness increases and visible striations are present. The best finish achievable on 10-mm plate is on the order of 10 µm.

Inert gas cutting, which requires high gas velocities, does not produce edges as smooth as oxygen cutting. A roughness of 3 µm on 1.5-mm material is typical.

Dross

Gas-assisted cutting works by expelling molten metal from the bottom of the cut. Under many conditions, some of this metal attaches to the workpiece and remains as dross or slag. This condition is often unacceptable.

In oxygen-cut carbon steel, dross appears when the focus is incorrect, the gas pressure is too low, or the travel speed is too high. Stainless steel cut with inert gas often has dross. This condition is eliminated by increasing gas pressure or kerf width. Antispatter coatings such as graphite or magnesium carbonate can be used to reduce the adhesion of recast material to the bottom of laser-cut metal.

ISBN 0-912035-15-3

Chapter 12: Laser Cutting

12.2.3 Laser Cutting of Specific Metals

Carbon Steel

CO_2 laser cutting of carbon steel is a standard industrial process. Thicknesses cut range from 0.5 to 20 mm, with most cutting being done on cold-rolled sheet 3 mm or less in thickness.

The use of an oxygen assist is standard. Optimum laser powers and travel speeds for several thicknesses are shown in Table 2. Note that when using an oxygen assist, increasing laser power has a limited effect on travel speed. Powers in excess of those noted will cause reduced cut quality. If the speeds noted cannot be achieved because of mechanical limitations, the laser should be operated at a reduced duty cycle.

Table 2. Recommended Powers and Speeds for Carbon Steel

Thickness (mm)	Power (W)	Travel speed (m/min)
0.5	250	3.5
1.0	300	4.0
1.5	400	4.0
3.0	600	3.0
6.0	1200	1.5

Inert gas is sometimes used for cutting thin (1-mm) carbon steel sheet. Using several kilowatts of laser power, one may achieve very high cutting speeds with good edge quality.

Alloy Steel

While there are hundreds of alloy steel compositions, only a few are commonly laser cut. Low-alloy steels such as 4140 or 8620 cut much like carbon steel, although cut uniformity is generally better because alloy steels usually have fewer impurities. Chromium, a common constituent of alloy steels, reduces the reactivity of the steel to oxygen and generates a thick, tenacious oxide coating. Steels, alloy or straight carbon, containing more than 0.3% carbon will have a hard, martensitic layer on the cut edge.

Stainless Steel

Stainless steels are iron alloys containing large amounts of chromium. Oxygen cutting of these materials results in a heavy oxide on the cut edge. High-pressure nitrogen gives much better results on these materials. Table 3 presents some recommended cutting conditions for stainless steels.

Table 3. Recommended Cutting Conditions for Stainless Steel (nitrogen assist gas)

Thickness (mm)	Power (W)	Travel speed (m/min)	Gas pressure (kPa)
1.0	1000	3.5	600
1.5	1500	3.5	700
3.0	1800	2.0	800
6.0	2000	1.0	1200

Aluminum

Aluminum, because of its high optical reflectivity and thermal diffusivity, requires high laser power to cut. Thicknesses greater than 3 mm are seldom cut in production. Most commercial aluminum alloys exhibit microcracking on laser-cut edges along with high surface roughness. Table 4 presents some recommended cutting conditions for aluminum.

Table 4. Recommended Cutting Conditions for Aluminum (nitrogen assist gas)

Thickness (mm)	Power (W)	Travel speed (m/min)	Gas pressure (kPa)
1.0	1200	3.0	600
1.5	1500	2.5	800
3.0	1800	1.0	1000

Titanium

Titanium and its alloys react strongly with oxygen and nitrogen. If they are laser cut with either as an assist gas, brittle compounds form on the cut edge. It is necessary, therefore, to use an inert gas as an assist.

Argon is satisfactory at pressures up to 750 kPa. Above this, a plume tends to form. This absorbs laser power and degrades the cut. For cutting titanium thicker than 3 mm, pressures above 750 kPa are needed to get clean edges. Mixes of argon and helium, such as 75% Ar/25% He, are then required. Table 5 presents some recommended cutting conditions for titanium.

Table 5. Recommended Cutting Conditions for Titanium (argon assist gas)

Thickness (mm)	Power (W)	Travel speed (m/min)	Gas pressure (kPa)
1.0	800	3.5	600
1.5	900	3.0	700

Reference

1. D. L. Carroll et al., 1997: Experimental Analysis of the Materials Processing Performance of a Chemical Oxygen-Iodine Laser (COIL) Proc. ICALEO'96, Laser Institute of America 1997, E19–E33.

LEONARD MIGLIORE

12.2.4 CO_2 Laser Cutting of Metals

General

CO_2 lasers usually are used to cut metals by one of two methods:
1. melt shear cutting (called fusion cutting in Section 12.1.1) and
2. oxidation cutting.

1. Melt shearing: The principle here is very simple and is illustrated in Figure 2. Basically the power of the laser beam is focused to a small spot (typically 0.2 mm diameter), and this melts the workpiece. A pressurized jet of inert gas (e.g., argon) incident coaxially with the laser beam ejects the melt and produces a cut. (Melt shearing is called *fusion cutting* by some workers in the field.)

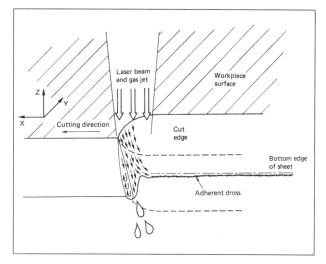

Figure 2. Melt shearing schematic.

2. Oxidation cutting: This is similar to melt shearing except that the gas used to eject the melt reacts chemically with it to generate extra heat and therefore increase cutting speeds. Usually oxygen is the gas employed although air can be used if oxygen is too reactive, such as with titanium alloys. The most common application of the technique is in the cutting of steels of all grades using oxygen.

One great benefit of laser cutting over such methods as plasma or water jet cutting is the fine cut (or kerf) width produced. The kerf width can range from approximately 0.1 to 1.0 mm depending on the application, but widths of between 0.2 and 0.3 mm are most common. With kerf widths as small as this and almost perpendicular edged cuts, it is possible to cut very fine detail such as saw teeth, etc. Penetration holes are also small, which means that internal details such as bolt holes can be profiled.

Penetration of the Workpiece

Before a component can be cut, the laser must (usually) penetrate the material to produce a hole. This can be the most troublesome part of the cutting process.

If the material is highly reflective or conductive, like aluminium or copper alloys, penetration is always more difficult to achieve than cutting. In some cases it may be worthwhile to mechanically predrill holes in the workpiece from which the cutting process may begin. The reasons for this difficulty in piercing are as follows:

1. The surface of the workpiece is solid, cold, and at an angle of 90° to the incoming laser beam. This is a much more reflective body than the liquid, hot, inclined cutting front that absorbs the beam during cutting.
2. Heat is conducted away from the hot spot created on the material surface more effectively than it is from a cutting front.

For certain highly reflective materials it may be necessary to roughen the surface with abrasives or to coat it with an absorptive medium. Paints are not usually successful because they burn off in advance of the cutting zone. Household cleaning fluids (like for cleaning windows), which dry to leave a powdery deposit, can be extremely effective.

One should beware of high-intensity reflections when carrying out trials or piercing/cutting highly reflective materials. As well as posing a hazard to the operator, reflections from the workpiece can damage the focusing lens or the laser optics. Scrap or cut components in the bottom of the cutting bed can also cause hazardous reflections as the cutting beam passes over them.

In cases where the conductivity/reflectivity is not such a problem (e.g., steels) penetration can still cause difficulties. During the cutting process, laser energy and pressurized gas enter the top of the cut zone and material is ejected from the bottom (see Fig. 2). During piercing, however, the material has no escape route because there is not yet a hole. The molten material generated therefore leaves the area in an upward direction and can easily contaminate the nozzle or lens. Such contamination can seriously affect the cutting performance of a machine. The amount of melt generated during the piercing operation can be minimized by utilizing the beam in its pulsed mode to "peck through" the material. Pulse frequencies of 50–100 Hz with an on-off ratio of 1–5 are suitable for this technique. Increase the off time to minimize the melt splash; decrease it to accelerate the piercing event.

Fatigue Life Considerations

When cutting low-carbon (mild) or stainless steels for general engineering use, there is rarely any need for concern about the effect of laser cutting on the fatigue life of the cut component. Certain applications, however, require care. Aerospace or automotive components cut from high-performance alloys might, for example, not be suitable to laser cutting if their fatigue life is badly affected.

Laser cutting is a thermal process capable of cutting fine detail. The cut edge undergoes a severe thermal cycle, which may be accompanied by a localized chemical reaction. Edge hardening as a result of the thermal cycle or chemical contamination of the resolidified melt must be considered a potential diminisher of the fatigue life of some materials. Titanium alloys are the clearest example of materials that could lose their ductility, although high-carbon steels are also affected in a similar way.

Laser cutting can also introduce stress increases on the cut edge either because of an injudicious choice of profile or the inherent micro-roughness of the edge itself.

ISBN 0-912035-15-3

Chapter 12: Laser Cutting

Most engineering components are designed so that the reduction in fatigue life associated with thermal cutting methods is not important. In certain cases, however, it may be best to check with the customer that, for example, cutting a titanium component with air assist is appropriate to the design.

A. Cutting of Carbon Steels (Mild and Low-Alloy Steels)

The Role of Oxygen

During the cutting of carbon steels an oxygen gas jet is used with the laser beam to generate a burning reaction. The oxygen has two beneficial effects on the process:

1. The burning reaction generates a great deal of heat and therefore accelerates the cutting process.
2. The burning reaction produces a liquid in the cut zone that does not stick to the solid steel. For this reason all the melt is clearly blown out of the cut zone and the resultant edge is dross free.

Cutting Speeds

Figure 3 gives typical cutting speeds for carbon or mild steels.

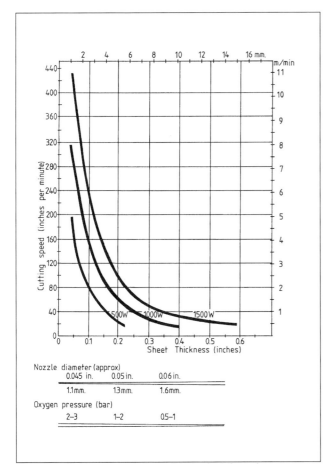

Figure 3. Cutting speeds for mild steel at three laser powers with guidelines concerning nozzle diameter and oxygen pressures (2).

A number of points are important when considering Figure 3:

1. The cutting speed decreases with increasing steel thickness. It is also true that for any CO_2 laser there will be a maximum carbon steel thickness that can be cut. At thicknesses above this maximum, the cutting process travels so slowly that widespread oxidation and burning of the workpiece take place instead of cutting.
2. The cutting speed generally increases with laser power. This is not always the case, as higher power lasers sometimes produce beams that do not focus as well as those of lower-power machines. In this case the resulting cut may be wider rather than faster. (Doubling the laser power does not always mean that the cut speed will be doubled.)
3. The nozzle diameter should be increased for cutting thicker sections and the oxygen pressure must be reduced. The idea is to allow an adequate oxygen flow to the cut zone without allowing the oxygen pressure in the zone to increase to a level at which the workpiece will experience widespread burning. The cut width for thicker steels will generally be larger than for thinner sections, and so larger diameter nozzles are appropriate.

General Notes on Cutting Quality

Cut edge qualities for carbon or low-alloy steels are similar to a milled finish. However, at the thickest sections for any particular laser the quality will deteriorate. The cut edge is covered by a regular series of ridges or striations similar to those shown in Figure 4.

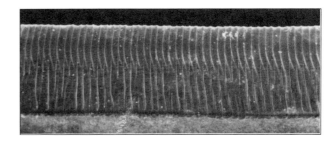

Figure 4. The regular striations observed on carbon steel cut edges. Sample is 2 mm thick (2).

These striations exist on the cut edge of mild steel even if the laser is producing a continuous-wave (CW) beam rather than operating in the pulsed mode.

Figure 5 (3) gives a clear depiction of how an unpulsed energy input can generate a pulsed-type cut edge covered in regular striations.

Although continuous laser outputs can be used to cut carbon steels, the oxidation process in the cut zone becomes more controllable if the laser is used in its pulsed mode. Cutting at frequencies in the range 200–500 Hz with on-off ratios of between 10:1 for standard cutting and 1:10 for fine detail can give superior cut edge quality (2).

ISBN 0-912035-15-3

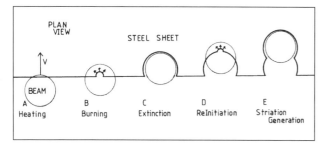

Figure 5. A schematic showing how striations can be generated (3).

Heat-Affected Zones

Because laser cutting is a thermal process, it produces a heat-affected zone (HAZ) next to the cut edge. In low-carbon steels the hardening effect is minor, but in medium- or high-carbon steel plate the edge will approach its maximum hardness for the material involved. This can have drawbacks if the cut product needs to undergo a bending operation. At the highest carbon contents (~0.8% or more) the severe thermal cycle can spontaneously generate cracks in the cut edge.

The depth of the HAZ is related to the cutting speed and therefore to the thickness of the steel involved. The depth of the HAZ toward the top of the cut edge is generally of the order of tens of micrometers. It becomes deeper farther down the cut edge and can be assumed to be between 10 and 30% of the material thickness at the bottom. Heat accumulation can occur when cutting a lot of detail in one area (e.g., saw teeth). In this case the HAZ can extend several millimeters. As long as the edge has not become microcracked during cutting, the HAZ can be removed by a suitable annealing cycle.

Oxide Coatings

Because the cut is generated by an oxidation reaction, it is not surprising that the cut edge is coated by a thin layer of oxide. This layer is generally not firmly attached to the underlying steel edge. In some cases this can cause problems if the items are to be painted. Loose oxide layers can be removed by abrasion, wire brushing, or pickling. In most cases, however, there is no need for oxide removal, and the paint holds firm.

Cutting Holes and Details

There is a minimum limit to the diameter of hole that can be cut in a given thickness of carbon steel. Unless special techniques are employed, a rule of thumb says that the minimum size hole that can be cut has a diameter equal to the thickness of the steel. This one-to-one relationship holds true for other details such as slots; that is, an 8 × 15-mm slot may be cut in 8-mm-thick carbon steel, but a 4 × 15-mm slot would present problems of uncontrolled burning. This burning can be reduced or eliminated if various precautions are exercised, such as:

1. Pierce the material using widely spaced low-power pulses rather than the full-power cutting beam. This "pecking through" produces a much smaller start-up hole with less heating of the surrounding area.

2. Use a pulse setting that minimizes overall heating of the workpiece. Once again this may mean low-power pulses with definite off times between them (for example, 50 or 100 Hz with an on-off ratio of 1:4 or more).

3. Spray a fine mist of water into the cut zone during piercing and cutting. The liquid will not interfere with the cutting process because it will be repelled by the heat and the oxygen jet. On the other hand, it will follow the cut (by capillary action) and cool the surrounding area.

Dirty optics widen the focus spot and make matters worse when cutting detail. Rusty or dirty steel will also have a negative effect.

Stop-Start Marks

When a cut line is completed, there is generally a stop-start mark on the edge of the workpiece. This becomes more pronounced as the material workpiece is increased. Figure 6 demonstrates how a stop-start mark can be produced. These marks can also be caused by poor CNC programming and by the weight of the component tearing it away from the steel sheet as the cut is nearing completion.

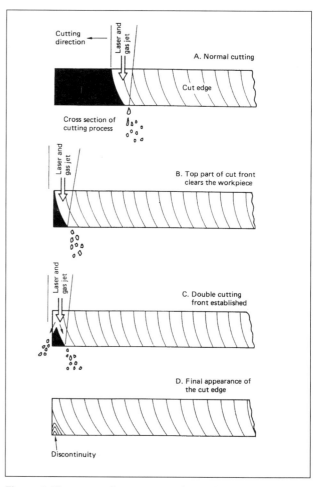

Figure 6. The cause of stop-start marks on thicker section materials.

Chapter 12: Laser Cutting

Steel Surface Condition and Oxygen Purity

Laser cutting of carbon steels depends on a pure iron reacting with pure oxygen. Surface coatings (e.g., paint or rust) allow impurities to enter the cut zone, which can affect the process. In the same way the process is very sensitive to contaminents in the oxygen supply.

The Effect of Surface Coatings

The following list gives details of the various surface conditions of carbon steel sheet and their influence on cutting:

1. Bright (cold-reduced or cold-rolled). This should present no problem.
2. Black (hot-rolled). The dark surface coating of oxides can be of varying thickness depending on the supplier or the position on the sheet. This material can interfere with the cutting process to give inferior cut quality (burning and dross). In some cases, however, it has a negligible effect. The oxide layer can be removed by pickling.
3. Pickled and oiled. This is a hot-rolled sheet that has had the oxide layer removed by chemical treatment. It cuts as bright mild steel but is covered in a layer of oil. Wipe surplus oil off sheets with a cloth before cutting; a residual thin layer does not affect cutting.
4. Zinc coating. Depending on coating thickness the zinc can slow the cutting process and result in dross on the lower cut edge.
5. Cadmium coating. The same as for zinc coating, however, the fumes given off are dangerous to health. It is not recommended to laser cut cadmium-coated steel.
6. Paint. Most paints interfere with the cutting process to give slower speeds and poorer quality. The paint is also damaged near the cut edge. Paints used for identifying steel sheets can interrupt the cutting process on an otherwise unpainted sheet.
7. Shot blasting. Shot blast particles (silica) can become imbedded in the steel surface and can result in drossy, poor-quality cuts. Remove particles by wire brushing.
8. Rust (corrosion). Rust and the moisture it often contains will interfere with the cutting process. Remove by wire brushing or sanding.

The Effect of Oxygen Purity

Commercially available oxygen is usually of a purity higher than 99.75%. At this purity it generates high-speed, high-quality cuts.

If even small amounts of impurities are present in the gas, the cutting speeds drop rapidly, and the resulting cut will be of poorer quality. Table 6 demonstrates the dramatic reduction of cutting speed with increasing impurity levels.

Some oxygen-producing companies now offer a high-purity oxygen (which is 99.99% pure) for laser cutting. This gives an increase in cutting speed between 10 and 20%, although it costs considerably more than standard grades. One area where the increased purity can be commercially beneficial is in the cutting of thicker sections. If, for example, a laser is only capable of cutting 10-mm carbon steel with standard grade oxygen, it should be possible to increase this limit to 11 or 12 mm by using higher-purity oxygen. The same sort of benefits can result from the use of low-impurity carbon steels.

Table 6. Optimum Cutting Speeds Over a Range of Oxygen Purities (4)

Oxygen purity	Impurity level	Relative cutting speed
99.75%	0.25%	100%
99.50%	0.50%	90%
99.00%	1.00%	70%
98.00%	2.00%	50% (dross on lower cut edge)

High-Purity Steels

A number of steel manufacturers are now producing high-purity carbon steels for laser cutting. The reduction of elements such as silicon improves cutting speeds and, perhaps more important, increases the maximum sheet thickness that can be cut.

B. Cutting of Stainless Steels

Cutting Speeds

Stainless steels of all grades can be cut with a CO_2 laser using either oxygen or an inert gas (usually nitrogen) as the cutting gas jet. Oxygen-assisted cutting is the most common of the two, and typical cutting speeds are given in Figure 7.

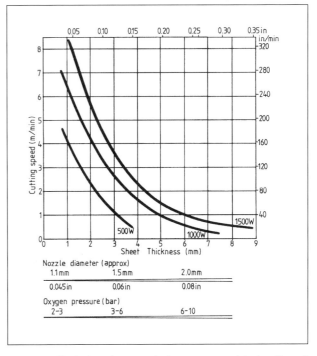

Figure 7. Typical cutting speeds for oxygen-assisted cutting of stainless steels at a number of laser powers. Guidelines are also given for oxygen pressures and nozzle diameters (2).

ISBN 0-912035-15-3

Nitrogen-assisted cutting is a slower process that produces a higher-quality product. Cutting speeds in this case are generally 30–60% of the oxygen-assisted cutting speed.

Cutting Quality

Oxygen-assisted cutting: Figure 8 shows a typical laser-oxygen cut edge in 4-mm-thick stainless steel. The edge is macroscopically flat but covered in microscopic ripples. There is a small amount of dross attached to the underside of the cut edge, which generally needs removal by grinding.

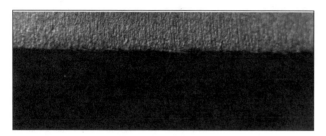

Figure 8. A typical example of a stainless steel cut edge cut with oxygen assist (4 mm thick).

The chemistry of the cut edge is rather more complicated than for carbon steels. There is an outer skin of hard oxide, which is only a few micrometers thick. Below this there is a thin layer of resolidified molten steel, which has a lower chromium content than the base material. The reason for this chromium depletion is that during the cutting process the iron, nickel, and chromium in the melt compete to react with the oxygen jet. Chromium is the most reactive of the three elements, and thus more of it becomes oxidized. This leaves the remaining solidified melt low in chromium. Because chromium is added to stainless steels to prevent them from oxidizing, this depletion of the chromium content of the cut edge means that it can be come corroded when exposed to water. The layer that can corrode is only a hundred or so micrometers thick, but this is enough to discolor the laser cut edges of stainless steels if the components are used in exterior environments. Fortunately most engineering products are not exposed to the weather, and if they are, discoloration is not necessarily a problem. Industries where this potential corrosion could cause a problem include the chemical, food, and sign-making trades. Work for such companies is usually carried out using nitrogen as the cutting gas.

For companies that require the lower prices of oxygen-assisted cutting but want to avoid edge corrosion, the susceptible layer can be removed by grinding or pickling. The problem can also be minimized by coating the cut edge with paint, lacquer, or oil.

Nitrogen-assisted cutting: Nitrogen-assisted cuts are bright silver in appearance and covered with microscopic ripples. If the gas pressure is high enough, the dross will be blown away during cutting, and the bottom edge of the cut will be clean.

The resolidified melt in this case has the same chemistry as the bulk material and is thus resistant to corrosion. This method of cutting is generally stipulated by users such as the chemical or food industries.

C. Cutting of Nonferrous Metals

Aluminum Alloys

Aluminum alloys can be cut by CO_2 lasers using either an inert gas jet or oxygen. Cutting speeds and maximum thicknesses are lower than they are for many other metals such as stainless steels because aluminum has:

1. A high reflectivity for CO_2 laser light
2. A high thermal conductivity
3. An oxidation reaction that is self-limiting because it creates an oxide that is impermeable to oxygen.

Figure 9 gives typical cutting speeds for aluminum for two laser powers with oxygen as the cutting gas. If nitrogen is employed, the cutting speeds and maximum thicknesses may be decreased by a factor of approximately two. Anodized aluminum cuts approximately 30% faster than what is indicated in the figure.

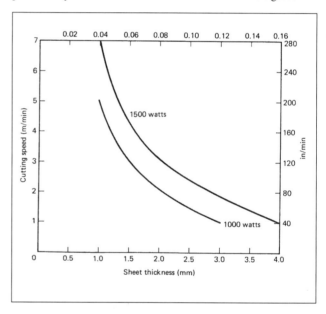

Figure 9. Typical cutting speeds for aluminum alloys at laser powers of 1000 and 1500 W. Cutting gas: oxygen at pressures of 2–6 bar.

With oxygen cutting, the cut edge will be covered by microscopic ripples with adherent dross on the lower edge. With nitrogen cutting, the edge will be smoother and, if sufficient pressure is employed, can be dross free.

There is a wide variation in the ease with which various aluminum alloys can be cut. Figure 9 must be taken only as a guideline. In some cases where the eventual customer does not stipulate the grade of aluminum to be cut, the laser cutter can choose a favorable grade or finish.

Anodized aluminum sheet cuts and can be pierced more easily because it is coated in a highly absorptive layer of aluminum oxide.

Titanium Alloys

Titanium alloys, like stainless steels, can be cut using an oxidizing or an inert gas. The use of pure oxygen is not common because the resulting chemical reaction with laser-heated titanium is extremely violent and results in poor-quality edges with broad (1 mm+) kerf width. This process can be used for thicker sections if edge quality is not important. The oxygen is absorbed by the workpiece near the cutting zone, which results in severe edge hardening and embrittlement. A better-quality cut is produced if compressed air is used as the cutting gas. Although this produces a much smoother cut, the edges are again severely embrittled by oxygen and nitrogen absorption. This embrittlement has a catastrophic effect on the toughness and fatigue life of the cut component but in some cases (like skids attached to the underside of racing cars) this is not important.

Inert gas cutting using argon gives a smooth cut edge, which can be clean of adherent dross if the jet pressure is high enough (10 bar). There is no embrittlement by gas absorption, but a certain amount of edge hardening is usual in the narrow heat-affected zone near the cut path. Although nitrogen can be used for "inert gas" cutting of stainless steels, this is not the case for titanium alloys. Titanium reacts chemically with nitrogen and can absorb it to generate an embrittled edge. For true inert gas cutting, only argon or helium may be used, although argon is far more common. If the pressure and flow of the inert gas is insufficient to keep air away from the cut zone, the cut edge may change color from bright silver to yellow or blue. Colors of this type on the cut edge indicate gas (atmospheric N_2 and O_2) absorption and embrittlement. Colors on the surfaces of the workpiece sheet do not necessarily indicate a problem if the cut edge is bright silver in appearance. The appearance of the cut edge is self-diagnostic as follows: grey and very rough indicates an oxygen cut, grey and slightly rough indicates an air cut, yellow and smooth indicates a nitrogen cut, silver and smooth indicates an argon cut.

All cut edges that are not silver in color should be treated as unweldable. This is because the absorbed oxygen or nitrogen will be mixed into the weld pool, resulting in a brittle weld and poor fatigue life.

Typical cutting speeds using oxygen, air, and nitrogen as the cutting gas are given in Figure 10 for a laser power of 1000 W.

Nickel Alloys

Nickel alloys include such materials as monels (nickel-copper), nimonics, inconels, and hastalloys (nickel-chromium-iron) and renes (nickel-chromium-cobalt-molybdenum). All these materials can be cut by CO_2 lasers using inert gas or oxygen as the cutting gas. The wide range of thermal conductivities and reflectivities covered by this group of alloys means that cutting trials may be necessary to establish cutting speeds or maximum possible thicknesses. However, as a rule of thumb, these alloys will have cutting speeds and maximum thicknesses between 50 and 90% of those of stainless steels.

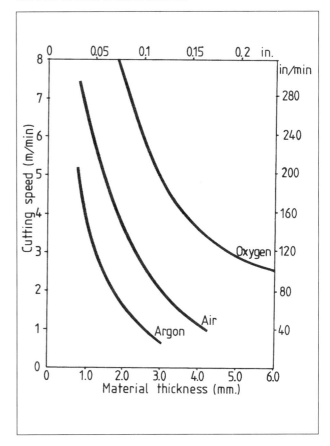

Figure 10. Guideline cutting speeds for titanium alloys with a laser power of 1000 W and a selection of cutting gases (argon, air, and oxygen). Notes: (1) If an unoxidized edge is required, argon must be used (3–10 bar) and the cut edge must be silver in appearance. Any blue or yellow colors indicate oxidation. High-pressure cutting can result in a dross-free edge. (2) Cutting with oxygen is potentially hazardous and can lead to an uncontrollable burning reaction, particularly when cutting thicker sections. The sparks are also highly energetic and can cause fires in the fume extraction system, etc.

The thermal and chemical cycles experienced at the cut edge are severe as they always are with laser cutting. In cases where the fatigue life of a component is important, a careful assessment of the cut edge must be carried out.

Copper Alloys

As in the case of aluminium alloys, copper alloys are cut slowly and with small maximum thicknesses because of their high reflectivity and conductivity. It is difficult to cut pure copper sheet, but profiling of brass is common. Brass has a thermal conductivity that is less than one-third that of copper (110 W/m/K compared with 385 W/m/K), and this allows the material to be cut more effectively. A typical cutting speed for 1-mm-thick copper using oxygen and a 1500-W laser would be 3 m/min compared to 5 m/min for the same thickness in brass. At a thickness of 2 mm, the cutting speeds would be 1 and 2 m/min, respectively. Cut edges tend to be microscopically rippled with adherent dross on the lower edge. A degree of zinc depletion may also be associated with the cut edge because zinc is volatile. Inert gas cutting would give smoother edges, but piercing and cutting are more difficult in the absence of oxygen.

Other Materials

Although the CO_2 laser cutting market is dominated by the profiling of steels, it is possible to cut most metals at commercially profitable rates. The only obvious exceptions to this rule are gold and silver, which are too reflective and conductive (although Nd:YAG lasers can cut them more effectively).

The choice of oxygen or inert gas cutting depends on the cut edge quality required. Cutting speeds depend on the following material properties:

- Thermal conductivity
- Reflectivity at a wavelength of 10.6 μm
- Surface condition (polished, etc.)
- Oxidation reactions
- Material thickness

Piercing the material is generally more difficult than cutting it. As a rule of thumb, if the material can be pierced by the laser, cutting will be possible.

Alloys of lead, zinc, molybdenum, silicon, etc. have all been cut successfully by CO_2 lasers, but applications are not common enough for there to be a library of cutting conditions and speeds.

References
2. J. Powell, 1993: *CO_2 Laser Cutting,* Springer Verlag, ISBN 3-540-19786-9.
3. Y. Arata, H. Maruo, I. Miyamoto, and S. Takeuchi, "Dynamic behaviour in laser gas cutting of mild steel," *Trans. Japanese Welding Research Institute* **8** (2), 15–26 (1979).
4. A. Ivarson, PhD Thesis: "On the physics and chemical thermodynamics of laser cutting," Lulea University of Technology, Sweden. 1993: 114D, ISS0348-8373.

JOHN POWELL

12.2.5 Nd:YAG Laser Cutting

General Notes

Nd:YAG lasers produce a high-intensity infrared light beam that can be focused to carry out cutting operations in a very similar way to CO_2 lasers. The general principles of cutting are the same for both types of laser and will not be repeated here. The following notes will explain the differences between Nd:YAG and CO_2 laser cutting.

Far fewer Nd:YAG lasers are sold as cutting machines compared with CO_2 lasers. This is because, for general cutting applications, CO_2 lasers are more cost effective. Nd:YAG lasers are preferred only in the following situations:

1. If very fine detailed work is required in thin section material
2. If highly reflective materials such as copper or silver alloys are to be cut on a regular basis
3. If an optical fiber is to be used to transport the laser beam to the workpiece

Although both CO_2 and Nd:YAG lasers generate infrared light, the wavelength of the CO_2 laser light is 10 times that of the Nd:YAG lasers (10.6 and 1.06 μm, respectively). Because the Nd:YAG laser light has a shorter wavelength, it has three advantages over CO_2 laser light:

1. Nd:YAG laser light can be focused down to a smaller spot than CO_2 laser light. This means that finer, more detailed work can be achieved (e.g., ornamental clock hands).
2. Nd:YAG laser light is less easily reflected by metal surfaces. For this reason Nd:YAG lasers are suited to work on highly reflective materials. A lower reflectivity for Nd:YAG laser light is actually more important to the piercing process than it is during cutting for the reasons outlined in Section 12.2.4.
3. Nd:YAG light can travel through glass, whereas CO_2 light cannot. This means that high-quality glass lenses can be used to focus the beam to a minimum spot size. Also quartz optical fibers can be employed to carry the beam relatively long distances to the workpiece.

If an optical fiber is used, the ability of the Nd:YAG laser light to be focused down to a very small spot may be lost, if the average power is above 100 W. The focused spot size after traveling through an optical fiber may be larger than a CO_2 laser spot.

In summary, Nd:YAG lasers can be used to cut fine detail or they can be used with an optical fiber, in which case fine detail will not be possible (except when cutting foils or thin masks at low power). They are particularly suited to cutting high-reflectivity alloys, but cannot cut many nonmetals.

Cutting Speeds and Cut Quality

Table 7 presents typical cutting speeds for metals cut by Nd:YAG lasers. The list must be used only as a general guideline, and as usual with laser cutting, specific production trials will be needed to confirm the performance of a machine. CO_2 lasers can be used close to their maximum power in either the continuous wave or pulsed mode. For this reason a machine's cutting speeds are easy to identify. In the case of Nd:YAG lasers, the situation is not so straightforward. Nd:YAG machines can be used in the CW mode, but pulsing is more common. The design of Nd:YAG lasers means that the pulse rates of these machines are much lower than for CO_2 lasers. CO_2 lasers can, for example, pulse at frequencies greater than 10,000 Hz. Nd:YAG lasers, on the other hand, are limited to hundreds of hertz. This can be a limit on the cutting speed because the pulses must overlap on the workpiece to be able to cut through it. If the pulses do not overlap, the laser will

Chapter 12: Laser Cutting

generate a series of unconnected holes. If we take, for example, a focused spot size of 0.3 mm and a laser with a maximum pulsing rate of 500 Hz, then the maximum cutting speed of the machine will be less than 0.3 x 500 x 60 mm/min, 9 m/min. The actual maximum cutting speed may be as low as half this value to ensure a good amount of overlap between pulses. Cut edges will have parallel ripples on them that show where one pulse started and the next one finished. At lower speeds the pulses get closer together, the ripples become shallower, and the cut edge becomes smoother.

If high-quality lenses are used without optical fibers, Nd:YAG lasers can cut finer detail than CO_2 machines. Cut widths smaller than 0.1 mm (0.004 in.) can be achieved. Cuts on this scale have a minimal amount of dross on the lower edge of the cut. Fine cutting of this type is generally restricted to low-average-power pulsed applications with a high level of pulse overlap. For this reason cutting speeds and workpiece thickness will generally be low.

The speeds given in this table were taken from data provided by the equipment manufacturers and should be treated as general values.

The Use of Optical Fibers

Optical fibers can be used to transport Nd:YAG laser light to the workpiece. Figure 11 (next page) shows that the beam from the fiber is expanded before being refocused onto the workpiece. The cutting head also includes a nozzle and pressurized gas system to remove melt from the cut zone. Optical fiber cutting systems of this type have a number of advantages and one main disadvantage.

Advantages:

1. The laser can be situated meters (or hundreds of meters) from the workstation. This can be of great benefit in automobile production line situations where space near the line is very limited.
2. One laser can time share between a number of fibers and cutting heads. Although this is possible with mirror-controlled systems, it is much easier when using fibers.
3. A number of cutting heads can work simultaneously in a confined area.
4. Robots that control the movement of an optical fiber head are less specialized and vibration sensitive than multiple mirror systems. This makes them less expensive and more reliable.

Disadvantage:

1. Except at the lowest powers (less than 100 W) optical fibers corrupt the laser beam and reduce its ability to be focused to a very small spot. Focused spot sizes after an optical fiber are generally in the range 0.3–0.6 mm. At these larger spot sizes cutting speeds are reduced, and more important, the machine cannot cut fine detail.

Table 7. Speed for Cutting of Metals by Nd:YAG Lasers

Material	Thickness (mm)	(in.)	Average laser power	Cutting Speed (m/min)	(in./min)	Gas
Mild steel	2.5	0.1	350	0.559	22.0	Oxygen
	5.0	0.2	350	0.127	5.0	Oxygen
	10.0	0.4	350	0.010	0.4	Oxygen
	10.0	0.4	500	0.10	4.0	Oxygen
	1.0	0.04	1000	4.5	177.0	Oxygen
	2.0	0.08	1000	2.5	98.0	Oxygen
	3.0	0.12	1000	1.5	59.0	Oxygen
	1.0	0.04	3000	20.0	790.0	Oxygen
	2.0	0.08	3000	11.0	433.0	Oxygen
	4.0	0.16	3000	5.0	197.0	Oxygen
	6.0	0.24	3000	2.0	79.0	Oxygen
	8.0	0.30	3000	1.0	39.0	Oxygen
	10.0	0.4	3000	0.8	31.0	Oxygen
	12.0	0.47	3000	0.5	20.0	Oxygen
Stainless steel	0.5	0.02	120	1.0	40.0	Oxygen
	2.0	0.08	120	0.45	18.0	Oxygen
	4.0	0.16	120	0.1	4.0	Oxygen
	1.0	0.04	400	0.9	36.0	Oxygen
	3.0	0.12	400	0.5	20.0	Oxygen
	5.0	0.2	400	0.25	10.0	Oxygen
	10.0	0.4	400	0.1	4.0	Oxygen
	1.0	0.04	500	3.0	120.0	Oxygen
	2.5	0.1	500	0.8	32.0	Oxygen
	10.0	0.4	500	0.16	6.4	Oxygen
	15.0	0.6	500	0.07	2.8	Oxygen
	2.0	0.08	3000	9.0	354.0	Oxygen
	4.0	0.16	3000	4.4	173.4	Oxygen
	6.0	0.24	3000	2.5	98.5	Oxygen
	8.0	0.3	3000	1.0	39.5	Oxygen
	10.0	0.4	3000	0.6	23.5	Oxygen
	2.0	0.08	3000	5.0	197.0	Nitrogen
	4.0	0.16	3000	2.8	100.5	Nitrogen
	6.0	0.24	3000	1.5	59.0	Nitrogen
	8.0	0.3	3000	0.5	20.0	Nitrogen
	10.0	0.4	3000	0.2	8.0	Nitrogen
Aluminum	1.0	0.04	120	0.5	20.0	Oxygen
	3.0	0.12	120	0.05	2.0	Oxygen
	2.0	0.08	500	0.75	30.0	Oxygen
	6.3	0.25	400	0.1	4.0	Oxygen
	2.0	0.08	3000	13.0	512.0	Oxygen
	3.0	0.12	3000	6.5	256.0	Oxygen
	4.0	0.16	3000	3.5	138.0	Oxygen
	6.0	0.24	3000	1.5	59.0	Oxygen
	2.0	0.08	3000	7.0	276.0	Nitrogen
	3.0	0.12	3000	4.0	157.0	Nitrogen
	4.0	0.16	3000	1.8	71.0	Nitrogen
	6.0	0.24	3000	1.0	40.0	Nitrogen
Copper	1.0	0.04	120	0.5	20.0	Oxygen
	3.0	0.12	120	0.05	2.0	Oxygen
Titanium	1.0	0.04	120	1.0	40.0	Argon
	3.0	0.12	120	0.3	12.0	Argon
	4.0	0.16	400	0.25	10.0	Argon

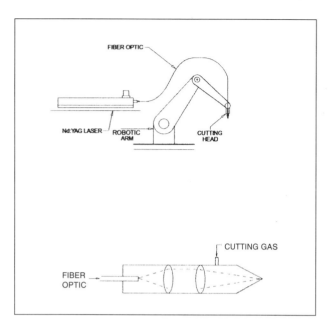

Figure 11. A schematic diagram of a robot-operated Nd:YAG laser cutting machine using an optical fiber to transport the laser beam to the cutting head.

JOHN POWELL

Thickness Versus Cutting Speed

Figures 12 and 13 show data on the cutting of two different types of steel with an Nd:YAG laser.

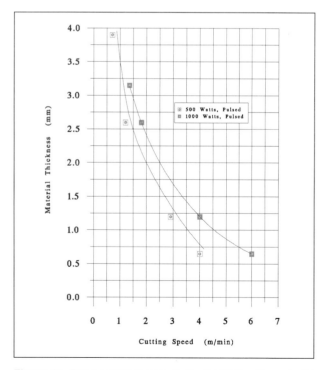

Figure 12. Representative speeds for Nd:YAG cutting of mild steel with oxygen assist.

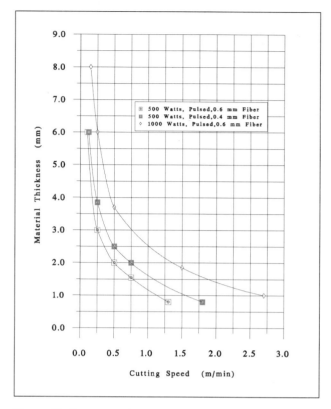

Figure 13. Representative speeds for Nd:YAG cutting of stainless steel with nitrogen assist.

DAVID HAVRILLA

12.2.6 Microcutting of Metals with Pulsed Nd:YAG Lasers

Laser microcutting can create many kinds of geometrical structures. The advantages of microcutting by means of pulsed Nd:YAG lasers are the flexibility and the higher production rate, as compared to electrical discharge milling (5). Moreover, there is no tool wear and the cutting edges are smooth (6). This section illustrates common microcutting applications and provides some characteristic cutting data in different metals.

Figure 14 shows the entrance surface of a laser cut spin nozzle, which is used for spinning of hollow polymeric fibers for the textile industry. An objective with a focal length of 50 mm and a 2x beam expansion is used to cut out the spinneret with two passes of the laser beam. This is necessary to achieve a cutting kerf width of 85 mm with a small radius in the corner. The thickness of the stainless steel is 0.5 mm. The cutting speed is 20 mm/min, and oxygen is used as a process gas. The taper of the spinnerets is smaller than 5%, and the standard deviation of the cutting kerf is 4 μm. With one laser pass it is possible to create a smaller cutting kerf width.

Chapter 12: Laser Cutting

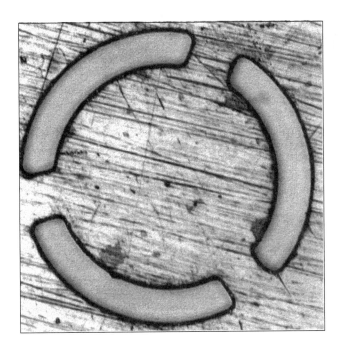

Figure 14. Spin nozzle in stainless steel. Photograph courtesy of LASAG AG Industrial Lasers.

Stents used in coronary surgery are another example of laser microcutting. Typically an objective with a focus length of 50 mm is used for this application to prevent damage of the opposite side of the small tube. A maximum cutting velocity of 300 mm/min can be obtained (see Fig. 15).

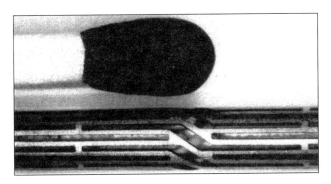

Figure 15. Laser-cut stent of stainless steel with an outer diameter of 2 mm. Photograph courtesy of LASAG AG Industrial Lasers.

Figure 16 shows a watch spring of 0.6 mm thickness. The width of the bar is only 0.1 mm. The heat-affected zone must be smaller than 2 µm to achieve a good spring suspension. The watch spring is cut with a velocity of 80 mm/min.

The influence of the pulse energy is shown with two metallographic sections in Figure 17. Both kerfs are cut with the same process parameters, except for the pulse energy. The material is 1-mm-thick stainless steel. The left kerf is cut with a pulse energy of 0.02 J and the right kerf with 0.20 J. A higher pulse energy widens the cutting kerf at the entrance and in the lower half of the material thickness. For the pulse energy of 0.02 J the kerf width is 50 µm at the entrance side and 40 µm at the exit side for a material thickness of 1 mm. Therefore, the taper of the cutting kerf is only 0.5%. Furthermore, the heat-affected zone is very narrow.

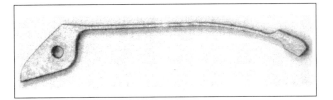

Figure 16. Watch spring. Photograph courtesy of LASAG AG Industrial Lasers.

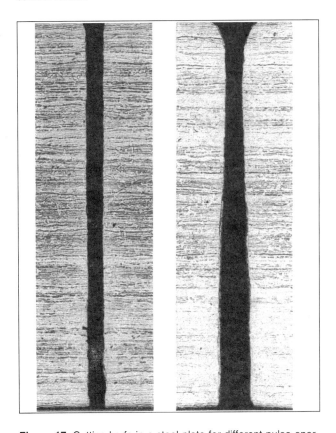

Figure 17. Cutting kerfs in a steel plate for different pulse energies. Left: 0.02 J. Right: 0.2 J. Photograph courtesy of LASAG AG Industrial Lasers.

The important role of the focal position on the geometry of the cutting kerf is illustrated in Figure 18 for a material thickness of 1 mm. The cutting velocity is 50 mm/min with a pulse frequency of 50 Hz. The material layers are measured from the entrance side of the laser beam. The first layers, up to a depth of 300 µm, have variable kerf width because of the variation of the focal position. Figure 18 indicates that the entrance has a minimum for the focal position at the workpiece surface. The smallest difference of the cutting kerf width for all layers is obtained with a focal position 0.2 mm beneath the workpiece surface. Consequently the smallest conicity of the cutting kerf is achieved with this focal position.

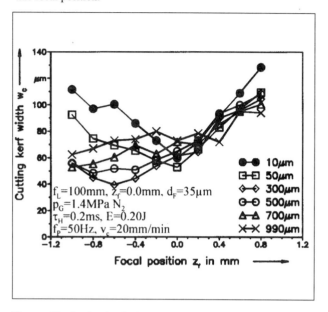

Figure 18. Cutting kerf width as a function of focal position.

Table 8 gives a summary of data for laser microcutting applications. In the table s is material thickness, E the laser energy, τ_H the pulse duration, f_p the pulse frequency, f_L the lens focal length, p_G the gas pressure, v_c the cutting velocity, w_{CE} the entrance size, and w_{CA} the exit size.

References

5. H. Rohde and P. Verboven, 1995: *Precision Cutting and Drilling with a Nd:YAG Slab Laser*. In: Proc. International Symposium for Electromachining ISEM XI, 777–83.
6. W. M. Steen and J. N. Kamalu, 1983: *Laser Cutting*, in: Laser Materials Processing, M. Bass (Ed.), Vol. 3, North-Holland Publ. Company, New York, 15–111.

HANSJOERG ROHDE

12.2.7 Cutting of Metals with Other Lasers

Cutting with a CO Laser

Because of its shorter wavelength, the light from a CO laser is absorbed better by metallic surfaces than that from CO_2 lasers (see Chapter 5). In addition to favorable absorption characteristics, the beam from a CO laser will have half the beam divergence of a CO_2 laser with the same value of M^2, since the wavelength of its beam is half that of the CO_2 laser.

Consequently, when a beam from each laser is focused by a lens system with the same $f/$ number, the CO laser should produce four times the power density of the CO_2 laser.

For equal power, the cutting performance of the CO laser is better than that of the CO_2 laser. Figures 19 and 20 (next page) show measured data on the cutting of two different types of steel using 1–5-kW CO lasers and CO_2 lasers (7). According to the theoretical work of Dausinger, the 5-μm CO laser provides better absorption characteristics than the 10-μm CO_2 laser (8).

Table 8. Typical Parameters and Results of Microcutting Performance

Material	s (mm)	E (J)	τ_H (ms)	f_P (Hz)	f_L (mm)	p_G (MPa)	Gas	v_C (mm/min)	w_{CE} (mm)	w_{CA} (mm)
Steel 1.4301	1.00	0.05	0.20	50	100	1.4	O_2	20	0.05	0.04
SUS 630	0.95	0.10	0.20	50	100	1.0	O_2	15	0.20	0.15
Stainless steel	0.70	0.13	0.15	300	100	1.8	N_2	300	0.13	0.10
SUS 304	0.55	0.13	0.14	50	100	1.0	O_2	20	0.05	0.05
Inconel 718	0.50	0.30	0.25	500	100	1.8	N_2	2000	0.25	0.20
Zirconium	0.49	0.11	0.20	150	100	1.0	Ar	400	0.18	0.13
Inox	0.30	0.06	0.15	300	50	1.0	O_2	500	0.10	0.10
Copper	0.10	0.12	0.10	500	50	1.0	O_2	1800	0.20	0.20
Tantalum	0.10	0.01	0.15	300	50	1.8	O_2	30	0.04	0.03
Molybdenum	0.05	0.05	0.16	50	100	1.0	O_2	4	0.01	0.01

Chapter 12: Laser Cutting

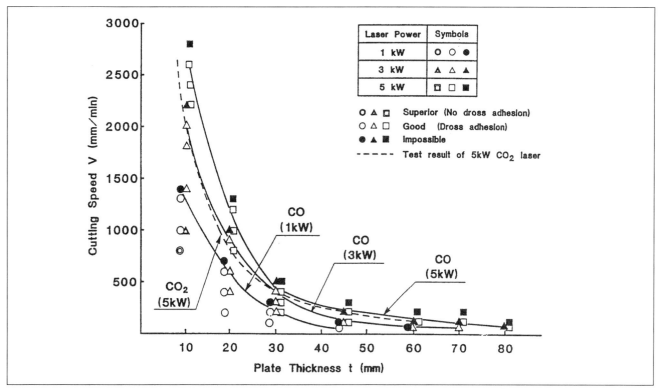

Figure 19. Laser cutting test results at various powers (SS41). Laser power: 1 ~ 5 kW. Material: SS41 (carbon steel). Plate thickness: 10 ~ 80 mm. Focal length: 190.5 mm. Focal point elevation: 0 mm. Assist gas: O_2, 3 kgf/cm², 85 l/min.

Figure 20. Laser cutting test results at various powers (SUS 304). Laser power: 1 ~ 5 kW. Material: SS304. Plate thickness: 6 ~ 60 mm. Focal length: 190.5 mm. Focal point elevation: 0 mm. Assist gas: O_2, 3 kgf/cm², 85 l/min.

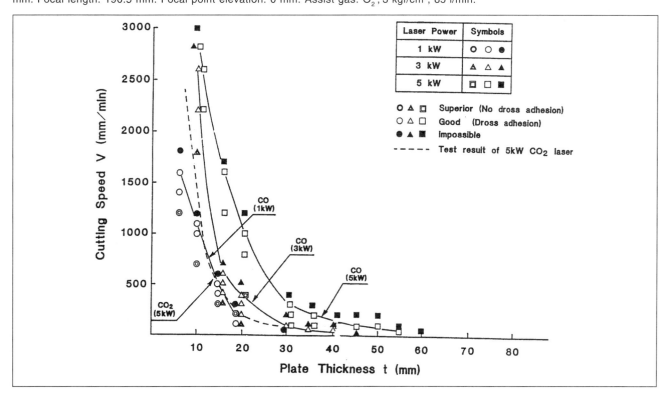

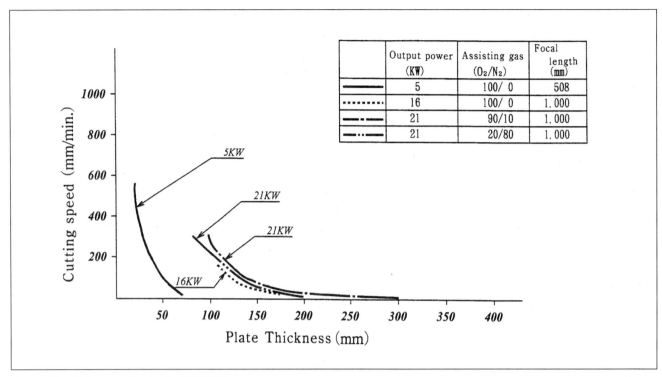

Figure 21. CO laser cutting in air (SUS304).

Figure 22. CO laser cutting in water (SUS304).

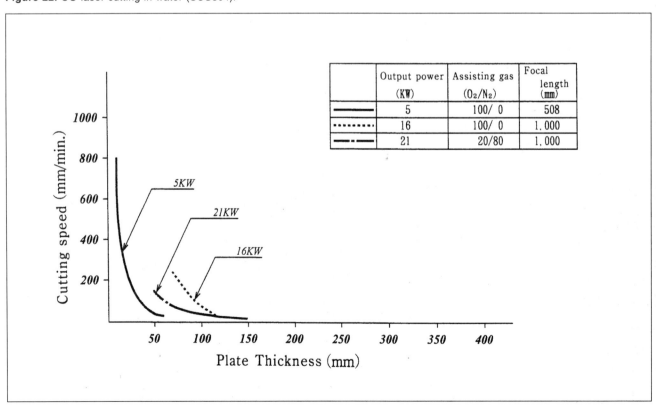

Figures 21 and 22 show data for a 20-kW CO laser developed for use in decommissioning nuclear reactors. It has been successfully used to cut 30-cm-thick steel in the atmosphere and under water.

A comparison of the welding performance of CO, Nd:YAG, and CO_2 lasers on aluminum also confirms the superior welding performance of the CO laser (9).

In terms of applicability, the CO laser has demonstrated its superiority to CO_2 and Nd:YAG lasers for materials processing. But because of issues involving reliability and maintenance, it has not been adopted widely for industrial materials processing (see Section 2.5.1). It remains to the future to produce a stable and industrially reliable CO laser.

References
7. T. Fujioka, 1989: *Proc. ICALEO* 89, Laser Institute of America, Orlando, FL.
8. F. Dausinger, 1990: *ECLAT* 90, 17–19.
9. M. Schellhorn et al., *Optics and Laser Tech.* **28** 405–7 (1996).

TOMOO FUJIOKA

Cutting with a Chemical Oxygen-Iodine Laser

The development and characteristics of the chemical oxygen-iodine laser (COIL) operating at 1.315 µm have been described in Section 2.5.5. Advanced lasers capable of high-power beam delivery through fiber optics potentially will revolutionize manufacturing techniques. High cutting speeds have been achieved for thick stainless steel using a 10-kW COIL. The rates measured were comparable to those predicted by a model developed by researchers at Japan's Applied Laser Engineering Center (ALEC) based on their measurements with a 1-kW COIL (10, 11). The fiber delivery of a 4-kW Nd:YAG laser beam has been reported (12). The potential for even higher power delivery has been demonstrated at ALEC with an irradiance of 1.4 MW/cm^2 achieved using a 300-µm fiber to deliver 1-kW COIL. With 1500-µm core fibers commercially available, this suggests that 25 kW could be delivered through a single fiber. Of the continuous wave lasers with wavelengths suitable for fiber delivery, only COIL has demonstrated the ability to scale to high powers (13, 14).

This scalability makes COIL suitable for new industrial applications such as shipbuilding, heavy machinery manufacturing, and nuclear power facility decontamination and dismantlement (15). Remote delivery of the beam has the advantage of removing the laser from the processing floor, thus addressing safety concerns associated with chemical laser operation while increasing the flexibility for work station layout to optimize production efficiency. This also allows for remote operations using robotic manipulators for materials processing in hazardous environments or confined spaces.

Metal Cutting Experiment Setup

A 10-kW Research Assessment, Device Improvement Chemical Laser (RADICL) device was used to measure the cutting capability of COIL with thick stainless steel. This laser was operated multimode with a stable resonator consisting of a 10-m radius of curvature high-reflectivity mirror and a flat outcoupler spaced 3.0 m apart. A dual lens focusing assembly was located 7.6 m from the outcoupler to produce a rectangular focal spot calculated to be approximately 1.2 mm wide by 1.7 mm long. The spot was horizontally oriented such that the length of the rectangle was oriented along the direction of target translation. The power on target ranged from 3.6 to 7.2 kW for different tests.

The targets consisted of stainless steel (400-series) plates. Scans were conducted at various speeds and laser powers to determine the maximum cutting thickness. Targets thicker than 25 mm were scanned through the beam at various speeds, and the depth of the cut was measured.

Assist gas nozzles were constructed from stainless steel tubes that were flattened and shaped to form rectangular nozzles. Three sizes of nozzles were used: the smallest with dimensions of 0.6 by 2.5 mm, the next with 0.6 by 14.5 mm, and the largest with 1.0 by 23 mm. The nozzles were oriented horizontally; so the long dimension was lined up with the kerf, and fixed at a 45 degree angle from normal to the target. The assist gas was inert, either helium at pressures up to 1400 kPa (~200 psi) or nitrogen at pressures up to 1000 kPa (~145 psi).

During the COIL metal cutting experiment, stainless steel sections were cut to depths up to 50 mm. The kerf width was measured and was found to average 1.5 mm. The narrowest kerfs were 1.0 mm wide and belonged to the thinnest-section, highest-speed cuts, while the widest kerfs averaged 1.9 mm wide. Figure 23 compares the experimental data with the results obtained from a model based on scaling law concepts and developed at Phillips Laboratories.

Figure 24 (next page) shows data points taken with powers between 6 and 7.2 kW. The kerf widths range from 1.1 to 1.9 mm. The solid line shows the calculated behavior at 7 kW with a kerf width of 1.5 mm.

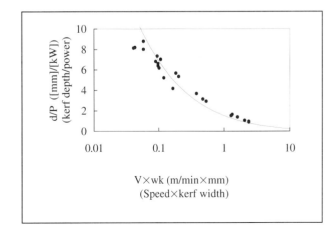

Figure 23. Fit of Phillips Laboratory model to experimental data.

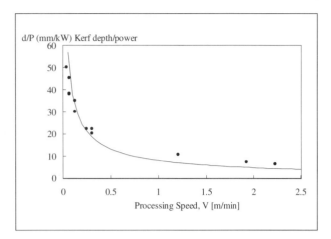

Figure 24. Experimental data for powers from 6 to 7.2 kW and kerf widths from 1.1 to 1.9 mm, with a calculation for 7 kW and a kerf width of 1.5 kW.

The results indicate that thick sections can be cut with a relatively low-power laser, but at a cost of greatly reducing processing speed. In order to increase the speed, it is possible either to decrease the kerf width, which may be limited in the ability of the assist gas to remove the melt, or to increase the power of the laser. With the demonstrated scalablility of COIL, the maximum power available for processing is no longer a limiting factor. Added to the scalability to high powers, COIL has a wavelength that is optimum for high-power beam delivery through fiber optics. With demonstrated capabilities, it may be possible to deliver as much as 25 kW through a single fiber.

References

10. T. Atsuta, K. Yasuda, T. Matsumoto, T. Sakurai, and H. Okado, 1994: Conference on Lasers and Electro-Optics (CLEO '94), 1994: OSA Technical Digest Series, Optical Society of America, Washington, D.C., **8**, p. 351.
11. H. Fujii, 1994: 25th AIAA Plasmadynamics and Lasers Conference, AIAA 94–2419.
12. Wordservice International, *Photonics Spectra* **32** (July, 1995).
13. W. E. McDermott, N. R. Pchelkin, D. J. Benard, and R. R. Bousek, *Appl. Phys. Lett.* **32**, 469–70 (1978).
14. K. A. Truesdell, C. A. Helms, and G. D. Hager, 1994: 25th Plasmadynamics and Lasers Conference, AIAA 94–2421.
15. J. E. Scott and K. A. Truesdell, 1994: Space Instrumentation and Dual-Use Technologies, Firooz A. Allahdadi, Michael P. Chrisp, Concetto R. Giuliano, William P. Latham, and James F. Shanley (Eds.), SPIE **2214**, 188–96.

WILLIAM. P. LATHAM
ARAVINDA KAR

Cutting with Photolytic Iodine Lasers

Photolytic iodine lasers (PILS) have been described in Section 2.5.5. To demonstrate materials processing, the PILS was combined with a five-axis machining center with x, y, and z linear axes and two rotary axes. In cutting and welding demonstrations, Ar, He, O_2, N_2, and air assist gases were used. The combining of gas mixtures into different ratios was used to explore effects of different assist gases with high-intensity PILS beams.

The optical delivery system, shown in Figure 25, consisted of a beam reduction telescope, beam delivery optics and tubes, and a 5-in. focusing lens. The entire optical train consisted of 12 optics, including 2 transmissive elements. Whereas the optical elements were of the highest quality, the telescope, because of its off-axis implementation of spherical elements, imparted approximately a full wave of stigmatism to the laser beam.

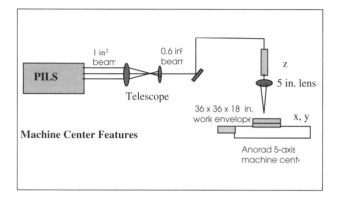

Figure 25. Optical delivery system of precision machining center used with PILS.

Cutting of Stainless Steel

Series 316 stainless steel with thickness from 0.004 to 0.020 in. thickness was cut with a 20-μm PILS beam. Good results were obtained with an assist gas. Cut widths were 20 μm top and bottom, and small HAZ were observed with little slag or flash as shown in Figure 26.

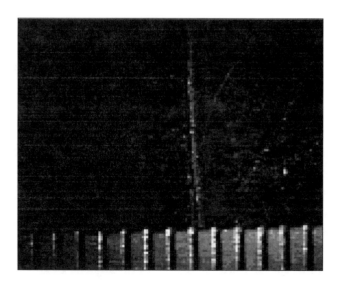

Figure 26. Photograph of cut using oxygen as assist gas and 5-in. standard focus lens (power 20 W, feed rate 0.02 in./s, and O_2 assist gas 35 psig).

Chapter 12: Laser Cutting

Because of the high-intensity PILS beams, much less power is needed for processing than with CO_2 and Nd:YAG (plasma-lamp-driven) laser beams. Figure 27 illustrates that 50 and 75% more power is needed from Nd:YAG and CO_2 lasers, respectively, to cut stainless steel from 0.004 to 0.020 in. thickness, using a 5-in. focal lens (f /7.5). Data from several sources were used for Nd:YAG and CO_2 systems and generally fall on the dotted lines above that of the PIL.

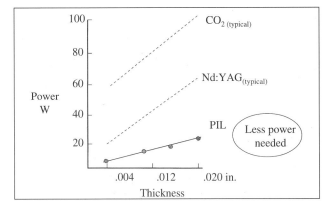

Figure 27. Cutting of 316 stainless steels using PILS, Nd:YAG, and CO_2 lasers and 5-in. focal lens.

Cut widths are graphically shown in Figure 28 to illustrate the much smaller feature size of the PILS, using the same optic train for PILS, Nd:YAG, and CO_2 lasers. This is due to very high intensities of the PILS versus other lasers.

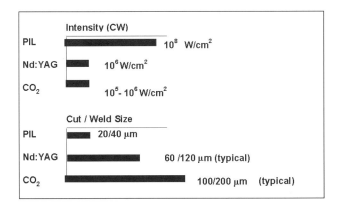

Figure 28. Cut widths and intensities at the focal spot using the same optic train for PILS, Nd:YAG, and CO_2 lasers.

Cutting of Aerospace Composites

Cutting of Kevlar was demonstrated using the high-intensity PILS beam, shown in Figure 29. A 20-µm beam was used to cut a 0.050-in.-thick Kevlar glass matrix. Assist gases utilized were Ar, N_2, and mixes of Ar/N_2 in these demonstrations. Results were reasonably good for processing; fine cuts were made, and there was not severe thermal damage to the material. Even at higher feed rates, the glass fibers were completely cut through.

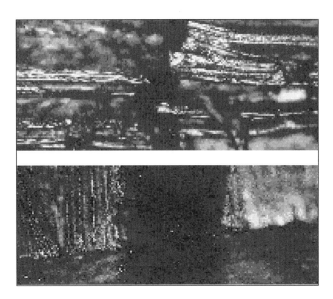

Figure 29. Cutting of 0.050-in.-thick Kevlar glass matrix using PILS (power 12.5 W, feed rate 0.02 in./s and Ar assist gas 13 psig): upper-cut top; lower-cut bottom.

Using Ar as the assist gas produced 100-µm wide cuts at the top and 20-µm wide cuts at the bottom. Results with N_2 were not so good, with 130- and 20-µm cut widths at the top and the bottom, respectively. The wider dimension at the top is assumed to come from scattering of the high-intensity beam sideways from the plume near the top of the cut. Similar results have been reported from processing of composite using high-power Nd:YAG beams. Essentially the same results were observed on a processing thicker 0.060-in. black Kevlar composite. Table 9 shows the effects of using various assist gases during processing with the PILS high-intensity beams. Cutting of materials with oxygen was excellent, and the use of air was good, as expected.

Table 9. Effects of Assist Gases on Cutting of Stainless Steels and Aerospace Composite Materials Using 10^7 W/cm² PILS Beams

	Assist Gases					
	He	Ar	N_2	5%O_2/N_2	O_2	Air
302 & 316 SS: Cutting	No cut	Poor	Poor	Fair	Exc	Good
Kevlar Cutting		Exc	Wide top cuts		Ignites	Ignites
Black Composite Cutting		Exc	Wide top cuts		Ignites	Ignites

PHILIP R. CUNNINGHAM
L. A. (VERN) SCHLIE

12.3 Laser Cutting of Nonmetals

12.3.1 Cutting Mechanisms and Cut Quality

Most nonmetallic materials are highly absorptive at the CO_2 laser wavelength, and many of them also absorb Nd:YAG laser light. For this reason a wide range of nonmetals can be laser cut.

The cutting process involves three mechanisms, one of which is usually dominant for any particular nonmetallic material:

- Melt shearing
- Vaporization
- Chemical degradation

The dominant cutting mechanism has a significant influence on the quality of the resultant cut edge. This is best explained by discussing them separately:

Melt shearing: The focused laser and a gas jet act together on the surface of a sheet of material. The laser produces a localized melt and the gas jet (usually air) continuously blows the liquid away to produce a cut.

Because the gas jet cannot separate all the liquid from the surrounding solid sheet, a small amount solidifies on the cut edge surface. In addition, a line of resolidified material can often be found adhering to the lower edge of the cut. The cut edges are generally macroscopically flat but are covered in microscopic ripples.

Materials that are cut by this mechanism include thermoplastic polymers (e.g., polypropylene, polyamide, polyethylene, ABS, etc.). Although ceramics can be cut by the melt shearing method, straight lines can be cut an order of magnitude faster if a pulsed laser is used to scribe a line across the material surface. The ceramic is subsequently broken along the scribed lines. Scribing is described in detail in Chapter 26.

Vaporization: In this case the material is boiled or vaporized by the laser, and the vapor is ejected from the cut zone by the air jet. Only materials whose vaporization point is close to their melting point respond well in this way.

The resulting edge is generally smooth and flat and has a polished appearance. There is no adherent melt on the bottom of the cut edge.

Two commonly encountered thermoplastics are cut by vaporization: acrylic (plexiglass or perspex) and polyacetal.

Chemical degradation: Nonmetallic materials that do not melt (e.g., wood or thermoset resins) are cut by a burning reaction set up by the laser. Such materials are degraded to their constituent chemical (carbon, water vapor, etc.), and this debris is blown away by the air/gas jet. The resulting cut edge will be smooth and flat and generally covered in a layer of carbon dust.

The generation of carbon dust cannot be avoided in carbon-based materials, and so the cut edge will be covered in a thin layer of carbon. The majority of this layer can be wiped off, but the cut edge is invariably darkened. It is also worth noting that the carbon layer is electrically conductive and needs to be completely mechanically removed in cases where the eventual cut component is intended to be an insulator.

Materials cut by this mechanism include: thermoset polymers (phenolic and epoxy resins, rubbers, etc.) and wood and wood-based products.

Safety note: Polyvinyl chloride (PVC) is cut by this method but generates clouds of highly toxic hydrogen chloride (HCl). For this reason PVC should never be laser cut (see Section 6.4).

JOHN POWELL

12.3.2 CO_2 Laser Cutting

Cutting of nonmetals with a CO_2 laser beam is very efficient because of very high surface absorption of these materials at 10.6 µm. It is feasible to use CO_2 laser for cutting glass cloth, different types of synthetic cloth, ceramics, wood, paper, plastic materials, artificial leather, etc. Because of low conductivity, cutting of such materials does not need high laser beam power to reach an irradiance necessary to ensure high-quality shaping. Fixturing for CO_2 laser cutting of nonmetals in general is similar to what is used for sheet metal cutting. For fabrics, a multilayer material package is usually fixed mechanicaly on the work table and the laser beam with the help of "flying optics" scans according to a prescribed program.

Cut width is mainly determined by cutting speed. At constant laser power, increase of the cutting speed leads to cut width reduction (see Fig. 1), but a laser power increase causes an increase of cut width (see Fig. 2). Cut width depends as well on material thickness, type of material, degree of laser beam defocusing, etc.

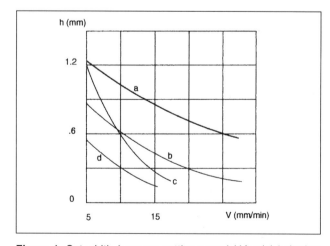

Figure 1. Cut width *h* versus cutting speed *V* for (a) imitation leather, (b) natural leather, (c) plastic film, and (d) kirsa (a domestic synthetic waterproof material) at P = 500 W, p = 0.2 MPa, f = 240 mm.

Chapter 12: Laser Cutting

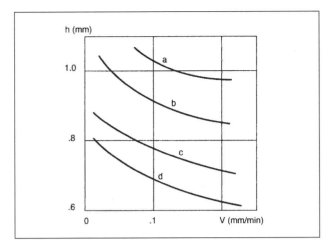

Figure 2. Cut width *h* versus cutting speed and laser beam power *P* for 18-mm-thick plywood (a: P = 290 W; b: P = 260 W; c: P = 200 W; d: P = 140 W).

Cut depth mainly depends on laser power, cutting speed, type of assist gas, and gas pressure. A power increase causes the cut depth to increase. For given laser beam power, there is an optimal cutting speed at which the cut depth is maximum. To prevent combustion when cutting flammable materials, it is preferable to use compressed air, argon, or nitrogen at pressure 0.2–0.25 MPa instead of oxygen. In cutting multilayer material, the cut depth determines the amount of layers that can be cut successfully. The number of layers may reach 10–15. To avoid edge welding when cutting synthetic materials, each layer is separated with thin paper sheet or the material is wetted.

Cut quality depends on the working conditions and may be improved be using special means as well. Table 1 shows that cut inclination increases with increase of cutting speed. At low speed (less than 0.5 m/min) the inclination is smaller, but edge burning is observed.

Table 1. Cutting Speed Influence on Cut Quality for Glass-Reinforced Plastic 2 mm Thick

Cutting speed (m/min)	Cut width (upper edge) (mm)	Cut width (lower edge) (mm)	Inclination (mm)
1	1.02	0.56	0.46
2	0.91	0.44	0.47
3	0.88	0.29	0.59
4	0.84	0.17	0.67

Choice of cutting conditions for CO_2 cutting of nonmetals may be a problem because not all thermophysical constants for such material are known. As a first approach, it is possible to use some recommended experimental data (Table 2), but to find accurate parameters, some actual trials need to be carried out.

Table 2. Working Conditions for CO_2 Laser Cutting of Nonmetallic Materials

Material	Thickness (mm)	Power (W)	Cutting speed (m/min)	Assist gas
Wood				
Poplar	10	500	5	air
	10	350	4.8	air
Yellow pine	10	500	3.2	air
Walnut	10	500	3.8	air
Oak	10	500	2.9	air
Ebony	10	500	1.2	air
Plywood	6.5	850	5.2	argon
	9	500	2.8	air
	12	500	1.4	air
	12	1000	4.0	air
	17.0	500	0.5	air
	25.4	8000	1.5	air
Cardboard	0.1	400	96.0	air
	1.0	360	60.0	air
	4.0	500	4.0	air
	19.0	200	0.1	air
Paper	0.25	4	1.2	oxygen
	0.1	500	500	air
	0.001	400	600	air

Table 2. Working Conditions for CO_2 Laser Cutting of Nonmetallic Materials (continued)

Material	Thickness (mm)	Power (W)	Cutting speed (m/min)	Assist gas
Leather	1.6	1200	18.0	air
	3.2	200	9.6	argon
Rubber	2.0	100	1.9	air
	3.0	400	12.2	air
	9.0	400	0.9	air
	12.0	400	0.6	air
Glass	1.0	500	1.5	air
	2.0	500	1.0	air
	3.0	500	0.5	air
	4.0	250	0.1	air
	9.53	20,000	1.52	air
Fiber glass	1.6	450	5.2	air
	1.6	1200	15.0	air
	2.0	1000	2.0	air
	2.4	200	0.64	air
	3.2	400	2.4	air
	4.5	400	1.5	air
Glass cloth	1.5	25	0.15	oxygen
Acrylic	1.0	500	35.0	air
	1.5	400	3.0	air
	3.0	500	8.0	air
	6.0	500	3.5	air
	8.0	500	2.3	air
	12.0	500	1.2	air
	12.7	20,000	4.6	air
Ceramic	1.5	230	1.5	nitrogen
	0.5	850	0.6	argon
	6.3	1200	0.6	air
Polyethylene	0.15	60	5.0	nitrogen
	1.0	500	11.0	air
	3.0	500	2.2	air
	6.0	500	1.0	air
	9.0	500	0.5	air
	12.0	500	0.3	air
Polypropylene	0.5	4	0.2	oxygen
	1.0	500	17.0	air
	3.0	500	4.0	air
	6.0	500	1.6	air
	9.0	500	0.9	air
	12.0	500	0.4	air
Quartz	1.0	500	1.52	oxygen
	1.2	100	0.5	oxygen
	2.0	400	1.0	air

Table 2. Working Conditions for CO_2 Laser Cutting of Nonmetallic Materials (concluded)

Material	Thickness (mm)	Power (W)	Cutting speed (m/min)	Assist gas
Asbestos				
Cloth	1.6	400	1.0	air
Board	6.0	400	1.5	air
Cement	5.0	500	1.2	air
Carpet	6.0	400	18.0	air
	6.0	1200	35.0	air
Wool cloth	0.7	500	50.0	air
Synthetic cloth	0.75	250	45.0	argon
Nylon	0.8	200	5.0	air
	1.0	500	20.0	air
Lavsan	0.25	4	1.2	oxygen
Felt	6.0	400	19.0	air
	6.0	1000	40.0	air
Ceramic tile	6.3	1200	0.6	–
	6.4	850	0.5	–
Concrete	38	8000	0.13	–

References

J. Powell, 1993: *CO_2 Laser Cutting,* Springer-Verlag, London, Chapter 4.

D. Belforte and M. Levitt, 1992: *The Industrial Laser Handbook,* 1992-1993 edition, Springer-Verlag, New York, Section 1.

V. S. Kovalenko (Ed.), 1985: *Handbook on Laser Technology,* "Technika," Kiev, Chapter 5.

V. S. Kovalenko, 1989: *Laser Technology,* "Vyscha schola," Kiev, Chapter 4.

VOLODYMYR S. KOVALENKO

12.3.3 Cutting of Nonmetals with Nd:YAG Lasers

General Considerations

Many organic materials (like plastics, wood-based products, leather, natural rubbers, etc.) are transparent to Nd:YAG laser light or at least have low values of absorption coefficient. For this reason they cannot be cut well by Nd:YAG lasers. If the laser power is low or the focused spot size is large, the light passes through the material without heating it enough to cut it. If the irradiance of the laser beam is increased by increasing the power or reducing the spot size, the material will eventually respond with a localized explosion, which may produce a tear or hole. This is not the result of thermal absorption but happens because the material cannot support the intense electric field generated by the focused laser. The material therefore experiences dielectric breakdown.

The situation with inorganic nonmetals (ceramics, glasses, carbon, etc.) is not so uniform. Some of these materials can be cut very successfully. For example, industrial sapphire or diamond sheet can be cut into drill tips and similar cutting blades. Ceramic substrates for the electronics industry are also profiled in large quantities by Nd:YAG machines. The addition of carbon dust to rubber (to make tires, etc.) makes the material suitable for Nd:YAG laser cutting. Inorganic fillers (e.g., marble dust) are also added to plastics to color or harden them. Once again this can make the material cut well. In these cases, however, the "cuttability" of the workpiece is heavily dependent on the type and amount of filler used. Adjustments to the mix can have catastrophic effects on the cutting process.

Table 3 (next page) presents some data on Nd:YAG laser cutting of inorganic nonmetallic materials.

Glass and quartz are not cut by Nd:YAG lasers because they are transparent at this wavelength.

Table 3. Nd:YAG Laser Cutting of Inorganic Nonmetallic Materials

Material	Thickness (mm)	(in.)	Average laser power	Cutting Speed (m/min)	(in./min)	Gas
Alumina (Al_2O_3)	2.0	0.08	100	0.18	4.5	Air
Silicon Carbide	2.0	0.08	100	0.10	2.5	Air

JOHN POWELL

Nd:YAG Laser Cutting Data

The Nd:YAG laser is mainly used to obtain precise cuts of relatively small dimensions in hard to machine materials, like diamonds, ruby, sapphire, ceramics, ferrites, etc. Workpieces are usually fixed on the work table mechanically or using vacuum fixturing. Both X-Y table movement or laser beam programmed scanning may be used for cuts or slots of desired configurations.

Cutting is usually performed using high-repetition pulsed lasers, so the cut is formed as a succession of holes obtained from the action of each pulse. Almost all the dependencies described for hole drilling in Chapter 13 are valid for this case as well. The main difference is the influence of every consequent pulse on the hole formed by the previous pulse, which is determined by the amount of overlapping. For the majority of cutting applications, the recommended value of the overlapping coefficient lies in the range 0.5–0.7. The quality of cut is better, but cutting speed is lower for higher overlapping and vise versa. The laser beam is focused with conventional optics or may be shared and transferred to the different working stations with fiber optics. To intensify the cutting process, the compressed flow of air or oxygen is coaxial with the laser beam. To suppress material flaming, inert gas may be used. Table 4 (next page) presents some conditions and results of nonmetal Nd:YAG laser cutting.

Cutting speed depends on material thickness and laser power. This dependence is shown in Figure 3.

Quality of cutting depends on many factors: material, power density, overlapping coefficient, etc. Figure 4 presents the influence of ceramic type and cutting speed on surface roughness (Ra). Figure 5 shows surface roughness versus overlapping coefficient for different types of ceramic at two levels of irradiance.

References

V. S. Kovalenko and A. V. Lavrinovich, 1991: *Laser Machining of Ceramic Materials,* "Technika," Kiev, Chapters 4–5.
D. Belforte and M. Levitt (Eds.), 1992: *The Industrial Laser Handbook,* 1992-1993 edition, Springer-Verlag, New York, Section 1.

VOLODYMYR S. KOVALENKO

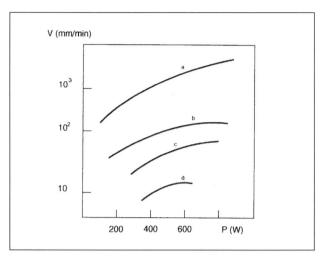

Figure 3. Cutting speed versus material thickness and laser power for silicon nitride ceramic of different thickness (h = 2–8 mm). The pulse frequency is 150 Hz; the assisted gas is nitrogen. (a) h = 2 mm; (b) h = 4 mm; (c) h = 6 mm; (d) h = 8 mm.

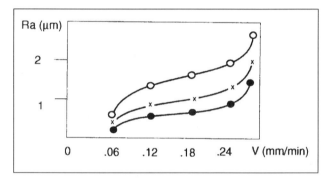

Figure 4. Surface roughness (Ra) versus cutting speed (V) for different types of ceramic: ° - Si_3N_4 - TiN - MgO; x - Si_3N_4 - MgO; • - Si_3N_4 - AlN - Al_2O_3.

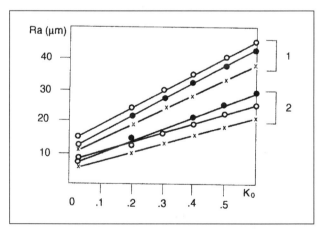

Figure 5. Surface roughness (Ra) versus overlapping coefficient (k_0) at two levels of irradiance: 1: 3×10^8 W/cm²; 2: 1.5×10^8 W/cm² for different types of ceramic: ° - Si_3N_4 - TiN - MgO; x - Si_3N_4 - MgO; • - Si_3N_4 - AlN - Al_2O_3.

Table 4. Conditions of Nonmetal Nd:YAG Laser Cutting

Material	Thickness (mm)	Power (W)	Pulse duration (ms)	Pulse frequency (Hz)	Assist gas	Cutting speed (mm/min)	Cut width (mm)	Other
Ceramic	0.6	120	0.5	100	oxygen	600	0.10	
	1.0	120	0.5	75	oxygen	300	0.10	
	5.0	100	0.6	21	oxygen	30	0.15	
Diamond (polycrystal)	2.5	100	0.3	42	–	60	0.15	
Diamond (natural)	0.8	8	0.002	1000	–	100	0.05–0.20	Q-switch
Borazon	2.0	200	0.2	100	air	240	0.08	
Al_2O_3	1.0	200	0.2	100	air	450–500	0.08	

12.3.4 Cutting Jewelry Materials

Unless otherwise specified, the CO_2 laser used produced 1500 W (3000 W peak). The cutting lens had a 7.5-in. focal length and the nozzle was 1.5 mm in diameter. The focal point was on the top surface of the material.

Jade

Jade is a semiprecious stone and is available in both green (most well known) and black. The material is diamond sawed to thickness. Slabs are usually 2 in. square or smaller. Table 5 presents some results.

Table 5. Cutting 0.25-in.-thick Green Jade, Nitrogen Assist Gas

Condition	Power (W)	Pulse rate (Hz)	Pulse ratio (%)	Duration/ speed	Gas pressure (psig)
Pierce	550	100	27	0.5 s	7
Cutting	750	100	34	12 ipm	55

Jade cuts easily, but there is a globular, glassy slag on the bottom that comes off easily. The kerf is about 0.025–0.05 in. The cut edge has a glassy, yet rough, sandpaper look. Since jade has different color intensities, the lighter-color areas cut better. There is some striation to the cut, also. The cut has some cupping. The first third or so of the cut is smooth and then it becomes much rougher. The part gets very hot. If the part is cut with oxygen, the edge is about the same, perhaps slightly rougher. Argon is about the same as oxygen. Lower assist gas pressures produce an incomplete cut; higher have no effect. Black jade cuts about the same power as green jade, but about 10% slower.

Marble

The base material was actual marble floor tile size (about 18 in. square), both imported and domestic. Table 6 presents some results.

Table 6. Cutting ½-in. Material, Oxygen Assist Gas

Condition	Power (W)	Pulse rate (Hz)	Pulse ratio (%)	Duration/ speed	Gas pressure (psig)
Piercing	350	200	28	2.0 s	7
Cutting	1500	100	65	5 ipm	30

The material cuts, but just barely. There is a lot of surface energy; the area around the point of cutting seems to glow. The pierce goes through nicely. There is no dross on the bottom, but there is a slight spalling on the top edge. The cut is filled with powder. The kerf is about 0.04 in. or wider. The color of the marble does not affect the cutting. If the material is not absolutely dry, the water will make cutting difficult to impossible because of spalling and blowouts. Oxygen, argon, or helium do not seem to make much difference to the cutting. The assist gas basically blows out the dust.

Sapphire

Sapphire is a semiprecious stone that is diamond sawed to thickness. Material slabs are small. Table 7 presents some results.

Table 7. Cutting 0.1 in. (Nominal) Material, Nitrogen Assist Gas

Condition	Power (W)	Pulse rate (Hz)	Pulse ratio (%)	Duration/ speed	Gas pressure (psig)
Pierce	550	100	27	0.5 s	7
Cutting	600	100	27	20 ipm	30

The pierce will sometimes cause some apparent burning on the back side. The dross on the bottom is globular and glassy, but is easily removed. The kerf is about 0.025 in. wide with the cut edges very rough. The top edges of the cut are usually spalled and rounded off. The cut edges are very wavy, almost as if the material was torn apart.

Man-made Stone

The material is used quite extensively as a substitute for precious stones of equivalent color, particularly in Southwest (so-called Indian jewelry) artifacts. The exact content of the man-made stone is difficult to determine because each manufacturer has its own trade-secret recipe. Basically, the material appears to be a resin-type binder that is filled with various materials, such as crushed stones, perhaps some real semiprecious stone, such as turquoise, and other crushed ingredients. There are about six different basic colors (turquoise, jet, red, coral, lapis, and sugalite). The material, in particular turquoise, can also have swirls and striations so that it visually matches the real stone. Jewelers and artisans often call the material "block." The material is often cut, polished, and used in imitation jewelry and, sometimes, as counterfeit material in expensive jewelry. It is sometimes difficult to tell the real from the man-made. Table 8 presents some results.

Table 8. Cutting 1/8-in. Material, Nitrogen Assist Gas

Condition	Power (W)	Pulse rate (Hz)	Pulse ratio (%)	Duration/speed	Gas pressure (psig)
Pierce	100	100	22	0.2 s	7
Cutting	150	100	27	25 ipm	20

The cutting produces much dust and debris. The cut edge is generally whitish in appearance and reasonably smooth. There is taper to the cut toward the wider bottom, and some material will cup the cut edge. Because of material density and composition differences within a given piece, complete through cutting may not always occur; this can leave a wide "tab" on the bottom. On smaller parts (less than an 3/32 in. wide) some materials will taper and cup very badly. Some of the materials, when cutting long thin parts, will actually warp and twist the resultant part.

The cutting conditions in Table 8 are basically correct for the different materials from many different manufacturers. For a given thickness, lot-to-lot power required will change. Some colors will require more or less power (usually a delta of less than 50 W, although turquoise may require as much as 100 W more). The material is often supplied nonuniform in thickness, often tapering as much as 1/16 in.; this is due to the difficulty of cutting/sawing the material by the supplier from the loaf (as it is called) as produced by the manufacturer. In general, a slab is about 1 x 4 to 3 x 4 in. in size. Thicknesses in excess of about 5/8-inches thick cannot be pierced or cut. Other assist gases (oxygen, argon, or helium) can be used but produce no measurable difference in the cut part except oxygen will sometimes produce greater cupping of the cut edge.

If one cuts parts from the various source materials that must fit together (such as parts of a figure), some editing of the various part files and cutting conditions may be in order to make everything fit together properly. Some, or a lot, of experimentation is required to make the parts interlock properly. Generally, a dark, filled epoxy is used during assembly to mask any discrepancies between the smaller pieces of a larger part.

Mother of Pearl

Mother of pearl is the shiny layer that is on the inside of a number of different mollusk shells. Although the shells are cut into "relatively" flat pieces, they do have a wide variety of thicknesses and top-surface shapes. Nothing is regular. Table 9 presents some results.

Table 9. Cutting 1/4-in. Material, Nitrogen Assist Gas

Condition	Power (W)	Pulse rate (Hz)	Pulse ratio (%)	Duration/speed	Gas pressure (psig)
Pierce	125	100	22	0.2 s	7
Cutting	175	100	28	28 ipm	20

There is a slight smell like cutting bone. The edge quality can range from rather rough to fairly smooth, depending upon which mollusk shell is used. The thickness of the shell has little effect on edge quality. The mother-of-pearl layer itself does not appear to have any affect on the cutting. On some shells, the cutting leaves a white, powdery residue. There is some tapering of the cut and some cupping of the cut edge. Oxygen seems to have the greatest effect on the cut edge, making more powder, a rougher edge, and a stronger smell. Argon and helium appear the same as nitrogen.

Real Turquoise

This is a semiprecious material. The material is usually sliced to thickness with a diamond saw. Just about any thickness is essentially impossible to cut.

The pierce basically blows the turquoise apart as it puts a small hole through the material. The laser is unable to cut for the same reason. Although the exact cause is not known, it is understood now that turquoise has a lot of water in its matrix; perhaps the water is vaporizing and causing the shattering.

German Silver/Nickel Silver

Nickel silver, or as it is loosely called, German silver, is an alloy. Table 10 presents some results.

Table 10. Cutting 22 ga, Oxygen Assist Gas

Condition	Power (W)	Pulse rate (Hz)	Pulse ratio (%)	Duration/speed	Gas pressure (psig)
Pierce	480	200	20	0.2 s	7
Cutting	425	150	25	40 ipm	35

German silver cuts very well with the laser, but leaves a rather rough edge. The material will cause some beam reflection off the surface, so a light scuffing is necessary. The HAZ is about 0.03 in. wide. There is a small burr on the bottom, but it comes off easily.

Gold

Pure gold is very difficult to cut with the CO_2 laser. However, alloys cut very well. Tables 11, 12, and 13 present some results for different thicknesses.

Table 11. Cutting 0.021-in. 14-karat Material, Argon Assist Gas

Condition	Power (W)	Pulse rate (Hz)	Pulse ratio (%)	Duration/ speed	Gas pressure (psig)
Pierce	1250	750	35	1.5 s	7
Cutting	1000	750	25	35 ipm	58

Table 12. Cutting 0.035-in. 14-karat Material, Argon Assist Gas

Condition	Power (W)	Pulse rate (Hz)	Pulse ratio (%)	Duration/ speed	Gas pressure (psig)
Pierce	1250	750	22	2.0 s	7
Cutting	1050	750	28	35 ipm	50

Table 13. Cutting 18 ga, 14-karat Material, Argon Assist Gas

Condition	Power (W)	Pulse rate (Hz)	Pulse ratio (%)	Duration/ speed	Gas pressure (psig)
Pierce	1250	750	35	1.8 s	7
Cutting	1100	800	25	28 ipm	73

The edge quality is reasonably smooth. If the laser nozzle is not well adjusted, the edge can be quite grainy in appearance. If possible, lightly scuff the surface with a green Scotch Brite pad. When cutting, the color of the light at the cut is greenish. Cutting seems much noisier than cutting other materials. Over 95% of the base material can be returned, rather than about 70% when the same patterns are cut by hand. The above conditions are for a 7.5-in. lens. Using a shorter-focal-length lens will increase the probability of success.

DAVID M. MARUSA

12.4 Costs of Laser Cutting

Laser cutting system operating costs can be estimated if the application data are known. One way to calculate cost is calculating it per hour (or per unit of length of cut), while amortizing some of the more significant maintenance costs into an hourly figure. The following examples are given primarily as an aid. They may be manipulated and enhanced to suit individual situations.

12.4.1 Conventional CO_2 Laser Cutting System

Typical cutting systems utilizing CO_2 lasers have operating costs generally falling into the categories listed in Table 1. However, recent developments in CO_2 laser technology has made available a CO_2 laser that does not use a continuous flow of laser gases, but rather uses a static volume of gas. For this style of laser, the laser gas consumption data and costs would differ from those listed.

Table 1. Operating Costs for CO_2 Laser Cutting

A 2000-W CO_2 laser (with $M^2 \cong 2.5$) cutting 3-mm-(0.12 in.) thick carbon steel with oxygen assist @ 2.5 bar (37 psi) with a 127-mm (5 in.) lens, and a 1.5-mm-(0.06 in.) diameter nozzle orifice:

Cutting speed	5.2 m/min (205 in./min)	
Laser electrical power	(25 kVA)(0.8 pf)($0.08/kW h) =	1.60
Laser gas, carbon dioxide	(0.15 scf/h)($0.12/scf) =	0.02
Laser gas, helium	(2.30 scf/h)($0.14/scf) =	0.32
Laser gas, nitrogen	(1.10 scf/h)($0.08/scf) =	0.09
Chiller electrical power	(10 kW)($0.08/kW h) =	0.80
Chiller additive	(0.35)(60 gal)($10/gal)/(6000 h) =	0.04
Laser optics	($2340)/(6000 h) =	0.39
Assist gas	(2.3 scf/min)(60 min/h)($0.03/scf) =	4.14
Focus lens	($400)/(1000 h) =	0.40
Nozzle tip	($30)/(200 h) =	0.15
Exhaust system power	(5 kW)($0.08/kW h) =	0.40
Exhaust system filters	($50)/(100 h) =	0.50
Maintenance labor (with overhead)	(12 h/2000 h operation)($45/h) =	0.27
Total approximate operating cost per hour		$9.12/h

Cost per unit length of cut (assuming 85% utilization)
[($9.12/h)/(0.85)(5.2 m/min)](h/60 min) = $0.034/m
($0.034/m)(m/39.37 in.) = $0.0009/in.

12.4.2 Conventional Nd:YAG Laser Cutting System

Typical cutting systems utilizing Nd:YAG lasers have operating costs generally falling into the categories in Table 2 (next page). Note that the laser arc lamp life is strongly dependent on laser power and duty cycle (assumed below 1000 h at full power and 100% duty cycle).

Table 2. Operating Costs for Nd:YAG Laser Cutting

A 2000-W CW Nd:YAG laser with 0.6-mm fiber optic beam delivery cutting 3-mm-(0.12 in.) thick stainless steel with nitrogen assist @ 7 bar (103 psi) with a 80-mm-(3.15 in.) focal length, and a 1.5-mm-(0.06 in.) diameter nozzle orifice

Cutting speed	1.8 m/min (71 in./min)	
Laser electrical power	(75 kW)($0.08/kW h) =	6.00
Chiller electrical power	(40 kW)($0.08/kW h) =	3.20
Chiller additive	(0.35)(75 gal)($10/gal)/(4000 h) =	0.07
Laser arc lamps	($250)(8)/(1000 h) =	2.00
Assist gas	(5.2 scf/min)(60 min/h)($0.03/scf) =	9.36
Cover slide	($50)/(1000 h) =	0.05
Nozzle tip	($30)/(200 h) =	0.15
Exhaust system power	(5 kW)($0.08/kW h) =	0.40
Exhaust system filters	($50)/(100 h) =	0.50
Maintenance labor (with overhead)	(5 h/2000 h operation)($45/h) =	0.11
Total approximate operating cost per hour		$21.84/h

Cost per unit length of cut (assuming 85% utilization)
[($21.84/h)/(0.85)(1.8 m/min)](h/60 min) = $0.237/m
($0.237/m)(m/39.37 in.) = $0.0060/in.

DAVID HAVRILLA

12.5 Comparison of Laser Cutting with Other Technologies

12.5.1 Advantages and Drawbacks of Laser Cutting

To determine whether to use laser technology, it is helpful to consider how laser cutting differs from other mechanized methods. In doing so, it is important to note that the laser effectively competes against the capabilities of a wide range of processing techniques and therefore possesses tremendous flexibility. Table 1 (next page) compares advantages and drawbacks of laser cutting to other methods.

DAVID HAVRILLA

12.5.2 Comparison of CO_2 Laser Cutting with Other Profiling Techniques

General

There are a large number of techniques that can be used to cut materials, ranging from mechanical milling to electric discharge machining. An exhaustive survey of techniques that could be employed instead of CO_2 laser cutting is beyond the range of this handbook. There are, however, four common cutting methods that are closely allied to CO_2 cutting because they use a high-energy beam;

1. Nd:YAG laser cutting
2. Plasma arc cutting
3. Abrasive water jet cutting
4. Oxygen-flame cutting

Potential users of CO_2 laser cutting are often familiar with one or more of the above techniques and may require information for comparison. The following brief notes should help. More detailed information may be found in Reference 1.

Each of the four "alternative" cutting techniques will be compared individually with CO_2 laser cutting under the following subheadings:

- Range of materials that can be cut
- Thickness of material that can be cut
- Cutting speeds
- Cut quality
- Capital costs
- Cutting costs
- General notes

Nd:YAG Laser Cutting

The subject of Nd:YAG laser cutting is covered in detail in earlier sections of this chapter. The following notes are a brief guide to the pros and cons of Nd:YAG laser cutting as compared with CO_2 laser cutting.

Very similar to CO_2 laser cutting; a high-intensity infrared light beam is focused onto the surface of a workpiece and penetrates it with the assistance of a coaxial gas jet. The jet may or may not be chemically reactive with the workpiece. The movement of this area of penetration across the workpiece surface results in a cut line.

The near-infrared light generated by the Nd:YAG laser has a wavelength of 1.06 μm as opposed to the 10.6-μm light produced by CO_2 lasers. This shorter-wavelength light has a number of benefits:

1. Glass is transparent at this wavelength. High-quality complex lenses can be used rather than the simple but expensive zinc selenide lenses used with CO_2 lasers. Also optical fibers can be employed to direct the beam.
2. Shorter-wavelength light focuses to smaller-diameter spots, and it should therefore be possible to produce higher irradiance at the workpiece surface.
3. Metals are more absorptive at shorter wavelengths; so reflectivity becomes less of a problem.

In spite of all these optical advantages, Nd:YAG lasers occupy only a small part of the general laser cutting market. The majority of Nd:YAG machines are sold for welding and drilling applications, which is a reversal of the CO_2 laser market. The reasons why CO_2 lasers dominate the field are as follows:

1. Although cutting speeds for most metals are similar for both Nd:YAG and CO_2 machines at any particular laser power, the usual range of powers for Nd:YAG cutting machines is much

lower (50–500 W) than it is for CO_2 machines (50–3000 W). At the highest powers (above 500 W) the mode of Nd:YAG lasers becomes complex, and this undermines the optical advantages as the beam becomes difficult to focus.
2. A major part of the cutting market involves the profiling of polymers. Carbon dioxide laser radiation is very effectively absorbed by these materials, but they are generally transparent, and therefore uncuttable at the Nd:YAG wavelength of 1.06 µm.

Nd:YAG laser cutting can be used for the following materials:

1. All metals
2. Ceramics
3. A limited number of other nonmetals

As the power and effectiveness of the machines gradually improve with time, the maximum thicknesses cut are increasing. Maximum thicknesses tend to be lower than those for CO_2 lasers except where high-reflectively metals are being processed.

Examples of cutting speeds for laser powers up to 500 W are given in Table 2 (next page).

Higher-power machines are available, and these can cut at higher speeds.

The cut quality for Nd:YAG laser cutting is usually similar or superior to the quality possible using a CO_2 laser. Adherent dross on the underside of cuts is less of a problem because only a small amount of melt is generated during cutting.

The kerf width for low-power (< 500 W) Nd:YAG cutting is the smallest of the five processes under discussion. Very detailed work can be carried out with kerf widths of the order of tens of micrometers. These small kerf widths are not possible if optical fibers are used. The optical quality of the higher-power lasers is inferior to lower-power machines, and this also results in larger kerf widths (e.g., 0.5 mm).

The capital cost of Nd:YAG laser cutting machines is higher than

Table 1. Comparison of Different Cutting Methods to Laser Cutting

Method	Material thickness practical maxima mm (in.)	Advantages	Drawbacks
Oxyfuel cutting (OFC)	1220 (48)	low cost, portable, easy to use	slow, accuracy limit, large kerf, large HAZ, thermal distortion, fumes, metals only
Plasma arc cutting (PAC)	50 (2)	lower capital cost, fairly portable	high consumable cost, accuracy limit, large kerf, large HAZ, thermal distortion, noise, ultraviolet rays, dust and fumes, metals only
Laser	20 (0.75)	high speed and accuracy, flexibility	high capital cost, material restrictions, thickness limitations, fumes
Water jet	150 (6) nonmetals 25 (1) metals	cut any material, cut stacked material, no HAZ, no recast, no dross, no fumes	high operating cost, disposal of metal contaminated abrasive, larger kerf, noise, tool wear
Punching (nibbling)	13 (0.5)	lowest cost per piece for high volume, accurate, reliable	shear edge distortion, requires fixed tooling and dies, setup time, noisy, nibbles arcs, metals
Blanking (stamping)	3 (0.12)	low cost per part, fast	high changeover cost and time, more material waste, metals only
Wire EDM	100 (4)	most accurate, high edge quality, noncontact	slow, electrode wear, wire cost, metals only

ISBN 0-912035-15-3

for a CO_2 laser device if the two are compared on a W-for-W basis. For example; a 1-kW Nd:YAG machine could cost 150–200% more than a 1-kW CO_2 machine.

Cutting costs for Nd:YAG lasers are generally higher than for CO_2 machines. This is largely due to the higher purchase price for the same power.

Table 2. Nd:YAG Laser Cutting Speeds

Material[a]	Thickness (mm)	Average laser power (W)	Cutting speed (m/min)	Frequency (Hz)	Pulse Length (m)
Mild steel	2.5	350	0.559	CW	
	5.0	350	0.127	CW	
	10.0	350	0.010	CW	
	10.0	500	0.10	CW	
Stainless steel	0.5	120	1.0	100	0.5
	2.0	120	0.45	60	0.5
	4.0	120	0.1	30	1.5
	1.0	400	0.9	CW	
	3.0	400	0.5	CW	
	5.0	400	0.25	CW	
	10.0	400	0.1	CW	
	1.0	500	3.0	CW	
	2.5	500	0.8	CW	
	10.0	500	0.16	CW	
	15.0	500	0.07	CW	
Aluminum	1.0	120	0.5	100	0.5
	3.0	120	0.05	30	1.5
	2.0	500	0.75	CW	
	6.3	400	0.1	CW	
Copper	1.0	120	0.5	60	0.2
	3.0	120	0.05	15	2.00
Titanium	1.0	120	1.0	100	0.5
	3.0	120	0.3	30	1.5

[a]Cutting gas is oxygen for all materials except titanium, where argon is used.

Nd:YAG lasers have found a market in applications where fine detailed work or highly reflective metals need to be cut. For this reason, Nd:YAG cutting machines generally have an XY movement of a few centimeters rather than the usual CO_2 stroke length of 3 m.

Although Nd:YAG lasers generally cannot cut polymeric materials, they can be used to cut ceramics with great success by scribing or full penetration cutting.

Plasma Cutting

An electric arc is struck between a nozzle and the workpiece. The workpiece is melted by the arc and the melt is propelled out of the cut zone by a gas jet. The gas jet is partially ionized and is a major constituent of the arc.

The process can be used to cut a wide range of metals, but interest is usually concentrated on steels and aluminum alloys.

A heavy-duty torch with a current capacity of 1000 A can cut through 150 mm of stainless steel or aluminum. In most applications, however, the plate thickness seldom exceeds 65 mm. The process is not generally used to cut carbon steels in sections above 50 mm because at this thickness oxygen flame cutting is a cheaper alternative.

Typical cutting speeds are given in Table 3.

Table 3. Typical Cutting Speeds for Plasma Arc Cutting

Material	Thickness (mm)	Cutting speed (m/min)
Mild steel	6	5.0
	13	2.5
	25	1.2
	50	0.6
Stainless steel	6	5.0
	13	2.5
	25	1.2
	50	0.5
	100	0.2
Aluminum	6	7.5
	13	5.0
	25	2.2
	50	0.5
	100	0.3

The edges of the cut are bevelled. Typically this bevelling can be of the order of 20–30° or more from the vertical (see Fig. 1). As a result of this a 25-mm-(1 in.) thick plate could have a kerf width of 7.0 mm at the top of the cut and 4.5 mm at the bottom. In some cases this bevelling can be an advantage if the cut product is subsequently to be welded. In most cases, however, it would be preferred if the cut edges were perpendicular.

The heat input to the workpiece is large, and this results in extensive heat-affected zones and thermal distortion on cooling.

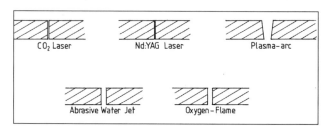

Figure 1. A generalized comparison of the kerf cross sections produced by each process (Ref. 1).

The capital cost of a plasma cutter is far less than a laser machine. The equipment can also be hand held, which reduces capital costs to a minimal level. If a large gantry machine is purchased, its productivity can be greatly increased at a small extra cost by the addition of extra nozzles.

Although the capital cost of the equipment is fairly low, running costs are higher than for most lasers. Cost comparisons must take into account the drilling of holes, etc., which may be necessary after plasma cutting but which can be drilled by the laser.

In summary, it can be said that plasma cutting is a very effective rough cutting operation for medium to thick sections. Cutting speeds are high for metals, but the process does not lend itself to the profiling of nonmetals. In cases where the cut components are to be welded, the bevel of the cut edge can be an advantage, but in general the cut edge quality is the major restriction on the use of this technology.

The new generation of "microplasma" machines have concentrated on the improvement of cut edge quality and the reduction of the kerf width. Some progress has been made, but CO_2 lasers are generally superior, especially where fine detail is involved.

Abrasive Water Jet (AWJ) Cutting

Fine particles of abrasive are mixed into a high-pressure water jet. Materials are cut by the abrasive action of these particles as they move through the cut zone at high speed.

An abrasive water jet can cut any material. In this respect it is the only one of the four techniques under discussion here that is superior to CO_2 laser cutting.

Given a powerful enough machine and enough time, abrasive water jet cutting can cut up to the limiting available thickness of most engineering materials.

Abrasive water jets are generally very much slower than CO_2 lasers when cutting metals (in the range of thicknesses where CO_2 lasers can compete). For example, for 1.6-mm-thick mild steel, typical CO_2 laser cutting speed is ~7.0 m/min; typical abrasive water jet speed ~0.5 m/min.

When cutting polymers, the two processes cut at similar speeds, although flexible materials can be distorted by the action of the high-pressure water jet.

Typical cutting speeds are presented in Table 4.

Cut edges are generally of high quality, although some laminated materials can delaminate. The surface of the cut edge is often covered by microscopic ripples similar to those seen on laser cut edges. There is no heat-affected zone associated with the cut edge, but the mechanical nature of the cutting process may have an equivalent negative effect on component fatigue life.

Table 4. Typical Cutting Speeds for the Abrasive Water Jet Method

Material	Thickness (mm)	Cutting speed (m/min)
Mild steel	1.6	0.50
	13.0	0.10
	50.0	0.038
	180.0	0.010
Stainless steel	5.0	0.40
	13.0	0.15
	25.0	0.076
Aluminum	1.6	1.30
	6.0	0.50
	25.0	0.13
	100.0	0.025
Titanium	3.0	0.50
	6.0	0.40
	12.0	0.10
Glass	13.0	1.3
	19.0	0.6
	25.0	0.13
Marble	50.0	0.4
Concrete	250.0	0.025

The cut (or kerf) width generated by abrasive water jets is considerably larger than that produced by laser cutting. Kerf widths between one and two millimeters may not sound large, but they do restrict the technique when fine detail is required.

The capital cost is similar to CO_2 laser cutting machine (both techniques are always CNC or DNC controlled). It is worth pointing out that for a relatively small additional cost, extra cutting heads can be fitted. This can of course improve productivity.

If a CO_2 laser can cut the material involved, it will generally do the job less expensively. This is particularly true when cutting thin section steels (15 mm thick or less). However, there are a wide range of materials and thicknesses where a CO_2 laser cannot compete, because it is incapable of cutting the material (e.g., several centimeters of aluminum, brass, glass, marble, etc.).

In the opinion of the author, abrasive water jet cutting is a complementary technique to laser cutting rather than a competitor. A review of the work carried out on both types of machine has rarely identified similar jobs. Basically the CO_2 laser has a range of materials and thicknesses it can cut. Within this range it generally outperforms abrasive water jet cutting. Outside this range the abrasive water jet technique takes over.

Oxygen-Flame Cutting

Oxygen and a fuel gas are ignited to produce a flame. Inside the center of this flame is a stream of pure oxygen. The flame is used to heat up carbon steel to a temperature at which it will spontaneously burn in oxygen. The core of the flame provides this oxygen, and the resulting burning reaction produces a cut.

This process is only suitable for carbon or low-alloy steels.

The process is not suitable for very thin sections (< 2 mm) but can be used for carbon steel thicknesses in excess of 1 m. It is most commonly used in the 5–100-mm range. The process can obviously cut far greater thickness of carbon steel than CO_2 laser cutting.

Examples are given in Table 5.

At thicknesses below ~12 mm, CO_2 laser cutting is considerably faster than flame cutting. As the thickness increases toward 25 mm, the two processes have similar speeds.

Cut surfaces are covered in striations, which are similar to, but coarser than, those observed on laser cut specimens. The surface roughness of cut edges becomes more pronounced as the thickness of the material increases. Heat-affected zones (HAZs) on each side of the cut can be extensive, particularly at thicker sections (e.g., ~5 mm HAZ at a section of 150 mm for a high-carbon steel). Tolerances of + 0.5 mm can be held up to ~50 mm, and there is a gradual decay in quality up to 150 mm, where tolerances can only be held to + 1.5 mm.

Table 5. Typical Speeds for Oxy-Flame Cutting of Carbon or Low-Alloy Steels[a]

Thickness (mm)	Typical cutting speed (m/min)
3	0.4–0.8
6	0.4–0.6
12	0.3–0.6
25	0.2–0.4
50	0.1–0.3
100	0.1–0.25
200	0.07–0.1
300	0.05–0.1

[a]Note that the lower speeds give the best quality.

Cut widths are always larger than laser cutting, ranging from 1–2 mm for thin sections (up to 4 mm thick) to 5–10 mm for thicker sections. This, of course, gravely restricts the level of detail that can be cut. Start holes in the middle of sheets will be several millimeters in diameter, which procludes the possibility of cutting bolt holes, etc.

Unlike laser cutting or abrasive water jet cutting, this process can be carried out with hand-held equipment. In this case the capital costs are trivial by comparison with laser cutting (~0.1% of the cost of a laser cutting machine).

A computer-controlled oxy-flame cutting machine is approximately half the cost of a similar-size laser cutter. As is the case for abrasive water jet cutting, a computer-controlled gantry can be fitted with multiple heads for a small extra cost.

Cutting costs for oxy-flame cutting are substantially lower than for laser cutting.

Operations involving hand-held equipment are an inexpensive option for rough blanking or small batch jobs. Multiheaded computer-controlled gantries are suited to bigger batches with higher tolerances.

Oxy-flame cutting can compete with CO_2 lasers only if the job satisfies the following conditions:

1. The material is carbon or low-alloy steel.
2. No bolt holes or fine details need to be cut.
3. Dimensional tolerances are relaxed.
4. The material thickness is not less than 2 mm (although stacked layers of thinner materials can be cut successfully).

Even if these constraints are satisfied, laser cutting can often compete on price as cutting speeds are higher. As with the other processes discussed in this section, the biggest disadvantage of CO_2 laser cutting is its inability to cut thick sections.

Table 6 summarizes the general conclusions of the earlier discussions by qualitatively comparing the four "alternative" cutting methods with CO_2 laser cutting.

Table 6. A Qualitative Comparison of the Four "Alternative" Cutting Methods with CO_2 Laser Cutting

	Nd:YAG laser	Plasma	Water jet	Oxygen-flame
Capital costs	S	G	S	VG
Running costs	S	S	S	G
Metal cutting				
Speed	P	G	VP	P
Quality	S–G	VP	VG	P
Max thickness	S	VG	VG	VG
HAZ	S–G	VP	VG	P
Kerf width	S–G	VP	VP	VP
Nonmetal cutting				
Ceramics				
Speed	P	N/A	P	N/A
Edge quality	S–G	N/A	G	N/A
Max thickness	S–G	N/A	VG	N/A
Kerf width	S–G	N/A	P	N/A
Polymers				
Speed	N/A–P	N/A	S	N/A
Quality	N/A–P	N/A	S	N/A
Max thickness	N/A–P	N/A	G	N/A
Kerf width	N/A–P	N/A	P	N/A

Source: Reference 1. *Key:* N/A, not applicable; VG, very good; G, good; S, similar; P, poor; VP, very poor.

Chapter 12: Laser Cutting

Table 7. Comparison of Laser and Alternative Methods of Nonmetal Cutting

Fabrics		Fabrics	
Laser	**Water jet**	**Laser**	**Knives**
Advantages	*Advantages*	*Advantages*	*Advantages*
Edge quality	No HAZ	Edge quality	Multilayer
Edge fixing	No fumes	Edge fixing	
Disadvantage	*Disadvantages*	*Disadvantage*	*Disadvantages*
	Material watering	Flexibility	Dust
	Edge quality		Accuracy
			Tool wear

Wood		Wood	
Laser	**Water jet**	**Laser**	**Router/sawing**
Advantage	*Advantages*	*Advantage*	*Advantage*
Accuracy	No HAZ	Cut quality	Low cost
	Thickness		
Disadvantage	*Disadvantage*	*Disadvantage*	*Disadvantages*
Edge char	Wet surface	Edge char	Tool wear
			Large kerf
			Poor edge quality

Plastic		Plastic	
Laser	**Router/sawing**	**Laser**	**Water jet**
Advantages	*Advantages*	*Advantage*	*Advantages*
Cut quality	Low cost	Edge quality	No HAZ
No swarf	Cut multilayer		Stacked parts
Disadvantage	*Disadvantages*	*Disadvantage*	*Disadvantage*
Single-layer cutting	Large kerf	Edge quality for	Operating cost
	Poor edge quality	certain materials	
	Tool wear		

Ceramics		Ceramics	
Laser	**Ultrasonic**	**Laser**	**Water jet**
Advantage	*Advantage*	*Advantage*	*Advantage*
Narrow kerf	High accuracy	Cut quality	No HAZ
Disadvantage	*Disadvantages*	*Disadvantage*	*Disadvantage*
HAZ	Tool wear	HAZ	Part intricacy
	Excess swarf		limitation
	Cut-shape limitation		

Ceramics		Rubber	
Laser	**Diamond wheel**	**Laser**	**Die punch**
Advantage	*Advantages*	*Advantages*	*Advantages*
Part intricacy	No HAZ	High accuracy	Low cost in high volume
	High accuracy	Low cost in low volume	No fumes
Disadvantage	*Disadvantage*	*Disadvantage*	*Disadvantages*
HAZ	Only straight cuts	High cost	Tool wear
			Edge quality

ISBN 0-912035-15-3

As the table shows, the performance of CO_2 lasers is equalled or improved on in some cases. From among these comparisons, it is clear that CO_2 laser cutting has two weak points when compared with the other techniques:

1. Capital costs are high. Although Nd:YAG and AWJ systems cost a similar amount of money, plasma and flame equipment is very much cheaper.
2. The maximum thickness of metal that can be cut is very low compared with all the other techniques except Nd:YAG lasers.

The table also makes it clear that there are a number of overall advantages to the use of CO_2 laser cutting, including:

1. Cutting speeds for thin section metals (particularly steels) are generally high and are exceeded only by the plasma arc process. (Very highly reflective metals such as gold, silver, and copper can be cut more effectively by high-power Nd:YAG lasers.)
2. The kerf width is very small (0.1–1.0 mm), and thus the amount of detail that can be profiled is high. In this respect the only superior method is Nd:YAG laser cutting (without fiber optics).
3. The range of materials that can be cut is very wide. In this respect the only superior cutting method is AWJ.

Reference
1. J. Powell, 1993: *CO_2 Laser Cutting,* Springer Verlag, ISBN 3-540-19786-9.

JOHN POWELL

12.5.3 Advantages and Limitation of Laser Cutting of Nonmetals

Among the main general advantages of the laser cutting process are the following:

- Noncontact processing
- Very high cutting speed (productivity) because of high absorption of infrared radiation by the majority of nonmetal materials
- Very narrow kerf width
- No need for strong fixturing
- Ability to use the same laser beam to cut entirely different materials
- High cut quality

General disadvantages include:

- High equipment cost
- Fume formation

For different groups of materials in comparison with alternative cutting methods there are some additional advantages and disadvantages (see Table 7). Among the alternatives to laser cutting of nonmetals there are the following methods: water jet (abrasive fluid jet), ultrasonic cutting, diamond wheel cutting, die punch, and router/sawing.

References
D. Belforte and M. Levitt (Eds.), 1992: *The Industrial Laser Handbook,* 1992-1993 Edition, Springer-Verlag, New York, Section 1.
J. Powell, 1993: *CO_2 Laser Cutting,* Springer-Verlag, London, Chapter 8.
V. Kovalenko and A. Lavrinovich, 1991: *Laser Machining of Ceramic Materials,* Technika, Kiev, Chapter 2.

VOLODYMYR S. KOVALENKO

Chapter 13

Hole Drilling

13.1 Basic Description of Laser Drilling

13.1.1 Surface Reflectivity

The first step in the laser drilling process is the absorption of laser radiation by the workpiece. The ratio of the absorbed laser energy to the incident laser energy is defined as the absorptivity, A. The incident laser energy can also be reflected and transmitted by the material, with the appropriate fractions defined as reflectivity, R, and transmissivity, T. Therefore, $A = 1 - R - T$. Because one deals mostly with opaque materials in this chapter such as metals, transmission is negligible, and $A = 1 - R$. Hence, to increase energy absorption, one must reduce the reflectivity.

Wavelength Dependence

Surface reflectivity of a material strongly depends on the incident light wavelength, as shown in Figure 1, for several metals with typical smooth surfaces.

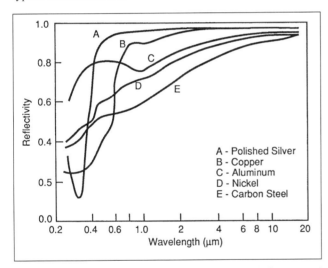

Figure 1. Reflectivity as a function of wavelength for several metals (1).

It is generally true that metals reflect less and thus absorb more at shorter wavelengths. In the case of nickel, for example, the absorptivity at 1.064 μm wavelength is about 4.5 times higher than that at 10.6 μm. This means that an Nd:YAG laser will have its energy coupled into the material more efficiently than a CO_2 laser at the same incident intensity or irradiance. These factors are described in more detail in Chapter 5.

Incidence Angle and Polarization Dependence

In many situations, holes are drilled at specific incidence angles required by the part design other than 90 degrees (normal incidence). In addition, the laser beam is often polarized as a result of the laser cavity design, or one might want to take advantage of the polarization effects described here. Therefore, the angle of incidence and laser beam polarization are also factors to consider. These dependencies are shown in Figure 2 for steel at the 1.064 μm wavelength of an Nd:YAG laser. These factors are described in more detail in Chapter 5.

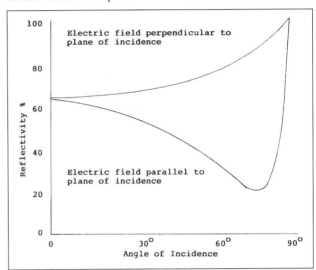

Figure 2. Reflectivity of steel for polarized 1.064-μm light (2).

Temperature Dependence

As the surface temperature rises, the reflectivity normally decreases, and the absorptivity increases, as shown in Figure 3. Therefore, during the initial stage of laser interaction, or even within a single pulse, the surface reflectivity may decrease significantly as the surface is heated up by the laser beam.

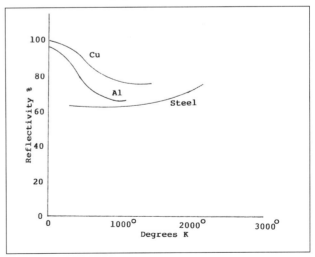

Figure 3. Reflectivity as a function of temperature for 1.064-μm radiation (2).

ISBN 0-912035-15-3

Surface Condition Dependence

Surface roughness is an obvious factor affecting reflectivity. Rough surfaces tend to introduce multiple reflections within the rough surface topography, giving the surface more opportunities to absorb and thus a reduced overall reflectivity. The existence of oxidized layers on metals also reduces reflection. The enhanced absorptivity of oxidized surfaces is shown in Table 1.

Table 1. Absorptivity of Some Metals at 10.6 µm Wavelength (3)

Metal	Absorptivity	
	Unoxidized surface	Oxidized surface
Au	0.010	–
Al	0.034	0.25–0.50
Fe	0.050	0.33–0.74
Zr	0.083	0.45–0.56
Ti	0.094	0.18–0.25

Once material removal starts, a fresh surface is exposed to the incoming laser beam, and laser interaction with the altered solid surface, or molten and vaporized material must be taken into account. It is well known that at high irradiance, typically above 10^7 W/cm², a laser-induced plasma can form a shield that inhibits laser delivery to the workpiece. Finally, after a crater is formed, the incident beam is likely to be trapped in the hole through multiple reflections, thereby improving the total absorptivity.

References

1. John F. Ready, *Industrial Applications of Lasers*, Academic Press, San Diego, CA, Chapter 12 (1997).
2. W. M. Steen, *Laser Material Processing*, 2nd Edition, Springer-Verlag, London, Chapter 2 (1998).
3. A. G. Grigoryants, *Basics of Laser Material Processing*, CRC Press, Boca Raton, FL, Chapter 4 (1994).

13.1.2 Thermal Properties

After the incident laser energy is absorbed by the workpiece, the next step in the hole drilling process is the heat flow inside the solid material, leading to the change of state (melting and vaporization) that results in material removal. Hence an understanding of the thermal properties and thermodynamic processes is necessary. Although complicated simulations can yield more accurate results, some simple analyses are presented here that can give a user the order-of-magnitude estimates for the feasibility of the process.

For the transient heat flow process in solids, the key thermal property is thermal diffusivity

$$k = K/\rho c$$

where K is the thermal conductivity, ρ is the density, and c is the specific heat. The diffusivity values of some metals are presented in Table 2.

Table 2. Thermal Diffusivity Value of Some Metals (1)

Metal	Thermal diffusivity (cm²/s)
Silver	1.70
Aluminum alloys	
Commercially pure	0.85
2024 alloy	0.706
A13 casting alloy	0.474
Copper alloys	
Electrolytic (99.95% pure)	1.14
Cartridge brass	0.378
Phosphor bronze	0.213
Iron alloys	
Commercially pure	0.202
303 stainless steel	0.056
Carbon steel (1.22C, 0.35Mn)	0.119
Nickel alloys	
Commercially pure	0.22
Monel	0.055
Inconel	0.039

From a simple one-dimensional diffusion theory, the depth of penetration in time t is given by

$$d = 2(kt)^{1/2}$$

where d represents the depth at which the temperature has risen to 1/e or 37% of the temperature at the heated surface. One can use the above equation to estimate heat penetration depth for certain pulse durations. Since d is proportional to $t^{1/2}$, longer pulse duration results in deeper penetration within a single pulse. This can be an advantage in providing efficient drilling, but it can also become undesirable because of the larger heat-affected zone produced by radial heat flow.

Let us use inconel as an example. For a typical free-running Nd:YAG laser pulse with a duration of 1 ms, the penetration depth is 0.1 µm, while a typical Q-switched Nd:YAG laser pulse of 100 ns results in 1 µm penetration. Although laser hole drilling with the 1 ms pulse regime has been in use for a long time, the Q-switched short pulses can make up the drilling speed by increased pulse repetition rate, and have been shown to reduce the depth of the heat-affected zone and recast layer thickness by about 10 times (4).

After energy absorption and heat diffusion, the next steps in the drilling process are melting and vaporization. Therefore, other important thermal properties include: melting and vaporization temperatures T_f and T_v, latent heats of fusion and vaporization L_f and L_v, and heat capacity at constant pressure c_p. The heat capacities of solid and liquid states are assumed equal in this approxi-

Chapter 13: Hole Drilling

mation. We further assume that all the absorbed energy is confined to a cylinder of diameter D equal to the diameter of the laser beam at the surface and depth equal to the depth of melting d_f or vaporization d_v. The energy balance equations below give us a first approximation of d_f or d_v for a laser pulse of energy E and reflectivity of R:

For melting: $[c_p(T_f - T_0) + L_f]\rho d_f \pi D^2/4 = (1 - R)E$

For vaporization: $[c_p(T_v - T_0) + L_f + L_v]\rho d_v \pi D^2/4 = (1 - R)E$

where T_0 is the ambient temperature.

Heat conduction away from the above mentioned cylinder is neglected; hence the above equations tend to overestimate the depths. However, the reduced reflectivity and possible expulsion of unvaporized material during drilling are also neglected, which tends to underestimate the depths.

References
4. X. Chen, W. T. Lotshaw, A. L. Ortiz, P. R. Staver, C. E. Erikson, M. H. McLaughlin, and T. J. Rockstroh, *J. of Laser Appl.* **8**, p. 233 (1996).

XIANGLI CHEN

13.1.3 Physical Processes: Melting, Vaporization, Flushing, Percussion

The physical processes of laser hole drilling are fairly simple. The solid material absorbs laser energy, and the photon energy is converted to thermal energy. When the temperature rises above melting and vaporization temperatures, melting and vaporization occur. At high laser irradiance (> 10^6 W/cm²), materials are removed mostly through vaporization. The vapor also builds up pressure that pushes molten material out of the hole, a phenomenon called flushing. In most practical applications, a high-pressure assist gas jet is directed toward the hole, further assisting material removal.

For certain materials, such as polymers, photon absorption by the solid material can lead to direct breaking of bonds between atoms or molecules. This leads to photo-fragmentation and direct vaporization or ablation without melting.

It is advantageous therefore to use pulsed lasers that heat up and remove a small volume of material very quickly with each pulse. To quantify such a statement, one can estimate the time t_v to reach the vaporization temperature as:

$$t_v = (\pi/4)(K\rho c/I^2)(T_v - T_0)^2$$

where I is the absorbed irradiance of the laser beam (in W/cm²). One would like to use a pulse duration that is longer than the t_v. This equation can be used as a rough guide to verify whether effective drilling can take place with certain laser pulse duration and irradiance.

For example, at 10^5 W/cm² irradiance, t_v is 1.84 ms for nickel; while at 10^7 W/cm² irradiance, the time shortens to 184 ns. Therefore vaporization happens very quickly for high irradiance. Note that these times are similar to typical pulse durations of free-running and Q-switched Nd:YAG lasers, respectively. Conversely, one can think of the irradiances mentioned above as the threshold irradiances above which effective vaporization and drilling occur using these pulse durations.

When a hole is drilled without relative motion of the laser beam to the workpiece, the process is called percussion drilling. The most popular drilling lasers are pulsed Nd:YAG lasers, and the maximum diameter of a percussion drilled hole is usually less than 1 mm. For holes that are larger, a technique called trepanning is used, which rotates either the workpiece or the laser beam to cut out a circular hole. Holes of rectangular or other shapes can also be pierced in this fashion. Percussion drilling and trepanning are described further in Section 13.1.5.

13.1.4 Appropriate Lasers: Power/Irradiance, Pulse Duration

The questions of what appropriate lasers and what process parameters to use can be partially answered with a simple analysis as described above, based on a material's thermal and optical (absorptivity) properties. In general, shorter pulsed lasers work better than longer pulsed lasers or continuous wave (CW) lasers. Higher irradiance is better as long as plasma effects are not significant.

One also prefers to use shorter wavelength lasers for the enhanced absorptivity. But visible and ultraviolet lasers do not have high enough average power at present to provide economic process throughputs, except for drilling small holes in thin materials such as in the electronic industry. Excimer lasers operating at between 193 and 308 nm and the second harmonic of the Nd:YAG lasers at 532 nm all have found wide applications in microelectronics manufacturing. Typical pulse duration of these lasers are 10–100 ns, with typical average powers of about 1–10 W.

For applications such as automotive and turbine manufacturing, average powers of 100–10,000 W are desired. Currently, only the CO_2 and Nd:YAG lasers can deliver this average power level with reasonable cost and performance stability. Most common CO_2 lasers are CW and not suitable for drilling, but pulsed CO_2 lasers are used for drilling in ceramics. Pulsed Nd:YAG lasers are by far the most popular in industrial drilling applications. Typical commercial Nd:YAG lasers are lamp-pumped and free-running, providing 0.5–10 ms pulse durations at a 1.064-μm wavelength and up to several kW in average power. This type of laser can typically percussion drill a hole of approximately 1 mm diameter through most metals up to several centimeters thick. Other solid-state lasers, such as ruby and Nd:glass lasers, can also be found in industrial use.

Pulse repetition rate is also a factor to consider, especially when a high drilling rate is required. One should consider this rate and the number of pulses it takes to drill a hole.

With recent developments in diode-pumped solid-state laser technology, high-power Q-switched Nd:YAG lasers are becoming commercially available. These lasers provide average powers in the kW range with pulses of 100 ns duration and excellent beam quality. The close to diffraction-limited beam quality means that one can focus the beam extremely tightly over a long depth-of-focus, thus providing very high irradiance. Second harmonic generation with these lasers has also been demonstrated with average powers at the 100 W level. Initial process tests have shown excellent drilling speed and quality with the higher irradiance and shorter wavelength (5, 6).

References
5. X. Chen, W. T. Lotshaw, A. L. Ortiz, P. R. Staver, C. E. Erikson, M. H. McLaughlin, and T. J. Rockstroh, *J. of Laser Appl.* **8,** p. 233 (1996).
6. X. Chen, A. L. Ortiz, P. R. Staver, W. T. Lotshaw, T. J. Rockstroh, and M. H. McLaughlin, *J. of Laser Appl.* **9,** p. 287 (1997).

XIANGLI CHEN

13.1.5 Percussion Drilling and Trepanning
There are two ways of generating holes: percussion drilling and trepanning. Percussion drilling is typically used for hole diameters less than 0.025 in. (0.63 mm), while trepanning is used for generating holes of larger diameter.

Percussion Drilling

Percussion drilling is accomplished by transforming a cylindrical section of material from a solid to a vapor. Holes are drilled by focusing the laser beam to the approximate diameter required, and exposing the material to one or more pulses of energy. Small changes in hole diameter can be made by increasing or decreasing pulse energy. Even though nonmetals are poor thermal conductors, too much pulse energy can cause excessive melting in materials that are not readily sublimated, or charring in those materials that are. Too much pulse energy can also distort the shape of the hole. Insufficient energy can cause the hole to be too small or tapered.

In some cases the material type and thickness allows for the percussion drilling of holes as high as 0.030 in. (0.8 mm). Examples of such materials are polyethylene and acetal.

Shape (roundness) of percussion-drilled holes is determined by the spatial characteristics of the laser beam. Even with lasers having very low M^2 values, devices such as spatial filters and stops can be used to improve roundness. Repeatability of percussion-drilled holes is as good as the repeatability of laser pulse-to-pulse energy output.

Percussion-drilled holes are typically small: < 0.020 in. (0.5 mm) diameter), although larger-diameter holes can be drilled through very thin materials.

Lenses used for percussion drilling are selected according to the diameter of the holes to be drilled. For a given beam diameter input to the focus lens, shorter focal length lenses focus the laser beam to smaller diameters. For most optical systems, a 2.5-in. focal length lens can be used when drilling holes 0.003 (75 µm) to 0.010 in. (0.25 mm) in diameter, and 5.0-in. focal length lenses can be used when drilling holes 0.008 (0.2 mm) to 0.020 in. (0.5 mm) in diameter.

Focal position can be optimal on, above, or below the material surface, depending on the desired hole characteristics. The best focus is determined empirically following an evaluation of the hole quality.

Percussion drilling can be accomplished with or without a gas jet. Most often, compressed air is used as the process assist gas. Nozzle designs vary, but typical orifice diameters range from 0.040 (1 mm) to 0.250 in. (6.25 mm), and nozzle standoff ranges from 0.020 (0.5 mm) to 1.0 in. (25.4 mm). If a gas jet is not used, an alternative lens protection method must be employed. Vapor produced by laser drilling will condense on the lens surface, creating a film that readily absorbs laser energy. The heat resulting from absorption will cause the lens to fracture spontaneously.

Trepanning

If one uses a rotating optical device, holes up to ≅ 0.250 in. (6.25 mm) diameter can be drilled. So-called "boring heads" rotate the focused laser beam at very high rates. Holes are drilled by either a single pass or multiple passes of the laser beam.

Drilling by trepanning is to cut a hole around its periphery. Depending on the hole diameter, a slug may be produced. Boring heads usually use 2.5-in. focal length lenses and are equipped with gas jets similar to those used for laser cutting applications.

Roundness of the holes produced by boring heads is exact, and repeatabilty of hole diameter is excellent. Boring-head-hole diameter is established either manually or by use of a programmable controller.

Trepanned holes can also be drilled by interpolation of linear axes, moving either the material or the laser focusing device. Speed of drilling by interpolation is dictated by the size of the linear axes. The linear axes servo system must be properly tuned to produce circular holes. Specialty beam-manipulation devices use very small linear axes to move the focusing device in a circle. The system controller can be programmed to establish desired hole diameters.

DANA ELZA
STEVEN R. MAYNARD

13.2 Drilling of Metals

13.2.0 Introduction
Laser hole drilling in metals has a variety of applications, such as producing cooling holes in aircraft turbine blades, fabrication of orifices for nozzles and controlled leaks, and making pinholes for optical applications. The Nd:YAG laser has frequently been

Chapter 13: Hole Drilling

used for hole drilling in metals. Because of the high reflectivity of metals in the far-infrared spectrum, the CO_2 laser is less often used. In addition, the copper vapor laser has proved to be an effective tool for drilling metals.

13.2.1 Nd:YAG Laser Drilling

Lasers are widely used in metal drilling applications because of the high processing speed, high tolerance and repeatability (1). Typically threshold irradiances in the range of 10^6–10^9 W/cm^2 are necessary (2). Such high values are best achieved by means of a pulsed Nd:YAG laser.

Table 1 presents typical results for Nd:YAG laser drilling of metals. Laser beam drilling may be considered in three different drilling strategies: single pulse drilling, percussion drilling, and trepan drilling.

Table 1. Typical Hole Dimensions in Metals Like Stainless Steel, Tool Steel, Cast Iron, etc., for Different Drilling Techniques and Nd:YAG Laser Systems

Beam quality	Rod-system multimode	Slab-system fundamental mode	Units
Single pulse drilling			
Maximum depth	3	2	mm
Hole diameter	0.1–0.9	0.01–0.1	mm
Taper	5–40	1–20	%
Max. aspect ratio	1:25	1:25	
Percussion drilling			
Maximum depth	30	10	mm
Hole diameter	0.1–0.9	0.006–0.1	mm
Taper	0.2–20	0.1–10	%
Max. aspect ratio	1:50	1:100	
Trepanning			
Maximum depth	15	3	mm
Hole diameter	0.15–∞	0.1–∞	mm
Taper	0.5–15	0.1–4	%
Max. aspect ratio	1:20	1:20	
Speed	10–150	2–50	mm/min

Single Pulse Drilling

In single pulse drilling, one laser pulse penetrates the material and creates the hole. The hole diameter can be larger or smaller than the beam diameter and depends decisively on the temporal and spatial intensity distribution in the focused laser beam and on the material thickness. The focal length of the objective and the beam expansion ratio of the beam expander determine the spot size at the focal point and the Rayleigh length. Therefore, it is very important for this application that the laser provide good beam quality together with a short wavelength (3). Figure 1 shows the influence of the focal position on the hole diameter for a thin metal foil.

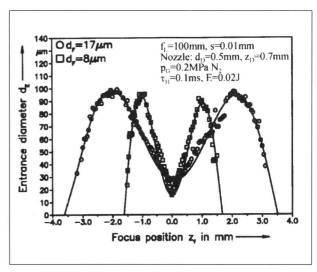

Figure 1. Hole diameter as a function of the relative focal position.

The selection of the pulse energy and of the pulse duration affects the hole taper (4). A pulse length adapted to the material thickness improves the hole quality (5). Furthermore, the hole taper can be minimized by proper focusing. If oxygen is used as a process gas with a nozzle coaxial to the laser beam, the drilling process achieves a higher ablation rate because of the exothermic reaction. Additionally the process gas improves the protection of the focusing optic. An aspect ratio of 1:25 is achievable in metals with a material thickness up to 1.5 mm. Single pulse drilling is used for applications where high processing speed plays an important role. Typical industrial applications for single pulse drilling are sieves or filters, in which holes are drilled while the part is continuously moved relative to the laser beam. Figure 2 presents such a sieve of stainless steel for the food industry, which was drilled by means of the rectangular spot slab laser. One slit was drilled with one laser pulse with a pulse duration of 0.12 ms. A production rate of 100 slits per second can be obtained with a material thickness of 0.5 mm.

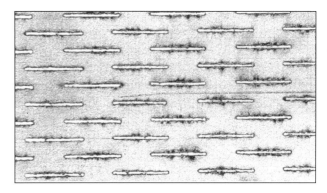

Figure 2. Sieve with slits of 0.06 × 2 mm^2 in stainless steel with a thickness of 0.5 mm.

Another example for an industrial application is the cracking of connecting rods. Blind holes are drilled at 45° in cast iron with a production rate of 140 holes per second, as Figure 3 shows. The depth of the holes is approximately 565 µm. After the drilling process the connecting rod is cracked. To achieve a good cracking process, the form of the blind hole plays an important role.

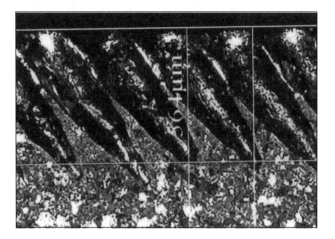

Figure 3. Metallographic section of blind holes drilled at 45° in a connecting rod after the cracking process.

Percussion Drilling

With percussion drilling several laser pulses create the hole. This technique achieves a larger hole diameter to hole depth ratio, up to 1:100 for through holes and 1:20 for blind holes. First the molten material is ejected from the bottom of the hole through the entrance side of the hole with the aid of the vapor pressure. It is necessary to adjust the pulse duration and the pulse frequency to the expulsion rate of the molten material. This avoids absorption and distortion of the incident laser beam by the vapor plume and the molten material. In the case of through holes the process gas expels the molten material through the exit side of the hole, after the melting front has reached the opposite side. Percussion drilling is used in applications in which numerous holes must be precisely located in a highly reproducible manner.

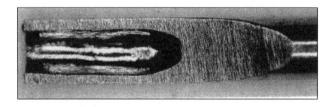

Figure 4. Blind hole in a surgical needle with a diameter of 100 µm and a depth of 425 µm.

Figure 4 shows a blind hole in a needle of stainless steel with a diameter of 100 µm. The diameter of the needle itself is 150 µm. Therefore, the wall of the hole is only 25 µm thick. The drilling rate is 1–10 blind holes per second. This hole was drilled without a process gas. A moving plastic film protects the focusing objective. It is possible to position the needles with a CCD-camera that looks through the Nd:YAG focusing objective.

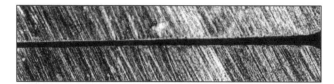

Figure 5. Lubrication hole with a diameter of 60 µm in a 4-mm valve lifter (hole entrance is on the right-hand side).

Lubrication holes of every description are another industrial application. Figure 5 typifies the appearance of a hole with a diameter of 60 µm that has been drilled in 100MnCr V4 steel plate 4 mm thick. This means that the diameter to length ratio is 1:65. The laser beam gets through the material after 4 to 5 pulses. It is important to drill these holes with more laser pulses to prevent contraction at the exit side from slag deposition. The time of the whole drilling process is 1 s.

One major laser application for percussion drilling is holes in turbine combuster parts or turbine blades for aircraft engines, which is shown in Figure 6 (see also Section 13.4). Hole diameters are achievable in the range 0.3–0.8 mm. A drilling time of 0.5–2 s per hole is necessary, depending on the angle of the hole and the material thickness.

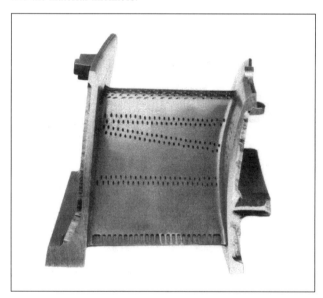

Figure 6. Turbine blade of Hastalloy X with laser drilled holes for an aircraft engine.

Further data concerning drilling applications by means of single pulse or percussion drilling are summarized in Table 2 (next page). In the table, s is the material thickness, E the pulse energy, τ_H the pulse duration, f_p the pulse repetition rate, f_L the lens focal length,

Chapter 13: Hole Drilling

Table 2. Characteristic Drilling Results for Pulsed Nd:YAG Lasers

Material	s (mm)	E (J)	τ_H (ms)	f_P (Hz)	f_L (mm)	z_F (mm)	No. of pulses	d_E (mm)	d_A (mm)
Stainless steel	43.0	45.0	2.00	10	150	-5.0	1200	0.90	0.80
Inconel 718	10.0	15.0	0.50	10	150	-4.0	70	0.90	0.86
Hastalloy X	6.0	16.5	0.98	12	150	-1.0	120	0.78	0.72
CrNi steel	2.2	0.07	0.10	35	100	0.0	350	0.03	0.03
Tungsten	2.0	0.10	0.10	20	50	-0.1	350	0.04	0.04
Titanium	1.0	0.19	0.10	80	100	-0.5	1	0.06	0.06
Nickel silver	0.9	0.12	0.10	20	100	0.0	10	0.06	0.05

z_F the relative focal position, with negative values below the surface and positive above it, d_E the entrance diameter of the hole, and d_A the exit diameter.

Trepanning

The trepan technique can drill holes only with a diameter larger than the laser beam diameter and offers a smaller conicity and a higher repeatability of the hole diameters. Furthermore, only through holes are possible with the trepan technique. The trepan process divides into two or more parts. First a starting hole is pierced by percussion drilling at the center or on the contour of the future hole (6). Second the first trepan drilling circle is cut out. Either the workpiece rotates or rotating optics moves the laser beam relative to the fixed workpiece. The diameter of the contour controls the diameter of the hole. With trepanning only, the movement itself determines the accuracy of the hole diameter. This is in sharp contrast to the other two drilling techniques, where the beam characteristic mostly influences the hole quality. It is possible to trepan holes with two or more circles to improve the hole quality (7).

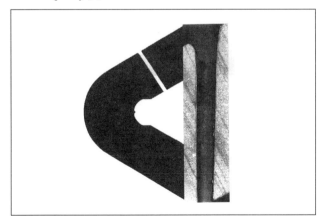

Figure 7. Tip of an injection nozzle and a metallographic section of a hole at 60° to the surface.

Most industrial applications for trepanning are nozzles, as can be seen in Figure 7. On the left-hand side there is a tip of an injection nozzle with one hole vertical to the nozzle surface. Holes at different angles are also possible, which illustrates the metallographic section on the right hand side. All holes were trepanned from the outside of the nozzle. So the entrance side of the laser beam is the exit side of the fuel and vice versa. The thickness of the wall, where the holes were drilled, is 1mm. The conicity of these double trepanned holes is in the range 1.9–3 % and is reduced by a factor of 2 in comparison to holes trepanned with one circle. One hole is drilled in 7–25 seconds, depending on the trepan velocity and the piercing time.

All these drilling strategies use a "direct beam." This means that only mirrors are used as a beam guiding system. In most cases an optical fiber cannot be used because the beam quality is too poor for drilling applications.

References

1. G. Chryssolouris, *Laser Machining, Theory and Practice*, Springer Verlag, New York (1991).
2. H. Hügel, *Strahlwerkzeug Laser*, Teubner 1992, Stuttgart (in German).
3. C. J. Nonhof, *Material processing with Nd-Laser*, Electrochemical Publications (1988).
4. B. S. Yilbas, *Study of affecting parameters in laser hole drilling of sheet metals*, Transaction of the ASME, **109,** 282–7 (October 1987).
5. H. Rohde and F. Dausinger, in "Investigation of the dynamical process during the formation of a micro through hole," *ECLAT'96*, F. Dausinger, H. W. Bergmann, and J. Sigel (Eds.), **2,** 675–82.
6. M. H. van Dijk, in "Drilling of aero-engine components: Experiences from the shop floor," *Industrial Laser Handbook,* D. Belforte and M. Levitt (Eds.), Springer Verlag, New York, 113–18 (1992).
7. H. Rohde and E. Meiners, "Trepan drilling of fuel injection nozzles with a TEM_{00} Nd:YAG slab laser," *J. of Laser Appl.* **8** (2), 95–101 (April 1996).

HANSJOERG ROHDE

13.2.2 CO_2 Lasers for Metal Drilling

High-peak-power CO_2 lasers have found a niche in drilling applications. These lasers typically operate with pulse durations that may range between 20 μs and 1 ms with pulse rates up to 20,000 Hz at a 50% duty cycle. The range of average powers for these lasers is 50–600 W, with peak power between 300 and 1,500 W. The beam quality (M^2) of high-peak-power CO_2 lasers that are good for drilling has $M^2 < 1.2$. Note that the "perfect" laser beam would have $M^2 = 1$.

$$M^2 = \pi w (w^2 - w_o^2)^{0.5}/\lambda z$$

where w_o is the waist, λ is the wavelength, and z is the distance between w_o and w. See Section 3.4 for more detail about M^2.

The beam parameter, M^2, is particularly useful for defining the quality of a laser beam since it is proportional to the focused beam diameter. The type of CO_2 laser that can best achieve the desired beam parameters and operating beam format is a sealed slab design.

The laser energy pulse shape is the primary reason that effective drilling applications can be realized. The most desirable laser pulse shape for CO_2 laser drilling would be a square wave. The sealed slab laser can generate such a pulse shape. Figure 8 contrasts a laser pulse from a flowing gas CO_2 laser and the sealed CO_2 system.

The rapid rise time of the leading edge of the pulse and its rapid fall time at the end of the pulse minimizes unnecessary heating or charring of materials that are being processed. The square wave pulse shape also reduces the heat-affected zone (HAZ).

In addition to the pulse shape, a sufficient laser energy level is required to affect the drilling process. The typical processing threshold (see Fig. 8) for drilling requires a laser irradiance between 10^6 and 10^8 W/cm^2. These levels are readily achievable with the sealed CO_2 laser because M^2 is very low. This low value of M^2 leads to a 2x reduction in focused spot diameter and, therefore, a 4x increase in irradiance over conventional flowing gas CO_2 laser beams. The magnitude of this processing threshold is material dependent.

The radio-frequency (RF) excited, sealed CO_2 laser is being used in several small hole drilling applications. One such application addresses drilling microvias in multilayered (copper and dielectric material) printed circuit boards. Microvia diameters from 50 to 325 μm can be achieved. Because of the laser high repetition rate, 300 microvias can be drilled in a second. CO_2 transversely excited-atmosphere (TEA) lasers are also used for drilling microvias.

The sealed laser is used for drilling and cutting (overlapping drilling spots at high frequency) thin metals. These metals include galvanized steel, mild steel, and stainless steel in the thickness range between 0.5 and 1.5 mm (9). One advantage of drilling/cutting with sealed CO_2 lasers is the high thickness-to-diameter/kerf ratios (e.g., 50:1).

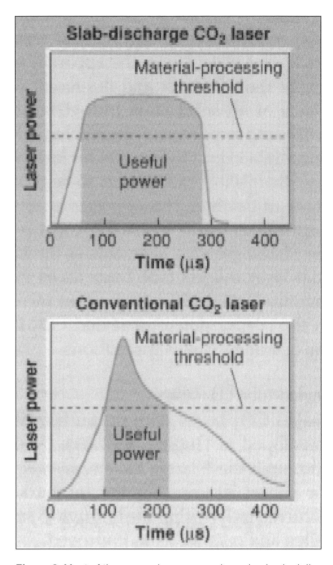

Figure 8. Most of the energy in a square-shaped pulse is delivered above the material-processing threshold (top), and little is wasted just heating the material. Conventional-design CO_2 lasers produce pulses with relatively slow rise times (bottom). Benefits of square-shaped pulses include faster processing with finer features for cutting and drilling and with a small heat-affected zone (8).

The sealed CO_2 laser is also good for other nonmetal applications (see Section 13.3), which include drilling pills for time-release drugs, perforation of 0.003-in.-thick carbonless paper, drilling blind holes in ceramic substrates for surface mount technology devices, drilling holes in latex nipples (see Section 13.3.3), and drilling vapor tap holes for dispensing products such as aerosols, paints, deodorants, etc.

References

8. K. Bondelie, "Sealed Carbon Dioxide Lasers Achieve New Power Levels," *Laser Focus World,* PennWell Publishing Co. (1996).

9. W. H. Shiner, "Sealed CO_2 Laser Opens Door to New Industrial Uses," *Industrial Lasers,* Photonics Spectra, Laurin Publishing Co., Inc. (1992).

MARSHALL G. JONES

13.2.3 CO_2 Laser Drilling
With CO_2 lasers, TEA or pulsed, the same three drilling techniques are possible, as described in Section 13.2.1, for Nd:YAG lasers. Since Nd:YAG lasers are available with a high beam quality, the importance of CO_2 lasers in deep micro hole drilling of metals is diminished. There are three reasons for this:

1. The wavelength of Nd:YAG lasers is 10 times smaller than that of CO_2 lasers. Therefore the focal spot is 10 times smaller for the same beam quality and focusing conditions.
2. The absorption of the laser radiation is for the most metals higher at the wavelength of 1.06 μm (Nd:YAG) then at the wavelength of 10.6 μm (CO_2). On the other hand, many nonmetallic materials have very high absorption at the wavelength of 10.6 μm. Therefore the CO_2 laser can be employed to advantage for nonmetals in comparison to Nd:YAG lasers, but the Nd:YAG laser usually has an advantage for the drilling of metals.
3. The drilling efficiency is strongly dependent on the phenomenon of laser-supported absorption waves. This is a problem specific to the long wavelength of CO_2 laser radiation, because the threshold intensity for the ignition of these waves decreases as the inverse square of the wavelength (10).

Depths of a few millimeters may be drilled through metallic plates, either by a single pulse of high energy or by a series of pulses of lower energy delivered to the same spot. The depth that each laser pulse penetrates depends on the pulse length, pulse energy, spot size and the material. The pulse length is usually set from 0.05 to 1 ms (11). Some drilling data are summarized in Table 3. The notation is the same as in Section 13.2.1.

Table 3. Typical Drilling Parameters for CO_2 Lasers

Material	s (mm)	E (J)	τ_H (ms)	f_L (mm)	d_E (mm)	Ref.
Stainless steel	0.6	0.10	–	100	0.07	(12)
Aluminum	1.0	2.72	0.50	–	–	(13)
Brass	1.5	2.72	0.50	–	–	(13)
Copper	0.2	2.72	0.50	–	–	(13)
Aluminum	0.5	–	–	100	0.10	(14)
Aluminum	1.0	–	–	100	0.12	(14)

The CO_2 laser is well used in drilling application on most nonmetals because many nonmetallic materials have very high absorption at the wavelength of 10.6 μm.

References
10. E. Stürmer and M. von Allmen, "Influence of Laser-Supported Detonation Waves on Metal Drilling with Pulsed CO_2 Lasers," *J. of Applied Physics,* **49** (11), 5648–54 (1978).
11. L. M. Heglin, "Introduction to Laser Drilling," in *The Industrial Laser Annual Handbook,* D. Belforte and M. Levitt (Eds.), 116–20 (1986).
12. D. C. Hamilton and D. J. James, "Hole Drilling with a Repetitively-Pulsed TEA CO_2 Laser," *Journal of Physics D: Applied Physics* **9,** L41–L43 (1976).
13. A. Cingolani et al., "Metal Drilling Investigation by Means of Different High Power Laser Radiation," in *Applied Physics Communication* **2** (1 and 2), 9–16 (1982).
14. E. Armon et al., "Metal Drilling with a CO_2 Laser Beam. II. Analysis of Aluminium Drilling Experiments," in *Journal of Applied Physics* **65** (12), 5003–6 (1989).

HANSJOERG ROHDE

13.2.4 Drilling with Copper Vapor Lasers
Laser beam material removal using copper vapor lasers (CVL) is a suitable technology for drilling of all kinds of metals. Different processes can be classified either according to the sequence of the pulses (single or multiple pulse drilling) or the process strategy (focusing, trepanning, or imaging). The achievable accuracy in laser drilling is limited by the properties of the laser system (e.g., pulse-to-pulse-stability, pointing stability) and the physical properties of the workpiece (e.g., composition, microstructure).

Laser Characteristics and Setup
The profile of a desired laser source for precision machining has been defined (15). The ideal source should provide a visible, pulsed and diffraction limited laser beam with pulse energies up to 200 mJ and repetition rates about 10 kHz. To achieve small heat- and mechanical-affected zones, a pulse length about 100 ps to 200 ns is advantageous. Typical properties of copper vapor lasers utilized for drilling of metals are summarized in Table 4.

Table 4. Properties of CVLs Suitable for Drilling Metals

Wavelength	511, 578 nm
Repetition rate	6.5 kHz
Pulse length	50 ns (FWHM)
Pulse energy	0.3–25 mJ
Pulse power	1–300 kW
Average power	10–100 W
Divergence	140 μrad
Focal spot diameter	10–150 μm
Irradiance	10^8–10^{11} W/cm²

An experimental setup of a CVL-MOPA system (Master-Oscillator-Power-Amplifier) used for material removal is shown schematically in Figure 9 (next page).

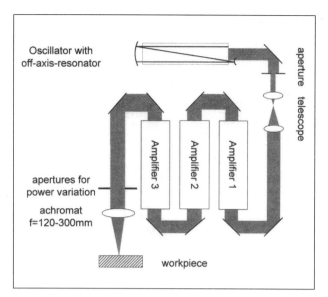

Figure 9. Experimental setup of a CVL-MOPA-chain.

Single Pulse Material Removal Process

With increasing pulse power, ablation of metals shows three distinct processes (Fig. 10). However, the generation of a thin film of molten material and its continuous displacement by the pressure of the produced metal vapor is the dominant ablation process. Hence, there is no need for the use of a gas jet to blow out the molten material. For metals, the drilling speed during a single laser pulse becomes steady after a few nanoseconds and can range up to 2 km/s (16). Consequently, as in aluminum, it is possible to drill a hole of 100-µm depth with a single laser pulse.

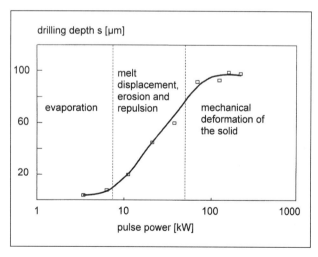

Figure 10. Effect of the pulse power on ablation depth in single pulse CVL-drilling of aluminum and identification of processes for material removal.

Material Dependence in Single Pulse Drilling

A systematic overview of ablation depths in pure metals produced by a single CVL pulse is given in Figure 11.

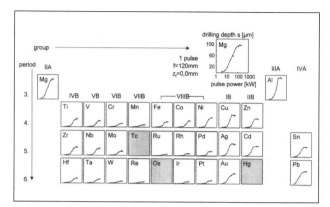

Figure 11. Ablation depths in pure metals as a function of the pulse power of a single CVL pulse.

The ablation behavior for pure metals and alloys has been empirically found to depend on only two material properties (17): melting temperature T_m (in K) and indentation hardness (in Vickers hardness values HV). The maximum drilling depth s_{max} achievable by single CVL pulses under standard focusing conditions (focal length: 120 mm, focal position: on the surface) follows the equation:

$$s_{max}(\mu m) = 16000\{1/[HV \cdot T_m(K)]\}^{1/2}$$

Material Dependence in Multiple Pulse Drilling

To achieve deeper holes in metals, repetitive CVL pulses on the same workpiece area (percussion drilling) are applied. An empirical description leads to a square root dependence of the depth with the number of pulses (Fig. 12).

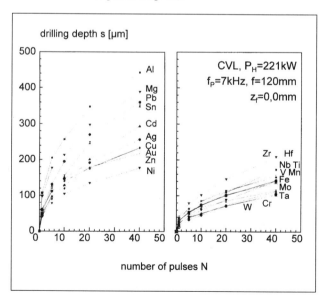

Figure 12. Drilling depth as function of the number of pulses for various pure metals.

Chapter 13: Hole Drilling

An estimate of the drilling depth s_N with a certain number of pulses N in a specific metal is possible using the following equation, which shows the mathematical connection between single pulse and percussion drilling depths. Single pulse depth s_1 and the index of the depth gradient n are material dependent and can also be calculated from the material's hardness and melting point values (17). Experimental values of n for different pure metals are given in Table 5.

$$s_N = s_1 \times N^n$$

Table 5. Values for the Index of the Depth Gradient n for Percussion Drilling of Various Pure Metals

Metal	n
Al, Mg, Ti, Ni, Cu, Ag, Au	0.3–0.4
V, Cr, Fe, Co, Zr, Nb, Mo, Ta, Pb	0.4–0.5
Zn, Cd, Sn, Hf, W, Mn	0.5–0.6

These empirical correlations are also valid for metal alloys and have been shown for the binary systems Cu-Al, Cu-Ag, Cu-Ni, Cu-Zn, Fe-Ni, and Fe-Cr (17).

Different Processing Strategies

In drilling with CVLs, various processing strategies can be applied, depending on the desired depth and hole diameter. Material can be removed either in the focal plane with or without relative movement between sample and laser beam (trepanning) or by mask projection via imaging optics. The kind of drilling technique most suitable for a certain removal depth and depth/width ratio is shown in Figure 13. The range of machining is restricted upward by plasma shielding and process ineffectiveness as well as downward through the optical resolution and removal of the molten material out of deep and narrow holes.

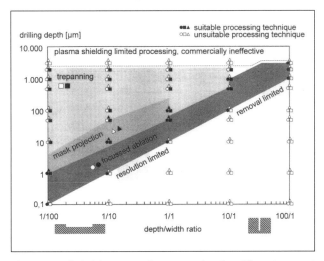

Figure 13. Suitable processing strategies for different aspect ratios (depth/width).

For CVLs, various drilling techniques have been experimentally investigated, and they have been quantified by the precision achieved and the processing speed (18). Some details on geometrical deviations are given in Table 6. Typical average powers used for the manufacturing of circular holes range between 0.2 and 1.6 W (focused ablation), 3 W (trepanning), and 23–56 W (mask projection).

Table 6. Geometrical Deviations in Drilling of 25-μm-Thick Copper with CVLs for Various Processing Strategies

Processing strategy	Focused (μm)	Mask projection (μm)	Trepanning (μm)	
Nominal drill hole diameter	10	100	100	1000
Measured diameter	9.6	92.4	93.5	1002.0
Concentric deviation	0.2	5.3	1.5	2.3
Right-angle tolerance	3.4	1.3	0.1	3.3
Ridge width beam entrance	5.3	1.6	7.5	19.4
Ridge width beam exit	0.7	1.9	2.3	5.0
Heat-affected zone width	< 1	< 1	< 1	< 1

Drill Hole Shapes

Copper vapor lasers are suitable tools for drilling of blind and through holes in all kinds of metals, metal alloys and metal-nonmetal compounds. The achievable drill hole diameter in focused drilling is proportional to the applied pulse power and ranges from about 10 to 150 μm (Fig. 14). Machinable workpiece thicknesses lie within some micrometers up to 5 millimeters.

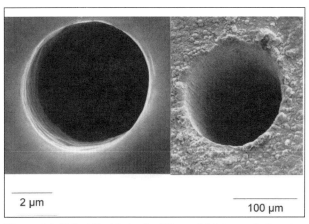

Figure 14. CVL-drilled holes in 100-μm-thick brass (left, pulse power 1 kW) and 400-μm-thick tungsten (right, pulse power 337 kW).

ISBN 0-912035-15-3

Normally, drill holes produced by focused ablation have circular shapes. Larger or noncircular cross sections can be produced by either mask projection or trepanning. Figure 15 shows differently shaped drill holes and slits in copper and copper alloy foils achieved by imaging and trepanning techniques.

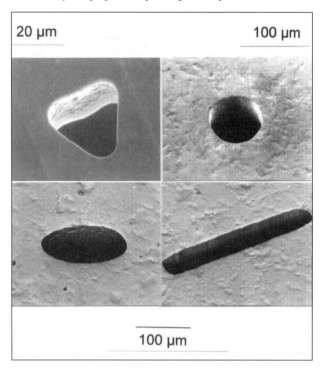

Figure 15. CVL-drilled holes in 100-µm-thick brass using different processing strategies; a: mask projection (pulse power 10 kW), b–d: trepanning (pulse power 3 kW).

The deposition of a melt layer at the drill hole walls or foil surface at the beam entrance side is observed if subliming products fail to combine with the surrounding atmosphere (e.g., tungsten oxide) during the ablation process. Melt layers have to be removed either by mechanical or chemical post-processing treatment.

Applications

Applications for CVL-drilled holes can be subdivided by their manufactured form (blind or through holes). Mainly, the latter form serves for the generation of a defined flow of gaseous, liquid and solid material, which includes the production of fuel injection nozzles as well as filters and screening plates (Fig. 16). Further possibilities also exist for the production of scan patterns for high-resolution imaging techniques.

Surface structuring of metals with high processing speed is feasible using single pulse drilled blind holes. One aspect of this kind of processing is the improvement of the tribological behavior of functional surfaces, for example the emergency running properties of cylinder liners in automotive engines (materials: grey cast iron, aluminum alloys). Oil-filled, several micrometers deep, single pulse drill holes serve as micro pressure chambers. Clear advantages compared to conventional techniques include the possibility to produce defined sizes and dispersions of the drill holes.

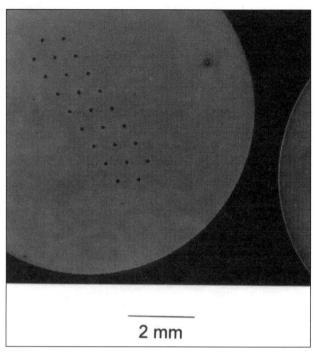

Figure 16. Nozzle plate with CVL-drilled holes (diameter 100 µm in 100-µm-thick brass).

Analogously, the tribological behavior of roller bearings can be improved using this technique. Another kind of surface structuring with laser drilled blind holes deals with the interconnection of different materials. Examples can be found for medical (titanium implant – human tissue) as well as microelectronic (chip – polymer isolation) applications.

References

15. C. E. Little and N. V. Sabotinov (Eds.), *Pulsed Metal Vapour Lasers,* Kluwer Academic Publishers, Dordrecht, 313–30 (1996).
16. C. Körner, R. Mayerhofer, M. Hartmann, and H. W. Bergmann, "Physical and Material Aspects in Using Visible Laser Pulses of Nanosecond Duration for Ablation," *Applied Physics* A **63,** 123–31 (1996).
17. R. Mayerhofer, *Mikromaterialbearbeitung mit Kupferdampflasern: Prozeßcharakterisierung und Werkstoffabhängigkeit des Abtrags,* Ph.D. Thesis, University of Erlangen-Nürnberg, Germany (1997).
18. H. W. Bergmann, M. Hartmann, R. Mayerhofer, and N. Bartl, *Kupferdampflaser für die effiziente und schädigungsarme Präzisionsbearbeitung von Metallen,* Proc. of the 6th European Conference on Laser Treatment of Materials ECLAT´96, Stuttgart, 741–50 (September 16–18, 1996).

ROLAND MAYERHOFER
HANS WILHELM BERGMANN

Chapter 13: Hole Drilling

13.2.5 Applications of Copper Vapor Laser Drilling

Diesel Injector Nozzles

Automotive engineers are under considerable regulatory pressure to reduce the level of emissions of internal combustion engines. One of the major contributors to high emissions is the fuel injector design. The current technique for drilling the fuel injector orifice is the wire electron discharge machining (Wire-EDM). This process produces excellent quality holes, but suffers from slow processing speeds. Hole diameters of less than 150 µm become increasingly difficult to achieve, and any change in hole diameter requires costly retooling of the device. Additionally, variations in hole geometry are not possible, e.g., tapered, oval, etc.

CVL micromachining has demonstrated the ability to produce nozzles with diameters in the range 50–200 µm (Table 7). Figure 17 is an SEM photograph of the exit side of a 150-µm hole in 1-mm-thick stainless steel. The hole has exceptional roundness and is completely dross free on the exit side. The entry side has minimal dross, which can be removed by light abrasion.

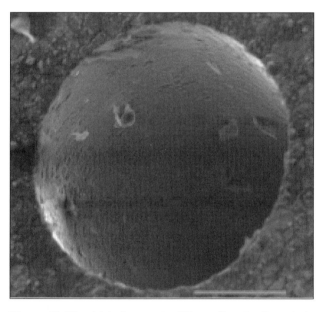

Figure 17. Diesel injector nozzle 150 µm diameter through 1-mm stainless steel.

The process speed, reproducibility, roundness, parallelism, and edge quality are well within the requirements for a production process. The laser has the ability to control taper, hole shape, and hole size, making it ideal as a development tool.

High Aspect Ratio Features

For the nuclear and aerospace industry, the ability to detect micro-cracks in reactor cooling pipes or turbine blades of jet engines is critical from a safety standpoint. In order to calibrate the detection equipment, precision high aspect ratio features are machined with copper vapor lasers to provide these simulated micro-cracks (see Fig. 18).

Table 7. Typical Specifications for a CVL-Drilled Diesel Injector Orifice

Material	Hardened steel
Thickness	1 mm
Hole diameter	70–200 µm
Taper	0 µm
Reproducibility	< 2 µm
Drill time	< 15 s

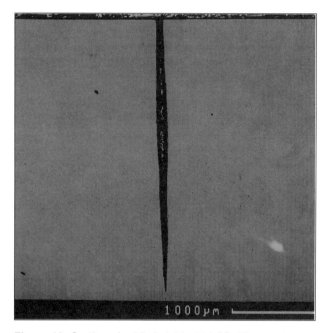

Figure 18. Section of a blind slot in 304 SS. 70-µm entrance width, 3500-µm depth, 50:1 aspect ratio.

High Density Hole Array

Because of the low thermal impact on the material, it is possible to produce hole spacings less than the diameter of the holes. This capability is being applied in a wide range of materials such as metals, carbon fiber composites, ceramics, and diamond (see Fig. 19).

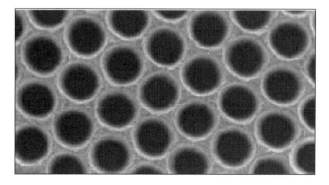

Figure 19. 200-µm-diameter holes on 230-µm pitch in copper.

ISBN 0-912035-15-3

Frequency Doubling for Machining Polyimids

In the production of printed circuit boards (PCBs), the miniaturization of components requires the size of via and through holes to be less than that capable of mechanical drilling processes. The visible output of the CVL is being used to drill small holes (25–150 μm) in the copper layer of PCBs. To process the polyimide layer, which absorbs ultraviolet wavelengths well, the output of the CVL is frequency-doubled to produce high-pulse-rate ultraviolet radiation. If one switches between the visible and frequency-doubled output, only one laser is required to produce PCBs in a single-step process. Table 8 presents typical specifications for such lasers.

Table 8. Typical Specifications for Frequency-Doubled Copper Vapor Lasers

Beam diameter	4 mm
Beam divergence	1.2 mrad
Pulse width	30 ns
PRF	6–10 kHz
Wavelengths	255 nm (freq. doubling 511 nm)
	289 nm (freq. doubling 578 nm)
	271 nm (sum mixing)
Power	1–6 W

Via drilling is described in more detail in Section 25.1.

The copper vapor laser, because of its high pulse rate and power, is increasingly being used for micromachining, particularly where high-aspect ratio (50:1), small feature size (= 2 μm) and high precision are required.

RICHARD SLAGLE

13.3 Drilling of Nonmetals

13.3.1 General Considerations

Most nonmetals are of one of two types, characterized by their response to exposure to high-energy radiation: those that transform from a solid directly into a vapor without significant liquefaction, and those that transform from solid state into a liquid state before vaporization. Paper is an example of the former; acrylic resin is an example of the latter.

When absorbed by a material, this energy is transformed into energy associated with the motion of atoms or molecules and is capable of being transmitted through solids or fluids by conduction, that is, as heat. Most nonmetals do not conduct heat effectively. Properly applied, the effect of short, high-energy laser pulses is localized to the area of exposure. As such, each pulse of laser energy affects a volume of material consistent with the irradiance of the focused beam and the specific heat of the material, with negligible impact to material adjacent to the area of exposure.

The total energy required to drill a hole comes from the specific gravity of a material and the volume of material which must be converted from solid to vapor. The rate at which holes can be drilled is determined by the rate at which energy can be input to the material without degrading hole quality.

Hole quality is quantified by the measures of: roundness and taper; recast (material that has resolidified in the hole or around the hole entrance); or charring (usually exhibited as a carbonaceous residue). These qualities affect the function of the hole, whether it be air flow, spray pattern, or part fit.

As described in Section 13.1.5, holes may be drilled by percussion drilling or by trepanning. Generally, trepanning is used to produce holes with diameter greater than 0.025 in.

DANA ELZA
STEVEN R. MAYNARD

13.3.2 Nd:YAG Laser Drilling

Solid-State Lasers for Drilling

The Nd:YAG laser is the most common solid-state laser used for drilling applications. In this laser, the host crystal material is neodymium-doped yttrium aluminum garnet. More recently, other crystal materials such as yttrium lithium fluoride (YLF), yttrium vanadate (YVO_4), lanthanum scandium borate (LSB) etc. have been used with appropriate neodymium doping concentrations to produce the fundamental laser wavelength. The gain medium is created by optically pumping the Nd:YAG crystal material using either flash lamps or laser diodes. The multiple harmonics of the fundamental wavelength are generated by introducing high quality, nonlinear crystal materials such as lithium triborate (LBO) and beta-barium borate (BBO) into the optical path of the original laser beam (1). The 2nd, 3rd, and 4th harmonic laser wavelengths, generated at 532, 355, and 266 nm, offer new opportunities in material processing applications. In particular, for drilling applications solid-state lasers can provide very high peak irradiance (in the range 10^8–10^{12} W/cm^2), good mode quality, low beam divergence, short pulse width in the nanosecond to femtosecond regime, and near diffraction-limited spot sizes. These attributes greatly contribute toward their superior performance in achieving precise tolerances and repeatability.

More recent developments in diode-pumped solid-state (DPSS) lasers have resulted in even better performance characteristics, such as higher efficiency, improved pulse-to-pulse reproducibility and beam quality, as well as long term reliable operation. Instant ablation or vaporization of the workpiece material with minimal heat-affected zone is possible with the available high irradiance. Solid-state lasers in general are particularly attractive for drilling hard-to-machine materials such as ceramics, diamond, carbides, and composites (2–4). Other drilling applications include a multitude of nonmetallic materials such as polypropylene, polyimide, enamels, and semiconductors along with organic and biological materials (5). Typical parameters for drilling several nonmetals are listed in Table 1 (beginning on page 488).

ISBN 0-912035-15-3

Drilling Process

In general, the drilling process is carried out by expanding the original laser beam using a beam expander and then focusing it using either a lens or a microscope objective onto the work surface. The hole depth generated by the beam–material interaction depends on the thermal properties of the workpiece material and on the incoming laser beam properties which include spot size, wavelength, pulse duration, pulse energy, and peak irradiance. Once the hole is created, additional laser pulses cause an increase in the hole depth. This is accomplished by means of reflections of the laser beam from the interior walls of the hole, the effect commonly known as the light pipe effect (6).

Depending on the workpiece material, the drilling process is carried out by direct vaporization, melting, or a combination of both. The process is optimized so that the holes show minimal traces of molten or re-solidified conditions in the processed zone. Specially designed fixtures to hold the workpiece accurately in place can be used. Integrated systems using computer-aided design (CAD) based design software allow on-the-fly changes in the laser, motion system, and other process control parameters. Use of galvanometric and/or scanning devices to steer the laser beam onto the work surface can facilitate the drilling process. In addition, recent developments in high-speed, high-accuracy positioning stages and control software can provide drilling rates as high as several hundred holes per second with resultant increase in the overall process efficiency.

Drilling Techniques

The conventional methods used to drill fine holes using solid-state lasers can be described as follows. These methods involve single pulse drilling, the superposition of a series of pulses over the same focal area (percussion drilling), and the rotation of the workpiece under the laser focal spot for producing larger-diameter holes (trepanning). The trepanning method involves direct scanning of the laser beam around the hole circumference. For smaller-diameter hole drilling, the optical trepanning technique can be used. In this case, the focusing lens is rotated in the beam path (7).

A slight variation of the percussion drilling technique is the drill-on-the-fly process. Here the pulses are delivered while the laser beam is moving relative to the workpiece. If multiple pulses are required to make a hole, the motion system and laser pulse repetition frequency are synchronized so that a predetermined number of pulses are delivered to the same location. The method is used to increase the hole production rate.

The edge quality, circularity and the aspect ratio of the holes depend on the method of drilling and the laser beam properties. Figure 1 shows typical percussion drilled hole patterns in silicon and aluminium nitride ceramic material using a femtosecond pulse, solid-state laser (8).

The high quality of holes apparent in Figure 1 is primarily due to the short pulse (250×10^{-15}s) laser interaction with the material, leading to the rapid creation of vapor and plasma phases, negligible heat conduction and the absence of a liquid phase. The latter allows better control during the drilling process with further enhancement in reproducibility.

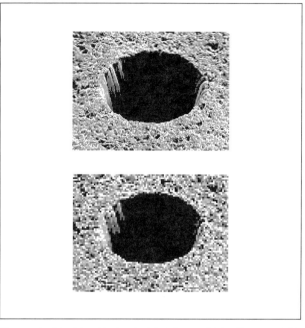

Figure 1. Machined holes in (a) 0.3-mm-thick silicon and (b) 0.8-mm AlN ceramic materials using a 250-fs pulse solid-state laser. Hole size ~ 150 μm (8).

Among newer drilling techniques is the use of diffractive optical elements (DOE) in the path of the laser beam to produce an array of micro-holes (9). When conventional beam focusing geometries are used, the beam intensity in the focal plane is so high that ionization, plasma formation and other nonlinear effects such as self-focusing, self-phase modulation, and filamentation can occur in the surrounding air. These effects are detrimental and cause a distorted spatial profile of the beam. Use of diffractive optical elements in the beam path can minimize these distortions and provide accurate beam delivery to the workpiece. In effect, significant improvements in the resultant quality of the holes can be obtained in terms of reproducibility, burr-free edges, and high-aspect-ratio drilling in a wide range of metals and nonmetals. Another benefit of using diffractive optical elements, is high-energy throughput compared to a typical masking-imaging system. A particularly challenging example of an application using this technique is quartz glass drilling. At pulse widths less than 200 fs, highly reproducible 20-μm diameter holes can be drilled in 1-mm-thick quartz substrates (10). Drilling of micro-hole arrays in polyimide material for ink-jet printers and micro-hole via drilling of glass-woven epoxy materials such as FR4 are some of the other applications where this method is particularly effective.

Table 1. Solid-State Laser Drilling of Nonmetals

Material	Laser type	Wavelength (nm)	Pulse length (s)	Pulse frequency (Hz)
Alumina (Al_2O_3)	Nd:YLF	1047	100×10^{-9}	1000
Alumina (Al_2O_3)	Nd:YAG	1064	630×10^{-6}	10
Alumina (Al_2O_3)	Nd:YAG (Trepan)	1064	630×10^{-6}	10
Al_2O_3/SiC_w	Nd:YAG	1064	2×10^{-3}	11
Aluminium nitride	Ti:Sapphire	780	250×10^{-15}	—
$BaTiO_3$	Q-Sw Nd:YAG	532	10×10^{-9}	20
Copolyester LCP	Nd:YAG	1064	$0.6–5 \times 10^{-3}$	10–40
Copolyester LCP	Nd:YAG	1064	$0.6–5 \times 10^{-3}$	10–40
CVD diamond	Q-Sw Nd:YLF	1047	100×10^{-9}	1000
Diamond	DPSS Nd:YLF	527	40×10^{-12}	1000
Epoxide woven glass fabric	Nd:YAG	1064	0.2×10^{-3}	20
Epoxide woven glass fabric	Nd:YAG	1064	0.2×10^{-3}	20
GaAs wafer	Nd:YAG	532	50×10^{-9}	2440
HDPE	Q-Sw Nd:YAG	532	7×10^{-9}	20
Hot pressed SiC	Nd:YAG	1064	630×10^{-6}	5
Hot pressed SiC	Nd:YAG (Trepan)	1064	630×10^{-6}	10
Human tooth enamel	Nd:YAG	1064	1×10^{-6}	10
Human tooth enamel	Q-Sw Nd:YAG	1064	10×10^{-9}	10
MgO-Al_2O_3-SiO_2	Q-Sw Nd:YAG	532	10×10^{-9}	20
$Nd_{15}Fe_{77}Be$	Nd:YAG	1064	0.2×10^{-3}	20
PE–PTFE	Q-Sw Nd:YAG	1064	12×10^{-9}	1000
Polyimide	Q-Sw Nd:YAG	1064	12×10^{-9}	1000
Polyimide	Nd:YAG	355	35×10^{-9}	500
Polyimide	Q-Sw Nd:YLF	1047	100×10^{-9}	1000
Polypropylene	Q-Sw Nd:YAG	1064	12×10^{-9}	1000
Reaction bonded Si_3N_4	Nd:YAG	1064	630×10^{-6}	5
Reaction bonded Si_3N_4	Nd:YAG	1064	630×10^{-6}	5
Hot pressed Si_3N_4	Nd:YAG	1064	2×10^{-3}	20
Si_3N_4	Nd:YAG	1064	40×10^{-12}	750

Chapter 13: Hole Drilling

Average power (W)	Material thickness (mm)	Number of pulses	Inlet hole diameter (mm)	Outlet hole diameter (mm)	Assist gas
10	6.35	—	0.110	—	—
40	3.3	10	0.279	—	N_2
50	3.18	230	0.457	—	Air
98	5	12	0.255	0.110	N_2
—	0.8	35,000	0.150	—	Vac
0.160	0.0355	—	0.090	0.085	—
120	16.4	—	—	—	Ar
120	20.7	—	—	—	Ar
10	0.50–0.70	—	0.11	—	—
0.0161	0.015	—	0.007	—	Air
300	0.836	1	0.110	—	Ar
300	1.636	1	0.110	—	Ar
0.04	0.060	1	0.028	—	—
0.022	0.63	—	0.050	0.016	—
40	2.87	10	0.254	—	Air
80	2.87	390	1.52	1.5	Air
5	3	100	—	—	—
35	0.75	2500	—	—	—
5	0.115	—	0.070	0.030	—
20	0.7	2	0.075	0.062	—
1	0.0125	—	0.0015	0.014	Air
3	0.025	—	0.020	0.018	Air
30×10^{-3}	0.25	—	0.0075	0.0025	—
10	—	—	0.025	—	—
2.45	0.35	500	0.082	0.020	Air
25	4.78	12.5	0.254	—	N_2
25	4.78	15	0.254	—	N_2
100	8.00	40	0.610	0.254	N_2
0.150	—	1000	0.0055	—	Air

Table 1. Solid-State Laser Drilling of Nonmetals (concluded)

Material	Laser type	Wavelength (nm)	Pulse length (s)	Pulse frequency (Hz)
SiC composite	Nd:YAG	1064	300×10^{-9}	5000
SiC composite	Nd:YAG	1064	0.6×10^{-6}	5
SiC composite	Nd:YAG	1064	0.6×10^{-3}	5
SiC composite	Nd:YAG	1064	2.1×10^{-3}	20
SiC composite	Q-Sw Nd:YAG	1064	260×10^{-12}	—
SiC composite	Q-Sw Nd:YAG	1064	300×10^{-9}	5000
SiC composite	Q-Sw Nd:YAG	1064	0.3×10^{-3}	20
SiC crystal	Nd:YAG	1064	15×10^{-9}	20
SiC crystal	Nd:YAG	1064	15×10^{-9}	20
SiC crystal	Nd:YAG	1064	15×10^{-9}	20
SiC crystal	Nd:YAG	1064	15×10^{-9}	20
SiC fiber in LAS glass	Nd:YAG	1064	630×10^{-6}	5
SiC fiber in LAS glass	Nd:YAG (Trepan)	1064	630×10^{-6}	5
SiC: sintered alpha	Nd:YAG	1064	630×10^{-6}	5
SiC: sintered alpha	Nd:YAG (Trepan)	1064	630×10^{-6}	5
Silicon wafer	Nd:YAG	1064	250×10^{-9}	—
Silicon oxide	Q-Sw Nd:YAG	1064	30×10^{-9}	11,000
Siliconized SiC	Nd:YAG	1064	630×10^{-6}	5
Siliconized SiC	Nd:YAG	1064	630×10^{-6}	5
Siliconized SiC	Nd:YAG	1064	630×10^{-6}	5
Siliconized SiC	Nd:YAG	1064	630×10^{-6}	5
Siliconized SiC	Nd:YAG (Trepan)	1064	630×10^{-6}	5
Siliconized SiC	Nd:YAG (Trepan)	1064	630×10^{-6}	5
Siliconized SiC	Nd:YAG (Trepan)	1064	630×10^{-6}	5
Sintered SiC	Nd:YAG	1064	250×10^{-6}	200
Slate tile	Nd:YAG	1064	0.5×10^{-3}	10
Slate tile	Nd:YAG	1064	1.0×10^{-3}	10
Slate tile	Nd:YAG	1064	2.0×10^{-3}	10
$SmCo_5$	Nd:YAG	1064	0.2×10^{-3}	20

Chapter 13: Hole Drilling

Average power (W)	Material thickness (mm)	Number of pulses	Inlet hole diameter (mm)	Outlet hole diameter (mm)	Assist gas
100	2	40,000	0.4	0.13	Air
50	2	60	0.5	0.2	Air
50	3	—	0.5	0.15	—
140	3	—	0.5	0.2	—
100	3.2	—	0.13	0.1	—
100	3	—	0.13	0.1	—
140	2	60	0.5	0.25	Air
110	0.5	100	0.07	0.03	—
110	0.5	1200	0.07	0.03	—
150	0.5	1	0.2	—	—
150	0.5	100	0.17	—	—
20	3.18	10	0.279	—	N_2
20	3.18	230	1.52	1.5	N_2
10	3.76	15	0.355	—	N_2
25	3.76	185	2	1.98	N_2
—	0.3	10,000	0.150	—	Vac
6	0.012	—	0.040	0.030	Air
25	3.18	5	0.254	—	N_2
40	3.55	12.5	0.457	0.229	N_2
42.5	3.4	12.5	0.254	—	N_2
45	6.35	30	0.457	0.203	Air
42.5	3.4	370	1.51	1.49	Air
45	6.35	1000	1.52	1.5	Air
80	3.18	220	1.52	1.5	N_2
100	3	—	0.25	—	N_2
100	5	30	0.5	—	N_2
200	12	120	0.85	1.14	N_2
100	2.7	10	0.6	0.95	N_2
20	0.7	2	0.080	0.070	—

Angled and Shaped Hole Drilling

The versatility of the laser as a tool provides a high degree of control to change process parameters. For example, pulse energy, pulse repetition rate and focal length of the lens can be varied to produce holes with less taper and better uniformity. Pulse shaping can also be used to improve tapering effects. Recent developments include use of a beam forming system, equipped with a slit stage or mask, that extracts the optimum part of the beam mode intensity distribution. The output laser beam available from such a system contains a uniform intensity distribution, which produces micro-fine holes with diameters as small as a few micrometers (11).

Another major advantage of laser drilling is its ability to produce a wide range of shapes and angled hole patterns in a host of materials. Hole drilling angles less than 10 degrees with respect to the work surface in ceramic and plastic materials are reported (12). Unusually shaped holes such as cup shaped, angular, square, elliptical, conical, funnel-shaped, and counter-bored holes can be engineered into difficult-to-machine materials. In addition, appropriate CNC programming can readily provide custom-designed 2-½D and 3D structures around the entrance side of the holes. An application of these types of holes can be found in nozzles with nonlinear tapered holes to aid the laminar flow of the droplet through the orifice or to create a rifled tapered hole that spins the droplet to aid its accuracy of trajectory (13). Chamfering the end-tips of the ceramic tubes for easy wire entry in wire bonding applications and around the circumference to prepare slanted edges are interesting approaches. More ingenious shapes such as these along with the beam splitting and hybrid systems comprising multiple laser sources are being employed for unique drilling applications.

References

1. W. Koechner, *Solid-State Laser Engineering,* Springer Verlag, Heidelberg, Germany (1996).
2. R. W. Frye and D. H. Polk, *Laser welding, machining, and material processing,* Proceedings of the ICALEO'85, 11–14 November 1985, San Francisco, CA, USA.
3. E. Tasev, G. Delacretaz, and L. Woste, Proceedings of the SPIE conference on Laser surgery: *Advanced Characterization, Therapeutics and Systems II* **1200**, 437–45, (1990).
4. M. U. Islam, *Advanced Performance Materials* **3**, 215–38 (1996).
5. E. Gofuku, et al., *Applied Surface Science* **64**, 353–60 (1993).
6. D. Belforte and M. Levitt (Eds.), *The Industrial Laser Handbook,* PennWell Books, Tulsa, Oklahoma, 116–20 (1986).
7. W. Duley, *Laser Processing and Analysis of Materials,* Plenum Press, New York, Chapter 2 (1983).
8. B. N. Chichkov, et al., *Applied Physics A* **63**, 109–15 (1996).
9. B. Craig, *Laser Focus World,* 79–88 (September 1998).
10. H. Varel, et al., *Applied Physics A* **65**, p. 367 (1997).
11. "YAG Laser Machining for Drilling Holes of Diverse Shapes," *New Technology Japan* **25:1**. 23–24 (1997).
12. J. J. Benes, *American Machinist,* 78–79 (July 1996).
13. M. Gower, *The Industrial Laser User,* 26–9 (August 1998).

SUWAS K. NIKUMB

13.3.3 CO_2 Laser Drilling

The CO_2 laser output is at 10.6 µm; most nonmetals absorb this wavelength very efficiently. When the output of a pulsed CO_2 laser is focused to a diameter of $\cong$ 0.005 in. (0.125 mm), extremely high irradiance is produced (on the order of 100 megawatts/cm^2).

Pulse energy is determined by laser pulse length and discharge current, and by pulse repetition rate. Typically, pulse lengths used in percussion drilling range from 100 µs to 1 ms. Table 2 gives examples of operating parameters for percussion drilling a variety of materials.

Examples

CO_2 lasers are used widely for drilling a variety of products, both common and esoteric.

When one drills with a CO_2 laser, there are many considerations that have to be taken into account. The size of the laser is determined by the total thickness of the material, and the material type. When one is percussion drilling holes in a single pulse, the en-

Table 2. Drilling of Nonmetals: Examples of Widely Used Processes

Description	Material	Thickness (in.)	Diameter (in.)	Hole drill rate (per sec)	Lens (in. f.l.)	Pulse length (µs)	Rep rate	Average power (W)
Baby bottle nipple	Si rubber	0.060	0.015	5	5.0	200	100 Hz	150
Cigarette filter tipping paper	Paper	0.003	0.002	10,000	2.5	30	10 kHz	200
Carbonless copy paper	Paper	0.005	0.010	5000	2.5	100	5 kHz	250
Aerosol nozzle	Acetate	0.030	0.010	2	5.0	300	200 Hz	150
Medical catheter	Si rubber	0.010	0.035	3	2.5	200	100 Hz	150
Pharmeceutical capsule	Proprietary	0.003	0.020	20	2.5	250	3 kHz	150
Sound abatement septum	Glass/epoxy	0.015	0.010	250	5.0	200	250 Hz	225
Drip irrigation tubing	Polyethylene	0.012	0.010	200	5.0	500	200 Hz	250

ergy per pulse is the determining factor. Energy per pulse is determined by dividing the average power by the repetition rate. The higher the energy per pulse, the deeper and larger the hole that can be produced.

Typical hole diameters for a number of materials and thicknesses can be seen in the table.

The focal position will also have an affect on the hole diameter. When one is drilling in sharp focus, the hole diameter will be the smallest obtainable for that given setup. If one defocuses, the hole diameter can be enlarged. Defocusing can also have an effect on the taper of the hole.

DANA ELZA
STEVEN R. MAYNARD

13.3.4 Excimer Laser Drilling

Excimer Laser Advantages

Excimer lasers offer three significant advantages for drilling applications over lasers that emit in the visible and infrared. First, the short ultraviolet wavelength excimer output can be imaged to a smaller spot size than visible or infrared light. This is because the minimum feature size that can be achieved by an optical system is limited by diffraction, and diffraction increases linearly with wavelength. Thus, excimer lasers offer the inherent capability for drilling smaller, more well defined holes than can be achieved with longer wavelength sources.

The second advantage of excimer lasers derives from the nature of the physical interaction between high energy ultraviolet photons and many solid materials, particularly organic materials. In this interaction, termed "photoablation," ultraviolet photons directly break the molecular bonds holding the material together (14). Surrounding, unilluminated material is virtually unaffected by this nonthermal ("cold") process, resulting in sharply defined, clean features, and virtually no heat-affected zone (HAZ). In contrast, visible and infrared lasers process material by heating it until it is boiled off or vaporized, resulting in peripheral thermal damage and much less precise process control.

Finally, most materials have extremely high absorption in the ultraviolet region. This, together with the short pulse length of excimer lasers, means that the penetration depth of the light is very small. Since each pulse removes only a thin layer of material, drilling depth can be precisely determined by controlling the number of pulses. The shallow penetration also causes underlying material to be unaffected by the laser.

Excimer Laser Drilling Methods

There are various approaches to drilling using excimer lasers; the most common is photomask imaging. In photomask imaging, the laser beam illuminates a mask (called a reticle) containing the pattern to be machined. An optical system images this pattern on to the worksurface, usually at a large reduction ratio, machining the entire pattern at once. The workpiece must usually be exposed to a number of laser pulses in order to achieve the desired effect, because each individual pulse ablates only a thin layer of material. The general advantage of this type of excimer laser processing is submicrometer depth control (by controlling the number of pulses used) as well as high process repeatability. Figure 2 shows the photomask approach.

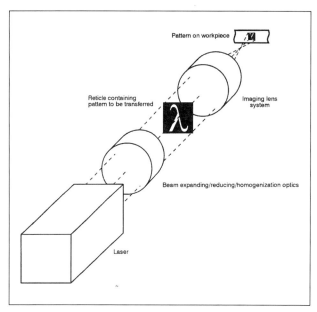

Figure 2. The photomask method of excimer laser drilling.

This drilling method is currently used on manufacturing floors on a high volume scale. The most important applications are the drilling of interconnection holes (vias) for electronic packaging, the drilling of very precise nozzle arrays for ink jet printer heads and in medical device manufacturing. Depending on the needs of the particular application, hundreds to tens of thousands of tiny holes can be drilled in parallel using this method without scanning the beam or moving the workpiece. Today, the precision of these holes, even in volume manufacturing, extends down into the micrometer and submicrometer range.

The key to reproducibly achieving this precision on a production basis is a well designed ultraviolet beam delivery system, consisting of an illumination and an imaging part. Depending on the size relationship between the raw excimer laser output beam and the photomask, the beam may have to be optically expanded or reduced before illuminating the mask. Inherent intensity variations across the profile of excimer laser beams can cause uneven material removal across the pattern being machined. As a result, specialized intensity homogenization optics also have to be incorporated into the mask illumination system. The most efficient design for a homogenizer is based on the "fly eye" principle. Other approaches use diffractive and/or reflective optical designs.

In another method of excimer laser drilling, the entire beam is simply focused or imaged down to a single spot to drill each hole sequentially. Beam and/or part movement is required to produce an array of holes. The primary advantage of this approach is its greater optical simplicity. It is primarily useful for lower throughput applications utilizing a low-energy/high-repetition-rate excimer laser, or for very special material processing applications, such as high precision drilling of ceramics, sapphires, and diamonds.

A third excimer laser drilling method is the multi-beam approach. In this case, the excimer laser beam is divided (by refractive, diffractive, or reflective optical elements) into many of individual beams, up to thousands, each of which drills separate holes.

Excimer Laser Drilling Parameters
Table 3 lists the threshold energy density needed to drill a number of common plastics, ceramics and glasses at one of more excimer laser wavelengths. The rate of material removal per pulse at a given energy density is also tabulated.

References
14. V. Mayne-Banton and R. Srinivasan, *Applied Physics Letters* **41** (6), 576–8 (1982).

M.C. Gower, 1993, *Excimer lasers, current and future applications in industry and medicine, Laser Processing in Manufacturing*, Chapman & Hall, London.

HEINRICH ENDERT
DIRK BASTING

Table 3. Excimer Laser Drilling Parameters for Various Nonmetals

Material	Optimum laser	Wavelength (nm)	Threshold drilling energy (J/cm²)	Rate of material removal amount (μm/shot)	Rate of material removal energy (J/cm²)	Comments
Polymers						
Polyacetylene	ArF	193	0.06	0.17	1.0	Smooth etch
Polyamide, PA (Nylon 6 and 66)	KrF	193	0.35	0.46	1.5	Smooth at both wavelengths
		248	0.75	1.40	1.6	
Polyetheretherketone, PEEK	XeCl	193	0.25	0.12	0.5	Similar at all wavelengths
(Stabar K)		248	0.20	0.40	2.0	Coned at threshold, smooth above
		308	0.20	0.46	2.0	
Polyetherimide PeI	XeCl	193	0.10	0.15	1.0	Similar at all wavelengths
		248	0.15	0.38	2.3	Coned at threshold, smooth above
		308	0.20	0.62	4.2	
Polyethersulfone PES	KrF	193	0.07	0.17	1.0	Similar at all wavelengths
(Stabar S)		248	0.09	0.55	3.0	Smooth at 0.5–1.0 J/cm²
		308	0.20	1.13	5.6	
Polycarbonate (Makrolon film)	KrF	193	0.10	0.14	1.1	Rippled surfaces, 248 nm
		248	0.10	0.54	1.7	Worse
Polycarbonate (Lexan)	KrF	193	0.05	0.18	1.2	Smoother than Makrolon
		248	0.12	0.32	2.0	
Polyethylene	ArF	193	0.25	0.45	1.6	Smooth etch
Polyethylene terephthalate	XeCl	193	0.03	0.16	0.3	Small surface structures. Poor
PET (Melinex, Mylar)		248	0.10	0.64	2.7	thermal effect at 308 nm
		308	0.20	1.76	2.8	
Polyimide, PI (Kapton)	XeCl	193	0.05	0.14	1.1	Similar at all wavelengths
		248	0.06	0.44	2.8	Coned at threshold, smooth above
		308	0.05	0.63	3.8	
Polymethyl-methacrylate, PMMA	ArF	193	0.05	0.44	0.8	Smooth above 0.6 J/cm²
		248	0.30	4.20	6.0	Melting at 248 nm
Polyparaxylylene	KrF	193	0.08	0.21	1.2	Smooth at both wavelengths
		248	0.10	0.65	2.6	
Polystyrene, PS	ArF	193	0.08	0.13	0.5	Highly structured
Polyurethane PUR	KrF	248	–	1.00	1.5	Smooth above 0.5 J/cm²
Polytetrafluoroethylene PTFE (Teflon)	F₂	157	0.2	0.30	1.20	
Polyvinylchloride PVC	ArF	193	0.05	0.30	0.8	Smooth etch above 0.25 J/cm²
		248	0.15	0.65	2.4	
Polyvinylidene chloride PVDC	ArF	193	0.08	0.38	1.1	Smooth above 0.15 J/cm²
		248	0.40	0.71	2.1	Highly structured
Polyvinylidene fluoride PVDF (Kynar)	ArF	193	0.30	0.60	2.0	Highly structured
Nitrocellulose	ArF	193	0.02	1.50	3.0	Smooth etch
Silicone rubber	ArF	193	0.30	0.30	1.2	Highly structured

Chapter 13: Hole Drilling

Table 3. Excimer Laser Drilling Parameters for Various Nonmetals

Material	Optimum laser	Wavelength (nm)	Threshold drilling energy (J/cm^2)	Rate of material removal amount (μm/shot)	Rate of material removal energy (J/cm^2)	Comments
Polymers (continued)						
Cellulose (paper)	ArF	193	0.20	1.80	2.0	Rough surface
		248	0.60	0.57	2.1	Damaged surface
Cellulose acetate	KrF	248	0.46	1.53	1.4	Smooth
Fiber/epoxy composites						
Glass fiber	XeCl	308	1.0	2.00	10	Clean etching
Carbon fiber	XeCl	308	2.0	1.20	11	Clean etching
Aramid	XeCl	308	1.0	2.00	9	Clean etching
Ceramics						
Alumina (Al$_2$O$_3$)	XeCl	193	1.0	0.08	32	At threshold highly structured,
		248	2.0	0.14	34	appears porous above
		308	3.0	0.22	36	
Alumina (hipped)	XeCl	193	1.0	0.08	30	Smooth for all wavelengths above
		248	2.0	0.16	40	10 J/cm^2
		308	3.0	0.23	42	
Lithium tantalate (LiTaO$_3$)	XeCl	193	2.0	0.18	50	Smooth etch at all wavelengths
		248	1.5	0.20	45	
		308	0.8	0.35	45	
Silicon carbide	XeCl	193	1.5	0.15	30	Cones at low fluences. Ripples
		248	2.0	0.16	34	at higher fluences
		308	2.5	0.32	42	
Silicon carbide (toughened)	ArF	193	1.5	0.15	34	Smooth etch at 193 nm only
		248	2.3	0.14	35	
		308	4.0	0.29	45	
Silicon nitride (Si$_3$N$_4$, hipped)	XeCl	193	1.5	0.21	34	Cones for 248 and 308 nm
		248	2.0	0.20	34	below 5 J/cm^2; ripples higher
		308	2.5	0.35	40	
Silicon nitride (reaction bonded)	KrF	193	0.8	0.26	38	Highly structured near threshold,
		248	1.5	0.27	40	rough at higher fluences
		308	2.5	0.36	38	
Silicon nitride (pressureless sintered)	XeCl	193	1.0	0.22	32	Smooth etches at all wavelengths
		248	1.5	1.00	33	
		308	2.5	0.35	42	
Silicon nitride (gas pressure sintered)	KrF	193	1.0	0.22	32	Highly structured for 248 and
		248	2.0	0.19	32	308 nm at low fluences
		308	3.0	0.33	42	
Silicon nitride (post reaction bonded)	XeCl	193	0.8	0.20	32	Good etches at over 9 J/cm^2
		248	2.0	0.20	34	Cones at lower fluences
		308	3.0	0.36	40	
Silicon nitride (hot pressure sintered)	XeCl	193	0.8	0.19	30	Smooth at low fluence at 193 nm
		248	2.0	1.60	30	
		308	3.0	0.36	44	
SiAlON (α + β)	XeCl	193	0.8	0.17	32	Cones below 5 J/cm^2, smooth
		248	2.0	0.22	38	above
		308	2.5	0.31	42	
Lead zirconate titanate PZT	KrF	248	4.0	0.30	40	Smooth etch
Zirconia (ZrO$_2$)	XeCl	193	1.0	0.14	30	Smooth at all wavelengths
		248	2.0	0.15	30	above 3 J/cm^2
		308	4.0	0.25	39	
Crystals and glasses						
Fused silica (SiO$_2$)	ArF	193	15.0	0.33	30	Poor at all fluences
Borosilicate glass	ArF	193	4.0	0.32	53	Smooth above 7 J/cm^2. Rough
		248	8.0	1.68	43	at 248 and 308 nm
		308	10.0	2.47	66	

Table 3. Excimer Laser Drilling Parameters for Various Nonmetals (concluded)

Material	Optimum laser	Wavelength (nm)	Threshold drilling energy (J/cm²)	Rate of material removal amount (µm/shot)	Rate of material removal energy (J/cm²)	Comments
Crystals and glasses (continued)						
Yttrium aluminum garnet (YAG)	ArF	193	2.0	0.06	13.5	Smooth above 3 J/cm²
Silicon	KrF	193	3.0	0.36	15.0	Smooth
		248	1.0	0.32	12.0	
GaAs	XeCl	193	0.05	0.26	19.0	Smooth etch at all wavelengths
		248	0.1	0.27	15.0	
		308	0.1	0.40	15.0	

13.3.5 Copper Vapor Laser Drilling

The drilling of all kinds of nonmetals is possible using copper vapor lasers (CVL) (see Section 13.2.4 for specifications), although restrictions may exist for the wavelength best suited for a certain material and irradiance.

Glasses

In the case of drilling highly transparent materials with visible laser light, a specific threshold has to be exceeded to achieve optical breakdown at the surface, which precedes the drilling process. For pure quartz glass and laser pulses of 50-ns duration, this threshold is about 2×10^9 W/cm² (corresponding to a focal spot diameter of 30 µm), which lies one order of magnitude above metal thresholds. In increasing the concentration of network transformers, impurities, and combined water molecules, glasses show a significant decrease in the ablation threshold (Table 4). However, the working range of the irradiance has an upper limit because of thermal and mechanical damage on the drill hole entrance as well as on the drill hole walls.

Table 4. Drilling of Different Glasses with Copper Vapor Lasers[a]

Glass	Ablation threshold (W/cm²)	Ablation rate (µm/pulse)
Fused silica	1×10^9	0.18
Soda-lime glass	7×10^8	0.3
Lead glass	5×10^8	0.22

[a]Focal length 120 mm, focal position on the surface

Using optimized parameters, i.e., selecting the appropriate irradiance and setting the focal position exactly on the surface, aspect ratios of more than 250:1 are achievable. One may obtain drilling depths exceeding 5 mm with a diameter of 20 µm. Figure 3 shows cross sections of CVL-drilled holes in quartz glass.

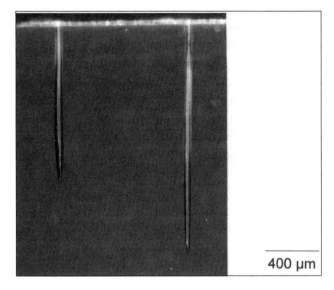

Figure 3. Cross section of CVL-drilled holes in quartz glass: (laser pulses: 5000 (left) and 10,000 (right), pulse power 22.6 kW, focal length $f = 120$ mm, rep. rate 6.5 kHz, focal position on the surface).

Drilling speeds for white sapphire and synthetic ruby typically range from 0.08–0.12 µm/pulse (15).

Ceramics

Compared to metals, drilling ceramics with focused ns-laser pulses with visible wavelength results in a different removal behavior because of the high hardness and brittleness of ceramic materials. Thus, maximum single pulse ablation depths s_1 in ceramics (fired condition) typically are in the range 8–12 µm. With an increasing number of pulses N, an almost linear increase of the drilling depth s_N is observable. According to empirically derived equations (for metals, see Section 13.2.4) a mathematical description of the drilling behavior is possible through an exponential function ($s_N = s_1 \times N^n$). Maximum values for single pulse depths s_1 and the index of the depth gradient n are summarized in Table 5.

Table 5. Drilling of Sintered Ceramics with Copper Vapor Lasers[a]

Ceramic	Max. s_1 (µm)	n
Al_2O_3	8	0.70
AlN	12	0.62
SiC	12	0.62
Si_3N_4	10	0.67
ZrO_2	9	0.71
WC/Co	9	0.65

[a]Pulse power 197 kW, repetition rate 7 kHz, f = 120 mm, focal position on the surface

Typical drilling speeds are in the range 1–5 mm/s when a copper vapor laser is used with a kHz-pulse repetition rate and an average power about 20 W. As is the case with metals, drill hole diameters scale with the pulse power and lie within a range of 20–150 µm for focused ablation. Depending on the focal point position and the Rayleigh-length of the laser beam, drill hole conicities as low as 1% are achievable and even negative values are possible. Small distances between laser drilled holes do not cause problems because the plasma induced mechanical deformation of the bulk material will not occur significantly in sintered ceramics (Fig. 4).

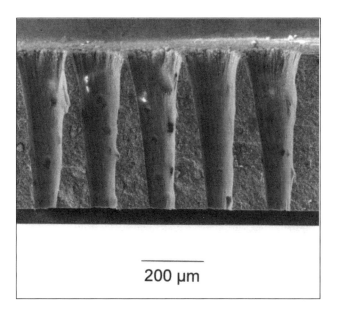

Figure 4. Cross sections of CVL-drilled holes in silicon nitride (thickness s = 500 µm, N = 800 pulses, pulse power 240 kW, focal length f = 300 mm, rep. rate 6.5 kHz, focal position on the surface).

The condition of the drill hole walls is determined by the formation and redeposition of products originating from reactions between the ablated material and the surrounding atmosphere. In the case of drilling silicon nitride, a layer of silicon oxide has been detected (16). Depending on the laser parameters, the layer thickness can vary from submicrometer (beam exit side) to 10 µm (beam entrance). Glassy films on drill hole walls lead to a smooth surface topography and may be removed using chemical etching techniques.

Polymers

Because of a poor absorption of visible radiation in polymers, material ablation with laser beams is generally carried out using infrared (e.g., TEA-CO_2 laser) or ultraviolet radiation (see Section 13.3.4). In the ultraviolet region, excimer lasers and frequency doubled copper vapor lasers (UV-CVL) are utilized for drilling polymers. Table 6 presents typical parameters for drilling of polymers with UV-CVLs (17).

Table 6. Properties of UV-CVLs for Drilling Polymers

Wavelength	255 nm
Repetition rate	4–20 kHz
Pulse length	10–35 ns
Pulse energy	0.03–0.4 mJ
Average power	0.6–1.7 W
Divergence	55 µrad
Focal spot diameter	≥ 10 µm
Energy density	0.08–2.2 J/cm²

Carbon-based and Natural Materials

Copper vapor laser drilling of carbon based materials in air benefits from the fact that ablation products will sublime to carbon oxides during the ablation process. Thus, redeposition of particles on the drill hole walls will not occur. Typical representatives belonging to this class of materials are graphite, diamond, glassy carbon, wood, fabric, and paper. Figure 5 shows a CVL-drilled hole in diamond (diameter 350 µm, percussion drilling) and wooden veneer (thickness 500 µm, drilling and cutting).

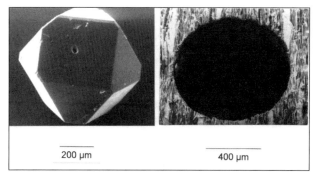

Figure 5. CVL-drilled holes in diamond (left) and wood (right).

Depending on the material structure, such as the bonding type, ablation mechanisms vary from sublimation to mechanical cracking, leading to a restriction of the maximum pulse power applicable for damage free processing of carbon-based materials. Table 7 gives limiting values of the irradiance for different materials.

Table 7. Drilling of Different Carbon-based Materials with CVLs[a]

Material	Irradiance limit (W/cm²)	Max. ablation rates (µm/pulse)
CVD-diamond	$> 2.5 \times 10^{10}$	6
Glassy carbon	$< 4 \times 10^9$	7
Graphite	$< 4 \times 10^9$	9

[a]Spot diameter 30 µm, pulse width 50 ns

As with metals, drill holes in hard carbon-based materials are applied for the production of a defined flow of solids, liquids, or gases. Low-temperature applications of diamonds include the manufacturing of wire drawing dies and printer nozzles for ink jets with monodispersed droplets. Drill holes in glassy carbon are utilized for pressure reduction in high-temperature analyzing systems (Fig. 6).

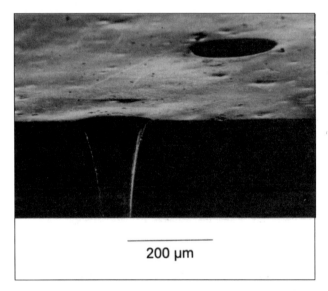

Figure 6. CVL-drilled hole in glassy carbon.

Composite Materials

Composites of different classes of materials (e.g., ceramics and polymers) are widely found as an intermediate stage of powder packed workpieces (e.g., magnets, ceramic substrates, microelectronic components). Generally, because of lower binding forces, drilling of composites in the green state with copper vapor lasers is advantageous as a result of higher ablation rates and superior particle ejection behavior from the drill hole. A promising industrial application is the drilling (and cutting) of low-temperature cofired ceramics for medical implants.

References

15. C. E. Little and N. V. Sabotinov (Eds.), *Pulsed Metal Vapor Lasers,* Kluwer Academic Publishers, Dordrecht, 359–64 (1996).
16. C. Körner, R. Mayerhofer, M. Hartmann, and H. W. Bergmann, "Physical and Material Aspects in Using Visible Laser Pulses of Nanosecond Duration for Ablation," *Applied Physics* **A 63,** 123–31 (1996).
17. A. C. J. Glover, E. K. Illy, M. J. Withford, and J. A. Piper, *Ablation Threshold and Etch Rate Measurements in High-Speed Ultraviolet (UV) Micromachining of Polymers with UV-Copper Vapor Lasers,* Proc. of the Conf. ICALEO´95, San Diego, USA, 361–70 (13–16 November 1995).

ROLAND MAYERHOFER
HANS WILHELM BERGMANN

13.4 Aerospace Applications

13.4.1 Hole Requirements

The dominant application of drilling in the aerospace industry is the drilling of cooling holes in turbine components – blades, vanes, outer air seals, and combustors. Typical requirements for these holes are summarized in Table 1.

Table 1. Typical Hole Requirements

Parameter	Typical value
Angle to surface	15–30 degrees
Diameter	8–40 mil (0.20–1.0 mm)
Configuration	Blind hole with passage or shoulder behind hole
Required metallurgy	Minimal recast, minimal heat-affected zone, no microcracks in parent metal
Hole geometry	Cylindrical or slightly tapered hole with minimal wall roughness and minimal surface burr
Diameter reproducibility	< +/-1% variation

Because the materials typically used in aerospace technology are difficult to machine and because of the inability of conventional drilling to meet the above requirements, laser drilling is widely used.

13.4.2 Laser Type

Pulsed Nd:YAG lasers are usually chosen for drilling of aerospace materials. This choice is driven by the following considerations:

- Good coupling of 1.06-µm radiation into the part (both in terms of material absorption and plasma avoidance).
- Availability of cost-effective, industrialized, pulsed Nd:YAG laser systems with compact laser heads, and with pulse energy (e.g., 10 J), pulse width (e.g, 0.2–1.0 ms) and average power (e.g., 200 W) well-suited to this application.

Chapter 13: Hole Drilling

13.4.3 Typical Focus-Head Arrangement

A typical drilling focus head is shown in Figure 1. In this case, the primary purpose of the assist gas is to protect the cover slide from spatter.

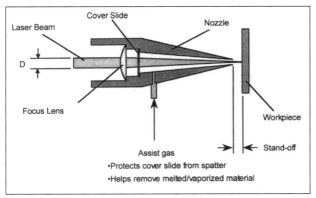

Figure 1. Typical focus-head arrangement for laser drilling.

13.4.4 Percussion Drilling

Hole Diameter: For small diameters (e.g., 8–30 mils), holes are usually percussion drilled, with the part maintained stationary relative to the focal spot and with multiple pulses used to create the hole through the part. For percussion drilling of high-aspect-ratio holes (large l/d), typical of aerospace applications, the hole size is determined by a rather complex combination of parameters, shown schematically in Figure 2.

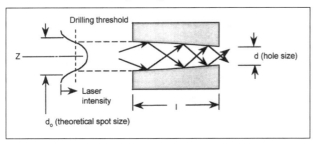

Figure 2. Hole size parameters.

The nominal hole diameter d depends on the following parameters:

- d_o (theoretical spot size)
- Beam intensity profile at focus
- Drilling threshold
- Number of pulses
- Attenuation characteristics of walls
- Waveguiding characteristics of walls
- Optical depth of focus
- Location of focus along Z
- Dynamics of material removal process

The theoretical spot size d_o is given by the expression

$$d_o = M^2 \frac{4}{\pi} \frac{f\lambda}{D}$$

where M^2 is the beam quality factor, and D is the beam diameter at the focus lens. The drilling threshold is the irradiance at which material is vaporized and is material dependent.

In practice, the hole size is set empirically by adjusting the various parameters in order to obtain the desired hole size while optimizing other hole characteristics such as recast and taper. Once an initial set of parameters is obtained, the hole size is typically fine tuned by adjusting D (e.g., with a variable-magnification beam expander) and/or by adjusting the pulse energy (peak power).

Metallurgy: Recent studies (1) have shown that laser hole quality (taper, recast, and parent metal damage) is significantly affected by the laser pulse duration and peak intensity. Plots of average recast in a high-nickel alloy versus peak power (1) are presented in Figure 3. The general trend is for reduced recast with increasing peak power. Figure 4 shows the relationship between average recast and pulse duration, independent of peak power. Pulse durations < 100 ns show a slight minimum in average recast.

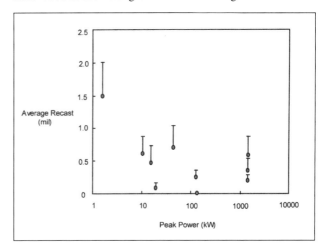

Figure 3. Average recast versus peak power.

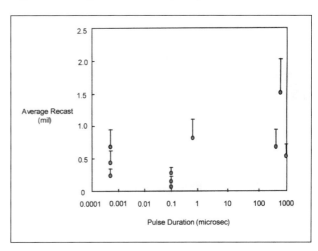

Figure 4. Average recast versus pulse duration.

Typical Parameters: While the majority of production drilling is currently carried out with pulse durations of 0.5–1.5 ms, recent studies have shown the advantages of using short, high-intensity pulses (1–4). Representative holes in high-nickel alloy (Waspalloy), obtained with a more advanced pulse format (2), are shown in Figure 5, with the laser pulse format and beam-focus geometry shown schematically in Figure 6. This pulse format was obtained by installing a commercial acousto-optic modulator in the laser optical cavity, with an intracavity aperture used to set the cavity Fresnel number. Detailed laser parameters are listed in Table 2.

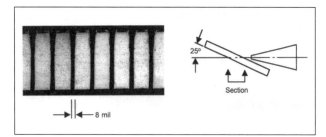

Figure 5. Percussion drilled holes.

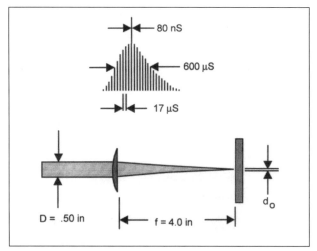

Figure 6. Laser pulse parameters.

Table 2. Drilling Parameters

Parameter	Value
Laser	Raytheon SS-500 pulsed Nd:YAG
Optical cavity	Stable cavity (2 m between cavity mirrors), with 6 mm intracavity aperture and an intracavity acousto-optic modulator (Neos)
Near-field beam profile	Round beam, "bell-shaped" intensity profile
M^2 (beam quality factor)	19
Total pulse energy	2.6 J (total energy in macropulse)
Micropulse energy	0.075 J (ave energy per spike)

Table 2. Drilling Parameters (continued)

Parameter	Value
Macropulse repetition rate	5 Hz
Theoretical spot size	8 mil
Nozzle stand-off	0.5 in
Assist gas	Shop air
Focus location	At surface of part
Number of macropulses	Approx. 20 for breakthrough, approx. 40 total
Surface preparation	No anti-spatter on front surface, no backer on back surface
Post-laser cleanup	None

Figure 5 illustrates holes with good reproducibility and with minimal recast where the laser exits the hole (bottom). In practice, the recast/burr seen at the hole entrance would be reduced by applying an anti-spatter coating to the surface (e.g., a boron-nitride solution) and by using post-drilling cleanup (e.g., grit blasting).

13.4.5 Trepan Drilling

For larger holes (e.g., > 30 mil), the part and focus spot may be moved relative to one another in order to "cut" the desired hole, a process known as trepanning. This motion can be achieved by articulating the part, by precessing the focus lens or by tilting the beam into the focus lens. For the fabrication of cooling holes in aerospace parts, trepan drilling is very similar to percussion drilling, with the addition of motion of the part relative to the beam focus. For the conditions of Table 1, pulsed, high-intensity pulses are desirable in order to achieve clean, high-aspect-ratio cuts (4), and pulsed Nd:YAG lasers are again used. In practice, the pulse energy must usually be increased over its percussion value in order to clear the material from the larger diameter hole. In addition, the gas assist jet plays a more important role, particularly for holes through open structures (e.g., combustor liners).

References

1. T. J. Rockstroh, X. Chen, and W. T. Lotshaw, ICALEO '96 Proceedings **81**, C/113–22 (1996).
2. R. T. Brown and R. W. Frye, ICALEO '96 Proceedings **81**, C/78–85 (1996).
3. X. Chen, W. T. Lotshaw, A. L. Ortiz, P. R. Staver, C. E. Erikson, M. H. McLaughlin, and T. J. Rockstroh, *Journal of Laser Applications* **8**, 233–9 (1996).
4. X. Chen, A. L. Ortiz, P. R. Staver, W. T. Lotshaw, T. J. Rockstroh, and M. H. McLaughlin, *Journal of Laser Applications* **9**, 287–90 (1997).

ROBERT T. BROWN

Chapter 13: Hole Drilling

13.5 Ultrashort-Pulse Laser Machining

13.5.0 Introduction

Conventional mechanical lathes and machine tools are effective for machining simplified shapes (cutting, drilling) in metals down to approximately 200 µm (8 mil) kerf width at depths of approximately 1 mm (aspect ratio < 5:1). For finer features or irregular shapes, electron beam, electron discharge (EDM), or conventional laser tools are typically used. Conventional laser tools such as those based on CO_2, Nd:YAG, or copper vapor lasers machine materials by localized heating. Both EDM and existing industrial laser technology heat the material to the melting or boiling point, resulting in thermal stress to the remaining material and often a heat-affected zone. Higher precision or higher aspect ratio (e.g., 100-µm holes through 1-mm steel) is difficult to achieve with these techniques. Furthermore, nonmetals (e.g., ceramics, SiC, diamond, sapphire, bone, etc.) are very difficult to machine using EDM or conventional laser processing. Laser processing by molecular dissociation in organic (and some inorganic) materials can be achieved with ultraviolet lasers (e.g., excimer lasers-KrF, XeCl), but this photodissociation mechanism is not applicable to metals.

By using ultrashort ($\tau < 10$ ps) laser pulses *any* material can be machined to very high precision. The ability to machine any material including high bandgap dielectrics such as SiC, diamond, etc., is a result of the fact that these ultrashort pulses interact by a mechanism that is very different from that of conventional longer pulse lasers. This interaction is independent of the usual linear absorption properties of the material and is applicable to materials that would otherwise be transparent to the laser wavelength. Machining to a micrometer scale (< 0.1 mil) precision with no collateral damage to the remaining material is achieved by removing material faster than heat can be conducted to the bulk. Ultrashort pulse lasers have been described in Section 2.5.9.

13.5.1 Dielectrics

By dielectrics, we are generally referring to materials with no free electrons and low thermal/electrical conductivity. Common materials such as fused silica, sapphire, SiC, diamond, SiN, AlTiC, ZrO_2, glass, plastic, bone, cornea, heart tissue, etc., would fall in this category. Semiconductors such as silicon and gallium arsenide would generally not be considered dielectrics by this definition. However, these materials behave similarly to dielectrics when machining with ultrashort laser pulses.

Attempts to machine dielectrics with lasers followed shortly after laser induced damage was observed in transparent solids (1). For pulses longer than a few tens of picoseconds, the generally accepted picture of damage to dielectrics involves the heating of seed electrons by the incident radiation and transfer of this energy to the lattice. Damage occurs via conventional heat deposition resulting in melting and boiling of the dielectric material. Because the controlling rate is that of thermal conduction through the lattice, this model predicts a $\tau^{1/2}$ dependence of the threshold fluence (energy/area) on pulse duration τ (2), in reasonably good agreement with numerous experiments that have observed a τ^α scaling with $0.4 < \alpha < 0.5$ in a variety of dielectric materials from

100 ps to ms (3). With these conventional lasers, material is removed by thermal ablation, wherein the material is locally heated to near the boiling point. Because the boiling point of these materials is very high (typically > 1000°C), this ablation mechanism is accompanied by a strong thermal shock to the remaining bulk material. This thermal shock often results in cracking of the remaining material and uncontrolled material removal. These effects can be observed in Figure 1, where the initial stages of hole drilling in a tooth using a conventional Nd:YAG laser are shown. In Figure 1a, linear absorption because of defects produces inhomogeneous energy absorption across the laser beam. Thermal stresses increase to the point where ablation begins first from the point with the least material strength.

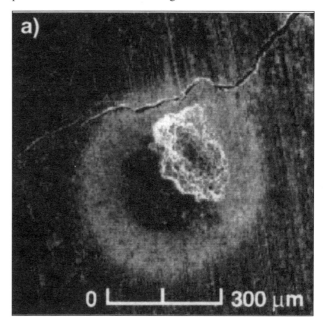

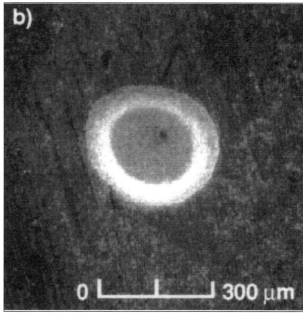

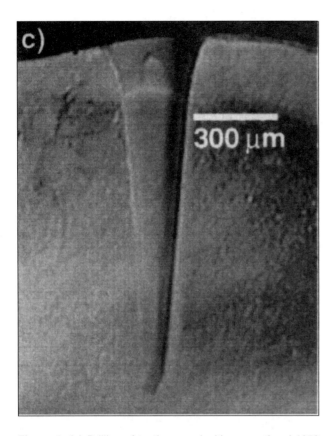

Figure 1. (a) Drilling of tooth enamel with conventional 1053 nm, nanosecond pulses (ablation threshold = 30 J/cm² for τ_p = 2 ns). (b) Same as in (a) but with the pulse duration reduced to the ultrashort regime (ablation threshold = 3 J/cm² for τ_p = 0.35 ps). In both cases, the laser spot size was 300 μm. (c) Cross section of hole made with 350-fs pulses.

It had been postulated that the $\tau^{1/2}$ dependence of the laser damage threshold for dielectrics would break down for pulse durations less than a few picoseconds as the probability of multiphoton ionization of the individual atoms within the dielectric became significant. To quantify the transition from a thermal mechanism of damage to one associated with direct ionization, the authors began a systematic study of the damage threshold in a variety of dielectric materials. In all dielectrics that were examined, a strong deviation from the $\tau^{1/2}$ dependence of the damage threshold was observed. This deviation occurred in a range 10 ps (SiO_2) to ≈ 20 ps (CaF_2) as shown in Figure 2 (4).

In all cases, the deviation was accompanied by a dramatic change in morphology of the damaged surface (Fig. 1b). With femtosecond pulses, all regions throughout the laser beam profile with sufficient intensity for multiphoton ionization will be removed resulting in extremely fine control of the position of material removal. In addition, the morphology of the surface drilled with femtosecond pulses is characteristic of the internal enamel and dentin. There is no evidence of heat transfer into the surrounding material and no thermal shock cracking in any of the surrounding material (Fig. 1c).

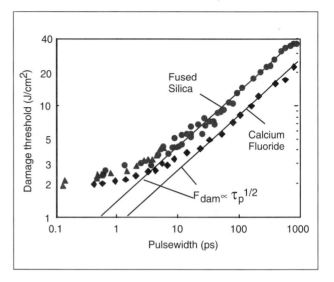

Figure 2. Observed values of damage threshold at 1053 nm for fused silica (●) and CaF_2 (◆). Solid lines are $\tau^{1/2}$ fits to long pulse results. Estimated absolute error in data is ± 15%.

Both the change in surface morphology and the deviation from the $\tau^{1/2}$ dependence of the damage threshold on pulse duration are predicted by a rapid ionization mechanism (4). Fused silica will be considered in greater detail in order to describe the model with a specific material.

Damage occurs at a threshold of ≈ 2 J/cm² for a 1-ps pulse (see Fig. 2). With an irradiance of 2x10¹² W/cm², there is no need to invoke some arbitrary number of initial "seed" electrons. Field-induced multiphoton ionization produces free electrons which are then rapidly accelerated by the laser pulse. For these very short, intense pulses, energy is gained by the newly free electrons from the laser field much faster than it is transferred from the electrons to the lattice. These electrons gain energy from the laser field until they have sufficient energy to collisionally ionize neighboring atoms thereby producing more free electrons. This process continues until a critical density plasma is reached wherein no further energy deposition from the laser occurs. The actual damage occurs after the pulse has passed, when the dense plasma expands away from the surface.

Plasma formation is quantitatively described by the time dependence of the electron energy distribution function.

Figure 3 (next page) shows the evolution of electron density for a 10-TW/cm², 100-fs pulse incident on fused silica as calculated based on the model. The temporal profile of the laser pulse and the electron density produced by multiphoton ionization alone are included for reference. Because multiphoton ionization is strongly intensity dependent, the electron production takes place principally at the peak of the pulse. For this 100-fs duration, multiphoton ionization produces a substantial amount of free electrons. When the electron density produced by multiphoton ionization approaches $\approx 10^{17}$ cm^{-3}, the collisional ionization rate begins to exceed the multiphoton ionization rate. Once a high free electron density is produced by mutliphoton ionization the material no longer has the properties of a dielectric. It is now a conductor and will absorb the laser via inverse Bremstrahlung (Joule) heating similarly to a metal. *It is for this reason that both dielectrics and metals have similar behavior and morphology when machined with ultrashort pulses.* In essence, the dielectric is converted to a metallic state within the first few tens of femtoseconds. As the laser intensity decreases past the peak of the pulse, the driving force for both multiphoton and collisional ionization ceases and the free electron density remains constant.

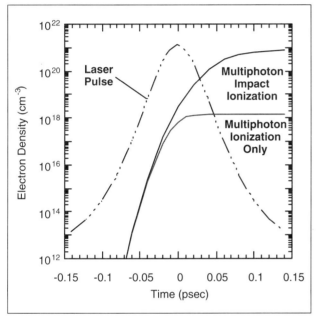

Figure 3. Calculated evolution of free electron density for a 100-fs, 1053-nm pulse (dashed curve) of peak irradiance = 10 TW/cm^2 in fused silica. The total electron density including impact ionization and that due to multiphoton ionization alone are shown for comparison.

For laser pulses of different duration, the relative fraction of multiphoton ionization to avalanche ionization will change. Multiphoton ionization will contribute a relatively greater fraction of the electron density with shorter pulses while avalanche ionization will dominate with longer pulses. In all cases, the electron density saturates at the critical density, N_c. The critical density is the density at which the plasma frequency, ω_{pe}(rad/s) = $(4\pi N_e e^2/m)^{1/2}$ = $[2.21 \times 10^8 \, N_e(\text{cm}^{-3})]^{1/2}$ is equal to the laser frequency, $\omega = 2\pi c/\lambda$. The critical density may be written as $N_c = (\pi m_e c^2/e^2\lambda^2)$. At a laser wavelength of 1064 nm, $N_c = 0.98 \times 10^{21}$ cm^{-3}. Note that the ratio $N_e/N_c = \omega_{pe}^2/\omega^2$. The critical density plays an extremely important role in the interaction of electromagnetic waves with plasmas. Once the electron density reaches the critical value, very little electromagnetic energy is transmitted.

Formation of a critical density plasma has an important effect in

materials processing with short pulse lasers. Once the critical surface is formed, laser energy is either absorbed at that surface or reflected from it. For most plasmas, there is strong absorption at the critical surface since the scale length, L, is equal to or greater than the wavelength of the incident light, $L > \lambda$. Now, the maximum scale length is $L_{max} = v_s \tau_p$ where the ion sound velocity, v_s = $(ZkT_e/m_{ion})^{1/2} \approx 6 \times 10^5$ cm/sec. Since the pulses of interest here are < 10 ps, the maximum scale length is $L_{max} \approx 0.1$ µm which is much less than the incident wavelength. In the limit that $L \ll \lambda$, electromagnetic waves are reflected from the critical surface and not absorbed. In Figure 4, we show the reflectivity of a normally transparent fused silica surface as a function of incident laser intensity. Near the damage threshold ($\approx 10^{13}$ W/cm^2), critical density is not produced until late in the pulse (Fig. 3). Only the last part of the laser pulse will experience any strong reflection. However, by operating high above threshold, critical density is achieved early in the pulse and reflectivities exceeding 90% can be obtained.

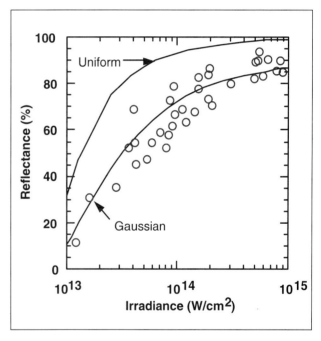

Figure 4. Reflectivity of fused silica surface as a function of laser irradiance for λ = 1053 nm and τ_p = 350 fs. Calculated reflectivities using the model described in the text for a Gaussian and uniform beam are shown for comparision.

The damage threshold of fused silica calculated according to the plasma model just described is compared to measured damage thresholds at both 526 and 1053 nm from 10 fs to over 10 ps in Figure 5 (next page). The theoretical damage fluence defining damage as the point at which the free electron density reaches the plasma critical density ($\approx 10^{21}$ cm^{-3}) is calculated with no adjustable parameters (see Fig. 5, solid lines). Because of the rapid avalanche following production of the seed electrons by multiphoton ionization, the predicted damage threshold is only weakly dependent on the actual free electron density at which damage occurs. A lower limit would correspond to the condition that the energy density of the conduction electrons equals the binding energy of the lattice ($\approx 10^{19}$ cm^{-3}). Use of this lower limit serves only to reduce the predicted damage threshold by $\approx$ 20%. In addition to the good agreement with the measurements presented here, experiments by Auderbert (6), von der Linde (7), Kautek (8), and Kraucsz (9), are also in good agreement with our calculations but not those of Du (5). For pulses less than 100 fs, the predicted damage threshold asymptotically approaches the multiphoton limit. In the long-pulse regime ($\tau > 20$ ps), the data fit well to a $\tau^{1/2}$ dependence, characteristic of transfer of electron kinetic energy to the lattice and diffusion during the pulse. The damage is thermal in nature and characterized by melting and boiling of the surface. For long pulses, heating of the lattice and subsequent thermal damage can occur without significant collisional ionization.

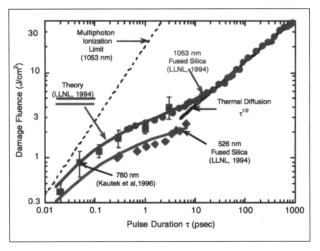

Figure 5. Measured and calculated damage thresholds of fused silica in the infrared and visible (526 nm). Deviation from $\tau^{1/2}$ scaling below $\approx$ 10 ps indicates the transition to an ionization dominated damage mechanism. The calculated threshold for ablation by multiphoton ionization alone is shown as the dashed line. Data is taken from References 4 and 5.

A significant feature of this nonthermal material removal mechanism is that since there is minimal energy deposition in the remaining material, there is a minimal increase in temperature. Thermal measurements show that when irradiated with conventional nanosecond laser pulses, the bulk temperature of a 1-mm slice of tooth increased by over 40°C while for femtosecond pulses the temperature rise was less than 2°C (Fig. 6). The fluence in each case was set to remove approximately 1 µm depth of material per pulse. This required 30 J/cm^2 for the nsec pulses and only 3 J/cm^2 for the fs pulses. The practical consequences in dentistry are substantial. In the case of existing laser systems, active cooling of the tooth is necessary to prevent permanent damage to the pulp and nerves, which occurs at an increase of $\approx$ 5°C over body temperature. With ultrashort laser pulses, no cooling would be necessary.

Another dramatic example is the machining of explosives with ultrashort laser pulses. Cutting and machining operations on energetic materials present significant safety challenges. With conventional machine tools, improper fixturing of the work, improper tool configuration and improper cutting speeds have resulted in violent reactions during machining operations. Conventional laser pulses are often used to ignite explosives. However, with femtosecond pulses, plasma formation and material removal occur too fast for significant energy transfer to the remaining material. Furthermore, since only a small amount of material is removed per laser pulse ($\approx$ 3 µm), there is negligible shock imparted to the remaining material. The shock wave that does exist decays to an insignificant level within $\approx$ 1 µm of the surface. The waste products from short-pulse laser cutting are, for the most part, solid carbon or benign gases, which can be released into the atmosphere.

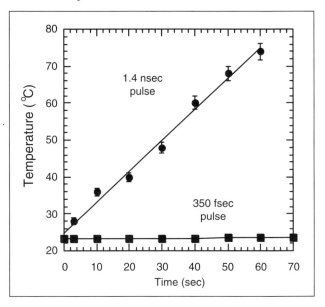

Figure 6. Temperature increase of bulk tooth due to drilling with 1.4-ns (circles) and 350-fs (squares) laser pulses. In both cases, the laser wavelength was 1053 nm, and the spot size was 300 µm. The fluence was adjusted to achieve a material removal rate of 1 µm/pulse at 10 Hz for both pulse durations.

We have machined a variety of high explosives including LX-14 (95.5% HMX/4.5% Estane), LX-15 (95% HNS/5% Kel-F), LX-16 (96%PETN/4%FPC 461), LX-17 (92.5% TATB/7.5% Kel-F), PBX-9407 (94% RDX/6% Exon 461), and pressed TNT. In some of the experiments, the beam first cut through the explosive and then into a stainless steel substrate, and in other experiments the beam first cut through stainless steel and then into the explosive. Figure 7 (next page) shows two cuts across a 1-cm diameter, 2-mm thick pellet made using a 1-kHz, 100-fs Ti:Sapphire laser system. Fourier Transform Infrared Spectroscopy of the laser cut LX-16 surface showed no evidence of any chemical reaction products. The laser cut surface was chemically identical to the original LX-16 material. We also observed very high aspect ratio cuts and holes ($\approx$ 1000:1) in high explosives. When we used pulses only modestly in the conventional regime

(600 ps) deflagration of the LX-16 pellet was immediately observed (Fig. 7b). Examination of the pellet afterward revealed that the edges of the cut were melted and contained a multitude of reaction products consistent with thermally induced ignition.

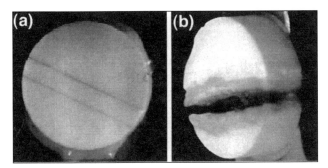

Figure 7. Cuts in explosive pellet (PETN) by a Ti:Sapphire laser operating at 120 fs (a) and 0.6 ns (b). Thermal deposition in the long-pulse case caused the pellet to ignite.

In summary for dielectric materials, there is a strong deviation from the usual $\tau^{1/2}$ scaling of laser damage fluence for pulses below 10 ps. The damage threshold continues to decrease with decreasing pulsewidth, but at a rate slower than $\tau^{1/2}$ in the range 0.1–10 ps. As the pulses become shorter than ≈ 0.1 ps, the increasing influence of multiphoton ionization results in a rapid decrease of the damage threshold. Multiphoton ionization provides an upper limit to the damage fluence for short pulses preventing any increase in damage threshold with decreasing pulse duration as might be predicted from a pure avalanche model. This new mechanism of damage (material removal) is accompanied by a qualitative change in the morphology of the interaction site. The damage site is limited to only a small region where the laser intensity is sufficient to produce a plasma with essentially no collateral damage. This process enables high precision machining of all dielectrics with no thermal shock or distortion of the remaining material. Although the absolute damage fluence varies, all pure dielectrics (oxides, fluorides, explosives, plastics, glasses, ceramics, etc.) exhibit similar behaviour. All dielectrics share the same general properties of slow thermal diffusion and an electron-phonon scattering rate slower than the rate at which energy is absorbed from the field by the free electrons. All dielectrics should therefore exhibit similar short-pulse machining characteristics.

13.5.2 Metals

Metals are machined either with abrasive techniques (lathes, saws, drills), or by localized thermal processing (conventional lasers, electron beam, plasma, or acetylene torch, etc.). The basic interaction in localized thermal processing is the deposition of energy from the incident beam in the material of interest in the form of heat (lattice vibrations). In the case of the laser, the absorption of energy is dependent on the optical properties of the metal. The laser energy that is absorbed results in a temperature increase at and near the absorption site. The magnitude and spatial extent of the temperature achieved during the laser pulse is strongly dependent on the thermomechanical properties of the metal. As the temperature increases to the melting or boiling point, material is removed by conventional melting or vaporization (10).

Depending on the pulse duration of the laser, the temperature rise in the irradiated zone may be very fast resulting in thermal ablation and shock. The irradiated zone may be vaporized or simply may ablate because of the fact that the local thermal stress has become larger than the yield strength (thermal shock). Plasma formation may even result in the vaporized plume. In all these cases, there is an impact on the material surrounding the site where material has been removed. The surrounding material will have experienced a large temperature excursion or shock often resulting in significant change to the material properties. These changes may range from a change in grain structure to an actual change in composition. Such compositional changes include oxidation (if cut in air) or, in the case of alloys, changes in composition of the alloy. This heat-affected zone may range from a few micrometers to millimeters depending on the thermomechanical properties of the metal, laser pulse duration, and other factors (e.g., active cooling). In many applications, the presence of the heat- or shock-affected zone may be severely limiting because the material properties of this zone may be quite different than that of the bulk. Furthermore, small scale devices (features on the order of a few tens of micrometers) cannot tolerate the thermal stress induced in the material during the machining process.

Another limitation of conventional laser or electron beam processing in certain applications is the lack of precision and the presence of redeposited or resolidified material. As mentioned previously, cutting or drilling occurs by either melting or vaporizing the material of interest. The surface adjacent to the removed area will have experienced significant thermal loading often resulting in melting. This melting can be accompanied by flow prior to solidification. This can result in the deposition of slag surrounding the kerf (Fig. 8a, next page), which in many high-precision applications is unacceptable. Also, the resolidification process is not uniform resulting in a lack of precision in the machined surface. In the cases where the deposition of conventional slag can be prevented, redeposition of vaporized material on the walls or upper surface of the kerf is common. This condensate often reduces the quality of the cut and decreases the cutting efficiency since the beam must again remove this condensate before interacting with the bulk material underneath. Many of these limitations can be reduced by the use of secondary techniques to aid the cutting process. The most common of these are active cooling of the material of interest either during or immediately following the laser pulse, and the use of high-pressure gas jets to remove vaporized or molten material from the vicinity of the cut. These techniques can be effective at improving the kerf at the cost of an increase in system complexity and often a decrease in cutting efficiency.

As in the case of dielectrics, ultrashort-pulses enable the laser cutting/machining of metals and alloys with high machining speed, extreme precision, negligible heat-affected zone, and no modification to the material surrounding the kerf. Unlike dielectrics however, there is no multiphoton ionization step necessary because the metal already contains "free" electrons in the conduction band. These electrons will absorb the laser light via inverse Bremstrahlung heating (collisional absorption) as described previously. A Fokker-Planck equation can be established to describe the energy transfer from the electrons to the lattice (electron-phonon coupling) and heat transfer directly by electron conduction away from the absorption site. Historically, this situation has been described by a simple two temperature model for the ion and electron temperatures (11). Since on the time scales of interest, the temperature gradients in transverse dimensions are negligible relative to that in the longitudinal dimension, a one-dimensional description is adequate.

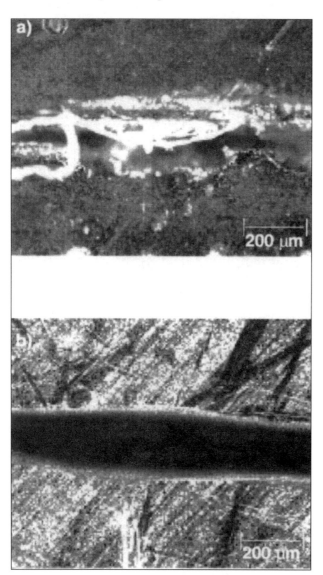

Figure 8. Cuts in stainless steel performed with 1054-nm laser pulses with a duration of (a) 1.4 ns at a fluence of 52 J/cm² and (b) 350 fs and 14 J/cm². The fluence was adjusted to achieve a material removal rate of 0.5 μm/pulse in both cases.

A solution based on this model in the limit of fast equilibration between the ions and electrons for gold irradiated at 1053 nm and 0.5 J/cm² is given in Figure 9. The thermal penetration depth achieved during the pulse $L_{th} = 2\,(\alpha\tau)^{1/2}$ is less than one micrometer. Here α is the thermal diffusivity. This leads to a very small amount of material (0.01–1 μm) heated to above the boiling point with extremely small transport of energy either by shock or thermal conduction away from the volume of interest. For pulses with a duration below the characteristic energy transfer time between electrons and the lattice, the model predicts a damage threshold that no longer scales as $\tau^{1/2}$ as is predicted by a conventional thermal mechanism of damage. Instead, the damage threshold is predicted to be *essentially independent of pulse duration* (12). This behavior is observed in all metals which we have investigated. Figure 10 (next page) shows the damage threshold of gold measured at 1053 nm. The essential constancy of the damage threshold below ≈ 80 ps is readily observed and the data is well fit by the two temperature model with the rate γ that energy is dissipated to the lattice via phonons is $\gamma = 3.5 \times 10^{11}$ W/cm³-K.

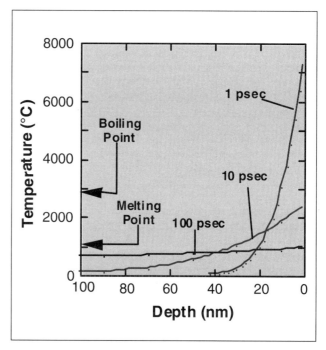

Figure 9. Calculated temperature profiles in gold irradiated at 1054 nm and a fluence of 0.5 J/cm² for 1, 10, and 100 ps pulses.

For real machining applications, the surface of the metal is heated far beyond its boiling point and the simple two temperature model breaks down. Instead, a full radiative hydrodynamic model which accounts for plasma formation, multiple ionization, material equation of state, and shock wave generation and cooling by radiation, conduction and plasma expansion is required. A one-dimensional Euler-Lagrangian code was developed for this purpose (14). The predicted pressure and temperature of aluminum irradiated in the ultrashort-pulse regime (350 fs) and the conventional (ns) regime are given in Figures 11–13. For the femtosecond pulse focused to 5 J/cm² (1.4x10¹³ W/cm²), the absorbed laser energy heats the a skin depth of the material to ≈ 12.5 eV (Fig. 11a). In the next few picoseconds, this energy is dissipated into the bulk by both shock and electron conduction and is also dissipated by the initial plasma expansion off the surface and radiation. A depth of ≈ 0.1 µm is heated to near 1 eV. This material blows off the surface with a static expansion velocity of 2x10⁶ cm/s over the next nanosecond (Fig. 12a). Note that the solid which is left behind remains essentially at room temperature even within ≈ 1 µm of the machined surface. The initial shock wave launched into the material is large reaching 2 mbar. This shock propagates with a velocity equal to 6x10⁵ cm/s but dissipates rapidly in magnitude. The pressure associated with the shock drops to less than 100 kbar (less than the yield strength of the material) within the first micrometer (Fig. 12). This offers extremely high-precision machining with no heat- or shock-affected zone extending beyond ≈ 1 µm of the machined surface. In the case of a 1 ns pulse, the majority of the laser energy is absorbed in the expanding plasma. The energy that strikes the surface heats a depth of ≈ 2 µm to the boiling point and a few micrometers to the melting point (Fig. 13). For the even longer pulses more typical of laser machining, the temperatures achieved are below the ionization threshold, and standard thermal models that only account for melting and boiling are adequate.

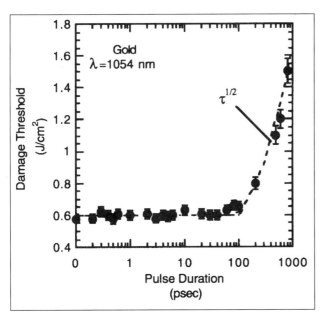

Figure 10. Damage threshold of gold at 1054 nm as a function of pulse duration, from Reference 13.

The lack of significant energy deposition beyond the volume of interest achieved by using ultrashort pulses enables the use of high repetition (0.1–100 kHz) lasers without the need for external cooling of the part being machined. Even though only a very small depth of material is removed per pulse, the high repetition rate enables extremely high cut rates (beyond 1 mm depth per second). Another feature of the very short pulse duration is the fact that there is no vaporization or transport of material during the pulse (Fig. 11). During the pulse, there is insufficient time for hydrodynamic expansion of the vaporized material. As a result, the laser encounters the solid surface for the duration of the pulse depositing energy into solid density material.

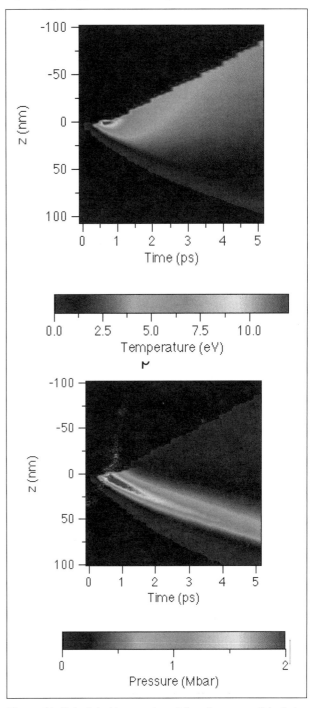

Figure 11. Calculated temperature (a) and pressure (b) of aluminum irradiated by 1053-nm, 350-fs laser pulses at a fluence of 5 J/cm².

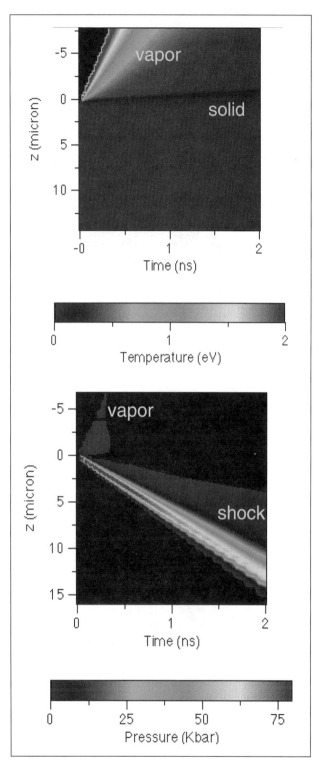

Figure 12. Calculated temperature (a) and pressure (b) of aluminum following irradiation by 1053-nm, 350-fs laser pulses at a fluence of 5 J/cm². The calculation is carried out to two nanoseconds showing plasma blowoff and decay of the shock wave.

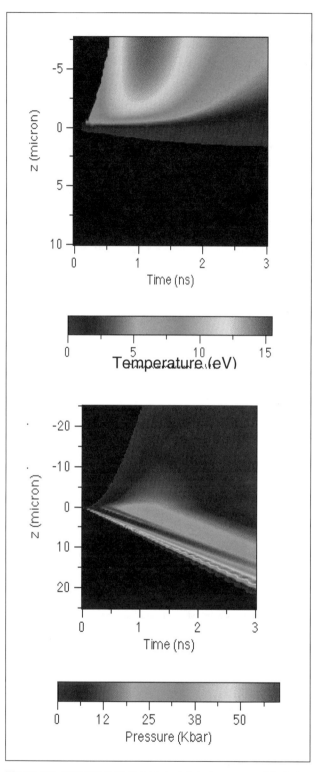

Figure 13. Calculated temperature (a) and pressure (b) of aluminum following irradiation by a 1053-nm, 1-ns laser pulse at a fluence of 20 J/cm² (same depth of material removed as in Figure 12).

While the typical temperatures achieved at the damage threshold may be only a fraction of an electron volt (1000–3000 K), those achieved for useful machining are between 1 and 100 eV. The temperature is determined by the product of the incident laser irradiance, $I(W/cm^2)$, the square of the laser wavelength, $\lambda^2(mm)$ and the absorption characteristics of the metal. The difference between the threshold and the fluence required for useful machining is illustrated for stainless steel in Figure 14. At threshold, only a very small amount of material (< 0.1 μm) is removed per laser pulse. As the laser fluence is increased, the depth of material removed increases rapidly and then saturates at ≈ 12 J/cm². For the 120 fs pulses used in these experiments, the peak irradiance was over 10^{14} W/cm² and produced an initial plasma temperature near 20 eV.

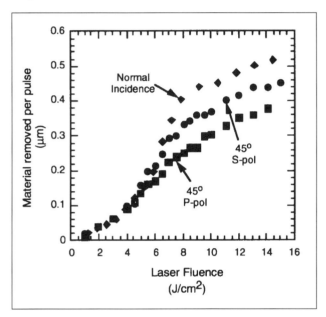

Figure 14. Depth of material removed *per laser pulse* for stainless steel and λ = 825 nm.

The high plasma temperatures associated with saturated material removal ensure that the vaporized material will be completely removed from the kerf without redeposition on the walls. For example, an expanding vapor with even a low expansion velocity of 10^5 cm/s will be 1 meter away from the surface before the arrival of the next pulse 1 ms later (operating at 1 kHz). With conventional nanosecond or microsecond lasers, the vapor will evolve during the laser pulse (Fig. 13). This reduces the coupling of the laser light to the solid surface since the incident laser light will be scattered and absorbed by the vapor.

The cross section of a 400-μm hole in 0.8-mm-thick stainless steel drilled at 45° with 120 fs pulses shows that metallic grain structure is unaltered up to the edge of the hole (Fig. 15). High-resolution microscopy indicates that there is no heat- or shock-affected zone extending beyond ≈ 1 μm away from the surface. The top (entrance) and bottom of the hole are typical of holes drilled with pulses having a Gaussian spatial profile. The shape of the hole is deterministic with no evidence of slag or heat-affected zone. Material is removed only in those regions where the beam intensity is sufficient to form a plasma. This deterministic nature of material removal makes possible the production of shaped cuts, holes or textured surfaces by shaping the spatial profile of the laser beam. Several researchers have used diffractive optics to modify the spatial profile of the beam to produce holes with very steep side walls (15, 16). A shaped fuel injector nozzle produced with 120 fs pulses and a diffractive phase plate to produce a nearly flat top, 0.2-mm-diameter beam is shown in Figure 16.

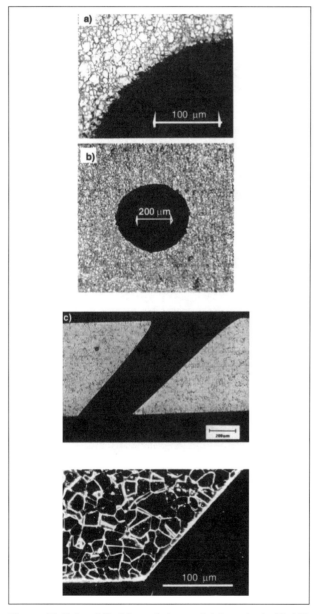

Figure 15. Holes drilled through 1-mm-stainless steel with 120 fs laser pulses at 1 kHz at 45°: a) Magnified section of top of hole, b) exit hole on bottom, c) cross section, d) magnified (bottom left) section of cross section.

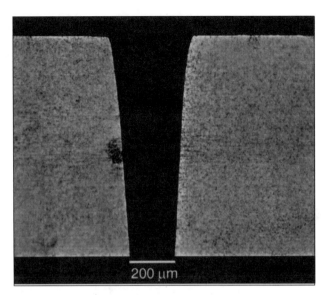

Figure 16. Holes drilled through 1-mm-stainless steel for fuel injector nozzles.

High-aspect ratio holes and cuts (0.05 mm diameter through 1.0) have been produced in numerous metals and dielectrics. Production of high-aspect ratio features requires consideration of the waveguide nature of the feature and associated beam shaping. Tailoring the beam to avoid possible condensation of the plasma plume on the walls must also be considered for the production of high aspect (> 8:1) ratio features.

References

1. *Laser Induced Damage in Optical Materials*, Proceedings of the Boulder Damage Symposium, **1–25,** 1969–93.
2. R. M. Wood, *Laser Damage in Optical Materials,* Hilger, Boston (1986).
3. J. H. Campbell, F. Rainer, M. Kozlowski, C. R. Wolfe, I. Thomas, and F.Milanovich, in *Laser Induced Damage in Optical Materials*, SPIE **1441,** p. 444 (1990).
4. B. C. Stuart, M. D. Feit, A. M. Rubenchik, B. W. Shore, and M. D. Perry, *Phys. Rev. Lett.,* **74,** p. 2248 (1995).
5. D. Du, X. Liu, J. Squier, and G. Mourou, *Appl. Phys. Lett.* **64,** p. 3071, (1994).
6. P. Audebert, Ph. Daguzan, S. Guizard, K. Krastev, P. Martin, G. Petite, A. Dos Santos, and A. Antonetti, *Phys. Rev. Lett.,* **73,** p. 1990 (1994)
7. D. von der Linde and H. Schuler, in Proceedings of Short Wavelength VI: *Physics with High Intensity Pulses*, St. Malo, France (1994).
8. W. Kautek, J. Kruger, M. Lenzner, S. Sartania, C. Spielmann, and F. Krausz, *Appl. Phys. Lett.* **69,** p. 3146 (1996).
9. F. Krausz, et al., *Phys. Rev. Lett.,* to be published.
10. J. F. Ready, *Effects of High-Power Laser Radiation,* Academic Press, New York (1971).
11. S. I. Anisimov, B. L. Kapeliovich, and T.L. Perlman, *Sov. Phys. JETP* **39,** p. 375 (1974).
12. P. B. Corkum, F. Brunel, N. K. Sherman, and T. Srinivasan-Rao, *Phys. Rev. Lett.* **61,** p. 2886 (1988).
13. S. Nolte, C. Momma, H. Jacobs, A. Tunnermann, B. Chichkov, B. Wellegehausen, and H. Welling, *J. Opt. Soc. Amer. B* **14,** p. 2716 (1997).
14. A. M. Rubenchik, M. D. Feit, M. D. Perry, and J. T. Larsen, *App. Surface Science* **127,** p. 193 (1998).
15. M. D. Perry, B. C. Stuart, H. Nguyen, M. D. Feit, and S. Dixit, OSA Annual Meeting, Portland (1996).
16. S. Nolte, C. Momma, et al., OSA Annual Meeting, Long Beach, CA (1997).

M. D. PERRY
B. C. STUART
P. S. BANKS
M. D. FEIT
J. A. SEFCIK

13.6 Comparison with Other Technologies

In this section we compare the benefits and disadvantages of the various manufacturing technologies for drilling. The comparison will be limited to the drilling of holes less than 1.0 mm (0.040 in.) in diameter. This is generally the upper limit for percussion drilling (fixed focal location) with a laser. Larger (and smaller) diameter holes can be "trepanned" which is technically a cutting process and will not be discussed in this section.

The previous chapters of this handbook have referred to the material dependence of laser processing. In this section, material dependencies will not be discussed except in the most general form. The annual ICALEO Proceedings (1) typically contains several material specific drilling papers and The Machining of Composite Materials Conference Proceedings has contained several drilling technology comparisons (2). This section will concentrate on two groups of components: a) hole quantity per part, few, hundreds and thousands; and b) hole diameter range, less than and greater than 0.025 mm (0.001 in.) diameter.

The first category, quantity of holes per part is typically the first limiting factor in selecting a drilling technology. The selection process is compounded by the quality of the hole required in the part.

13.6.1 Consideration of Quantity of Holes Drilled

Small Number of Holes per Component

An example of a part with a small number of holes is a fluid metering hole, such as a fuel injector port. The injector hole requires a high degree of uniformity in geometry, which mandates a low level of laser "damage" to the side walls. The contrasting part is for example an oil bleed hole, as found on engine connecting rods, which does not have the critical quality requirements and thus may be more tolerant of the variation of laser drilling. It should also be noted at this point, that several advances in laser technology, as reported in the literature (2), have been making progress on the quality issues.

Moderate Number of Holes per Component

An example of a part with a moderate number of holes is an aircraft engine turbine airfoil. Airfoils typically have between a few dozen and several hundred drilled holes. The drilling technology selection process is largely governed by the significant cost benefits achievable by a "fast" drilling process while balancing a manageable quality level. Laser drilling is typically chosen as the best combination of speed and quality for these applications. A more detailed analysis of the part performance may identify a few critical holes within the larger pattern, that should be drilled with a higher quality process such as electron discharge machine (EDM), mechanical drilling or advanced laser.

However, advanced lasers and advanced machine tool control architectures are continually making advances in better management of quality while maintaining speed.

Large Number of Holes per Component

Examples of parts with a large number of holes are sound suppression panels in aircraft (typically composites), combustors, ducts, and liners in aircraft engines and laminar flow panels on aircraft. These parts typically have tens of thousands of holes that require various levels of quality but are largely driven by the speed of the drilling technology. Lasers have been used in all of these types of parts with various levels of success.

Sound suppression panels made of composite materials have been drilled at thousands of holes per second by carbon dioxide lasers. The process is an "on-the-fly" drilling operation in which the part is in continuous motions (typically rotational) and synchronized with the laser pulsing rate to perforate the part in a controlled pattern. The holes are usually drilled normal to the surface and can be drilled in a single laser pulse. Hole quality varies with the material properties and hole depth.

Combustors, ducts, and liners are metal/coated metal components and have been successfully drilled with Nd:YAG lasers. These parts are less amenable to on-the-fly processes, but laser drilling has been successful from the standpoint of reasonable cost (throughput) at a reasonable quality. Electron beams could be used for faster throughput, but the parts can be too large for standard vacuum chambers and the geometry of the parts is not conducive to electron beam "compensating" techniques (see the following discussion specific to electron beam).

Laminar flow panels are the "stretch" component for the application of any drilling technology. Aircraft wing leading edge sections may have millions of holes of relatively small diameters. In addition, the hole quality is critical to minimizing blockage from the drilling process byproducts or post-drilling process cleaning operations. The components will require in excess of hundreds of holes per second to be produced to become commercially viable. Advanced laser systems and electron beams have been the primary drilling technologies considered to date.

13.6.2 Large Diameter Holes, > 0.025 mm (0.001 in.)

Large diameter holes, per this definition, are the oldest and most widespread application of laser technology. The aerospace industry has employed this application of lasers for over 20 years. The electronics industry has also utilized lasers for drilling via holes in this range in printed circuit boards. The following are the primary competing technologies for this range of hole drilling and are summarized in Table 1 (next page).

Mechanical

Mechanical drilling is the oldest and most established form of drilling. The lower end diameter limit is a few hundredths of a millimeter. Mechanical drilling is also sensitive to material; it is applied generally to steels and common automotive alloys. It is not applied to aerospace alloys, such as nickel and cobalt-based materials. Drill tool wear can lead to large cyclic process variation and potentially high tooling costs and disposal costs.

Electron Beam (EB)

Electron beam is not as widespread in drilling as it is for joining and cutting. The primary benefit of EB is its potential speed for producing thousands of holes per second in thinner materials. EB is generally a higher-quality process, with respect to recast and material damage. The drawbacks of EB are the capital equipment costs and the cost of maintenance of vacuum chambers. EB can only be used on conductive materials. The down side to EB drilling is that the process relies on eddy currents generated within the material being drilled to guide the beam through to the exit point. As the beam nears the exit location at some non-normal angle to the exit surface, the eddy currents are disrupted and are no longer symmetrical around the hole circumference. This disruption in the eddy "focusing" circuits will cause the beam to hook or bend to the shallow side of the hole. Several techniques have been applied to correct the hook, which involve adding parent or coated material to the exit side to envelop the "hook" portion. The down side to these technologies is the generation and disposal of waste material generated from removing the hooked material and machining time required.

Electro-discharge Machining (EDM)

EDM is largely utilized to drill components with moderate amounts of holes. The advantages of EDM are the high drilled hole quality, with recast levels typically an order of magnitude less than laser drilling and the overall straightness of the side walls of the hole. An EDM electrode can also be shaped to create noncircular and nonsymmetric hole geometries. EDM is typically limited to metallic components, but recent work has shown that doping ceramic materials with small amounts of metals can enable the application of EDM (2). The disadvantages of EDM include relatively slow drilling times: minutes per hole. EDM also is limited to line of sight, but can be ganged into a group of several electrodes to drill a cluster of holes in parallel. The ganging of electrodes requires a relatively flat component surface to enable multiple hole drilling along a single electrode plunge axis. EDM also utilizes an oil bath, which needs to be replenished frequently. The cost of the oil and the disposal of contaminated oil can be prohibitive, although the initial equipment cost is relatively low.

Laser

Laser drilling is utilized to drill components with a moderate to large number of holes. A laser is generally selected as the best overall compromise between capital cost (high), throughput (high) and drilled hole quality (medium). Laser drilling may require the use of insert materials to prevent overdrilling internal cavities. The costs to remove and dispose of these insert materials can be significant. The details of the cost of ownership of a laser drilling machine are covered in Section 13.6.4.

Water Jet (WJ)

Water jet (WJ) has primarily been used in cutting applications, but has recently progressed into the drilling arena. WJ utilizes a high-pressure water jet with and without abrasive particle additives to abrade the material away from the parent material. The advantages of WJ include the athermal nature of the abrasion, with little or no heat generated in the material causing material transformations. The hole geometry is moderately smooth and uniform. The disadvantages of WJ include the capital cost, focusing nozzle wear leading to hole variation, and the disposal costs of abrasive laden slurries. WJ also suffers from the "skidding" at the hole entrance, that is, overspray at the onset of hole drilling which produces a gouge along the part surface at the hole entrance. The high-pressure jets can also produce mechanical damage in some layered or composite materials.

Table 1. Large Hole Drilling Technologies

Type	Quality	Speed
Mechanical	high	medium
Electron beam	m-high	highest
Electro-discharge	high	slow
Laser	medium	m-high
Water jet	high	medium

13.6.3 Small Diameter Holes, < 0.025 mm (0.001 in.)

Drilling small diameter holes, per this definition, is a newer application for lasers. These smaller holes are typically found in more delicate applications where extremely small holes (<< 0.025 mm) and/or extremely high-quality holes are required. The various alternative small hole drilling technologies were reviewed by Hayes and Wallace (3). This section will summarize the technologies.

In general, these drilling processes are slow, removing micrometers of material per second and are relegated to extremely precise and high-cost components, such as silicon manufacturing.

Chemical Milling

Chemical milling is the selective etching of material, and requires the material to exhibit metallic properties. Spraying chemical enhancers can speed the chemical etching process to speeds similar to pulsed laser drilling. Chemical milling requires maskants, which can result in under/over cutting and is limited to depth/diameter ratios of two or less. Chemical milling, as the name implies, also involves the cost of chemicals, chemical handling equipment, and disposal.

Electro-forming and Plating (EF)

Precision small diameter holes have been achieved by plating material onto a mandrel. The mandrel is later removed mechanically or chemically. Holes with ± 1 µm diameter tolerances have been manufactured in this manner. EF is extremely slow and has not been implemented on large, nonmicroscopic scale components to date. EF can also require maskants, chemicals, and the associated costs.

Electron Beam (EB)

EB has also been used to drill small diameter holes. However, the small diameter hole quality is affected more severely by small variations in the electron beam parameters and its use is not widespread.

Electro-Discharge (EDM)

EDM has been used in the small hole drilling arena. EDM is limited to about 125-µm diameter holes utilizing state of the art EDM systems. EDM, when used to drill small holes, is limited to a depth/diameter ratio of approximately 10:1. Roundness can be maintained to within ± 1.0 micrometer and surface roughness can be as small as 0.1 micrometer. The disadvantages of EDM, are, again, the oils used, and cost of disposal. EDM, when applied to small diameter holes, is much slower than larger diameter hole EDM processes because of the need to protect the electrode filaments from damage and off-axis "wander" during the plunge through the material.

Ion Milling

Ion milling has been successfully applied to high-precision holes in thin films. It is limited to depth/diameter ratios of five or less. Ion milling is relatively slow, removing material at rates of 300 angstroms per minute.

Mechanical Drilling

Mechanical drilling has been applied to drilling holes as small as 250-µm diameters. Flexibility of the drill bit and friction heating of the bit are limiting factors.

Mechanical Punching/Broaching

A combination of punching and broaching has been used to drill holes on the order of 25 µm in diameter. The resulting hole quality has been shown to be superior. The broaching operation is used to create a tapered pilot section of the hole, effectively thinning the material in the through hole section. The punch is then used to finish the through hole section of the hole. Alignment between the broach and punch operations and potential mechanical damage has limited its application.

Glass Fiber Forming

Glass fibers, in a controlled geometrical pattern or in a totally random pattern, have been used to create holes in "cast-like" components. Procedurally, the glass fibers are laid out into a mold. The component material is injected into the mold where is solidifies around the glass fiber matrix. After the mold is removed, the glass fibers are etched out of the component. In most cases the fibers have soluble cores, surrounded by glass. Therefore the glass "tubes" remain in the component, a potentially limiting factor.

Laser

Lasers, conventional and advanced, have been used to drill smaller and smaller diameter holes, competing with the etching processes listed above. Laser drilling is material independent and can produce repeatable holes down to approximately 30 µm in diameter. However, laser drilling suffers from relatively large diameter variations, on the order of ± 25 µm in diameter or ± 10% of the hole area. There remains a significant amount of taper, even on these microscopic scales, as compared to the chemical processes. Table 2 compares drilling technologies for small holes.

Table 2. Small Hole Drilling Technologies

Type	Quality	Speed
Chemical milling	high	low
Electro-forming	medium	med
Electron beam	med	high
Electro-discharge	med	med
Ion milling	high	low
Mechanical drilling	med	med
Punching/broaching	high	med
Glass fiber forming	high	low
Laser	med	high

13.6.4 Laser Costs and Other Factors

All of the technologies discussed above have similar factors that go into the decision to apply the technology on demonstration of the drilling process. The following is a more detailed assessment of the cost of implementing a laser drilling system (4). Table 3 lists the primary elements associated with the cost of owning a laser drilling machine.

Table 3. Cost Elements of Laser Drilling

A. *Equipment costs*
  i. initial investment
  ii. water (if not closed loop)
  iii. maintenance of filters, etc.
  iv. downtime

B. *Process costs*
  i. lens and lens covers
  ii. flash lamps
  iii. nozzle assist gas(es)
  iv. overdrill protection and inserts
  v. inspection costs
  vi. spare parts/inventory
  vii. floor space
  viii. temperature and humidity (scrap)

Equipment Costs

The initial investment for a 50- to over 250-W laser driller is $100,000 to over $250,000 for the laser only. Complete turnkey multi-axis machine tools with the laser integrated can be procured for $500,000 to over $1 million per machine, depending on the machine volume and laser chosen. An estimate for a complete laser drilling machine is approximately $150,000 per machine axis. Several vendors offer lower-cost systems that may not be sufficiently robust for two- or three-shift operation.

In addition to the cost of water usage, there can be a charge for disposal, depending on local ordinances. Generally, the water is simply carrying heat. Most installations utilize in-house chilled water supplies to provide cooling to the laser. Alternatively, the laser can be equipped with a refrigerated cooler, which entails a heat load to the air and an increase in maintenance costs.

Maintenance on filters, oil traps, and deionizing cartridges are relatively low-cost items. Providing the planned downtime, one half to one day each month or quarter, for maintenance is a primary stumbling block. However, the planned downtime will result in an overall uptime improvement and lessening of process variation. As the filter elements become less efficient, the temperature variation in support equipment will increase and cause the laser to drift in beam quality from thermal lensing. The resulting change in focused spot size will change the fluid flow characteristics and must be watched carefully by inspecting the components drilled.

Process Costs

Lenses can cost from around $50 to over $300 each. A high-quality lens is generally preferred, utilizing a high quality anti-reflection multilayer coating. From the standpoint of beam absorption, ultraviolet grade fused silica or Infrasil are preferred. It is better to spend more money on a high-quality lens and utilize lower-cost cover windows to protect the lens from spatter. It is also recommended to utilize a standard or custom lens, cover slide, nozzle assembly from original equipment manufacturer (OEM) vendors versus standard designs from the laser machine builder. Most of the OEM vendors can assemble a custom flexible lens holder from standard subassemblies without the cost of a design effort at the machine builder.

Flash lamps are typically replaced every few million pulses; the replacement rate is highly dependent on the laser parameters. Lamps can be replaced as frequently as once per month and cost $100 to over $300 per pair per laser head. It will require between thirty minutes and one day for maintenance personnel to change the lamps and technical personnel to re-establish the process parameters. The drilling process also utilizes a flowing gas stream to protect the lens assembly and aid in the removal of material in the hole. The gas can be shop air, argon, oxygen, or more exotic combinations and 150 ft^3/hr can be required for laser drilling.

When drilling components with hollow, closed internal passages, materials must be utilized to protect the internal cavities from laser scarfing and over drill. Plastic, rubber, ceramic bead, and wax-based materials are commonly employed. The initial cost of these materials can be expensive, especially for the design of a preformed insert or a pressurized wax injection machine. A secondary cost that can be prohibitive is the disposal of used material, which can be considered hazardous, depending on local ordinances and the material being drilled, which is retained in the insert.

As noted before, the variation of laser drilling, from inputs and the laser medium, hole quality can result in the need to inspect a significant number or all components drilled. The inspection may require another machine such as an air flow stand, an x-ray machine and some form of cleaning machine(s) to remove the insert material and/or clean up the external laser spatter. Figure 1 depicts a laser drilling flow line. Some or all the equipment in Figure 1 will be required to maintain a high process quality level. The cost of these support machines can be significant. However, a complete set of support equipment is typically sufficient to support several laser drilling machines. The cost of scrap components, from the inherent laser parameter variation, can also be significant, particularly at the beginning stages of a new process.

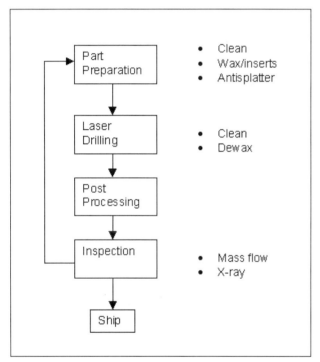

Figure 1. Processing methodology for laser drilling cost consideration.

To minimize down time for maintenance and repair, many companies will chose to stock many or all of the recommended spare parts from the laser vendor. Power supply modules, capacitors, laser rods, mirrors and optics, and alignment tools can be a substantial cost. The cost to keep these materials in inventory can also be significant. The cost of floor space can be a significant factor in choosing laser drilling over other technologies. The laser machine tool can be significantly larger than more conventional tools because of the need for system stability and vibration isolation.

Most important, laser systems are designed to operate in a stable environment and tight control of HVAC; accounting for all laser accessory loads is a must. The laser should be operated in a controlled environment that can be held to a ± 3-degree temperature throughout the year. Temperature and humidity control is critical to minimizing process variation. Several industries have reported achieving 6-sigma process quality (one defect per million holes/parts drilled) by carefully laying out and controlling the laser environment.

13.6.5 Summary

Laser drilling can be successfully implemented in a production shop if the proper environment is established to operate and control the laser machine. The overall cost of acquisition and installation can be significant but generally is recovered by throughput of the laser process relative to competing drilling technologies. The competing drilling technologies all have similar elemental considerations for process quality, speed, inspection and costs of operation. Table 4 summarizes some of the more critical considerations in owning the various technologies.

Table 4. Drilling Technology Challenges

Technology	Challenge
Laser	Process variation
	Insert materials
	Disposing materials
EDM	Oils and electrodes
	Disposal of oil and electrodes
E beam	Vacuum chamber maintenance
	Drill barrier materials
Water jet	Process variation
	Disposal of grit stream
Chemical processes	Acquisition and disposal of chemicals

Regarding laser parameter variation, several new laser products are offering improved shot to shot repeatability from solid state power supplies, high brightness resonators, diode pumping, and advanced control features. Much work has been done to model and control the laser drilling process without much success in implementing control. The lack of control depends largely on the accurate monitoring of the laser condition, which affects the validity of the model input parameters.

References

1. International Conference on Lasers and Electro Optics Proceedings (ICAEO), 1994, 1995, and 1996, Laser Institute of America, Orlando, FL.
2. T. S. Sriratsan and D. M. Bowden (Eds.), *Machining of Composite Materials Conference Proceedings,* November 1992, ASM International.
3. D. J. Hayes and D. B. Wallace, *Overview of Small Holes,* Nontraditional Machining Conference, Orlando, FL, October 1989.
4. K. Withnall, "Calculating the Cost of Nd:YAG Laser Ownership," *Industrial Laser Review,* April 1997.

TODD J. ROCKSTROH

Chapter 14

Balancing

14.1 Basics of Balancing

14.1.0 Introduction

Balancing is a "procedure, by which the mass distribution of a rotor is checked and, if necessary, adjusted to ensure that the residual unbalance or the vibration of the journals and/or forces on the bearings at a frequency corresponding to service speed are within specified limits" (1).

Typical metal working machines apply the same CNC program for all parts of a type. Balancing machines have to treat each part (rotor) separately, since unbalances are individually created by scattered tolerances in dimensions, materials, and fits.

A single unbalance can be described as a mass on a radius, with dimension g•mm. It has an amount and, given by the radius, a direction: The unbalance is a vector quantity.

A rotor typically has many sources of unbalance along its axis, of different amounts and radial directions, but they can accumulate to produce:

- A resultant unbalance
- A resultant couple unbalance
- Modal unbalances

Resultant unbalance and resultant couple unbalance together describe the position of the mass axis of the rotor relative to the shaft axis (Fig. 1). Modal unbalances influence the flexure of the rotor at high speeds. This will be discussed later.

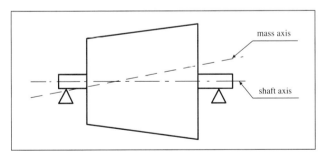

Figure 1. Shaft axis and mass axis of a rotor (deviation enlarged).

The aim of balancing is to let the shaft axis (given by the bearings) and the mass axis (principal axis of inertia near to the shaft axis) coincide within a permissible error, the balance tolerance. This may be performed either by moving the shaft axis toward the mass axis or by moving the mass axis toward the shaft axis (see Fig. 2).

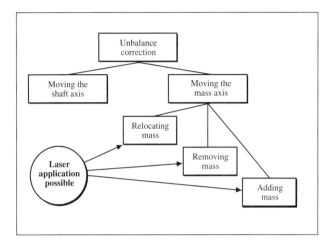

Figure 2. Principles of unbalance correction.

Moving the Shaft Axis

Based on a measurement of the unbalance around the given shaft axis, a new shaft axis with reduced unbalance is defined. This procedure is called "mass centering."

For this new shaft axis surfaces often have to be remachined, for example, shafts and seals. Thus systematic changes in unbalance will occur later on; they have to be considered properly when defining the new shaft axis.

Moving the Mass Axis

The mass axis is moved by relocating masses on, by removing masses from, or by adding masses to the rotor.

Today almost everything that rotates or is supported on bearings, which allow it to rotate, is balanced. The rotors may vary in:

- Mass: from a fraction of one gram to hundreds of tons
- Speed: from a few rpm to one million rpm
- Balance tolerance (permissible rotor mass center displacement from shaft axis): from some nanometers to some millimeters
- Unbalance correction: from some micrograms to some hundred kilograms mass

According to this variety of conditions, very different solutions and procedures are applied for balancing.

14.1.1 Conditions for Balancing

There are two different conditions under which balancing of rotors/assemblies may be performed:

- With balancing machines, using balance tolerances as permissible limits
- In situ conditions, using vibration tolerances as permissible limits

On a Balancing Machine

Both principles of unbalance correction are applicable. In special cases the shaft axis is moved. In all other cases the mass axis is moved.

The balancing machine indicates the necessary unbalance correction. On hard bearing machines with permanent calibration this occurs after input of the position of correction planes relative to the bearing planes; on soft bearing machines this occurs after a calibration procedure with test masses.

In Situ

This condition does not allow for a variation of the shaft axis; only the movement of the mass axis is applicable.

Typically portable measuring equipment is used. The once-per-revolution vibrations without and with test masses in the correction planes are used to obtain the influence coefficients and to transform the vibration data into information on the necessary unbalance correction.

14.1.2 Balancing Procedures

The balancing procedure is chosen according to the behavior of the rotor. Mainly the initial unbalance, balance tolerance, operational speed, and support condition determine the state of the rotor, if it is in a constant (rigid) or variable state. Figure 3 shows a decision tree for selection of an appropriate balancing procedure.

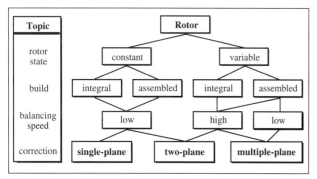

Figure 3. Decision tree for an appropriate balancing procedure (simplified).

Rotors in a Constant (Rigid) State

These rotors can be balanced at any low speed (below operational speed). Unbalance correction is done in one plane (single-plane balancing) or two planes (two-plane balancing) (2).

For full information on unbalance and thus for the necessary unbalance correction, only one speed is needed. This is important for possible application of laser balancing.

Rotors in a Variable State

Typical for these rotors is a movement of their components relative to each other at higher speed (up to the operational speed). Among possible different states, the flexible state, the component-elastic state, and the seating state, the flexible one is the most important. In this state the rotor flexes because of modal unbalances. Some important topics of the flexible state are detailed below.

Integral Rotors

If rotors in a flexible state are integral rotors (not assembled), balancing has to be performed using multiple speeds, for example:

- A speed, where the rotor is still in its constant (rigid) state
- A speed near to each (relevant) resonance speed
- Possibly the operational speed

Each speed gives specific (partial) information on the unbalance and its distribution along the rotor. Correction is done in more than two planes (multi-plane balancing) (3).

Important for a possible application of a laser is the fact that for full information on unbalance more than one speed is needed. Only after acquisition of all data can the necessary unbalance correction be calculated, indicated, and performed.

Assembled Rotors

For assembled rotors—although in a flexible state—sometimes modified low-speed procedures are applicable. Each part, module, assembly step is corrected for unbalance individually. As a result a correction in multiple planes is performed, but at low speed only.

It is important for a possible application of a laser that for full information on unbalance and thus for the necessary unbalance correction, only one speed is needed, but this information is needed separately for each part, module, and assembly step.

14.1.3 Balancing Process

Various activities needed to balance a rotor are sketched in Figure 4. Lasers may be applied to acquire vibration (unbalance) data or for unbalance correction.

Two aspects of a balancing solution must be considered, depending on whether unbalance correction is done:

- At standstill or under rotation
- In the same or a different station as the measuring of the unbalance

Rotor Speed during Correction

Most rotors are corrected for unbalance at standstill. But sometimes it may be advantageous to have the rotor surface moving or even staying at balancing speed. This is true in the following cases:

- For the correction process itself, e.g., in order to spread it over a certain angular range
- To cut out deceleration and acceleration times.

Chapter 14: Balancing

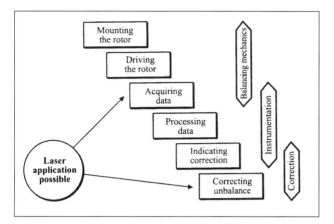

Figure 4. Individual steps of a balancing process.

If correction is performed under rotation, it must be an intermittent process, properly synchronized with the rotation of the rotor.

A pulsed laser, triggered to the rotor speed and adjusted to the angle of correction, may be applicable.

Number of Stations

Often the rotor is placed into a balancing machine, measurement and correction of unbalance are performed in turn, until the rotor is in balance tolerance, then it is removed; balancing is performed in a single station.

In other cases the unbalance is measured in one station, and the correction is done in another one. Reasons may be:

- Saving time with overlapping cycles, in manually operated machines or in transfer lines
- Avoiding pollution of the balancing section by the unbalance correction process
- Using standard or existing machine tools for the unbalance correction instead of an integrated special solution

Sometimes up to 10 stations are lined up in order to distribute individual tasks and to reach extreme short cycle times.

14.1.4 Example: A Typical Balancing Task

To illustrate a typical example of a small rotor, the main balancing data for an aircraft gyro is given below.

Mass	85 g
Maximum balancing speed	22,500 rpm
Correction radius	113 mm
Circumferential velocity	
at the location of correction	26.6 m/s

For the initial unbalance it can be assumed that:
Maximum initial mass center excentricity	8 µm
i.e., initial unbalance mass, max.	60 mg
per correction plane, max.	30 mg
Volume of material (high density)	
to be removed, max	2 mm^3

For the balance tolerance, it can be assumed that:
Permissible center of gravity displacement	0.01 µm
i.e., permissible unbalance mass	0.07 mg
per correction plane	0.035 mg
corresponding to a volume of	0.002 mm^3

The balancing system - measuring and correction sections - must be capable of handling all unbalances properly, from the initial to the permissible residual unbalance. It has to be more accurate by a factor of 3 to 10; that is, an unbalance mass with a volume below 0.001 mm^3 has to be detected and corrected for. To remove these extremely small quantities an appropriate laser would be suitable.

References

1. ISO Standard 1925: Mechanical vibration—Balancing vocabulary.
2. ISO Standard 1940: Mechanical vibration—Balance quality requirements of rigid rotors—Part 1: Determination of permissible residual unbalance.
3. ISO Standard 11342: Mechanical vibration – Methods and criteria for the mechanical balancing of flexible rotors.

(See Section 6.5 for ISO contact information.)

HATTO SCHNEIDER

14.2 Laser Balancing Procedures

14.2.0 Introduction

Laser balancing can be applied to a wide range of applications, including low-speed balancing on a balance machine, and in situ balancing of finished assemblies to reduce final vibration levels. Typically either pulsed Nd:glass, pulsed Nd:YAG, or CO_2 lasers are used as the means to remove required balance corrections. The method used to calculate the correction and verify the effectiveness of the installed correction is primarily independent of the laser material removal process. Lasers provide a means to remove very accurate amounts of material from a rotor at precise locations while it is spinning. This offers significant advantages in many balancing applications such as the one described in Section 14.1.4. Manual balancing of such a rotor requires a series of runs to the operational speed to calculate remaining unbalance that must be corrected with a precision down to fractions of a milligram. While the low-speed balancing machine is very capable of calculating an accurate two-plane balance solution, such as: 32 mg at 10° in Plane 1 and 20 mg at 43°, there is great difficulty involved in the removal of such precise amounts with a drill press with the rotor stopped. Each was run up to 22,500 rpm as a check on how well the correction was installed, a process that is very operator-skill dependent.

The laser is used to vaporize material by application of focused laser energy for a short pulse (or time) duration. The timing of the firing circuit provides the ability accurately to control the phase angle of the installed correction. The laser pulse duration for most laser balancing applications is in the range from 150 µs to a few milliseconds. High-speed applications where the rotor is spinning at speeds up to 30,000 rpm require short pulse durations so that the laser energy is delivered to a small enough area on the spinning rotor to achieve the necessary energy density to vaporize material. Lower-speed applications are typically in the 1000 to 2000 rpm range and are able to use the longer pulses from 1 ms up that can offer more laser energy and therefore higher material removal rates. Typically pulsed lasers can remove material in the range from a few milligrams per shot down to small fractions of a milligram per shot when required.

In the gyroscope balance example, removal of the 32- and 20-mg corrections at precise angular locations is ideal for a laser application. The typical procedure to balance the gyroscope would be to operate at a low speed typically around 6–12,000 rpm to acquire initial balance data and calculate a balance correction. The manual correction process then requires stopping the rotor and using some means, typically drilling, to attempt to remove the required amount of material. In a laser system the correction is calculated in terms of laser shots instead of grams as in the manual case, and the correction can be applied with the rotor running. The entire correction is often not performed initially in order to recalculate the answer based on progress achieved. That simple recalculation that requires only a brief pause in the firing can help achieve precise balance specifications in substantially reduced times compared to manual material removal.

Once the unit has been balanced at the initial speed, the speed is typically increased to the maximum operating speed. The balance process is then repeated to achieve the final balance specifications. In the gyro overhaul industry the average balancing time can be reduced from upwards of one to two hours for a highly skilled technician to 10–15 min with a reduced skill level requirement and training period for operators.

14.2.1 Advantages/Limitations of Laser Balancing

The main advantages of laser balancing are: precise control of the material removal process and ability to perform the removal while the part is spinning. Most applications use these capabilities to achieve very precise balance levels. The more demanding the balance specification, the more attractive lasers are as a means to achieve the required precision. Some applications achieve productivity or unit throughput improvements due to the removal of material at speed. This is most often the time when the precision requirements drive the manual balancing process into an iterative cycle. Advances in high-repetition-rate lasers and in burst operation of high-energy CO_2 lasers open up more applications to potential improved system productivity, such as high-volume production balancing for many parts in the automotive industry.

One disadvantage of an advanced laser balancing system is its cost. An automated laser balancing system is an advanced package integrating motion control, laser control, balancing, and safety requirements. With the cost of typical lasers being from $40,000 to $200,000, a full production system ranges from $250,000 to more than $1 million. To justify these costs usually the manual balance process must be made to achieve the required precision in an acceptable time cycle. One definite trend in industry is downward pressure on balance specifications to achieve reduced noise and vibration in products from rotating components in automobiles, refrigerators, laser printers, and many others. As required balance precision becomes more challenging, more applications will be able to benefit despite initial capital costs.

Two other disadvantages that apply in certain applications are possible reduction in fatigue life of the laser-balanced component and debris control. Debris control pertains to the fact that when the material is removed, most of it is ablated (transition from solid to vapor directly), but a small percentage at the end of the laser pulse is melted and must be controlled to avoid redeposition on the rotor. Taking advantage of the rotor speed, it is straightforward in many applications to trap the molten debris with a debris collection device.

Since most balancing is performed on sacrificial material in a low-stress region, the reduction in fatigue life is not an issue. Applications such as automotive turbocharges and gas turbine applications have to be carefully evaluated to determine if the fatigue life reduction is a factor in component life.

14.2.2 Balancing Systems

A typical laser balancing system is illustrated in block diagram form in Figure 1. The major elements of the system are:

- Laser with power supply and appropriate beam delivery hardware
- Motion control electronics and tables
- Data acquisition equipment, including the necessary vibration instrumentation and signal conditioning electronics
- Mechanical balancing hardware, including the balance machine, debris collector, and safety enclosure
- Gyro rotor power supply electronics
- Microprocessor for overall system control, balance correction, and operator interface
- Video display terminal with touch control

Operator Control Station

The operator control station is designed for straightforward production balancing. It houses the microprocessor, motion control electronics, gyro rotor power supply, signal conditioning subsystem, video display terminal (VDT), and control panel. The VDT is a standard color monitor with an accompanying touch control panel. Production operator interaction with the system is primarily by means of the touch control. The control panel provides a system power switch and an emergency stop button. Activation of the emergency stop will suspend all laser operation and motion immediately. A standard keyboard is provided on a slideout tray for use during the setup and test modes of operation.

ISBN 0-912035-15-3

Chapter 14: Balancing

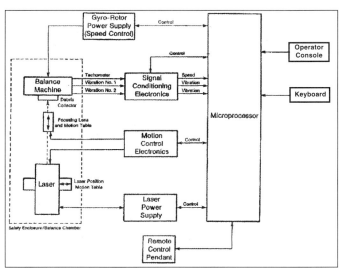

Figure 1. Automated Laser Balancing System.

Balance Chamber

The balance chamber includes the gyro rotor balance machine and the laser. The balance chamber provides for easy installation of the gyro rotor and fixture. Likewise, the laser head and beam delivery hardware are easily accessed for routine servicing. Construction of the balance chamber conforms to the requirements of ANSI standard Z-136 as a Class I system (see Section 6.5). This means that the laser beam is fully enclosed, which allows the installation of the system in a production environment without impacting surrounding workstations. Interlocks prevent system operation with the door unlatched.

The balance chamber includes a vacuum-assisted collector into which particulates and debris generated in the process of material removal are deposited. This collector ensures that the rotor bearings are not subjected to direct contamination from the material removal process, and that debris does not attach to the rotor.

Laser Power Supply

The laser power supply stores and regulates the energy used to pulse the laser. A front panel power-on switch is used during routine production-mode operation at the beginning and end of a shift. Other switches, controls, and indicators used only during servicing of the laser are located on the power supply cabinet, which is a free-standing 19-in. rack constructed of heavy-gauge steel. The cabinet access doors and panels are electrically interlocked to protect against accidental exposure to high voltage. The laser head cooling assembly is located in the lower section of the power supply cabinet.

The following paragraphs describe the functions, features and capabilities of the laser balancing system, highlighting the operator interface, modes of operation, and system control equipment.

Operator Interface

The automated laser balancing system is simple to operate, yet flexible. The production operator controls the system by using five interface elements. These are the master on/off switch, the laser power switch, the emergency stop, the touch control video monitor, and the remote control pendant. The master on/off switch is used to turn the system on and off at the start and conclusion of each day's shift. This switch applies power to all system electrical hardware elements, with the exception of the laser power supply. The laser power switch is used to activate the laser power supply.

For the most part, the production operator will interface almost exclusively with the touch control in the automatic mode (described below). In this mode, system prompts, directions, and the status of operations are reported on the video screen. Examples of input required from the operator include selection of a specific rotor model to be balanced, positive indication that the rotor is loaded and that the balance operation is to begin. The remote control pendant permits operator control over the laser system motion hardware for alignment and focus verification checks prior to the start of the balancing operation. An emergency stop switch is included in the system, giving the operator the ability to override the microprocessor and stop all system operations, if necessary.

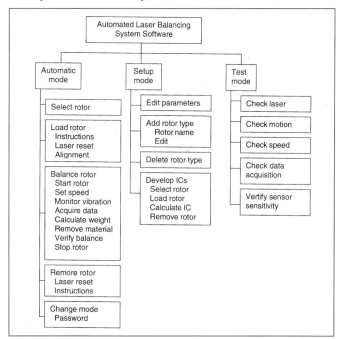

Figure 2. Showing Modes of Operation.

Modes of Operation

An automated laser balancing system software supports three modes of operation; these are automatic, setup, and test (Fig. 2). Summaries of each mode are provided in the following subsections.

Automatic Mode. This mode allows the production operator (via the touch control) to select, load, balance, and remove the rotor. The change mode, which appears last on the main screen, is used only by a qualified system operator having a valid password that will then allow access to the setup and test modes.

At the beginning of the automatic balancing mode, the system is in its idle state and the select function screen is displayed on the video monitor. Activating the select rotor region on the video screen presents the operator with a list of twenty rotors that can be balanced. The *previous*, *next*, and *select* functions on the select rotor type screen allow the operator to select one of the twenty rotor types.

Rotor loading steps are then displayed. Verification of laser alignment is possible at this point through the align laser function. On the balance status screen are shown the desired and current rotor speed, the balance specifications and current vibration levels, and the current number of laser shots fired and number needed to achieve the specification. The following operations are then automatically performed under microprocessor control:

1. All status indicators checked to verify that the system is operational and that all safety interlocks are closed
2. Speed control unit activated, which spins the rotor to the first balance speed
3. Vibration data acquired and conditioned
4. Amount of material to be removed and its precise location determined for each balance plane to achieve the balance limit specified in the rotor setup file
5. Laser firing control pattern loaded
6. Laser activated and material removed from the rotor
7. Balance condition monitored during the material removal process and balance correction updated to ensure that rotor is balanced precisely without repeated iterations
8. Steps 2 through 7 repeated for the second balancing speed
9. Electronic rotor brake activated to stop rotor after completing all balancing operations

Directions for unloading the rotor are displayed and the operator is then returned to the main screen.

Setup Mode. This mode is used by a system operator (primarily interfacing with the slide-out keyboard) to modify, add, or delete the rotor configuration files, as well as to develop the rotor influence coefficients (IC), which are the balance correction parameters needed by the microprocessor to control the laser material removal process. An easy-to-use, full-screen editor permits the interactive and selective change of parameters such as rotor description, drive power, weight, and bearing pedestal span. The individual parameters of each balance plane and balance speed can be separately defined. The balancing system gives the user maximum flexibility in defining both existing and new rotor types.

Test Mode. This mode is available if there is need for troubleshooting and diagnosis of difficulties with basic system functions. The major functions/hardware that can be tested include the laser, the motion system, speed control, and the data acquisition system.

During laser testing, all major laser control functions, such as shutter position, high-voltage activation, power level variations, and laser firing can be exercised. Similarly, the motion, speed control, and data acquisition systems can be tested independently to verify their proper operation.

MICHAEL MARTIN

14.3 Some Applications of Laser Balancing

14.3.1 Timing Wheel Balancing

Task

The timing wheel in question is an extremely lightweight construction - a rim connected by two spokes to the shaft. On the inside of the rim, the material is formed into teeth, which can be removed for unbalance correction (Fig. 1). The structure is characterized by an extremely light rotor, a very flexible assembly, a large number of pieces, and a short cycle time. Table 1 presents the parameters for the timing wheel.

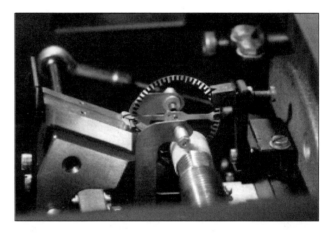

Figure 1. Timing wheel in a balancing station (Schench, G., GSI Lumonics, UK).

Table 1. Data for the Timing Wheel

Mass	0.1 g
Tooth pitch	36
Number of teeth	32
Number of pitches per spoke	2
Initial unbalance, typically	2 teeth
Balance tolerance	1 tooth
Corresponding to an eccentricity of	20 µm

Solution

A twin-station balancing machine with automatic correction in an overlapping cycle is used. While one station is manually

Chapter 14: Balancing

loaded, in the other station a rotor automatically is measured, corrected, and checked.

A Nd:YAG laser is used, with one fixed and one movable mirror, together with two optical systems. Table 2 presents the laser parameters.

Table 2. Laser Parameters

Wavelength	1064 nm
Maximum energy per pulse	1 J
Pulse duration at maximum energy (approx.)	100 µs
Average pulse power (approx.)	10 kW
Irradiance (approx.)	10^6 W/cm^2
Repetition rate	10 Hz

Unbalance correction is done at balancing speed. The measured unbalance is vectorially distributed to different teeth, avoiding the spokes. Each tooth is removed by a series of 9 pulses, all applied in slightly different angles. Total correction time for 2 teeth is 3 to 5 sec.

This laser application is similar to a drilling process (see Chapter 13).

14.3.2 Clutch Disc Balancing

Task

A converter lockout clutch disc is corrected for unbalance by material removal along the periphery. The nearby friction material and its bonding must not be affected. Initial unbalance is up to 800 g•mm; the permissible residual is 50 g•mm.

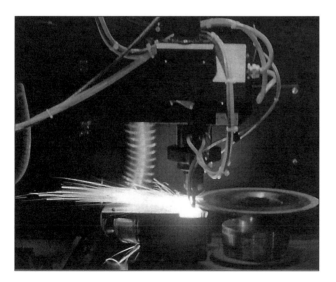

Figure 2. Balancing machine for clutch discs with laser correction (SCHENCK TURNER / Rofin-Sinar).

Solution

A balancing machine with a vertical axis is combined with a CO_2 laser for unbalance correction by cutting out a stripe from the periphery using a one-station system (see Fig. 2).

Table 3 presents the laser parameters.

Table 3. Laser Parameters

Wavelength	10.6 µm
Output power	700 W
Lens, focal length	127 mm
Irradiance (approx.)	3×10^6 W/cm^2
Assist gas	oxygen
Two-axis positioning system	radial, vertical

One of the different possible unbalance correction processes is explained below.

Unbalance correction is performed at standstill, but the ability to turn is used for that purpose. The rotor is indexed to the starting position according to the amount and angle of the unbalance measured. The laser beam is then delivered radially to the rotor to a set depth and the rotor turned slowly (25 mm/s) to its final position.

With an average laser cutting time of 3 sec for a cut of 50 mm length, the total machine cycle time for one rotor is approximately 15 s (from loading to unloading).

The laser application is similar to a cutting process (see Chapter 12).

14.3.3 Frequency Spindle Balancing

Task

A high-frequency spindle must be corrected under rotation. Material removal must be spread over a large area with limited depth. The operation must provide excellent appearance, a smooth, clean surface, and no burrs.

Solution

Processes have been developed with a pulsed Nd:YAG laser with additional Q-switch capabilities for different materials and conditions. One example is given below:

The laser beam is focused by a 125-mm lens slightly above the rotor surface (+3 mm). Each laser pulse is transformed into 80 Q-switched pulses, 120 ns duration each (see Fig. 3).

The laser pulse (1 ms) gives 9.5-mm surface length on the rotor at 9100 rpm. The repetition rate (triggered by the rotor) is approximately 35 Hz. To control the width of material removal, the rotor is moved in the axial direction repeatedly, with 0.1 mm/s velocity.

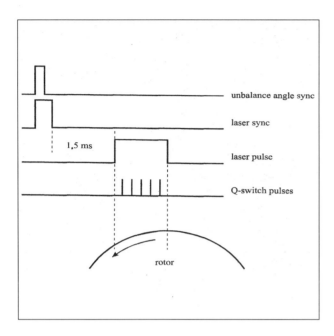

Figure 3. Schematic of process with Q-switched pulses (Fraunhofer IPM / Innovat / SCHENCK RoTec).

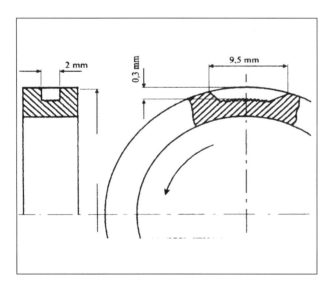

Figure 4. Schematic of material removal (Fraunhofer IPM / Innovat / SCHENCK RoTec).

Gases are coaxially fed, oxygen for fast material removal, argon for finishing. With a total of 3000 pulses and a total time of 90 s approximately 50 mg were removed from steel (90 MnCrV8) (see Figs. 4 and 5).

The laser parameters are presented in Table 4.

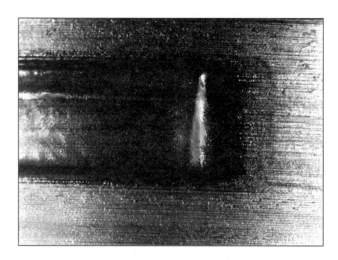

Figure 5. Photograph of machined rotor surface (Fraunhofer IPM/ Innovat / SCHENCK RoTec).

Table 4. Laser Data

Wavelength	1064 nm
Energy per pulse	2 J
Pulse duration	1 ms
Average pulse power (approx.)	2 kW
Repetition rate (approx.)	35 Hz
Data for Q-Switched Operation	
Frequency	80 kHz
Number of pulses per sequence (1 ms)	80
Energy per pulse	20 mJ
Pulse duration	120 ns
Average pulse power (approx.)	160 kW
Irradiance (approx.)	10^{10} W/cm^2

14.3.4 Other Applications

Lasers may be used not only for removing mass but also for other unbalance correction methods, such as for relocating mass and for adding mass (welding).

Compared to many other applications of lasers, in laser balancing the rotors are more or less finished, ready to be used. So special care has to be taken to avoid contamination of the rotor with the material removed, and to avoid unwanted and possibly destructive material transformations.

In most cases it will not be sufficient simply to replace a given unbalance correction method (e.g., drilling, grinding, milling, welding, or soldering) by an equivalent laser process. In order to gain the full benefit of this technology, possibly totally new approaches will be needed, even changes in design and/or in assembly. This is a real challenge for modern laser technology.

HATTO SCHNEIDER

Chapter 15

Marking

Laser marking of manufactured parts has become common in industry. Product marking is performed to identify parts, to provide product information, to imprint distinctive logos, and to aid in theft prevention.

15.1 Basic Principles

General Description

Using a laser to mark or code information on a product – *laser marking* – is one of the most common industrial applications of lasers. Laser marking often takes the form of an alphanumeric code imprinted on the label or on the surface of the product to describe date of manufacture, best-before date, serial number or part number, but the mark can also be a machine-readable bar code or 2D symbol (ID matrix). As well as coding, laser marking sometimes takes the form of functional marking (such as gradation lines on a syringe) or decorative marking (such as a logo or graphic image on an integrated circuit). Laser marking is often one of the final processes in the assembly of a product, taking place during the final filling cycle at a brewery, for example, or on a finished product before it is boxed for shipment. Compared to other on-line marking techniques, such as inkjet, hot stamping, or mechanical scribing, laser marking offers many advantages: indelibility, reliablity, no consumables, cleanliness and high speed. Laser marking is usually the best marking solution with one proviso: Not all materials mark well with every laser.

What Is a Laser Mark?

Laser marking (1) can take a number of forms: 1. black carbonization, 2. bleaching or changing the color of the material, 3. physical modification of the surface finish, 4. scribing a shallow groove into the material by vaporization, 5. highly controlled modification of the surface by melting, or 6. a combination of any of the above. In some cases, a surface mark by color change with little material removal is desired. On the other hand, noncolored marks that scribe a shallow groove into the material are sometimes desired to provide resistance to abrasion.

Laser marking is a surface process. Typically, the light absorbed during the optical pulse (which can be very short, e.g., < 0.1 μs) is transformed into heat, thereby creating a high "instantaneous" temperature rise in the material, resulting in surface melting and resolidification, carbonization, chemical decomposition, or explosive ejection of the material. The resultant mark consists typically of a crater of shallow depth, surface modification within the crater and around the heat-affected zone, a raised ridge or kerf around the crater, and debris scattered nearby (see Fig. 1).

Absorption of light in dielectrics follows an exponential form such that the absorbed energy E (per unit volume) at depth z is given by

$$E(z) = I_0 \, a \, e^{-az} \, \Delta t$$

where a is the absorption coefficient at that wavelength for the material being marked, I_0 is the laser irradiance incident on the material, and Δt is the time duration of the laser pulse. A simple description of the heating process and temperature rise ΔT (per unit mass) for a volume of material at depth z is

$$\Delta T = \frac{\text{(heat added)} - \text{(heat conducted away)}}{\text{(specific heat of material)}}$$

where the heat added is determined by the light absorbed in the material at depth z, and the heat lost is determined by the thermal conductivity of the material. Since the laser pulse is finite in duration, this description must be integrated over time.

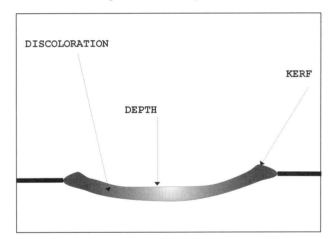

Figure 1. Schematic representation of a laser-marked surface. A kerf may be present only for cases where melting and material flow has occurred. Depending on the laser and beam delivery process used, the depth of the crater can be negligible or as much as 0.005 in. Although subsurface marking is possible on some materials, it is not a common application.

This simple thermal description helps to explain laser marking qualitatively. However, it is evident that melting and material removal would add other terms to the energy balance. Absorption may be strongly temperature dependent, as, for example, in silicon marking at wavelength 1.06 μm, or strongly time dependent, as, for example, in marking metals reflective at the laser wavelength (where plasma formation and initiation of surface damage may occur before a significant portion of the energy can be absorbed). Absorption of radiation from lasers such as pulsed CO_2 lasers with very high peak power can be highly nonlinear. In fact, the marking interaction of light at various wavelengths with different materials can be quite complex (2–5).

Reasonably strong absorption of the laser light is the key not only to efficient, cost-effective marking, but also to aesthetically attractive marking. Light that penetrates too deeply will either not raise the surface temperature enough to have any effect, or it may cause incomplete or noncontinuous marking (e.g., bubbling in plastics). For this reason, it is important to choose the laser wavelength to interact best with the material to be marked. For example, radiation from the Nd:YAG laser at 1.06 µm passes through a transparent PET (polyethylene terephthalate) water bottle, but radiation from the CO_2 laser at 10.6 µm marks clear PET bottles very nicely. Excimer lasers have extremely shallow penetration depth in most organic materials such as plastics; so they can provide very shallow marks in white fluoropolymers with relatively low laser energy.

Acceptability of the Mark and Marking Process
Many techniques are available to evaluate the readability of the laser mark. Often a subjective evaluation by the customer is all that is required. However, quantitative techniques are available to aid in this evaluation and also to ensure that the marking process quality is maintained from run to run. The use of an optical contrast meter to measure the contrast between scattered light from the marked region compared to the unmarked region of the samples provides a simple quantitative estimate of readability. However, for marks that cut a shallow groove into the surface, edge sharpness and depth can also have a strong effect on readability. In this case, it may be necessary also to use surface profiling equipment such as an optical interferometer or a profilometer to evaluate the depth of the mark, the edge sharpness, and the change in surface texture. This equipment would also be essential if the depth of the mark must be carefully controlled, for example, in the case of very thin integrated circuit packages.

Bar codes are commonly coded using lasers. Bar codes are sensitive to edge quality and line thickness; so issues such as dot overlap (in the laser writing technique) and surface roughness can have a major effect. Bar code readers will not use light at the same wavelength as room light; so mark contrast must be optimized for the bar code reader wavelength. Because bar codes can be difficult to mark reproducibly in some situations with lasers, some users, particularly in the electronics sector, have moved to two-dimensional identification codes, such as a matrix.

Laser marking systems are often chosen because they provide an indelible and durable mark. Testing procedures such as scratch resistance, lifetesting for ultraviolet degradation in plastics, and testing for mark permanence under various environmental conditions are standard.

One major factor in the acceptance of laser marking systems has been their inherent reliability. In applications such as marking integrated circuits, lasers provide the only potential route to very high marking reliability. At the other environmental extreme,

CO_2 laser marking systems used in breweries are subjected to daily water washdowns along with the whole bottling line, but the lasers must continue to work year after year. In many cases, sophisticated microprocessor-based controls now provide the means to collect statistics about unscheduled downtime, and also to provide remote service diagnostics via modem.

In order to ensure a repeatable marking process month after month, companies that use laser marking equipment expect the lasers to perform reproducibly and reliably within a specified operating range. However, it should not be forgotten that the material being marked represents another important factor. Material properties of the part being marked must also be controlled to ensure mark repeatability from batch to batch.

15.2 Materials

Practically every material can be marked with a laser of one kind or another. The key to cost-effective, cosmetically attractive laser marking is to have the laser light absorbed very near the surface of the material to be marked. In many cases, the proper choice of laser wavelength will ensure adequate absorption and good marking. Occasionally, however, it is necessary to use additives, coatings, and other schemes to achieve adequate absorption at the surface.

Plastics
Laser-marked plastics include both the thermoplastic polymers used to make extruded parts for almost every application imaginable and the thermoset materials used as encapsulants in the electronics sector. Lasers are used not only for on-line coding of plastic parts, but also increasingly for custom decorating applications. Depending on the additives used, visually stunning laser marks can be obtained under certain situations, primarily in thermoplastics.

Plastics are rarely seen in their pure state because a plethora of additives are commonly used as fillers, colorants, release agents, ultraviolet retardants, etc. Because it is strongly absorbing at 10.6 µm even in its pure state, polyvinyl chloride (PVC) is one polymer that always marks well with CO_2 lasers to produce a characteristic yellow/orange colored mark. As well as bulk PVC, vinyl films used in labels are often CO_2 laser marked. Another polymer that always marks well using CO_2 lasers is PET (polyethylene terephthalate).

The marking of other plastics such as ABS (acrylonitrile butadiene), polycarbonates, polyamides (e.g., nylon), PBT (polybutylene terephthalate), and polyolefins (polyethylene, polypropylene) depends primarily on what laser is used and what additives are present. Of the above materials, all except the polyolefins usually mark to some degree with the Nd:YAG laser; however, the mark may be unattractive because of too-low absorption. Bubbling and roughness of the mark indicate too low absorption of the laser light. Colorants in particular have a marked effect on absorption, as would be expected because the Nd:YAG laser wavelength at 1.06 µm is very close to that of visible light. Some inert additives that are used to improve laser marking are carbon black, mica, kaolin, and titanium dioxide. Figure 1 shows an example of laser-marked polyester.

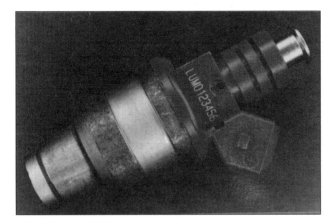

Figure 1. Laser-marked black polyester cap of fuel injector.

Some chemical companies that supply the bulk polymer materials and intermediary companies that supply the colored concentrates have recently undertaken research programs to identify additives to enhance the laser markability of their products. For example, Hoechst Inc. offers laser-markable grades of black Celcon® acetal copolymer, which allows Nd:YAG marking with contrast as high as 0.95. GE Plastics offer laser-markable grades of Valox® PBT polymer. BASF Inc. offers laser-markable grades of their engineering plastics such as Ultramid® nylons. These companies and the companies below are mentioned as illustrative examples, and not as an endorsement.

Until recently, polyethylene and polypropylene had been virtually unmarkable with lasers in their commonly used forms. However, mica additives such as the the Afflair® series offered by EM Industries (Iriodin® in Europe by E. Merck) now allow these materials to be marked using either CO_2 lasers or Nd:YAG lasers (6). Polyethylene and polypropylene are very important polymers used frequently in packaging and bottling applications.

Excimer laser marking of fluoropolymer-insulated aircraft wire has become common. Fluoropolymers provide a very effective lightweight insulation that must be marked indelibly without any penetration that could reduce the insulating properties of the wire. The use of 1–2% titanium dioxide colorant in this wire facilitates very shallow laser marking by the ultraviolet excimer laser. Du Pont Inc. now offer specially formulated grades of their fluoropolymer resins with additives (7) for excimer marking of aircraft wire.

Recently, colored marking of polymers has been demonstrated. This has taken two forms: 1. colored marking of black or dark substrates via foaming, and 2. colored marking via photochemical change of the colorant itself (8). M. A. Hanna Corp recently announced dark polymer concentrates that allow color marking using lasers.

The vast majority of thermoset epoxy encapsulants are black. Carbon black is the additive most widely used, and it is also a strong absorber of laser radiation at all wavelengths (9). For this reason, integrated circuits and other electronics components are easily marked using either CO_2 or Nd:YAG lasers. However, since the laser-induced color change is largely a function of controlled pyrolization of the underlying resins using carefully controlled application of the laser energy, the marks tend to be golden rather than white in color. Once the carbon black content exceeds 1%, it can very effectively reduce the contrast obtained via laser marking (10). Similar results are obtained for phenolic thermoset materials. Figure 2 shows an example of laser-marked phenolic.

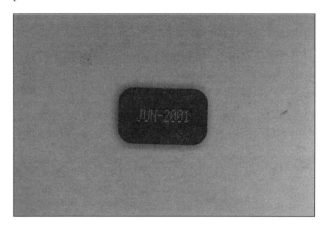

Figure 2. Laser-marked phenolic 9-V battery cap.

The major suppliers of thermoset encapsulants offer "laser-enhanced" grades of their materials. Another approach has been the use of clear coatings to improve laser markability.

Metals

Metals are commonly marked using Nd:YAG lasers at 1.06 µm wavelength. Lasers with wavelengths < 1.2 µm typically have reflectivities between 85 and 95% for polished metals while longer-wavelength infrared lasers (like CO_2 at 10.6 µm) may have reflectivities approaching 99%. For this reason, CO_2 lasers do not mark polished metal. With Nd:YAG lasers, enough energy is absorbed to initiate surface damage, which then results in more efficient coupling of the energy in the remainder of pulse to mark the metal. Successive pulses can overlap each other to remove material more deeply to form a groove. Because heat deposition is usually high, a heat-darkened region may result around the groove, and a kerf or raised ridge may be present on the edge of the marked region. Fine dust particulates of some metals can be health hazardous.

Painted metal and anodized metal mark exceptionally well using either CO_2 or Nd:YAG lasers. Since aluminum oxide is a very strong absorber of radiation at 10.6 µm, it is easy to remove a dark-colored anodized layer to make a very attractive mark (e.g., polished aluminum against black). Sequential laser marking/

colored anodizing of aluminum can result in attractive and robust multicolored marking. Ink-washed metal (e.g., toothpaste tubes), are frequently date-coded using dot matrix CO_2 markers. Figure 3 shows an example of dot matrix marking on metal.

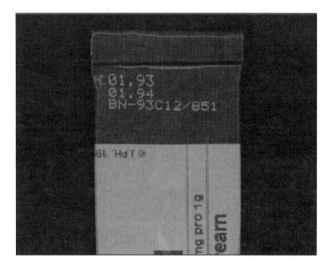

Figure 3. Dot matrix CO_2 laser mark on ink-washed metal tube.

Gold-coated lids of microelectronics packages are marked using Nd:YAG lasers. Usually the lids consist of a thin gold layer plated onto a thin nickel layer on a thick kovar lid. The laser makes an attractive black mark against gold. Frequency-doubled green lasers are sometimes used to mark gold.

Ceramics

Ceramics are another class of materials that are rarely seen in their pure state. In the electronics sector, ceramics are used to encapsulate and also to act as capacitors or inductors by virtue of added electronically active impurities. Most ceramic materials can be laser marked, but it is difficult to predict in advance which of the excimer, Nd:YAG, or CO_2 lasers will provide the best wavelength for any given sample. In some cases, depending on the laser processing parameters used, the Nd:YAG laser can make both black and white marks on ceramic materials.

Semiconductors

Silicon wafers are commonly marked at rates up to 250 wafers per hour using Nd:YAG lasers at the beginning of the fabrication process. Although silicon actually has a linear absorption depth > 250 µm at 1.06 µm (right at the band edge of silicon), nonlinear effects dramatically change the absorption process (11) so that a shallow mark of consistent depth about 2.6 µm results (the SuperSoftMark®). Laser parameters can be adjusted to optimize the absorption in the case of doped silicon so that consistent marks are obtained on any wafer. If one maintains the laser pulse energy constant to ± 0.2% pulse to pulse to just melt the surface without imparting any extra kinetic energy to the molten silicon, ejection of any dust or debris from the marked region is minimized. The diameter of each marked spot is 70 ± 10 µm, and characters are made using lines of nonoverlapping dots. The prime criteria are 1. debris-free marking, and 2. a readable mark even after successive process steps in the wafer fabrication process.

The back side of diced silicon wafers (backside die marking) is also done using Nd:YAG lasers. This process occurs after the die is bonded to a conductor substrate; so debris-free marking is not as strict a requirement. Backside die part line speeds are significantly faster than wafer marking speeds.

Other semiconductor materials such as III-V compounds are also marked using lasers. For example, GaAs wafers can be marked using frequency-doubled Nd:YAG green lasers. Extremely careful ventillation is essential for safety.

Glass

Glass television tubes and glass bottles are frequently marked using CO_2 lasers. The characters marked in clear glass are visible via room light scattered from numerous small discontinuities or microcracks. The absorbed laser light causes very shallow melting near the surface, which, when it solidifies, results in a region of shallow microcracking. Extensive measurements (5) have shown that microcracking is essentially defined to the melted region of depth about 18 µm. Time-resolved measurements show that microcracking takes place about 120 ms after laser irradiation. Soda-lime glass marks easily, but heat-resistant glasses such as borosilicate glass do not mark.

Ultraviolet ArF and KrF excimer lasers have been used to etch glass, for example, to mark flat panel displays. Very fine features can be precisely etched using the excimer laser with no evident effect to the glass outside the marked region (see Fig. 4).

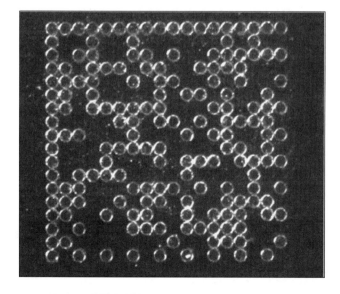

Figure 4. ID matrix 2D code marked on glass using an excimer laser (dot diameter 0.1 mm; dot spacing 0.125 mm).

Paper

Inked paper labels are commonly marked using CO_2 lasers. Typically the ink layer is thin enough that the infrared radiation passes through it but is strongly absorbed by the paper. A thermally-induced temperature rise causes ablation of the ink and/or surface layer of the paper. Very attractive marks can be achieved on colored inks such that the mark is white against color. Marking paper labels was the first laser marking application, and it is still among the most common.

Nd:YAG will also mark inked paper labels, although the selection of inks and colors becomes more important. Blue and black inks usually mark well.

Celcon® is a trademark of Hoechst Celanese (Summit, NJ); Valox® is a trademark of GE Plastics (Pittsfield, MA); Ultramid® is a trademark of BASF (Parsippany, NJ); Afflair® is a trademark of EM Industries (Hawthorne, NY); Iriodin® is a trademark of E. Merck (Darmstadt, Germany); SuperSoftMark® is a trademark of Lumonics (Oxnard, CA).

References

1. T. J. McKee, *Plastics Form. & Comp.* **1** (2), 27–32 (November, 1995); T. J. McKee, *Electrotechnology* (UK) **7** (2), 27–31, April 1996.
2. J. H. Bechtel, *J. Appl. Phys.* **46**, 1585 (1975).
3. S. C. Hu et al., *Metallurgical Trans.* **11B**, 29 (1980).
4. D. A. Hill and D. S. Soong, *J. Appl. Phys.* **61**, 2132 (1987).
5. G. Allcock et al., *J. Appl. Phys.* **78**, 7295 (1995).
6. J. Babich, Proc. RETEC 94 SPE, Decorating Div., Chicago, (September, 1994), 210–7; T. J. McKee, *Packaging Tech. & Eng.* **4** (6), 48–52 (August, 1995).
7. J. N. Birmingham et al., U.S. patent No. 5,560,845 (October 1, 1996).
8. G. Graff, *Modern Plastics* **73** (13), 30–4 (December 1996); T. McKee, L. Toth, and W. Sauerer, *Packaging Tech. & Eng.* **6** (11), 26–9 (November, 1997).
9. K. Spanjer, U.S. patent No. 4,654,290 (March 31, 1987).
10. C. Bosnos et. al., *Adv. Packaging* **6** (2), (February 1998).
11. J. Scaroni and T. McKee, *Solid State Technology* **40** (7), 245–51 (July, 1997).

TERRY MCKEE

15.3 Appropriate Lasers

15.3.1 CO_2 Lasers

Introduction

Two types of pulsed CO_2 lasers are commonly used for marking applications: TEA (transversely excited atmospheric-pressure) lasers and RF (radio frequency) excited lasers.

TEA lasers are characterized by low repetition rate, and high pulse energy operation and are typically used for single-shot stencil marking. RF excited lasers operate at high repetition rate and low pulse energy and are used to make dot-matrix marks.

A complete marking system is composed of a laser and beam delivery optics. Industrial systems are highly reliable and are modular in design for easy maintenance. Built-in micro-processors provide maintenance diagnostics and the capability of host computer control.

TEA CO_2 Lasers

The properties that make the TEA CO_2 laser suitable for single-shot marking are its high pulse energy and high peak power. Table 1 shows the output characteristics of a typical range of commercially available marking lasers. The choice of laser for a particular application depends on the marking speed required and the size of the mark. Pulse energy determines mark size.

Table 1. Performance Characteristics of Typical TEA CO_2 Marking Lasers

Parameter	Low speed	Medium speed	High speed
Repetition rate (pps)	15	30	150
Pulse energy (J)	5	2.5	0.5
Beam size (mm²)	25 x 25	14 x 16	14 x 11
Average power (W)		75	
Pulse duration (µs)		3–8	
Wavelength (µm)		9.3 or 10.6	

Low- and medium-speed lasers generally make a complete mark, composed of several characters, with a single pulse. High-speed lasers generate a single character per pulse, and the beam is scanned to make a complete mark.

The optical pulse, which is characterized by a gain-switched spike and a tail of several microseconds, is shown in Figure 1.

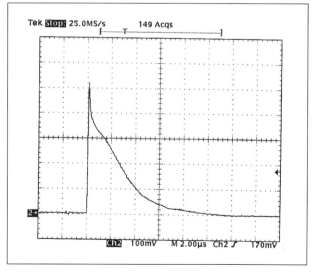

Figure 1. TEA CO_2 laser optical pulse shape. Time scale=2 µs/division.

The output beam is multimode and typically has a top hat profile in one dimension and a somewhat rounded top profile in the other dimension. The beam divergence is about 6 mrad.

The laser beam is delivered to the target by steering mirrors inside beam tubes. A field lens is used to focus the beam onto a stencil mask. A second lens images the mask, at reduced size, onto the part to be marked.

The physical characteristics and facilities requirements of a typical TEA CO_2 laser are given in Table 2.

Table 2. Physical Characteristics and Facilities Requirements of Typical TEA CO_2 Marking Lasers

Parameter	Specifications
Cabinet size	121 cm x 66 cm footprint x 41 cm high
Weight	130 kg
Cabinet material	Aluminum or stainless steel
Cabinet sealing	IEC 529 (IP66) water and dust tight
Electrical service	100–120 or 200–240 V, 50/60 Hz
Power consumption	2.0 kVA
Cooling water	90 L/h at 10–25°C
Cooling air	Not required
Laser gas mixture	0.5% H_2, 4% CO, 8% CO_2, 16% N_2, bal He
Laser gas consumption	0.5 L/h: large cylinder (7500 standard liters) lasts 2 years

Modern TEA CO_2 lasers use solid-state modulator technology to generate an electrical discharge in the laser gas. Early TEA CO_2 lasers used spark-gap and thyratron high-voltage switches, which are inherently unreliable and have high operating costs.

The high-voltage switch in the solid-state modulator is a silicon controlled rectifier (SCR). This is a long-life solid-state device. The rest of the modulator is composed of reliable passive components: capacitors, inductors, and transformers. Table 3 lists the expected lifetimes of the high-voltage components.

Also shown in Table 3 are the lifetimes of the laser cavity optics. The rear total reflector is typically diamond-turned aluminum, which may have a gold coating. The front partial reflector is usually germanium.

The cavity optics are mounted directly on the laser vessel and are in contact with the laser gas. Fine dust particles that are present in the laser gas can contaminate the optics and shorten their life. However, a dust filtering system may be used to prevent optic contamination, resulting in the long optic lifetimes shown in Table 3.

Table 3. Component Lifetimes of Typical TEA CO_2 Marking Lasers

Component	Component lifetime, 150 pps laser	
	Laser pulses (millions)	Years (16-h shift, 5 d/wk)
Solid-state modulator	10,000	4.4
Discharge electrodes	2,500	1.1
Rear cavity optic	5,000	2.2
Front cavity optic	2,500	1.1

RF-Excited CO_2 Lasers

The RF-excited CO_2 laser operates at high repetition rate and is therefore suitable for dot-matrix marking. Table 4 gives typical output characteristics for the laser.

Table 4. Performance Characteristics of Typical RF-Excited CO_2 Marking Lasers

Parameter	Specification
Repetition rate	Up to 16 kHz
Pulse energy	6 mJ to 1 J
Average power	100 W
Dot size	0.1 to 0.3 mm diameter
Character size	2 to 20 mm high
Pulse duration	30 µs to 5 ms
Wavelength	10.2 to 11.2 µm

The output beam mode is TEM_{00}, which gives the lowest beam divergence. The beam is circularly symmetric and has a Gaussian intensity profile. Low divergence is required to achieve small dots in the mark, because the laser beam is directly focused onto the target rather than imaged through a mask.

The laser beam is delivered to the target by a spinning multifacet mirror. Laser triggering is computer controlled and is synchronized with the mirror to generate successive columns of dots on the target, which ultimately result in the dot-matrix mark. Character generation rates up to 430 characters per second are achieved.

The physical characteristics and facilities requirements of a typical RF-excited CO_2 marking laser are given in Table 5.

The laser tube is permanently sealed and has a service life of over 10 years (16 h/d, 5 d/wk use). The laser cavity optics are an integral part of the tube. The RF power supply, which excites the laser, uses long-life solid-state switching components.

ISBN 0-912035-15-3

Table 5. Physical Characteristics and Facilities Requirements of Typical RF-Excited CO_2 Marking Lasers

Parameter	Specifications
Cabinet size	35 cm x 51 cm footprint x 114 cm high
Weight	129 kg
Cabinet material	Stainless steel
Cabinet sealing	IP56
Electrical service	100–120 or 200–240 V, 50/60 Hz
Power consumption	1.2 kVA
Cooling water	Not required
Cooling air	Ambient temperature 5–35°C
Laser gas	Not required (sealed tube)

ROBERT K. BRIMACOMBE

15.3.2 Nd:YAG Lasers

Nd:YAG is the most widely used solid-state laser material. Nd:YAG lasers have been described extensively in Section 2.2. They are frequently used in marking applications.

This laser resonator determines the beam quality of the laser, which determines how narrow a line can be marked. When running multimode the beam will have a diameter a little smaller than the laser rod. The intensity profile would be flat topped with numerous hot spots. This would produce wide marks when focused onto the workpiece in an engraving application. Multimode lasers provide the flat intensity profile required for image micromachining.

The laser can also be operated in the TEM_{00} mode at lower power. This is achieved by restricting the angle of rays propagating between the laser mirrors, either by introducing an aperture or by increasing the distance between the mirrors. The profile of a TEM_{00} beam is smooth and Gaussian and when focused onto the workpiece will produce very narrow lines.

Pulsed Lasers

Most laser marking applications require relatively low average power (1–20 W) but require high irradiance (> 10^6 W/cm^2); so the peak power needs to be enhanced by either pulsing or Q-switching. Pulsing means flashing the pump lamps or diodes to high peak power levels, but the pulses are still relatively long (100–2000 µs) and pulse repetition frequencies are limited and peak power may still not be high enough. Table 6 shows typical pulse and beam parameters used in laser marking.

Q Switching

Q switching is the most widely used method of producing the laser power required for marking applications. The so-called Q of a laser cavity is the ratio of stored energy to cavity loss per round trip. In Q switching, energy is stored in the laser rod by optical pumping. The laser is prevented from oscillating by introducing a controllable loss. When this loss is removed the combination of the high gain and low round trip loss results in the stored energy being discharged in a very short (< 100 ns) pulse with a peak power of > 10^4 W. In continuously pumped lasers Q switching can be achieved at rates > 50 kHz. Because energy is stored in an energy level that has a lifetime of ~230 µs, the maximum pulse energy and peak power is achieved at pulse repetition frequencies up to 4 kHz.

Table 6. Typical Laser Pulse Parameters for Marking Applications

	Image micromachining	Engraving
Pulse energy	2–10 J	0.5–2 mJ
Pulse duration	50–2000 µs	50–200 ns
Pulse repetition frequency	5–20 Hz	2–20 kHz
Output beam size	6–10 mm	0.5–1.0 mm
Beam divergence	Typically > 3 mrad	1–3 mrad
Focused spot size	Imaged mask	50–200 µm
Focused power density	> 10^4 W/cm^2	> 10^6 W/cm^2

CW-pumped marking lasers use acousto-optic Q switches almost exclusively. In an acousto-optic switch an ultrasonic wave is launched into a block of transparent material, usually fused silica. This wave produces a traveling compression in the material, which, because of the photoelastic effect, produces a grating that diffracts a portion of the light traveling along the axis of the laser resonator out of the cavity and introduces a loss. This loss is sufficient to prevent the laser from oscillating. The acoustic wave is launched by bonding a piezoelectric transducer to the fused silica block. These devices typically run at frequencies from 27 MHz upwards.

When the radio frequency drive to the transducer is removed, the loss returns to a very low value, and the laser oscillates normally.

The pulses produced in this way possess enough peak power when focused onto the material to melt and vaporize the surface and thus produce a visible mark.

Harmonics

Most marking applications use light at 1064 nm or the fundamental wavelength of Nd:YAG. There are materials, however, that respond better to light at shorter wavelengths. For instance, aluminum and copper are reflective at 1064 nm, but light at green wavelengths (~500 nm) is coupled well into those materials. Some plastics will discolor rather than burn or vaporize when exposed to high-intensity ultraviolet light.

Frequency conversion extends the wavelength range of high-power lasers. This is achieved by exciting harmonics of the fundamental wavelength in special types of crystal using nonlinear effects produced in high-intensity optical fields (see Chapter 2). Doubling the frequency (halving the wavelength) produces green light at 532 nm. By mixing green light and fundamental light in a crystal, ultraviolet light at 355 nm is produced. If one doubles the frequency of green 532 nm light, ultraviolet light at 266 nm is produced.

MARTIN MATTHEWS

15.3.3 Excimer Lasers for Marking

In terms of output parameters, the optimum choice of excimer laser for a given task depends upon the material to be marked and the marking technique to be employed. In general, however, there are two basic approaches used for excimer laser marking. These are summarized in Table 7.

Table 7. Excimer Laser Marking Methods

Method	Optimum laser
Mark each digit or part of pattern separately	High repetition rate/low energy
Mark entire pattern at once	High energy/low repetition rate

Table 8 lists actual typical operating parameters for each type of marking situation.

Table 8. Typical Marking Laser Parameters

	ArF 193 nm	KrF 248 nm	XeCl 308 nm	XeF 351 nm
High-energy/low-repetition-rate laser				
Pulse energy	400 mJ	600 mJ	400 mJ	320 mJ
Repetition rate	100 Hz	100 Hz	100 Hz	100 Hz
Average power	32 W	56 W	38 W	28 W
Pulse duration (FWHM)	23 ns	34 ns	28 ns	30 ns
Low-energy/high-repetition-rate laser				
Pulse energy	100 mJ	300 mJ	125 mJ	100 mJ
Repetition rate	200 Hz	200 Hz	200 Hz	200 Hz
Average power	20 W	60 W	25 W	20 W
Pulse duration (FWHM)	17 ns	17 ns	20 ns	14 ns

In the real world of industrial marking applications, laser reliability, ease-of-use, and cost of ownership characteristics are just as important as output performance. Significant advances in excimer laser technology have been made in all these areas over the past few years.

Lifetime

One of the leading problems limiting excimer laser performance and reliability was the corrosive effect of the laser gases with the laser tube and tube components. The contaminants created through this corrosion quench laser action, thereby reducing laser operating efficiency, which can significantly limit the lifetime of a gas fill. Reduced efficiency also negatively impacts laser beam quality and pulse energy stability. In addition to limiting tube lifetime, corrosion also increases the frequency of routine component cleaning and replacement.

To address this problem, laser manufacturers have adopted an all metal/ceramic tube construction that virtually eliminates corrosion. All insulators and high-voltage feed-throughs in the plasma tube are constructed from corrosion-resistant ceramics (1). The metal parts of the laser tube are made from specialized carbon- and silicon-free alloys to avoid the production of common contaminants, such as SiF_4 and CF_4. The construction involves a multi-step passivation process to eliminate all traces of water from the components, ensuring that exposed surfaces will remain inert. Also, all assembly is performed under clean room conditions to prevent exposure to external contaminants.

Maintenance

Industrial excimer lasers must be constructed so as to minimize the time required for various maintenance procedures. Modular construction of both the laser tube and electronic components has recently aided in achieving this end. The discharge unit, high-voltage power supply, gas handling, and computer control may all be in separate modules for easy replacement. In order to shorten the time needed for routine optics cleaning, a slide valve mechanism is used. When optics are pulled out for cleaning, this slide valve seals the laser to avoid internal contamination by air or moisture.

Typical mean time to repair (MTTR) values for industrial excimer lasers are on the order of less than eight hours today (see table 9). For specificity, model numbers of a particular manufacturer are named; this does not constitute an endorsement.

Integrated Gas Generator

A significant item connected with the use of excimer lasers is the storage and handling requirements for the halogen gases used. Technical and legal requirements may demand such precautions as safety cabinets, earthquake proofing, and passivated gas lines. To alleviate these problems sealed internal units that generate HCl or F_2 on demand, from all solid, inert materials, have been developed.

Ease of Use

Successfully integrating an excimer laser into an industrial production line is greatly facilitated if all functions of the laser can be controlled both internally and externally through software. For example, all operating parameters in industrial excimer lasers can be set through software menus. Diagnostics of all systems can be accessed, and the laser can keep a running electronic log of operating parameters to aid in process control. The laser can communicate with production line control systems through a standard computer interface.

Chapter 15: Marking

Typical Reliability and Cost Data

Based on these various design innovations, excimer lasers now demonstrate the reliability and cost characteristics to make them useful in a wide variety of industrial processing tasks. Table 10 lists typical values, obtained under real world industrial operating conditions, for mean time between failure for excimer lasers used in marking operations. Again, for specificity, model numbers of a particular manufacturer are listed; this does not constitute an endorsement. Table 11 lists consumable and component lifetimes; the same cautionary note applies to mention of a particular manufacturer.

Table 9. Mean Time To Repair (MTTR) Data of Industrial Excimer Lasers

Laser type	MTTR[a] (h)
LPX 200i series	< 12
LAMBDA 1000/2000/3000/4000 series	< 8
NovaLine 100	< 4
NovaLine LITHO	< 2

[a]With a trained service staff and spare parts management conducted according to recommended procedures. These times include a worst-case scenario of complete tube exchange (necessary after 1–5 billion pulses).

Table 10. Mean Time Between Failure (MTBF) Data of Industrial Excimer Lasers

Application	Laser type	MTBF[a]
SMD marking	LPX 210i	> 2000
Ink-jet nozzle	LAMBDA 1248	> 2000
MCM drilling	LAMBDA 3308	> 1500
Wire stripping	LPX 220i	> 1500

[a]Unscheduled downtime is < 0.5%.

Table 11. Measured Component and Consumables Lifetime of Industrial Excimer Lasers for Micromachining (60 W, KrF)

Component	Without NovaTube	With NovaTube
Gas lifetime @ 200 Hz	10 - 56 x 10⁶ pulses	77 - 168 x 10⁶ pulses
Window cleaning interval	50 - 150 x 10⁶ pulses	150 - 450 x 10⁶ pulses
Laser tube lifetime	0.7 - 1.2 x 10⁹ pulses	1.2 - 2.3 x 10⁹ pulses

Reference

1. D. Basting, H. Endert, R. Pätzel, M. Powell, and U. Rebhan, New KrF and ArF excimer lasers for advanced deep ultraviolet optical lithography, *Japanese Journal of Applied Physics* (**34**), 4050–4, 1995.

HEINRICH ENDERT
DIRK BASTING

15.4 Dot Matrix Marking

15.4.1 Techniques

General Description

Dot matrix marking is a technique used for applying indelible codes to a wide variety of materials and material surfaces. In dot matrix marking, a pattern of tiny holes defines the desired characters or figures. The laser beam is focused on the surface, scanned in the desired pattern, and pulsed when a mark is needed. The marking system utilizes a continuous-wave (CW) laser and optical scanning mechanism (see Fig. 1).

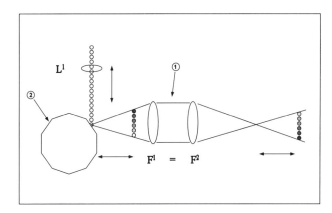

Figure 1. Typical optical configuration of a polygon dot matrix marker. ← Unity magnification telescope, ↑ polygon.

The laser is used to generate a continuous beam of infrared light that is then modulated to produce a train of laser pulses. When one directs the pulse train at an optical scanner, a vertical column of dots (raster scan) can be produced. The numbers of dots in a column are adjustable to suit the character style and number of lines of text.

Laser Sources

The most commonly used laser source is a sealed continuous-wave carbon dioxide laser, operating in the infrared at a wavelength of 10.6 µm. Average power between 70 and 100 W is typical in single-source dot matrix marking systems. Lower-average-power lasers can be used when operating in an array.

The Nd:YAG laser has also been employed for dot matrix marking, because many materials to be marked absorb well at the 1.06 µm wavelength and because it offers short pulses of high peak power, capable of vaporizing a mark on the surface. Dot matrix marking using *Q*-switched lasers have often been used on metals and anodized surfaces.

Scanning Techniques

There are a number of scanning techniques currently being used to create dot columns. The most common techniques are polygon, acousto-optic, and piezoelectric scanning (see Fig. 2).

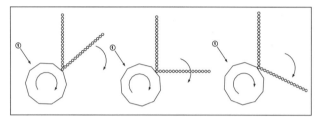

Figure 2. Example of a polygon-generated raster scan.

The simplest and most cost-effective scanning technique utilizes a rotating optical polygon. The polygon containing a number of optical facets rotates at a fixed speed; the speed is determined by the width of the character and the number of dots in a particular column. The modulated laser beam is directed at the rotating facet, and the resultant reflected angle changes at a rate determined by the number of facets and the facet speed. The resultant dot matrix scan is then reproduced on the target and forms one column of a character per facet scan. In the generation of a typical character, six facet scans are used to create the complete character (five vertical scans plus one scan space between characters).

15.4.2 Results

Energy Density

The visibility of a mark is very much dependent upon absorption of laser light into the product surface. Energy density, therefore, plays a key part of the process. Spot size, even distribution of energy, and laser peak power are important factors for successful marking. Peak power is particularly important when marking harder materials such as glass. A peak power at least twice the laser average power is generally sufficient to mark a wide range of materials. Figure 3 shows and example of dot matrix marking.

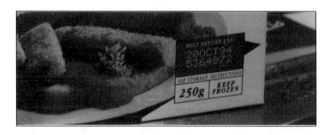

Figure 3. Typical dot matrix marking application. Best-before date and internal batch code on printed cardboard. Photograph courtesy of Lumonics.

ANDREW JOHN CHAMBERS

15.5 Engraving

15.5.1 Techniques

Basic Methods

In laser engraving, the laser etches grooves into a workpiece. There are two basic engraving methods for reproducing artwork on an object. These are raster engraving and vector engraving.

Raster

A raster image is an image composed of dots. This is similar to the dot matrix marking discussed in Section 15.4. Pictures in a newspaper or a television screen are examples of a raster image. The data used to create a raster image are divided into rows: A row describes a one-dot-high strip of the image. These dot rows are then stacked top down to create the image. In a black and white image each dot in the row is given a value to define its color, with 1 being black and 0 being white. The binary image would then appear as shown in Figures 1 and 2. The image may be filled and colored, for example, with paint.

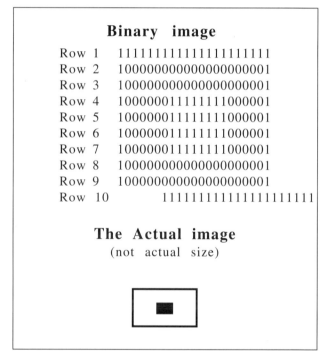

Figure 1. Raster engraving.

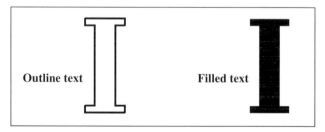

Figure 2. Outline and filled engraving.

Graphics are not limited to simple shapes, just as television images are not limited. Complex patterns can be created using simple graphic packages. Artwork can be scanned into a computer using a flatbed or hand scanner. Digital images can be imported in a graphics package and manipulated as desired. Images can also be made up of different colors. These colors can be used to change the power on the laser or converted into a halftone. The most common approach to this is to dither the image. The resulting images appear as shown in Figure 3.

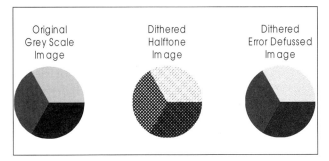

Figure 3. Original and dithered graphics.

Resolution Effects

Resolution is defined as the number of dots per inch (DPI). Placing more dots per line and more lines per inch can give a raster image more definition. The edges of an image become smoother as the resolution increases (see Fig. 4).

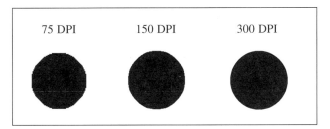

Figure 4. Resolution.

Increasing resolution while giving better definition will also increase the engraving time. An engraving machine can put down only a finite number of lines per minute. Increasing the number of lines to be reproduced will increase the amount of time it takes for engraving the image.

Vector (Scribing)

Vector scribing is another way to produce an image. The scribing process consists of tracing a line around an object using the laser as the pen. The difference between scribing and cutting is that in scribing an image is produced in the material to a limited depth. This depth could be as thin as few thousandths of an inch to cutting almost through the material. The artwork can be produced in a graphics program or manually written. The advantage of scribing is that some images can be more efficiently reproduced using a vector scribe than a raster image. The image is drawn using point-to-point moves rather than produced by one line of dots at a time.

Simple Line Art

Some examples of simple line art that are more efficiently produced by a scribing technique are shown in Figure 5.

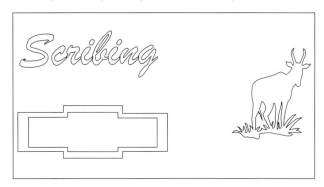

Figure 5. Line art.

Complex Graphics

Complex graphics can best be accomplished using a combination of raster and vector engraving. By rearranging the 1s and 0s in the above example, many different types of graphics can be created. An example would be filled text. The 1s and 0s can be arranged to outline the letter or to fill the letter. The latter approach is called filled text.

15.5.2 Lasers

CO_2 Lasers

CO_2 lasers are used to engrave items to depth and to surface engrave. Items made of nonmetals such as wood, plastic, leather, or rubber absorb the 10.6 μm wavelength of the CO_2 laser very well. They have a low enough vaporization temperature that the vapors can be removed from the cut area easily. It is easy to engrave a deep image into these materials.

Surface engraving with a CO_2 laser typically involves removing a thin surface coating applied to a different type of substrate. This may be paint on a metal surface or a thin plastic coating on a plastic or metal substrate. Surface engraving also can be accomplished on a solid material by changing the surface color or texture but not engraving to any significant depth.

Engraving into metal is not a strong point of the CO_2 laser because the 10.6 μm wavelength does not couple well into the surface of metals. Ferrous metals such as stainless steel can be effectively marked with higher-power CO_2 lasers, however.

Nd:YAG Lasers

Nd:YAG lasers are good for surface engraving many types of materials. The 1.06 μm wavelength couples much more effectively into metals than the CO_2 wavelength and is typically the laser of choice for metal engraving.

Many nonmetal materials, such as wood and some plastics, do not engrave effectively with an Nd:YAG laser because the wavelength is not absorbed well. The surface of these materials may be slightly changed by the laser beam, but typically no material removal will occur. This can be used to advantage because one can engrave inside materials such as plastic or glass. The beam is focused inside the material, and the material is not affected until the energy density gets high enough at the focal point to microfracture the material.

15.5.3 Surface Effects

Nonmetals

The majority of nonmetallic materials can be readily engraved. The composition of each material will determine the engraving depth. Materials that have the best ability to absorb the laser beam will engrave the best. These include, but are not limited to, wood, plastic, leather, rubber, and variations of each.

Metals

As previously mentioned, the Nd:YAG laser is the laser of choice for engraving metals. The CO_2 laser will not couple into metals well but can be used for removing a coating from metals, which will provide a form of engraving.

15.5.4 Beam Motion Systems

X-Y

An *X-Y* system is one type of system that can be used to engrave objects. This type of system typically moves in two axes and modulates the laser beam to produce engraving. In an *X-Y* system, the part can be moved in both axes, the beam can be moved in both axes, or a combination of both motions can be used. An advantage of moving the part is that the beam path and delivery system always stays the same and can be very rigid. An advantage of a system where the beam moves in both axes is that the part is stationary and does not need to be clamped. The motion system is usually smaller and lighter. Some disadvantages of moving the part are that the part typically needs clamping and the motion system is large and heavier. A disadvantage of the moving beam is that the beam path may change, causing problems with alignment and changing focal point size.

Galvo

Galvo (galvanometer) systems are moving beam engravers. They tilt two mirrors, one for each axis, in order to position the beam on the part surface. An advantage of the galvo-type systems is that they are very fast because they are moving only a mirror. One disadvantage can be that the beam typically hits the surface at an angle, and if the part is engraved to depth, the angled cut can be very noticeable.

Another thing to note is that the bigger the area that can be engraved, the bigger the focused spot size is. Fine-resolution engraving typically cannot be accomplished over a large area.

15.5.5 Masking

General

The main purpose of a mask is to protect the unengraved portions of an item. Color filling by painting is one of the most common examples for using a mask. After applying the paint, one must pull off any pieces of the mask that remain in the area that is not colored. One may choose to apply the paint to the engraved areas either with a brush or by spraying. There is a wide variety of paint options to choose from. Oil-based enamels are one choice. One may prefer the easy clean-up associated with water-based acrylic latex paint.

After the paint has dried, the mask is peeled away, taking any excess paint along with it. The engraved images will be highlighted with color, and the surface (unengraved) areas will usually require no additional cleaning.

Masks are also convenient when using materials that are sensitive to heat, such as some types of plastics. The mask will absorb the excess heat and protect the material from heat and/or smoke damage. There are three types of masks that are commonly used for laser engraving, which will be discussed in the following.

Liquid Masks

Liquid masking materials are water-based latex products. They are applied as a liquid and dry into a flexible, rubbery coating. The manufacturer may suggest a sprayer to apply the material in an even manner, or it may be practical to brush the liquid on. The masking material should be applied in a thick, even coating. Too thin a coat will be difficult to peel. After engraving, a liquid mask will peel off nearly any material, except porous materials such as unfinished wood. A liquid mask may take up to 12 hours to dry before engraving can take place.

Film Masks

This mask is a polyester film material. The film masking material is wound in a roll, similar to single-sided tape. To use the film, simply apply it over the material, smoothing any bubbles by hand or with a squeegee. The silicone adhesive provides good contact with the surface of virtually any laser-engravable material. However, after engraving and peeling away the excess masking material (from outline images that will be painted) and before applying any paint, it is recommended that a finger be run along the edges of the engraved images. This will reseal any edges that may have been pulled up during the processes and will prevent paint seepage that might occur as a result. For similar reasons, it is recommended that one apply paint to the material using a spraying device, such as an air brush, inexpensive spray gun, or cans of aerosol spray paint. If one prefers a brush, a foam brush should be used, dabbing paint on rather than actually brushing it on. Polyester film masking materials will not tear or rip easily and can usually be removed in one piece. It is recommended that the film be removed as soon as the paint has dried, or the mask may become more difficult to peel off. Film mask should not be used on film-covered press board.

Paper Masks

Paper masking material has a self-adhesive backing and comes in various tack grade levels. The less aggressive adhesive can be used on mylar, which will protect it from smoke damage. The more aggressive adhesive is recommended for unfinished wood.

Chapter 15: Marking

It will adhere to the material better. Paper masks do not adhere as strongly to the material surface as either a film or a liquid mask. Paint can sometimes bleed through the paper onto unengraved areas.

Miscellaneous Masking Tips

If one is engraving acrylic deeply, one may want to mask it first. A mild nonabrasive liquid soap is recommended. Apply a liberal coating of soap before engraving. The soap will prevent engraved areas from fogging. Masking materials can also help prevent damage to heat-sensitive items. Also it can save considerable time and effort when color filling.

15.5.6 Engraving Recommendations

Wood (1/4-in. Hardwood)

If one chooses to use unfinished wood, it must be masked to prevent the residue from staining it. A high-adhesion mask is recommended so that it will adhere better to the raw wood. It will also stay on better if one wants to paint fill later. If one does not use a mask, the residue must be sanded off. When one works with a finished wood that has a lacquer or sanding sealer for a top coat, a damp cloth (lint free) will remove the residue. During cutting one should use a vacuum box or elevate the part off the table so the heat will not affect the part. Also using air will help reduce heat-affected areas. For paint filling one can use a spray paint if the part is masked. Acrylic-based marker works well if the engraving area to be filled is fine.

Table 1 presents recommendations for power and speed for engraving 1/4-in. 114-1N hardwood.

Table 1. Recommendations for 1/4-in. Hardwood

	Raster	Vector cut	Vector scribe
Power (W)	100	100	15
Speed (ips)	22	1	4

Acrylic (1/4-in.)

Two types of acrylic generally used for laser engraving are cast and extruded. Cast acrylic such as lucite will turn white or frosted when engraved. The edge quality will not look as polished as extruded acrylic. In many applications the cast material will be a finished product and ready for shipping when the engraving is complete. The extruded material may need to be paint filled, because it has a clear look after engraving. If one is not sure of the material, do a sample cut to see how it appears, clear or frosted. The factory mask on the bottom should be left to avoid scratches from handling and focusing on the part. The factory mask should be removed from the top surface. If one is planning to paint fill, one should use a low tack adhesive masking. It is also recommended that one use an acrylic- or water-based paint. After paint filling, the part should be thoroughly dry before one removes the mask. Past experience suggests using low power and a fast speed setting. This will cause less heat, which can leave a white film around the engraving and can also cause the edges to craze. Table 2 shows guidelines for different power and speed for 1/4-in. acrylic.

Table 2. Recommendations for 1/4-in. Acrylic

	Raster	Vector cut	Vector scribe
Power (W)	100	100	15
Speed (ips)	22	5	4

Glass

Glass will vary depending on the manufacturer and type of glass used. Lead content of glass is a major factor. Lower lead content glass is better for engraving. Domestic glass seems to engrave best. When engraving flat glass or when removing the coating from the back of a mirror, note that the artwork is usually reversed. It is important to work on a clean surface; dirt and oil can vary the appearance of the engraving. The glass should be cleaned after engraving to remove small particles of glass adhering to the engraving. Steel wool and a little soap is recommended to lightly rub the particles off. One should not rub too hard, or the glass will be scratched. Table 3 shows recommendations for glass.

Table 3. Recommendations for 1/4-in. Glass

	Raster	Vector scribe
Power (W)	100	8
Speed (ips)	22	4.5

Coated Metal

Low-powered engravers will not cut through metal, but will remove a coating. One may have to adjust the power so the heat does not affect the adjacent coating. As an example, black anodized material will turn white when engraved. Colored markers may be used to color the engraved area to achieve variety. The excess material is then wiped off and the engraving finished with a coat of acrylic spray for protection. Table 4 shows recommendations for coated metal.

Table 4. Recommendations for 1/4-in. Coated Metal

	Raster	Vector scribe
Power (W)	100	8
Speed (ips)	22	4.5

PETER BECHER
PHIL DEBOER
ARLENE ZDRAZIL

15.6 Image Micromachining

15.6.1 Techniques

General Description

Image micromachining is a method for generating marks on a variety of substrate materials using a pulsed laser and a simple optical imaging technique. The technique is also called mask imaging.

In its simplest form, the pulsed laser beam illuminates some form of stencil mask, and the transmitted laser radiation is reduced in size and imaged onto the substrate. This is shown schematically in Figure 1.

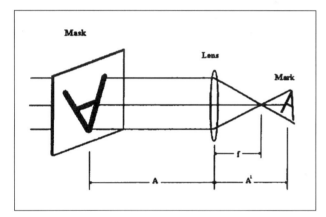

Figure 1. Basic stencil mask imaging configuration.

The content of the mark can consist of alphanumeric characters, logos or symbols, bar codes, or two-dimensional codes.

Laser Sources

The most commonly used laser source is the pulsed TEA CO_2 laser, with pulsed Nd:YAG lasers and excimer lasers also being used. Typical laser parameters are given in Table 1.

Table 1. Typical Pulsed Laser Parameters

Parameter	TEA CO_2	Nd:YAG	Excimer
Pulse energy	2–6 J	2–10 J	0.1–0.5 J
Pulse duration	1–2 µs	50–2000 µs	0.02–0.05 µs
Wavelength	10.6 µm	1.06 µm	0.308 µm
Repetition rate	10–150 pps	5–20 pps	10–200 pps

Mask Techniques

The simplest type of mask is a thin stainless steel or beryllium copper plate with the mark information chemically etched onto the mask. These are called leaf masks. The drawback of this technique is that the characters on the mask require small webs to hold the centers in place, and the resultant mark shows these webs.

Nd:YAG and excimer masks can also be fabricated from thin glass plates with a reflective surface coating on one face. The mark information is etched into the reflective coating and eliminates the requirement for webs in the characters.

Single leaf masks can contain all the mark information, which means that the mask has to be changed each time the mark information changes. A more flexible configuration is to use a set of "stackable" masks, with each mask containing only one part of the total mark.

Even more flexibility can be achieved by using a set of up to eight overlapping discs. Each disc can contain up to 40 different characters. The position of each disc is controlled by a stepper motor, and by controlling all eight discs, random number or character codes can easily be generated.

One other technique that has been developed for pulsed Nd:YAG systems is to use a liquid crystal mask. The mark information is input to the liquid crystal display, which can be changed on a random access basis.

15.6.2 Results

There are three primary processes that result in laser marking. The first process requires the removal of a surface layer to expose an underlying layer of contrasting color. The second requires bulk absorption of the laser radiation and a resultant thermochemical or photochemical reaction in the material to produce a color change. The third process requires a modification of the surface reflectance of the material to produce a contrasting surface finish. Several review articles (1, 2) have been published that discuss the laser marking process in detail.

Energy Density

The visibility of the resultant mark on the material is strongly dependent on the energy density of the laser radiation transmitted by the mask and imaged by the lens. If the energy density is below the marking threshold, then no mark is produced. If the energy density is above the marking threshold, the process will create visible marks.

The energy density at the material is determined by the energy density of the laser beam at the mask and the amount of demagnification introduced by the imaging lens.

Typical systems are designed to ensure that the actual energy density at the material is approximately 20% higher than the marking threshold energy density to ensure consistent marking quality, and to account for small variations in the laser output energy.

Some typical energy densities for different substrate materials are shown in Table 2.

In all cases the threshold energy density is determined by performing a series of tests on the actual material that is to be marked.

Table 2. Typical Marking Threshold Energy Densities

Substrate material	Laser source	Threshold energy density (J/cm²)
Inked Paper	CO_2	2 to 4
Plastics/Epoxies	CO_2	6 to 16
Glass	CO_2	15 to 25
Ceramic	CO_2	15 to 25
Plastics/Epoxies	YAG	1 to 8
Ceramic	YAG	5 to 16
Cable Insulation	Excimer	1 to 3
Ceramic	Excimer	6 to 15

References

1. T. J. McKee, *Physics in Canada* **51**, 107–14 (1995).
2. T. J. McKee, *Packaging Technology and Engineering* **4**, 48–52 (1995).

BRIAN NORRIS

15.7 Applications

The approximate breakdown among the major laser types used for industrial marking is:

CO_2 lasers	35%
Nd:YAG lasers	60%
Excimer lasers	5%

Utilizing about 40% of the installed laser marking base, the electronics sector has historically been the largest market. The applications of lasers for marking of electronic devices and components will be described in Chapter 18. Other important markets are consumer packaging, and the automotive, medical, and aerospace industries. Table 1 shows major applications arranged by laser type.

Table 1. Major Marking Applications by Laser Type (1)

Laser type	Market/application	
CO_2	electronics:	integrated circuits (ICs) transistors, capacitors TV tubes
	packaging:	beverage containers, paper labels cosmetics, soaps, pharmaceuticals
Nd:YAG	electronics:	integrated circuits (ICs) keyboards, molded parts, switches control panels, consumer items
	automotive:	metal parts, dashboard displays
	medical:	molded parts, syringes, containers
	aerospace:	displays, metal parts, wire
Excimer	electronics:	capacitors aircraft wire

15.7.1 CO_2 Lasers

CO_2 lasers mark most materials except metals. CO_2 lasers are widely used to mark packaged goods using both the imaged-mask and the dot matrix formats (2). The most common application is to code a date or batch code on an inked paper label, whereby the laser removes a dark ink showing the white paper underneath; thus the characters are seen as white against dark (see Fig 1).

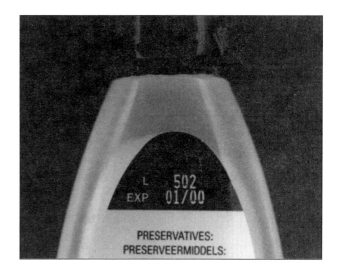

Figure 1. Imaged-mask CO_2 laser marks blue paper label.

Other examples of consumer packages marked with the CO_2 laser include plastic bottles marked directly with the laser, anodized or inked metal containers such as toothpaste tubes, glass parts such as vacuum tubes where the CO_2 laser marks the glass directly, plastic film labels, and thermoplastic elastomer items such as wiper blades. Figure 2 shows an example.

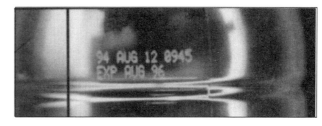

Figure 2. Dot matrix CO_2 mark 94 AUG 12 0945 EXP AUG 96 on a transparent PET (polyethylene terephthalate) water bottle.

Line speeds as high as 1800 parts per minute are obtained in beverage marking applications.

Applications of CO_2 laser marking in the electronics industry are presented in Chapter 18.

15.7.2 Nd:YAG Lasers

Nd:YAG lasers are most often employed in the directed beam (laser writing) marking format (1). In this case, the marking process is somewhat slower because the sample is usually stationary during the marking process. However, since the marking process is computer controlled, cosmetically attractive marks including alphanumerics, bar codes, 2D codes, logos, and graphics are possible. Also, if the material marks easily, multiple samples can be marked simultaneously.

The Nd:YAG laser wavelength marks most materials except for visually transparent materials such as clear plastics and glass; sometimes, however, if the absorption is not high enough, the laser may penetrate too deeply into the material, making a rather unattractive mark. Often with plastics, additives such as colorants and fillers can dramatically increase the absorption, leading to better marks.

The largest market for Nd:YAG laser writing systems is to mark integrated circuits. This is described further in Chapter 18.

The Nd:YAG laser writer is the best system to mark bare metal, including aluminum, copper, brass, stainless steel, nickel, and most alloys (3). Marking often is in a dot matrix format, because the energy per unit area must be relatively high. It is important with metals to ensure that particulates are vacuumed from the air at the source because some metal particulates can be health hazardous. Also, this marking system can produce a very attractive mark on painted metal. If desired, the Nd:YAG laser can cut or scribe a groove of depth up to 0.005 in. in metal, although the time to mark will vary substantially with the metal being marked and the depth.

One issue that can arise is the kerf or raised edge that often occurs around the marked area because of flow of molten metal to the edge of the mark. The kerf can usually be minimized by careful control of the marking process, that is, dot placement. The Nd:YAG laser writing system is used to mark metal parts in the automotive, aerospace, and medical industries, and in the electronics industry to code metal leadframes (see Fig. 3 for an example).

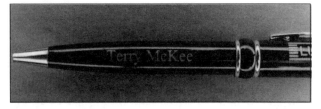

Figure 3. Nd:YAG laser writer enscribes a blue-enamelled pen where the mark shows gold against blue.

In some cases when the Nd:YAG wavelength is not effective for marking the desired sample, the wavelength can be harmonically multiplied in nonlinear crystals to produce shorter wavelengths which are then used to mark via the laser writing technique (see Chapter 2). Examples include some ceramics and plastics, which are best marked with ultraviolet wavelengths (tripled Nd:YAG at wavelength 0.355 μm) (see Fig. 4 for an example).

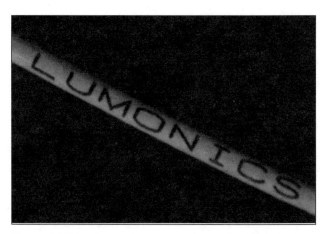

Figure 4. White fluoropolymer-coated aircraft wire marked using a frequency-tripled Nd:YAG laser writing system.

References
1. T. J. McKee, *Plastics Form. & Comp.* **1** (2), 27–32 (November 1995); T. J. McKee, *Electrotechnology* (UK) **7** (2), 27–31 (April 1996).
2. J. Hunter, *Good Packaging Magazine,* April 1994, 30–2.
3. J. Scaroni, *Design News,* July 1985, 17–20.

TERRY MCKEE

15.7.3 Excimer Lasers

Excimer Laser Marking Methods

Excimer laser marking systems are typically more complex than those used with CO_2 or Nd:YAG lasers, so their use is preferred in applications where they offer a distinct functional advantage. The most important advantages are related to the color change marking approach (without any material removal) and the submicrometer ablation precision for engraving. The various methods of marking possible using excimer lasers are listed in Table 2 (next page), along with the benefits of each.

Excimer laser marking is typically accomplished using a photomask. In this technique, the laser beam illuminates a mask (called a reticle) containing the pattern to be marked. An optical system images this pattern on to the worksurface, usually at a high reduction ratio, marking the entire pattern at once, or by scanning the beam over the mask (if it is larger than the beam). This has already been shown as Figure 1 of Section 15.6.1.

The requirements of many marking applications call for high resolution, contrast, and depth control. Therefore, advanced beam delivery systems, including homogenizers and high-quality imaging lenses, are preferred.

When marking large patterns, such as 16- or 32-digit alphanumeric patterns on aircraft cables, there are two different methods that can be used. These are summarized in Table 3 (next page).

Table 3. Large Pattern Excimer Marking Methods

Method	Optimum laser
Mark each digit or part of pattern separately	High repetition rate/low energy
Mark entire pattern at once	High energy/low repetition rate

In order to produce marks in which digits change from part to part, such as serial numbers, various schemes are employed to combine multiple masks in stacks or side by side.

The most popular industrial excimer laser marking applications using color change are for aircraft cables, ceramics, and cosmetic and medical devices. Submicrometer precision material removal is used for optical lenses (glasses, contact lenses) and lens molds.

Excimer Laser Marking Parameters

Table 3 in Section 13.3.3 lists the excimer laser ablation threshold for a number of nonmetals. The laser would be operated below this threshold energy for methods that involve no material removal (color change or surface modification), and above it for methods that that do require material removal (ablation or engraving).

HEINRICH ENDERT
DIRK BASTING

15.8 Comparison with Other Techniques

Other Techniques

In the majority of applications, laser marking is an on-line process. Laser coding is often one of the final steps in the manufacture of a product, taking place during the final filling cycle at a brewery or on a finished product before it is boxed for shipment. Competitive on-line coding techniques include 1.) inkjet printing, 2.) thermal transfer printing, 3.) pad printing, 4.) stick-on decals, 5.) mechanical stamping, 6.) hot stamping, 7.) nameplates, 8.) mechanical scribing, 9.) chemical etching.

Lasers are less frequently used for decorating or preproduction run applications because speed is less important for these applications. If speed is not important, there are a number of other cost-effective techniques. Still lasers often find a place when reliable, easily customized, and indelible marking is desired. Com-

Table 2. Excimer Laser Marking Techniques

Marking mechanism	Example	Characteristics	Typical applications	Advantages over other marking methods
Color Change		Laser produces photochemical color change (usually a reduction of titanium dioxide)	High visibility, excellent contrast	Electronic components, airplane wires, chemical, cosmetic, and pharmaceutical industry	No material removal. Does not affect surrounding or underlying material
Ablation		Laser removes a thin layer of a different color from a substrate	High visibility, excellent contrast	Automotive, consumer products	Can be precisely controlled
Engraving		Laser removes a thin layer with submicrometer depth resolution	"Hidden" marks possible for product identification and security	Eye glasses, contact lenses, glass molds, optical lenses	Does not affect surrounding or underlying material
Surface modification		Laser induces local surface modification, e.g., melting with recrystallization or phase transition	Visibility dependent upon number of pulses	Metals, polymer fibers	No material removal; minimal effect on surrounding material

petitive decorating techniques include: 1.) silk screen printing, 2.) dry offset printing, 3.) clear and colored film labels and decals, 4.) postmold painting, 5.) in-mold film, 6.) colored anodizing (metals) or coatings, 7.) chemical etching.

Advantages of Laser Marking

The advantages provided by laser marking over competitive techniques include: 1.) high reliability, low downtime, 2.) an indelible mark, 3.) high speed, 4.) noncontact processing, 5.) low operating and consumable costs, 6.) easily changed message, 7.) high technology, 8.) environmental friendliness. Two notable disadvantages of laser marking include 1.) not all materials mark well with each laser, and 2.) lasers rarely provide marking in color except on some plastics and metals.

Laser marking is often the highest capital cost solution, although the payback in added speed and reliability will more than compensate for high initial capital cost over the lifetime of the product. The technology that competes most often with laser marking for the customer who wants fast and attractive on-line coding is inkjet (1).

Inkjet Markers

Both inkjet marking and lasers address the high-speed, high-end marking market in both packaging and electronics. Inkjet marks can be modified to address high-speed on-the-fly applications such as aluminum beverage can labeling with a low-quality dot matrix mark, or to address lower-speed electronics applications with a better-quality filled-in font. Inkjets can mark in a variety of colors, although not all colors (e.g., white) are available for all materials to be marked. Inkjet machines are small and portable. The dot matrix CO_2 laser markers are designed to compete head-to-head with inkjet in terms of size and portability.

Because inkjets are prone to clogging when inactive, lasers have a deserved reputation for better reliability, that is, less unforecast downtime. Reliability is usually the key reason to choose laser marking over inkjet.

In comparison with lasers, the capital outlay for inkjet markers is significantly lower; this is often the key reason to choose inkjet. However, buying the inks then becomes a large operating cost that more than balances the initial lower capital outlay during the lifetime of the equipment. The profits for companies that make inkjet markers come primarily from selling the inks, and a large fraction of their research and development costs are spent to design inks. Figure 1 shows a comparison of costs versus production run time.

As customers have become more sensitive to environmental issues, the organic solvents used in the inks have come under scrutiny. To maximize adhesion and minimize drying time, the solvent of choice has overwhelmingly been MEK (methylethylketone); however, most customers are now attempting to restrict or ban the use of this solvent in their manufaturing plants because of health concerns. In order to address this issue, inkjet suppliers are moving to other solvents, such as water, which are environmentally friendly but take longer to dry, do not adhere as well, and tend to smear. Although this is not an insurmountable problem, it has tended more toward laser marking, especially in large, multiple-unit facilities such as breweries.

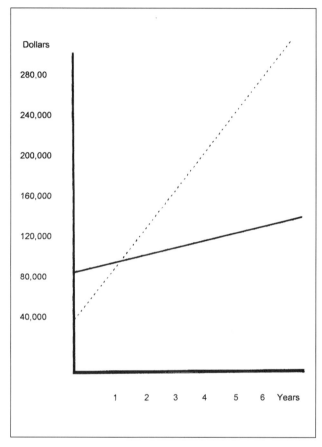

Figure 1. Cost comparison: inkjet versus laser marking. Dotted line: inkjet; solid line: CO_2 laser (2).

Thermal Transfer Printing

In thermal transfer printing, the solid ink is coated onto a ribbon that contacts the product to be marked. An array of tiny thermal sources (e.g., resistors or even microlasers) behind the ribbon melts the ink onto the product. In this way, the use of dangerous solvents is minimized, but the advantages of inks are retained. Very attractive marks including graphics can be obtained. However, the process is too slow to compete with lasers, even for the relatively modest speeds typical of electronics component marking (e.g., 500 parts per minute). And the inked ribbon represents a high operating cost for the process. For small facilities, however, where the line speed may be low, thermal transfer printing is an alternative to both laser marking and injet marking. Heat transfer labeling is similar in concept to thermal transfer printing.

Pad Printing

In pad printing, a soft pad inscribed with the desired message first picks up an inked image from a plate, then stamps the message onto the product. To change the message, it is necessary to stop the machine to install another pad. Because mechanical contact is made with the product, it is essential that the product be rigid and sturdy to withstand the force. Pad printing is slow. Nevertheless, pad printing equipment is widely used because it is low cost and simple.

Mechanical Stamping and Etching

Etching with a vibrating tip is commonly used to mark metals. For a soft material like plastic, simple mechanical stamping can be used to imprint a message directly. In hot stamping, a heated metal die serves to press the desired shape into a soft sample while also transferring a decoration from an intermediary foil. As with pad printing, stamping techniques are slow, and it is difficult and expensive to change the message. However, because many applications do not require frequent message changes, stamping is a common on-line marking technique.

Off-Line and Decorating Applications

Lasers are at a disadvantage for decorating applications. Labels, bottles, cans, and consumer items can be decorated off-line, sometimes at a different location than the final production facility. When there is no need to change the decoration frequently, printing techniques in particular produce attractive results cost effectively (3). In this case, lasers compete only in niche areas.

Lasers provide an indelible mark which does not wear off. For this reason, lasers are often used to mark letters onto keyboards or electronic remote controls. Although inks stick well, they and even their protective coatings wear off in time. Because the laser actually cuts a groove into the plastic, the letter does not wear away. Plastic money or credit cards are marked using lasers (including images for some banks in Europe) because the decoration is permanent and not easily conterfeited. Glass bottles can be decorated with distinct graphics using CO_2 lasers.

Lasers can be used to decorate below the surface of a transparent upper layer or film. This can be accomplished easily if the upper layer does not absorb the laser radiation or, alternately, if the laser beam can be focused at the desired depth without affecting the upper surface. This technique is most common for clear glass or plastics.

Sometimes laser decorating is used for small, previously silk-screened decorated items that need to be modified, for example, to announce a sale of a small batch. It may be cheaper to inscribe a small batch logo in-house rather than send the bottles out to be re-silk-screened.

Lasers provide a very accurate marking process that is sometimes advantageous to mark graduated items such as syringes or rules.

References
1. *Packaging Technology & Eng.,* February 1994, 32–3.
2. *Effekte,* **3**, p. 2 (published by E. Merck GmBh, Darmstadt, Germany).
3. *Plastics Technology,* April 1996, 68–71.

TERRY MCKEE

Notes

ISBN 0-912035-15-3

Chapter 16

Rapid Prototyping

16.0 Introduction and Glossary

Rapid prototyping (RP) has emerged as a powerful tool to quickly bringing new products to market. It is a fast and economical way to generate three-dimensional solid models of new designs. RP enables designs to be finalized in a fraction of the time formerly required.

RP is not one technology. It is a family of technologies that have two fundamental elements in common: they begin with electronic data and use an additive process to build the items, one layer at a time.

Most of the important RP technologies are laser based and these are the subject of this chapter.

Each technology has different strengths and weaknesses. The appropriate one to use will be a function of your application. One application may require that the part be made of metal; in this case, selective laser sintering (SLS) may be the best technology. Another application may require the part to be ceramic; laminated object manufacturing would be a clear choice here.

If one intends to produce numerous prototypes on an ongoing basis, one may wish to consider installing an in-house RP facility. However, it might be best to first work with one of the many service bureaus that have available the whole spectrum of laser based RP technologies. In this way you can gain experience with RP strategies on a contract basis before investing in equipment.

While many companies find it advantageous to use an outside service on an ongoing basis, whether or not this approach is best depends on what the laser-based RP needs are and which of the technologies meet those needs within the framework of a given economic structure.

This chapter serves two purposes: It provides hard-core information for people who work in laser-based RP, and it gives information about its limitations, capabilities, and costs for people who want to utilize laser-based rapid prototyping.

Most terms used in this chapter are defined at the point where they are introduced. There is, however, a glossary provided to assist the reader in browsing through the chapter.

TERRY FEELEY

Glossary

1. *Actinic:* Radiation capable of initiating a chemical reaction in a photopolymer.
2. *DLF (Directed Light Fabrication):* A technique developed at Los Alamos National Laboratories that uses a high-power laser to create a melt pool, into which metal powder is deposited. As the laser spot, directed by a computer, moves past a given location the melt pool cools, solidifies, and leaves an essentially fully dense solid.
3. *Dp (Depth of Penetration):* The "1/e absorption depth" (mm, or thousandths of an inch) of the actinic radiation used to cure a stereolithography photopolymer.
4. *Ec (Critical Exposure):* The minimum incident laser energy per unit area (mJ/cm^2) necessary to initiate solidification (i.e., "gelling") of a stereolithography photopolymer.
5. *F#:* A dimensionless optical ratio, equal to the focal length of a lens divided by its diameter.
6. *FDM (Fused Deposition Modeling):* An RP&M technique using CAD data to selectively extrude a molten thermoplastic through a nozzle moving over the work area under computer control. The result is a bead of solidified thermoplastic material deposited according to the cross-section data for that layer. While solidifying, the bead on the current layer adheres to the material of the previous layer. The process continues on a layer-by-layer basis until the part is complete.
7. *Green Strength:* The strength of an RP&M part after initial fabrication, but prior to postprocessing (e.g., in SL, after laser polymerization but before postcure, and in SLS, after laser sintering, but before binder elimination and infiltration).
8. *LENS (Laser Engineered Net Shaping):* An RP&M process developed at Sandia National Laboratories that uses a high-power infrared laser to generate a moving melt pool. Metallic powder is dispensed into the melt pool. Upon cooling, the melt pool solidifies and adheres to the material below, enabling the direct layer-by-layer fabrication of solid metallic objects from a CAD file.
9. *LOM (Laminated Object Manufacturing):* An RP&M technique that uses laser cut sheets (typically paper) coated with an adhesive. A given sheet is cut according to the computer file for that layer; a subsequent sheet is registered above one below, mechanically adhered to the lower layer, and laser cut in accord with the computer file for that layer. The sequence continues layer-by-layer until the part is completed.
10. *RP (Rapid Prototyping):* The general term for those processes that build physical, three-dimensional models or prototypes from CAD data, on a layer-by-layer, additive basis.
11. *RP&M (Rapid Prototyping & Manufacturing):* An extension of RP where the articles being built can now be used as patterns, mandrels, or tooling inserts, for the generation of objects in "end use engineering materials" (e.g., investment casting patterns to produce functional metal parts, or patterns to generate rapid tooling inserts).
12. *SL (Stereolithography):* An RP&M technique where CAD data is used to direct a scanned actinic laser beam onto the surface of a liquid photopolymer, resulting in the solidification of the resin in the form of a specific cured cross section on a given

layer. The process is then repeated on the next layer, with sufficient exposure to ensure adhesion to the previous layer. The green part is then completed on a layer-by-layer basis.

13. *SLA (StereoLithography Apparatus):* Refers specifically to the *apparatus*, or machine used to generate SL parts. The term SL, (*not* SLA) should be used to describe both the SL process and parts produced by the SL process.
14. *SLS (Selective Laser Sintering):* An RP&M technique where CAD data is used to direct a scanned infrared laser beam onto the surface of a powder/binder, resulting in the sintering of the powder in the form of a specific cured cross section on a given layer. The process is then repeated on the next layer, with sufficient exposure to ensure adhesion to the previous layer. The green part is then completed on a layer-by-layer basis.
15. *STL (STereoLithography file format):* A data format where the surfaces of a CAD object are represented by an array of triangles obeying a specific set of rules. Currently the *de facto* data standard of the RP&M industry, CAD-to-STL file translators now exist for all major CAD systems
16. *SLI (SLIce file format):* After an STL file has been mathematically sliced into thin layers, the data describing each of the layer cross sections and its relationship to the layers above and below form an SLI file.

PAUL F. JACOBS

16.1 Basics of Laser-Based Rapid Prototyping

16.1.1 Rapid Prototyping: An Overview

Rapid prototyping (RP) is a description applied to a set of technologies that fabricate components through layered manufacturing (i.e., one layer at a time, succeeding layers adhered to preceding layers (1). Not yet in commercial use are systems that may overcome the layering restrictions (e.g., vapor deposition). RP systems form solid material only where it exists in the component. In comparison, traditional manufacturing starts with a block of material and cuts away all the excess material. This section will be concerned with layering techniques and limited to laser photopolymerization: sterolithography (SLA) and laser sintering (SLS). Another laser-based technique, laminated object manufacturing, is a hybrid RP system. Later sections of this chapter are devoted to each.

The most common technique to provide spatially selective material formation is to use a laser to initiate gross material solidification (photochemical, photothermal, etc.) at only the locations specified. The laser material interaction generates a solid primitive (unit cell) and the primitives are subsequently joined together, first in one dimension then in the cross dimension, to form the layer. The most common processes, SLA and SLS, sweep the laser beam forming a line (Fig. 1).

The laser is then "turned off" while it is moved to the next starting position. The primitive formed (both cross section and depth) bears characteristics of the laser beam. The scanner permits vector scans, usually employed for boundary definition. Interior material is typically formed using raster scanning. Thus, as RP dimensional accuracy becomes more precise, control of the layer formation will require that knowledge of the three-dimensional laser intensity profile be incorporated into the laser beam motion. Also, incorporation of the laser–material interaction will be critical. Beer's law absorption profiles may not be valid and the impact of bleaching, scattering, etc., will need to be taken into account.

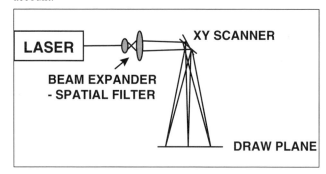

Figure 1. Laser scanning system drawing a line.

16.1.2 Lasers Parameters for RP

The lasers most commonly used in current RP systems are listed in Table 1. Other lasers have been used in the past; no doubt more will find application in the future.

Table 1. Lasers Used in Current RP Systems

Laser	Wavelength (nm)	Mode (temporal, spatial)
HeCd	325	CW, TEM_{mn}
Ar	351–365	CW, TEM_{00}
CO_2	10,600	CW/pulsed, TEM_{00}
Nd:YAG (third harmonic)	355	Q-switched, TEM_{00}

The Ar and CO_2 are gas lasers operated in their fundamental mode, TEM_{00} (see Chapter 1), but they may go multimode if the operating conditions change. The operating mode of the laser should be checked periodically. The 30x wavelength factor for CO_2 laser is significant when focusing is considered.

The HeCd is a metal vapor laser that requires heating to achieve stable operation. The trade-off between suitable Cd density, excited state population distribution, and pumping results in high-order multimode operation, TEM_{mn}.

Nd is a metal distributed in a host solid matrix (YAG, YLF, and YVO are common). The Nd ions can be excited by broad-band illumination (flashlamp) or by diode pumping. Flashlamps contribute excess energy that heats the matrix, causing thermal distortions. Using the diode pump, tuned to the Nd absorption, considerably reduces the thermal loading. Nd:YAG lases at 1060 nm, which is then frequency tripled to 355 nm. The exact laser wavelength depends on the host matrix. Efficient frequency tripling usually requires TEM_{00} operation.

The laser's mode structure impacts RP operation in several ways. Two important effects of the interaction are the primitive shape formed by the laser exposure, and the beam's operational depth of focus. The primitive's shape usually reflects the laser footprint. Higher-order laser modes are not centrosymmetric (2), consequently the solidified material's profile may depend on the direction of laser sweep relative to the mode structure. This may also affect the downfacing surface profile and the shape in corners. The depth of focus becomes important as the accuracy increases. The laser's intensity profile has minimum spatial extent at the focus point, broadening away from the focus (above and below). The centerline intensity (fluence) decreases away from the focal point. The rate of change depends on several factors, one of which is the laser mode which is discussed in the next section.

16.1.3 Scanning Exposure Factors

Achieving a precision of 25 μm requires precise control of laser exposure, which impacts the maximum allowed scan angle and the minimum laser footprint. The dimensions of the material primitive formed are proportional to the laser fluence and the radiation pattern. Precision determines the ability to locate an edge. It is not the primative's size, which may be 10x larger. As the laser is scanned from the center, several factors come into play that will cause the primitive's dimensions to change. For example, the laser footprint will elongate by a amount given by the product of $(1/\cos q_x)(1/\cos q_y)$ (see Fig. 2).

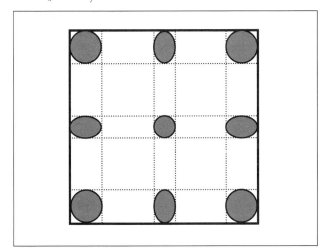

Figure 2. Laser spot variation.

Also, if the medium is nonscattering the solid primitive formed will be aligned along the laser direction; this is typical of nonfilled epoxy and acrylate photopolymer resins. To get the required depth, the exposure will need to be increased by the factor $(1/\cos q_{xy})$ (see Fig. 3).

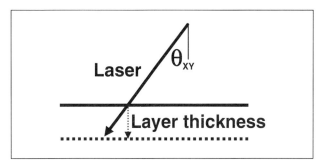

Figure 3. Additional penetration required to compensate for oblique incidence.

As the scanner sweeps the laser, if the focus is fixed, the locus of minimum diameter will lie in a circle on the build layer. Inside the circle, the laser hits the surface before the focus, and outside the circle the laser–surface intersection is after the focal point. This can be accommodated either by continually adjusting the focus to maintain the focus at the surface, or by adjusting the beam's F# so that the beam's dimensions do not vary outside of prescribed limits during the sweep (see Fig. 4).

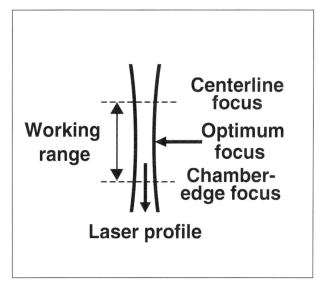

Figure 4. Laser profile during focus (boundary is locus of e^{-2} x laser centerline intensity).

The $\cos\theta$ factor is problematic because it depends on the direction of the sweep relative to the principle axes of the laser footprint. In general, this factor will vary from $(1/\cos\theta)^2$ to more than $(1/\cos\theta)^3$ along the sweep. The simplest method to account for this factor is to make it a nonfactor, i.e., limit the maximum sweep angle so that the maximum change is within the limits of precision. For example, consider the typical laser that is focused to provide a footprint with a cross section of 250 μm (0.010 in.). To hold the footprint dimension to an accuracy of 25 μm (0.001 in.) requires that $(1/\cos\theta)^3 < 1.10$, i.e., $\theta < 0.25$ rad (14°). (For simplicity, assume all angles are the same. Although this overestimates the maximum allowed angle, it gives results that are close enough to illustrate the effect.) Taking into account the maximum scan dimension determines the minimum distance from the build layer to the scanner. For the common 250 x 250 mm platform (SLA), under the circumstances described above, this requires that the scanner be more than 700 mm away from the surface.

The next factor that needs to be accounted for is the laser intensity variation as a function of distance from optimal focus. In practice the spot dimension, the projection angle, and the intensity variation are all coupled in their impact on the solid primitive formed. Consequently, they need to be considered together and not separately as done here for illustration. A TEM_{00} beam will focus to (2):

$$d = (2/\pi)\lambda F\#_{eff} \quad (1)$$

where d is the beam diameter, λ the laser wavelength, and $F\#_{eff}$ is the effective $F\#$ for the focused beam (i.e., lens focal length / laser beam diameter at the lens). The intensity distribution along the laser direction is given by:

$$I(0,z) = I_0 / [1 + (z/z_0)^2] \quad (2)$$

and

$$z_0 = \pi W_0^2/\lambda \quad (3)$$

where $I_0 = I(0,0)$ and W_0 is the minimum beam radius (d/2). z_0, usually referred to as the Rayleigh range, is the distance over which the laser's footprint is within a factor of 2 of its minimum dimension and the centerline intensity is, also, within a factor of 2 of I_0. Thus, at a distance z_0 from best focus, the laser fluence has decreased by 50% and the footprint has increased substantially. The effective solid primitive increase in dimension does not depend linearly on the actual laser footprint. Currently, precision demands require that the laser maintain its fluence within 10%. Using Equation 2

$$z_{0.1} = 0.33 \, z_0 \quad (4)$$

For higher-order mode structures the minimum focus diameter will increase for the same $F\#_{eff}$ and $z_{0.1}$ will decrease, both a result of the increase in beam divergence as the mode order increases.

Using the example developed earlier with $d = 250$ μm, the working distance away from best focus can be developed as shown in Table 2.

Table 2. Working Range for TEM_{00} Operation Assuming $d = 250$ μm

λ (nm)	z_0 (mm)	$z_{0.1}$ (mm)
325	151	50
365	134	45
10,600	4.6	1.5

From Equation 1, one can also determine the effective $F\#$ required. Once these values are computed, they will give the lens stand-off distance and laser beam dimension at the lens needed for a particular vat dimension. For example, consider the popular 250 x 250-mm vat and 325-nm laser. If the laser were TEM_{00} as with an Ar laser, then from Equation 1 $F\#_{eff} = 1200$. If the focusing lens has a focal length of 1 m, the laser diameter need only be 0.8 mm diameter at the lens. As a result, the XY steering mirrors can be kept relatively small. Using Equations 3 and 4, $z_{0.1} = 50$ mm. The actual change in length from centerline to corner from a stand-off of 1 m is 7 mm, well within the allowed working range. The operating parameters would need to be recomputed to account for higher-order mode structure in the laser, as with the HeCd laser, different wavelength, altered geometry, e.g., a more compact design, or any of the other parameters described.

16.1.4 Small Spot Systems

The goal of achieving small-spot operation RP is driven by several needs. Small-spot operation will permit finer feature definition, a goal of the current scale systems. It will also permit fabrication of smaller scale devices, perhaps achieving mesoscale features suitable for integration with micro-electro-mechanical system (MEMS) devices. As the lateral dimensions shrink, the goal is to also reduce the layer thickness and the resulting stair-stepping associated with build-by-layer systems. The reduced dimension goal impacts the laser and scanner requirements and this can be examined using the parameters developed above. A cautionary note needs to be made: As the primitive dimensions shrink in each direction, the number of primitives required to build a unit volume increases as the cube of the shrink factor. If the laser power is kept constant, the fluence will increase as the square of the shrink factor. The layer thickness also decreases, so the exposure control-precision requirements escalate as the cube of the shrink factor. This can be compensated for by:

- Reducing the laser power, with an ensuing increase in build time
- Using faster scanners, which may compromise pointing accuracy
- Implementing some other factor

The choice will require an engineering compromise between the dimensional requirements and the need for "rapid" parts.

It is worthwhile to consider the system parameters one of the commonly used lasers, for example the frequency-tripled Nd:YAG. In Table 3, the system parameters are computed for spot demagnification by 3× and 10× compared with the current standard.

Table 3. Small-Spot System Parameters

Spot diameter (μm/in.)	$F\#_{eff}$ (355 nm)	$Z_{0.1}$ (mm)	Vat (max) (mm)
250 / 0.010	1100	46	600
75 / 0.003	330	4.1	180
25 / 0.001	110	0.46	60

The vat maximum dimension (diagonal) is computed assuming a

fixed-focus system, scanning from 1 m distance, and keeping the scanned beam within the working range as determined by z_{01}. As noted in Section 16.1.2, the footprint dimension limitations may be more restrictive. The lower F#s will impact the size of the scanner mirrors and may result in the geometry becoming unworkable; a complete system parameter computation will be needed. There are at least a couple of options that may be considered to overcome engineering obstacles. However, these may introduce other issues and a complete system analysis will be needed. If a shorter wavelength laser can be used the decrease in λ will affect the system parameters. The Nd:YAG laser's fourth harmonic is available and it lases near 265 nm. Caution is recommended as this is beneath the breakdown wavelength of oxygen, and the region in which the laser is transmitted will need to be purged with a nitrogen flush. Another option is to use a gantry delivery for the laser beam. This will permit positioning the focusing lens in close proximity to the build layer and eliminates the need to consider the scanner. This option is used by Denken Engineering (Japan), for small-spot operation, and by Helisys (USA), using a CO_2 laser while achieving 250-μm operation.

References

1. P. F. Jacobs (Ed.), *Rapid Prototyping & Manufacturing: Fundamentals of Stereolithography*, Society of Manufacturing Engineers, Dearborn, MI (1992).
2. B. Saleh and M. Teich, *Fundamentals of Photonics*, Wiley-Interscience, NY (1991), (in particular, Chapter 3 and Figure 3.3.2).

ALLAN LIGHTMAN

16.2 Stereolithography

16.2.1 The Stereolithography Process

Stereolithography (SL) builds physical, three-dimensional objects directly from a computer-aided designed (CAD) model. The part is generated in a layer-by-layer manner, using a scanned ultraviolet laser beam to locally solidify a liquid photopolymer resin.

The rapid prototyping and manufacturing (RP&M) field began in 1988 with the introduction of the first commercial Stereolithography Apparatus (SLA). Note that the system is known as an SLA, but the process is referred to as SL. The four commercial SLA units sold since 1989 are listed below. Their build volumes are nearly cubic. The CW equivalent ultraviolet laser output power values are typical.

SLA	Build volume (mm cube)	Laser	Wavelength (nm)	Power (mW)
SLA-190	190	He-Cd	325	15
SLA-250	250	He-Cd	325	30
SLA-350	350	Nd:YVO	355	160
SLA-500	500	Argon ion	351	250

The SL process begins with a CAD model of the object. A surface model can be used, but a solid model is preferred. The CAD surfaces are then *tessellated*, or formed as a connected array of triangles. The specifications for the .stl file format are explained in detail in Reference 1. The result is a "stereolithography," or .stl file. Virtually every CAD vendor has developed CAD to .stl translators, and the .stl file has become the *de-facto* RP&M standard.

The .stl file is then mathematically "sliced" into a series of thin layers, typically 100 to 200 μm thick. Each slice generates a 2-D cross section of the object at a given Z level. The final result is a layered representation of the CAD model.

As a consequence, *all* RP&M systems produce *stair-stepping* or inclined surfaces. This is an inevitable result of building 3-D objects with finite layer thickness. The heavy outline of Figure 1 shows the desired part geometry. The lighter line shows the result of building the same object with finite layer thickness. Because the resulting inclined surface resembles a tiny staircase, this effect is often referred to as "stair-stepping."

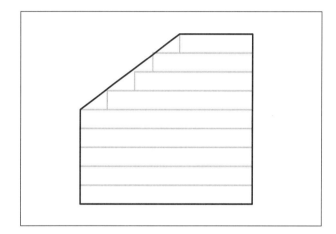

Figure 1. Building an object with finite thickness layers.

Stair-stepping may be acceptable for concept models, but SL parts serving as master patterns for Rapid Tooling (RT), require superior accuracy and surface quality. Thus, SL tooling patterns still demand skilled finishing, which adds both time and cost.

SL involves precise, geometrically controlled, actinic laser exposure of a photopolymer. That is, the radient energy/cm² capable of initiating photo-polymerization. The exposure is controlled using a scanned, focused laser beam. If the laser wavelength matches the photoinitiator absorption bands, a chemical reaction can occur resulting in cross-linked polymerization of the resin monomers.

However, the photo-polymerization process is fundamentally nonlinear, as discussed in Reference 2. Below a critical exposure threshold, F_e, (typically 5 to 15 ml/cm²), the resin remains liquid. Conversely, where the laser beam yields an exposure above F_e, the resin will undergo a transformation from the liquid phase to the solid phase. Simply stated, wherever sufficient actinic laser exposure is provided, the resin will locally solidify.

The fundamental elements of a SLA system are as follows:

1. A vat of photopolymer resin.
2. An actinic laser with an output wavelength selected for optimum photoinitiator absorption.
3. An accurate, high-speed, software-controlled servo-actuated, galvanometer-driven, laser-scanning system utilizing twin orthogonal rotating mirrors.
4. A precision motor-driven Z-stage, to move both the build platform and the attached part downward during build, and upward upon completion of the last layer.
5. A resin leveling sub-system.
6. A laser power, peak irradiance and spot-size-measuring subsystem.
7. A drift correction subsystem.
8. A resin recoating subsystem.
9. A workstation to execute the various software tasks involved in part preparation.
10. A process control computer to regulate the entire sequence of events involved in part building.

The SL process is fully automatic, requiring no attending personnel until the object is completed. The key steps are described in the following subsections.

Part Prepartion
Part preparation requires the following steps:

1. Start with a CAD model of the desired object.
2. Translate the CAD file into a .stl file.
3. Select a desired layer thickness. Thinner layers reduce stair-stepping and improved surface quality, while increasing the number of layers and extending the build time.
4. Select the desired SL build style from the SLA software menu (see also Section 16.2.4 under the heading Prototypes of Injection-Molded Plastic Parts for a further description of the processes that follow). The QuickCast™ build style directly generates quasihollow patterns that can be used to quickly and economically produce small quantities of fully functional metal components through the investment casting process. This allows the end user to bypass the typically expensive and often time-consuming requirement for wax pattern dies. Thus, QuickCast can significantly reduce the time to market. Alternatively, the ACES™ (Accurate Clear Epoxy Solid) build style can be used for (1) concept models, (2) patterns for sand casting, (3) transparent flow models, (4) test parts for photo-optic stress analysis, (5) accurate models for vibration analysis, (6) rapid soft tooling masters to form silicone rubber molds for vacuum casting up to 30 parts in polyurethane, (7) rapid bridge tooling core and cavity inserts for CAFE (Composite Aluminum Filled Epoxy), or direct AIM™ (ACES Injection Molding) cores and cavities yielding 50 to 200 functional prototypes, and (8) as master patterns for such rapid hard tooling processes as 3D Keltool™ ExpressTool™ and Nickel Ceramic Composite™ (NCC) electroformed inserts, to produce fully functional injection molded parts in a wide range of engineering plastics. The ultimate goal is rapid manufacturing, getting products to market faster.
5. Develop the required support structure. While this can be accomplished manually, there are now automatic support generation software packages commercially available to SL users, such as: 'Bridgeworks' from Solid Concepts, Valencia, CA, 'MAGICS' from Materialise, Heverlee, Belgium, and 'VISTA' from 3D Systems, Valencia, CA. These software modules provide rapid, effective, automatic, support generation. Some editing may still be appropriate for unusual geometries where excess default supports are occasionally generated.
6. Select appropriate process parameters such as border, hatch, and fill cure depths, etc. Thoroughly tested, optimum default values are provided in the SLA system software menu.
7. Merge the support file with the part file.
8. Slice the merged files, generating a build file.
9. Execute the build command.

Part Building
Part building requires the following steps:

1. The SLA proceeds through a number of self-calibration steps. These determine laser power, peak laser irradiance, laser spot size, scanning systems pointing accuracy as well as the resin level in the vat. If the level is too low, the system alerts the operator to add resin to the correct level. When all these checks are properly satisfied, the SLA will automatically begin to build the desired physical part.
2. The build platform is positioned just below the liquid resin surface. The SLA then scans the laser spot at the precise speed required for optimum exposure to promote adhesion of the first layer of supports to the platform surface. This step firmly secures the new part to the platform.
3. A fresh coating of resin is then formed at the desired layer thickness. The Zephyr recoater is a recent advance that uses a double-edged hollow blade and a vacuum system to enable resin release during recoating. Accurte, uniform, and rapid recoating of viscous resins in 50 unit layers over arbitrary part geometries, has proved to be a formidable task.
4. The support layers continue to build, one atop another, to a minimum Z height of 8 mm. If the part geometry includes "roofs" or cantilevered sections, some supports will continue to still higher Z levels.
5. The SLA now automatically builds the part. If QuickCast is used, the pattern builds in a quasi-hollow manner, enabling drainage of internal uncured resin. The result is a strong, lightweight structure, 80–90% hollow. QuickCast patterns greatly reduce thermal expansion stress in the ceramic shell during pattern burnout, relative to solid ACES parts. To date, over 50,000 high-quality aluminum, stainless steel, inconel, and titanium investment castings have been produced from QuickCast patterns. Substantial cost and time savings are documented in Reference 3.
6. The ACES build style is described in detail in Reference 4.

The laser beam initially scans the border of each slice cross section. The enclosed region is first scanned as a series of parallel vectors in the X direction, each about 100 μm apart. A cure depth » 25 μm (0.001 in.) less than the layer thickness is generated on the first exposure. ACES allows the shrinkage inherent in this polymerization process to occur while producing minimal distortion to the previous layer since the two are not yet connected. After shrinkage relaxation, a second, orthogonal laser scan is performed in the Y direction, resulting in: additional cure depth, adhesion to the previous layer, and improved green strength.

7. With the new Zephyr recoater, the platform moves down one layer thickness after each cross section is cured. The recoater then applies another layer of liquid resin. For SLAs using the earlier doctor blade, a series of Z stage motions known as *deep dipping* are described in Reference 5.
8. A "Z-wait" of 10 to 25 seconds, is typically sufficient for fluid dynamic relaxation to form a quasi-planar resin surface, depending on the resin viscosity and surface tension.
9. The laser spot is moved to pinhole sensors positioned just outside the SLA working area. The measured laser beam centroid is compared to the known center of the pinhole. The scanner servo is then "drift corrected" per Reference 6. This procedure enables repeatable laser scanning layer-after-layer, with » ± 8 μm, at laser scan speeds up to 5 m/sec.
10. The system now checks the resin level, which must be located near the focused laser beam waist, otherwise the spot size would vary as the resin surface moved up or down relative to the waist, adversely effecting part accuracy. The resin level is measured with a visible indium gallium aluminum phosphide laser diode. The diode beam strikes the resin surface at a shallow angle and its reflection is sensed with a silicon detector. The entire resin vat is then moved up or down, until the resin level is within tolerance.
11. The system now scans the next layer's cross section. This *recoat, Z-wait, drift correct, resin level, scan* process occurs on every cross section. After the final layer scan, the system raises the build platform/part above the free resin surface. Subsequent to draining excess liquid resin, the build platform/part can be removed from the SLA.

Post Screening

Post screening requires the following steps:

1. An operator wearing rubber gloves removes the platform and the attached part from the SLA. If the part is especially large or heavy, assistance may be required.
2. An ACES part is first wiped of excess liquid resin with paper towels. The platform and part are then oscillated in a bath of cleaning solvent. Based on test results, Tri-Propylene Glycol Monamethyl Ether, or 'TPM' is recommended. After fifteen minutes, nearly all exterior uncured liquid resin will be removed. Next, the part is rinsed in cool water and dried with compressed air. As all SL epoxy resins are somewhat hydrophilic, one must dry the part thoroughly and keep it in a controlled environment. High relative-humidity values can compromise the accuracy of SL epoxy resin parts.
3. With a QuickCast pattern, uncured interior liquid resin should be gravity drained, and uncured exterior resin wiped from the part surface with paper towels. QuickCast patterns should *never* be cleaned with TPM and then rinsed with water, as their high surface to volume ratio promote water absorption. This leads to swelling and hence degraded pattern accuracy. Nearly complete drainage of uncured liquid resin from the interior of QuickCast patterns is best performed using the low-speed centrifuge system originally developed for extracting honey from beehives.
4. Next, the part is separated from the platform. Long, thin, serrated bread knives work especially well.
5. The supports can now be removed. Formerly this was a very tedious task. However, support removal has become easier since the advent of automatic support generation software. Structures utilizing novel castle, saw-tooth, or Sierra geometries provide reduced support-to-part contact. Despite recent improvements, care must still be taken to avoid damaging fragile QuickCast patterns.
6. The cleaned, support-free part is now placed in a post curing apparatus (PCA). Laser cured green parts require only cross-linking sufficient to maintain accuracy until post curing. The PCA-250 and PCA-500 utilize low-cost, long-lifetime, and actinic fluorescent ultraviolet lamps optimized to complete the cross-linking process for the relevant resins. For small SLA-250 parts, about one hour in a PCA-250 will achieve asymptotically full strength and a tack-free surface. Larger parts require longer postcure intervals, but even very large SLA-500 parts can be cured overnight in a PCA-500.
7. After postcure, SL parts can be finished with progressively finer sandpaper, to eliminate stair-stepping, and subsequently polished to achieve a mirror-like finish for such applications as photo-optic stress analysis, transparent flow models, and especially, as master patterns for Rapid Tooling.

Over 40,000 CMM UserPart measurements have been made since 1989. *ACES parts built with Ciba epoxy resin SL 5170 set the accuracy standard for RP&M systems.* Masters up to 241 mm now yield σ acrs $\cong$ 42 μm. Thus, 95% of all SL dimensions to 241 mm should now lie within ± 84 μm (± 0.0033 in.) tolerance. These results approach typical CNC machining accuracy ($\sigma \cong 20$ pm) However, including errors from subsequent RP processes, further work is needed to rival the accuracy and surface finish of CNC production tooling.

References

1. G. O. Floyd, "Software Architecture," Chapter 5 in P. F. Jacobs', *Rapid Prototyping & Manufacturing: Fundamentals of Stereolithography*, Society of Manufacturing Engineers, Dearborn, MI 1992.
2. M. Hunziker and R. Leyden, *Basic Polymer Chemistry*, Chapter 2, Jacobs, 1992, op. cit.
3. Andre L. Daniels, S. Kennerknecht, and B. Sarkis, "QuickCast Foundry Experiences," Chapter 5 in P. Jacobs', *Stereolithography and Other RP&M Technologies,* SME & ASMF, Dearborn, MI 1996.

ISBN 0-912035-15-3

4. B. Bedal and H. Nguyen, *Advances in Part Accuracy*, Chapter 5, Jacobs, 1996, op. cit.
5. R. P. Fedchenko and P. F. Jacobs, *Introduction*, Chapter 1, op. cit.
6. D. Kaliaz and J. Thayer, *SL Hardware Technology*, Chapter 3, op. cit.

PAUL F. JACOBS

16.2.2 Materials for Stereolithography

The stereolithography process utilizes ultraviolet radiation to cure (selectively solidify) a liquid photopolymer resin. After curing a layer, a second liquid layer can be applied by a recoating process. This second layer can then be selectively cured just as the first. Materials used for stereolithography must be capable of undergoing photo-polymerization. A number of liquid photopolymers can be solidified by exposure to ultraviolet radiation.

Resin Parameters

The photospeed of a stereolithography resin is characterized by two resin specific parameters: Dp and Ec. The semi-log plot of the laser exposure versus depth of resin cured is called a working curve. Dp, or depth of penetration is given by the slope of the working curve. The Dp of a resin is the depth below the resin surface at which the power of an incident laser beam is attenuated to $1/e$ of its incident power. Ec, or critical exposure, is the minimum laser exposure required to cure a finite amount of resin. This is the intercept of the working curve with the x-axis. A typical working curve is shown in Figure 2. The speed of a resin is often judged by the Ec alone. Since the thickness of a layer that can be cured is determined by the Dp, this parameter must also be considered. In addition, other parameters (i.e., recoating speed, and liquid leveling time) are also involved in determining its overall productivity of a stereolithography resin.

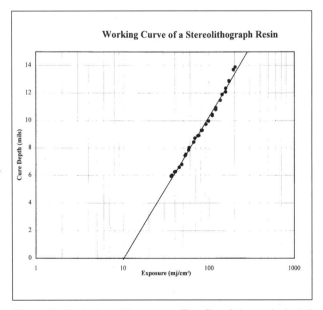

Figure 2. Typical working curve. The Dp of the resin is 4.5 mils, and the Ec is 10.5 mJ/cm².

Resins for Stereolithography

Initially only acrylate resins were available for stereolithography. The acrylate resins generally have high photospeeds but suffer from curl-related distortions due to large effective linear shrinkage. This limits the achievable accuracy in the produced stereolithography part, and the production of flat parts was difficult. In addition, acrylate resins typically are higher in viscosity than other resin classes. This reduces the resins' ability to be drained from models prepared for investment casting using the QuickCastä build style. QuickCastä is a quasi-hollow build style used for shell investment casting. The quasi-hollow pattern can be burned out of a ceramic shell. In order to do this, however, the liquid photopolymer must be of low enough viscosity to be drained from the interior of the pattern. Poor drainage can result in thermal expansion of the pattern during burnout, and thus fracture of the ceramic shell.

There are several major materials companies involved in the production of resin specifically tailored for stereolithography. The recent advances by these companies have focused on epoxy and vinylether chemistries to produce low viscosity photocurable resins with lower curl distortion. These resin systems are capable of producing models exhibiting significantly lower curl-related distortions than can be produce in the acrylate-based resins. The lower curl allowed the introduction of a more accurate build style, ACES™ (Accurate Clear Epoxy Solid).

This build style is designed to provide a uniform exposure to the material so that shrinkage is minimized, a transparent part is produced, and the vast majority of the material is cured in the vat. The ACES™ build style is not compatible with acrylate resins. The advent of the epoxy materials and this build style allowed stereolithography to make tremendous gains in the production of highly accurate prototypes usable as master patterns for investment casting or for secondary tooling processes. The SLA 250 using Ciba Specialty Chemicals' SL 5170 epoxy resin is capable of producing prototypes of up to 10 in. with an RMS accuracy of ± 0.0019 in. In addition, the low viscosities of epoxy and vinylether materials allow for the resin to be drained easily from the internal structure of patterns built using the QuickCastä build style.

Some manufacturers have focused on expanding the applications of stereolithography through materials. One example is a photocurable acrylate resins by Zeneca Specialties. They have produced selectively colorable material for stereolithography. Their resins, H-C 9100R and A-C 9200R, can produce models that are colored only in areas where high laser exposure is applied. This colorability opens up a variety of new applications for SL materials, such as the production of colored medical models.

Mechanical Properties

Stereolithography materials have a wide range of mechanical properties. True functional prototypes, however, must eventually be made in the method of manufacture, using the production material. There is no RP equipment available that can produce prototypes with characteristics that match injection molded engineering thermoplastics. Epoxy and vinyl ether resins produced by Ciba Specialty Chemicals and epoxy resins produced by DuPont, can be used to form highly accurate rigid models having excellent surface finish, high tensile and flexural strengths. Many of these materials are also humidity and/or heat resistant.

Some of the acrylate, and urethaneacrylate resins produce more durable, high-impact, and high-elongation models. These materials, however, may not offer the ultimate accuracy of epoxy patterns, but allow for the production of more flexible parts that are better suited for some applications. Ciba Specialty Chemicals and DuPont each have durable epoxy resins. These flexible materials are characterized by having high elongation at break, and high impact strength. The Cibatool SL 5520 is a clear durable epoxy resin, while the DuPont Somos 8100 series produce translucent prototype models. These materials are characteristic of the growing move in the stereolithography materials market to develop more end-use/applications focused polymers.

Table 1 compares the mechanical properties of typical stereolithography resins. Table 2 shows the properties of some typical thermosets and engineering thermoplastics for comparison with SL materials.

Special Applications of SL Materials

The materials available for stereolithography offer a wide range of properties appropriate for many different applications. Unlike other rapid prototyping systems, stereolithography can produce parts that are optically transparent by using epoxy resins in tandem with the ACES™ build style. This makes stereolithography models ideally suited for applications, such as flow visualization testing, or photoelastic stress analysis. Such studies cannot be done without the benefit of a model with the high optical clarity afforded by these materials.

Table 1. Properties of Some Post-Cured Stereolithography Materials

Material	Somos 3100	Somos 7100	Somos 8100	SL 5149	SL 5210*	SL 5510	SL 5520	Stereocol A-C 9200R
Chemistry type	Acrylate	Epoxy	Epoxy	Urethane acrylate	Vinyl ether	Epoxy	Epoxy	Acrylate
Liquid viscosity (cps at 30°C)	900–1000	800	620	2000	305	180	444	1090
Tensile strength (KSI)	3.0	8.6	3.4–3.9	5.1	6.5	11.1	3.8–4.8	6.5
Tensile modulus (KSI)	117	331	68–102	160	438	478	150–200	190
Elongation at break (%)	9.2	4.5	18–30	11–19	1.6	5.4	23–43	7
Flexural strength (PSI)	N/A	13.9	3.6–4.0	4	10.7	14.4	4.2–6.0	N/A
Flexural modulus (KSI)	45	404	91–105	N/A	444	443	100–130	N/A
Impact strength (ft-lb/in.)	0.4	0.5	0.9–1.1	0.4	0.5	0.5	1.1	N/A
Heat deflection temperature (°C at 66 PSI)	N/A	64	60–63		99*	62	44	
Shore hardness (Shore "D")	80	84	75–78	78	85	86	80	75

*After a two-hour 120°C thermal post cure.

Table 2. Properties of Thermoplastic Materials

Material	Urethane thermoset	Polypropylene	Nylon 66	ABS	Polycarbonate
Manufacturer	M.C.P.	Amoco	DuPont	G.E.	G.E.
Product name	SG95	PP 51 S12A	Zytel 101	GMP 5500	Lexan 141
Tensile strength (KSI)	8.7	4.7	12.0	6.9	10.0
Tensile modulus (KSI)	288	210		360	
Elongation at break (%)	7.0	> 100	60	20	130
Flexural strength (KSI)	7.23			12.3	14.0
Flexural modulus (KSI)	396	200	410	380	340
Impact strength (ft-lb/in.)	0.35	3.4	1.0	5.0	15.0
Heat deflection temperature*		218	235	100**	280
Shore hardness (Shore "D")	79		89		

*Heat deflection temperature (°C) at 66 PSI
**Heat deflection temperature (°C) at 264 PSI

In addition, there are resins available that can be selectively colored so that particular areas can be identified. These resins have been very useful for a number of applications, specifically for the production of medical models.

Despite their apparent brittleness, epoxy resins can be used to produce accurate "bridge tools." These tooling inserts can be used directly to produce as many as 500 functional injection molded prototypes in a variety of engineering thermoplastics without having to do costly and time-consuming hard machine tooling. These prototypes are produced using the method of manufacturing in the final material. In addition, the newest generation of epoxy stereolithography resins allow for the production of durable and flexible models suitable for snap fit and other forms of functional testing.

Stereolithography allows for the curing of a wide variety of liquid photopolymers to produce accurate models in a variety of materials in a fraction of the time that would be required to produce similar parts by conventional approaches (such as machining). Materials are available that allow for the production of rigid, flexible, or thermally resistant models. In addition, stereolithography is the only rapid prototyping equipment capable of producing optically transparent models that can be useful for fluid flow visualization, photoelastic stress analysis, and other purposes. Stereolithography materials allow rapid exploration of design concepts and functional testing.

References
1. P. F. Jacobs (Ed.), *Rapid Prototyping & Manufacturing: Fundamentals of Stereolithography*, Society of Manufacturing Engineers, Dearborn, MI 1992, Chapter 2.
2. P. F. Jacobs (Ed.), 1996: *Stereolithography and Other RP&M. Technologies: From Rapid Prototyping to Rapid Tooling,* Society of Manufacturing Engineers, Deerborn, MI, Chapter 2.

STEPHEN D. HANNA

16.2.3 Lasers for Stereolithography
A criteria for a stereolithography resin curing source is that it reliably generate the correct wavelengths. Most commercially available resins are ultraviolet cured, but resins that cure in the visible range are becoming available. In addition, the process requires localization of the light–resin interaction, which effectively eliminates incoherent lamp sources at the power levels required. In the current stereolithography systems, the laser is focused with a long focal length telescope to a waist at the surface of the resin. The diameter of the beam waist, D_0, which in large part determines the lateral resolution of the system, is determined by the wavelength λ of the laser, the M^2 of the beam and the convergence angle θ given by the focal length of the lens system, $D_0 = 4\lambda M^2/\theta\pi$.

The direct-write, vector-scanning nature of the process demands that any optical source be continuous (CW) on the time scale of the writing speed. At present there are only two commercially viable CW sources of ultraviolet light at these wavelengths; the HeCd laser and the Argon ion laser. There has been progress in the development of high-repetition-rate, Q-switched, diode-pumped solid-state lasers (DPSS) that are quasi-continuous for low scan speeds. Other common sources of ultraviolet light, such as Rare Gas Halide (Excimer) lasers, are of insufficient repetition rate to be considered quasi-continuous for all practical scan speeds.

The choices for stereolithography users are therefore quite limited. The most appropriate laser to use is determined primarily by cost and by the trade-off between the throughput or production rate of the system and the precision of the parts being processed.

Scan Speed and Throughput
The laser power P_1, scan speed V_s and beam diameter D_0 at the surface of the resin are related by $V_s = k\, P_1 / D_0$, where k is resin dependent. Because the rotational scan speed of mirrors is limited by current scanner technology, the linear scan speed of the laser beam over the resin is typically increased by extending the distance from the scanners to the resin surface. This allows for faster linear scans as well as increased depth of focus to produce larger models. It also results in larger beam waist sizes and, therefore, lower precision parts.

Despite the increasing size of stereolithography systems, throughput is typically not limited by laser power. In addition, the current trend to use stereolithography as a part of the production process, tends to favor smaller beam waists for high-precision parts and surface finish. With currently available scanning systems, the requirements on stereolithography laser sources are therefore less to increased power levels and more to mode quality and stability. See Section 16.1.2 for a further discussion of this topic.

Mode Considerations
The interaction zone at the surface of the resin is determined by the focused spot size of the laser beam and the cure depth. For precision components, the laser beam mode can be a limiting factor in the resolution of the process. Typical HeCd lasers for stereolithography, for example, have M^2 values in the region of 3.5–5.0. Where precision processing is required, it may be necessary to reduce the mode of the laser to TEM_{00}. Although a reduced-mode laser typically has lower power, the smaller beam waist more than compensates for this. Consequently, a TEM_{00} mode laser requires higher scan speeds than a multimode laser. The maximum scan speed V_s^{max} of the overall system is related to the M^2 and output power P_1 of the laser by $V_s^{max} = (P_1/M^2) \times$ (Constant). It is important to understand the trade-off between mode, power, and scan speed to optimize a stereolithography system for either precision or throughput. In practice, this trade-off only exists in smaller stereolithography systems. All large systems use an optical delivery train that prohibits process dimensions below about 200 μm. For small stereolithography systems fabricating precision parts, HeCd lasers provide the short wavelength, narrow linewidth, and low M^2 value required to form the smallest focal spot size at the resin. However, the HeCd laser is inherently low power at practical sizes, and limits the throughput of larger and lower resolution systems. Larger stereolithography systems use TEM_{00} mode Ar-ion lasers to enhance throughput.

Chapter 16: Rapid Prototyping

In principle, solid-state sources, such as high-repetition-rate DPSS lasers, can be used to replace either HeCd or Ar lasers in any stereolithography system. The principle barrier to the wider use of solid-state lasers is the technical immaturity of the product as well as the cost of system components. Table 3 tabulates a comparison of laser types.

Table 3. Comparison of Laser Types

Laser type (wavelength)	Power (mW)	Mode (M^2)	Typical process dimensions (µm)	Principle benefit
HeCd (325 nm)	10–40	TEM_{00} (< 1.1)	65–80	Precision
HeCd (325 nm)	20–100	Multimode (2.0–5.0)	200–300	Low cost
Ar-ion (351 nm)	200–500	TEM_{00} (< 1.1)	250	Throughput
DPSS (354 nm)	> 150	TEM_{00} (> 1.1)	> 250	Efficiency

HeCd Laser

HeCd lasers are true CW laser sources at a wavelength of 325 nm; the shortest wavelength used by commercial stereolithography systems. In addition, they may be configured as single mode (TEM_{00}), or multimode (TEM_{mn}) systems with M^2 values varying from 1.05 to 5. The combination of short wavelength and low M^2 allows the HeCd laser to be focused to the smallest spot size of any commercial stereolithography laser to fabricate high-precision parts. Typically, multimode HeCd lasers produce a spot size of 250 µm in, for example, the popular SLA250. A single-mode laser may have a corresponding spot size of only 65 µm, greatly enhancing the precision of processed parts. HeCd lasers, however, tend to be relatively low power; they range from 10 to 40 mW for TEM_{00} mode systems and from 20 to 100 mW for multimode. As the throughput of a stereolithography system is partly determined by the power of the laser source, HeCd lasers are used extensively only in processing smaller parts in small resin volumes. Small-volume systems ensure that the distance from the resin surface to the focusing optics is minimized for faster lenses to produce the reduced spot size. In small systems using a TEM_{00} mode laser, the maximum scan rate V_s^{max} effectively limits the useful power of a laser to about 15–20 mW. Now available are upgrades and new systems using a 13-mW TEM_{00} HeCd laser for high-resolution (< 100 µm) parts processing.

Ar-ion Laser

Ar-ion lasers are currently the highest-power commercial sources of CW ultraviolet light. To process larger parts in a stereolithography system, it is necesary to increase both the power of the laser source, and the rate at which the beam is scanned over the resin surface. Increasing the maximum linear scan rate V_s^{max} usually involves increasing the distance from the scan mirrors to the resin surface, as the rotation rate of the mirrors is limited by the mirrors inertia and the torque of the galvanometers. The increased scan distance, and therefore focal length of the system, leads to larger focus spot dimensions. For the largest stereolithography systems, the laser source must have a TEM_{00} mode even to maintain the 250-µm interaction zone typical for multimode lasers in small systems. Argon-ion lasers are capable of up to several watts of output power in the ultraviolet. Unlike HeCd lasers, however, the output of Ar-ion lasers is not a single wavelength, but a discreet set of wavelengths between 350 and 365 nm. Multiple-wavelength operation, even if all wavelengths are TEM_{00} mode, tends to increase the size of the focus region. Argon-ion lasers suitable for high-power stereolithography at a modest resolution of 250 µm still need to be operated at a single line and TEM_{00} mode. Even in such a single line, single mode, configuration however, it is still possible to produce hundreds of mW output power from an Ar-ion laser. The excellent mode characteristics and high power of Ar-ion lasers are well suited to high throughput stereolithography systems for the fabrication of either large parts or simultaneous fabrication of smaller parts.

Diode-Pumped Solid-State (DPSS) Lasers

DPSS lasers use diodes as the main energy sources to pump a solid-state laser material. In principle the technology is compact, efficient, rugged, and reliable. Compare the 1% electrical to optical conversion efficiency of a DPSS laser to the 0.01% efficiency of a typical Ar-ion laser. DPSS lasers have been available in longer wavelengths for some years in both CW and pulsed configurations. However, in order to achieve the short wavelengths required for stereolithography, all known solid-state sources require nonlinear optical processes, such as third harmonic generation (THG), to frequency convert the longer wavelength fundamental laser to an ultraviolet output.

The most common DPSS lasers are based on an Nd:Host crystal material (usually Nd:YVO$_4$ for lasers used in stereolithography), with a fundamental wavelength of approximately 1.05 µm and third-harmonic wavelength of some 350 nm. Although the principles of nonlinear optics are well understood, the high optical fields required for efficient THG can easily lead to long-term material damage of the nonlinear crystals, especially at surfaces and on coatings.

This requirement for high fields for efficient THG means that, unlike gas lasers, DPSS lasers are most efficient when the lasers are running in a TEM_{00} mode, so there is no trade-off between the mode and the power of a solid-state ultraviolet laser source. It should be noted however that the beam quality of the ultraviolet output of DPSS lasers used for stereolithography does not typically match that of gas lasers apertured to a true TEM_{00} mode, because of the birefringence properties of the nonlinear materials. High optical fields are very expensive to produce in a CW laser. As a result, all high-power ultraviolet DPSS lasers are operated in the Q-switched mode, where the output is a low duty cycle pulsed form.

As the stereolithography process requires some scanning technique to draw a part, any pulsed system must be quasi-continuous on the time scale of the drawing motion; which means having a pulse repetition frequency (PRF) that is high enough to ensure that successive pulses remain overlapped on the resin surface even at the highest scan speeds of the system. For larger SLA systems where the economic use of DPSS lasers is most apparent, linear scan speeds are high, and require a PRF of 30–100 KHz from the laser to ensure part integrity. Current commercial ultraviolet DPSS lasers fall into two categories: those using external cavity THG and those using internal cavity THG to produce the ultraviolet output. Extra-cavity THG is optically more simple, as the laser cavity and the nonlinear processes are decoupled. However, the optical fields intra-cavity are 10–20 times higher than outside, making the intra-cavity THG process more efficient and allowing for higher ultraviolet power, more collimated beams, and a higher repetition rate. At present, extra-cavity based lasers are specified in the 200–300 mw power range at 30 KHz, and are used for mid-range stereolithography systems. Intra-cavity based lasers are 1000 mW at 30 KHz, or 500 mW at up to 100 KHz, and are increasingly used to replace Ar-ion lasers on the highest-performance stereolithography machines.

Solid-state laser technology and nonlinear optics are developing very rapidly. The combination of size, efficiency, and long-term reliability suggest that all future stereolithography systems will likely use solid-state laser sources.

Cost of Ownership

The major costs of ownership for lasers used in any stereolithography system may be divided into immediate running costs associated with facilities such as power and water, and the maintenance costs of the laser over the long term. All of the currently available ultraviolet lasers suitable for stereolithography have significant maintenance costs that typically outweigh the immediate running costs. In the case of HeCd and DPSS lasers the running costs are insignificant as the lasers typically use < 1 kW electrical power and no cooling water services. This is not the case with an Ar-ion laser, where the cost of power may be as much as $20,000 per year for high-use systems. (Consider 16 hours per day as high use.) The long term maintenance cost of gas lasers is determined primarily by the cost of replacement discharge tubes. Laser tubes have a typical life of 3000–5000 hours for a HeCd laser and 5000–8000 for an Argon laser. In both cases, the higher-power versions of the lasers tend to have a reduced life; users must determine whether the productivity of a higher-power laser results in sufficient economic value to warrant the added costs. With replacement prices of approximately $10,000 for HeCd laser tubes and $30,000 for Argon laser tubes, a high-use stereolithography system requires between $20,000 and $70,000 operating costs for the laser alone. The cost of running DPSS lasers is not yet clear. However, all the evidence to date points to reduced costs. The required maintenance includes replacement of diodes and nonlinear materials, both of which currently deteriorate over time. The cost of maintenance is estimated to be $10,000 per year for moderate-power, 150-mW lasers, as shown in Table 4.

Note: Someone new to RP may find these costs higher than those for basic laser components. This is so because the lasers are part of the RP system and are integral to the system's warranty, and because the lasers are often purchased from the supplier rather than the laser's manufacturer.

Table 4. Annual Running Cost of High-Use Lasers: Upper Estimates*

Laser type	Operation	Maintenance
HeCd	< $ 1000	$ 20,000
Ar-ion	> $ 20,000	$ 50,000
DPSS	< $ 1000	$ 10,000

*Since prices increase with time, we have taken $10,000 as the cost for a replacement HeCd laser tube as our baseline, and all dollar amounts are relative to that figure.

References

P. F. Jacobs (Ed.), 1996: *Stereolithography and other RP&M Technologies,* ASME Press, New York.

Kenneth G. Ibbs and Norma-Jean Iverson, "Rapid Prototyping: New Lasers Make Better Parts," *Photonics Spectra,* June 1997, Laurin Publishing, Pittsfield, MA.

KENNETH G. IBBS

16.2.4 Stereolithography in Product Development

Introduction

In the 10 or so years since it was first introduced, the application of stereolithography in the development of mechanical components has become commonplace. The fact that companies such as Motorola and Hewlett Packard routinely use stereolithography in the development of new products is testimony to the value it provides. Stereolithography is used in a variety of ways, from initial concept development to preproduction models, and is used in different ways for different prototyping applications. Following are brief descriptions of the major applications.

Concept Models

Concept models are simply three-dimensional representations of a design. They are not made of the production material, they are most likely not functional, and they may not be dimensionally accurate. They are simply a model of the design that can be used to communicate the design to others. Even though the concept model is extremely limited in what it can do, it is of great value in the development process, often bypassing the need to visualize a component from looking at an engineering drawing. That ability to accurately convey a design early in the development process enables aesthetic and design problems to be identified long before investing in tooling and before expensive design commitments are made. Although any of the rapid prototyping methods can be used to create concept models, stereolithography generally produces models with the best accuracy and surface finish.

Presentation Models

Presentation models are a step above concept models. Like concept models, they are not of the production material and are usually not functional. Unlike concept models, they are finished and painted to look like the finished product and in many cases are difficult to distinguish from production components without close inspection. Presentation models can be used to accurately convey the appearance of the finished product to nonengineering personnel: senior management, marketing personnel, and customers. Many companies use presentation models as photography prior to the finished product being available. They are also used as trade show and marketing samples. Presentation models can be made available long before the finished product and usually at relatively low cost. Consequently, they provide a low-risk way to evaluate the appearance of the finished product.

Prototypes of Injection-Molded Plastic Parts

Because of the high cost of production tooling in the injection-molding process and the long lead times required for acquiring tooling, prototyping provides a high level of value in the development of injection-molded parts. Prototyping helps to identify any design issues prior to creating tooling. Correcting design issues via RP is far less expensive and time consuming than if corrections have to be made to the tooling.

Rapid prototyping is used in three different ways in prototyping injection molded parts: RP parts are used directly as prototypes; they are used to make master patterns, which in turn are used to make molds in which duplicates of the master can be made in materials that more closely approximate the intended production material; and finally, RP methods are used to make injection molds in which prototype parts in the production material can be molded.

Until recently, SLA parts have rarely been used directly as prototypes of injection molded parts because the resins were in general too brittle to survive functional testing (see Section 16.2.2). Selective laser-sintering and fused-deposition modeling were more often selected because they were able to make parts in materials that more closely approximated the material properties of injection-molded components. Recently, however, new resins have been introduced that provide increased flexibility and toughness for SLA parts compared to previous resins. SLA parts made from certain types of plastics, such as polypropylene, will reasonably approximate the characteristics of the molded parts. However, for higher durometer materials, SLA parts do not provide a good approximation.

For such materials, and in applications where the number of prototypes required make SLA parts economically unfeasible, a better solution is to create a master pattern and use it to build a mold. To make a master pattern, an SLA model of the part to be molded is built. The pattern may be scaled up to compensate for shrinkage in the duplication material. The pattern is worked to the level of finish desired on the duplicates.

Typically, the SLA part is first primed. A coat of primer makes minor surface flaws much easier to see. Surface flaws are filled and the surface is sanded to the level desired. Some areas may be polished if a gloss finish is required. Textured paint may be used to apply a light texture to the surface of the master.

The most common use of master patterns is to create silicon rubber molds in which polyurethane castings can be made.

The most straightforward method of making a mold is to suspend the pattern in a vat of liquid room-temperature vulcanizing (RTV) silicon rubber and allow the rubber to cure into a solid block. Once cured, the block is cut into two halves with scalpels and the pattern is removed. The block can then be taped back together to form a mold.

Duplicates of the pattern can then be created in a two-part polyurethane material. Polyurethane materials are available in a range of stiffnesses and can therefore approximate the stiffness of most common injection molded plastics. Appropriate proportions of the two components of the material are mixed together and poured into the mold, typically under a vacuum to assist in filling and to minimize any air that might be trapped in the mixture. The casting is then allowed to cure. Cure times range from less than a minute to several hours, depending on the urethane used.

Once cured, the casting can be removed from the mold and be used as a prototype of the molded part. Urethane castings can provide a good simulation of the molded part. The process is the fastest, least expensive way to prototype injection molded parts. The urethane is not the material that will be used in production. Since it may not be able to simulate the production material closely enough to fully verify the design, prototypes might have to be molded in the production material.

Rapid prototyping methods can also be used to create tooling for injection molding so that prototypes can be molded; stereolithography is one of the leading methods for doing this. Stereolithography is often used to directly create cavity and core inserts for the mold. This process is known as Direct AIM (an acronym of ACES Injection Molding where ACES is a build style for stereolithography). Although the SLA resin falls far short of the material properties of aluminum or tool steel, it typically is adequate to allow several parts to be molded. Those few parts may be adequate to verify design adequacy.

In addition to the AIM process, there are a number of alternative methods for creating injection mold tooling which are pattern based. Examples of such tooling include cast epoxy tooling, electroformed tooling, and cast metal tooling. Each of these processes require a master pattern in the shape of the part to be molded scaled to compensate for shrinkage of the plastic. Stereolithography is by far the first choice among RP methods for creating master patterns, because of its superior accuracy and surface finish.

Prototypes of Investment Cast Metal Parts

Stereolithography has been a significant innovation in the development of investment castings. It is used in two ways in prototyping investment cast parts. The first is in the creation of direct patterns, stereolithography parts which can be used in place of wax patterns. The second is in the creation of prototype wax pattern dies.

Direct patterns are achieved by using a build style called Quickcast, a style that builds hollow SLA parts. The part is built with all surfaces complete, but the interior of the part consists only of a truss structure of thin ribs to provide strength to hold the walls in place. The entire part is 70% or more void. The hollow structure enables the pattern to be burned out quickly. In addition, because the structure can collapse inwardly as it expands when the shell is fired, it minimizes chances that the shell will crack.

Modern SLA resins have been shown to burn out cleanly with a minimum of residue. The use of stereolithography patterns for prototype investment castings has gained wide popularity in the last few years. Although a number of other RP methods can also be used to create direct patterns, including SLS, FDM, and LOM, stereolithography is by far the most popular method because of its superior accuracy and surface finish.

Two limitations prevent the complete takeover of prototype investment casting patterns by stereolithography.

The first is ensuring that the pattern has no leaks. A leak in the skin of the pattern will likely allow slurry to enter the pattern during the shell building process. That infiltrated slurry will result in an inclusion in the casting, weakening the casting at that point.

The second issue is the difficulty of removing supports in internal cavities; stereolithography requires the use of supports in the build process which are later removed. Small internal cavities will, by necessity, have supports in them that must be removed after the build. It is critical that the supports be removed completely and the surface completely smoothed. If even a remnant of a support creates a notch in the ceramic shell, a point at which stresses will be concentrated and from which a crack is likely to propagate during the burnout portion of the process. Once the shell cracks, there will likely be a failure of the shell. It is difficult to completely remove supports completely in small internal cavities of a number of parts, such as the water jacket in a water cooled internal combustion engine. For those types of parts, other processes are more likely to be used, particularly the SLS process with either the trueform or polycarbonate materials.

Prototypes of Die Cast Parts

The cost of tooling for die casting ranks among the highest of any manufacturing process because of the high temperatures and pressures of die casting involved. Consequently, it is especially important to minimize any chances of design errors which would require reworking of the tooling. Unfortunately, the nature of the process makes it difficult to prototype die castings without actually creating machined tooling. Reasonable simulations of die castings can be obtained, however, with the plaster mold casting process. In recent years, the process has become faster and less expensive with the introduction of rapid prototyping.

The process of creating prototype die castings using rapid prototyping and the plaster mold casting process involves four major steps: 1) creation of a master pattern, 2) creation of tooling for the plaster mold casting process, 3) creation of the plaster mold, and 4) casting the prototype. Rapid prototyping is involved only in the first step.

Stereolithography is used more than any other RP method to create the master pattern because of its superior accuracy and surface finish. However, the pattern must be scaled to compensate for the shrinkage of the metal involved. The pattern is finished to the level of surface finish desired on the castings.

In the second step of the process, the master pattern is used to create tooling for the plaster mold casting process. Two tools must be created, one for each side of the plaster mold. The first step is to define the parting line and this is done with the creation of a device known as a parting line block. It often simply is a block of modeling clay in which the pattern has been imbedded up to the parting line. The geometry of the pattern is then reversed into dummy molds and tooling is cast against the dummy molds. Tooling for plaster mold casting can be either rubber or a more durable material like epoxy. The tooling typically can be used to create from 50 to several hundred plaster molds, depending on the tooling material used.

Once the tooling has been created for both sides of the tool, the plaster mold can be poured. The tooling is placed on a platform and a frame is set on top of the tool to contain the plaster. Wet plaster is poured into the frame and allowed to set up, usually in 30 minutes or less. After the plaster has set, the mold can be lifted off the tool. The mold is dried in an oven to eliminate as much moisture as possible. The cope and drag sections of the dried mold can then be assembled and it is ready to pour.

Molten aluminum, zinc, or magnesium is poured into the plaster mold, depending on the production intent material. The casting is allowed to cool for several hours to ensure it is completely solidified and to minimize warpage. The mold is then broken apart to extract the casting.

THOMAS J. MUELLER

16.3 Selective Laser Sintering

16.3.1 The Selective Laser Sintering Process

Selective laser sintering (SLS) is a versatile rapid prototyping technique capable of producing complex parts from a variety of powdered materials. SLS can produce functional parts from polymers as varied as nylons, polyamides, and thermoplastic elastomers. SLS can be used to produce patterns for sand and investment casting from various materials, and metal composites and ceramic/metal composites suitable for injection molding, electrical discharge machining, die-casting, and other applications. SLS uses a laser as a heat source that is scanned across the surface of a powder bed, melting or *sintering* the powdered material where scanning occurs.

The SLS Machine

A typical SLS machine layout can be seen in Figure 1. The major components of a SLS machine include: 1. a CO_2 laser, 2. two mirrors connected to precision galvanometers used to direct the laser beam, 3. two feed cartridges containing fresh, powdered material, 4. a part cylinder to contain the powder and part being processed, 5. a roller that distributes powder between the feed cartridges and the part cylinder, and 6. heaters located above the feed cartridges and the part cylinder (not shown in Fig. 1). These components are controlled by a dedicated computer through various programmable logic controllers (PLCs), sensors, and electronic apparatus. It should be noted that the roller in the SLS machine rotates in the opposite direction of the roller movement (just as up-milling in a machining operation). This type of roller movement evenly distributes the powder by "pushing" it ahead of the roller rather than "compressing" it below the roller.

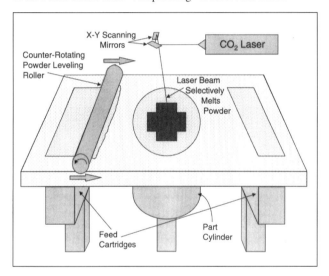

Figure 1. SLS machine components and their general layout.

Oxidation is a significant problem for most heated powder materials, therefore the powder heating and melting in SLS occurs in the presence of nitrogen gas. The powder, cartridges, and heaters are enclosed in a "process chamber" that is filled with nitrogen gas and maintained at a slightly positive pressure, to separate the process from oxygen in the atmosphere.

The SLS Process

Selective laser sintering requires a CAD solid model of the part to be built. That model must be supplied to the machine in the .stl file format (see Section 16.1). If multiple parts are to be built at one time, they can be combined into a single file prior to fabrication. This will cause the different parts to be scanned at the same time, as if they were separate features of the same part, increasing the speed of the scanning process. Conversely, if multiple files are kept as separate files they will be scanned one at a time, which gives the operator flexibility to prescribe different laser and/or scanning parameters for each part. This flexibility is particularly useful for laser and scanning parameter optimization studies.

Consumables in the SLS process include nitrogen gas and the desired powdered material. Nitrogen gas usage can be significant for certain materials and must be factored in as a cost of operating the machine.

After the SLS machine is loaded with the appropriate files and powder for the desired build, the operator starts the building process, which runs unattended. Depending on the material used, a long warm-up period may be required to fill the process chamber with nitrogen and preheat the material in the feed cartridges and the part piston, to bring the process chamber to a steady-state temperature. Typically the higher the melting point of the material being processed, the longer it takes for the warm-up stage, and the more uniform the temperature in the part bed must be. In order to achieve part bed temperature uniformity quickly and successfully, a bed of powder is built up in the part piston layer-by-layer as the powder is being heated. This warm-up stage can last anywhere from a couple of minutes to more than an hour depending on the material being processed, the starting temperature of the process chamber, and the temperature uniformity desired.

When the warm-up stage is complete, the machine begins to create the part using the following steps:

1. The feed cartridge corresponding to the side the roller is currently on rises and introduces fresh powder
2. The part piston lowers to receive the fresh powder; the distance the part piston lowers determines the layer thickness of the part which is typically 0.005 in.
3. The roller distributes the powder from the feed cartridge to the part piston and continues moving until it reaches the far side of the process chamber (just past the opposite feed cartridge)
4. The computer downloads the bottom slice of the part to the laser scanning system and the laser scans the bottom layer of the part
5. Steps 1–4 are repeated for each successive layer until the entire part has been fabricated

After the part is complete, it is sometimes necessary to allow the machine to go through a cool-down stage. This stage is designed to minimize the distortion of the part that might occur because of uneven cooling and shrinkage. In most cases materials with higher melting temperatures require more careful cooling. During the cool-down stage, the temperature in the part piston is lowered to room temperature over a period of time. This is accomplished by reducing the temperature of the heaters and continuing to place on top of the finished part successive layers of fresh, cooler powder from the feed cartridges (build steps 1–3 are repeated to lay down powder over the part). The time necessary for cool-down is dependent on the material used, the size of the part, and the propensity for the geometry that was created to distort. Cool-down times can range from a couple of minutes to more than an hour.

Once cool-down is complete, the part is removed from the SLS machine. The part is encased in loose powder that may clean off easily or, depending on the material being used, may require brushing, forced air, or bead-blasting to remove all of the loose powder from its surface. Once clean, the part can immediately be used as a visualization model, a functional prototype, or a pattern for secondary processes. If the desired finished product is a metal or ceramic/metal composite, post-processing in a furnace is required.

Reference
P. F. Jacobs (Ed.), *Rapid Prototyping & Manufacturing*, Society of Manufacturing Engineers, Dearborn, MI (1992).

BRENT STUCKER

16.3.2 Materials for SLS

A distinctive feature of SLS is the wide range of materials that can be used for the fabrication of prototypes. Examples of these materials are provided in Table 1.

Table 1. Some Materials Used in SLS

Polymers: poly(methyl methacrylate), acrylic-styrene, acrylonitrile-butadiene-styrene, polycarbonate, polyamide, glass-filled polyamide, poly(vinyl chloride), polyethylene, paraffin wax
Metals: Cu, Fe, Ti-6Al-4V, 17-4 PH stainless steel, inconel 625, 89 Cu-11 Sn, 59 Ni-41Al, tool steel, 50 Cu -50(70Pb-30Sn), Mo, 90 Cu-10 Sn, Cu-Ni, Fe-Co, W-Mo
Ceramics: Al_2O_3, Si_3N_4, SiC, $ZSiO_4$, hydroxyapatite, quartz, glass
Cermets: WC-Co, ZrB_2/Cu, Al_2O_3- Al, SiC/Al, Al_2O_3-Co, Al_2O_3-Ni, Al_2O_3-Cu, $YBa_2Cu_3O_{7-x}$/Ag

The diversity in materials allows the fabrication of parts of direct relevance to specific applications. Accordingly, operating conditions, in terms of input power, part throughput, and post SLS processing vary considerably.

Polymers are commonly used because of their low laser-energy requirements as compared with metals or ceramics. While low melt viscosity materials such as waxes and polyamides can be used to make full density parts, injection molding grade polymers are used to make porous parts that can be infiltrated with epoxy, polyester, or phenolic resins if necessary.

The use of metals and ceramics allows access to improved thermal and mechanical properties, as well as a wider range of functional attributes. Heated powder beds are often used to facilitate sintering of metals or ceramics. Depending on the material being processed as well as temperature, vacuum, or an inert atmosphere may need to be used. Also, polymers such as poly(methyl methacrylate), poly(methyl methacrylate-co-butyl methacrylate), poly(ethylacrylate-co-styrene), and phenolics are used to coat ceramic and metal powders to reduce SLS power requirements and fabrication times. These coatings can be applied by a solution technique, spray drying, or in a fluidized bed (1). Additives such as zinc chloride and ammonium dihydrogen phosphate are also occasionally used to reduce energy input in the processing of metals and ceramics, respectively.

Material Properties

The use of SLS materials in the form of particulates requires the practitioner to be familiar with several principles of powder metallurgy (2). These principles impact material selection as well as process design. In particular, distortion and surface finish are significantly affected by the particle characteristics of the material. Table 2 lists some important properties that need to be considered. Details of these properties and their effects on processing are common to a number of shape forming techniques that use powders and are extensively covered in the literature (2–6).

Table 2. Some Material Properties and Their Relevance to SLS

Property	Effect on processing
Particle size distribution (mean and width)	Sinterability, packing efficiency, surface roughness
Particle shape	Packing efficiency
Apparent and tap densities	Packing efficiency
Flowability	Uniform spreading of powder layer
Melting point	Indicator of energy requirements
Green strength	Facilitates component handling prior to thermal processing (debinding, sintering, infiltration)
Burnout	Decomposition temperature and ash content of binders
Specific heat, thermal conductivity	Heat transfer in powder bed
Void fraction	Residual porosity in prototypes

Post SLS Processing

Except in the case of polymers, several stages follow the SLS processing of polymers and are listed in Table 3 (next page). Details of these procedures can be readily found in works related to powder metallurgy (2–6).

One of the key issues in post SLS processing concerns component distortion. Distortion relates to anisotropic changes in the original shape. Reduction in accuracy, in terms of reproducing geometric detail and targeted dimensions, in SLS particularly occurs when the extent of shrinkage is high. A common method to minimize distortion is to limit the extent of interparticle neck growth during sintering to improve mechanical properties without undergoing significant shrinkage. The extent of sintering is controlled by several possible transport mechanisms which in turn depend on a number of parameters including time, temperature, density, particle size, grain size, and external pressure. Additional densification and strength can be achieved if necessary by infiltration with materials described earlier in this section.

Table 3. Post Processing

Process step	Description
Debinding	Binder removal from coated metal or ceramic powders
Sintering	Fusing of powders to enhance densification and mechanical properties accompanied by shrinkage and decrease in surface area
Hot isostatic pressing (HIP)	Densification
Infiltration	Densification with minimal shrinkage
Grinding	Obtain final dimensions
Polishing	Improve surface finish

Applications

Some applications of frequently used SLS materials are described in Table 4. This list can be expected to grow rapidly over the next few years (7).

Table 4. Selected Applications

Material	Application
Polyamide	Functional models
Polycarbonate	Expendable investment casting patterns
1080 carbon steel/ copper infiltrated	Metal mold inserts
Silicon carbide/ aluminum infiltrated	Prototypes for automotive parts
Zirconium diboride/ copper infiltrated	EDM electrodes
Zirconium silicate	Investment casting cores
Hydroxyapatite	Artificial bone implants

Examples

The mean particle size of some commercially available materials as well as their tensile strength following fabrication by SLS are listed in Table 5.

Table 5. Typical Properties with Selected Commercial SLS Materials

Material	Mean particle size (μm)	Tensile strength (MPa)
Polyamide, unfilled	120	36
Polyamide, glass-filled	50	49
Polycarbonate	90	23
Acrylic-styrene	33	10
1080 carbon steel[a]	55	475[b]
Zirconium silicate	105[a]	3.3[c]

[a]Polymer coated
[b]Following debinding, sintering, and copper infiltration
[c]Following curing of phenolic polymer

References

1. H. S. Hall and R. E. Pondell, "The Wurster Process," in *Controlled Release Technologies: Methods, Theory and Applications,* **2,** A. F. Kydonius (Ed.), CRC Press, Boca Raton, FL (1980).
2. R. M. German, *Powder Metallurgy Science,* Metal Powder Industries Federation, Princeton, NJ (1994).
3. R. M. German and A. Bose, *Injection Molding of Metals and Ceramics*, Metal Powder Industries Federation, Princeton, NJ (1997).
4. R. M. German, *Powder Injection Molding*, Metal Powder Industries Federation, Princeton, NJ (1990).
5. R. M. German, *Sintering Theory and Practice,* John Wiley and Sons, New York, NY (1996).
6. R. M. German, *Particle Packing Characteristics*, Metal Powder Industries Federation, Princeton, NJ (1989).
7. J. J. Beaman et al., *Solid Freeform Manufacturing: A New Direction in Manufacturing,* Kluwer Academic Publishers, Boston, MA (1997).

SUNDAR V. ATRE
RANDALL M. GERMAN

16.3.3 Lasers for Selective Laser Sintering

Introduction

The laser choice in commercial selective laser sintering (SLS) machines has historically been limited to the CO_2 laser and the Nd:YAG laser. These choices were based on price, commercial availability, and the material being processed in the machine. The CO_2 laser is by far the most popular choice because of its good coupling efficiency to most materials and low price per watt. The Nd:YAG laser is used with specialty materials, such as metals, which exhibit high reflectance with the CO_2 laser. Economic reasons limit commercial machines to these lasers at the moment. Table 6 shows a listing of lasers that could be used in SLS applications, along with the advantages and disadvantages of each.

Table 6. Lasers for Selective Laser Sintering

Laser	Wavelength (μm)	Advantages	Disadvantages
CO_2	10.6	Low price/watt; fairly efficient; couples well to most materials; commonly available	Long wavelength requires semi-fragile optics and makes large focus spot; harder to power control
Nd:YAG	1.064	Couples well to metals; commonly available	High price/watt; does not couple well to most plastics; generally poor beam quality
CO	5.0–5.5	Good compromise between CO_2 and Nd:YAG lasers	High price/watt; not commonly available; requires semi-fragile optics; hard to power control
NIR diode	0.7–1.6	Easy to power control; very efficient	Very poor beam quality
Fiber	1.55	Easy to power control; easy to scale; excellent beam quality	Low power; high price/watt
MIR SS/OPO	3–5	Combines advantages of CO_2 and Nd:YAG	Output power low; under development

The choice of a laser for a particular SLS application comes down to the answers to the following questions:

1. Does the laser heat the material efficiently?
2. Is the laser low in cost initially and in use?
3. Is the laser power easy to control?
4. Can the laser power be changed fast enough?
5. Can the laser be focused to a small enough spot size?

CO_2 Laser

The CO_2 laser couples well with almost everything. In addition, its price per watt is very competitive with nearly any other laser type in the 50- to 100-W power range. Accessories are available commercially that allow the laser to achieve the required bandwidth. Beam quality is marginal to excellent, varying with the manufacturer and laser model. An M^2 of about 1.3 or better is usually adequate for SLS. This is based on a final lens-to-part bed distance of about 600 mm, a 30-mm final aperture, and a $1/e$ spot diameter of 400 μm.

Nd:YAG and Other Near-Infrared Solid-State Lasers

The Nd:YAG laser is most useful in metals selective laser sintering operations. Most polymers are transparent to it. It is a fairly simple matter to put an absorber in the polymers so that the Nd:YAG would work with them. But, since the CO_2 laser is less expensive and works well, there is little commercial reason to do so.

Nd:YAG power control for flashlamp pumped models is about as complex as that of the CO_2; power control is very simple for diode-pumped models. The diode-pumped models have a definite edge in low down-time, as well. Diode-pumped Nd:YAGs are currently more expensive than flashlamp pumped ones, and this will probably be true for a few more years. Beam quality is poor to excellent, depending on the model chosen. Due to the much shorter wavelength of the Nd:YAG compared with the CO_2 laser, this poses only a minor problem. An M^2 of 10 or less is usually sufficient, based on the assumptions given in the CO_2 section.

The above comments about the Nd:YAG apply to most other solid-state lasers with lasing wavelengths in the near-infrared.

Other Lasers

The CO (carbon monoxide) laser can be used in much the same way as the CO_2 laser. The laser's efficiency is less, thus the cost per watt is higher. However, its use may be warranted if a halving of spot size relative to the CO_2 laser is necessary and the lower power is not a problem.

Diode lasers can be used directly, and show similar properties to the diode-pumped Nd:YAG. However, the beam quality of high-powered diode lasers is very poor compared to CO_2 or even Nd:YAG lasers. Currently, diode lasers are suitable only for SLS applications with a small part area, since the beam quality is so poor that an acceptable spot size cannot be achieved with a large final aperture to part bed distance. Advances in using fiber coupling with these lasers are resolving these difficulties.

Excimer lasers couple well with most materials but suffer from two problems. First, most high power excimer systems are pulsed. Commercial systems are now reaching the 5-kHz minimum repetition frequency needed for SLS operation. In addition, excimer lasers process material by photoablation, not vaporization. The primary interaction is the dissolution of the molecular bonds of the substance. The SLS process requires heat deposition. This makes excimers unsuitable for SLS applications.

Fiber lasers/amplifiers may be used in the future for the same applications as Nd:YAG lasers. The most common wavelength for these lasers is 1.55 μm. These lasers are rugged, easily scalable in power up to the fiber limit, and have excellent mode quality, because they are typically generated in a single mode optical fiber. High-power versions have not been commercially developed because of the lack of need and suitable inexpensive alternatives, such as the Nd:YAG laser.

Solid-state lasers with "optical devices" operating in the 3–5μm wavelength range will be very useful. The shorter wavelengths allow smaller spot sizes and better coupling with metals materials. Most polymers have overtone absorption bands in the mid-infrared. For example, polyamide (nylon) and polycarbonate have absorption bands at about 3.1 μm. Current commercial lasers in the 3–5μm wavelength range do not have the power necessary to perform selective laser sintering at reasonable speeds.

Conclusions

Currently, there is no pressing reason to use any type of laser other than a CO_2 or an Nd:YAG in a selective laser sintering machine. These two lasers are commonly available, relatively inexpensive, and complement each other very well. An SLS machine containing both CO_2 and Nd:YAG lasers can efficiently process almost any known powder. A machine with only a CO_2 laser can also process most everything, but its efficiency with metal powders is low.

DAMIEN F. GRAY

16.3.4 Directed Light Fabrication

Directed Light Fabrication (DLF) is a rapid fabrication technology developed and patented at Los Alamos National Laboratory that produces fully dense metal components from a computer design. Unlike a sintering process, defined by solid-state diffusion across a powder particle interface, the input metal powders are fully melted and resolidified to achieve full density. Hence, functional metal parts with mechanical properties equivalent to conventionally processed metal can be produced (8).

The process, requiring a computer workstation, a laser integrated with a motion system, and a powder delivery system, is shown schematically in Figure 2.

The process begins by designing a model of a required part on a computer which is used to define the motion commands that move a laser focal spot throughout the solid volume of the part. Metal powder particles are fed into the laser focal spot, creating a molten pool of material that solidifies just behind the moving molten zone. Typically the motion path establishes sets of planar layers that are traced and successively stacked to form a portion or all of the part. Layers are typically 0.08–0.508 mm (0.003–0.020 in.) thick.

The microstructure of DLF deposited 316 stainless steel is shown in Figure 3. Layer boundaries melt back into previously deposited material and cellular solidification structure, seen in the image, are characteristic of DLF deposits. Maintaining a continuous molten pool ensures that all powder input material has been melted and resolidified such that no powder particle boundaries or pores are observed in the microstructure. Adjustment of laser power, velocity, powder feed rate, overlap from pass to adjacent pass, and layer depth are necessary to assure fully dense microstructures.

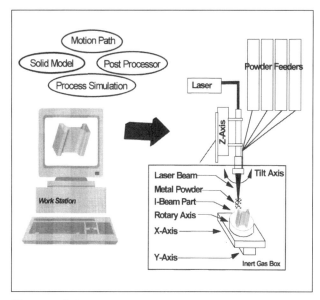

Figure 2. Schematic representation of the DLF process with five axes of motion and four powder feed systems attached.

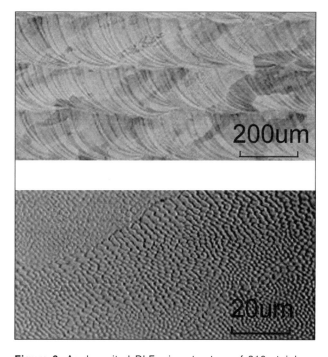

Figure 3. As-deposited DLF microstructure of 316 stainless steel material showing deposition layers (top) and cellular microstructure (bottom).

All layers do not have to be in the same planar orientation. Appendages attached to the parent feature can be produced with layer orientation at nearly any angle to that of the parent provided appropriate axes of motion are present in the DLF system. Simple one-dimensional parts requiring one axis of motion, and complex three-dimensional parts requiring five or more axes of motion, can be produced by the DLF process.

The hemisphere shown in Figure 4 is an example of an out-of-horizontal-plane deposition that requires four axes of motion. The deposition head is always kept normal to the deposited planar layers. It is tilted horizontally at the start of the hemisphere and changes angular orientation as the wall is built toward the equator where head orientation is vertical. Position commands for the four axes and a velocity command to maintain constant surface velocity as the radius from the axis of revolution increases are given for every revolution of the part. Wall thickness typically can be varied from about 0.5 mm (.020 in.) using a single pass per revolution to thicknesses greater than 0.5 mm by multiple side-by-side passes.

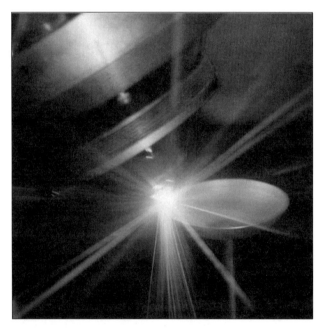

Figure 4. Fabricating an out-of-horizontal-plane part using four axes of motion.

Multiple powder feeds (Fig. 2) can be used to feed more than one material into the laser produced molten pool, either successively or simultaneously, and vary the composition of the deposit zone. The DLF process has proven the feasibility to deposit many metals or intermetallic compounds, and is applicable to any particulate material that can be melted by the laser beam and then allowed to solidify. Metals ranging in melting point from that of Al to W, the highest melting point metal, have been processed. Intermetallics such as molybdenum disilicide, nickel aluminide, and titanium aluminide have been processed.

Fully dense components are produced with properties (9) equivalent to or better than conventionally processed material of the same composition. Table 7 compares the properties of a DLF deposited material to conventionally processed material. Yield strengths of DLF processed material are equal to or higher in all cases to those of cast and wrought material. These strength levels are achieved in a single step compared to the casting and themomechanical processing steps of the conventional materials.

Table 7. Properties of DLF Deposited Materials Compared with Conventionally Processed

Material	0.2% YS[a] (MPa)	UTS[b] (MPa)	Elong. (%)
DLF 316 ss	296	579	41 (46)
316 ss (cast)	269	517	39
316 ss (wrought)	262	572	63
DLF inconel 690	448	669	49
Inconel 690 (wrought)	372	738	50
DLF Ti-6Al-4V	958	1027	6
Ti-6Al-4V (cast)	889	1014	10
Ti-6Al-4V (wrought)	827–1000	931–1069	15–20

[a]Yield strength; [b]Ultimate tensile strength

Figure 5 shows a 0.3-m-long part made from inconel 690 using the DLF process. The dimensional accuracy of this part illustrates the current capability to build parts close to net shape requirements in a single step. The hole diameters were produced throughout the length to within 0.05 mm and placement was within ± 0.13 mm of the specified bolt circle centered on the center hole. Radial distance to the center of the hexagonal faces was within ± 0.076 mm. Surface finish was measured at 10 μm arithmetic average and mechanical properties are those shown in Table 7.

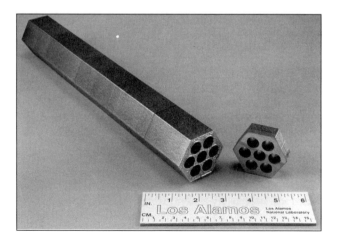

Figure 5. A 0.3-m hexagon with hole array was fabricated out of inconel 690, a high-temperature alloy.

Chapter 16: Rapid Prototyping

The most important aspect of the DLF process is its capability to control microstructure and material composition (10, 11) throughout a part as it is built; whereas processes such as casting or forging rely on control of the bulk volume of the entire metal component by metal mold or die design. The tooling design not only has to account for dimensional specifications, but the resultant microstructure and properties that are determined by thermal and stress/strain management during processing. DLF processing provides localized control of the laser power and velocity throughout the part at a resolution close to that of the molten pool size. These parameters determine molten pool size (ranging from 0.25–2.5 mm in width), cooling rate, and solidification rate of the molten pool, which in turn determine microstructural feature size and composition. This makes control of microstructural feature size, and/or placement of desired alloy composition possible so that material properties are matched to variable service requirements such as stress or strain within the part.

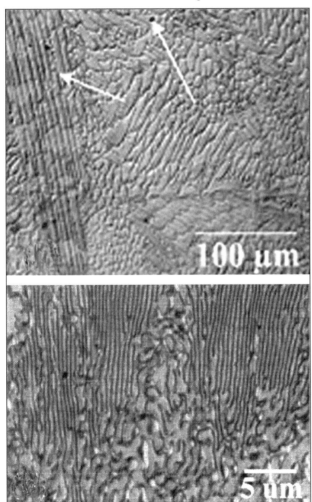

Figure 6. Microstructures of Fe-25%Ni alloy (top) show secondary dendrite arm spacing averaging 3 µm that correspond to cooling rates of 104 K/s, and Al-33Cu eutectic alloy (bottom) show lamellae spacing of 300 nm that correspond to calculated growth velocities of 1.2 mm/s.

Measurement of secondary dendrite arm spacing and eutectic lamellae spacing are input into calculations that provide the cooling rate and solidification velocity information relative to the DLF processing parameters. Figure 6 shows two representative alloys that have been used to measure these microstructural features to demonstrate the range of control possible. Cooling rates ranging from 102 to 104 K/s and solidification velocities ranging from 1 to 50 mm/s have been calculated for DLF processing as currently practiced.

The DLF process gives the designer the advantage of a one-step process that converts a three-dimensional design on a computer into a functional metal component. This allows design iterations to be tested without the need of die or mold fabrication and that allows materials to be varied within a single part. Fabrication of entire assemblies to be made without welding or joining.

References
8. G. K. Lewis, D. J. Thoma, J. O. Milewski, and R. B. Nemec, *Directed Light Fabrication of Near-Net Shape Metal Components,* World Congress on Powder Metallurgy and Particulate Materials, Washington, D.C. (June 16–21, 1996).
9. G. K. Lewis, J. O. Milewski, and D. J. Thoma, *Properties of Near-Net Shape Metallic Components Made by the Directed Light Fabrication Process,* 8th Solid Freeform Fabrication Symposium, University of Texas, Austin, TX (August 11–13, 1997).
10. D. J. Thoma, G. K. Lewis, J. O. Milewski, K. C. Chen, and R. B. Nemec, *Rapid Fabrication of Materials Using Directed Light Fabrication,* Thermec '97, Wollonging, Australia (July 7–11, 1997).
11. D. J. Thoma, G. K. Lewis, E. M. Schwartz, and R. B. Nemec, "Near Net Shape Processing of Metal Powders Using Directed Light Fabrication, Advanced Materials and Technology for the 21st Century," *Journal of the Institute of Metals,* 1995 Fall Annual Meeting (117th), Hawaii, (December 13–15, 1995).

GARY K. LEWIS

16.3.5 The Laser Engineered Net Shaping Process

The laser engineered net shaping (LENS) process is technology that uses a high-powered Nd:YAG laser to fabricate solid metallic objects directly from a computer aided design (CAD) solid models. The process, evolved from rapid prototyping (RP) techniques, provides several significant advantages over the existing RP processes. Providing the ability to create a functional mechanical component in a single operation is one key advantage. In addition, the unique thermal history produced by the laser source has been shown to improve material properties as compared to conventionally processed materials of similar composition. Mechanical properties for several of the materials processed using the LENS process are included in Table 8. Note that for all three of these materials, the tensile strength increased significantly and the ductility was as good or better than the conventionally processed materials.

Table 8. Mechanical Test Data from LENS Manufactured Tensile Specimens

Material type	Ultimate strength (ksi)	Yield strength (ksi)	Elongation (% in one inch)
316 stainless steel	115	72	50
316 ss anneal bar	*85*	*35*	*50*
Inconel 625	135	84	38
625 annealed bar	*121*	*58*	*30*
Ti-6Al-4V	170	155	11
Ti-6Al-4V annealed bar	*130*	*120*	*10*

The process is driven directly from data derived from a CAD solid model. The CAD solid model is first sliced into thin layers electronically on the computer. From the layer data, patterns are generated to outline both the external and internal surface features of the object and to produce a hatching pattern to direct the LENS process for filling in the featureless regions of the object. A schematic representation of the LENS process is shown schematically in Figure 7. The laser is focused onto a substrate to create a molten puddle and powder is injected into this puddle (analogous to filler metal application during welding) to increase the volume of the material in this localized area. Computer-driven relative motion between the substrate and laser source provides a means to create patterns from the deposited metallic materials.

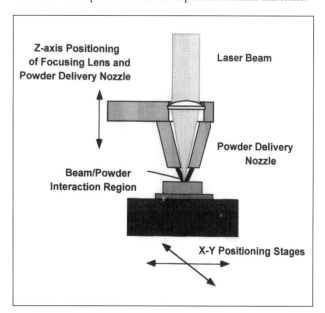

Figure 7. Schematic representation of the LENS process.

The LENS process relies heavily on control software to drive the process and create an object that is both fully dense and accurate. For a better surface finish, it is preferred to first outline the contours defining the internal and external surfaces. Then the featureless regions between the outlined surfaces are filled by depositing a series of parallel metallic lines that overlap to create flat uniform layers. Alternating the direction of the hatching is generally incorporated into the process to attempt to create a more homogeneous macrostructure within the LENS fabricated components. A series of algorithms have been incorporated into the software to compensate for the ability of the finite width of the laser beam to create an accurate part. Table 9 presents the typical process parameters used in depositing various iron- and nickel-based materials.

Table 9. Typical Process Parameters Used in Depositing Iron- and Nickel-Based Alloy Materials

Process variable	Condition
Laser power	250 W
Travel velocity	0.85 cm/s
Hatch line separation	381 µm
Laser spot size	600 µm
Line offset	191 µm
Powder feed rate	0.003 kg/min

The specific process recipes developed for fabricating a solid object will have some variation with respect to the above process values given in Table 9. These general values given have been shown to produce exceptional material properties within the solid structure. The improvement in material properties is attributed to the fine grain structure obtained using the LENS process. In many materials a simultaneous increase in yield strength and ductility, as compared to conventionally processed materials of similar composition, can be obtained using the LENS process. Using process conditions similar to those of Table 9, a two-fold increase in yield strength and a 30% increase in ductility has been obtained for 316 stainless steel materials (see Table 8). Similar results have been other LENS processed materials as well.

The accuracy of the final fabricated components is a critical issue when fabricating mechanical hardware. It is generally believed that a smaller laser spot size will provide the best accuracy. However, this accuracy is obtained at the expense of processing speed. Therefore, in developing processing recipes, the user must compromise between these generally conflicting requirements. For the process conditions given in Table 9 an accuracy of ± 127 µm can be obtained in the deposition plane with an accuracy of ± 381 µm in the growth direction.

Other laser sources, such as CO_2 lasers, can be used for this process as well. In general, a continuous laser source is preferred to a pulsed source to optimize processing speed and, more important, to avoid cracking of the hot crack sensitive alloys such as inconel 718. However, there are times when a pulsed source can also provide an advantage. Pulsed laser sources have been shown to provide an advantage over a continuous laser source when high-reflectivity materials such as copper are being processed.

A variety of materials can be processed using the LENS method including 303 and 316 stainless steel, inconel 625, 690 and 718, tungsten, titanium-6 wt.% Al-4 wt.%V, H13 and Micromelt 10 tool steel, Haynes 230 and copper. In addition, liquid phase sintering between tungsten and titanium carbide particles mixed with a nickel or cobalt binder can be achieved. It is expected that the LENS technology will play an increasingly significant role in manufacturing applications.

More recent advances in LENS technology allow multiple materials to be deposited. This advancement provides an enabling feature for the LENS process in fabricating multiple material structures including both abrupt and gradient transitions from one material to another.

DAVID M. KEICHER

16.3.6 Results

Currently, commercial selective laser sintering systems are available from several manufacturers. Some of these systems can process a broad range of materials, while others are material specific. The majority of commercial SLS systems use CO_2 lasers, although high-powered Nd:YAG lasers are employed in commercial LENS systems (see Section 16.3.5). The maximum available work area is approximately 700 mm X 700 mm. Since sintered volumes are supported by unsintered powder, it is not usually necessary to anchor parts to a reference surface. This allows parts to be "nested" and stacked in the vertical direction. As a result, productivity is good and highly complex parts can be built.

Plastic Parts

Materials flexibility provides selective laser sintering with a significant technological advantage. The commercial challenge has been to exploit this advantage while minimizing limitations associated with finite particle size. Materials capabilities have increased significantly since selective laser sintering systems were commercialized in late 1992. An important commercial focus has been plastic part applications. The methods for producing plastic parts using selective laser sintering are summarized in Table 10.

Table 10. Routes to Plastic Parts Using Selective Laser Sintering

Laser sintering powder(s)	Conversion process	Final part material	Typical number of parts
Polyamide polymer, glass-filled polyamide polymer	None	Laser sintered material	1–5
Nickel-bronze, stainless steel-bronze	Injection molding – metal mold insert	Choice	100–50,000 +

Functional plastic test models are fabricated directly from polyamide (nylon) powders and glass-filled polyamide powders. These models have good strength, toughness, and densities that approach theoretical values. Historically, the direct creation of such functional models has been a unique and important laser sintering application. Figure 8 shows an example of a laser sintered polyamide test model.

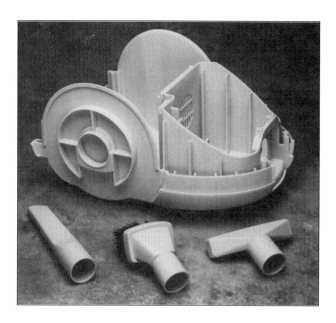

Figure 8. A laser sintered polyamide model.

The polyamide models are also used as durable masters for silicone rubber molds. Limited quantities (20–50) of urethane-based plastic models can be cast from these molds. This has become an increasingly important laser sintering application as the resolution and surface finish of polyamide parts has improved.

Metal-based powders have been used to create mold inserts for plastics molding. Porous nickel-bronze metal tools are prepared by sintering the metal powder directly using a 200 W CO_2 laser. These mold inserts enable users to injection mold test quantities of true prototype parts from the production material. Fully dense stainless steel-bronze tools are prepared by sintering a polymer coated steel powder and then infiltrating the resulting "green" preforms with bronze in a furnace. In some cases, mold quality and durability are sufficient to allow preproduction or production requirements to be addressed.

Metal Castings

The other important application has been metals casting, in particular, investment casting and sand casting. Table 11 (next page) summarizes the methods for producing metal castings using selective laser sintering.

Expendable patterns for investment casting are built from a number of amorphous polymers. These patterns are porous and do not expand and crack shells during the pattern removal and shell firing processes, although nonstandard heat cycles are often required. Cores and molds for sand casting are fabricated directly from phenolic-based shell sands. These laser-sintering materials allow prototype castings to be prepared without tooling. Limited production runs are also possible.

Table 11. Routes to Metal Parts Using Selective Laser Sintering

Metals production process	Laser sintering powder(s)	Application for laser sintered parts
Investment casting	Acrylic, styrene, and polycarbonate polymers	Expendable patterns
Sand casting	Shell foundry sand	Cores and molds
Pressure die casting	Stainless steel-bronze	Limited-run mold insert

In addition, the design freedom available with layer manufacturing allows castings to be made that would not be feasible using conventional technology. Figure 9 shows an example of a laser sintered sand core that would be nearly impossible to produce if individual pieces had to be molded with core boxes.

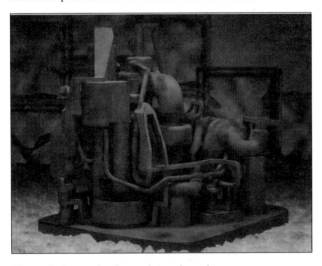

Figure 9. A complex laser sintered sand core.

Finally, the stainless steel-bronze mold inserts can also be used to mold limited quantities (100–300) of pressure die cast parts.

Research

Laser sintering of complex three-dimensional metal shapes is an ongoing research area. One approach is to create green preforms in the laser-sintering machine and then sinter the parts to high density in a furnace. A second approach is to sinter metal powders directly, typically with an Nd:YAG laser. Methods include conventional selective laser sintering as well as directed light fabrication (see Section 16.3.4) and laser engineered net shape (see Section 16.3.5). The densities of these sintered metal parts can approach theoretical values and a wide variety of metal powders can be processed. Typically, the parts are welded to a base plate to reduce distortion due to thermal stresses. There are a number of possible applications for sintered metal parts. They can serve as functional test models early in the design cycle. More importantly, however, limited quantities of parts can be manufactured without tooling, including those that would be difficult or impossible to create using material removal processes. Durable tooling for processes such as plastics molding and pressure die-casting is also of interest.

Laser sintering of ceramic systems for tooling and medical applications is an active area of development.

Reference
J. J. Beaman, J. W. Barlow, D. L. Bourell, R. H. Crawford, H. L. Marcus, and K. P. McAlea, *Solid Freeform Fabrication: A New Direction in Manufacturing,* Kluwer Academic Publishers, Norwell, MA (1997).

KEVIN P. McALEA

16.4 Laminated Object Manufacturing

16.4.1 The LOM Process

Laminated object manufacturing (LOM), as the name implies, creates complex three-dimensional objects by electronically slicing the intended object into planar cross sections, and sequentially reconstructing the object by laminating sheet materials and cutting the corresponding cross sections with a focused laser beam. Figure 1 (next page) illustrates the commercially reduced process. Lamination of each layer is achieved by way of a heated roller traveling across the top surface in one single reciprocal motion. The heat-sensitive adhesive under the top sheet of paper is then activated momentarily and provides the necessary tack for adhesion. The power of the laser beam is adjusted so that the depth of cut is limited to the thickness of each layer. The excess material, which supports the model during the fabrication process, is cross-hatched to facilitate its removal after the entire object has been constructed.

Materials

Potentially, any sheet material can be utilized in LOM. Research has shown that the LOM process is well suited to handle a wide variety of materials, including paper, plastics, polymer composite prepregs, metals, ceramics, and even ceramic matrix composites. Paper, however, has been the most popular because it is inexpensive and possesses many of the same properties of wood, the most popular pattern material.

The choice of material depends on the application. For visualization and form-fitting, paper would be the ideal choice. For snap-fit and limited functional testing where flexibility and high interlaminate strength are needed, plastics would be superior. For intermediate temperature and pressure tooling applications, such as injection molding, polymer composites may provide a solution. High-temperature (> 1000°C) structural parts and tooling will necessitate ceramic or metal materials.

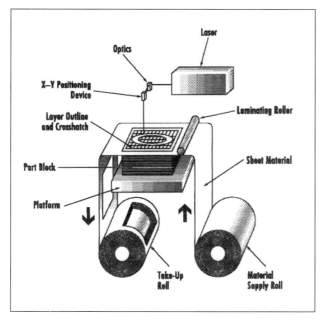

Figure 1. Schematic of the laminated object manufacturing (LOM) process.

Equipment

Two models are in commercial use. Model LOM 1015 Plus and 2030H whose working envelopes are 10" W X 14.5" L X 14" H, and 22" W X 32" L X 20" H, respectively.

16.4.2 Applications

Visualization

An LOM part's wood-like composition allows it to be painted or finished as a true replica of the product. These replicas can be used for a variety of functions, including consumer testing, marketing product introduction, packaging studies, and samples for vendor quotations.

Form, Fit, and Function

In addition to viewing the prototype as a finished product, LOM parts can also be used for design verification and performance evaluation. In low-stress environments, LOM prototypes can be used to evaluate the functionality of the design in its total environment. If the original design warrants a change, it can easily be modified by conventional machining.

Investment Casting

Investment casting is a process by which metal duplicates are created from an expendable master. The master, typically wax, is repeatedly dipped in a ceramic slurry and dried until a thick shell is created. The master is then extracted from the shell by heating the assembly in an oven beyond the melting point of the wax. The empty shell is then densified by further heating. Next, a molten metal is cast into the empty shell. The metal duplicate is obtained by breaking open the shell.

LOM paper masters can be used as a one-to-one replacement of wax masters (direct investment casting) or as a tool into which up to 100 wax patterns can be injected (indirect investment casting).

Indirect investment casting is used when more than several duplicates are needed. It is much more economical to fabricate a single LOM mold, and inject wax to create hundreds of duplicates. The wax patterns can then be taken through the normal investment casting process described above.

Sand Casting

Sand casting is a metal-forming process in which objects are produced by casting molten metal directly into sand molds. Sand molds have traditionally been created from meticulously hand-crafted wooden patterns by highly skilled workers. The detail and artistry required for these patterns involve several weeks of preparation. With the advent of LOM and its ability to quickly and inexpensively produce wood-like sand casting patterns, the traditional, labor-intensive pattern making is being drastically refined.

When just a few castings are needed, an LOM pattern is used to make direct impressions in sand. First, an LOM pattern with appropriate shrinkage factors and draft angles is created. It is then sealed (with epoxy or lacquer), filled, coated with a primer, and sanded until an acceptable surface finish is obtained. Finished patterns that are simple in shape and contain a flat surface are mounted onto a flat, wooden board. This is called a lost pattern. For more complicated patterns, a special wooden follow board is created by boring out a cavity in a wooden plank up to the depth of the parting location. The follow board thus determines the parting line. The top half of the pattern is placed into the follow board so that the bottom half is exposed above the board's surface.

The bottom half of the sand mold, called the drag, is formed first by placing sand in the volume defined by the bottom half of the pattern and surrounding flask. The drag is turned over and the board is removed. The top half of the sand mold called the cope is then formed by packing sand over the drag. Next, the two halves are separated and the pattern is removed. The mold is completed by creating gates and risers, which is typically accomplished by manually cutting into the mold. The mold is then ready for pouring molten metal.

Rubber Plaster Casting

Similar to sand casting, rubber plaster casting is used to manufacture highly complex aluminum components that have a better surface finish than sand cast components. This process is often used to simulate die cast parts. LOM parts are used in this technique as patterns around which a rubber sheet is pulled. The plaster is packed into a rubber sheet which is then removed. After the plaster is set and dried, metal is poured into the plaster cavity, and later removed to expose the metal part.

Silicone Rubber Molding

Silicone rubber molding is a quick process used to create duplicate plastic components using an LOM master. Room temperature vulcanizing (RTV) silicone is poured around an LOM master and after setting, the mold is cut in half. The LOM master is removed and plastic urethane or epoxy is poured into the mold.

Spray Metal Tooling

With spray metal tooling, a metal of relatively low melting point is used to coat the surface of an LOM master. The resultant tooling is used for short run prototype injection molding. Most thermoplastic materials can be injected into this prototype tooling.

SUNG S. PAK

16.4.3 Laser Cutting-Based Rapid Prototyping Options for Metal and Ceramic Components

Introduction

Many rapid prototyping (RP) systems are beginning to offer more in the way of build materials, beyond the traditional plastic material offerings. Other engineered material options such as advanced ceramics and metals are being offered. High-density metal and ceramic prototypes have been produced using the laminated object manufacturing (LOM) rapid prototyping process. Research groups investigating laser-based RP processes for ceramics include University of Dayton and Case Western Reserve University. And, as you might expect, at the company the author is with.

Rapid prototyping processes have several features in common. They all begin with a computer-generated model of the part. The computer model is electronically sectioned into layers of predetermined thickness. The individual layers collectively define the shape of the final part. Information about each layer is transmitted to the rapid prototyping machine where the part is built layer by layer. In a true RP approach, no tooling is required to produce the part.

Modified LOM Process

The LOM system normally uses thin sheets of paper to build wood-like components. The basic laminated object manufacturing rapid prototyping technique must be modified to build prototypes from metal and ceramic materials. For example, single sheets of flexible metal or ceramic tape is used in place of the paper. The tape can be fed into the LOM by hand, semi-automatically or by a totally automated system that works in conjunction with the LOM machine.

Only a few organizations have successfully modified and adapted the LOM machine to ceramics and metals. One commercial LOM system for ceramics and metals is currently on the market; a limited variety of tape compositions are available.

To adapt ceramic and metal materials to the LOM system, flexible, tape-cast metal and ceramic sheets are produced that are suitable for the LOM process. A limited variety of tape compositions are available. Single tape-cast sheets are fed into the LOM machine one at a time using a single-sheet feeder. The system picks up a single sheet of tape using a vacuum chuck. The tape is wrapped around the roller and secured by a second vacuum chuck. The tape is coated with a lamination aid. The coated, tape-wrapped roller moves into the LOM machine, where the loader laminates the tape to the stack of previously cut and laminated tapes. The loader retreats back to its home position to wait for the LOM to complete the cutting operation.

The LOM's CO_2 laser, controlled by the machine's software, cuts the part cross section out of the top layer of tape. Figure 1 of Section 16.4.1 presents a schematic of the LOM machine. A new layer of tape is laminated to the previously cut layer. The computer-directed laser then cuts the next layer and the process is repeated until the part is finished. The excess material around the part area supports the part as it is built. The laser cuts tiles into the support material to facilitate the removal of the part at the end of the build cycle.

After the part has been built, the support material is removed. Ceramic and metal parts built by these processes have similar appearances and strengths to green parts formed using ceramic or metal injection molding techniques. In these processes, the built parts undergo heat treatments in conventional furnaces to remove the binder and sinter the parts to high density. Typical green and sintered properties for prototypes created using these processes are presented in Table 1.

Table 1. Green and Sintered Densities of Ceramic and Metal Prototypes[a]

	Green density (g/cm^3)	Sintered density (g/cm^3)	(%TD[b])
Ceramics			
Alumina	2.50	3.80	95.2
Zirconia	3.05	5.67	96.2
Ce-TZP	2.77	5.92	97.8
Silicon nitride	1.92	3.16	96.2
Metals			
Stainless steel	3.45	7.63	95.0
Titanium-6Al-4V	2.07	4.14	93.5

[a]Courtesy Lone Peak Engineering, Inc.; [b]Theoretical density

Engineered ceramic materials used to build parts in the system include: alumina, zirconia, silicon carbide, aluminum nitride, silicon nitride, and various titanates. Metals successfully used include 316L stainless steel and titanium-6 aluminum-4 vanadium alloy.

The LOM machine by itself can build very large parts, up to 81 x 56 x 51 cm high. However, the size of the metal and ceramic parts that can be produced practically by the LOM process is

Chapter 16: Rapid Prototyping

smaller and mainly limited by the part geometry such that each geometry must be evaluated on a case-by-case basis. On the small end, parts less than 1 mm in size have been built using the LOM process.

The primary use of rapidly prototyped metal and ceramic components is as functional prototypes wherever ceramics and metals are used such as in medical, wear/erosion resistant, high-temperature, automotive, and aerospace applications. Some customers use these RP processes to produce production parts when the quantities are small. The RP process described above can be used to produce metal tools for injection molding.

References
H. Marcus and D. Bourell, "Solid Freeform Fabrication," in *Advanced Materials and Process,* 28–32 (September 1993).
C. W. Griffin, J. Daufenbach, and S. McMillin, "Desktop Manufacturing: LOM Versus Pressing," *Bulletin of the American Ceramic Society* **73** (8), 109–13 (August 1994).
C. W. Griffin, J. Daufenbach, and S. McMillin, "Solid Freeform Fabrication of Functional Ceramic Components using Laminated Object Manufacturing Techniques," *Proceeding of the Solid Freeform Fabrication Symposium,* 17–24, Austin, Texas, University of Texas Press, Austin, TX (1994).

CURTIS W. GRIFFIN
ALAIR GRIFFIN

16.5. CAM-LEM Processing of Ceramic and Metal Parts

16.5.0 Introduction
Computer-aided manufacture of laminated engineering materials, or CAM-LEM, is a cut-then-stack implementation of laminated object manufacturing.

The goal of the process, common to all of RP, is to produce a faithful physical realization of a 3D-CAD design. In CAM-LEM, this is accomplished by computationally slicing the part to define a set of contours, using laser cutting to sequentially prepare a set of psuedo-two-dimentional outlines that are assembled by stacking, laminating or fusing together to form the part, and then postprocessing to achieve the desired final state and concomitant properties. These steps are illustrated in Figure 1.

The cut-then-stack motif is an important distinction, and it may be exploited in at least three distinct ways. First, because the preprocessing of the sheet stack is separated from the shaping operation, great flexibility of composition is possible. A wide variety of materials have been successfully employed, including model materials such as polystyrene foam, paper, cardboard, polyester, and plexiglass, but the central focus of CAM-LEM is the production of engineering prototypes and parts from ceramics or powder metallurgy using green tape as sheet stock. In this context, the term *green* indicates that the material has not yet been fired, or densified, by sintering.

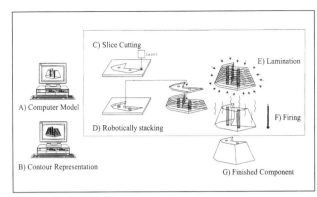

Figure 1. Schematic outline of the steps involved in the CAM-LEM process. The boxed steps are the essence of the process; in addition there can be important preprocessing steps carried out on the CAD data.

Second, cut-then-stack also allows each layer to be assembled in a manner similar to a jigsaw puzzle, i.e., many individual parts of different composition can be placed in a given layer by repeatedly feeding, cutting, and stacking. This allows the composition within a given layer to be varied as a function of position. One obvious use of this is the production of composite materials. Another very useful application is the fabrication of parts with complex internal geometry by placing a "fugitive" material in the space ultimately to be a void, during assembly, such an application is illustrated in Figure 2.

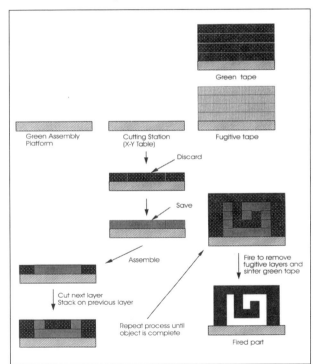

Figure 2. Schematic illustration of the use of CAM-LEM with a multimaterial feed stream to produce a composite assembly from which one phase can be selectively removed, using leaching or burnout, etc., to yield complex internal features.

Third, individual handling of each sheet prior to fusion to the partially completed object allows the laser beam to be readily inclined relative to the sheet permitting tangent cutting, which permits the more faithful approximation of curvature in the stacking direction (see Fig. 3).

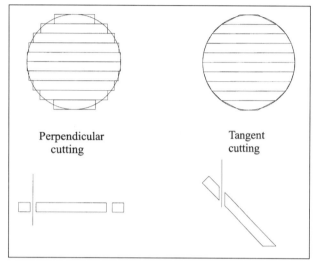

Figure 3. Illustration of the substantial improvement in surface finish possible when curved surface elements are approximated by tangents rather than normals.

Successful implementation of the CAM-LEM process to produce parts that are faithful to the original CAD representation requires all process steps to be executed well. Of particular importance is the precision and accuracy of laser cutting, i.e., the degree of taper, kerf width, and roughness of the cut. Each affects the ability to achieve a cut outline that is a precise replica of that which is desired, and the relative effects are additive. Systematic experiments have demonstrated that these features are sensitive to both laser cutting parameters and the material properties of the feedstock itself.

Before discussing machine variables, it would be useful to review the mechanism of low-power cutting of the materials most commonly used for CAM-LEM.

In the context of CAM-LEM and LOM, in general, the goal of laser cutting is to produce an outline of arbitrary geometry, both in terms of the nominal outline and the angle of inclination for the laser. Almost by definition, this requires a variable cutting velocity. To achieve maximum precision and simplicity of machine design, the combination of stationary optics and a moving table is preferred. To minimize deviations from the intended trajectory due to inertial effects, it is desirable, for example, to reduce the velocity to move around tight corners. Thus, how cutting characteristics vary as a function of cutting velocity is an important question.

16.5.1 Material Properties

The microstructure of the green tape differs depending on the process used in its fabrication. There are three classes of phases that are important to consider: the inorganic powders (which are densified during firing); the binders (which aid in flow during tape manufacture and provide green strength, but are removed during the initial stages of firing); and porosity (which provides compressibility in the green state, and vents the system during binder removal).

Two types of feedstock that present very different characteristics are tape-cast green sheets of ceramic and compression molded sheets of powder metallurgy steel. Typical properties of three tapes are given in Table 1 (next page).

The porous and amorphous polymer in the tape cast systems yield flexible material that has a broad softening range (Tg of roughly 40°C). In contrast, the crystalline binder of the compression molded sheet stock gives a stiff material with a sharply defined melting range (approximately 110°C). It was expected that the crystalline binder would give better laser cutting, but the reverse proved to be true. The markedly higher thermal conductivity of the pore-free and crystalline binder leads to appreciable lateral heat conduction during low-speed low-power cutting.

The poor cutting behavior can be seen in the data set presented in Figure 4, which shows the kerf width measured on the top and bottom surfaces of a piece of laser cut 316L sheet.

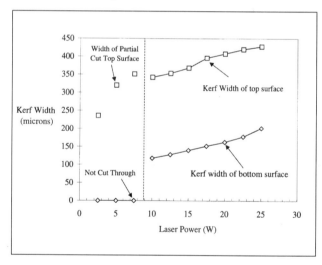

Figure 4. Plot of the kerf width measured on the top and bottom surfaces of a compression-molded sheet of green stainless steel P/M with polyacetal-based binder. For laser power settings lower than that indicated by the dotted vertical line, through cuts are not produced. Kerf widths are large compared to the laser beam diameter and strongly tapered ($\approx 20°$).

The kerf width is substantially wider than the laser diameter (200 μm), indicating conduction of heat took place, and the big difference between the values for the top and bottom indicates that there is significant taper (taking into account the thickness of the tape, a taper of 20° is calculated). The tape cast material typically cuts with a much narrower kerf with significantly less taper.

Table 1. Physical Characteristics of Green Sheet Feedstock for CAM-LEM Processing

Material	Process	Solids loading (vol. %)	Binder content (vol. %)	Binder type	Porosity (vol. %)
Al_2O_3[a]	Tape cast	55	20	Amorphous	20
Si_3N_4[a]	Tape cast	55	20	Amorphous	18
316L ss[b]	Compression molded	64	36	Crystalline	none

[a]Plasticized poly(vinyl)butyral (Butvar 76, Monsanto Chemical, St. Louis, MO)
[b]316L stainless steel feedstock based on a polyacetal resin and manufactured by BASF (Wyandotte, MI).

A particular advantage of the tape cast material is that there is an additional degree of control; i.e., the amount of porosity can be varied by changing the slurry formulation used during casting.

For example, decreasing the binder concentration from 37 to 21 vol. % gives smoother and straighter walled cuts as seen in the photomicrographs shown in Figure 5.

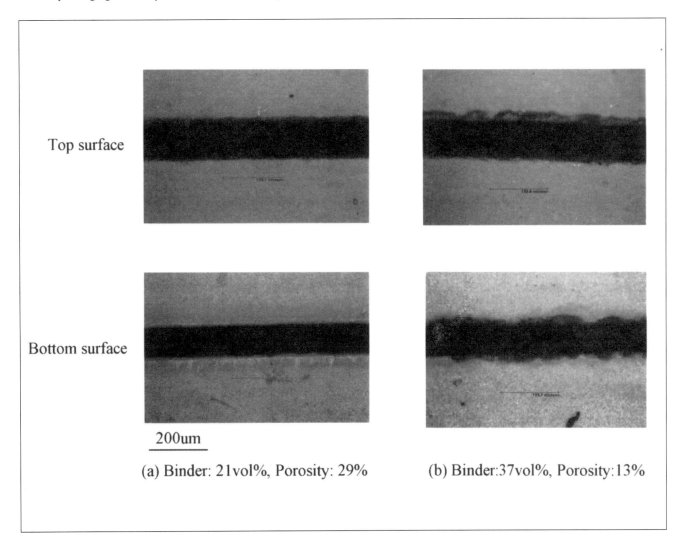

(a) Binder: 21vol%, Porosity: 29%   (b) Binder: 37vol%, Porosity: 13%

Figure 5. Scanning electron photomicrographs of the top and bottom surfaces of a laser-cut tape-cast silicon nitride tape with a poly(vinyl) butyral-based binder for two different tape formulations that contain different amounts of binder.

Choice of binder type and amount are very important variables in controlling laser cutting of green tape.

16.5.2 Machine Variables

For a given material, machine variables can have important consequences. There are four that are key: laser power; cutting velocity; mass flow rate through the cutting nozzle; and venting around the kerf. These will be discussed in reverse order.

A schematic of laser cutting (a) and laser drilling (b) is shown in Figure 6.

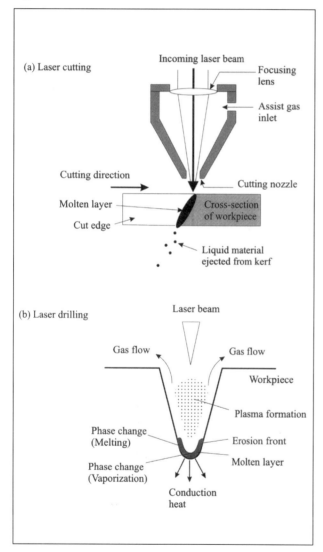

Figure 6. Schematic of the mechanisms for material removal during laser cutting and laser drilling. Key points include the fact that removal involves two steps, melting and ejection by gas jet, and that for cutting the gas jet and laser are both directed down, but for drilling the gas jet must reverse direction and removal is accomplished by upward motion.

In both cases, material removal is affected by producing a molten layer that is induced to flow by the action of the gas jet. In the case of cutting, essentially all of the material flows out of the bottom of the kerf and the gas jet suffers only a mild angular deflection. In contrast, for drilling (or scribing) the tape remains intact and the flow field of the gas jet is required to reverse direction so that the material is carried out of the top of the tape. In this latter case, significantly higher shear forces can be produced that increase the extent of material removal. This is clearly evident in the data set graphically represented by Figure 7.

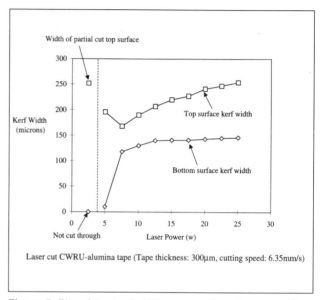

Figure 7. Plot of the kerf width measured on the top and bottom surfaces of a tape-cast aluminum oxide sheet with a poly(vinyl) butyral binder. Top surface kerf width for scribing is substantially wider than the minimum observed for power settings just able to produce complete smooth through-cuts.

The vertical dotted line represents the separation of power levels that produce through-cuts from lower values that only scribe the tape for the given velocity. The upper curve gives the kerf width on the top side of the tape measured by optical microscopy. It is immediately evident that piercing the tape so that there is through venting gives much narrower kerfs. (The narrowness of the kerf can determine the degree to which it is possible to follow a complicated outline that has concave elements.) This was observed in all feedstocks although the degree of the effect can vary. Cutting surfaces that permit ready flow of gasses are necessary. For CAM-LEM, an aluminum honeycomb, commercially available as a low-mass stiffener, is used. A photograph of the cutting surface, which is greater than 90% open, is shown in Figure 8 (next page).

Because this effect is always observed at the start of any cutting operation, it is necessary to account for it when designing the cutting trajectory to produce a given feature. Often the best solution is to employ the standard technique of starting and stopping cutting off the outline, as illustrated in Figure 9 (next page).

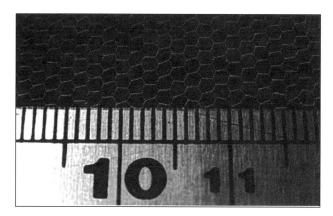

Figure 8. Photograph of the aluminum honeycomb used as a cutting table, with a centimeter scale. The small cell size allows small parts to be well supported. The narrow wall size means that the overwhelming fraction of the surface area is available for gas flow to carry debris away from the kerf.

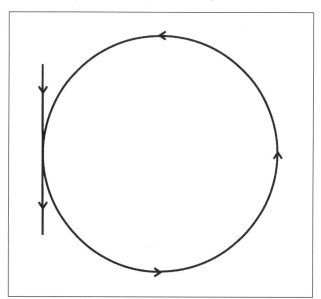

Figure 9. Typical "on-ramp/off-ramp" trajectory used so that the wide kerf width observed during initial drilling does not occur on the perimeter of the desired cut-part.

Mass flow rate and stand-off distance of the cutting nozzle is empirically optimized to produce the best cuts. Higher pressures are generally preferred. The high flow rate produced by the high pressure ensures that the molten material is completely ejected from the kerf; some recondensation of molten material is observed at lower values, which can cause roughness or, in extreme cases, welding.

The ratio of laser power to cutting velocity gives the amount of energy deposited per unit line length. If all of the energy deposited goes into material removal then the minimum energy necessary to cut through a tape would be independent of cutting velocity, and directly scaling the instantaneous laser power to the cutting velocity would be sufficient to give constant cutting characteristics. However, this is not the case. Heat conduction always carries some of the energy away from the kerf and into the body of the tape. At the lower speeds necessary for CAM-LEM, heat conduction can be appreciable. This has two consequences, the first is that the material immediately adjacent to the kerf must not be seriously degraded by heat conduction. A general rule of thumb is that the composition of the polymer must be such that there are no particularly volatile species so that boiling within the tape, which causes distortion, does not occur. Second, it means that the scaling between laser power and cutting velocity is not necessarily linear.

Shown in Figures 10a and 10b are three-dimensional plots of kerf width (top and bottom, respectively, on a same samples) for a variety of power–velocity combinations.

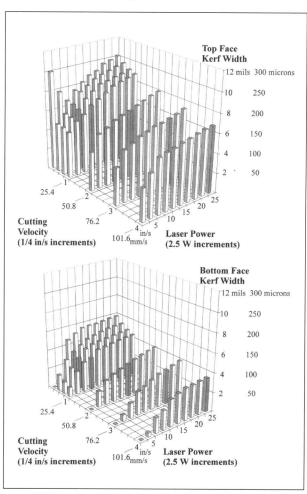

Figure 10. Psuedo-three-dimensional plot of the measured kerf width on the top and bottom surfaces of tape-cast aluminun oxide sheet. Variations occur both for constant velocity and variable power as well as constant power and variable velocity. Nevertheless, it can be seen that it is possible to keep very nearly constant properties if the power is systematically varied with velocity as indicated by the set of shaded columns.

Several trends are visible. The region that shows the strongest sensitivity is that of low-power and low-velocity. For the top side of the tape, the value of power that gives a minimum in kerf width is not at either the low or high power extreme. Experience has shown that a minimum kerf width is obtained when the power level is just slightly above the smallest value necessary to cut through the tape. At higher values of power, the variations are modest. This is attributed to the fact that the once a certain speed is reached then heat conduction becomes so modest that its continued variation becomes increasingly unimportant.

The highlighted columns in each graph show that it is possible to scale the laser power to keep the kerf of constant geometry, i.e., a constant 170 μm for the top and 90 μm for the bottom which corresponds to a $\cong 4°$ taper for a 600-μm-thick tape.

JAMES D. CAWLEY

16.6 Coating of Rapid Tools by Pulsed Laser Deposition

Pulsed laser deposition (PLD) is a thin-film deposition technique that has been pursued for more than twenty years. This section is concerned with the specific application of PLD to the coating of rapid tooling. Other aspects of the technique are discussed in Section 27.1.4.

The basic equipment required for a PLD is a high-peak power-pulsed laser source, a high-vacuum chamber to perform the deposition, target and substrate manipulation fixturing, and appropriate diagnostics to monitor vacuum parameters, laser parameters, and the deposition process. The laser is usually an Nd:YAG laser or an excimer laser. The Nd:YAG laser is operated at the fundamental wavelength of 1064 nm or one of the harmonics (532, 355, or 266 nm). The excimer is typically operated at either 248 (KrF) or 193 nm (ArF).

PLD is performed in vacuum and uses a high-peak-power laser to ablate a target composed of the material that is desired for the coating. After traveling a short distance, the ablated material impinges on the substrate with sufficient kinetic energy to embed into the surface. This results in growing a thin film (0.5 to 1.0 micrometer) on the surface of the substrate that has superior adhesion properties over other coating techniques. In addition to the better adhesion, the coatings are nearly fully dense and have optimized crystal structure and morphology. Perhaps the most important attribute of the PLD process is that the coating retains the stoichiometry of the target during the film growth process in most cases. Coatings grown in this manner are thin enough to cause virtually no dimensional change to the surface making them ideal for mold coating applications.

The most convenient way to evacuate the PLD chamber is with a turbomolecular pumping station. A pressure of less than 10^{-5} torr must be reached for effective deposition. However, in some cases, it may be desirable to introduce a reactive gas into the chamber during the deposition process to influence the reaction dynamics and stoichiometry of the thin film. This can develop experimental conditions that result in a trade-off between the desired film chemistry and the film adhesion and deposition rate because of the increased number of collisions of the material ejected from the plume encounters prior to impacting the substrate.

The laser pulse is focused onto the target with optics placed either external or internal to the PLD chamber. To provide the most uniform coating, some type of scanning technique is employed to randomly expose the target surface to the laser pulses. One such method employs two galvanometer-driven scanning mirrors that scan the focused beam across the face of the target in two orthogonal directions while the target is rotated. The frequency, amplitude, and zero position can be adjusted for each mirror to cover as much of the target surface as possible. The scanning mirrors are placed external to the chamber, and a long focal length lens is used to focus the beam at the target surface. The entrance aperture of the chamber limits the scan angle in this arrangement, but targets on the order of 3 in. in diameter can readily be scanned. Another method that can be employed if the PLD chamber is sufficiently large is to simultaneously rotate and translate the target through the focused laser beam. The position of the focal spot remains at a fixed point in space in this method, which has the advantage that the focal spot size remains a constant diameter. The focusing lens can be placed inside the chamber in this configuration, and permits the use of shorter focal length lenses for increased power density. The surface of a target 3 in. in diameter or larger can be randomly scanned under these conditions.

Manipulating the substrate in the plume ejected from the target also ensures the uniformity of the coating. PLD is a line-of-sight technique, and to adequately coat all surfaces of a three-dimensional part such as the core and cavity of a mold, the substrate must be oriented properly in the plume. This can be accomplished by rotating the substrate, if the contours are simple, or using a multi-axis robotic arm to manipulate the substrate in the plume, if the geometry is more complex.

Often PLD coatings require the substrate be heated to promote appropriate chemistry and crystal growth for the film. Elevated substrate temperatures are typically achieved either by radiant heating or by resistive heating. Radiant heating also elevates the temperature of the surroundings as well as the substrate. Resistive heating is typically applied only to small samples. However, rapid tools can readily be coated at room temperature. Numerous types of thin films have been grown by PLD, and many can be applied to the specific application of tooling. For example, materials such as Ni-200, silicon carbide, and stainless steel can readily be deposited.

One of the challenges facing PLD is scaling the process to coat large areas such as those encountered in the rapid tooling industry. In order to coat such tools, a large PLD chamber and appropriate pumping station is required, as well as appropriate fixturing within the chamber to appropriately position the tool pieces. PLD has the restrictions of a line-of-sight technique, but these restrictions can be circumvented with appropriate sample and/or target manipulation within the large chamber.

There are advantages and disadvantages to any technology, and PLD is no exception. The major advantages of PLD are summarized below, and relate primarily to improved adhesion and control of the film chemistry.

Advantages of pulsed laser deposition:

- Excellent adhesion
- Stoichiometry of the target material is maintained in most cases
- Stoichiometry can also be modified through the use of an appropriate atmosphere
- Film is nearly fully dense
- Reaction chemistry during the deposition process can be controlled
- Process can be monitored and controlled

The disadvantages of PLD are summarized below and are primarily related to cost and complexity.

Disadvantages of pulsed laser deposition:

- Not a turnkey operation
- Large capital investment
- Costly support hardware
- Often requires frequent access to analytical techniques such as SEM and auger spectroscopy
- High level of training and experience required in lasers, vacuum, and chemistry or physics

The thinness of a film grown by PLD can be both an advantage and a disadvantage. In the case of mold applications, a film that is 1 µm thick has no affect on dimensional tolerances of the mold. However, if the coating wears appreciably, a 1-µm film can be abraded away quickly. One problem that all coating techniques face is failure of the substrate. If this happens, the coating will simply move with the substrate material.

PLD represents an exciting and practical way to coat rapid tools of appropriate size for improved wear resistance. The advantages of the technique in terms of improved adhesion and control of coating chemistry make this a technology to be considered for other types of coating applications as well.

Reference
D. B. Chrisey and G. K. Hubler (Eds.), *Pulsed Laser Deposition of Thin Films,* John Wiley & Sons, NY (1994).

LARRY R. DOSSER

16.7 Adaptation of RP Technology to the Manufacture of Die Casting Tools

Die Casting Tooling (Dies)

Pressure die casting (or simply, die casting) is a century old process of injecting molten metal under high pressure into reusable metal dies. The injected metal, either aluminum, zinc, magnesium, or sometimes copper based alloys, is held under pressure until it solidifies into a net shape metal part. No other metal casting processes allow for a greater variety of shapes, intricacy of design, or closer dimensional tolerance.

Typical production of die casting tooling or dies is facilitated by machining part features into blocks of H13 steel, a process with a turn around time that ranges from weeks to months. It follows that for large production runs, where multiple sets of dies are required, the time associated with tool acquisition can escalate rapidly. On the other hand, if one were able to adapt RP's additive building process and vast material selection (a selection that includes both metallics and ceramics), dies could be produced more quickly as well as have superior material properties.

Although die casting and injection molding are very similar processes, both inject liquid materials into a die under pressure, the required die material characteristics are different. The construction of dies is almost identical to that of molds for injection molding. However, molten die casting alloys are much less viscous than the polymer melt in injection molding and have a greater tendency to flow between the contacting surfaces of the die. This phenomenon, referred to as flashing, tends to jam molding machines. The combination of flashing and high injection temperatures (> 300°C for polycarbonates versus > 950°C for copper alloys), requires that die casting dies be more robust. Hence, pressure die casting tooling using RP techniques requires the development of appropriate material systems.

Two of the RP processes being developed for making die casting inserts are Selective Laser Sintering (SLS is covered in Section 16.3)(1) and Laser Engineered Net Shaping (LENS is covered in Subsection 16.3.5); powder materials can be processed either directly or indirectly. Since almost any material can be made into a powdered form, the selection of materials is nearly unlimited.

Selective Laser Sintering

SLS is highly flexible. It can use any powdered material with a viscosity that lowers as heat is applied; for a material whose viscosity does not lower when heat is applied, such as a ceramic, this can be overcome by coating it with a polymer that does.

These polymer coatings act as adhesive agents for the sintering of both ceramics and metal materials and are often referred to as "binders". The combination of being an additive building process and being able to use powder materials and various binders to coat the particles gives RP the potential of producing virtually any shape.

SLS employs a low-energy laser beam to selectively bind particles to form a "green" shape. Once formed, the part is extracted from the power bed and the excess or nonfused powder is removed.

The part at this stage is generally termed a green part and is very fragile. Green parts require post processing to remove the polymer binder and to impart greater strength. Since ceramic green parts produced by SLS currently exhibit low relative densities, on the order of 40 to 50%, the shrinkage required to achieve full density would be large. Hence, binder burnout and slight sintering is used to impart some strength without significantly changing the dimensions thereby converting the green part into a "brown" part.

Infiltrating the brown structure with a lower melting point metal produces parts with good strength and little dimensional change. The final microstructure of the "fully dense" part will be that of a bi-material or more specifically, a particulate composite (see Fig. 1). The fully dense part is ready for polishing or post build machining and then placement directly into the base for die-casting.

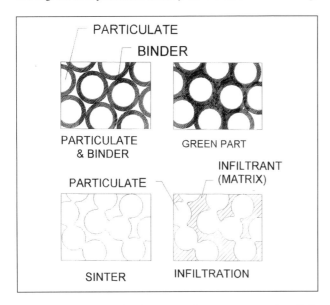

Figure 1. Powder bed prior to sintering; green part after SLS; porous structure after debind/sinter; dense part after infiltration (shown clockwise from top left) (1).

Composite tooling offers the advantages of both RP techniques and composite materials, along with the ability to create robust tools in 5 to 10 working days. The resulting molds, which range in size up to 150 x 250 mm, can then be used to create die-cast parts. The development of new material systems can be expected to lead to improved production numbers.

LENS' great advantage is in creating a fully dense component from a powder material with no further heat-treating, the latter attribute being unusual in RP (see Fig. 2). Furthermore, varying compositions of powder can be used (i.e., metal particles mixed with ceramic particles) which allows cermets, multi-metal, and gradient materials to be produced. This process allows for producing parts that meet the specific material and property requirements of die cast tooling (see Fig. 3).

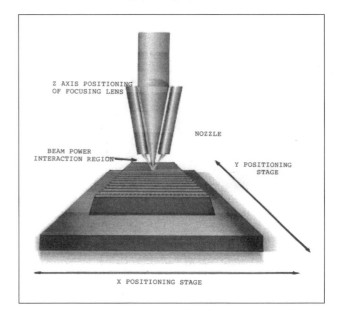

(a)

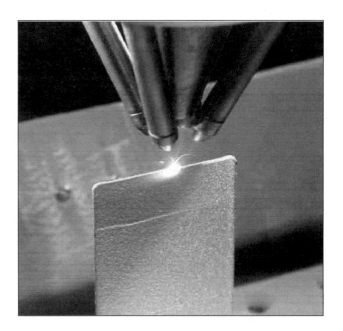

(b)

Figure 2. Schematic of LENS process (a) and actual build (b) (2).

ISBN 0-912035-15-3

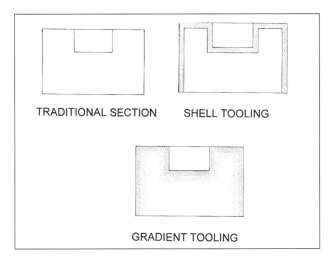

Figure 3. LENS capability to create shell and gradient structures.

With die casting, an increase in tool complexity means that the time and cost to manufacture a traditional H13 tool will increase greatly. With rapidly manufactured tools, the time and cost will increase marginally (see Fig. 4) with the caveat that the process is used only when the part's dimensional accuracy is directly achievable and that there is no additional time or costs associated with finish machining operations. Rapidly manufactured tools are typically unaffected by complexity; setup, build rate and most post processing operations are independent of the intricacy of the geometry.

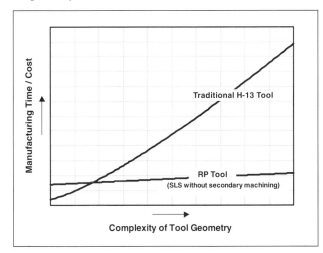

Figure 4. General trend in manufacturing time/cost based on tool complexity, neglecting secondary machining (3).

The major shortcoming of the process is the limited accuracy of the final part. Tolerances can be held only to a range of .005 to .010 in. across the part-building envelope. The typical tolerance associated with machining die cast tooling inserts is on the order of ± 0.002 in. Hence, some advances in RP are required in order to produce shapes with surface finish and tolerances comparable to machined parts.

Examples of RP Die Casting Inserts

The so-called RapidSteel 1.0 Metal™ material system is the first generation of material systems designed for metal mold inserts. To determine its tool life, approximately 1,000 magnesium parts were pressure die cast into RapidSteel 1.0 Metal inserts created using SLS (4). This was followed by producing pre-production tooling for pressure die casting of aluminum parts. Slight heat cracks were discovered on the surface of the die after the first 40 parts. After 300 parts the tool was deemed unusable because of extensive wear from the heat cracks. One can say that the RapidSteel 1.0 Metal material system is viable for short run or pre-production tooling when die casting magnesium and aluminum alloys.

With the second generation RapidSteel 2.0 Metal a benchmark insert was constructed (5, 6); compared to RapidSteel 1.0, the use of SS316 in RapidSteel 2.0 increases the mold wear resistance, while the decrease in average particle size (55 to 34 μm) allows for a smaller layer thickness with a reduction in stair stepping and a better surface finish (7). Additionally, modifications to the material and binder system have allowed for decreased processing time and increased dimensional accuracy.

Once the RapidSteel 2.0 insert was manufactured, it was mounted in a hot chamber zinc pressure die casting machine. The tool was used to produce 1,000 parts with no visible or measurable wear of the cavity (see Fig. 5). However, RapidSteel 2.0 is a relatively soft material and is not nearly as durable as other cermet or composite material systems yet to be investigated. The fact that RapidSteel 2.0, in spite of its lack of optimum material properties, has worked in initial zinc die casting studies and that RapidSteel 1.0 has been shown to have usefulness even when die casting magnesium and aluminum indicates that material systems can be developed for die casting tooling for long production runs.

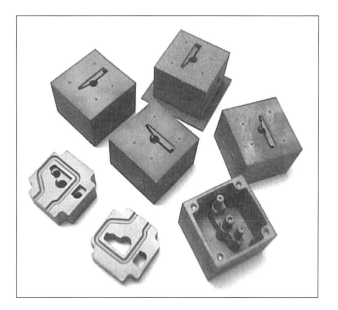

(a)

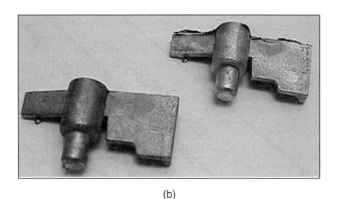

(b)

Figure 5. Die Cast tool inserts from various laser manufacturing methods (a) and Parts produced in an RP tool before vibratory cleaning (right) and after vibratory cleaning (left) (b) (5).

References

1. P. Hardro, *Manufacturing by Selective Laser Sintering,* Industrial & Manufacturing Engineering Department, University of Rhode Island, Kingston, RI, Material Fabrication and Properties, Report 3, December 1998.
2. Optomec home page, http://www.optomec.com, Optomec Corporation, Albuquerque, NM.
3. P. Hardro, *Comparison of Manufacturing Time, Cost and Accuracy of Rapidly Manufactured Tools to a Traditional H13 Tool,* Industrial & Manufacturing Engineering Department, University of Rhode Island, Kingston, RI, Die Cast Tooling, Report 5, October 1999.
4. DTM Corporation, *Case History: Prototype Tooling for Aluminum Die Casting made by the RapidTool Process*, DTM Corporation, Austin, TX, 1997.

Table 1. Comparison of Rapid Prototyping Systems

Methods: Lasers/Other Sources	Materials Processed
Stereolithography (SL): Laser Photolithography Lasers used: • 25–30 mW Helium-Cadmium Ultraviolet (325 nm) • 300–400 mW Argon-Ion Ultraviolet (351 nm) • 800 mW Tripled Solid State Nd:YVO$_4$ Ultraviolet (355 nm) Photomask* Source used: • Broadband UV Source	• Acrylate Photopolymer (early resins) • Acrylate-Epoxy Photopolymer, SL 5170, SL 5180 • Epoxy Photopolymer, SL 7540, SL 7520, SL 7510, SL 5210, SL 5220, SL 5410, SL 5530
Selective Laser Sintering (SLS): Laser Sintering, Powder Bed Lasers used: • 50 W CO$_2$ (10.6 µm) • 100 W CO$_2$ (10.6 µm)	• Polyamide, DuraForm PA & Glass-Filled Polyamide, DuraForm G • CastForm Polystyrene • Wax • Copper Polyamide • Elastomer, Somos 201 • Nylon

5. P. Hardro and B. Stucker, *Die Cast Tooling from Rapid Prototyping*, Proceedings of the Rapid Prototyping and Manufacturing '99 Conference, Society of Manufacturing Engineers, Dearborn, MI, April 20–22, 1999.
6. T. Woodiel, *Tri/Mark Corporation Die Casts more than 11,800 Zinc Parts with Tooling made from DTM's RapidSteel 2.0 Material*, http://www.rapid-discussion.com/Trimark.html, September 9, 1999.
7. D. Pham, S. Dimov, and F. Lacan, *Technological Aspects of the RapidTool Process*, Proceedings of the Time-Compression Technologies '98 Conference, Communication Technologies, Inc., Doylestown, PA, 343–50.

PETER J. HARDRO

16.8 Comparison of Rapid Prototyping Systems

Table 1 compares a number of the rapid prototyping systems discussed in this chapter, in terms of the lasers used, the materials processed, the applications, the process characteristics, and the limitations. The table also includes some nonlaser systems.

PETER J. HARDRO

Applications	Process Characteristics	Limitations
• Design Visualization, Verification, Iteration, and Optimization • Form & Fit • QuickCast • Investment Casting Patterns • Patterns for Sand Casting • Flow Analysis • Design Analysis • Mechanical Operation and Low Stress Function Testing • CAD Verification • Tool Development • Patterns for Soft Tooling and Bridge Tooling • Improved Design for Manufacturing & Assembly (DFMA) • Low & Medium Volume Production Parts • Patterns for Silicone RTV Rubber Tooling • Direct Tooling (DirectAIM) • Patterns for Epoxy Mold Tooling • Patterns for Electroforming and Metal Spray Tooling • Patterns for Composite Tooling • Optical Components • Photo-Optical Stress Analysis	• Maximum Processing Volume: 20" x 20" x 23.6" (3-D Systems) 20" x 14" x 20" (Cubital) • Relative Build Rate: Medium to Fast • Relative Accuracy: Good (Considerable detailed data available) • Relative Surface Finish: Excellent on up-facing surfaces; stair-stepping on sloped surfaces; moderately rough on down-facing surfaces • Easily repaired with photopolymer resin • Support structures are required on all down-facing surfaces • Post Processing: flood ultraviolet curing in a Post Curing Apparatus (PCA)	• Limited Material Selection • Limited Mechanical Property Range • Limited Elevated Temperature Resistance
• Design Visualization, Verification, Iteration, and Optimization • Form & Fit • Investment Casting Patterns • Patterns & Sand Cores for Sand Casting • Design Analysis • Mechanical Operation and Low & Medium	• Maximum Processing Volume: 15" x 13" x 16.7" (DTM) 27.5" x 15" x 15" (EOS) • Relative Build Rate: Medium • Relative Accuracy: Good (Limited data available) • Relative Surface Finish: Fair to good	• Features must be larger than 0.040" to allow for part breakout • Intrinsic roughness due to particle size

Methods: Lasers/Other Sources	Materials Processed

• 2 x 50 W CO_2 (10.6 µm)
• 250 W CO_2 (10.6 µm)
	• Zircon, SandForm Zr, and Silica, SandForm Si, Sands Coated with Phenolic Binder
	• Polymer-Coated Metals & Ceramics
	  – Metal Matrix Composites, RapidSteel 2.0
	  – Epoxy Matrix Composites

Laser Engineered Net Shaping (LENS): Laser Fusion, Powder Injection Lasers Used: • 600 W Nd:YAG (1.064 µm) • 1100 W Nd:YAG (1.064 µm) • 2400 W CO_2 (10.6 µm)	• 304, 316, & 420 Stainless Steel • Iron-Nickel Alloys • H13, P20, S7, D2, & MM10 Tool Steels • Inconel • Titanium Alloys (Ti-6Al-4V) • Tungsten • Haynes 230 • Nickel Aluminide • Copper (OFHC pure copper) • CuNi alloys • CuSn alloys (bronze) • TiB_2 (titanium di-boride)
Layered Object Manufacturing (LOM): Lamination, Laser Cut Lasers used: • 25 W CO_2 (10.6 µm) • 50 W CO_2 (10.6 µm)	• Paper • Alumina • Silicon Nitride • Zirconia • 316L Stainless Steel
Fusion Deposition Modeling (FDM): Extrusion A nonlaser process	• ABS, P400 • ABSi, P500 • Elastomer, E20 • Investment Casting Wax, ICW 06 • Polyester Compound, P1500

Chapter 16: Rapid Prototyping

Applications	Process Characteristics	Limitations
Stress Function Testing • CAD Verification • Tool Development • Patterns for Soft Tooling and Bridge Tooling • Improved Design for Manufacturing & Assembly (DFMA) • Low & Medium Volume Production Parts • Patterns for Silicone RTV Rubber Tooling • Direct Tooling (RapidSteel) • Patterns for Epoxy Mold Tooling • Patterns for Electroforming and Metal Spray Tooling • Composite Tooling • Prototype Gaskets, Seals, etc.	on up-facing surfaces; stair-stepping on sloped surfaces; fair to good on down-facing surfaces • No support structures required • Some materials must be processed in a relatively inert atmosphere (Nitrogen) • Post Processing: breakout part from loose powder • Furnace debinding and infiltration required for composites (RapidSteel) • Wax infiltration required for CastForm polystyrene	
• Functional Metal Parts • Form, Fit, & Function • Excellent Mechanical Properties (due to rapid cooling rate of the melt pool) • Able to generate functionally gradient materials (by varying the powder type with position) • Overhaul and Repair (especially turbine components and tools) • Joining of metals with dissimilar coefficients of expansion through gradient transition • Production Tooling • Design Analysis • Mechanical Operation and High Stress Function Testing • Improved Design for Manufacturing & Assembly (DFMA) • Low Volume Production Parts of Highly Engineered Parts • Composite Tooling	• Maximum Processing Volume: 18" x 18" x 42" (OPTOMEC) 24" x 24" x 24" (POM) • Relative Build Rate: Slow • Relative Accuracy: Moderate • Relative Surface Finish: Poor • Support structures are required on all down-facing surfaces • Must build on a substrate • Post Processing: Removal of substrate • Must be processed in an inert atmosphere (Argon)	• Minimum feature size, which is material dependent, generally must be larger than 0.040" • Intrinsic roughness due to particle size and build process • Currently cannot build a part with a geometry having an overhang greater than a 45° angle (from the vertical) • Part geometry affects build and material properties
• Design Visualization, Verification, Iteration and Optimization • Form & Fit • Patterns for Sand Casting • Limited Use for Investment Casting • Design Analysis • Mechanical Operation and Low Stress Function Testing • CAD Verification • Patterns for Soft Tooling and Bridge Tooling • Improved Design for Manufacturing & Assembly (DFMA) • Patterns for Silicone RTV Rubber Tooling • Patterns for Epoxy Mold Tooling • Patterns for Electroforming and Metal Spray Tooling • Patterns for Composite Tooling	• Maximum Processing Volume: 32" x 22" x 20" (Helisys) • Relative Build Rate: Fast • Relative Accuracy: Moderate • Relative Surface Finish: Moderate • Support Structures Not Required • Post Processing: Removal of extraneous material	• Limited Material Selection • Limited Mechanical Property Range • Minimum feature size generally must be larger than 0.040" (due to breakout limitations)
• Design Visualization, Verification, Iteration, and Optimization • Form & Fit • Investment Casting Patterns • Patterns for Sand Casting • Design Analysis • Mechanical Operation and Low Stress Function Testing • CAD Verification	• Maximum Processing Volume: 23.6" x 19.7" x 23.6" • Relative Build Rate: Slow to Medium • Relative Accuracy: High • Relative Surface Finish: Good on all surfaces • Support structures are required on all down-facing surfaces	• Limited Material Selection • Limited Mechanical Property Range • Limited Elevated Temperature Resistance

ISBN 0-912035-15-3

Methods: Lasers/Other Sources	Materials Processed
Multi-Jet Modeling (MJM): Liquid Jetting onto Substrate A nonlaser process	• Thermoplastic • Wax • Photopolymer
Three-Dimensional Printing (3DP): Liquid Jetting onto Powder Bed A nonlaser process	• ABS Plastic • Starch/Cellulose, ZP11, infiltrated with Elastomer, Urethane, ZR10 Resin, or Wax • Plaster, ZP100, can be infiltrated with Urethane, Sicomet 9000, or Wax • Stainless Steel/Copper Composite • Tool Steel/Copper Composite

This table offers some representative numbers based on systems from: Row 1 – 3D Systems, CA; 3D Systems GmbH (Germany); (Germany); Cubital America, Inc. (MI). Row 2 – DTM Corporation (TX); EOS GmbH (Germany). Row 3 – OPTOMEC MACRO Row 5 – Stratysis (MN). Row 6 – 3D Systems (CA); Sanders Prototype, Inc. (NH); Objet Geometries Ltd. (Israel). Row 7 – The citing of the above companies is not to be interpreted as an endorsement of their products.

ISBN 0-912035-15-3

Applications	Process Characteristics	Limitations
• Tool Development • Patterns for Soft Tooling and Bridge Tooling • Improved Design for Manufacturing & Assembly (DFMA) • Low Volume Production Parts • Patterns for Silicone RTV Rubber Tooling • Patterns for Epoxy Mold Tooling • Patterns for Electroforming and Metal Spray Tooling • Patterns for Composite Tooling • Prototype Gaskets, Seals, etc.	• Post Processing: WaterWorks or Break-Away support system allows easy support removal	
• Design Visualization, Verification, Iteration and Optimization • Form & Fit • Investment Casting Patterns • Patterns for Sand Casting • Design Analysis • CAD Verification • Tool Development • Patterns for Soft Tooling and Bridge Tooling • Improved Design for Manufacturing & Assembly (DFMA) • Patterns for Silicone RTV Rubber Tooling • Patterns for Epoxy Mold Tooling • Patterns for Composite Tooling	• Maximum Processing Volume: 10" x 7.5" x 8" (3D Systems) 12" x 6" x 9" (Sanders) 10.6" x 12.6" x 7.8" (Objet) • Relative Build Rate: Medium to Fast • Relative Accuracy: Medium to High • Relative Surface Finish: Fair to good on up-facing surfaces; stair-stepping on sloped surfaces; fair to good on down-facing surfaces • Support structures are required on all down-facing surfaces • Support material is easily removed with a solvent for sanders	• Limited Material Selection • Limited Mechanical Property Range • Limited Elevated Temperature Resistance
• Design Visualization, Verification, Iteration, and Optimization • Form & Fit • Investment Casting Patterns • Patterns for Sand Casting • Design Analysis • Mechanical Operation and Low Stress Function Testing • CAD Verification • Tool Development • Patterns for Soft Tooling and Bridge Tooling • Improved Design for Manufacturing & Assembly (DFMA) • Low & Medium Volume Production Parts • Patterns for Silicone RTV Rubber Tooling • Direct Tooling (ProMetal) • Patterns for Epoxy Mold Tooling • Patterns for Electroforming and Metal Spray Tooling • Patterns for Composite Tooling • Prototype Gaskets, Seals, etc.	• Maximum Processing Volume: 8" x 10" x 8" (Z Corp.) 12" x 12" x 10" (Extrude Hone Corp.) • Relative Build Rate: Fast • Relative Accuracy: Low to Medium • Relative Surface Finish: Fair to good on up-facing surfaces; stair-stepping on sloped surfaces; fair to good on down-facing surfaces • Support Structures Not Required • Post Processing: breakout part from loose powder • Furnace debinding and infiltration required for metal composites • Infiltration required for ZP100 and ZP11 composites	• Limited Material Selection

CMET (Japan); D-MEC (Japan); DENKEN (Japan); Fockele and Schwarze (Germany); Meiko (Japan); Teijin-Seiki (Japan); MicroTEC Group (NM); AeroMet Corporation (MN); Precision Optical Manufacturing (MI). Row 4 – Helisys, Inc. (CA); CAM-LEM, Inc. (OH). Z Corporation (MA); Extrude Hone Corporation (PA). Contact these or other equipment manufacturers for exact or updated figures.

Notes

Chapter 17

Trimming

17.0 Introduction

Resistors for use in electronic circuits are characterized as thick-film or thin-film resistors. Thick-film resistors are printed on a substrate from a liquid ink and then fired and dried. Thin-film resistors are fabricated by vacuum deposition of metals, like nickel-chromium.

In most cases, it is difficult to control the value of the resistance to within the tolerance required by the circuit. To improve the yield of the process, the resistors are fabricated with intentionally low values of resistance. Then material is removed from the conducting path to increase the resistance. This process is called trimming.

17.1 Basics of Laser Trimming

Laser trimming involves an understanding of several technologies in addition to those required initially to fabricate a hybrid circuit. The thick-film process of screening a wet paste onto a ceramic (96% alumina) substrate and then firing it in a furnace is very inexpensive, but very inexact. There is a variation in paste content, paste thickness, and *x* and *y* dimensions of the screened paste. There are also variations in firing temperatures.

Therefore, accuracies better than ±10% are difficult to achieve on passive components. Laser trimming is primarily concerned with the physics involved in material removal and the measurement means to monitor the material removal process. Circuit layout and geometry further define an assortment of cut patterns, which can be applied to meet objectives of circuit performance. Following is a review of the key aspects of laser trimming technology.

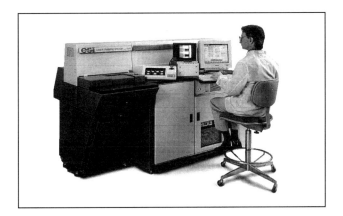

Figure 1. Typical laser trimming system.

17.1.1 Physical Processes

The process of laser trimming involves connecting a resistor to be trimmed, via probes and wires, to a high-speed tracking measurement system. The laser is guided by a beam positioning device to micromachine a cut in the resistor material. When the resistor reaches its target value, the measurement system signals the laser to stop cutting.

Commercial equipment for resistor trimming has become highly sophisticated, containing automated parts handling equipment, a laser beam positioning system, a high-speed measuring system, closed circuit television monitoring, automatic alignment, and a control computer. An example of such a system is shown in Figure 1 (see also Fig. 9).

Material is actually removed with the laser by creating a short duration (less than 100 ns) high-intensity coherent light pulse. This pulse, impinging on a material that absorbs the light energy, causes the material to heat rapidly and vaporize. The amount of material removed by one laser pulse is typically one to two mils in diameter, although this value will vary widely depending on power level, focus, and composition of the material. A laser "cut" (kerf) is created by a succession of overlapping laser pulses, as shown in Figure 2.

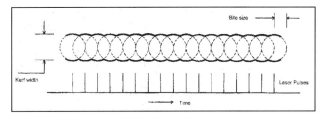

Figure 2. Characteristics of a laser "cut."

Certain relationships become obvious. For example, for a fixed hole size, a ragged kerf results if bite size is too large, as shown in Figure 3.

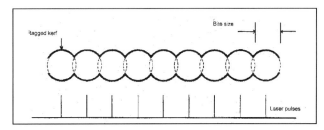

Figure 3. Example of a "ragged" kerf.

If the hole size is small, as would be desired in high-resolution circuits, the bite size must be lowered to achieve a quality cut.

This results in a lower cutting speed if the same pulse repetition rate is maintained.

Sufficient overlap of holes must be maintained to assure a "clean" kerf. A "clean" kerf is one that has all the material within the kerf removed. Almost all trimming requires hole overlap. Excessive overlap, as would occur if bite size were too small for the hole size, results in "overpowering" the cut. This may assure a smooth clean kerf, but generates excessive heating, which can cause drifting of the resistance value, or microcracking of the uncut material after the trim is complete.

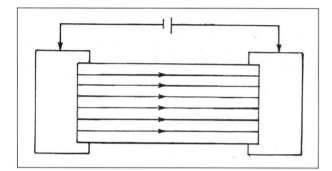

Figure 4. Untrimmed resistor showing current flow lines.

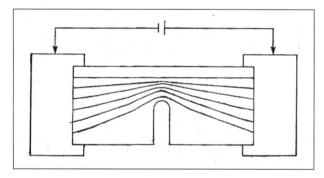

Figure 5. Trimmed resistor showing current flow lines.

The laser is pulsed very quickly. This rapid pulsing allows the high power required to vaporize the resistor paste to be delivered in a very short period of time. The energy must be delivered in a time short enough not to allow thermal spreading, because thermal spreading reduces energy available for vaporization and causes heating and, therefore, drift of resistance value.

When one trims high-accuracy parts, it may be necessary to utilize very small bite sizes for reasons other than good kerf characteristics. Because measurements are made prior to each laser pulse, the amount of change in value for the material removed by one bite must be less than the desired accuracy tolerance. Otherwise, one laser pulse may yield a value below tolerance, while the next pulse removes enough material to place the value well above its tolerance.

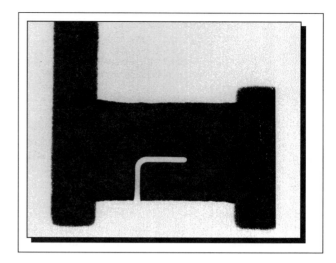

Figure 6. Thick-film trim on ceramic.

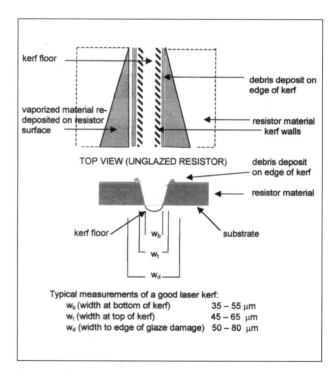

Figure 7. Typical measurements of a good laser kerf on an unglazed resistor.

During the trimming process, current flow changes and the current flow lines crowd together as material is removed. This is shown in Figures 4 and 5. If current flow is crowded into a damaged region near the end of the cut, the value of the resistance may be unstable. The trimming process should avoid creating narrow damaged regions through which high current density must flow.

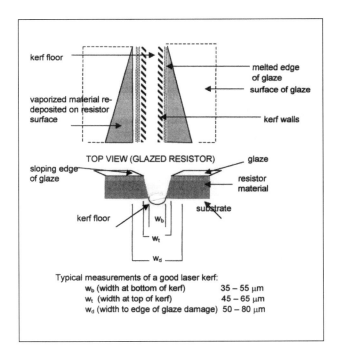

Figure 8. Typical measurements of a good laser kerf on a glazed resistor.

Many geometries have been used for cutting. One frequently employed geometry is the L-shaped cut, shown in Figure 6. The resistor is cut part way across, and then the direction of cutting is changed by 90 degrees. Thus the cut is in the form of a letter L. This procedure yields finer control of the final resistance. If one simply continued to cut straight across the resistor, control of the resistance value would become poor when the cut reached almost all the way across the resistor. The percentage change in resistance per unit length of cutting would become very large. The L-shaped cut permits a more gradual approach to the final desired resistance.

The characteristics of a good laser-trimmed kerf include nearly vertical walls, a clean floor with no remaining material, an undamaged ceramic substrate, and a sharp edge definition. Figures 7 (previous page) and 8 show typical measurements for good laser trimming cuts.

Thermal shock and damage along the cut have been problems that cause drift of the resistance after trimming. Keeping the laser power down to the minimum needed for a clean cut will reduce problems of damage and post-trim drift. With careful control, the change in resistance after the trimming can be in the range of 0.1 percent.

17.1.2 Overview of a Laser Trimming System

The evolution of the laser as a production tool enabled the development of laser trimming systems for a variety of production and engineering uses. These systems are used primarily by the electronics industry to remove material or to "trim" components (usually resistors) of a circuit to some specified condition. Trimming with a laser offers dramatic advantages of speed, precision, and ease of automation over manual adjustment, abrasive trimming, or milling techniques. Because of these advantages, laser trimming manual adjustment systems have been widely accepted and are well established in the industry.

Generally, a laser trimming system consists of a laser, a mechanism to move the laser beam, an optics path, a control system, and a measurement system. Viewing and parts handling systems may also be included. The control system is driven by a computer, which allows for a major increase in system utility through its computational and data gathering power, its intelligent interaction with the operator, and increased flexibility. Figure 9 shows a diagram of a laser trimming system.

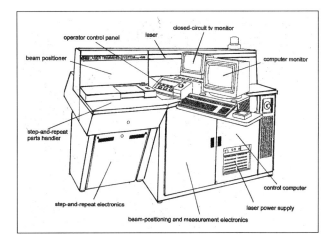

Figure 9. Diagram of a laser trimming system.

Laser trimming software, resident on the system, makes it easy for the operator to follow a menu to develop a new program or call up an existing stored program for each device to be laser trimmed. In run-time mode, the system is ready to trim parts at production rates with parts being fed either automatically or manually to the system parts handler.

17.1.3 Types of Laser Trims

The majority of laser trims made on resistors consist of three types of cuts — straight cuts, L-cuts, and double cuts. The last category, double cuts, can also include a double reverse cut or serpentine cut. Table 1 (see next page) lists characteristics of some different cut types.

17.1.4 Appropriate Lasers

In the early days of laser trimming, both CO_2 and Nd:YAG lasers were investigated. After extensive experimentation, it was concluded that the Nd:YAG, with a Q switch, produced the optimum trims. The high-energy, very short duration pulses give maximum trimming speed with minimum average power. The high repetition rate of the laser is also necessary to achieve adequate trim rates. If a spot size of two milli-inches with a 50% spot overlap is used, the laser is removing one milli-inch per

Table 1. Summary of Cut Types

Cut Type	Name	Application	Resistor Geometry	Tolerance Expected	Stability	Speed
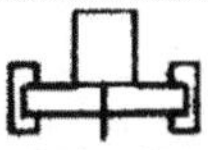	Plunge	Medium value change; 10 – 30% range of adjustment	Top hat or square	1%	Fair	Fast
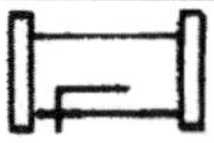	L-cut	Medium - high value change; 10 – 60% range of adjustment	Rectangle	< 1%	Very good	Medium
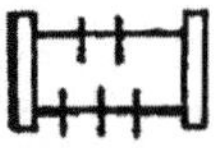	Serpentine	High-value change	Rectangle	1%	Poor	Slow
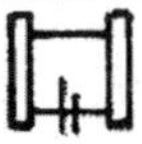	Double plunge	Medium value change; good accuracy	Rectangle	< 1%	Good	Medium
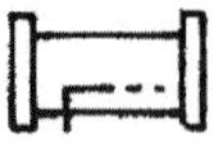	Measure predict L-cut	Medium – high value change; high accuracy	Rectangle	0.5%	Very good	Slow
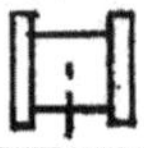	Measure predict plunge	Low – medium value change with good accuracy	Top hat or square	< 1%	Fair	Slow
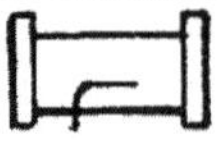	Curved L	Medium value change; reduced hot spots at turn	Rectangle	< 1%	Very good	Medium
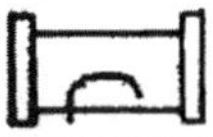	Curved J	Similar to curved-L; high accuracy	Rectangle	< 1%	Very good	Medium
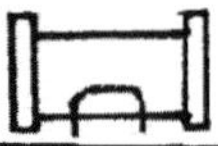	Curved U	Medium value change	Rectangle	1%	Very good	Slow
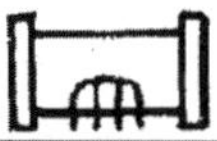	Curved U with isolation cuts	Used in high-voltage applications	Rectangle	1%	Good	Slow
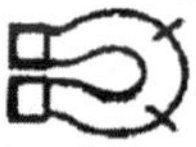	Non-orthogonal plunge	Pot trimming	Circular		Fair	Slow

pulse. For an eight inch per second removal rate, the laser must have a repetition rate of 8,000 pulses per second.

For many years, lamp-pumped Nd:YAG lasers operating at a wavelength of 1.06 µm were employed for resistor trimming. More recently, as diode-pumped solid-state lasers with relatively high average power have become available, those lasers have replaced lamp-pumped devices because of their smaller size, higher efficiency, and reduced cooling requirements. In modern trimming equipment, diode-pumped Nd:YAG lasers (1.06 µm) and Nd:YLF (1.047 µm) lasers are most often used. If very fine cuts and small kerf are required, frequency-doubled Nd:YAG (532 nm) and Nd:YLF (523 nm) lasers may be employed. As we shall see in Section 17.2.4, Nd:YAG or Nd:YLF lasers operating near 1.3 µm may be used for trimming of thin-film resistors on silicon.

RODGER DWIGHT

17.2 Trimming Techniques

17.2.1 Thick-Film Trimming

Laser processing in microelectronics production began in thick-film resistor trimming, where it proved to be faster, cleaner, noncontacting, and more accurate than previous techniques like sand blasting and mechanical abrasion. In addition, because laser trimming lends itself to computer control and automation, it is the method of choice for volume manufacturing of thick-film hybrid microcircuits.

Even though laser control and beam positioning are constantly being refined, thick-film trimming applications have not changed that much in recent years. The laser trimming systems themselves, however, continue to add new technologies like diode-pumped lasers, machine vision, automated parts handling, and dual high-speed processors.

The trimming operation may be characterized as passive or active (functional). Passive trimming refers to the trimming of the resistors to a specific predetermined value. The resistance is monitored during the trimming, and when the desired resistance is reached, the trimming is terminated. In functional trimming, the circuit is operating during the trimming. The performance of the circuit is measured during trimming and the trimming is terminated when the circuit is operating properly and within specification. Functional trimming improves device performance and increases yield. It does require fully automatic testing.

Table 1 presents some typical laser parameters for the trimming of thick-film resistors.

Table 1. Typical Laser Parameters for Thick-Film Resistor Trimming

Laser	Diode-pumped Nd:YAG
Wavelength	1.064 µm
Mode	TEM_{00}
Repetition rate	to 20 kHz
Average power	< 6 W
Pulse energy	0.6 mJ at 10 kHz
Pulse duration	70 ns

17.2.2 Thin Film on Ceramic Laser Trimming

An alternative resistor technology uses thin-film resistors, like nichrome or tantalum nitride, on 99% alumina substrates. These resistors are more expensive, but have better stability and a lower temperature coefficient of resistance than thick-film resistors. The laser trimming processes are similar to those for thick-film resistors except that the geometries are typically smaller and the focal spot sizes of the laser beam are smaller.

With the development of stable, reliable diode-pumped, frequency-doubled lasers, the second harmonic (532 nm) of Nd:YAG can be used for trimming of thin-film resistors, to provide better stability and a smaller kerf.

The use of the wavelength near 1.3 µm preserves the capability of focusing the beam to a small size. It is also well absorbed by nickel-chromium thin-film resistors, so that the resistors do not need to be changed.

Table 2 presents typical laser parameters used for trimming thin-film resistors on silicon.

Use of the wavelength near 1.32 µm allows functional trimming at higher throughput rates than use of the 1.067- or 1.047-µm wavelengths.

Use of the 1.32-µm Nd:YLF laser wavelength has been shown to eliminate the troublesome photoelectric response in the trimming of thin-film resistors on silicon. At the same time it preserves the trim quality and resistor stability obtained with functional trimming at the shorter wavelengths.

Table 2. Laser Parameters Suitable for Trimming of Thin-Film Resistors on Silicon

Laser	Diode-pumped Nd:YLF
Wavelength	1.3 µm
Mode	TEM_{00}
Repetition rate	Up to 20 kHz
Average power	48 mW at 1.2 kHz
Pulse energy	40 mJ at 1.2 kHz
Pulse duration	16 ns

17.2.3 Chip Resistor Laser Trimming

Chip resistors are predominantly thick-film resistors ink screened on a ceramic substrate, with wraparound metal terminations attached to facilitate easy mounting to a printed circuit board. This segment of the hybrid microelectronics market is differentiated from thick-film and thin-film laser trimming by the large volume of parts that must be processed. Individual resistors are arranged on pre-scribed ceramic substrates in rows and columns and, depending on their size, can be trimmed and measured at very high speeds in the order of milliseconds per resistor.

Typical commercial laser systems for chip resistor trimming use diode-pumped Nd:YAG lasers, operating at an average power around 6 W at a pulse repetition rate of up to 20 kHz.

17.2.4 Thin Film on Silicon Resistor Trimming

Functional trimming of thin-film resistors on silicon has been carried out for many years. Most early work employed Nd:YAG lasers pumped by arc lamps and operating at a wavelength of 1.06 µm. More recently, diode-pumped Nd:YLF lasers operating at a wavelength of 1.047 µm have been favored.

Functional trimming of thin films on silicon has been difficult because the wavelengths of 1.06 and 1.047 µm are both absorbed by the silicon and produce free electrons and holes in the silicon. This generates a photoelectric response, and this response interferes with the performance measurement of the circuit. The photoelectric response must be allowed to dissipate before the performance measurement is carried out. Thus functional trimming has usually been a relatively slow process, because of the time needed for the device to recover after each laser pulse.

The use of a Nd:YAG laser operating at 1.32 µm (or a Nd:YLF laser operating at 1.30 µm) eliminates this problem. Such lasers are commercially available and may be incorporated in trimming systems intended for use with silicon devices. This wavelength is long enough that the corresponding photon energy is smaller than the energy band gap of silicon; so the laser light will not generate free carriers in the silicon.

PHILIP DELUCA

17.2.5 Interference Effects

Most thin-film structures on silicon consist of an overlying passivation layer above the thin film and an underlying passivation layer between the thin film and silicon. The laser beam is highly coherent. When the beam hits the structure, the reflected beams at all the interfaces of these layers will interfere with each other. This interference will affect the amount of laser energy effectively absorbed by the film, thus the trimming quality. The interference effects are dependent on the thickness of these layers, the materials, and laser wavelength used. A bad choice or variation of passivation layer thickness across the silicon wafer will result in poor or inconsistent trimming quality. To maximize the amount of laser energy absorbed by the film and reduce the sensitivity of the trimming quality to the variation of the passivation layer thickness, the interference effects have to be simulated and optimized by choosing the right thickness for these passivation layers.

For a film thinner than the optical absorption depth of its material, the interference has to be simulated with both the overlying and underlying passivation layers included. When the thin film is much thicker than the optical absorption depth of its material, the interference optimization has to be carried out in two steps.

1. Optimizing the layer structure above the material when the resistor is intact.
2. Optimizing the layer structure below the resistor assuming that the remaining thickness of the film after being partially trimmed is less than the optical absorption depth.

Figures 1 (a) and (b) show the results of simulations for layers above and below the resistor material, respectively. The interference effect has a periodic nature with multiple optimized values for absorption in the material. The best choice among those optimized values is made considering the specific manufacturing process.

In summary, laser trimming of resistors is now standard in the electronics industry. It has essentially replaced older methods, such as abrasive trimming. Laser trimming offers the advantages of cleanliness and better control over the final resistance. The use of laser trimming also results in a higher yield.

YUNLONG SUN

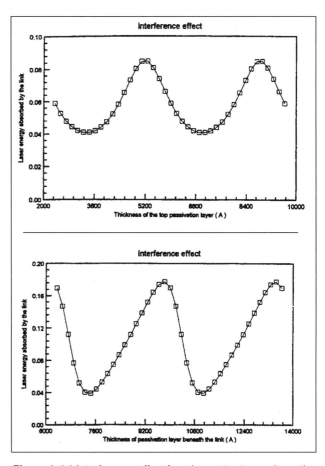

Figure 1. (a) Interference effect from layer structures above the material being vaporized. (b) Interference effect from layer structures below the material being vaporized.

Chapter 18

Laser Marking/Branding

18.0 Introduction

The techniques and applications of laser marking have been described previously in Chapter 15, along with a discussion of lasers used for marking. This chapter discusses some applications of laser marking as they are employed in the electronics industry, specifically the marking of packages, components and integrated circuits, and the serialization of wafers.

18.1 Package Marking and Branding

18.1.1 Laser Marking in Production

Laser marking or branding is used to mark the complete range of integrated circuit packages manufactured by the semiconductor industry. Major benefits are permanence of the mark, ease of programmability of the marking information, and compatibility with computer integrated manufacturing (CIM) environments. Laser-based systems are reliable manufacturing tools and provide consistent process control with low maintenance and service requirements. Lasers are also environmentally friendly and reduce or eliminate regulatory requirements over existing processes.

Packages and Systems

Virtually all package types can be marked. Plastic mold compounds, ceramics, metals, and silicon have been successfully marked in production. All types of information can be easily marked including text, logo or graphic files, barcodes, and 2D symbologies. Most of these are marked with Nd:YAG or CO_2 lasers, using both galvanometer deflection (beam steered) and mask (stencil) beam delivery technologies. Figure 1 illustrates the two most common approaches to beam delivery, and Table 1 provides a basic comparison of the various laser types and related specifications.

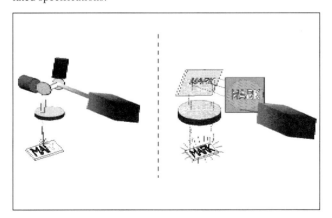

Figure 1. Common approaches for beam delivery for marking applications. Left: galvanometer deflection; right: mask projection.

Table 1. Comparison of Laser Types for Marking Applications

	CO_2 mask (TEA)	Nd:YAG mask (flash lamp)	Nd:YAG steered beam CW-pumped, Q-switched
Wavelength	10.6 µm	1.064 µm	1.064 µm
Spot size	NA	NA	100–200 µm
Field size	12 x 12 mm	50 x 50 mm typical (75 x 75 mm maximum)	200 x 200 mm (500 x 500 mm maximum)
Laser repetition rate	100 Hz (typical)	100 Hz (typical)	0–80 Hz
Peak power	5 MW	28 kW	50 kW
Average power	60 W	500 W	150 W
Laser transverse mode	Multimode	Multimode	Low order / multimode
Polarization	Random/ circular	Random/ circular	Random/ circular
Cost	Low	High	Medium
Depth of focus	Shallow	Shallow	Deeper
Contrast	Low	High	High

18.1.2 The Marking Process

The marking process is the result of laser energy interacting with the substrate to produce a mark. Lasers can be used to vaporize and remove material to produce the mark, or burn it to produce a color change. A visible mark can be a color change due to the energy burning the substrate material, removing a surface layer to expose a difference in color, or inducing a heat-related or photochemical effect in the substrate to produce a different color. The laser energy can be used to change the reflectivity of the part surface to produce a readable mark as a result of differences in surface reflectivity. Laser branding is the actual removal of material to engrave a mark in the substrate. Some materials allow for a combination of effects.

Peak Power

Differences in mark appearance can be made through variations in peak power. High peak power tends to vaporize the material and produce an engraved style of mark while lower peak power tends to burn or melt and produce a color change. Lasers can produce different power levels and can be operated for best results for the material in question. A CW Nd:YAG laser can be Q-switched to produce high peak power. Higher peak power is delivered at the lower repetition rates, and more average power is available at the higher repetition rates. This flexibility gives the laser an opportunity to mark a wider range of materials with the same tool. See Figure 2 for a typical graph of Nd:YAG laser output at the different pulse repetition rates.

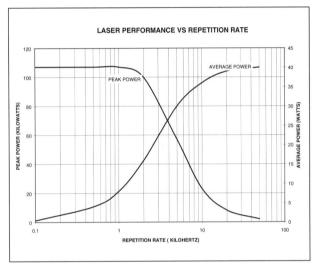

Figure 2. Peak power and average power as a function of pulse repetition rate for Q-switched Nd:YAG lasers.

18.1.3 Mark Quality Criteria

Contrast

The most common goal of laser marking is to produce the highest contrast mark possible on a wide variety of materials under various process conditions. Most lasers have programmable characteristics that can be used to optimize contrast for a given material.

Wavelength Dependencies

Mark readability or visibility to the naked eye can be affected by several factors. The most prominent of them are the material being marked and the specific wavelength being used to supply the energy. Both CO_2 and Nd:YAG lasers can be used to obtain different effects based on the wavelength of their respective outputs. Both can supply the energy required, but the absorption at the different wavelengths can produce different reactions in the material. For example, some plastic mold compounds marked with a CO_2 laser produce a light grey mark, while an Nd:YAG laser can produce a light brown or tan mark with potentially higher contrast on the same material. Other materials will have higher or lower absorption peaks at standard marking wavelengths, or, if more reflective, will not absorb much energy, limiting their ability to be marked.

Supplemental Factors

Additives can be used to improve the contrast of laser marks in some mold compounds, but this process belongs to the domain of the chemical manufacturers. Transferable media can also be used but are not as desirable, given the higher consumable cost and increased complexity of the process equipment.

Readability

Readability is affected by the width of the mark being made (kerf) and the surface finish of the part. The human eye tends to "integrate" information, and "blend" the mark into the background. This effect can be countered by making wider marks. Usually line widths of 100–200 μm are sufficient for character heights of 1 mm, with wider lines being easier to read. If the line width grows too large, it tends to fill in details on the characters being marked.

Surface Finish

Surface finish has a significant effect on the final result. Rougher surfaces tend to scatter reflected light and smoother surfaces provide a more consistent background. One technique for marking materials that provide little or no contrast is to alter the existing surface texture with a laser. This can produce contrast through the difference in reflected light between the background and the marked area. Nickel-plated transistors are a good example of where a rough finish can be used to produce a readable mark on a shiny surface. Unpolished silicon uses the opposite approach to marking by melting a rougher surface into a smooth finish.

Mark Depth

Another important consideration is the depth of the mark. The device reliability must not be compromised by the laser marking process. The newer thinner plastic packages are particularly vulnerable because of the low marking thresholds of the mold compounds. Extra care must be taken to monitor and control delivered power and maintain constant beam velocity with the beam steered models.

DONALD V. SMART
JOSE DOWNES

18.2 Wafer Serialization

18.2.1 Techniques

General Description

Wafer serialization is the distinguishing mark applied to silicon wafers at the beginning or during the wafer fabrication process. The laser mark is typically applied to the right or left of the fiducial axis on flatted or notched wafers. The mark usually consists of a string of alphanumeric OCR characters (optical character readable), but symbols, bar codes, two-dimensional codes, or logos can also be used. Unique indelible marking must be impervious to the various chemical etching, deposition, ion etching, cleaning, polishing, and die cutting steps applied to the silicon wafer during the fabrication process; the marking process must be noncontact and not generate impurities or dust in the cleanroom environment. Figure 1 shows serialization marks on silicon wafers.

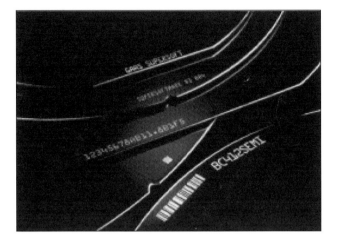

Figure 1. Typical serialization marks on silicon wafers.

The wafer marking station consists of an enclosed module designed to handle wafers under cleanroom conditions. The laser, beam delivery optics, and wafer handling equipment are enclosed within the single module. Wafers are transported using a pick and place robotic arm, and aligned to within ± 200 µm accuracy relative to the primary fiducial. Up to 240 wafers per hour can be marked.

Laser Sources

The most common form of wafer serialization is laser writing using continuously pumped, Q-switched Nd:YAG laser (wavelength 1.064 µm). Excimer lasers or harmonically multiplied Nd:YAG lasers can in rare instances be used, typically to mark other semiconductor materials such as GaAs. Although the laser power required is modest, very reproducible pulse-to-pulse output is essential to producing clean visible marking. The use of diode-pumped (rather than lamp pumped) Nd:YAG lasers has dramatically improved the ability to achieve excellent pulse-to-pulse stability (1). Table 1 shows typical parameters for Nd:YAG laser serialization of silicon wafers.

Table 1. Typical Laser Parameters

Parameter	Nd:YAG laser
Pulse energy	1–2 mJ
Energy reproducibility	< 0.2%
Average power	2 W
Pulse length	200 ns FWHM
Repetition rate	1000 pps

Marking Techniques

In the standard laser writing technique, each laser pulse focused onto the sample creates a dot. The laser beam is scanned using two computer-controlled, galvo-driven mirrors to write lines and characters as series of dots. In silicon marking, adjacent dots do not overlap with each other because this would result in unnecessary disruption to the wafer surface and excessive debris. The primary criterion in wafer serialization is to produce a clear, debris-free mark which remains readable throughout all fabrication processing. In a quantitative context, debris-free means less than 0.02 particles/cm^2 for a particle size of 0.17 µm, although this specification is arbitrary and will be modified as fabrication feature sizes decrease.

18.2.2 Results

Because 1.064 µm is very close to the band gap of silicon, the absorption depth can be accurately controlled by adjusting the energy density of the focussed laser beam (1, 2). This requires very reproducible laser pulses shot-to-shot, but also provides useful control over the depth and extent of the mark being made.

Although some older fabrication lines still use the 20-µm-deep "hard" mark, as lithographic feature size has decreased below the 2-µm level, virtually all modern fabrication lines now employ an industry standard, which is sometimes called a SuperSoftMark® laser marking process that makes a debris-free mark having a reproducible dot diameter of 70 (± 10) µm and a depth of 2.6 (± 0.4) µm. During the process, the absorbed laser radiation from each pulse heats up and melts a shallow region of the silicon at the surface of the wafer. When this melted region cools, a crater of reproducible diameter and depth is formed. If one carefully controls the deposited energy per pulse to just melt the silicon, no debris is ejected and the crater formed for each pulse has reproducible properties. Figure 2 shows such a mark.

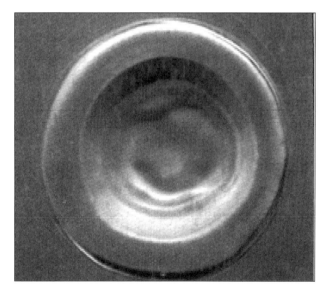

Figure 2. SEM view of single dot on a silicon wafer using the SuperSoftMark® process.

ISBN 0-912035-15-3

Variations of this marking process are sometimes used, such as multiple pulses per dot to make deeper marks but still without any debris formation. Laser parameters can be adjusted, depending on whether the marking process takes place at the beginning of the fabrication process on the base silicon wafer, or whether marking is done after one or more wafer processing steps have been completed.

Backside wafer marking of diced silicon wafers is a new marking process also done using the Nd:YAG laser. This process usually occurs after the die is bonded to a conductor substrate so debris-free marking is not a strict requirement, and marking speeds are significantly faster than wafer serialization.

SuperSoftMark® is a trademark of Lumonics (Oxnard, CA).

References
1. J. Scaroni, et al, Solid State Tech. **40** (7), 245–51 (July 1997).
2. F. Kuhn-Kuhnenfeld, et al., U.S. Patent No. 4,522,656.

JIM SCARONI
JERRY BECKER
TERRY MCKEE

18.3 Marking of Electronic Components

Pulsed carbon dioxide lasers, using the mask imaging technique, are very effective for marking electronic components encapsulated in thermoset epoxy such as integrated circuits, transistors, capacitors etc., when a relatively small mark is needed on-the-fly at high speed. Typical speeds for low-cost electronics parts are 500 parts/min.(1) (see Fig. 1).

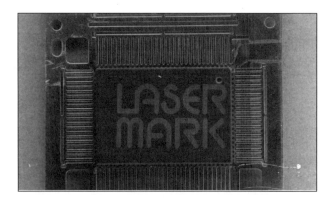

Figure 1. Pulsed CO_2 laser marked integrated circuit.

Because the imaged mask technique uses optical imaging, very sharp marks can be made, depending primarily on the surface smoothness. Characters as small as 0.012 in. in height are possible for very small parts, such as ceramic chip capacitors. The "webs" in each character caused by the supportive elements in the metal mask are indicative of the imaged-mask technique.

For marking larger parts, the maximum size of the marked area is typically restricted to 1/4 x 3/4 in., and possibly even smaller if the material does not mark easily. Additives and coatings can dramatically reduce the energy density required to achieve an acceptable mark, so that larger marks can then be made (see Fig. 2).

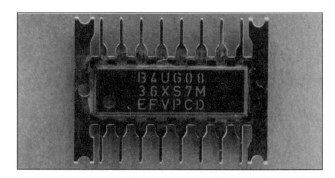

Figure 2. Marking of integrated circuit with clear coating by CO_2 laser (photo courtesy of Nippon Kayaku).

The largest market for Nd:YAG laser writing systems is integrated circuits marking (1). Black thermoset epoxy IC encapsulant material marks easily and typically a tray of ICs is marked within the 12 x 12-in. field of view of the marker. As well as alphanumerics, 2D symbologies, such as IC matrix and decorative logos, are commonly marked on the more expensive ICs such as computer processors (see Fig. 3).

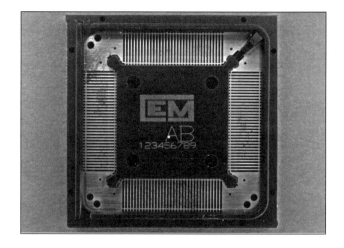

Figure 3. Nd:YAG laser writer marks IC package.

The Nd:YAG laser is used to mark ICs and other electronic components packaged in ceramic as well as plastic. These systems are also used to mark meters, switches, and other electronic components made from thermoset polyesters.

Another important application of the Nd:YAG laser writer in the electronics industry is marking thermoplastic items such as keyboards, control panels, enclosures, and displays. In many cases, additives are used in the thermoplastic materials to enhance the markability (2), and to allow gray-scale decorative marking (3). Although plastics such as PVC, ABS, and polyesters usually mark, it is not possible to provide a strict rule of markability for thermoplastics because their absorptions depend strongly on what additives they contain (see Fig. 4).

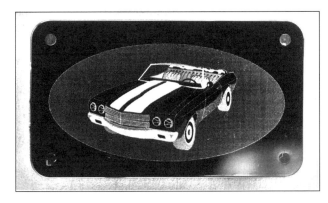

Figure 4. Decorative marking on black nylon containing the mica-based additive LS 830 (photo courtesy of EM Industries).

Excimer lasers are frequently used for package marking because of the high absorption at the excimer laser wavelengths. They are often employed for making identification marks on components, such as capacitors.

References
1. K. Koller, et al., *Semiconductor International*, 106–107, June 1994; C. Bosnos, *Electronics Engineer*, p. 146, July 1996.
2. T. McKee, *Packaging Tech. & Eng.* **4** (6), 48–52 (August 1995); G. Graff, *Modern Plastics* **73** (4), 24–5 (April 1996).
3. G. Graff, *Modern Plastics* **73** (13), 30–4 (December 1996); T. McKee, L. Toth, and W. Sauerer, *Packaging Tech. & Eng.* **6** (11), 26–9 (November 1997).

TERRY MCKEE

Notes

ISBN 0-912035-15-3

Chapter 19

Link Cutting/Making

19.1 Basics of Link Processing with Lasers

19.1.0 Introduction
Laser-based cutting and formation of electronic connections has been widely used in the repair of integrated circuit chips and for customization. The cutting of links by laser vaporization of a connecting link is very easy. It was the first of these two approaches to be used and has been more widely employed. The technology for making of interconnecting links has also matured and is of importance for both repair and for the fabrication of complex structures.

Link disconnect processing of high-density devices requires careful consideration of the interaction between device design and laser system capability. Design characteristics such as semiconductor process type, link material and geometry, link grouping, and alignment targets directly affect wavelength selection, pulse requirements, the mode of system operation, and system throughput.

This chapter offers insights into the laser–material interactions needed for applications such as the repair of redundant memories.

DONALD V. SMART

19.1.1 Basics of Link Cutting
The number of elements in an integrated circuit has increased rapidly with time. Now wafer scale integration is being developed. But there is a problem with yield, as circuit size continues to increase. A small defect can cause an entire very large circuit to be defective. This makes the yield of the large expensive circuits unacceptably low. Wafer scale integration with reasonable yield is accomplished by cutting out defective circuit elements and interconnecting operative circuit elements.

Laser cutting of links is accomplished by vaporization of the conducting lines which connect the circuit elements. The links are polysilicon or metals like gold, copper, and aluminum, with thickness of a few micrometers. Lasers that have been used for link cutting have included the argon ion laser, the Nd:YAG laser, and excimer lasers. Table 1 presents typical laser parameters for a link cutting operation.

Table 1. Typical Laser Parameters for Link Cutting

Laser	Nd:YAG
Wavelength	532 nm
Pulse energy	0.3 mJ
Pulse duration	50 ns

The metal links which are to be cut often have vaporization temperatures higher than the melting temperatures of the dielectric substrates. Also, to provide clean removal of the metal, the area irradiated is larger than the width of the link, so that some of the substrate is exposed to the laser light. To avoid damage to the substrate, the process parameters must be carefully chosen.

The laser irradiance must be high enough to vaporize the metal completely in the irradiated area. To minimize thermal damage, the pulse duration is kept very short, often a few tens of nanoseconds. Also the wavelength of the laser may be chosen so that absorption in the substrate is relatively low.

Applications for laser link cutting have included customization and personalization of circuits and the enhancement of the yield of memory devices.

One example (1) to illustrate how link cutting can be used involves link cutting for fast personalization of a multi-chip module (MCM). The MCM is designed with its personality confined to the two top layers, of which the uppermost layer consists mostly of bond pads. These layers are built on top of several generic design-independent wiring patterns. The top two layers are interconnected through vias.

The processing is maskless. The conductor lines are gold or gold-plated nickel, with a typical thickness of 5 μm and width of 15 μm. Cutting of the lines is done cleanly with two pulses from a 532-nm frequency doubled Nd:YAG laser. The underlying polyimide is not damaged.

Reference
1. H. G. Muller, et. al., Laser process for personalization and repair of multi-chip-modules, SPIE Proceedings, Vol. 1598, p. 132 (1991).

JOHN F. READY

19.1.2 Memory Repair Goals
Laser-based memory repair systems direct pulsed, highly focused energy at conductive components that lie beneath transparent layers of insulating materials on silicon wafers. These systems are used to selectively sever small links ("fuses") on memory wafers.

The goal of a memory repair system is to substitute spare rows (or columns) in DRAM or SRAM devices for defective ones by cutting closely spaced links. These links have two purposes: They are used to disable defective memory rows (or columns), and they are used to reprogram substitute circuits.

Individual links, identified by automatic test equipment (ATE), are cut by a focused laser. Because die space is precious and memory designs are continually shrinking, repair systems must undergo continual refinement to improve: spot size, accuracy, energy control, and adaptability to wafer materials. All these characteristics contribute to a system's ability to avoid adjacent feature damage and achieve maximum wafer throughput while still adapting to ever-shrinking link and pitch dimensions.

Memory circuits are constructed as a series of layers upon a silicon substrate. The substrate and the silicon dioxide layer immediately above it are patterned to form electrically active components. These components make up the memory circuits. Above them lie layers of metal interconnects separated by insulating oxide. Figure 1 shows a typical arrangement for layer structures.

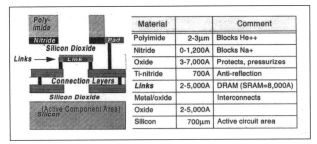

Figure 1. Memory layers.

The link layer lies above the interconnect layers. Most current memory designs use metal links (aluminum), but some still use polysilicon and silicides. A thin antireflective film on the aluminum links improves their ability to absorb energy. Another oxide layer isolates the links from a final metal layer that provides the pads that connect the die to a carrier. A final oxide layer offers scratch protection and inhibits oxidation. These oxide layers play an important role in link blowing.

A thin layer of silicon nitride (Si_3N_4) usually caps the outer oxide to protect the underlying structures from sodium (Na^+) contamination.

Polyimide is often added as a final layer to protect memory cells from disruption by alpha particles (He^{++}), which are emitted by trace radioactive elements in ceramic packages.

Additional processes etch away material to expose the bonding pads and to remove polyimide from link areas. Lasers have trouble penetrating the polyimide, which tends to carbonize at high power.

The oxide thickness above the links is critical for two reasons: First, it must be thick enough to contain a link until the link superheats, yet it must be thin enough to yield when the link reaches a critical temperature. Second, the oxide must be uniformly thick to ensure consistent energy absorption in all wafer areas. Absorption varies with oxide thickness because interference effects between surface and subsurface reflections can significantly alter the pulse energy setting needed to remove a link.

19.1.3 Processing Concerns

The ability of a system to process wafers depends on the optical properties of wafer materials, laser technology, spot size, interference effects, process control, die layout (links and alignment targets), and alignment strategy.

Every material possesses a unique combination of three optical properties that affect the way links are blown: reflectance, absorption, and transmittance. If every wafer layer possessed ideal optical properties for link processing, pulses would pass unimpeded through the upper layers, be fully absorbed in the target material, and have no effect on the underlying structures. Target material would superheat until it exploded its oxide covering and ejected the vaporized link material. The result would be an ideal cut, clean and localized, with no effect on surrounding structures.

Real materials and real processing problems are more complicated than idealized scenarios suggest. Silicon dioxide, which has nearly perfect transmittance at working wavelengths, allows all the energy that is not intercepted by the link to reach the substrate. Consequently the interaction between the laser light and the substrate is very important.

Silicon is subject to a phenomenon called "thermal runaway." In thermal runaway, the more a material (substrate) heats up, the more it absorbs; the more it absorbs, the more it heats up. This results in an accelerating process that is increasingly sensitive to further energy additions. As a result, any un-intercepted energy can cause substrate damage.

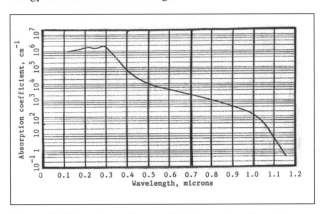

Figure 2. Silicon absorption coefficient as a function of wavelength.

Figure 2 shows how light is absorbed in silicon. Note that silicon absorbs heavily throughout the visible region and into the near-infrared. At 1.1 μm, silicon has an "absorption edge" where absorption falls off rapidly. The absorption difference between silicon and the link material makes link blowing possible at wavelengths longer than the absorption edge.

The monochromatic and coherent attributes of laser light make it susceptible to interference effects between top surface and subsurface reflections in a wafer stack. Top surface reflections come from the oxide, while subsurface reflections come from the aluminum links. When these reflections are in phase, the total reflection is enhanced and less light reaches a link. When they

Chapter 19: Link Cutting/Making

are out of phase, the reflections combine destructively and less light reflects, so more light reaches the link.

Bare aluminum links have a nominal absorption of 6.6%. With just two surfaces, that value can vary between 6.6 and 13.8% as oxide thickness increases. Figure 3 shows how the absorption varies in an oscillatory fashion with oxide thickness. This type of behavior has been discussed previously in Chapter 17 with reference to absorption of laser energy in resistor trimming.

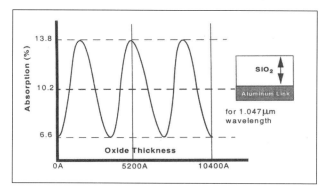

Figure 3. Aluminum absorption.

This represents a drastic change in the laser energy coupled to a link: ± 36% variation from a mean absorption of 10.2%. The main implication of this is that identical wafers, which differ only in oxide thickness, may require different laser power settings to achieve the same link removal results.

The optimum oxide thickness for a typical aluminum link is 5200 Angstroms. This thickness offers optimum absorption and is not too thick to contain the link for easy removal.

Energy studies should be performed for each new batch process. Individual wafers should also be visually inspected at periodic intervals to ensure the system is at its best power setting for the current wafers.

Wafer processes should be designed with energy windows that exceed the interference-induced energy variations.

19.1.4 Lasers for Link Cutting

System designers are not free to select just any wavelength that suits their purpose. This is because laser wavelengths are derived from energy state transitions within specific elements or molecules. The number of lasing materials is limited. Wafer fabrication facilities use laser wavelengths from all three regions of the optical spectrum: infrared, visible, and ultraviolet.

Infrared wavelengths are often used for link cutting. Standard wavelengths (in micrometers) are: 1.047, 1.064, 1.320, and 1.343, from Nd:YLF, Nd:YAG, and Nd:YVO$_4$. These wavelengths can be reflected and focused just like visible light. Visible laser wavelengths are usually derived from infrared lasers whose frequencies have been doubled. Their shorter wavelengths offer the possibility of a proportionally smaller spot size. Ultraviolet wavelengths can also be generated through frequency multiplication (tripled and quadrupled infrared). Recent advances in this type of laser technology are showing potential in the ultraviolet (355 and 266 nm).

Most memory repair systems use neodymium-doped YLF lasers or neodymium-doped vanadate lasers. Both are yttrium-based. "YLF" (YLiF$_4$) and "vanadate" (YVO$_4$) describe host materials used for different laser rods (see Section 2.3). The host material determines the energy storage and gain capability of a laser. The combination of host and neodymium dopant determines wavelength. Nd^{3+}:YLF lasers operate at 1.047 or 1.32 μm, while Nd^{3+}:vanadate lasers operate at 1.064 or 1.34 μm.

The high storage capacity of a YLF laser produces very high-energy pulses at low repetition rates. These same characteristics also cause the pulse width to increase significantly and pulse energy to decrease dramatically with increasing laser repetition rate.

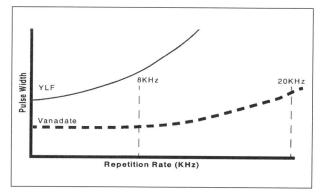

Figure 4. Pulse width versus repetition rate for Nd:YLF and YVO$_4$ lasers.

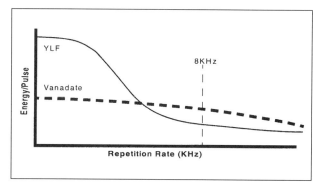

Figure 5. Pulse energy versus repetition rate for Nd:YLF and YVO$_4$ lasers.

Vanadate lasers have a higher gain that produces shorter pulse widths than YLF lasers, but they also produce lower-energy pulses. The lower pulse storage capacity enables vanadate lasers to maintain pulse width and pulse energy across a broader range of repetition rates (beyond 20 kHz).

The longer pulse widths from YLF lasers are better suited to processing thick links, while thinner metal links, including tungsten and titanium, are best served by narrow-pulse vanadate lasers that can couple energy into a link before it dissipates to the surroundings.

Figures 4 and 5 compare relative pulse width and pulse energy for Nd:YLF and Nd:YVO$_4$ lasers.

19.1.5 Positioning Systems

Lasers systems need to deliver focused energy to specific wafer features. There are many possible positioning system configurations, but all use some combination of three basic movements: moving stage, moving optics, and moving beam. Figures 6, 7, and 8 show schematic sketches of these three types of systems.

Moving Stage

A moving-stage system uses a stage table to move selected components into the path of a stationary beam, where they can be irradiated. This approach allows the simplest optical design but is likely to suffer from low throughput when relative motion is achieved by moving a relatively massive stage table. Large masses take more time and effort to move than small ones.

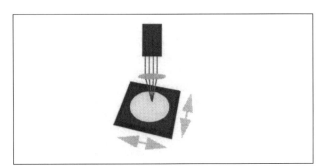

Figure 6. Sketch of moving-stage system.

Moving Optics

A moving-optics system moves the system optics above a stationary workpiece. When the optics are lighter than a stage table, a moving-optics system is likely to be faster than a moving-stage system. Moving-optics assemblies can be made lighter by moving the optics independently of the laser source. This can be done by having the optical assembly ride along a collimated beam path. An orthogonal mirror directs the collimated beam to the optical assembly, which moves about within an *X-Y* plane.

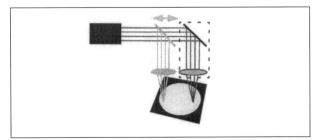

Figure 7. Sketch of moving-optics system.

Moving Beam

A moving-beam system holds both the workpiece and optical path stationary. Positioning is achieved by a pair of galvanometer-driven mirrors that direct a collimated beam onto a special lens. The properties of this lens cause it to offset the spot position within a reticle-sized scan field by an amount that varies with incident beam angle. Since this system needs only two rotating mirrors (no sliding movement), it is very precise, very reliable, and extremely fast.

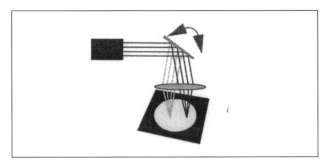

Figure 8. Sketch of a moving-beam system.

Early implementations of the moving-beam system moved a spot to each position and stopped there while the laser irradiated its link. "Stop and cut" operations can process a few hundred links per second. Current implementations cut a whole series of links with a beam that is in continuous motion. "Linksprint" operations are capable of cutting links at the laser Q-switch rate (20,000 Hz and beyond).

19.1.6 Optics

Competitive economic pressures have steadily forced memory links and link spacing to shrink so much that one-micrometer wavelength technology is now approaching the limits of optical physics with respect to spot size.

Spot size is proportional to the product of lens speed (focal length/aperture) and wavelength. The smaller the wavelength, the smaller the spot size.

$$\text{spot size} = k\lambda(f/D)$$

A standard spot size is defined by the $1/e^2$ points on a Gaussian distribution curve. The perimeter bounded by these points encloses 86.7% of the beam energy. Note that there are other measures of spot size that result in larger or smaller numbers for the same energy distribution.

Lasers may produce holes larger or smaller than the specified spot size. This is possible because actual hole size depends on the ablation *threshold* of the material being blasted and on the laser pulse energy setting. Figure 9 (next page) shows an example where the hole size is smaller than the beam spot size as defined by the $1/e$ points.

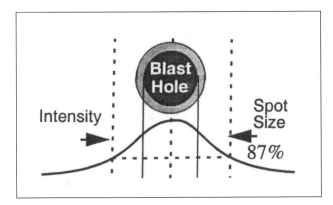

Figure 9. Blast hole size compared to spot size.

Commercial systems for link cutting systems offers spot size selections from 2 to 10 μm. As spot size decreases, energy density increases but depth-of-field (DOF) decreases. Precision chucktops and frequent focus checks ensure that these systems maintain optimum focus at even the smallest spot size. Figure 10 shows how DOF varies with spot size.

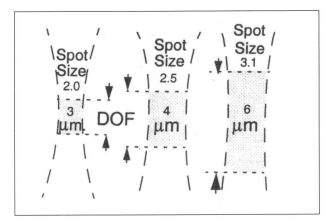

Figure 10. Depth of field variation with spot size.

19.1.7 Pulse Control

The delivery of appropriately sized laser pulses through the oxide layers is just the beginning of a link blowing process that should end up with completely severed links and no collateral damage. Success here requires precise control of pulse power and pulse energy. The ability of a pulse to transfer energy depends on its shape and duration as well as the link design.

Memory links are evaporated in the sudden release of superheated material. This process begins with the rapid laser heating of a memory link beneath an oxide layer. The restraining oxide causes a sudden pressure rise because of the thermal expansion of the link material. As the confined link superheats, pressure rises to extremely high levels. Eventually the oxide weakens and cracks. The abrupt pressure release vaporizes the link and blows away both it and the oxide.

The energy setting for link blasting is critical. Too little energy will fail to sever the link, or will leave debris (incomplete vaporization), while too much will damage the substrate. The right amount produces a clean round hole.

An energy study reveals the optimum pulse energy for a particular process. A typical study blasts several links on a representative wafer beginning with an energy level that is too low to affect the wafer. Subsequent links are blasted at successively higher levels until a pulse causes substrate damage.

The range between the lowest-energy pulse that blows a link and the highest-energy pulse that did not damage the substrate is the "energy window." Its width should accommodate normal process variations, and its integrity should be based on the worst-case upper and lower limits from several energy studies performed on different wafer batches that use the same process.

A good starting point for selecting a nominal energy is the energy window midpoint. Most user interfaces allow manufacturing engineers to make small energy adjustments within this range. Those adjustments are based on periodic visual inspections of blown links on production wafers.

Effective spot size changes with energy setting and may differ from the standard spot size ($1/e^2$). A vernier run reveals the effective spot size for a specific power setting by blasting a series of evenly spaced links with a laser step size slightly larger than the link pitch. This is illustrated in Figure 11. The pitch difference times the number of links affected by the laser equals the sum of the spot size and link width. Because three of the four parameters are known, the effective spot size may be obtained.

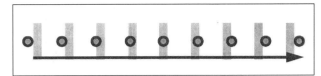

Figure 11. Determining effective spot size.

19.1.8 Energy Coupling

The ability of a system to deliver the right amount of energy to a link depends on how well energy is coupled from the laser to the link, and on how rapidly heat flows from a link to surrounding structures. More specifically, it depends on link absorption, pulse profile, link mass, link geometry, and thermal conduction.

Absorption, which describes the efficiency of radiant energy coupling, varies with link temperature and with material phase changes. Like the silicon substrate, polysilicon links have an absorption coefficient that increases with temperature and is subject to thermal runaway. Aluminum links do not exhibit thermal runaway.

Pulse profile refers to the energy and energy transfer rate (power) of a pulse. It strongly influences link removal.

If the pulse width is too long, heat transfer is slow and energy has time to diffuse into the surrounding material, where it can damage neighboring links or the substrate. This is illustrated schematically in Figure 12.

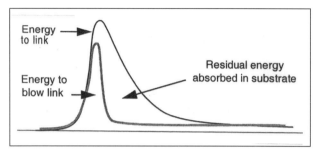

Figure 12. Pulse energy profile.

If the pulse width is too short, heat transfer is fast and does not have time to diffuse completely through the link. If it is too fast, it could vaporize the top half of a link and leave the lower half intact.

Pulse width can be reduced by decreasing pulse repetition rate. But this is not a good solution because it sacrifices system throughput. A better solution is to exploit the continual advances in laser technology by upgrading to shorter-pulse-width lasers as they become available.

One way to lengthen the time it takes for a link to blow is to reduce its thermal rise time. This can be done by altering link material, mass, and/or geometry. Each of these elements affects the temperature buildup in a link. This can be desirable if a laser with a short pulse is not available.

19.1.9 Link Materials
Common link materials are: polysilicon, polysilicides, and aluminum.

Polysilicon is a common link material with a high melting point. Although easy to fabricate, polysilicon has the disadvantages of low absorptance and high resistance. Polysilicides have higher absorptance than polysilicon and are more readily removed. They also have lower electrical resistance than doped polysilicon.

Aluminum is the most common link material for new memory designs. Its low link resistance allows faster circuit speed with less power consumption, but high reflectivity (92%) and high thermal conductivity make it harder to couple energy into a link. Antireflection films (titanium nitride) improve absorption.

Aluminum's high surface tension, low melting point (640°C), and high vaporization temperature (2400°C) can cause uncovered links, or links with defective oxide, to splatter. But its high coefficient of thermal expansion works to its advantage when the link is covered by oxide because oxide containment promotes rapid pressure buildup. When the link finally blows, the aluminum is superheated well beyond its vaporization temperature (2400°C). The sudden pressure release that occurs when the oxide yields causes the complete removal of the vaporized aluminum.

Refractory metals such as tungsten have higher melting points, better absorption, and lower thermal conductivity than aluminum, which make them useful link materials. Other link materials include platinum, gold, and refractory metal silicides.

19.1.10 Link Design
Energy that is coupled to a link begins to flow away as soon as the pulse begins. Short links dissipate energy to surrounding structures more readily than long links, so the temperature rise in a short link is slower than in a long one. Long links blow sooner than short links.

Typical link dimensions are a length of 7–10 μm, thickness of 0.5 μm, and width of 0.8–1 μm.

Narrowing a link at its center flattens the temperature profile because the heat dissipates faster.

Broadening the center of a link by adding tabs has the opposite effect: It steepens the temperature profile because the tab intercepts more pulse energy while the heat flow (rate) to adjacent structures remains relatively unchanged. Pads also absorb more of the pulse energy that would otherwise be dissipated in the substrate.

The term *energy window* refers to the useful energy range for blasting links. Its lower limit is the minimum energy that will blow a link, and its upper limit is the maximum energy that will not damage a wafer. These limits typically represent the worst case from a set of test wafers. Wafer-to-wafer oxide variations make it necessary periodically to check link blast quality.

A wide energy window helps to ensure good repair results. Designs can be optimized to widen the window at its upper and lower limits.

Substrate isolation helps to widen the energy window at the high end by reducing the thermal diffusion from link to substrate. About 300 nm separates polysilicon links from the substrate. Metal links have even more separation (about 1 μm) because they are laid down several layers above the substrate.

Energy dissipation in the substrate can also be reduced by adding a metal shield, preferably tungsten, between link and substrate.

Via isolation helps to widen the low end of the energy window by placing tungsten plugs/vias at each end of the links. The high thermal resistance of tungsten restricts thermal diffusion to adjacent metal interconnects. Since this causes a more rapid rise in link temperature, the laser pulse energy can be set lower, which widens the window. Figure 13 shows a design for tungsten plugs.

Chapter 19: Link Cutting/Making

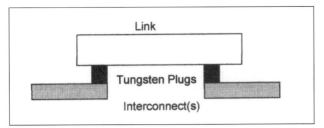

Figure 13. Tungsten plugs.

Link pitch is subject to periodic shrinks as process engineers try to squeeze more chips onto a given wafer. Designers would like link areas to be as small as possible, but link pitch must be large enough to avoid adjacent link damage during repair. Minimum pitch is affected by: spot size, link width, and positioning error.

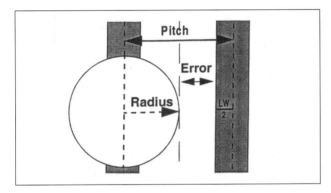

Figure 14. Link pitch.

Minimum link pitch equals the sum of half the effective spot diameter plus the system positioning error, plus half the link width. Figure 14 illustrates this relation. For example, a system with a 0.3-μm positioning error and a 3.4-μm spot diameter is capable of blasting 0.8-μm links on 2.4-μm centers.

Tabbed links can be spaced more closely if they are staggered as illustrated in Figure 15. Staggering, however, doubles the time needed to blast links in a group because the laser must make two passes. The minimum pitch for staggered links is twice the normal minimum pitch.

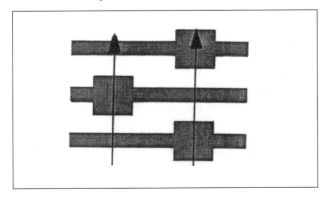

Figure 15. Staggered links.

While traditional links allow laser systems selectively to cut circuit conductors, recent technology makes it possible for lasers selectively to *connect* closely separated aluminum conductors in a circuit. Each "connect link" consists of two orthogonal conductors separated by an oxide.

The top conductor has an aperture that allows a laser pulse to pass through the upper conductor and impinge upon the lower conductor. As the lower conductor gains heat, it expands. This heating and expansion continues until fracture lines propagate through the oxide from lower to upper conductors. Molten metal then flows along the fracture lines to connect the conductors. This is illustrated schematically in Figure 16. Making links in this fashion is discussed in more detail in Section 19.3.

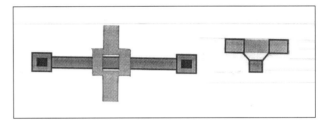

Figure 16. Connect links.

19.1.11 Link Groups

Links are arranged in groups that reflect the rows and columns of the memory elements in a die. There are two types of link groups: those that must be cut to sever the connections to a defective memory area (row or column), and those that must be cut to establish the logical address to a spare circuit. Depending upon design, a die could have 20–200 link groups with from four to one hundred links per group. The arrangement of groups, along vertical and/or horizontal axes, has a major impact on system throughput.

A typical 8-in. memory wafer holds about 250 die, roughly half of which need to be processed. Process time is divided into wafer handling, die alignment, and blast times. Blast time includes time spent cutting links and moving between groups. Most of the time it is moving between link groups.

As a beam sweeps across the links, an extremely fast optical "shutter" opens and closes to either blast or preserve individual links within a group. Software maintains the coordination between laser pulses and galvo and link positioning during these operations.

Link pitch (L_p) consistency has a huge influence on wafer throughput because of the system's ability to synchronize laser pulses with link pitch. In general, laser systems operate at a fixed pulse rate to ensure consistent pulse width and pulse-to-pulse energy. The combination of fixed pulse rate (time) and constant galvo velocity results in fixed blast intervals (distance). Blast intervals are set equal to the required pitch by supplying appropriately sized step increments to the beam positioner (galvos, in a moving beam system). Once the appropriate step size has been established, the system maintains its corresponding velocity.

Note that large pitch settings move a beam at higher velocity than small pitch settings but do not process links any more rapidly. This is because link processing speed depends on laser pulse rate, not velocity.

Throughput is directly related to laser pulse rate. Laser technology improvements that offer higher pulse rates translate directly into higher system throughput.

A typical memory repair system may blast 20,000 or more links per die, but since these blasts occur "on the fly," as the beam passes over them, the number of links to be blasted is of little consequence. More significant is how often a system must stop its uniform movement and synchronize to the start of a new link group.

Ideally, all link groups should lie on a common axis. If designers maintain this discipline, memory repair systems can coalesce the groups on an axis into the same supergroup. This allows a system to blast coalesced links in one galvo sweep. Coalescence offers major throughput improvement.

Throughput is dramatically reduced when a memory design uses more than one pitch in the same area. Mixed pitches are undesirable.

Consider an example where five pairs of links of 10-μm pitch are separated by 28-μm in a repeating pattern, as shown in Figure 17.

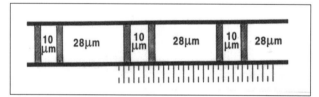

Figure 17. Mixed pitch example.

The smallest common pitch between these links is 2 μm, which means the system wastes four blast pulses between 10-pitch links, and 13 pulses between 28-pitch links (10/2 = 5; 28/2 = 14) if it tries to blast the links in the same sweep. Since the laser requires 82 blast opportunities to cover these, the sweep requires 8.2 ms at a 10 K pulse rate.

Lengthening the 28-μm pitch to 30 μm significantly increases the common pitch (10 μm) which provides a ratio of three galvo steps to one (30/10 = 3; 10/10 = 1). Now there are no more wasted pulses between 10-μm links and only two wasted pulses between the 30-μm links. This allows the system to cover all 10 links in 18 pulse intervals, which takes 1.8 ms at a 10 K pulse rate.

The relative efficiencies for the preceding pitch combinations are:

28/10 pitch = 8.2 ms = 12.5% efficiency

30/10 pitch = 1.8 ms = 56% efficiency

all on same pitch = 1.0 ms = 100% efficiency

Low efficiency means low throughput because the system wastes pulses.

Mixed Phase

A more likely example can occur when designers use the same pitch within adjacent groups but fail to preserve pitch synchronization between groups. This calls for a choice: combine groups into a super group and operate at reduced efficiency (50% in Fig. 18), or treat each group independently and spend time synchronizing the system to each of the groups.

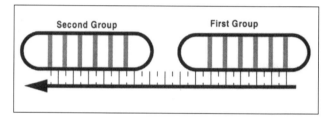

Figure 18. Groups with pitch alignment not preserved between groups.

19.1.12 Accuracy

Positioning errors come from two general sources: instrument and die alignment. These errors, however, are usually described in terms of "accuracy."

Instrument accuracy is determined by: optics, galvos, calibration grid quality, environment (temperature, vibration, etc.), and calibration quality. It is the subject of instrument design and system maintenance.

Alignment accuracy refers to the ability of a system to transfer its calibrated positioning accuracy to a die. This depends on alignment targets and how they are used.

Alignment targets (scan targets) are special reflective edges on a die that provide position references for locating other die features within the scan field coordinate system. Positions must be established as accurately as possible to avoid partial link blasts or adjacent link damage.

Reference edges may be located by monitoring the reflected energy from a series of overlapping, low-energy, laser pulses as they cross a contrasting edge (or stripe). Intensity change is usually gradual. A correlation function is used to establish the edge positions of an alignment target in the coordinate system. Position accuracy is affected by target material, geometry, location, and alignment strategy.

Chapter 19: Link Cutting/Making

Alignment targets can be made from different types of reflective materials, but they are almost always made of aluminum. Targets are laid down in the same process layer as memory links to eliminate registration errors.

Aluminum, a highly reflective material, is subject to irregular edge quality, which can affect alignment accuracy. Two types of redundancy can be used to minimize these effects: extra marks or extra scans. Extra marks need more space, while extra scans need more time. The best choice depends on die layout and on the alignment strategy.

To use extra marks, the system notes the scan field coordinate positions of several known edges and takes their average to obtain a reference position.

To use extra scans, the system makes several passes at different points along the same edge; it then averages them to obtain a reference position.

Alignment targets always consist of one or more sharp edges in a featureless background. Since each target defines one axis location, it takes two orthogonal targets to establish a point. Related pairs of targets are often combined into a single "L"-shaped feature.

Target Design

Alignment targets consist of reflective features on a contrasting but featureless background. The dimensions of these features and their backgrounds depend on spot size, system accuracy, and edge quality. Applicable dimensions include: target width, scan length, clear area, and target length. Because aluminum targets are susceptible to edge defects, they need to be long enough to support redundant scans.

A target should be wide enough to achieve maximum reflection. This can only be achieved if the target diameter is wide enough to contain 100% of the spot energy. A practical limit is 99.9% of the energy, which corresponds to a spot size 1.5 times the diameter of a standard ($1/e^2$) spot. This is called a "scan spot."

Scan length is the distance a spot must travel to acquire a target. The minimum scan length for a minimum target, excluding errors, is two scan spot diameters. This distance allows reflected intensity to go from minimum to maximum and back to minimum. This is illustrated in Figure 19.

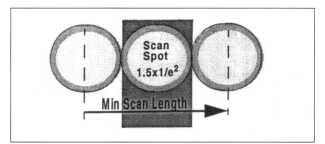

Figure 19. Theoretical minimum scan length.

Practical scans use wider targets (10 μm) and do not begin with a perfectly placed spot (4 μm). So, allowances must be made to accommodate initial position uncertainty. This uncertainty arises from table error (± 6.5 μm), theta error (± 10 μm), and beam error (0.3 μm).

The theta error contribution varies with radius. A positioner with a 100-μrad theta error will introduce a 10-μm translation error at the edge of a 200-μm wafer. The minimum *practical* scan length equals: spot diameter plus link width plus the sum of all positioning errors. In this example, the practical scan length is 4 + 10 + (13 + 20 + 0.3) = 47.3 μm (see Fig. 20).

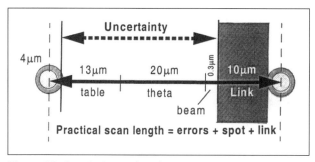

Figure 20. Practical scan length.

Scan targets need enough surrounding clear area to prevent the laser scan from sensing adjacent die features. The minimum clear area depends on the uncertainty of the initial spot position.

The clear area should be larger than the worst-case positioning error. Its dimensions should at least equal the positional uncertainty of the system plus one spot diameter (see Fig. 21).

The opposite edge should also have a clear area of equal dimensions.

Memory designs can conserve die space by arranging target pairs (x, y) so they share a common clear area. This results in distinctive "L"-shaped targets.

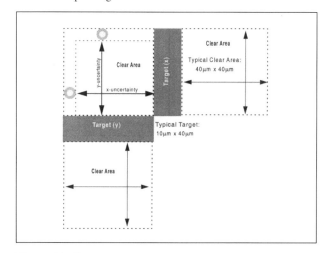

Figure 21. Clear area.

ISBN 0-912035-15-3

Targets can be placed anywhere on a die, but the recommended practice is to put a pair of targets in each corner of every die. This allows a system to align any die individually if needed.

19.1.13 Alignment Strategy
The goal of an alignment strategy is optimal wafer throughput. This calls for minimum die alignment time consistent with accuracy requirements. Die size and target design influence strategy.

The most accurate die alignment occurs when the system uses targets in all four corners of a die that is centered in the scan field. From these eight targets, it can derive x/y offset, rotation, and scaling corrections. Not all of these corrections, however, may be needed.

A small die, or a large die whose links are close to alignment marks, can get by using fewer alignment targets. For these links, the minimum requirements are x offset, y offset, and theta.

Widely spaced link groups on a large die usually need corrections for scaling as well as for theta and x-y offset. Extra alignment targets support these corrections. Systems usually accommodate up to eight targets (four pair).

A properly calibrated memory repair system is capable of extraordinary resolution and accuracy. Both are on the order of a few parts per million. At this resolution, even the smallest temperature change ($< 1°C$) can influence beam positioning components. Repair systems monitor these small but significant accuracy variations by applying a "least-squares fit" (LSF) to several alignment target determinations. The weighted results are used to establish the best alignment between die and scan field coordinate systems. The system performs a least-squares fit alignment during every die/reticle alignment.

Large-die setup considerations apply to small die when the small die are processed in a multidie alignment (MDA). MDA improves system throughput by fitting several small die within the same scan field. The same MDA setup can serve all these die. If eight die are in a setup, MDA has saved seven die alignment times. This offers a significant improvement in system throughput.

Scan field size is the main MDA setup limitation. This limitation is easy to calculate. It is simply the number of die that can fit in a scan field.

The fix-to-attempt (FTA) ratio is a measure of the overall effectiveness of the memory repair process. As the name implies, it indicates the percentage of memory die that have been repaired compared to the number of die that the system tried to repair. Good die, unrepairable die, and partial die are excluded from this calculation. FTAs are usually better than 99%.

FTA encompasses all concerns addressed by this section, including wavelength selection, oxide control, laser energy window setting, link design, system accuracy, die alignment, and alignment strategy.

DONALD V. SMART

19.2 Redundancy for Memory Yield Enhancement

19.2.0 Introduction
One of the most important applications for laser link cutting has been to increase the yield of memory chips, both dynamic random access memories (DRAM), and static random access memories (SRAM). As memory capacity increases, approaching the range of hundreds of megabits per chip, the chip yield would be low unless there were a way to bypass inevitable defects introduced in the manufacturing process. The approach to yield enhancement has been to design and fabricate chips with extra rows and columns of memory elements, test the devices and identify faulty elements, and then vaporize the interconnecting lines to the rows and columns containing those elements.

As a specific example, a 1-Mbit DRAM chip contains 32 spare rows of 512 bits and 32 pairs of spare columns of 256 bits. The links consist of doped polysilicon film. Links are cut with a 1.06-μm Nd:YAG laser to remove rows or columns with defective elements. Typical repairs may require cutting of several tens of links on a chip.

The evolution of laser-implemented redundancy, or simply "laser redundancy," as a production process used to improve semiconductor DRAM and SRAM yields, has gained unanimous industry acceptance. Increasingly demanding process requirements and associated implications for laser equipment have been met with continuously improved solutions. Laser redundancy is now being used to improve the yields on microprocessors with imbedded memories and other semiconductor circuits.

19.2.1 Development of Redundancy
The concept of laser-implemented redundancy had its genesis in research investigating the connection of different layers in a semiconductor device. This research suggested the laser could be used to disconnect electrical conductors, thereby modifying circuits after completion of most fabrication steps. Such modification has been implemented in the manufacture of large memory circuits, dramatically increasing the output of production facilities. Today, nearly all-dynamic and static DRAMs and SRAMs have been designed to be repairable by laser. A typical repair consists of testing the memory circuit to determine faulty elements in the array, then substituting available spares built into the circuit. The laser is used to vaporize electrical links, disconnecting the array row or column, which contains a faulty element. Subsequently, other links are opened in the decoding circuitry of a spare row or column, giving it the address of the one disconnected (see Fig. 1).

ISBN 0-912035-15-3

Chapter 19: Link Cutting/Making

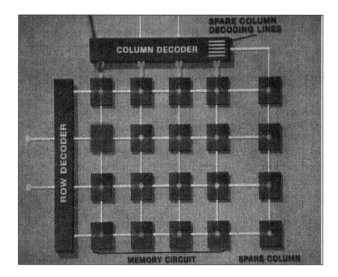

Figure 1. Use of redundant cells to replace defective cells by cutting relevant links.

In the late 1970s, a group at Bell Labs in Allentown, Pennsylvania undertook the development of a laser-redundancy process intended to increase production yields of 64K DRAMs. During startup production of such large memory arrays, typical yields without redundancy had been less than 10%; many of the rejects were due to a small number of defects. To overcome such low yields, Bell tested the fabricated memory array at the wafer level (during wafer probe) and replaced rows and columns containing faulty cells with some set of the four spare rows and columns provided in the circuit design. The addition of spare elements to the layout increased the size of a device by 3–5% — a small penalty to pay for the 1.4–30 times increase in yield that was achieved.

Before implementing the process, Bell extensively researched material and equipment requirements. Several potential link materials were evaluated, including aluminum and polysilicon structures compatible with Bell's MOS technology. Polysilicon links were selected for their lower contamination potential and higher probability of being successfully disconnected.

A Q-switched Nd:YAG laser was used to "blow" these links because of its ability repeatably to produce very brief, very sharp pulses of energy at kilohertz repetition rates and its proven reliability in years of hybrid microcircuit production. Even so, the standard pulse width of commercially available Nd:YAG lasers (typically 150 nsec) had to be reduced to fewer than 50 nsec to provide an acceptable process window.

In 1989 the diode-pumped YLF laser (1.047 µm) was introduced, and quickly replaced the lamp-pumped YAG lasers. The smaller, more compact diode-pumped lasers have pulse durations in the 4–15 nsec range.

Early circuit geometries determined two major equipment parameters: laser beam diameter and positioning tolerance. A beam diameter of approximately 8 µm was needed to remove each link with a single laser pulse, and the center of the beam needed to be positioned within 2.5 µm of the center of the target to accomplish the task a very high percentage of the time. A commercial laser system can provide the desired beam diameter and can meet requirements for positioning resolution and repeatability.

The systems capabilities have kept pace with the continued shrinking of the link pitch. Today the systems are accurate to ± 0.25 µm over a 35-mm field and can achieve spot sizes of less than 2 micrometers at 1.047 µm and handle 150-, 200-, and 300-mm wafers. All systems are required to have autofocus.

Production evolution has moved toward little or no human involvement and divides testing and laser processing into two separate process steps allowing maximum equipment utilization. As a corollary, automatic load and unload stations with automatic alignment, wafer identification, and tracking (by serial number) have been developed. A central management system communicating with the test and laser systems as necessary controls the entire process.

19.2.2 Laser Choice

Traditional "link blowing" has been accomplished using Nd:YAG or Nd:YLF laser sources operating at 1.064 or 1.047 µm, respectively. These conventional wavelengths perform extremely well for polysilicon link materials but can have serious limitations when cutting metal-based links.

The current development efforts for DRAM have included a search for new link materials useful in smaller geometries. To compete in the speed/power tradeoff, designers of these larger memory arrays have required lower interconnect resistances and, therefore, lower sheet resistances than possible with highly doped polysilicon. Polysilicon-silicide sandwiches, or other refractory metals systems, are being used to reduce interconnect resistance. As links become more metal-like in physical properties, the need has grown for an alternate wavelength better suited for metal structures, which led to the introduction of 1.3-µm laser technology, which will be described in Section 19.2.4.

The choice of the laser wavelength and pulse width depends on the link structure and the spot size required. General guidelines are:

1. 1.047 µm is the wavelength of choice for polysilicon links and for the smallest possible spot sizes. The pulse width is generally 9 ns, but 15 or 4 may provide a larger process window depending on the particular link structure.
2. The 1.3-µm wavelength is generally used for metal links or metal sandwich structures. Early work was done with the Nd:YLF laser at 1.321 µm with a pulse width of 27 ns. Currently, the laser of choice is the Nd:YVO$_4$ (vanadate) operating at 1.343 µm with a pulse width of 6 or 9 ns depending on the link structure. A further discussion of this point will be found in Section 19.2.4.

EDWARD J. SWENSON

19.2.3 Hardware Description

Commercial equipment available for memory yield improvement offers automatic wafer handling and positioning accuracy better than 0.35 µm. The wafer is first tested on a separate probe facility which identifies the defective circuits and prepares a map locating the defects with respect to fiducial marks. The map is stored in a computer.

A cassette of wafers is transferred to the repair machine. A diagram of a repair machine and its optics is presented in Figure 2. The machine loads each wafer, identifies it and retrieves the map of defective elements, positions the wafer and vaporizes the appropriate links. This removes defective cells and allows the redundant circuit to function. This procedure allows for maximum utilization of the equipment, because the repair system does not have to wait for the testing to be completed on the same machine.

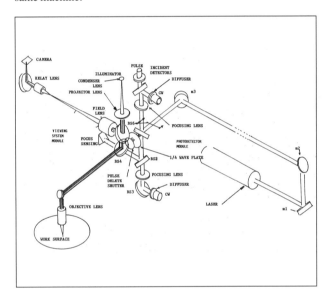

Figure 2. Diagram of optics of memory enhanced system.

Table 1 presents typical laser parameters for each of the two wavelengths, 1.047 and 1.3 µm.

Table 1. Representative Laser Parameters for Memory Yield Enhancement

Laser type	Conventional Nd:YLF	Longer wavelength Nd:YLF
Wavelength	1.047 µm	1.3 µm
Pulse duration	4–13 ns	6.5–9.5 ns
Pulse rate	to 6000 Hz	> 6000Hz
Energy/pulse	6 µJ	6 µJ
Spot size	2.1–8 µm	2.3–6 µm

19.2.4 Absorptivity Considerations

If one selects the laser parameters properly, almost all practical link structures should be cut cleanly. An important issue is that the underlying silicon substrate should not be damaged. The low end of the processing window, that is, the ability to cut the link, should fall well below the high end, which is damaging the silicon.

In order to optimize the process of link cutting, the contrast in absorption between the link material and the silicon underneath it should be maximized. The absorption of most link metals varies only slowly in the range from 1 to 1.3 µm, whereas the absorption of silicon decreases substantially as one goes from 1 to 1.3 µm. If one uses a laser wavelength near 1.3 µm, one may obtain a much wider process window.

Using a laser wavelength near 1.3 µm instead of the more conventional 1.047 µm leaves the low end of the processing window essentially unchanged, while the high end is raised by a factor of three to ten. The exact value depends on the doping level of the silicon.

Figure 3 shows results for cutting of links using a 1.047-µm laser just below the damage threshold and using a 1.32-µm laser operating in the middle of the process window.

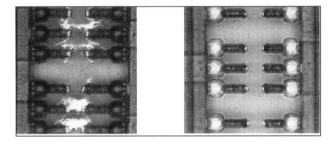

Figure 3. Link cutting results at 1.3 µm compared to 1.047 µm. Left: cutting just below damage threshold at 1.047 µm. Right: cutting centered in the process window at 1.3 µm.

Thus cutting of links on silicon substrates is now often performed using a laser operating at a wavelength near 1.3 µm, such as Nd:YLF at 1.321 µm or Nd:YVO$_4$ at 1.343 µm. Another method for increasing the energy absorption in the region where it is desired is the use of interference effects. This is discussed in Chapter 17, but will be reviewed here for completeness.

Figure 4 shows a typical link structure for laser processing. Both the dielectric layers consist of a single layer or multiple layers of films. A typical link may be one or two micrometers thick.

The effect of interference on processing of multilayer structures allows the energy absorbed by the link material to be maximized, and simultaneously reduces the energy reaching the substrate.

An important issue for high-quality link cutting is the ability to remove the very bottom part of the link material without damaging the substrate in order to realize a "high"-resistance open state.

ISBN 0-912035-15-3

For most link structures, the original link thickness is large enough compared with its optical absorption depth effectively to block the laser energy from going through it to reach the structure beneath. Thus there is no contribution by the structure beneath on the interference effect. But during the processing, as soon as the remaining link becomes thin enough, as material is removed from the structure, the laser energy penetrates through to the substrate and the interference effect by the film layers beneath the link starts to play a significant role in whether the remaining bottom portions of the link can be efficiently cleaned away.

The optimization, from the viewpoint of interference, is carried out in two steps:

1. Optimizing the layer structure above the link when the link is complete
2. Optimizing the layer structure below the link material, when the remaining thickness during trimming is less than the optical absorption depth

Calculations have indicated that the absorption in the link material is an oscillatory function of the thickness of the two dielectric layers, with periodic maxima. Examples have already been presented in Chapter 17 and in Section 19.1. One chooses the thickness of the layers so as to work near one of the maxima. This allows the energy to be deposited in the link material that is to be evaporated and reduces the energy reaching the substrate.

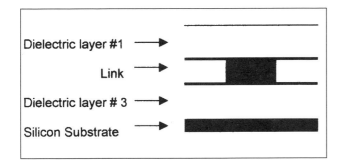

Figure 4. Typical link structure.

EDWARD J. SWENSON

19.2.5 Spot Size Consideration

There are two steps to choosing the most appropriate spot size for a link cutting application. The first step is to determine the theoretical range of spots that can physically fit in the areas targeted for link cutting. After determining a valid range, the second step is to base the final spot size selection on the observed quality of the cut. These two steps will be explained in detail.

In this section we will assume the energy distribution of the laser beam is Gaussian and that the term *spot size* refers to the diameter of the focused beam measured across the center of the beam between the "$1/e^2$" points (points where the energy density drops to 13.5% of the maximum energy at the beam's center).

Link Geometry

Spot size (S) selection is fundamentally constrained by the link's width (W), length (L), and pitch (P), as well as by the placement accuracy (A) of the laser beam delivery system. Figure 5 is a graphical representation of all the factors involved.

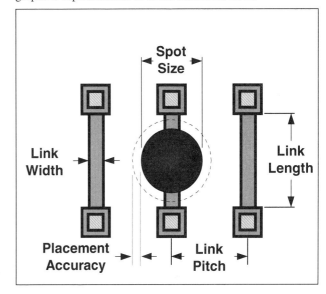

Figure 5. Factors used when computing spot size range.

The objective is to choose a spot size that is large enough to cover the desired link,

$$S \geq W + (2A)$$

yet small enough to prevent damage to adjacent links or active devices

$$S \leq (2P) - (2A) - W$$

and small enough not to exceed the length of the link

$$S \leq L - (2A)$$

The spot size range includes all sizes that fall within the bounds set by these three criteria.

Example: $L = 8.0 \, \mu m$, $W = 0.8 \, \mu m$, $P = 4.0 \, \mu m$, $A = 0.35 \, \mu m$

$S \geq 0.8 \, \mu m + (2 \times 0.35 \, \mu m) = 1.5 \, \mu m$

$S \leq (2 \times 4.0 \, \mu m) - (2 \times 0.35 \, \mu m) - 0.8 \, \mu m = 6.5 \, \mu m$

$S \leq 8 \, \mu m - (2 \times 0.35 \, \mu m) = 7.3 \, \mu m$

$1.5 \, \mu m \leq S \leq 6.5 \, \mu m$

Cut Quality

Once the theoretical spot size range is calculated, one must decide what size within the range is most beneficial. This requires some experimentation. Choosing the best spot size within the range involves balancing opposing constraints:

On the one hand, a larger spot:

- Allows for looser focusing accuracy (larger depth of field);
- Expands the range of pulse energies that will produce reliable link cuts. The pulse energy range is used to gauge the sensitivity of the laser process to variations in the link structure. In this sense, a larger range of acceptable pulse energies represents a more tolerant laser process.

On the other hand, a larger spot:

- Has a more gradual change in irradiance from center to edge, subjecting the area immediately surrounding the link to irradiance nearly the same as that over the link — areas that are preferred to remain unaltered. Historically, links that were composed completely or in part of polysilicon could be removed with such low energy settings that the surrounding areas could easily withstand damage. Today, links with higher vaporization thresholds (composed of various metals) require higher energy settings. Surrounding areas have difficulty withstanding these intensities. A smaller spot forces the irradiance to drop more quickly so that surrounding areas are exposed to lower irradiance than the link, lessening the chance of damage.
- Generates a greater volume of molten link material at the edges of the cut. This material, if it exists, can be found surrounding or streaming away from the cut and is often referred to as "slag." The existence of slag raises concerns of forming unintended conductive connections. A smaller spot forces the transition between melting and vaporizing to occur in a shorter space. Therefore, smaller spots limit the area of link exposed to melting temperatures, which in turn reduces the volume of material contributing to the formation of slag (see Fig. 6).

Spot Selection Process

The objective is to choose the spot that maximizes energy range and positioning tolerance. The procedure is to start with the largest spot size in the range and cut some links with a range of energies. Note the range of energies that produce acceptable cuts without damaging the surrounding area. Test for effects caused by mispositioning the spot because any laser delivery system will include some error, causing higher values of irradiance to fall off the link and into the surrounding areas. Positioning tolerance is measured as the range of offsets tolerated without damaging surrounding areas or neighboring links.

Then reduce the spot size and repeat the tests, again noting the acceptable energy range and positioning tolerance. Continue reducing the spot until the whole range of spot sizes has been tested. Finally, review the results and choose the spot size that maximizes these two criteria. This spot will provide for the most robust laser process for this particular link geometry and material.

Repeat this test for each link design. What may appear as a subtle process change may result in a different spot size choice.

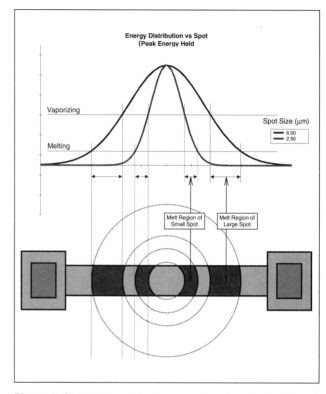

Figure 6. Comparison of "melt regions" produced with different spot sizes.

JAMES A. DUMESTRE

19.3 Link Making

19.3.0 Introduction

Lasers have been used to form electrical connections in electronic circuits for a number of years. Previous make-link technologies are explained in an article by S. S Cohen and G. H. Chapman (1). The most reliable type of link that can be formed works on the principle that two adjacent lines of metal can be exposed to a short laser pulse and thermal expansion of the metal fractures the dielectric separating them. At the same time, the rapidly expanding material flows through the crack to connect the lines with a low-resistance metallic short. The process works between adjacent lines on the same level of metallization or between two levels of metal. The means of forming links between lines, as described here, has been shown to work reliably with the most common metallization system for semiconductor manufacture, aluminum metal, and SiO_2 insulator.

Potential applications of a laser make-link are at least as extensive as the laser break-link. The ability to both make and break links allows for a much broader range of repair algorithms. If repair is the goal, many more combinations of replacing nonfunctioning circuitry with functional circuitry can be achieved. Furthermore, a design that incorporates additive as well removable circuit elements can be made very large, which is the goal of wafer scale integration (WSI) and is well described in Reference 2. It has been found that the metal make-link process is more reliable, has much greater yield, and is more compatible with CMOS fabrication than metal break-link.

19.3.1 Earlier Work

Many ideas have been proposed in the past to make connections between two otherwise insulated interconnect lines. The earliest attempt can be traced back to 1976, in which orange laser pulses were used to make links between metal and semiconductor substrates (3). However, the technique involved an uncontrollable micro-explosion of the target materials; so the process was not satisfactorily robust. Later, in 1984, an alternative method for making a link was disclosed in a patent (4). This method proposed creating two back-to-back bipolar junctions on a polysilicon (poly) island. The poly could then be heated with a laser, causing the thermally isolated block of material to heat up. The n^+ diffusions would then extend across the bar, resulting in an n-doped polysilicon link. The resistance of this link will be higher than an in situ doped poly line, and the process requires a modified CMOS process; thus it did not gain commercial acceptance.

Another problem with these process is the narrow energy range over which efficient heating and dopant diffusion could occur without damaging or blowing out the link. This "blow-out" phenomenon was recognized as a problem with the polysilicon make-link, and in the same patent, the authors suggested that the diffusions could be placed in the silicon itself. This has become known as a diffused link, and it meets the standard process compatibility requirement, but it requires that the circuit be restructured on a processed silicon device. It also requires a specially designed long laser pulse that is highly absorbed in the silicon surface, such as an argon ion laser. This process results in intolerable substrate leakage for most commercial applications (1–4).

Other means of making connections included the use of alternate materials, such as amorphous silicon between two levels of metallization, which is not compatible with standard process methods. Large pads of metal have been connected with an excimer laser, but the yield and reliability has never justified the expense of processing. In the end, laser-formed connections have not been found in commercial applications, until the advent of the laser-induced cracked-passivation make-link, which is described in the following section.

19.3.2 Principles

The formation of a laser-induced metallic make-link is based on a set of coincidental properties relating to the materials used in microelectronics manufacture (5). Metallization in silicon circuitry almost universally consists of aluminum-based alloys.

More advanced metallization schemes use copper, but the fundamental properties required to form the links are the same. The following properties are all salient to the creation of metallic links:

1. The metals are highly thermally conductive and thermally expansive.
2. They are plastic and easily conform to the shape of their surroundings.
3. They have low melting temperatures relative to the surrounding dielectric, which is primarily an amorphous ceramic such as SiO_2 or Si_3N_4.
4. Molten metal has a low vapor pressure, allowing a large energy tolerance between the onset of melting and evaporation.

All these properties contrast to the very low thermal expansion coefficient and thermal conductivity of the dielectric. The dielectrics are also highly brittle. Thus the metal, which is encased by dielectric, can absorb focused laser energy and expand within the time of a Q-switched laser pulse. However, the brittle dielectric will not be able to support the expansion without fracturing. Once a fracture occurs, the molten metal is able to expand and flow through the resulting crack.

One characteristic of dry-etched metallization manufacturing is a sharp corner along the side wall of the metal line. These corners represent mechanical stress concentration points for thermally expanding metal, heated by the laser, contained within the dielectric. The amorphous nature of the dielectric removes any consideration of grain boundaries associated with a crack trajectory. Thus a crack will form generally between points of greatest stress concentration and follow an energetically favorable path.

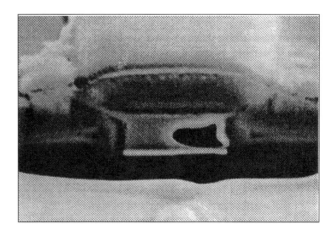

Figure 1. FIB cross section of a 2-μm-wide metal line after absorption of 0.33 μJ of laser energy showing ejected metal at the surface and a void remaining in the line.

The phenomenon of dielectric fracture and metal flow is seen in Figure 1. This is a cross-sectional image, taken with a focused ion beam (FIB), of a 2-μm-wide metal line that was exposed to a 15-ns Nd:YLF laser pulse. The energy was 0.45 µJ, and the spot size was 3 µm ($1/e^2$) diameter. The metal was passivated by a 1.2-µm-thick layer of plasma-deposited Si_3N_4, which cracked from the upper corners of the metal line to the upper surface. At the surface of the passivation is the metal that escaped and flowed through the cracks and resolidified at the surface.

Vertical Links

The most straightforward type of direct metallic connection that can be made to take advantage of the dielectric fracture phenomenon would employ a vertical link configuration. An upper layer of metal crosses over the lower level with an opening for the laser to heat up the lower line. Shown schematically in Figure 2 is the first metallic link that was reported (6, 7). The upper level of metal must overlap the region where the crack would terminate. The laser spot must also be small enough to impinge mostly inside the annular opening so the crack will be sure to terminate on both lines.

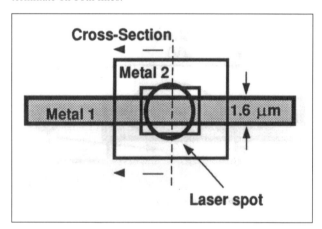

Figure 2. Schematic of the laser spot and cross-sectional image of a vertical link between lower metal 1 and upper metal 2, showing the 2.2-µm round spot and cross-section plane.

The major advantage of the vertical link is that the cracks are completely terminated on metal lines. Since the metal is plastic, any stresses induced in the structure will be absorbed in the metal without causing additional pressure on the dielectric. This results in a broad process window and a robust link. A cross section of a vertical link is shown in Figure 3. In this structure, the metallic link is visible as the light-colored line between the lower and the upper metal layers.

The link is formed mostly from extruded metal from the lower level, which flowed in the cracks originating from the one lower layer. This results in a deficit of metal, which remains in the line. The dark regions in the middle of the lower line are voids that result from the displaced metal. Metal flows due to the thermal expansion while it is molten. Then, as it cools, there will be voids left in the metal, as seen in Figure 3. The presence of these voids may pose a reliability problem, since there is a divergence in the current path. Electromigration experiments have been conducted to investigate the lifetime of the vertical links at accelerating stress conditions. A detailed discussion can be found in Section 19.3.3.

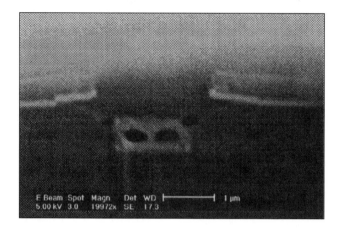

Figure 3. FIB cross section of a vertical link between the lower metal and two sides of the hole in upper-level metal.

Lateral Links

A lateral link between two adjacent lines of metal on the same level of metallization can also be formed. There are constraints, however, that must be applied to make a successful lateral link:

1. The lines must be wide enough to allow metal to flow into a crack.
2. There must be sufficient overlap of the lines.
3. The passivation on top of the metal must be made planar and thicker than half the gap between the lines.

One example layout is shown schematically in Figure 4.

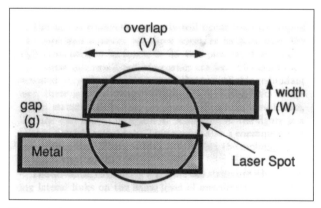

Figure 4. Schematic of the layout and laser position for a symmetric lateral link between two lines of metal (seen in the plane of the chip).

The size of the gap, g, is determined by the minimum allowable design rule space between metal lines. Typically this is between 0.5 and 2.0 µm, depending on the technology used. If the minimum allowable space is greater than 2.0 µm, a lateral link technology may not be practical for standard on-chip silicon circuitry. If, however, the dielectric layers are known to be thicker, the gap width can be increased accordingly. The metal line widths, W, should be at least 1.5 g and the overlap, V, should be at least 4 g. The $1/e^2$ laser spot diameter should be approximately equal to V plus the positioning error of the laser system.

Thermal expansion, cracking, and metal flow occur equally on both sides of the link in the lateral configuration, which is favorable from a reliability point of view. There will be less metal lost in each line as compared to the vertical link. The lateral connection will be secure as long as the energy chosen does not cause the outside edge cracks to propagate to the surface. This leads to a density consideration, since a second link cannot be placed at a minimum distance without there being a probability of an unintentional link. The lateral link process considerations are explained in Reference 8 and its references.

In the case of the symmetric link, the laser is positioned between the two lines. This assures that the fractures will be generated from the inside corners simultaneously. Both the thermal mass and edges are guaranteed to be symmetric in this configuration, which allows a connection between two ends in the same level of metallization. In order to implement a lateral link between two levels of metal, one of the layers must be brought to tabs adjacent to the other layer, as shown in Figure 5.

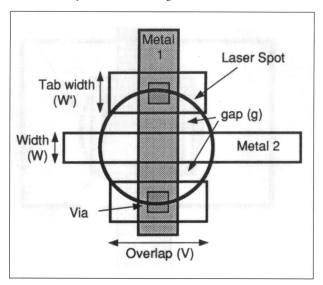

Figure 5. Schematic of the layout of a redundant lateral link implementation to connect two perpendicular metal line crossings.

In this configuration, the laser should be aimed over the center line with a spot wide enough to encompass both tabs. Since the tabs are finite in length, less laser energy is required to reach the same temperature as the line, which dissipates heat through the conductor. As a rule of thumb, the tab width, V, should be approximately equal to the full-width at half-maximum (FWHM) diameter of the laser spot size, which is approximately 0.6 of the $1/e^2$ diameter. The gap, g, should also be of minimum dimension, as should be the center conductor. Since metal flows from the center line as well as from the tabs, there should be sufficient metal in the link to avoid electromigration concerns.

The actual connection usually will occur from the top of the lines and connect all three together, as seen from the FIB cross section in Figure 6. In this picture, it is evident that there are small outside corner cracks. The cracks are arrested very close to the metal. Because of this redundant line, there is little worry of making accidental links to adjacent structures, as may happen with simple metal links, like the one shown in Figure 4. Also seen in the figure is a void in the left metal tab. This void is also a consequence of extruded metal. These voids occur within the molten region of the heated metal.

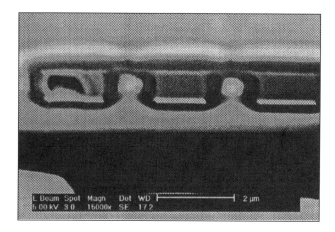

Figure 6. FIB cross section of a double lateral link between two metals and the center length of upper-level metal.

The advantages of using a double tab structure when making lateral links on the same level of metallization include a relaxed positioning accuracy requirement and more metal available to form reliable links. This structure allows the links to be formed with a laser spot that is larger than a comparable vertical link structure. The availability of extra metal also ensures that less metal will be lost from the line, leading to better electromigration resistance. Furthermore, there is inherent link redundancy, so if one side fails to form a link, the second one will.

19.3.3 Reliability

As mentioned in the earlier sections, the remaining voids in the lower metal after laser irradiation could invoke electromigration failure because of the high current density. Accelerating experiments have be performed to investigate the failure mechanisms and the related lifetime.

Vertical link samples employed for this experiment had a 4-μm-wide lower metal line aligned to a 6 × 6 μm upper metal opening, which were zapped by a 1047-nm Nd:YLF laser with a 15-ns pulse and 3.0-μm FWHM spot diameter. Then the samples were stressed at a fixed current density and different temperatures. The current density in the links was approximately 3.0 mA/cm^2. The temperature dependence of the mean time to failure (MTF) for a double-link structure is plotted in Figure 7, from which the activation energy is found to be 0.66 eV. A lifetime of 38 years is obtained by extrapolating the line back to room temperature (300 K) at the accelerating current density. It is noticed that the activation energy is in the range that can be associated with electromigration failure, although it is a little larger than the reported values (0.55–0.60 eV) for Al-Si-Cu alloy.

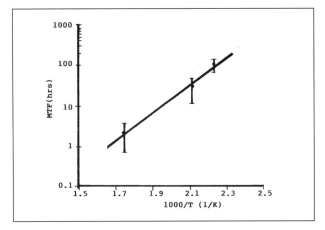

Figure 7. Arrhenius plot of vertical links with 4 µm lower metal and 6 × 6 µm upper opening.

Further experiments suggested that the lifetime is a function of laser energy as can be seen in Figure 8. Shown in comparison is the energy dependence of the electrical resistance of individual links. As expected, the lifetime and resistance show opposite trends over the range of laser energy, and the maximum lifetime corresponds to the lowest electrical resistance at the optimal energy of 0.7 µJ.

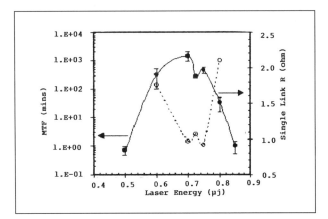

Figure 8. The link lifetime and the electrical resistance as functions of laser energy.

The above results indicate that electromigration may not be a major reliability concern if both structural parameters and laser conditions are well optimized. As a matter of fact, the link sheet (in 3D view) and the connecting upper and lower metal consists of a Blech structure. The mass flux at one boundary of the link sheet is blocked by the bottom TiN layer of the upper metal frame and largely alleviated at the other boundary by the abruptly decreasing current density in the lower metal line. Consequently, electromigration in the link sheet, which is much shorter than the critical length, is effectively restrained by the so-called backflow (Blech effect). Therefore, the apparently thin link sheet itself is relatively reliable. What needs to be considered is the lower metal line, since the remaining voids exacerbate electromigration. One structural solution has been proposed to restrain electromigration in the lower metal and improve the overall reliability. This will be discussed in detail in the following section.

19.3.4 Implementation

Strucutal Optimization

If a link site is desired between a lower and an upper level of metal, either for an on-chip repair purpose or to program a multi-chip module, the ideal implementation for the most reliable link is the vertical configuration. Simply place a second-level metal crossing over a first-level metal with an opening large enough to have the laser spot mostly absorbed by the first-level metal. This way, no vias need to be prefabricated, and the link itself will connect the two levels of metal at the crossover point.

The first consideration is the size of the hole that is needed to expose the lower metal to the laser. This size is limited to the FWHM diameter of the focused laser spot, plus an acceptable positioning accuracy. With today's infrared laser systems, the smallest spot size is approximately 1.5 µm, and the positioning accuracy is 0.3 µm (3 sigma). Thus a 1.8-µm opening is about the smallest acceptable hole for very high yield. Figure 9 shows a vertical link with a 2.3-µm opening. The lower level of metal was 1.2 µm wide beneath the opening, and the pulse diameter was about 2.3 µm.

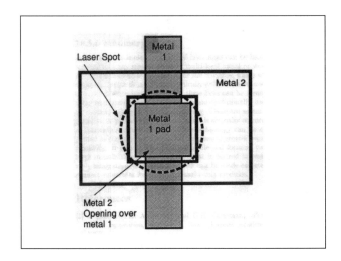

Figure 9. Schematic of another vertical link implementation with enlarged lower metal outside the link annulus.

The purpose of the design shown in Figure 9 is intentionally to build up a mass gradient. A backflow effect can then be induced in the lower metal line to block electromigration. As a rule of thumb, it is suggested that the line width be designed to ensure the primary reliability of lower metal, while introducing backflow by enlarging the two wings outside the link formation area, so that it would not increase the severity of electromigration in the lower line.

Scalability

These dimensions of the vertical link are completely scalable. If a wider laser spot is needed because of the equipment, the hole and all the other line widths must also be increased to accommodate. For wafer scale or multichip module dimensions, the lines may be as wide as 10 µm with a hole in the upper level as large as 16 µm. In a multichip module (MCM) application, the metal should be at least 2 µm thick, perhaps as thick as 5 µm, to accommodate much displaced material. In high-density designs, like memory repair or programmable gate arrays, it is preferred to have link sizes as small as possible; the scalability also largely depends on the mass of the lower metal near the link. In principle, reducing the interlayer dielectric thickness would also broaden the downward scalability since the crack path would be reduced.

An Example

A sample layout of an interconnect array using vertical links is shown in Figure 10. There are two links per crossing to maintain parity of metal pitch in both vertical and horizontal directions. Of course, the lines can be broken up to have single metal 1 tracks, all 4 µm wide, running perpendicular to the metal 2 tracks. The actual sizes of the lines depend on the density requirement of the interconnect and the design rules of the fabrication process. Lines this wide would be appropriate for chip-to-chip routing. The metal thickness in this example should be 1–1.5 µm. If metals as thick as 2–3 µm are to be used, the dimensions should be scaled up by 1.5, so the minimum metal width would be 6 µm.

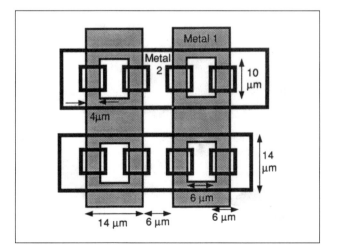

Figure 10. Schematic of a 20-µm metal pitch interconnect layout with two vertical links per crossing.

19.3.5 Laser Energy

The energy required to link connecting lines depends on the volume of material being melted and the time frame of the laser pulse. An infrared laser is recommended so that the energy is not absorbed in any of the dielectric layers. The wavelength is not a critical parameter, since the metal is well shielded and there is no chance of any significant radiation penetrating to the substrate.

What is needed is to have enough energy absorbed at the surface of the metal to heat up the metal line to the point of melting, in a time short enough that the surrounding dielectric remains near room temperature. Since the thermal diffusion in aluminum and copper is at least 50 times greater than SiO_2, laser pulses between 5 and 20 ns should meet this criterion. Thicker metals may require longer pulses. Surface reflection must also be taken into account, so the energy dose will vary based on surface coatings and the nature of the dielectric thicknesses on top of the metal.

The laser absorption in the line for making links is determined in the same way as the energy required to cut the lines, except the energy for linking is much lower. A good approximation for the ideal vertical link energy is approximately 1/4 the energy used for reliable cuts on the same metal thickness and width with the same spot size. For lateral links, the energy used is approximately half the cut energy, but the spot area should be at least doubled to accommodate the tabs on either side of the line. The upper energy limit is determined by the upper metal edges cracking to the surface.

19.3.6 Summary

In summary, metal laser links can be incorporated into any standard silicon multilevel metal process. Accommodations have to be made for the link area, which will always be larger than a lithographically defined via between two metallization levels. However, these links can be formed using commercial laser systems that are traditionally used for memory repair. There are no extra materials or processing steps than what is normally required to fabricate a silicon circuit, so this technology can be exploited in place of or even to complement cutting for purposes of greater flexibility. It also enables pretesting the die and forming very large monolithic circuits, such as what is desired in wafer scale integration. Furthermore, links can be made on interconnect substrates for routing of multichip modules.

References

1. S. S Cohen and G. H. Chapman, "Laser Beam Processing and Wafer-Scale Integration," from *Beam Processing Technologies*, E. G. Einsprich, S. S. Cohen, and R. N. Singh (Eds.), Academic Press 1989.
2. J. Raffel, A. H. Anderson, and G. H. Chapman, 1989: *Wafer Scale Integration*, Kluwer Academic, Chapter 7, p. 363.
3. Nicolaos S. Platakis, "Mechanism of Laser-induced Metal-Semiconductor Electrical Connections in MOS Structures," *Journal of Applied Physics,* **47** (5), (May 1976).
4. U.S. Patent No. 4,455,495, Programmable Semiconductor Integrated Circuitry Including a Programming Semiconductor Element.

5. U.S. Patent No. 5,861,325, Technique for Producing Interconnecting Conductive Links.
6. J. B. Bernstein, T. M. Ventura, and A. T. Radomski, "High Density Laser Linking of Metal Interconnect," *IEEE Trans. on Comp., Pack., and Manuf. Tech.*, **14,** 590–3 (December 1994).
7. J. B. Bernstein, Wei Zhang and Carl H. Nicholas, "Laser Formed Metallic Connections," *IEEE Trans. Comp. Pack. and Manuf. Tech., Part B: Advanced Packaging,* **21** (2), p. 194 (May 1998).
8. R. L. Rasera and J. B. Bernstein, "Laser Linking of Metal Interconnect: Linking Dynamics and Failure Analysis," *IEEE Trans. on Comp., Pack. and Manuf. Tech., Part A,* **19,** 554–61 (December 1996).

J. B. BERNSTEIN
WEI ZHANG

19.4 Personalization

19.4.1 Definitions and Basic Terms

Personalization

Personalization is the process of customizing a logic integrated circuit device for a specific application. The starting material for laser personalization is usually a gate array device on which all transistors are prefabricated in rows of uncommitted gates. The gates are interconnected via a metal grid comprising two or more metal layers (1). In the personalization process the connectivity of the metal grid is modified so as to interconnect the gates per a predefined logic net list, which determines the logic functionality of the device. Laser personalization can be realized by metal link cutting, by link making, or by laser direct write of the metal interconnect grid. Laser-based personalization systems and laser-programmable gate array devices (LPGAs) have been commercially available since 1990.

Damage Diameter

Damage diameter refers to the overall diameter that undergoes a phase transformation as a result of the laser pulse. When link cutting is employed, a certain radius of damage is associated with each laser pulse. The radius of damage is a function of the laser pulse energy, pulse width, film thickness, and heat conductance of the target material. For example, when cutting a narrow aluminum metal line 1 µm thick and 1 µm wide deposited over an insulator with a Nd:YAG laser pulse of energy 6 J/cm^2, pulse diameter of 1 × 1 mm^2 and pulse duration of 70 ns, the metal cut will extend 1.5 µm in length and the metal will be melted (and resolidified) over a total diameter (length) of 3.5 µm, which defines the damage diameter. The radius of damage of such aluminum lines increases by approximately 0.25 µm per each J/cm^2.

Diameter of the Personalization Spot

If we denote the critical dimension of an integrated circuit by δ (the critical dimension of a device is the dimension of the smallest drawn geometry on the silicon – usually it is the gate length), the pitch of the contacted metal grid of the device will be about 4δ. To achieve a dense personalized device, the personalization spot size must be of smaller diameter than 4δ. The damage diameter has to be even less. Presently, for state of the art devices, δ = 0.25 µm. As technology advances, this number decreases by a factor of two approximately each 4 years.

19.4.2 Personalization by Link Cutting: Choice of Laser

State of the art laser-programmable logic devices comprise well over 100,000 gates, with 100 to 200 laser cut points per gate. To achieve laser personalization of a device in less than an hour, the laser system must treat about 10,000 points per second at a random sequence, with precision better than 0.15 µm. A Q-switched Nd:YAG laser can generate this pulse rate, but it requires a pulse energy stabilization mechanism, because this rate exceeds the inverse lifetime of the population inversion energy level. Without pulse energy stabilization, the first pulse in a row will have a much higher energy than the next in the sequence, and pulses at a random sequence will all vary in energy beyond the allowed energy process window.

The energy density for material processing at the relevant dimension range is between 2 and 8 J/cm^2. To account for various energy loss mechanisms, the average laser power commonly used is about 1 W. The commonly used wavelength is 532 nm. Shaping the beam through a rectangular aperture can form laser pulses of dimensions as low as 0.7 × 1.4 µm^2, which is adequate for submicrometer device personalization.

Ar$^+$ lasers have also been used, particularly for mixed link-cutting/link-making personalization applications, and for laser direct-write applications.

19.4.3 The Personalization Process

Personalization by Link Cutting

Theoretical calculations and practical experiments show that given the thermal conductivity of aluminum, which is the main constituent of the metal system of the interconnect grid of integrated circuits, the aluminum latent heat, and its temperature of evaporation, and given the thickness of metal lines in ICs, which are between 1 and 0.5 µm, the amount of energy needed directly to cut a metal line is such that the damage diameter will extend over at least 3 µm. While this was acceptable at times where the critical dimension δ was 1.5 µm and above, and may still be acceptable for processing of multichip substrates where metal lines and spaces are above 5 µm, this large damage diameter is unacceptable for devices of submicrometer dimensions with δ 0.25 µm or less.

The modern process of laser personalization by link cutting is based on a combined laser ablation – dry etching process. The metal grid is coated by a laser-sensitive etch-resistant material with high absorption coefficient, low vaporization heat, and low thermal conductivity (2). The laser-sensitive coating is ablated by laser pulses, followed by a dry reactive ion etching process of the device in a chlorine-based plasma. In the personalization process, a series of apertures are opened in the laser-sensitive coating over the metal segments to be removed. The device is then transferred to a low-pressure reactive ion etch chamber, where the metal is etched, and the rest of the laser-sensitive coating is stripped by a fluorine-based plasma chemistry. The device is then ready for electrical measurement.

References

1. M. Janai, *Solid State Technology* **36-3,** 35–8 (March 1993).
2. U.S. Patent No. 5,329,152.

MEIR JANAI

Notes

ISBN 0-912035-15-3

Chapter 20

Repair

20.1 Repair Needs

Today's computing systems, with their application of high-density packaging and VLSI devices, represent a marked change from the electronic printed circuit boards made only a few years ago. The development of multilayered wiring, very large scale integration and CMOS technology has created new opportunities for microelectronic applications, but has also created a range of new issues in the area of repair, rework, and modification of microelectronic assemblies and devices.

Historically, corrective processes were considered a subset of the troubleshooting or diagnostics process. It was a simple matter to clip the leads of a failed component and solder a new one in place. With the advancements in microelectronics described above, the nature of microelectronic repair has dramatically changed, as have the techniques needed to make reliable corrections.

There are a wide variety of reasons to repair circuits or conductors. A circuit can be modified for design or optimized for performance. Yield problems can be resolved and new sections of wiring added or deleted for testing purposes. Typical repairs involve the connection of broken or missing metal sections omitted either because of faults in the masks or in the processing. Removal of unwanted metallization, typically as shorts or near shorts, is also common.

Techniques to repair defective conductors are strongly dependent on the size of the features and the materials used. Components built with thin film technologies, which include almost all semiconductor and high performance packaging devices, and where conductor dimensions are normally less than 25 micrometers, require a much different set of repair technologies than components built with "thick film" technologies, where circuit dimensions typically exceed 100 micrometers.

The demands of thin film dimensions limit the techniques available for repair of defective conductor patterns, and it is common to find lasers playing an important role in restructuring and repair of microcircuits. Localized deposition of conductive films and local removal of thin film material using these sources are now commonplace, especially for repair purposes of microelectronic substrates. Repairs of larger dimension circuit elements, like those used on printed circuit boards or multilayer ceramic substrates, still rely on more traditional, mechanically oriented procedures. Although some laser-based techniques have been described, they have not yet found widespread usage.

The repair of memory arrays through the removal of connections to rows or columns containing defective elements, with associated increase in yield, is described in Chapter 19. This chapter discusses the repair of substrates and repair of photomasks.

20.2 Substrate Repair

20.2.1 Repair of Shorts

Thin Film Structures

The use of laser cutting for removal of metal films has become a very important processing operation in the production of electronic components (1), and this technology has been extended to the repair of extraneous metal defects in thin film circuitry (2). Many conductors used in thin film packaging possess vaporization temperatures higher than the melting temperatures of the dielectric substrate. This is especially true for polymers, which are finding increasing utilization as the interlayer dielectric. Selection of the optimum processing conditions for repair requires an understanding of the practical considerations controlling the laser removal process (3).

To guarantee clean metal removal, it is desirable to use laser spots larger than the features being ablated, so the dielectric is irradiated by some portion of the incoming beam. Since most polymers are only weakly absorbing in the visible and infrared, transmitted laser radiation can create catastrophic damage in thin film structures when it is absorbed by subsurface structures (4). Additional damage can be created by direct absorption of the laser radiation by the dielectric or through the transfer of thermal energy from the irradiated region to the underlying substrate. To avoid thermal damage during laser metal removal, short duration laser pulses, such as those obtained from Q-switched solid-state or excimer lasers are commonly used, especially when the dielectric is thermally sensitive, as is the case for most polymers. Longer duration pulses are usually used only with inorganic dielectrics, such as glasses and ceramics. Besides being stable to higher temperatures, these materials tend to have higher thermal diffusivities than polymers, and can more readily dissipate the heat transferred during microsecond or millisecond laser pulses. Other critical laser parameters, such as wavelength and pulse energy, are chosen to minimize thermal or absorption damage to the irradiated areas while providing sufficient intensity to completely sever the conductor. For example, the ultraviolet radiation of the excimer laser is strongly absorbed in most microelectronically useful polymers. This interaction typically results in ablation of the polymer in the irradiated area and can produce a loss of dielectric integrity unless carefully controlled.

Short laser pulses from a Q-switched Nd:YAG laser were successful in removing copper lines from a polyimide surface (5). Excimer lasers are also well suited to this application because of the low reflectivity of metals in the ultraviolet and their short pulse widths. A variety of thin film metals can be easily removed from various dielectrics using a XeCl excimer laser (6). Figure 1 shows optical micrographs of a residual metal defect in a thin film packaging substrate repaired using the excimer laser.

ISBN 0-912035-15-3

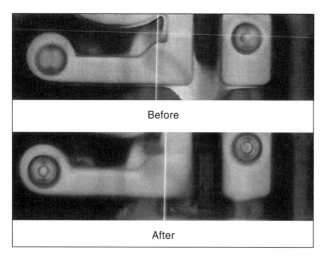

Figure 1. Metal defect repaired by excimer laser ablation. Note the clean removal of the metal with minimal damage to the underlying polymer dielectric. The micrographs show both the original defect and the same site after repair.

Typical laser pulse width conditions used for clean metal removal from thin film dielectrics are summarized in Table 1. Pulse energy and wavelengths are typically application specific.

Table 1. Typical Laser Pulse Width Conditions for Clean Metal Removal

Dielectric	Laser type	Pulse width
Polymers, ceramics	Excimer, Nd:YAG	20–50 nsec
Ceramics	Nd:YAG, ruby	μsec–msec

Laser irradiation can also be combined with chemical etchants to cut thin film circuits. This technique has been used to restructure circuits by severing discretionary aluminum interconnects with localized laser heating of a surface immersed in a liquid etchant (7).

20.2.2 Repair of Opens

Laser-induced deposition processes have been an area of extensive research over the last decade, with most activities centered around applications in the microelectronics industry.

Laser Chemical Vapor Deposition

The method most discussed for repair of thin film circuitry is laser chemical vapor deposition (LCVD), including deposition from both gas-phase and condensed phase precursors (8). LCVD and its applications are described in more detail in Chapter 27. The application of LCVD to a specific manufacturing need typically depends on a number of key elements: the deposition rate must be suitably fast, the deposit must have appropriate electrical and material properties as well as good adhesion to the substrate, and the overall process must be compatible with pre-existing structures. LCVD is being successfully used in a number of microelectronics applications, with localized gas-phase pyrolytic deposition the favored system.

Laser chemical vapor deposition (LCVD) is accomplished by focusing a laser beam into an area in which the vapors of an organometallic species are present. The number of materials capable of being laser deposited is large, covering almost all of the metals commonly used in the microelectronics industry, including aluminum, copper, gold, platinum, tungsten, chromium, titanium, cobalt, nickel, lead, tin, and palladium. Successful film formation requires optimization of the nucleation and growth conditions within the constraints imposed by the thermal environment established by the substrate. Localized laser deposition may be accomplished photochemically, using the laser to induce photochemical reactions of deposition precursors, or thermally, using a laser or directed energy source to locally heat a substrate surface, permitting pyrolysis of the gas-phase species on the surface.

In a typical gas-phase process, the substrate is immersed in a vapor environment containing organometallic molecules to be dissociated, and the system is exposed to the laser beam. While photochemically stimulated deposition reactions may provide superior resolution, the deposited films are typically contaminated with carbon and have poor electrical properties. In some cases, the photodeposition products must be decomposed further by conventional heating to obtain pure deposits. This method, therefore, has limited value in direct repair metallization schemes, and the pyrolytic process is almost exclusively used for repair activities.

Deposition of gold and copper from the beta-diketonates has been extensively studied (9). This work, along with specific process optimization assessments, has shown that the pyrolytic gas-phase deposition process can produce very pure metal films (> 95%) with film resistivities typically 3–5 times that of the bulk material. The result of structural imperfections and entrapped porosity in the film, these higher resistivities can be improved by annealing. (Photolytically deposited films rarely achieve this purity, containing high levels of carbon, oxygen, and other impurities.) The deposited film shows good adhesion to a range of dielectric and metal surfaces, with cross-sections showing good, intimate contact. It was this base technology that led to the usage of LCVD for repair of defective substrates in IBM's thin film packaging programs (10).

Figure 2 (next page) shows a thin film line repaired by this process under conditions developed specifically for the thin film polyimide structure used in one of IBM's MCM programs. Modification of these process conditions allows repairs to be made over a wider range of dielectrics and metallurgies, permitting the tailoring of a repair or deposit to a specific set of characteristics or requirements. With this approach, open defects can be consistently repaired in the manufacturing of substrates with thin film conductors or dielectrics.

The LCVD conditions required to produce high-quality deposits on various materials are dependent on the thermal and optical properties of the substrate, as well as the properties of the LCVD precursor. Nonetheless, useful ranges of laser powers and scan speeds have been established which provide good deposits on different substrate materials. The ranges for deposition with an argon ion laser operating at 514 nm with a 5 micrometer spot size are summarized in Table 2.

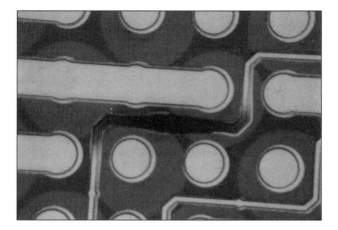

Figure 2. Thin film open repaired using laser chemical vapor deposition of gold.

Table 2. Representative LCVD Conditions for Substrate Materials

Material	Power range (mW)	Scan rate (μm/sec)	Number of scans
Polyimides	0.5–150	1.0–25.0	4–20
Glass ceramic	250–1000	5.0–25.0	1–12
Alumina	320–2000	5.0–25.0	1–12

A typical repair uses parameters similar to those shown in Tables 3 and 4, depending on the dielectric involved. In Table 3, the initial scan conditions are used to induce deposition without damaging the thermally sensitive polymer dielectric. This is followed by additional scans at increasing laser powers to build the deposit to the desired thickness. Actual scanning conditions are determined by the defect type and structure being repaired. With inorganic substrates, the risk of thermal damage is minimal and higher power conditions can be used to create the optimum repair thickness directly. Representative conditions for this type of repair are shown in Table 4.

Table 3. Representative LCVD Conditions for Repairs on Polymers

Pass	Power (mW)	Scan rate (μm/sec)	Number of scans
1	5–8	2	2
2	40–50	2	2
3	150–175	10	4

The resulting deposit has high chemical purity, low resistivity, and good intimate contact to both the substrate and the existing metal features. The films are typically granular, with some trapped porosity. Although the quality of the deposited film is high, it can be difficult to create a good electrical connection between the newly deposited metal and the existing circuit. For example, the metallurgy in the existing thin film circuit may consist of multiple layers, where the top layer is a barrier metal that is oxidized, forming a protective, insulating layer. Before a good connection can be made, this top protective layer must be removed. One method of doing this is to use a pulsed laser to partially ablate the metallurgy at the point of interconnection prior to depositing the repair patch. The partial ablation can be readily controlled by adjusting the fluence of the laser beam and by varying the number of pulses.

Table 4. Representative LCVD Conditions for Repairs on Ceramics

Pass	Power (mW)	Scan rate (μm/sec)	Number of scans
1	600	25	2

An alternative method for achieving good-quality laser deposited metal films on thermally sensitive dielectrics involves switching from a CW source to a high-repetition-rate pulsed laser. The ability to produce high-quality gold lines from dimethyl-Au-acetylacetonate and its trifluorinated analog has been demonstrated using this approach. Using a rectangular-shaped, scanned beam from a high repetition rate, frequency doubled Nd:YAG or copper vapor laser (pulse widths from 20–70 nsec), chemically pure films up to 10 mm thick and with resistivities as low as 2x bulk have been formed on polyimide dielectrics, with negligible thermal damage to the polymer.

Because of the thermal and chemical nature of the process and the relatively low temperatures at which deposits are created, there are some limitations in LCVD's flexibility and usefulness:

- Deposition parameters are affected by the geometric characteristics of the thin film line
- Repairs are not easily reworked since it is grown on the surfaces
- It forms a metallurgically weak bond to the thin film line and substrate surface. Therefore, a localized polyimide passivation is required to mechanically protect the repair
- Processing is not easily adaptable to substrates with components

In addition, the vapor phase process requires that the deposition be carried out in a pressure controlled vessel or vacuum chamber, or utilize specially designed gas systems that create localized concentrations of the organometallic species, while maintaining the capability to admit the laser beam. Additionally, care in the handling of organometallics is required, as a number are toxic, corrosive, and/or pyrophoric.

Laser Sonic Bonding

This repair technique is based on transfer-bonding a metal match over a defective area using a bonding tip energized by a combination of laser energy and ultrasonics (10).

The basic components of a lasersonic bonding system are an ultrasonic bonder, the bonding tip, a laser unit, and a grid containing the repair elements. The bonder is a thermosonic gold-wire ball bonder with dial set controls to vary ultrasonic power, pulse duration, and force. Force is applied by a ramping force generator. The ultrasonic horn is powered by a transducer operating at 60 KHz. An optical microscope attached to the bonder is used to align the grid wire element, the open line defect requiring repair, as well as allowing observation of bonding and inspection of the repairs made.

The tip is fabricated from tungsten or titanium carbide and contains a cylindrical hole where the diameter tapers down to a closed end. The tip end is closed to comply with the laser safety requirements of the production environment and to prevent energy losses from the bottom end of the tip. A capped tip provides a highly efficient laser beam trap and the capping covers the entire footprint of the tip. The tip footprint can be dimensioned to a rectangular or circular shape of a desired size. Moreover, the cap is polished to create a fairly flat footprint.

The laser is an Nd:YAG laser operating at 1.06 micrometers. The laser power is delivered to the bond tip through an optical fiber inserted into the tip. Laser pulses are delivered by action of a shutter that is activated by a trigger mechanism connected to the bonder.

The grid is mounted on a 2.5-cm rectangular holder with a 1.25-cm opening, which in turn is mounted on an x-y-z micro stage. The grid holder stage unit is used to align a wire from the grid with the line containing the open-defect. Then, using an x-y pantograph manipulator, the wire and thin film line are aligned to the tip. Soft repair grid elements consist of gold lines of any shape and dimensions embedded in a polymer. The metal slug is suspended by the sidewalls of the carrier opening to form a conductive segment. Figure 3 shows a top view of a defect before and after it is repaired.

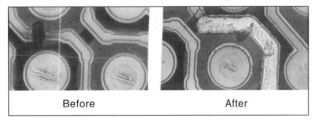

Figure 3. Thin film open repaired using laser sonic bonding repair methodology.

Other Laser-Based Techniques

Lift-Off Methods: Repair schemes can use local photoresist processing techniques, but without the use of masks. The area to be corrected is first covered with a layer of photoresist. This is followed by optical pattern exposure of the defective area using an appropriate optical source and development of the resist. A focused laser is used to locally expose the photoresist during fabrication to create new lines on a semiconductor device (11). Another variation of this process uses an excimer laser to ablate the openings directly in a resist or other suitable polymer film (12). Metal patches are then deposited by conventional evaporative or sputter techniques. Standard photolithographic lift-off techniques are used to remove the undeveloped resist or polymer and its unwanted overlying metallization, leaving the repair metallurgy behind.

Spin-On Deposition: Laser writing using solid thin films of metallo-organic precursors can be an attractive alternative to gas-phase processes. The selection of a suitable precursor for laser-writing is based on several criteria, including the ability to form homogenous films, the capability for high metal loading, sufficient optical absorption, and the ability to produce clean decomposition and volatilization of by-products at low decomposition temperatures.

A metallo-organic complex may meet these requirements, but most materials lack good film formation characteristics. In those cases, the metal complex is combined with a compatible organic film former, typically a polymer. A wide variety of metals complexes, including Pd, Pt, Ag, Cu, and Au, are available and have been used to form metal films (13). A variation of this technique has been used for the repair of open conductors by creating a conductive connection from a spin-on film across an open prior to completing the repair using another method (14). In this method, a seed layer consisting of palladium acetate in chloroform is spray deposited, dried, and laser pyrolyzed using a focused argon ion laser operating at 514 nm. The laser pyrolysis leaves a thin palladium film between the open circuit ends and provides electrical continuity from 10–30 ohms. The remainder of the nonpyrolyzed material is rinsed off in an appropriate solvent.

Liquid Phase Laser Deposition: Laser deposition from liquid phases has also been reported (15). This work has shown that a focused laser beam can enhance local electrodeposition or electroless plating rates by factors of 1000–10,000 over background rates, providing the capability for very high speed, highly selective deposition operations, including circuit repair.

References

1. M. I. Cohen, R. A. Unger, and J. F. Milkovsky, *Bell System Technical Journal* **47**, 385–407 (1968).
2. T. F. Redmond, C. Prasad, and G. A. Walker, *Proceedings of the 41st Electronic Components Conferences,* 689–92 (1991).
3. G. R. Levinson and V. I. Smilga, *Soviet Journal of Quantum Electronics* **6**, 885–97 (1976).
4. T. A. Wassick, *Proceedings of the 42nd Electronic Component Conference* 759–62 (1992).
5. P. B. Perry, S. K. Ray, and R. Hodgson, *Thin Solid Films* **85**, 111–17 (1981).
6. J. E. Andrew, P. E. Dyer, D. Forster, and P. H. Key, *Applied Physics Letters* **43** (11), 717–19 (1983).
7. D. J. Ehrlich, J. Y. Tsao, D. J. Silversmith, J. H. C. Sedlacek,

R. W. Mountain, and W. S. Graber, *IEEE Electron Device Letters* **EDL-5** (2), 32–5 (1984).
8. D. J. Ehrlich and J. Y. Tsao, 1989: *Laser Microfabrication: Thin Film Processes and Lithography*, Academic Press, San Diego, CA.
9. T. T. Kodas, T. H.Baum, and P. B. Comita, *Journal of Applied Physics* **62** (1), 281–6 (1987).
10. T. A. Wassick and L. Economikos. IEEE Transactions on Components, Packaging and Manufacturing Technology — Part B, **18** (1), 154–62 (1995).
11. J. C. Logue, W. J. Kleinfelder, P. Lowy, J. R. Moulic, and W. Wu, *IBM Journal of Research and Development* **25** (3), 107–15 (1981).
12. D. A. Chance, C. W. Ho, P. A. Leary, T. D. McCarthy, T. C. Reiley, and R. Srnivisan, *IBM Technical Disclosure Bulletin* **04**, 6481–2 (1985).
13. M. E. Gross, *Chemtronics* **4**, 197–201 (1989).
14. J. Partridge, B. Hussey, C. Chen, and A. Gupta, *IEEE Transactions on Components, Hybrids and Manufacturing Technologies* **15** (2), 252–7 (1992).
15. R. J. von Gutfeld, R. E. Acosta, and L. T. Romankiw, *IBM Journal of Research and Development* **26** (2), 136–44 (1982).

THOMAS A. WASSICK

20.3 Laser-Based Photomask Repair

Photomasks used in integrated circuit production are formed by patterns of chromium metallization on clear glass substrates. Photomasks may contain a variety of different types of defects. Defects include both excess chromium metallization, either as isolated spots or as extensions of metal from a feature, and also areas with missing metallization. The ability to repair such defects provides a cost-saving alternative to discarding the defective mask. Repair leads to higher productivity and faster turnaround in the mask making process.

Laser-based commercial systems for photomask repair are available. A mask is scanned and the image of the mask features is displayed on a television monitor. An operator can locate and identify the mask defects, and then repair them.

Areas with excess chromium metal are repaired by vaporization of the metal with a frequency-doubled Q-switched Nd:YAG laser beam. It is possible to remove excess chromium within feature spacings less than 1 µm.

Areas with missing metallization are repaired by a pyrolytic deposition process. See Chapter 27 for more details on such processes. A gas mixture containing chromium and molybdenum hexacarbonyls is introduced into a vacuum system containing the mask. Laser irradiation at selected locations decomposes the gas molecules, depositing chromium metal in the selected areas. A typical system uses an acoustooptically modulated continuous argon laser beam which is scanned over the area of missing metallization. The irradiation results in the deposition of a metallic film which fills in the missing metallization. An example is shown in Figure 1. The left portion of the figure has a missing 10-micrometer-square area of metallization. The right portion of the figure shows the metallization that has been filled in through the laser process. The laser deposited films are suitable for use in the photolithographic fabrication.

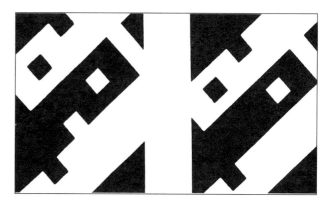

Figure 1. Repair of missing metallization by laser deposition. The left photograph shows a 10-micrometer-square area of missing chromium. The right photograph shows the area filled in by laser deposition. (Photographs courtesy of Quantronix Corp.)

The repair of masks by laser processing reduces waste and increases profitability in integrated circuit fabrication.

JOHN F. READY

Notes

ISBN 0-912035-15-3

Chapter 21

Applications in Photolithography

21.1 Overview

Lasers are used as an illumination source for deep ultraviolet ($\lambda < 0.25$ μm) lithography, where the i-line of a Hg lamp ($\lambda \cong 365$ nm) is not sufficiently short to produce semiconductor chips with critical feature sizes smaller than 0.25 μm. A typical application concerns photolithography for manufacturing 256 Mbit DRAM (dynamic random access memory) chips (1). Fabrication of chips with critical geometries down to 0.18 - 0.15 μm is carried out with a band-narrowed KrF excimer laser ($\lambda = 248$ nm). The general characteristics of a KrF laser used for deep ultraviolet photolithography are (2):

Laser energy: ~10 mJ/pulse
Repetition rate: 1000 Hz
Spectral width: < 0.8 pm at FWHM

Integrated circuits with geometries smaller than 0.15 μm require shorter-wavelength photolithography, such as that based on ArF ($\lambda = 193$ nm) and F_2 ($\lambda = 157$ nm) lasers. It is expected that ArF-based photolithography will be in production plants in the year 2000 or shortly thereafter (3).

References
1. H. L. Levinson and W. H. Arnold, "Optical Lithography," in *Handbook of Microlithography, Micromachining and Microfabrication*, **Vol. 1**, Edited by P. Rai-Choudry, SPIE Optical Engineering Press, 1997, 111.
2. P. Das, H. Heinmets, C. Maley, I. Fomenkov, R. Cybulski, and D. Larson, *Proc. SPIE* **3051**, 933–9 (1997).
3. P. Das and K. Rebitz, "Excimer Lasers Enable Next Generations IC's," *Laser Focus World*, June 1997, pp. 89–96.

J. J. DUBOWSKY

21.2 Laser Sources for Microlithography Exposure Tools

The microlithography exposure tool is a semiconductor manufacturing tool that performs a step in the creation of microelectronics circuit patterns on the surface of a silicon wafer. Microlithography is the process that determines design rules of microchips. At the time of publication of this book, the semiconductor industry was in the midst of switching from the mercury lamp i-line steppers with wavelengths of 365 nm to the excimer laser based deep ultraviolet (DUV) steppers and scanners with wavelengths of 248 nm. The first generation of microchips produced by the DUV lithography process were 64M DRAM and other microprocessors that require similar design rules.

There are two types of exposure tools currently used for mass production of high-density microchips: the stepper and the scanner. The stepper, or step-and-repeat machine, exposes the entire exposure area with lens, wafer, and mask still. The light is shaped to the size of the exposure area. After each exposure, the wafer moves to the next position so that the next area can be exposed. The stepper repeats step-and-exposure sequences until the entire wafer surface is exposed.

The scanner, or step-and-scan machine, performs exposure by moving a narrow slit of light over the mask and the wafer. The mask and the wafer move in opposite directions during the exposure. This difference in exposure methods imposes different requirements on the light source.

A simple illustration of the refractive lens stepper is shown in Figure 1.

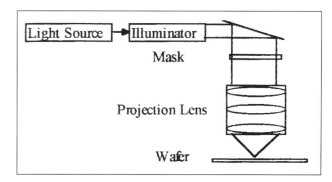

Figure 1. Schematic of a refractive lens stepper.

The beam from the light source is homogenized and collimated by the illuminator. The mask is patterned by transparent areas and opaque areas. The diffraction pattern produced by the mask is focused on the wafer surface, and the mask image is imprinted inside a resist film. The projection lens is designed to minimize optical distortion to produce the image of the mask pattern correctly on the wafer surface. The 4x and 5x magnifications are used to relax the requirements of the smallest feature size on the mask. Projection lenses that meet the microlithography requirements can have a maximum length of 1 m for high-numerical-aperture (NA) large-field lenses.

The design rules and the exposure tool light source wavelength are closely related, and the relationship is shown by the following equation:

$$R = k_1 \times \lambda / NA \quad (1)$$

where R is the resolution of the projection lens, k_1 is a process factor, λ is the wavelength of light source, and NA is the numerical aperture of the projection lens.

The k_1 factor depends on the illumination scheme, the object feature size, the resist, and other lithography processes. Under research conditions, a k_1 value of 0.5 ~ 0.6 is typically achieved. Resolution is improved by using shorter-wavelength radiation sources. Choice of the wavelength affects the depth of focus (DOF) of the projection lens, as shown in the following equation:

$$DOF = k_2 \times \lambda/NA^2 \qquad (2)$$

where k_2 is a process factor.

The k_2 factor is empirically determined by actually processing wafers. For a constant NA, progressively shorter-wavelength light sources are required to improve the resolution while keeping a usable depth of focus.

The only radiation sources available for microlithography in the deep ultraviolet region below 350 nm with high enough intensity are lasers. Light sources that have been used in the past or are considered to be used in the near future are listed in Table 1.

Table 1. Light Sources for Microlithography Exposure Tools

g-line (Hg lamp)	436 nm
i-line (Hg lamp)	365 nm
KrF Laser	248 nm
Nd:YAG harmonics	212 nm
ArF laser	193 nm
F_2 laser	157 nm

The practical resolution limit of the i-line stepper for semiconductor production is 0.35 µm. The KrF stepper can produce as small as 0.18 µm features with special optical techniques such as phase shift mask and off-axis illumination.

In addition to the short-wavelength requirement, lasers for microlithography exposure tools must satisfy other requirements. Table 2 defines the relationships between exposure tool performance parameters and corresponding laser parameters for the DUV scanner.

Below 300 nm, there is only one suitable optical material available for building the microlithography projection lens, fused silica. Other high ultraviolet transmissive materials, such as CaF_2 and MgF_2, have undesirable properties for use with a microlithography projection lens. With only one type of optical material available, it is not possible to design an achromatic lens. Therefore, the laser spectral bandwidth must be reduced to minimize dispersion effects. Although the lasers currently used or considered as microlithography light sources are homogeneously broadened devices, the spectral narrowing substantially reduces lasing efficiency. For instance, a gain generator that provides 10 mJ of highly spectrally narrowed KrF laser pulse can put out 40 mJ in a broadband laser pulse. If an additional material with a different dispersion characteristic is available to design a color corrector, the spectral bandwidth requirement will be relaxed, and more laser power will be available to increase the wafer throughput.

Table 2. DUV Scanner Requirements vs. Laser Performance Requirements

Scanner parameters	Laser parameters
Resolution	Spectral purity (bandwidth)
Focal plane stability	Relative wavelength stability
Magnification and distortion	Absolute wavelength stability
Illuminator efficiency	Beam profile, beam pointing and position stability, polarization stability
Exposure uniformity	Beam profile, beam pointing and position stability, pulse energy stability, repetition rate, misfire rate
Dose accuracy	Repetition rate, pulse energy stability, pulse energy dynamic range, misfire rate
Wafer throughput	Output power, pulse energy stability, repetition rate

The following equation relates the laser spectral bandwidth, $\Delta\lambda$, the laser wavelength, λ, the numerical aperture, NA, the wavelength dispersion of index of refraction, $dn/d\lambda$ the magnification, m, and the focal length, f, for a refractive lens.

$$\Delta\lambda = \lambda(n-1)/2f(1+m)\,(dn/d\lambda)(NA)^2 \qquad (3)$$

The laser for microlithography must have a very narrow spectral bandwidth. The 0.6 NA 248-nm projection lens requires a KrF laser bandwidth of less than 0.8 pm. The required bandwidth will be smaller for 212- and 193-nm light sources because λ is smaller and $dn/d\lambda$ of fused silica is larger at shorter wavelengths.

The laser wavelength must be controlled within a fraction of the laser spectral bandwidth to stabilize the focal plane. The typical wavelength stability requirement for a KrF laser is less than ±0.1 pm.

Beam profile and divergence stability both in the short and long term affect exposure uniformity and illuminator efficiency. More optical elements may be required to accommodate laser beam instabilities, and consequently reduce optical throughput. For scanner applications, laser pulse energy stability also affects the dose uniformity in the scan direction.

The exposure dose needs to be within very small ranges for critical dimension (CD) control because high-contact resists used for DUV lithography are very sensitive to the exposure dose. Typically, dose is controlled within ±1%. The following equation relates dose accuracy and laser performance parameters.

Eq. 4 $\delta D = \dfrac{\delta E}{\sqrt{N}}$

where δD is the dose accuracy, δE is the pulse energy stability of the laser, and N is the number of pulses used for exposure.

Lasers for microlithography must have good pulse energy stability and a high repetition rate to achieve the exposure dose accuracy required. The high repetition rate will increase the number of laser pulses per exposure without sacrificing wafer throughput.

References
- William B. Glendinning and John N Helbert (Eds.), 1991, *Handbook of VLSI Mircolithography, Principles, Technology and Applications,* Noyes Publications, Park Ridge, NJ, Chapter 4.
- Larry F. Thompson, C. Grand Wilson, and Murrae J. Bowden, 1994, *Introduction to microlithography,* 2nd Ed., American Chemical Society, Washinton, DC.
- M. Bigelow, J. Greeneich, and P. Jenkin, "Optical Strategies for Achieving 0.25 μm Design Rules," *Microlithography World* **2**, 9–14 (1993).
- M. van den Brink et al., "Step-and-scan and step-and-repeat, a technology comparison," *Optical/Laser Microlithography, Proc. SPIE* **2726**, 734–53 (1996).

TOSHIHIKO ISHIHARA

21.2.1 Excimer Lasers

The excimer laser for microlithography must meet a set of special optical requirements. High spectral purity is required to reduce undesirable effects of the wavelength dispersion of the index of refraction. The center wavelength must be very stable. Typically less than ±0.1 pm of stability is required. Other standard requirements for material processing lasers such as beam stability, energy stability, and high repetition rate are also required.

Figure 2 is a schematic diagram of an excimer laser designed for microlithography. The laser consists of the following key components:

- Gain generator
- Optical cavity with spectral narrowing elements
- Wavemeter with an absolute wavelength standard
- Pulse power module
- High-voltage power supply
- Computer control module
- Electrical, mechanical, and optical interfaces

The gain generator contains a pair of discharge electrodes to generate a laser plasma. The excimer laser gas is a mixture of a halogen gas, fluorine, a rare gas, krypton for KrF lasers and argon for ArF lasers, and neon as a buffer gas. The typical gas mixing ratio is 1–4 % of rare gas, 0.1% of fluorine, and neon at 3–4 atm.

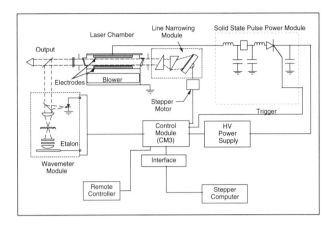

Figure 2. Schematic of excimer laser for microlithography.

The pulse power module typically consists of solid-state switch elements, capacitors, pulse compression elements, and a stepup transformer. The pulse power module generates short (~ 100 ns) high-voltage (15–20 kV) pulses, and the electrical discharge creates the laser plasma. The thyratron has been traditionally used as a high-voltage switching element of many gas discharge pulsed lasers. Because of the thyratron's short lifetime, they have been replaced by solid-state switches in semiconductor applications.

The bandwidth (FWHM) of a free-running KrF laser is approximately 300 pm. The bandwidth is reduced to less than 1 pm for high NA lenses. Figure 3 shows a typical spectral profile of a highly line-narrowed KrF laser. Spectral narrowing is normally accomplished by a combination of a prism beam expander and a diffraction grating. A high dispersion grating is used in a Littrow configuration. Prisms form a beam expander to reduce the divergence of the light hitting the grating surface, and to lower the beam intensity. Photons with the wavelength selected by the spectral narrowing module are fed back into the gain medium and amplified as they propagate through the medium. The center wavelength is controlled by the grating angle.

The laser output wavelength is monitored by a wavemeter. An etalon is used most often as the optical element to monitor laser output wavelength. The wavelength stability in an absolute sense is important for stepper focal plane stability. The laser monitors etalon fringes and determines wavelength. To ensure the absolute stability, an atomic reference is included in the wavemeter. Most commonly used KrF lithography lasers use an absorption line of the iron hollow cathode lamp. This particular reference calibrates wavemeters at 248.3271 nm.

The lasers also have interfacing hardware and software for system integration with steppers and scanners. Often a tool's beam matching unit is attached to the laser optomechanical interface. The exposure tool takes control of the laser via electrical interface carrying power, control, and safety interlock signals.

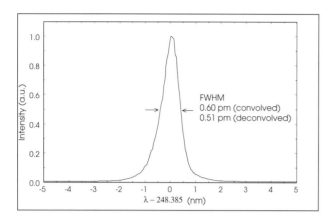

Figure 3. A spectral profile of a KrF Laser for NA 0.6 stepper.

The 1-kHz KrF excimer laser for microlithography is about 2 ft x 6 ft x 5 ft (WxLxH), and weighs about 800 lbs.

Table 3 shows typical KrF laser performance specifications for the refractive microlithography exposure tool.

Table 3. Typical KrF Laser Performance for Refractive MicroLithography Exposure Tools

Average power	10 W
Repetition rate	1 kHz
Pulse energy	10 mJ
Pulse energy stability	2% (1σ)
Dose accuracy	±0.6%
Spectral bandwidth	0.6 pm
Wavelength stability	±0.1 pm
Beam pointing stability	100 μrad
Beam size stability	±10%

Further improvements in KrF laser performance are expected, and KrF lithography will likely be extended to below 0.18 μm design rules.

As more KrF laser based microlithography exposure tools are installed in semiconductor manufacturing plants for production, laser engineers and researchers are rapidly improving line-narrowed ArF lasers, which are considered to be the next laser light sources for microlithography exposure tools. Rather recently, 1000 Hz, 5w, 0.67 pm line-narrowed ArF lasers have become commercially available for prototype ArF exposure tools.

As compared to KrF lasers, the performance of ArF lasers has been significantly inferior in the past. ArF lasers have lower gain, shorter upper-state lifetime, and increased optical damage problems. Recent advances in ArF laser technology have included modifications of the discharge chamber, pulsed power, and optics to yield line-narrowed prototype ArF lasers suitable for process development of 193 nm photolithography.

Properties of the ArF laser for photolithography are presented in Table 4.

Table 4. Properties of ArF Lasers for a Microlithography Exposure Tool

Average power	5 W
Repetition rate	1000 Hz
Linewidth	0.6 pm
Pulse duration	25 ns
Energy stability	8% (continuous)
Lifetime	> 600 million pulses

It is anticipated that when laser photolithography moves from the 248 nm wavelength to 193 nm, ArF lasers will have adequate performance to serve as exposure tools.

References
- U. Sengupta, "Krypton fluoride excimer laser for advanced microlithography," *Optical Engineering* **32,** 2410–20 (1993).
- R. Morton et al., "Design considerations and performance of 1-kHz KrF excimer lasers for DUV lithography," *Optical Microlithography IX Proc. SPIE* **2726,** 900–9 (1996).
- T. Ishihara and I. Fomenkov, "Excimer laser design for step-and-scan exposure tools," *Microlithography World* **6,** 21–5 (1997)
- J. H. Sedlacek et al., "Performance of excimer lasers as light sources for 193-nm lithography," *Optical Microlithography X Proc. SPIE* **3051,** 874–81 (1997).

TOSHIHIKO ISHIHARA

21.2.2 Diode-Pumped Harmonic Nd:YAG Lasers

Recent rapid development of nonlinear optical techniques for the ultraviolet now show that solid-state alternatives to the ArF laser could be a superior choice, but the solid-state laser must meet certain stringent requirements, as shown in Table 5. A tremendous investment in optical design and resist development has already been made to provide solutions working with 0.193-μm light, and the industry will not abandon this wavelength for the convenience of the laser technologists. This eliminates from consideration the 213-nm fifth harmonic of the Nd:YAG laser, and several other wavelengths readily produced by converted solid-state lasers. The excellent spatial coherence of converted solid-state lasers is a disadvantage for lithography; interference effects lead to speckle at the wafer, which disrupts the desired pattern being printed. Although current excimer lasers operate at 1 kHz pulse repetition rate, much higher repetition rates are desirable to counteract the speckle by averaging many pulses. Higher repetition rates also permit superior control of the radiation dose. The laser must be extremely reliable and have low life-cycle costs (called costs of ownership in the industry). Mean time between failures should be in the many thousands of hours, with system lifetimes of several years. Typical costs for the excimer laser systems now in use are about

Chapter 21: Applications in Photolithography

$500,000 to purchase the laser, plus several tens of thousands of dollars per year in maintenance and laser gases.

Table 5. Industry Goals for 193-nm Lithography Lasers

Wavelength	193.3 ±0.1 nm
Output power	5 W minimum, 10 watts desirable
Spectral bandwidth	0.6 pm
Repetition rate	5 kHz minimum, 10-20 kHz desirable

Advances in technology now make possible a solid-state 193-nm laser with inherent characteristics desirable for lithography. Solid-state lasers readily achieve repetition rates in the tens of kHz range. The solid-state laser typically can provide one-tenth the peak intensity compared to an excimer laser, reducing the peak power density on the stepper optics and extending their lifetime. Achievement of spectral linewidths < 0.1 pm for use with refractive lens systems is straightforward in solid-state laser systems, a significant advantage in wafer steppers with refractive optics.

Technical Approaches

It is comparatively simple to achieve efficient conversion at reasonable average power by using hundreds of Hz repetition rate pulses with high peak power. Such an approach would avoid the difficulties presented by walk-off and diffraction in nonlinear optics, because with high peak power, large beam diameters can be used while maintaining the required peak power per unit area needed to drive nonlinear conversion.

A favored technical approach (1) for a 5-10 W 193-nm laser is shown in Figure 4. This concept is based on generating the fifth harmonic of a Nd:YAG pump laser. The fifth harmonic is then frequency mixed with the output from an optical parametric oscillator (OPO) operating at 2.1 µm to produce light near 193 nm. Lithium borate (LBO) or cesium lithium borate (CLBO) (see Chapter 2) may be used in the final 193-nm stage to provide a material that has high optical transmission at 193 nm. Although the overall concept includes an OPO, this added complexity enables the 193-nm power to be scaled up since all nonlinear crystals are used in wavelength regions where they have good transmission. LBO is transmissive to 160 nm, and CLBO is transmissive to 180 nm, as shown in Figure 5. Both LBO and CLBO are acceptable for the final mixing stage, and their deep-ultraviolet transparency bodes well for handling substantial ultraviolet power. In fact, a recent study (2) achieved 4 W of 213-nm output power by mixing the 1064-nm Nd:YAG fundamental with its fourth harmonic at 266 nm in CLBO.

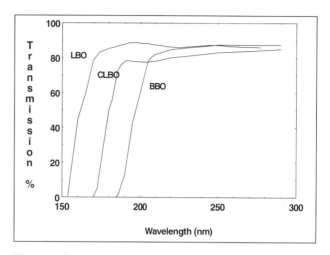

Figure 5. Spectral transmission of nonlinear optical materials. LBO: lithium borate, CLBO: cesium lithium borate, BBO: beta barium borate.

An especially desirable approach (3) would use a PPLN (periodic-poled lithium niobate) OPO. The very low threshold of the PPLN OPO would require a small fraction of the pump energy, leaving most of the power for conversion to the fifth harmonic and subsequently to 193 nm. This means nearly all the 1064-nm pump energy could be used to increase the 193-nm output. Low-pulse-energy OPOs constructed of bulk phase-matched nonlinear materials like KTP have low overall efficiency due to their relatively high pump pulse energy threshold.

Test results now show that the nonlinear wavelength concept can provide good conversion efficiency even with small 1.064-µm pulse energies. With a low-threshold OPO, the tests also show that the required 1-µm pump laser power is within the current state of the art. These conversion efficiency tests show that a 150-W, 10-kHz, 1.064-µm laser should be able to generate 5 W of 193-nm output.

The primary technical challenges that must be met relate to achieving efficient conversion for low-peak-power pulses, maintaining conversion at high average power in the nonlinear optical system, and achieving long life in the nonlinear optical sys-

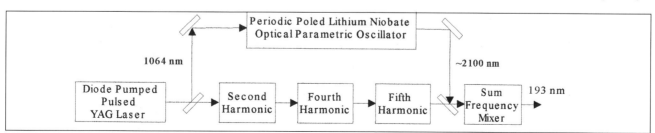

Figure 4. Diagram of solid-state laser source of 193-nm light.

tem components. Perhaps the greatest technical challenge for a solid-state laser is providing output power of order 10 W at 193 nm. The combination of high power in the nonlinear optics and low pulse energy – high-rep-rate pulse format is especially challenging (4). The power goal must be achieved at high repetition rate, to minimize optical damage and to facilitate speckle averaging, and with good efficiency, to allow scaling to higher power.

There is concern that the intense ultraviolet light will degrade the transmission of the nonlinear optical crystals. MIT Lincoln Laboratories has conducted lifetime testing on LBO, in which an LBO crystal was exposed to millions of pulses of 193-nm light from an ArF excimer laser, while its optical transmission was monitored. The exposed crystal's ultraviolet transmission was better than that of the unexposed crystal, even after 500 million pulses. On the basis of these tests, LBO looks better than excimer grade fused silica, although not as damage resistant as calcium fluoride.

Other Applications

Solid-state 193 nm lasers of only tens of milliwatts also have application in the semiconductor processing industry. Optical diagnostic, testing, and alignment lasers at 193 nm are needed, especially with narrow bandwidth.

References
1. R. D. Mead, C. E. Hamilton, and D. D. Lowenthal, "Solid-state lasers for 193 nm lithography," in *Optical Microlithography X*, Gene E. Fuller, Editor, *Proc. SPIE* **3051**, 882–9.
2. Y. K. Yap, Y. Mori, S. Harajura, A. Taguchi, T. Sasaki, K. Deki, and M. Horiguchi, "High-power all-solid-state ultraviolet laser by CLBO crystal," in *Advanced Solid-State Lasers,* Technical Digest (Optical Society of America, Washington, DC, 1997), 152–3.
3. U.S. Patent No. 5,742,626.
4. D. D. Lowenthal, M. S. Bowers, and C. I. Miyake, "Low pulse energy OPOs," *Lasers and Optronics*, p. 17 (October 1994).

ROY D. MEAD

21.3 Advantages of Laser Microlithography Compared to Other Sources

Exposure Source

Laser sources provide two great advantages for microlithography: unparalleled brightness and a narrow spectral bandwidth. The first allows the highest possible dose to be applied to the photosensitive resist of the wafer. The second simplifies the design of refractive lenses by minimizing the amount of chromatic correction needed. Table 1 compares an excimer laser, the laser of choice for microlithography, with a mercury xenon lamp having an approximate working wavelength of 248 nm. Because of its broad spectral output, the lamp produces unwanted energy and generates heat in the optics and the photoresist. Spectral filters are needed to constrain the output to achieve the spectral bandwidth shown for the lamp in Table 1.

Interferometer Source

The laser is also used in microlithography to measure position accurately. The helium-neon laser is usually selected for this purpose and is relatively unchallenged by other sources for this application. The position information is generated by counting fringes and interpreting differences to interpret the position to 1/20th of a wave or smaller. This allows for position resolution of approximately 30 nm and smaller.

Table 1. Comparison: Excimer Laser and Mercury Xenon Lamp Source

Source parameter	Excimer laser source	Mercury xenon lamp source
Dose at wafer	60 mJ/cm^2	30 mJ/cm^2
Pulse rate	1000 Hz	Continuous
Center wavelength	248 nm	248 nm
Spectral bandwidth	1–100 pm	8000 pm

A single-axis application of the interferometer is shown in Figure 1. The incoming laser beam reflects off the interferometer mirror and creates fringes at the interferometer output. The fringes and the phase information is processed by a photodetector, and the position of the interferometer mirror is determined very accurately. Since the interferometer mirror is attached to the wafer chuck, the position of the wafer in the X direction is determined. Additional interferometers are added to determine the Y position of the wafer as well as rotation.

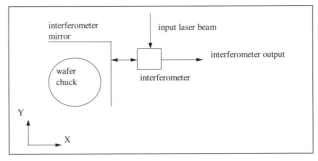

Figure 1. Single-axis position measurement by interferometer.

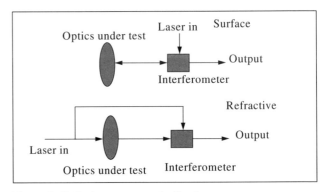

Figure 2. Optical measurement with a laser.

The laser is also used for measurement of the lithographic optics at the exposure wavelength. Once again interferometers allow the measurement of the glass radii and the index of the glass; so the tolerances specified by the optical designer can be accomplished by the optical fabrication and test people.

An example of how the laser is used to measure the optics surface and the optics refractive surface is shown in Figure 2. In the case of surface measurement the laser beam reflects off the optics surface and interferes with itself in the interferometer. The same process as is used in the position applications occurs. The only difference in the refractive case is that the incoming laser beam is passed through the optics.

JOHN J. SHAMALY

21.4 Laser-Based Photolithography System Issues

The laser is used for may types of photolithography systems. One of the most challenging applications, of course, is for the microlithography systems used by the semiconductor industry to make microprocessors, memory, and ASIC (Application Specific Integrated Circuit) chips.

The laser source for the microlithography systems are excimer lasers having the characteristics shown in Table 1.

Table 1. Excimer Lasers Characteristics for Microlithography Systems

Parameter	Value
Output power	15 W
Repetition rate	1000 Hz
Pulse to pulse stability	10%
Center wavelength	248.356 nm
Spectral bandwidth	1–300 pm

Requirements of the optical system:

1. The system must be able to compensate for focus as a function of wavelength.
2. The optical system must be designed to focus the narrow spectral bandwidth of the laser without significant loss of power.

Figure 1 shows the change in focus as a function of spectral frequency for a refractive optical system and a catadioptric system.

The sensitivity of the refractive system is such that a laser is the only source that will allow the design to work. The intrinsic spectral bandwidth of the excimer laser is 300 pm so bandwidth-limiting optics are normally required. Experience has shown that the proper bandwidth can be accomplished with a power loss of approximately 50%. The catadioptric system can use a filtered-mercury xenon lamp but only for designs with numerical apertures below 0.5. For higher-numerical-aperture systems such as 0.6 numerical aperture, the

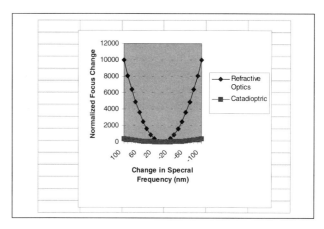

Figure 1. Focus as a function of spectral frequency for two optical forms.

full spectral bandwidth (300 pm) of the excimer laser can be used with no loss of output power.

JOHN J. SHAMALY

21.5 Deep Ultraviolet Laser Photolithography

21.5.1 Overview

The general term *lithography* refers to a process in which a surface is patterned by first coating it with a material called "resist," then forming a desired stencil pattern in the resist coating, and finally transferring the pattern into the surface. A variety of energy sources can be used for exposing the resist pattern, such as X-rays or electron beams. When optical photons are used, the process is referred to as photolithography. In recent years, photolithography has become an economically important process around the world. Table 1 lists a variety of devices that are manufactured via photolithographic processes.

Table 1. Applications of Photolithography

Device	End use
Silicon integrated circuits	DRAMs, SRAMs, microprocessors, CMOS circuits
Gallium arsenide devices	High-frequency wireless communication
Thin film heads	Hard disk drives
Active matrix liquid crystal devices	Computer monitors/televisions
Microelectromechanical systems (MEMS)	Inkjet print heads, air bag accelerometer sensors

The lithographic process can be thought of as a flow of information, as illustrated in Figure 1, beginning with the imagination of a designer and ending up as a physically patterned device layer. This information is subject to noise and distortion at each

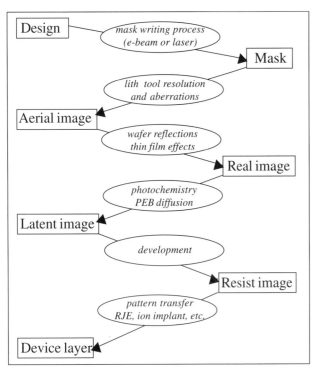

Figure 1. Information flow in the lithography process.

step along the way. The fabrication of a mask from the designer's CAD file is a full lithographic process in itself, which can be patterned via an e-beam tool or via the laser pattern generation tools described in Section 21.2. The mask is used by an exposure tool, which projects an image of the mask pattern onto the wafer. Diffraction effects, as well as lens aberrations and other optical imperfections, limit the resolution of the wafer exposure tool. The process films on the wafer cause reflections which further disrupt the image within the resist through standing waves and thin film interference effects. Chemical diffusion effects within the resist further degrade the sharpness of the photochemical latent image. The wet development process serves preferentially to remove either the exposed area (for positive resist) or the unexposed area (for negative resist). Finally, the resist pattern is transferred into the device layer by processes such as RIE (reaction ion etching) or ion implantation, and the resist is stripped away.

The amount of information to be transferred in each exposure can be measured as a pixel count, where a pixel is a small square whose side is equal to the minimum printable linewidth. Gigabit DRAM patterns need roughly 10^{10} lithographic pixels per chip, an amount of information equivalent to 10,000 megapixel computer monitor screens. Furthermore, to fabricate such a chip may require roughly 20 individual pattern layers to be properly aligned with each other.

We now consider the requirements for a lithographic process to be used in volume production of IC devices:

◆ Working resolution, that is, small pixel size
 • Ability to print all desired patterns to within linewidth control specification, for example, ±0.15 pixel.
 • Tolerance to small process variations, most important focus and exposure dose. The *process window* must be large enough to tolerate the inevitable process variations in production.
 • Adequate pattern fidelity when printing over wafer topography from previous levels.
◆ Overlay capability
 • Ability to overlay current layer to previously defined layers, for example, to within ±0.30 pixel.
 • Compensate for wafer size changes due to processing.
 • Overlay matching of different exposure tools in factory, such that any available tool may be used for any layer.
◆ Productivity
 • High throughput, for example, 100 wafers/h.
 • Highly accurate patterns – 1 bad pixel can kill chip.
 • Reasonable equipment cost, footprint, reliability.
 • Mask availability and cost.
 • Resist process cost.

The basic steps in a lithographic process are shown in Table 2.

Table 2. Lithographic Process Flow

Process step	Tool	Typical parameters
Coat resist	Spin coater	5000 rpm
Bake resist	Hot plate	110°C
Expose resist	Stepper exposure tool	20 mJ/cm² exposure dose
Postexposure bake	Hot plate	120°C
Develop resist	Spray development track	0.12 N tetramethyl-ammonium hydroxide solution for 60 sec
Transfer pattern	Reactive ion etcher or ion implanter	For example, CF_4 plasma to etch silicon dioxide layer

21.5.2. High-Resolution Lithography

The fundamental limits of the resolution of optical lithography are captured by the well-known Rayleigh scaling equations

$$W_{min} = k_1 \lambda / NA \qquad (1)$$

$$DOF = \lambda / NA^2 \qquad (2)$$

where W_{min} is the minimum linewidth, k_1 is a process dependent parameter, DOF is the Rayleigh depth of focus, λ is the exposure wavelength, and NA is the numerical aperture of the projection optics. High-resolution lithography has been achieved by attention to the three factors on the right-hand side of Equation 1, and we now briefly consider each of them.

Chapter 21: Applications in Photolithography

Exposure Wavelength

There is a strong motivation to shrink wavelength, since minimum linewidth scales proportionally. Table 3 lists several wavelengths of interest to optical lithography, as well as the resolution and DOF for NA = 0.7 optics at k_1 = 0.5. The fraction $\Delta\lambda/\lambda$ represents the driving force to jump to a given wavelength from the previous wavelength. The 47% drop in wavelength is a strong motivation to move from I-line to KrF excimer laser lithography, and over the past few years (1995-1998) KrF excimer lithography has been solidly established as a mainstream IC production process.

Table 3. Wavelengths of Interest to Optical Lithography

	λ (nm)	$\Delta\lambda/\lambda$ (%)	W_{min} (nm)	DOF (nm)
G-line	436		311	850
I-line	365	19	260	730
KrF excimer	248	47	175	500
ArF excimer	193	28	140	400
F_2 excimer	157	23	112	320

ArF excimer lithography, at λ = 193nm, appears to be well poised for applications in the near future. Pilot line tools are now available, and full production is likely to begin in the 2002 to 2005 time frame. Current technical issues that engage the 193nm development community include:

- Lens material radiation damage, especially damage to the main projection lens
- Pellicle lifetime
- Resist processes with high resolution and adequate resistance to typical RIE processes
- Laser source stability and cost

The F_2 laser, at 157 nm, may offer yet another incremental advance for optical lithography. But fused silica, the well-understood mainstay of 248-nm and 193-nm optics, has unacceptable transmission at 157 nm. Calcium fluoride, CaF_2, is the most promising material for refractive elements in this wavelength regime. While large pieces with the required optical quality are not currently available, advanced 193-nm optical systems will drive CaF_2 material quality improvements as well as polishing improvements. Other difficulties include:

- Absorption in air and ozone production forces the use of dry nitrogen or inert gas atmospheres.
- Current fused silica mask substrate is too absorbing. CaF_2 mask substrates are expensive and change dimension with temperature, leading to pattern placement errors.
- No practical pellicle material known for 157 nm.
- Single-layer resist processes may not be possible because of very high absorption of 157 nm in all organic polymers.

These barriers are significant, and may well prevent or delay widespread application of F_2 excimer lithography.

Numerical Aperture

The numerical aperture of an optical system in air is defined to be the sine of the angle of the most oblique ray incident on the wafer allowed by the optics, and therefore has an obvious limit of NA<1. Figure 2 illustrates the trend in the information content, as measured by a pixel count, of exposure tool lens fields. The lithographic pixels per field double every two years, yet another manifestation of Moore's Law. The progress has been built out of several contributions:

- Increases in NA from 0.28 (circa 1979) to 0.70 (circa 1999)
- Changing to shorter wavelengths.
- Larger image fields, currently limited by the mask size divided by the optical reduction factor, typically 4x or 5x.
- Improved optical design, fabrication and test methods enabling high-NA, large-field optical systems.
- Moving from step-and-repeat to step-and-scan tools.

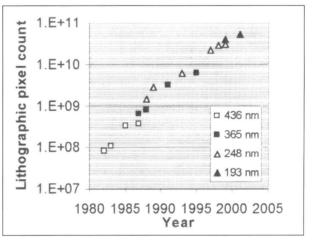

Figure 2. Information in exposure tool lens field.

Increasing NA to improve resolution is fundamentally tied to decreasing DOF, since the Rayleigh DOF decreases as the square of NA according to Equation 2. The continuous progress shown in Figure 2 has been enabled by the continuous improvement of all aspects of process focus control, including field flatness of the projection optics, wafer flatness, autofocus/autoleveling and decreased process topography via chemical mechanical polishing (CMP) and other advanced processing methods. The practical limits of NA are probably in the 0.7 to 0.8 range, considering the difficulty of lens fabrication with the required low aberrations over large field sizes. Shrinking DOF will continue to be an issue, since the Rayleigh DOF is only 2λ for NA = 0.71.

k_1 Factor

The k_1 factor, defined in Equation 1 as the linewidth in units of λ/NA, is a useful measure of the degree of difficulty of printing a particular feature. When k_1>0.8, the printing process is relatively easy. One can use conventional imaging techniques, for example, a binary chrome-on-glass (COG) mask with σ = 0.6, and assume that the exposure process simply replicates the mask pattern. The process is relatively tolerant of lens aberrations and mediocre resist performance, and process windows are large. As k_1 shrinks, the imaging process becomes less tolerant of any imperfections, and process windows decay. The assumption that the exposure process simply replicates the mask pattern begins to break down, and optical proximity correction (OPC) methods become necessary. When $k_1 \geq 0.5$, it becomes necessary to use resolution enhancement technology (RET) approaches such as phase shift mask (PSM) and off-axis illumination in combination with OPC. There is a fundamental limit to shrinking k_1 that applies to line grating structures, requiring that the grating half-pitch must have $k_1 \geq 0.25$. The limiting value can only be approached for "two-beam imaging," such as alternating PSM with very low σ illumination. Figure 3 shows the trend of k_1 in IC production lines. Within several years we expect to cross into the $k_1 < 0.5$ regime in full manufacturing, as many pilot line processes have already encountered.

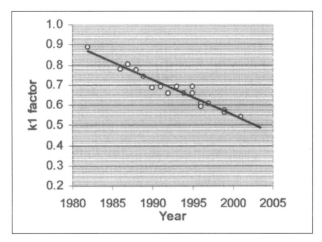

Figure 3. Trend of k_1 factor for manufacturing.

The use of advanced RET methods is necessary to sustain the trend toward lower k_1, and this presents many challenges to production applications. Many RET methods are superb at printing grating test patterns, but become much more complicated when used with real circuit patterns. The lithographer now has many choices, including:

- Variable NA setting
- Variable illumination setting, which includes high σ, low σ, and various annular and quadrupole shapes
- COG, attenuated PSM, or alternating PSM
- Mask bias and OPC designs

A vast parameter space must be searched for optimum printing strategies, and lithography simulation is playing an increasingly important role. Figure 4 shows a scanning electron microscope photograph of an advanced process that can produce lines and spaces with dimensions of 137.5 nm, corresponding to $k_1 = 0.33$.

For Further Information

Refer to the references at the end of 21.5.3. However, the field of microlithography is large and interdisciplinary. A lithography handbook contains useful collections of information on basic optical lithography (1) and DUV resist processing (2). The rapid progress in lithography means that conference proceedings are particularly valuable sources of the latest information. The most important conference is the annual SPIE Micro Symposium, which includes four individual conference proceedings on optical/laser microlithography, metrology, resist processing and non-optical lithography techniques. Information on this symposium can be found at the SPIE web site: www.spie.org/info/ml. Other valuable conference proceedings are published in the December issue of *the Journal of Vacuum Science and Technology B* and the December issue of the *Japanese Journal of Applied Physics B*.

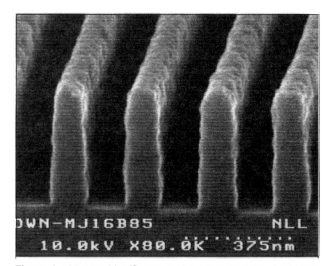

Figure 4. 137.5 nm Line/Space grating structure printed using an attenuated Phase Shift Mask exposed with a 0.6 NA DUV step & scan tool using off-axis illumination. The resist was 500 nm thick, and was coated on top of a 60 nm thick organic anti-reflective coating. This corresponds to k_1=0.33.

21.5.3. Deep Ultraviolet Lithography Issues

In the world of microlithography, Deep Ultraviolet (DUV) refers to wavelengths between roughly 250 and 150 nm. In the 1990s, DUV lithography has become established as a manufacturing technology, especially at the 248-nm wavelength. We now consider some of the characteristics of DUV lithography that distinguish it from the more traditional G-line or I-line mercury arc steppers.

DUV Exposure Tools

An exposure tool must have an illumination system that can deliver high intensity, uniform illumination over a spectral band which is acceptable to the projection optics. Some early DUV exposure tools were based on a mercury arc lamp, utilizing a few-nanometers-wide spectral band near 250 nm. The projection optics of such systems utilized catadioptric designs, that is, a combination of mirrors and lenses, to achieve the necessary

ISBN 0-912035-15-3

broadband characteristics. The excimer laser has emerged as a practical source for advanced DUV exposure systems. It is straightforward to narrow the spectral bandwidth to less than 1 pm, while maintaining sufficient power for high throughput. This is sufficiently monochromatic that pure refractive projection optics with no chromatic correction can be used. In addition, the multimode nature of the excimer laser output is quite useful in designing an illumination system with controlled partial coherence. Over time, the excimer laser has evolved from a laboratory research tool to a reliable industrial light source with acceptable total cost.

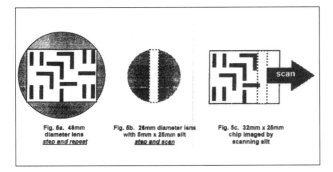

Figure 5. Comparison of a step and repeat optical system with a step and scan optical system to print a 32 mm x 25 mm chip. The step and scan system can use optics with smaller lens field than those required for a step and repeat sytem.

All optical projection systems depart from perfection because of various lens aberrations, especially when large image field size is combined with high NA. Table 4 lists some of the most important aberrations, each of which degrades the image in a characteristic way. In recent years, the step-and-scan approach has emerged as a practical method to ease the burden of increasingly complex optical designs. Figure 5 compares different methods to pattern a chip with area 25 x 32 mm. In the step-and-repeat method (Figure 5a) the chip must be wholly contained within the image field, and therefore an image field diameter of 48mm is required. Figure 5b illustrates a smaller 26mm diameter image field, with a 5mm x 25mm imaging slit defined within. The step and scan concept is to pattern the chip by scanning the image slit across the wafer, as illustrated in Figure 5c. Such an approach requires very accurate mechanical motion so that the wafer and the mask move in precisely 1:4 ratio (for 4X reduction optics). The smaller image field of the step-and-scan system dramatically simplifies the task of building high-NA optics with acceptable aberration control.

A unique aspect of DUV projection optics is their susceptibility to degradation. As the wavelength decreases, the energy carried by each photon grows, and thus shorter-wavelength radiation tends to be more damaging to optics. One damage mechanism comes from the combination of airborne organic contamination with the high-intensity DUV radiation, causing the gradual growth of an absorbing coating on the optical surfaces. This is most pronounced on the last optical surface, which is near the organic resist-coated wafer. Ozone generation can also damage optical coatings. Clean, dry nitrogen gas is sometimes employed as a purge gas to protect coatings. But more fundamentally, the fused silica lens material itself can be damaged by exposure to DUV radiation via two distinct mechanisms. The first damage mechanism is due to the formation of color centers, which decreases the transmission of the damaged area. The second and more important damage mechanism is a densification, which changes the optical path length and therefore the overall lens aberrations. Since both damage mechanisms are due to two-photon processes, any means of reducing the peak laser power can reduce optics damage, such as pulse lengthening or increasing the repetition rate. The damage problem is much more severe at 193 than 248 nm. Concerns about the lifetime of 193-nm projection optics are driving the development of high-quality CaF_2 optical materials and polishing methods. Besides having much higher resistance to radiation damage, CaF_2 has useful transparency down to about 150-nm wavelengths.

Table 4. Important Lens Aberrations

Name	Imaging consequence
Lens distortion (X, Y)	Shift of image, independent of pattern, causing overlay errors
Defocus	Image degrades in resolution
Astigmatism	Shift of focus, which depends on orientation of line
Coma (X, Y)	Image asymmetry and pattern-dependent shift of image
Three-leaf clover	Imaging anomalies with threefold symmetry
Third-order spherical	Pattern-dependent focus shifts

DUV Photoresist
Early DUV lithography was severely limited by inadequate resist processes. The diazoquinone-novolak polymer materials that have been so successfully applied to G-line and I-line lithography do not work for DUV wavelengths. The fundamental problem is that these materials absorb DUV radiation such that the bottom of the photoresist layer is severely underexposed relative to the top of the photoresist. Materials such as PMMA have the necessary DUV transparency, but were found to require impractical large exposure doses and had poor etch resistance.

Many modern DUV resists are based on *p*-hydroxystyrene, which is quite transparent at 248 nm and has adequate etch resistance. Virtually all modern DUV resist processes are based on the key idea of chemical amplication, where a photoreaction creates an acid catalyst that drives many subsequent chemical reactions. Since one photon can drive many individual chemical reactions, highly sensitive processes are possible. For example, a typical nonamplified resist process might require roughly 150 mJ/cm^2, while a typical chemically amplified process might require only 10 mJ/cm^2. Chemical contamination is a general problem with this approach. Airborne base molecules can neutralize the acid catalyst, which causes the developed linewidth to depend on how long it was exposed to the air. Special filters have been developed to cleanse the air inside a DUV process and thereby achieve stable linewidths. A related problem occurs when residual chemicals on the wafer surface cause the bottom of the resist to be contaminated, typically leading to bulges at the bottom of the resist profile called "feet." Optimized processes have been developed for 248-nm lithography, as shown in Figure 4, which have good sensitivity, excellent profiles, and adequate etch resistance, and are suitable for general purpose applications.

Resist processes for 193-nm lithography are the focus of intensive research and development, since most 248-nm materials such as *p*-hydroxystyrene are not sufficiently transparent. Concerns about the finite lifetime of 193-nm projection optics due to radiation damage are also driving the need for highly sensitive resist materials; so it is virtually certain that chemical amplification approaches will be employed. At 157 nm, almost all organic materials are highly absorbing, and it appears unlikely that a single-layer resist process will be possible.

References

1. H. Levinson and W. Arnold, "Optical Lithography", Chapter 1 in *Handbook of Microlithography, Micromachining, and Microfabrication,* **Vol. 1**, edited by P. Rai-Choudhury, SPIE Press, 1997. Chapter 7, on optical lithography modeling, is also of particular interest.
2. R. Allen, W. Conley, and R. Kunz, "DUV Resist Technology," Chapter 4 in *Handbook of Microlithography, Micromachining, and Microfabrication,* **Vol. 1**, edited by P. Rai-Choudhury, SPIE Press, 1997.

TIMOTHY A. BRUNNER

Chapter 22

Flat Panel Displays

22.0 Introduction

Laser processing has become essential for the economical fabrication of large flat panel displays. Lasers are used in a variety of processing operations. Some of the more important applications are discussed in this chapter.

The applications include the use of lasers for repair of the high-value display panels, both for the removal of shorts and for the replacement of missing metallization. These operations, similar to the repair of photomasks described in Chapter 20, are essential for the economical production of displays that have 100% of the pixels operative, a requirement for the displays to be visually acceptable.

Other applications include marking, similar to what has been described in Chapters 15 and 18, the use of laser vaporization to create patterns in indium tin oxide, a transparent conductor commonly incorporated in displays, and the annealing of polysilicon to produce drivers for liquid crystal displays. This last application is significant because it represents one of the first uses of laser annealing of semiconductors, which has been the subject of much research work.

22.1 Repair

As the density and overall size of flat panel displays (FPD) have grown, it has become more economical to develop techniques to repair them. A single pixel that is always on is very objectionable and must be repaired, or at least turned off. Other common defects are opens that leave part of an entire line inoperable or shorts between elements that make entire lines operate continuously. Thus it has become essential to have methods of repairing both types of defects.

22.1.1 Short Removal

FPD short removal by laser traces its origin to xenon laser systems developed for photomask repair in the early 1970s. These lasers were developed to remove opaque chrome defects from photomasks (and are still used today for the same purpose). Typically photomask and LCD display processes are set up so that shorts tend to occur more often than opens. This is because shorts are easier to fix than opens. (Opens typically call for deposition of a conductor.) Laser repair of shorts is applicable to nearly all types of displays in use today. Laser repair of FPDs is becoming more necessary as the size of displays increases and line and space dimensions become smaller. The investment in each panel for a 40-in. screen can be quite significant. It is typically very economical to spend the time repairing it. Additionally, laser repair is indispensable in prototype development. Figure 1 shows the typical optical schematic of a laser repair system.

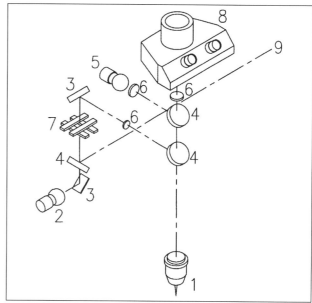

Figure 1. Optical schematic of a typical laser repair system. 1. Microscope objective lens; 2. Spot marker lamp; 3. Mirror; 4. Beam splitter; 5. Illumination lamp; 6. Focusing lens; 7. Square aperture; 8. Microscope; 9. Laser beam path.

The basic optics change little with the type of laser used. The laser source and a collimated illumination system illuminate an adjustable *X/Y* blade aperture. The aperture image is then projected onto the substrate by a projection lens and the final objective. Figure 2 shows how the illuminated aperture allows the laser to be targeted to cleanly remove a short without damage to the display conductors.

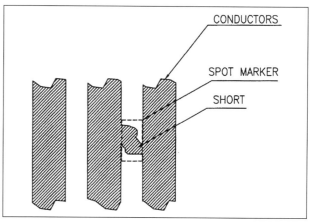

Figure 2. Illustration of the spot marker to allow precise location of the area to be removed.

A beam splitter and overhead illumination system complete the optics. This design can produce spots of any size within the power of the laser and the limitation of the optics. Typical spot size ranges of laser systems for FPD repair are 1 to 100 μm and can include square or rectangular areas.

It is important to have enough power to be able to remove most shorts with one shot of the laser. Many times the material is too thick, or the short too long to do this, and multiple or overlapping shots must be used. The problem with multiple pulses is they tend to increase the probability of a high-resistance short from the conductive material being fired into the glass. Typical energy requirements for FPD repair are 10 to 250 μJ.

Most FPD production lines are set up with a laser repair station as part of the production equipment. Lasers are useful for removing shorts with dimensions as small as 0.5 micrometers, depending upon the material involved. Generally 1-micrometer-thick aluminum is difficult to repair below 2-micrometer spacing, although many shots with an excimer laser operating at 308 nm have been used successfully.

A common problem that can develop in short removal is melting the metal being removed onto the glass, leaving residual conduction. This typically is not a problem with short-pulse ultraviolet Nd:YAG and excimer lasers. However, often the short removal requires the laser energy to be transmitted though the glass. Since glasses commonly used do not transmit ultraviolet light, this reduces the choices of a laser to those in the visible or near infrared. Therefore, excimer applications are limited to unassembled panels. Excimer lasers have the advantage of removing uniform amounts of material and stopping at a desired level, without damage to the underlying structure.

Lasers used include: visible lasers like xenon and Nd:YAG operating at 532 nm, near-ultraviolet lasers like Nd:YAG at 355 nm, and near-infrared lasers like Nd:YAG at 1064 nm. Xenon lasers (480-540 nm) seem to work best on short repair of completed liquid crystal dislpays with the liquid inside. When a short is removed with a laser pulse, a large bubble will form in the liquid crystal medium. This bubble formed with a xenon laser will always disappear within 24 hours. However, the same repair with a Nd:YAG laser operating at either 355, 532, or 1064 nm may sometimes form a permanent bubble. Energy requirements are in the 50–300 μJ range depending upon the size of the defect. The 355 nm laser may not be usable on some substrates because of low transmission.

22.1.2 Open Repair

FPD open repair also traces its origin to early photomask repair of clear or transmission defects. The difference is that not all photomask repair techniques used conductive material. Conductive material is required for FPD repair. Typical materials are gold, chromium, and nickel.

There are two basic techniques for repair of opens. The first is to have a few, typically 3 to 5, unconnected spare lines around the periphery of the FPD active area. These unconnected lines run underneath the array connections, just before fanout to the edge connectors, on each side of the display. Then on opposite ends of a defective open line, a laser-drilled hole in the middle of the crossover will connect each end to the drive line, thus saving the display. This method works because the underlying metal melts and forms a ridge around the laser hole, folds up across the middle insulating layer and onto the top metal. This makes a connection as shown in Figure 3.

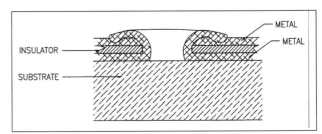

Figure 3. Cross-sectional view illustrating metal wraparound connection from laser-drilled hole.

The second method, which is rarely used, is to deposit a conducting layer over the short, either by chemical vapor deposition (CVD) or metallo-organic deposition. A major problem with these methods is getting the required degree of conductivity. Also the metallo-organic deposition requires additional cleaning steps, which are costly and may create more defects. The material is typically spun on or deposited with an ink jet type nozzle. Once deposited, the material has to be baked at 100°C to drive off the volatiles. Usual materials are gold and silver. An ordinary cw 500 mW multiline argon laser does a good job of depositing the metal onto the substrate. Depositions will be adherent, capable of passing the familiar "Scotch tape test."

22.2 Marking

Laser marking of FPDs is a relatively new area. The use of laser marking in electronics is surveyed in Chapter 18. For FPDs, the aim is to mark each glass plate, as it comes in, with a serial number, so that it may be tracked by a read station at each process of manufacture. This gives the ultimate in traceability.

Requirements for the laser marks on glass FPD substrates are generally quite different than typical laser marking applications. FPD manufacturers are very concerned about particles. A 1-μm particle is very undesirable in fine-pitch applications. Therefore, the glass needs to be marked without creating particles and microcracks that may yield particles at a later processing stage. This poses significant problems for the laser. First, the mark must be easily machine readable; this implies a change in the glass contrast. So the problem is to create a mark with good contrast and no loose particles or microcracks. Second, the marks must survive the etching and high-temperature baking steps in creation of the FPD without loss of contrast. This can be difficult in certain types of displays that have acid etch and high-temperature bake cycles.

A number of lasers have been used in marking FPDs. Nd:YAG lasers (1064 nm) and CO_2 lasers can make an easily readable mark, but they leave microscope damage to the substrate. Major particle generation and microcracking are unavoidable. Also, there is a concern about the microcracks propagating with process temperature cycles. If the marking area is outside the active display area, and marking is performed before initial cleaning, then there is less concern about the microcracks in some lower-resolution applications. Hand diamond scribing is even used in some areas.

Practical high-resolution, high-volume laser FPD marking has been limited to two laser types. Frequency-quadrupled Nd:YAG lasers (266 nm) and excimer lasers (248, 222, or 193 nm) can leave good machine-readable marks and keep up with the desired throughput of one panel per minute (for each assembly line) that the FPD industry hopes to achieve. Panel serial numbers up to 20 characters and with an error-correcting code are desired targets. Currently a 2D dot matrix code is the most widely accepted. It consists of a two-dimensional matrix of dots and blanks that lend themselves to easy laser generation.

Contrast of the laser marks can be quite different for the Nd:YAG and excimer. The Nd:YAG laser tends to leave a mottled mark, whereas the excimer laser removes a minute amount of material that leaves a clean, nearly polished hole with a distinct lip around the edge. Each of these marks can be machine read, but the off-axis lighting and camera angle is critical for good contrast. The Nd:YAG mottled mark has high contrast, but the laser parameters must be consistent to avoid microcracking. Excimer marks have little or no microcracking problems but present more of a challenge in proper lighting techniques for good contrast.

FLOYD R. POTHOVEN

22.3 Laser Patterning Indium Tin Oxide Coated Flat Panel Displays

22.3.1 Nature of Indium Tin Oxide
This section describes laser patterning of indium tin oxide (ITO) coated glass and plastic plates as typically used in the manufacture of flat panel displays (FPD).

ITO is a thin optical coating and functions as a transparent conductor. It is transparent to allow viewing through the FPD. It is electrically conductive so as to serve as "wires" for the grid pattern and as electrodes. Patterning ITO is a process step in the fabrication of most FPDs.

22.3.2 Maskless Pattern Generation
The conventional method of patterning is chemical etching, a wet chemistry process. Conventional patterning consists of etching to remove ITO not protected by a mask. By contrast the laser method is a dry process performed in ambient atmosphere. Additionally, laser pattern generation is maskless. Bypassing the photomask step as well as the entire photolithographic process saves both time and money. Laser pattern generation is therefore useful for prototyping and for quick turnaround jobs. It can be price competitive with chemical etching in low-line-density plate generation.

Perhaps the most important characteristic of the laser process is the ability to generate large area patterns greater than 14 x 14 in. Laser patterning competes well with photolithography in large plate generation. Yet another attribute is patterning down to features as small as 10 μm lines. Linewidths down to 5 μm have been achieved, but this size presents a problem for applications with large travel because of the small depth of focus. The typical range of laser cuts is 12–75 μm. From this discussion it is readily apparent that a (fine) viewing pitch of 0.2 mm on a computer monitor or digital (HDTV) television is easily achievable.

Patterning involves generating grid lines, fanouts, fiducial marks, borders, and alignment aids. Digital file downloads from diskette or e-mail are readily accomplished. By way of comparison, the term *laser scribing* usually refers to rectilinear *X-Y* patterns only. A fanout pattern is not rectilinear; therefore, we call it laser pattern generation, not laser scribing.

Basically, laser patterning of ITO involves drilling a series of overlapping holes in the thin film. One laser pulse drills one hole. The holes are overlapped at linear speeds up to 10 inches per second.

ITO is an unusual material for laser cutting. In all other materials the thicker the material, the more difficult it is to cut by laser. With ITO it is the reverse: the thinner, the more difficult it is to cut. This follows from the inverse relationship in ITO between thickness and transmission. The thinner the coating, the higher the transmission (1). This means the laser beam is more readily transmitted in thinner ITO and does not cut easily.

ITO patterning has been shown to work in production. For many years the lasers produced transparent membrane switches by patterning ITO on plastic substrates. This production laser was also capable of patterning chrome and gold films, also on plastic substrates.

22.3.3 Laser Choices

Lamp-Pumped Nd:YAG Lasers
The equipment used for ITO patterning is a high-power arc lamp pumped *Q*-switched Nd:YAG laser equipped with a computer-controlled *X-Y* linear translation stage and beam delivery optics. The laser is optically pumped by an arc lamp. Since these arc lamps are continuously on, not flashing, the usual descriptor is continuous wave or cw pumped. A more complete descriptor is optically pumped solid state laser. The lasing crystal is Nd:YAG. The *Q* switch is of the acousto-optic type and is capable of repetition rates to 20 kHz. It demonstrates excellent pulse-to-pulse stability of ±5%. Laser stability is important in ITO plate generation throughput due to the amount of overlap

required to cover any instability. An unstable laser would require slowing down the cutting speed in order to cut a straighter line. Further downstream from the laser are the focusing lens and X-Y stage.

Green Nd:YAG Lasers

The Nd:YAG laser is capable of operation at both its fundamental wavelength and frequency doubled. Converting the infrared laser output at 1.06 µm to green at 0.53 µm carries a cost of over 50% reduction in laser average power. But the laser focal size is also reduced. Using the same laser beam delivery optics, the linewidth of the cut is reduced by one-half. For example, if the minimum linewidth of the infrared beam is one mil, green will provide one-half mil. As a plus, the green light cuts cleaner on certain materials because of its higher absorption. On the negative side, the green Nd:YAG laser is more difficult to maintain. The doubling crystals are both temperature and alignment sensitive. They are also sensitive to laser mode structure, requiring the laser to operate in its lowest order TEM_{00} transverse electromagnetic mode. But if very fine lines are required, it is generally worth working with the green output.

Diode-Pumped Nd:YAG Lasers

Another candidate is the diode-pumped Nd:YAG laser. In the future when the price and performance of diode-pumped Nd:YAG lasers become competitive, it will undoubtedly be used for this application.

Comparison of Pulsed Nd:YAG, CO_2, and Excimer Lasers

Flashlamp-pumped pulsed Nd:YAG lasers are used for welding and thick metal cutting. They typically are limited to pulse rates of hundreds per second. By contrast, the cw pumped Nd:YAG, when Q-switched, produces upwards of 25,000 pulses per second. Processing speed is critical to laser patterning. Thus pulsed Nd:YAG lasers are not suitable for this application.

Other types of industrial lasers, such as the gas lasers, CO_2 and excimer, are also not suitable. The former is a powerful source of far-infrared laser energy at 10.6 µm while the latter is a high-energy ultraviolet source with wavelength less than 308 nm. The far-infrared source's wavelength is too large to focus to the small spots required for ITO. The excimer laser, has a limited repetition rate and suffers optical difficulties with focusing ultraviolet.

Thus the cw pumped repetitively pulsed Nd:YAG laser is the best choice for this application.

22.3.4 Laser Cutting

When the almost parallel laser beam is focused by a lens to a spot of about one thousandth of an inch on the ITO film, the high-power Q-switched pulse vaporizes the ITO in a round circle or blind hole of diameter one mil. Overlapping these spots by, say, 50% produces a laser-scribed line of one mil width. With a laser repetition rate of 20,000 pulses per second, a laser spot size of 0.001 in., and a spot overlap of 50%: the linear patterning rate is 10 in. per second. This is the speed at which the motion system must move in a production environment.

Table 1. Conservative Q-switched Nd:YAG laser parameters for patterning ITO

Laser wavelength	0.532 nm
Laser pulse repetition rate	8 kHz
Laser average power	0.5 W
Laser pulse duration	100-200 ns
ITO thickness	150-1000 nm
Linewidth/hole diameter	0.0005 in.
Hole overlap	50%
Hole penetration in ITO	Complete
Linear speed	2 ips

A cw-pumped Nd:YAG laser without a Q switch produces tens of watts of cw output power. Putting the Q switch in the laser cavity generates peak pulse powers on the order of 50,000 W. Focusing 50,000 W on ITO creates an irradiance on the order of a billion watts per square centimeter. This vaporizes the ITO.

Table 1 presents some relatively conservative parameters for the patterning of ITO.

One desirable feature of laser patterning is repairability. Defective plates failing testing for shorts may be repaired with nearly 100% yield. Laser patterning of ITO is a dry maskless process, ideal for quick-turnaround prototyping and production of large plates.

Reference
1. C. Barratt, C. Constantine, D. Johnson, and W. Barrow, *SID Digest,* p.68 (http://www.display.org/sid) (1995).

RODNEY WATERS
TERRY POTHOVEN

22.4 Annealing of Thin-Film Transistors

Characteristics of Excimer Laser Annealing

Laser annealing of polysilicon for thin-film transistors (TFTs) in the fabrication of flat panel displays is a significant application for exicmer lasers. In this instance, the excimer laser is used to change a material's surface characteristics. This application is in addition to well-established excimer laser uses for precise material ablation, as have been described in earlier chapters.

In the structure of active matrix liquid crystal displays (AMLCDs), driver circuitry is formed using thin-film silicon transistors in close proximity to the display pixels. The amorphous silicon material used in most active matrix liquid crystal displays in the past places fundamental limitations on device resolution, brightness, size, and cost. LCDs based on polycrystalline-silicon (poly-Si) thin-film transistors offer a number of advantages, as presented in Table 1.

Chapter 22: Flat Panel Displays

Table 1. Advantages of poly-Si TFTs over amorphous Si

Over 100 times greater carrier mobility
Faster charging times
CMOS process compatibility
Enables integration of display drivers into the display
Avoids use of numerous TAB-bonded interconnects
Screen pitch not limited by interconnection pitch
Improved brightness, aperture ratio, and refresh rates

In the traditional poly-Si process, amorphous silicon is deposited on a quartz substrate. This layer is then transformed into poly-Si by furnace heating it to over 600°C until it melts, and then allowing it to recrystallize. This extreme temperature cycling necessitates the use of quartz or special heat resistant glass substrates. Unfortunately this material is costly and difficult to obtain with the right quality in very large sizes.

In excimer laser annealing, amorphous silicon can be deposited onto a standard, low-cost glass substrate (1). The excimer laser melts the amorphous silicon on a nanosecond time scale, without heating the underlying material. The use of inexpensive, standard glass substrates is especially considered to be a major breakthrough for TFT flat panel manufacturing.

The primary features of excimer laser annealing are shown in Table 2.

Table 2. Primary features of excimer laser TFT annealing

High process quality and reproducibility
Uniform, high carrier mobility (>300 cm^2/Vs)
Uniform grain size
Uses inexpensive glass substrates
Decreased processing time
Reduced production costs
Increased reliability and yields

Laser and Optical System Requirements

To accomplish this annealing process on a production basis requires a laser with highly consistent operating characteristics, superior reliability, and minimal downtime. Industrial excimer lasers fulfilling these criteria are in the range of 200 W stabilized output power; we cite as an example one produced by the author's company; the LAMBDA 4000/5000, with 670 mJ at 300 Hz or 1 J at 200 Hz (2). This laser model is mentioned for illustrative purposes and does not constitute an endorsement. These energies are not sufficient to expose big flat panel displays (e.g., 720 x 600 mm) with one pulse. Therefore, an optical system transforms the excimer laser's original rectangular output beam into a long, thin line of high uniformity that can scan across the active substrate surface. This transformation requires highly specialized optics that must be matched to the particular output characteristics of the laser in use (3). Typically, the resulting line beam profile is "top hat" (uniform) in the length direction and either Gaussian or "top hat" in the width direction (see Fig. 1).

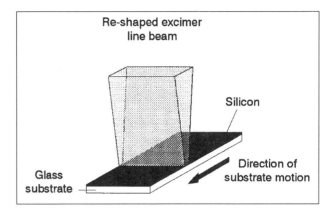

Figure 1. Schematic diagram of excimer laser annealing.

Table 3 presents typical operating parameters for an annealing laser and optical system:

Table 3. Typical annealing system output characteristics

Wavelength	308 nm
Maximum stabilized output energy	670 mJ
Repetition rate	300 Hz
Beam dimensions	0.1 x 300 mm
Beam homogeneity (2s)	±5%
Short axis (scanning direction) edge steepness (10 to 90%)	<50 μm

The line beam optics used in the system described in Table 3 utilize the "fly's eye homogenizer" approach. The homogenizer consists of two lenslet arrays; the first subdivides the beam, and the second recombines it so that intensity variations in the original beam are averaged out. A condenser lens relays this light to the objective lens, which focuses the shaped and homogenized beam onto the substrate.

The complete, fully automated system for performing TFT annealing includes the excimer laser and optics to shape the beam into a line and to scan the line, as well as an automated substrate handling and annealing chamber, cassette loading and unloading chambers, fully automated steppers, handling robots, and a main system controller. This "cluster type" configuration, shown in Figure 2, requires only one central transfer chamber, as opposed to a linear system that would involve the cost and complexity of multiple intermediate transfer chambers. Depending upon the throughput requirements, the system can be configured to perform the entire process, through the cooling cycle, at one station. Alternately, two chambers can be used for loading/unloading and preheating of the panels.

Process Considerations

The exact electrical properties of a poly-Si film depend upon the average grain size of the polycrystals. In general, larger poly

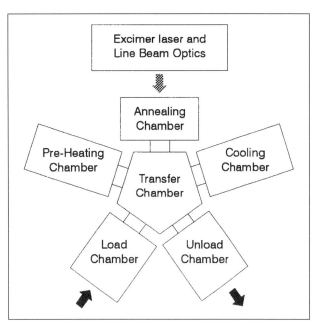

Figure 2. Schematic diagram of a fully automated TFT annealing system.

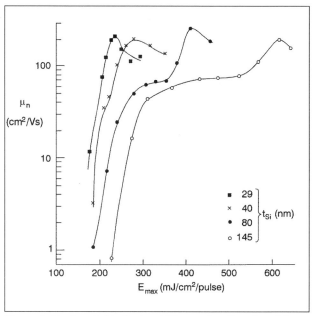

Figure 3. Electron field effect mobility as a function of peak laser energy density for poly-Si films of various thickness.

crystals lead to higher electron mobility, as well as other desirable characteristics. The three main parameters that control grain size during excimer laser annealing are the substrate temperature, film thickness, and the number of laser pulses used.

In general, higher substrate temperature leads to larger polycrystals. Best results have been found by heating the substrate to 400°C, the maximum that lower-cost glass can withstand. Thinner films have also been found to yield larger polycrystals; thickness values of less than 50 nm are typical.

Multiple shot laser irradiation leads to dramatically increased grain sizes. Furthermore, under near melt-through conditions, a "super lateral growth" regime of crystallization has been observed with significantly enhanced properties. The near melt-through condition, together with a thin layer, also largely eliminates stratification in the final poly-Si film.

Figure 3 (4) demonstrates recent results for electron mobility as a function of laser energy density and clarifies the interrelationship of film thickness and exposure conditions. Electron mobility as high as 300 cm^2/V s has been obtained.

References

1. James Im, Robert Sposili, and M. Crowder, *Applied Physics Letters* **70**, 1 (1997).
2. B. Becker-de Mos, D. Basting, H. Endert, U. Stamm, V. Pfeufer, and F. Voss, Optimization of 200 W excimer laser for TFT annealing, *Excimer Lasers, Optics and Applications*, SPIE 2992-05, 35-44, 1997.
3. Microlas GmbH, *Beam Homogenizer and Beam Forming Modules for Excimer Lasers*, Göttingen, 1996.
4. S. Brotherton, D. McCulloch, J. Gowers, J. Ayres, and M. Trainor, Influence of Melt Depth in Laser Crystallised Poly-Si TFTs, *J. Appl. Phys.* **82**, 4086 (1997).

HEINRICH ENDERT
DIRK BASTING

Chapter 23

High-Temperature Superconductors

23.0 Introduction

In the 1980s, high-temperature superconductors, that is, superconducting materials with transition temperatures of the order of 100 K, were first prepared. These materials, in thin-film form, represented a significant advance in science and technology. Lasers have played an important role in the fabrication and modification of high-temperature superconductors.

This chapter describes the use of lasers to deposit high-temperature superconductor films. It also describes the properties of the resulting materials, the comparison of laser-based deposition with other deposition techniques, and the use of lasers to treat and modify such materials.

Most of the discussion in this chapter emphasizes $YBa_2Cu_3O_{7-\delta}$ (YBCO) superconductors. This material is possibly the most important of the high-temperature superconductors, although it does not have the highest transition temperature. It can serve as a representative material for the other compositions of high-temperature superconductors that have been demonstrated.

23.1 Procedures

Pulsed laser deposition (PLD) is one of the most popular techniques for the growth of high-quality high-temperature superconducting (HTSC) thin films (1, 2). This is due to the simplicity and ease with which such multicomponent thin films can be synthesized by this technique, where the stoichiometry of a multicomponent target is reproduced reasonably well in the film.

The schematic of a typical PLD system is shown in Figure 1.

The incoming rectangular laser beam from an excimer laser that has a Gaussian energy profile along the short axis is passed through an aperture such that the beam emerging from the aperture has a uniform energy profile; a typical laser beam is 25 x 12 mm, and a typical aperture is 15–18 x 6–8 mm.

The laser beam then passes through a quartz or fused silica spherical lens (focal length 300–400 mm) and vacuum port (generally made of fused silica for ultraviolet transmission) before falling on the target material (e.g., $YBa_2Cu_3O_{7-\delta}$). The target is kept at the image plane so that a miniaturized aperture is imaged on the target (typical spot size is 3–4 x 0.8–1.2 mm). This is easily achieved if one follows the simple geometrical optics equation:

$$1/u + 1/v = 1/f \text{ and } v/u = \text{demagnification factor}$$

where u is the object distance (aperture to lens); v the image distance (lens to target), and f the focal length of the lens. This equation allows one to get the correct spot size on the target. The beam "hits" the rotating target (10–20 rpm) and the target material is "ejected" in the shape of a visible "plume." This plume is directed perpendicular to the target and condenses onto the heated substrate to form the required stoichiometric thin film.

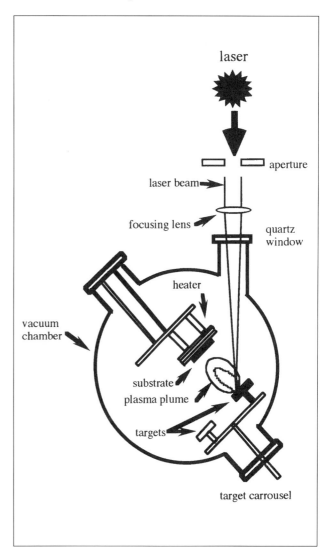

Figure 1. A typical PLD system schematic.

23.1.1 Targets and Ablation

Targets

The characteristics of a typical target for PLD are as follows:

Composition: $YBa_2Cu_3O_{7-\delta}$ (YBCO)

Size: 16 to 25 mm diameter and 3 to 6 mm thickness

Preparation: a) Calcined, pelletized, and sintered from precursors
b) Commercially purchased

Ablation

The following are the typical steps in the deposition of YBCO.

1. Sand the heater flat using smooth (#600) emery paper.
2. Clean the substrate (e.g., LaAlO$_3$) using organic solvents: trichloroethylene, acetone, and methanol (in this order) and blow dry with dry nitrogen. (Note: In a nonoxidizing deposition ambient DI water rinse is a recommended last cleaning step).
3. Mount the substrate using Ag paste (see vendor list at the end of this section) on the heater plate and slowly raise the temperature of the heater to 100°C for curing the Ag paste.
4. Sand the target (YBCO) flat using (#600) emery paper. Note: Without this step the plume emerging from the target will not be normal to the target and hence will deviate from the sample (3).
5. Fix the target on the target holder either mechanically or with Ag paste. A curing time of 15–30 min at 100°C is required for the Ag paste.
6. Mount the target with holder on to the target carrousel.
7. Mount both substrate and target flanges on the vacuum chamber and pump the chamber to a base vacuum of below 10^{-5}–10^{-6} Torr.
8. Allow the required gas (e.g., oxygen) into the chamber by throttling the vacuum system to get the required deposition pressure (100–300 mTorr).
9. Heat the substrate to the required temperature (750–800°C).
10. Predeposition: With a shutter (movable from outside through a vacuum feedthrough) in between the target and substrate ablate the rotating target for 2000 to 3000 shots (10 Hz, 3–5 min). This is required to remove impurities from the target surface as well as modify the target for a uniform deposition rate.
11. Film deposition: Once the temperature is stabilized, the shutter is removed from the path and deposition is continued until the required thickness of the film is realized (0.033 nm/shot is typical).
12. At the end of the film deposition the laser is switched off and the chamber vented (with oxygen) to 200–500 Torr before switching of the heater.
13. When the heater is cooled down, the chamber is vented (with oxygen) and the substrate removed with a sharp blade.

Pointers

1. The spot size is selected such that the energy density is 1.5 to 2.5 J/cm^2 and the visible plume during deposition covers about 2/3 to 3/4 of the target-substrate distance.
2. The spot should fall away from the center of the target to use the target more efficiently without making a hole at the center.

23.1.2 Appropriate Lasers and Systems

Usually a 248-nm KrF excimer laser is used. The laser parameters include:

Pulse width 20–25 ns
Repetition rate 1–50 Hz
Pulse energy 400–1000 mJ

The deposition is carried out in a high-vacuum system. The system includes:

Vacuum chamber with proper ports
UV optics and port
Target carousel and controls
Oxygen-compatible heater with temperature controller
Pumps and gauges

Some Sources

These sources are listed to aid the user in locating specialized items; no endorsement of the suppliers over other possible vendors is intended or implied and no representations are being made on their behalf.

Systems and accessories	Neocera, Beltsville, MD Kurt J. Lesker, Clairton, PA Thermionics, Hayward, CA
Optics	Esco Products, Oak Ridge, NJ Heraeus Amersil, Duluth, GA CVI Laser Corporation, Albuquerque, NM Rocky Mountain Instruments, Longmont, CO
Targets	Seattle Speciality Ceramics, Woodville, WA Micro Ceramics, Elmira, NY Cerac, Milwaukee, WI Superconductive Components, Columbus, OH
Substrates	Advanced Technologies, Forest Hills, NY Commercial Crystal Laboratories, Naples, FL Superconductive Components, Columbus, OH
Ag paste for target mounting	Structure Probe, Westchester, PA
Ag paste for substrate mounting	Aremco Products, Ossining, NY Ted Pella, Redding, CA

23.1.3 Film Growth

The processing conditions that affect YBCO film growth include a variety of factors, including laser wavelength, laser fluence, type of substrate, oxygen pressure, and substrate temperature.

Laser Wavelength

Laser-wavelength-dependent ablation of YBCO and the properties of the deposited superconductor films have been studied by various researchers (4). The superconducting properties of the films as well as the film microstructure and morphology have been correlated with the laser wavelength used for the ablation of superconducting materials. The YBCO films have been deposited using laser wavelengths of 193, 248, 308, 355, 532, and 1064 nm. It has been reported that the normal-state resistivity is lower, and T_c and J_c are higher for the films deposited at shorter wavelengths. The films deposited with a laser wavelength of 1064 nm are rough and have a high density of particulates, as compared to the films deposited by 193 and 248 nm. The optics as well as the atmospheric absorption problems are simpler at 248 nm, and the lasers are more energetic at 248 nm than at 193 nm.

Laser Fluence and Angular Dependence

The laser energy density used for the ablation influences the stoichiometry of the deposited films. At relatively low energy densities, it is found that the target material does not evaporate congruently. As the energy density is increased, the composition of the film more closely approaches that of the target. At a very high energy density, the ejection of molten matter or particulates tends to increase. Noticeable lateral nonuniformity of the composition and film thickness of the PLD films as well as angular variation in the stoichiometry of the flux of the ablated species from the YBCO target have been observed by Venkatesan et al. (5). Two distinct regions in the deposited films with different thickness and compositions have been observed. These regions are correlated with the angular distribution of the flux of the ablated species, that is, narrowly and widely dispersed components around the target surface normal. The composition of the outer region of the film corresponds to the deposition from the widely dispersed ablated flux component attributed to thermal vaporization and does not correspond to the stoichiometric composition of the target, whereas the forward-peaked component of the ablated flux appears to yield a film composition close to that of the target. Typically at a wavelength of 248 nm for YBCO the lower window for energy is 900 mJ/cm^2, the higher window is about 2 J/cm^2, and the collection angle is less than 20 degrees with respect to surface normal.

Substrates

The substrate type, structure, surface defects, lattice mismatch between YBCO and the substrate, thermal expansion coefficient, chemical reactivity of the substrate material, and orientation influence the characteristics of the PLD YBCO films. The list of selected substrates for the YBCO film growth is given in Table 1.

Oxygen Pressure

The oxygen background gas has two major effects on the film formation: It reduces the energy of the flux and provides a high flux of oxygen for oxidation of Y, Ba, and Cu. This pressure corresponds to approximately 1 x 10^{20} oxygen atoms/cm^2/s striking the substrate and the growing film. This arrival rate compares well with typical peak arrival rates of the ablated atoms ~10^{18}–10^{19}/cm^2 per pulse.

Substrate Temperature

The substrate temperature is crucial for the deposition of high-quality epitaxial or single-crystal YBCO thin films. The growth temperature influences the crystallization kinetics, phase stabil-

Table 1. Some Important Properties of the Selected Substrate Materials for YBCO Thin-Film Growth

Substrate	Crystal structure	Lattice constants (Å)	Thermal expansion coefficient (°C^{-1})
Film: YBCO	Orthorhombic	a = 3.82, b = 3.89, c = 11.68	a axis: 13 x 10^{-6} c axis: 20 x 10^{-6}
LaAlO$_3$	Pseudocubic	3.79	10.0 x 10^{-6}
SrTiO$_3$	Cubic	3.905	10.8 x 10^{-6}
LaSrGaO$_4$	Tetragonal	a = 3.84, c = 12.68	a axis: 10 x 10^{-6} c axis: 19 x 10^{-6}
MgO	Cubic	4.22	9.7 x 10^{-6}
Yttrium stabilized zirconia (YSZ)	Cubic	5.13	7.8 x 10^{-6}
MgAl$_2$O$_4$[a]	Cubic	8.085	8 x 10^{-6}
Gadolium gallium garnet (GGG)[a]	Cubic	12.38	8 x 10^{-6}
LiNbO$_3$[a]	Hexagonal	a = 5.15, b = 13.86	10 x 10^{-6}
Sapphire (Al$_2$O$_3$)[a]	Rhombohedral	a = 4.75, c = 12.99	8 x 10^{-6}
Silicon (Si)[a]	Cubic	5.43	3 x 10^{-6}

[a]These substrates require ~400–500 Å thin buffer layer of LaAlO$_3$, SrTiO$_3$, or YSZ in order to minimize the chemical reactions of the YBCO film and the substrate, and to accomodate the lattice and thermal strains in the YBCO films.

ity, film orientation, microstructure, defects, as well the final oxidation state of the film. At a relatively high substrate temperature, the depositing species possess a higher surface mobility that promotes growth of epitaxial or single-crystalline YBCO films. However, at very high temperatures, the bulk diffusion and chemical reactions between film and substrate area are also significant (6).

Typically, high-quality YBCO films are fabricated using ultraviolet lasers (λ = 248 nm, τ = 20–25 ns, E = 1–2 J/cm^2, oxygen pressure 100–300 mTorr), substrate temperature 700–760°C, followed by cooling in a few hundred Torr of oxygen. Orthorhombic YBCO films are typically grown on nonreacting substrates such as MgO, SrTiO$_3$, and LaAlO$_3$ (001). In general, substrate temperatures in the range of 720–780°C favor growth of c-axis films (7), whereas a-axis oriented films are observed at low temperatures (600–650°C) (8). Films that are c-axis oriented have a T_c of 88–91 K and a J_c of > 10^6 A/cm^2 at 77 K. Purely a-axis films are grown on LaSrGaO$_4$ (100) substrates. The in-plane alignment of the a-axis films characterized by XRD-Φ scans reveal two-fold symmetry, indicating a complete b- and c-axes separation on these substrates (9). The electrical resistivity measurements along the b and c crystallographic axes of the films show an anisotropic resistivity ratio (ρ_c/ρ_b) of ~ 20 near the transition and a T_c of ~90 K. The films consist of YBCO grains of the order of 1000–5000 Å. The PLD YBCO films have mean surface roughness of 10–20 nm for 25 μm^2 area as measured by atomic force microscopy.

Growth Kinetics

As far as the growth kinetics are concerned, the major stages of the film growth are: 1. thermal accommodation of the energetic and hot vapor species, 2. binding on the substrate surface, 3. surface diffusion, 4. cluster formation, 5. growth of supercritical clusters to islands, 6. coalescence of islands, and 7. growth of the continuous film. In general, film formation occurs via three basic growth modes: 1. island (or three-dimensional or Volmer-Weber), 2. layer (or two-dimensional or Frank-van der Merwe), and 3. planar growth followed by island growth (or Stranski-Krastanov). The growth characteristics are mainly derived by the factors such as a high degree of supersaturation (10^5 J/mole), a high degree of ionization (50%), and a high mean kinetic energy (~100–1000 eV) of the laser-ablated vapor species, and gas-phase collisions of the evaporated species between the target and the substrate. The most dominating factor controlling the growth mode is an instantaneous high rate arrival of a background gas and target atoms. This high flux of depositing species causes rapid nucleation of clusters, which are very small compared to those at steady-state deposition at the same average rate. Growth studies have indicated that YBCO films deposited by PLD exhibit a planar growth up to a few 100 Å followed by island growth (10–12). AFM studies have revealed spirals of YBCO islands on MgO substrate, which is evidence of screw dislocations (13).

References

1. *Pulsed Laser Deposition of Thin Films,* Douglas B. Chrisey and Graham K. Hubler (Eds.), Wiley-Interscience, NY, 1994.
2. T. Venkatesan and Steven Green, "Pulsed Laser Deposition: Thin Films in a Flash," *Industrial Physicist,* **2** (3), 22–4, (September 1996).
3. R. E. Muenchausen, S. R. Foltyn, N. S. Noger, R. C. Estler, E. J. Peterson, and X. D. Wu, *Nucl. Instrum. Meth. Phys. Res.* **A303,** 204 (1991).
4. G. Koren, A. Gupta, R. J. Baseman, M. I. Lutwyche, and R. B. Laibowitz, *Appl. Phys. Lett.* **55,** 2450 (1989).
5. T. Venkatesan, X. D. Wu, A. Inam, and J. B. Wachtman, *Appl. Phys. Lett.* **52,** 1193 (1988).
6. X. D. Wu, D. Dijkkamp, S. B. Ogale, A. Inam, E. W. Chase, P. F. Miceli, C. C. Chang, J. M. Tarascon, and T. Venkatesan, *Appl. Phys. Lett.* **51,** 861 (1987).
7. D. M. Hwang, T. Venkatesan, C. C. Chang, L. Nazar, X. D. Wu, A. Inam, and M. S. Hegde, *Appl. Phys. Lett.* **54,** 1702 (1989).
8. A. Inam, C. T. Rogers, R. Ramesh, L. A. Farrow, K. Remsching, D. L. Hart, X. X. Xi, and T. Venkatesan, *Appl. Phys. Lett.* **57,** 2484 (1990)
9. Z. Trajanovic, I. Takeuchi, P. A. Warburton, C. J. Lobb, T. Venkatesan and S. B. Ogale, *IEEE Transactions on Applied Superconductivity* **5,** (1995).
10. X. X. Xi, Q. Li, C. Doughty, A. Walkenhorst, S. N. Mao, C. Kwon, S. Bhattacharya, A. T. Findikoglu, and T. Venkatesan, *Proc. of SPIE Conf. on Progress in High Temperature Superconducting Transistors and Other Devices* (San Jose, CA, September 12–13, 1991) SPIE Vol. 1597, 118 (1992).
11. C. Kwon, Q. Li, X. X. Xi, S. Bhattacharya, C. Doughty, T. Venkatesan, H. Zhang, J. W. Lynn, J. L. Peng, Z. Y. Li, N. D. Spencer, and K. Feldman, *Appl. Phys. Lett.* **62,** 1289 (1993).
12. C. Doughty, A. Walkenhorst, X. X. Xi, C. Kwon, Q. Li, S. Bhattacharya, A. T. Findikoglu, S. N. Mao, T. Venkatesan, and N. G. Spencer, *IEEE Trans. Appied Superconductivity* **3,** 2910 (1993).
13. H. U. Krebs, C. Krauns, X. Yang, and U. Geyer, *Appl. Phys. Lett.* **59,** 2180 (1991).

S. P. PAI
R. D. VISPUTE
T. VENKATESAN

23.2 Results of HTSC Deposition

23.2.1 Characterization

Thin-film YBa$_2$Cu$_3$O$_{7-x}$ (YBCO) is the primary HTSC material studied and used in the fabrication of Josephson junctions, superconducting quantum interference devices (SQUIDs), microwave devices, and other active/passive devices. This discussion will concentrate on YBCO thin films and their related properties.

Superconducting Properties

The critical temperature, T_c, is the temperature at which a superconductor shows zero electrical resistance. The critical current density, J_c, is the maximum current density carried by a super-

Chapter 23: High-Temperature Superconductors

conductor at a given temperature before the loss of superconductivity. For most applications, both high T_c and high J_c values with a weak dependence on applied magnetic fields are required.

Figure 1 shows the resistivity versus temperature of a YBCO film on $LaAlO_3$ deposited by PLD. The inset in Figure 1 is the result from an inductive T_c measurement. Both measurement techniques give a T_c above 90 K. For good-quality YBCO films deposited by PLD, the transition width from an inductive T_c measurement is about 0.3 K.

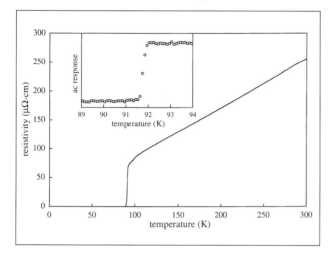

Figure 1. Electrical resistivity as a function of temperature for a YBCO film grown on $LaAlO_3$ by PLD. The inset is an inductive critical temperature measurement from the same film.

The J_c value is directly related to the chemical composition and microstructure of the films. Films with c-axis orientation out of the plane and small-angle grain boundaries in the plane usually show high J_c at self-field, the magnetic field produced by the current. High-quality YBCO films deposited by PLD typically show J_c in the range of 3–6 × 10^6 A/cm² at 77 K at self field. The current-carrying capabilities of YBCO films in high external magnetic fields and temperatures are more closely related to the pinning mechanisms for magnetic flux present in the materials. Twin boundaries, stacking faults, edge dislocations, low-angle grain boundaries, and cation nonstoichiometry can act as effective pinning centers. Figure 2 shows the critical current normalized by the current at self-field of a YBCO film deposited on CeO_2-buffered yttria-stabilized zirconia (YSZ) by PLD as a function of external magnetic field. The inset in Figure 2 shows a four-probe measurement on a patterned YBCO bridge at self-field.

Structural Properties

The structural properties of YBCO films have direct influence on the superconducting properties of the films. For most applications, it is preferable to use epitaxial YBCO films having highly oriented grains with the c-axis normal to the substrate and small-angle grain boundaries in the plane.

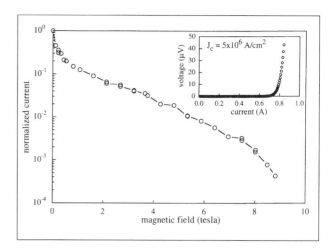

Figure 2. Normalized critical current as a function of magnetic field for a YBCO film deposited on CeO_2-buffered single crystal of YSZ by PLD. The external magnetic field is parallel to the c axis. The inset is the current versus voltage characteristic of the same film. The temperatures are both 76 K.

X-ray diffraction is the simplest and most commonly used technique to characterize the structure of YBCO films. Figure 3 shows typical x-ray diffraction data for a YBCO film on $LaAlO_3$ by PLD. The full width at half-maximum (FWHM) both from a rocking curve and a φ scan is used as a measure of the film quality. The smaller the value of the FWHM, the better the structural perfection of the film is. Typical values of FWHM from a rocking curve of the (005) reflection and a φ scan of the (103) reflection are in the range of 0.2° and less than 1°, respectively, for YBCO films grown on $LaAlO_3$ by PLD. A close match of lattice parameter between the YBCO and the substrate is important to achieve the lowest possible FWHM values.

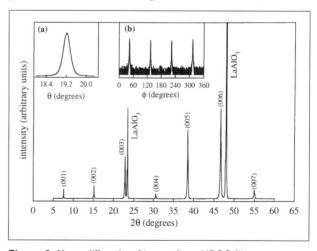

Figure 3. X-ray diffraction 2θ scan for a YBCO film grown on a $LaAlO_3$ substrate by PLD. The film is c-axis oriented. The insets show (a) a rocking curve from YBCO (005) reflection and (b) a f-scan from YBCO (103) reflection. The narrow rocking curve (FWHM ~ 0.2°) shown in (a) and the high degree four-fold symmetry in the plane (FWHM < 1°) shown in (b) indicate high-quality epitaxial YBCO thin films.

ISBN 0-912035-15-3

Microwave Properties

Low surface resistance is a prerequisite for applications of HTSC films in microwave devices. The value of surface resistance is an indicator of the power dissipation per unit area of the film. The properties of both the substrates and the HTSC films play roles in the design of microwave devices and circuits. Superconducting YBCO thin films with the lowest possible microwave loss are those high-quality epitaxial films. Evidence also shows that surface roughness can result in extra losses at microwave frequencies. The low-angle grain boundaries in the plane, which may not affect the superconducting properties at low frequencies, can serve as weak links between grains and increase the surface resistance of YBCO films at microwave frequencies. Surface resistances near 20 $\mu\Omega$ at 4 K and 200 $\mu\Omega$ at 76 K, both at 10 GHz, have been achieved for a YBCO film on single-crystal $LaAlO_3$ by PLD. Surface resistances close to 500 mW at 76 K and 150 mW at 4 K have been obtained for YBCO films with an in-plane full width at half-maximum value of about 7° on buffered polycrystalline substrates.

23.2.2 Comparison with Other Techniques

Epitaxial HTSC thin films can be deposited by physical vapor deposition (thermal evaporation, electron-beam evaporation, molecular-beam epitaxy, PLD, on- and off-axis sputtering, and inverted cylindrical sputtering), metalorganic chemical vapor deposition (MOCVD), and liquid-phase epitaxy (LPE). Except for the cost of the deposition equipment, the main considerations in selecting the deposition techniques are the deposition rate, the uniformity of the film (both thickness and composition homogeneity), the capability to grow multilayer structures with very smooth surfaces, and the deposition of large area. No single deposition technique currently can provide HTSC thin films with the best specifications for all possible electrical/electronic applications. The following discussion compares the most commonly used techniques for deposition of YBCO thin films.

Pulsed Laser Deposition

The relative ease of control of chemical composition of multicomponent materials and the capability to carry out the deposition in a background of high-pressure reactive gases make PLD one of the most attractive techniques to deposit complex compound metal oxide thin films including HTSC films. The growth of HTSC films in a two-dimensional nucleation process by PLD (or by many other physical vapor deposition and chemical vapor deposition techniques) results in many defects in the films such as twin boundaries and dislocations. These films show higher T_c and lower field-dependent J_c values. PLD is the most commonly used technique to deposit single-layer and/or multilayer YBCO thin films on $SrTiO_3$, $LaAlO_3$, $NdGaO_3$, MgO, YSZ, sapphire, Ni-based alloy, and semiconductor (Si and GaAs) substrates. The high-quality YBCO films deposited by PLD are being used for fabrication of active/passive devices and coated conductors. The relatively rough surface of YBCO films by PLD is a problem, although the density of the particles can be reduced by the careful design of the preparations.

Sputtering

Conventional sputtering performed by arranging the substrate facing the target (on-axis) does not routinely provide high-quality YBCO films because of preferential resputtering effects. The most commonly used sputtering configuration to deposit YBCO is off-axis sputtering, in which the substrate is perpendicular to the target. This sputtering technique is relatively insensitive to the processing parameters and has produced very good-quality YBCO thin films. The disadvantage of this arrangement, however, is its relatively low deposition rate. On the other hand, high gas pressure sputtering and inverted cylindrical magnetron sputtering have produced device-quality YBCO thin films.

Metalorganic Chemical Vapor Deposition

The ability to deposit large-area and double-sided HTSC films with a high deposition rate makes MOCVD one of the very attractive deposition techniques. Thin-film YBCO with high T_c and J_c has been produced by MOCVD. Nevertheless, transporting the precursors within the deposition chamber of a multiple-source CVD system introduces difficulties in controlling the composition of the metal components. A single-source MOCVD system, in which the gas vapor is produced from a single source of fixed composition, may solve the above-mentioned problems and provide more uniform film composition over a large substrate area. In addition, more work is needed to reduce the substrate temperature used in MOCVD processes.

Thermal Coevaporation

The high growth rate on a large deposition area makes thermal coevaporation a very promising technique for industry scale-up production of HTSC thin films. With this technique, the metals Y, Ba, and Cu are evaporated from resistively heated boats. The rates from each element have to be controlled within 1% accuracy to ensure high-quality films. Very good YBCO films on substrate areas up to a 9-in. diameter have been produced by this technique. Nevertheless, the deposition needs to be interrupted roughly every 1 μm of film thickness in order to refill the metal sources. This may generate some problems for deposition of thick films. The use of stockpiles kept in the vacuum chamber for refilling has been developed recently to solve this problem. Also, the deposition of multilayer thin films may become very complicated if one uses thermal coevaporation.

References

A. T. Findikoglu, P. N. Arendt, S. R. Foltyn, J. R. Groves, Q. X. Jia, E. J. Peterson, L. Bulaevskii, M. P. Maley, and D. W. Reagor, *Appl. Phys. Lett.* **70**, 3293–5 (1997).

Q. X. Jia, S. Y. Lee, W. A. Anderson, and D. T. Shaw, *Appl. Phys. Lett.* **59**, 1120–2 (1991).

Q. X. Jia, X. D. Wu, D. Reagor, S. R. Foltyn, C. Combourquette, P. Tiwari, I. H. Campbell, R. J. Houlton, and D. E. Peterson, *Appl. Phys. Lett.* **65**, 2866–8 (1994).

J. C. Miller (Ed.), 1994: *Laser Ablation*, Springer-Verlag, New York, Chapter 4.

N. Newman and W. G. Lyons, *Journal of Superconductivity* **6**, 119–60 (1993).

C. H. Stoessel, R. F. Bunshah, S. Prakash, and H. R.

Fetterman, *Journal of Superconductivity* **6**, 1–17 (1993).
B. Uts, R. Senerad, M. Bauer, W. Prusseit, P. Berberich, and H. Kinder, *IEEE Trans. Appl. Supercond.* **7**, 1272–7 (1997).

QUANXI JIA

23.3 Laser Treatment of HTSC Films

Laser treatment of HTSC films is applied to:

- Structuring including (a) local ablation (scribing) and (b) local modification (decomposition or amorphization);
- Synthesis, crystallization and modification of structure orientation including laser annealing during or after deposition of a film;
- Polishing.

Advantages of laser irradiation compared with other methods of treatment of HTSC are spatial and temporal localization that enable one to achieve micrometer and submicrometer resolution and also to prevent harmful effects on thermally sensitive layers and elements (1, 2). Also, the rapid laser heating and the following fast cooling allow one to obtain new metastable phases and compositions that cannot be obtained by common techniques (2). Tables 1 and 2 present typical procedures for HTSC films treatment using pulsed and CW lasers (1–5).

Structuring

The formation of microstructures in HTSC films is based either on a local removal of the film or on its local modification. The processes of producing superconducting tracks on a semiconductor film or of conductive or insulating tracks on HTSC films are the simplest microstructurization operations. The necessary pattern on the film is produced either by means of a mask or by

Table 1. HTSC Film Treatment Procedures Using Pulsed Lasers

Procedure	Laser	Wavelength (μm)	Pulse duration (ns)	Power density (MW/cm^2)	Thickness (μm)	Results
Scribing	KrF	0.248	20–30	1–3	0.2–1.0	Trace width of 1–5 μm
Scribing/patterning	Nd:YAG	1.06	50–70	2–4	0.3–2.0	Trace width of 4–20 μm
Modification	CO_2	10.6	100–400	0.5–1.5	0.1–3.0	Increase in absorptance; Decrease in reflectivity
Modification	KrF	0.248	20–30	0.3–0.5	0.05–0.15	Loss of superconductivity
Modification	Nd:YAG	1.06	50–70	0.4–1.0	0.05–0.20	Decrease T_c or loss of superconductivity
Polishing	KrF	0.248	20–30	0.2–0.3	0.05–0.1	Decrease in roughness
Polishing	XeCl	0.308	40–50	0.3–0.4	0.01–0.15	Decrease in roughness; Increase in J_c
Synthesising	CO_2	10.6	10^6	4×10^{-5}	~1	T_c = 60–80 K
Additional irradiation during deposition	KrF	0.248	20	0.2	0.1–0.5	Decrease in deposition temperature; increase in T_c and in the proportion of α-oriented grains

Table 2. HTSC Film Treatment Using Continuous-Wave Lasers

Procedure	Laser	Wavelength (μm)	Power density (kW/cm^2)	Conditions	Results
Reversible modification	Ar^+	0.488	100–400	in N_2/O_2 atmosphere	Decrease/increase in absorptivity; Deterioration/restoration of superconductivity
Modification	Nd:YAG	1.06	400–800	in air	Amorphization and reversible loss of superconductivity
Annealing	Ar^+	0.488	20–50	in O_2 at 400 °C	Restoration of superconductivity; T_c = 60 K
Annealing	CO_2	10.6	40–100	multistep in O_2 at 450 °C at 810 °C	Restoration of superconductivity; T_c = 62 K; T_c = 86 K
Annealing and patterning during deposition	CO_2	10.6	0.5	in O_2 at 700 °C	T_c = 90 K, J_c = 2.5×10^6 A/cm^2; Superconducting strips of 1 mm in width

scanning the film surface with a sharply focused laser beam. The latter method is capable of producing structures with micrometer- and submicrometer-size elements.

The technique of laser film deposition with CO_2 laser heating of the growing film makes it possible to deposit an HTSC film close to thermally sensitive elements and to carry out microstructurization concurrently with deposition. The film shows superconducting properties only in regions subject to an additional laser irradiation. The rest of the film possesses semiconductor properties (5).

23.3.1. Modification

Laser modification of HTSC is a purposeful change of the superconducting properties of a material, carried out by exerting a local laser effect on the structure and chemical composition of the material, which originally is (or is not) a superconductor.

Chemical Stability of HTSC Phase

The processes of decomposition and synthesis of HTSCs are thermochemical reactions involving either the liberation or absorption of oxygen (2). Typical reversible reactions of the decomposition of $YBa_2Cu_3O_7$ (123 phase) are presented in Table 3. The direction of such reactions is determined by the sign of the Gibbs thermodynamic potential $\Delta F = \Delta H - T\Delta S$. The kinetics depend on the intensity of the oxygen mass transfer through the solid reaction products. Here T is temperature, and ΔH and ΔS are enthalpy and entropy differences whose values are also shown in Table 3.

According to chemical equilibrium theory, the oxygen pressure at the interface is given by the relation

$$P = P_0 \exp(-\Delta H/RT_d), \quad P_0 = P_1 \exp(-\Delta S/R), \quad P_1 = 1 \text{ atm} \quad (1)$$

where R is the universal gas constant. The functions $T(P)$ for reactions 1–4 describe the area of stability of the 123 phase. There is a range of temperatures (T_1, T_2), whose limits depend on the external oxygen pressure, in which all the four reactions 1–4 lead to the synthesis of the 123 phase (2). Outside this region, at least one of the reactions leads to the decomposition of the HTSC material, and the dominance of decomposition or synthesis (as well as the formation of some or other phases) is governed by the kinetics of the heat and mass transfer processes involved. Where the temperature of the material changes rapidly enough, various phases may be superheated (supercooled) significantly (2). The conditions of HTSC stability could be varied by changing the external oxygen pressure or when laser treatment is curried out in atmosphere of nitrogen or other gases (3).

Conditions for Modification of HTSC Films

The reverse modification of superconducting films can be obtained using various types of lasers (Tables 1 and 2). The limitation for laser-induced nondestructive modification of HTSC films may be due to the cluster-type ablation of a film as a result of a sharp increase in pressure of gases involved into HTSC decomposition process (2). This ablation mechanism dominates at certain laser power density and only when film thickness is more than one light absorption depth α^{-1} where α is an absorption coefficient. The values of α for the 123 phase and for KrF, Nd:YAG, Ar$^+$, and CO_2 lasers are 1.5×10^5, 10^5, 5.5×10^4, and 3×10^3 cm^{-1} respectively (1–3). Therefore, HTSC films of hundreds of nanometers in thickness could be easily modified with a CO_2 laser or with an Ar$^+$ laser.

Over a long period of time all attempts to modify YBaCuO (YBCO) films with excimer lasers failed because the ablation threshold F_a was several times 0.1 J/cm^2. No changes were observed in the films at laser fluences below this threshold value. When the film thickness is small enough, the value of F_a increases because of a change in the ablation mechanism (Fig. 1). The process of smooth thermal decomposition of the HTSC material without its ablation by means of pulsed (of tens of nanoseconds in duration) excimer or Nd:YAG laser is possible for films thinner than 100 nm.

Irradiating a YBCO film with a CW Nd:YAG laser at low power density (about 15 W/cm^2) made the film amorphous. It then lost its superconducting properties, its electrical resistance showing temperature dependence characteristic of semiconductors. Annealing the modified film in oxygen at 970°C recovered its superconducting state with the original critical temperature value.

Table 3. Chemical Reactions of Decomposition/Synthesis of $YBa_2Cu_3O_7$

Chemical reaction	ΔH (kJ/mole)	ΔS (kJ/mole K)	No
$4YBa_2Cu_3O_7 = 6BaCuO_2 + 2Y_2BaO + 6CuO + O_2$	175	131	1
$4YBa_2Cu_3O_7 = 6BaCuO_2 + 2Y_2BaCuO_5 + 4CuO + O_2$	-3.6	-3.5	2
$4YBa_2Cu_3O_7 = 6BaCuO_2 + Y_2BaCuO_5 + 6CuO + Y_2O_3 + O_2$	-15.6	39.3	3
$4YBa_2Cu_3O_7 = 6BaCuO_2 + Y_2Ba_2O_5 + Y_2Cu_2O_5 + 4CuO + O_2$	-6.4	-25.0	4

Chapter 23: High-Temperature Superconductors

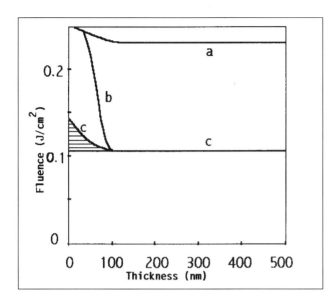

Figure 1. Modification, ablation, and polishing regions for YBCO films of various thickness treated with a KrF laser (a) evaporation threshold, (b) cluster-type ablation threshold, (c) modification boundary, polishing area (dashed).

Monitoring of Modification

The optical properties of HTSC films are quite sensitive to the structural and phase transformations taking place in the material under the effect of laser radiation (3). Figure 2 presents the laser fluence dependencies of optical density (measured at a wavelength of 550 nm) and reflectivity for 123 films of 500 nm thickness modified by means of a TEA CO_2 laser (2). When HTSC films lost their superconductivity, their transparency increased, and the reflectivity decreased.

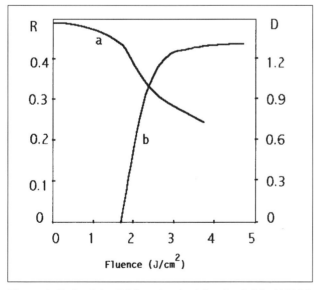

Figure 2. Reflectivity R (a) and optical density D (b) of YBCO film (of 500 nm thickness) as a function of CO_2 laser fluence for a pulse duration of 1.5 μs.

Synthesis and Formation of Film Structure

Superconducting tracks on YBCO ceramic were produced by irradiating the material in oxygen. Depending on the laser power and conditions of saturating the tetragonal structure of the material with oxygen, various HTSC phases were obtained, their critical temperatures being 55 and 88 K. The synthesis of the 123 phase was also demonstrated by exposing a tab consisting of Y_2O_3, BaO, and CuO to a Nd:YAG laser.

The orientation of the crystallite structure is one of the most important characteristics of the HTSC film. An amorphous film possesses no superconducting properties. A nonoriented polycrystalline structure has a lower critical temperature T_c and current density J_c (1, 2). If the crystallographic c axis of the film lattice is normal to the surface of the substrate, the electrical properties of the 123 film are typically as follows: $T_c = 90–92$ K, $J_c = 10^6$ A/cm² (2).

A disadvantage of c-oriented films is the small coherency length along the crystallographic c axis and the possibility of a sharp increase of their surface roughness as a result of formation of inclusions of a different orientation. This can make them useless in the manufacture of multilayer elements operating on the Josephson junction principle. The a-oriented films grown at somewhat lowered temperatures has a greater coherency length and a smoother surface, but were low in oxygen and possessed a lower critical temperature. On the other hand, fine a-phase crystallites, as well as the Moire network of grain boundaries, are additional pinning centers and may, with a certain spatial distribution, increase J_c several times.

The film orientation depends on temperature, gas pressure, and heating and cooling rates. In the case of rapid cooling, a predominantly a-oriented structure could be fixed. Films with a thermodynamically more advantageous c-oriented structure are produced on slow cooling. Therefore, laser annealing to modify film structure offers few advantages over conventional furnace heating.

Laser Annealing during Growth

An additional laser treatment of HTSC films in the course of growth provides control of their structures and properties. Irradiating the films additionally with KrF laser pulses ($F = 0.1$ J/cm²) smoothes them and increases the proportion of a-oriented grains in them, c-oriented films growing in the absence of such additional treatment.

An additional laser irradiation of the growing film allows the deposition temperature to be lowered. The degradation of the HTSC material associated with the diffusive film-substrate interaction can be reduced by using laser instead of furnace heating. The parameters of YBCO films obtained as a result of laser annealing during deposition are $T_c = 90$ K, $J_c = 2.5 \times 10^6$ A/cm² (5).

The laser annealing technique also allows amorphous films previously deposited to crystallize by local and rapid heating the surface in the chosen region without destruction of other areas. CW Ar, CO_2, Nd:YAG, and pulsed CO_2 lasers have been used for this purpose (2, 4). The multistep laser annealing in O_2 allows one to obtain superconducting YBCO films deposited by a N_2 laser on Si substrate (4). During the first step a film was heated by CW CO_2 laser radiation to 650°C for 1 s. Then the temperature was held at 450°C for 2 min. This was followed by a second increase up to 650°C for 1 s and then reduction to 450°C for 2 min. After that the film was heated to 650°C for 2 s, and then the temperature decreased to 450 °C for 2 min. Again, laser heating raised the temperature to 650 °C for 1 s and then the film cooled down to room temperature in O_2. This annealing cycle results in transformation of the disordered phase to orthorhombic 123 structure with T_c of about 80 K (4).

23.3.2 Polishing of Thin HTSC Films

Surface roughness is one of the most important characteristics of HTSC films. Surface irregularities not only lower the critical current density of the films, but make it difficult to produce multiple-layer structures and conduct the subsequent lithographic operations on them. Laser-induced evaporation of a bulk target or a thick film can be accompanied by a reduction of surface irregularities. Another possibility for polishing thin YBCO films (about 100 nm in thickness) was realized (2) by means of excimer laser radiation. It was found that an ablation mechanism and the ablation threshold F_a of the films depended on their thickness (Fig. 1). For thin films, the cluster-type ablation mechanism is impossible, so that their destruction requires evaporation, a process requiring much more energy. In thin films, ablation occurs by evaporation, and in thick ones, by a cluster-type mechanism under the pressure exerted by the evolving oxygen.

For relatively thick films ($h > 300$ nm), at $F_a = 0.11$ J/cm². The ablation of thinner films started at higher threshold fluence values, namely, $F_a = 0.14$ J/cm² for $h = 160$ nm and $F_a = 0.28$ J/cm² for $h = 60$ nm. Laser treatment under subthreshold conditions ($F < 0.1$ J/cm²) caused no perceptible changes in the optical properties and surface roughness of the films. Laser treatment at $F > 0.11$ J/cm² caused a material reduction of surface irregularities, but treating films at F fixed in the range 0.11–0.3 J/cm² yielded different results. For films differing in thickness, irradiating thin films ($h = 60$ nm) at $F = 0.12$–0.14 J/cm² reduced their roughness by a factor of over 20. There was no surface ablation, whereas thicker films ($h > 160$ nm) suffered ablation to a depth of 15–40 nm. Raising F to the range 0.14–0.24 J/cm² increased only insignificantly the ablation depth of "thick" films, but caused films with a thickness of $h = 60$ nm to undergo modification that manifested itself in a sharp increase of the film transparency. Increasing the thickness of films at a constant fluence led to their ablation accompanied by an increase in transparency and a reduction of surface roughness (2).

The effect of thin films being polished without ablation is explained by the fact that the presence of a projection measuring over 0.1 μm on the smooth surface of a film makes it "thick" at this spot and thus subject to the oscillatory ablation regime resulting in the removal of this projection (2). The rest of the film surface suffers no damage, its irradiation conditions being of a subthreshold character. To achieve low-energy ablation with a CO_2 laser requires a film thickness over 5 μm, and so the CO_2 laser polishing of HTSC films proves impossible. The characteristic roughness height is of the order of 1 μm.

Reversibility of HTSC Film Modification

The HTSC films (modified with both excimer and CO_2 lasers) recover their optical properties after being annealed in oxygen. This indicates that the modification and polishing processes are reversible and are not associated with changes in the concentration of the basic metals contained in the HTSC material. Where irradiation conditions are such that the film material partially undergoes evaporation, the chemical composition of the film changes, and this makes it impossible for the film fully to recover its optical and superconducting properties (2).

References
1. D. Bäuerle, *Applied Physics A* **48**, 527–42 (1989).
2. E. N.Sobol, *Phase Transformations and Ablation in Laser Treated Solids*: 1995, Wiley, New York, Chapter 6.
3. M. Rotshild, J. H. C. Sedlacek, J. G. Black, and D. J. Ehrlich, *Appl.Phys.Lett.* **52**, 404–6 (1988).
4. V. S. Serbesov, P. A. Atanasov, and R. I. Tomov, J. *Materials Science: Materials in Electronics* **5**, 272–4 (1994).
5. E. Von der Burg, M. Diegel, H. Stafast, and W. Grill, *Applied Physics A* **54**, 373–9 (1992).

EMIL N. SOBOL

Chapter 24

Laser-Produced Microstructures

24.1 Basic Laser Microstructuring Procedures

24.1.0 Introduction

Laser microstructuring is a method of fabricating small feature size structures, typically 100 μm, or less, using laser beams from the near infrared (1.06 μm, Nd:YAG) to deep-ultraviolet (157 nm, F_2 excimer). Laser beams of Raman shifted radiation at wavelengths below 150 nm have also been applied for microstructuring. The interaction of short duration pulses (100 ns or less) with solids results in a relatively confined heat-affected zone. Precision micromachining with few exceptions is carried out with ns, ps, or fs pulses. Microstructuring that involves material conditioning (annealing, surface texturing, hardening, etc.) and/or laser-assisted growth is typically carried out with longer pulses or with CW lasers.

The high absorption of solids in the ultraviolet is critical for processing with high lateral resolution and for achieving high-precision laser ablation rates (depth removed per pulse). Consequently, processing of materials with lateral resolution in the micrometer or submicrometer range typically requires short wavelength radiation. Excimer lasers are well suited for high-speed microstructuring of a wide range of materials, from polyimides and oxides to glass, various ceramics, and diamond, because of their particular characteristics (high-energy nanosecond pulses in the ultraviolet region, large beam size). Higher harmonic beams from Nd:YAG (532, 355, 266 nm) and Ar+ (244 nm) are also used for microstructuring applications where high-speed processing of large areas is not of a primary concern. The two most popular methods used for micromachining and microstructuring (patterning) are laser writing and laser projection lithography. They are schematically illustrated in Figure 1.

A laser writing approach makes use of a tightly focused beam (Nd:YAG, Ar+, HeCd, excimer) that is delivered to the surface of a processed piece with a focusing lens (Fig. 1a). Beam expansion and spatial filtering are applied to achieve diffraction-limited spots. Complicated 3D shapes can be obtained by moving the workpiece on a digitally controlled x-y-z stage and/or by steering the laser beam with numerically controlled mirrors.

Projection laser lithography, which has already been described in Chapter 21, is based on the application of large-size beams primarily provided by excimer lasers. Required patterns are projected on the surface of processed wafers with the use of a mask (Fig. 1b). Conventional masks, which are either absorbing or reflective, make use of a small portion of the energy carried by the laser beam. Thus, the corresponding cost of operation per photon is high. More economically favorable results are obtained with holographic masks that act as large single diffractive elements (analogous to lenses) with a complex amplitude-modulation pattern in the focal plane (1). A well-designed holographic mask can use 80% or more of the incident laser light. To achieve a uniform illumination of the mask the laser beam has to be shaped and homogenized. One of the most successful methods of homogenization employs a pair of fly's eye arrays (2).

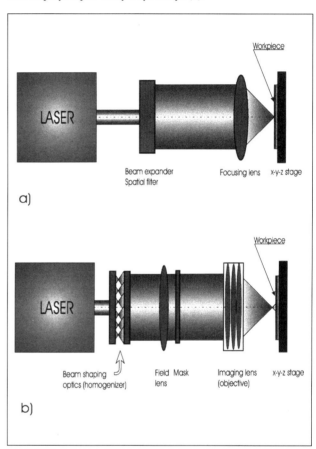

Figure 1. Schematic configurations of laser-beam delivery optics used for, (a) writing and, (b) projection laser lithography.

24.1.1 Microstructuring by Laser Direct Ablation

Focused laser beam pulses are used to ablate material in a vacuum, an inert gas, or an air environment. Typical applications of the laser writing approach include photomask repair (3), laser digital and analog data recording (4), production of submicrometer application-specific integrated circuits, abbreviated as ASIC (5, 6), and rapid fabrication of diffractive optical elements (7). Projection lithography that employs excimer lasers allows areas of 25 x 25 mm, or greater, to be processed in one step. This approach is the primary via formation technology (small hole with sloping walls) used in microelectronics for thin-film packaging and multichip modules (MCM) (8, 9). Large-size excimer laser beams also allow the fabrication of some regular 3D topologies, e.g., mirco-lens arrays, and sloped or stepped surfaces with a contour or gray scale mask technique (10). Some typical examples of microstructure fabrication obtained by direct laser ablation are listed in Table 1.

24.1.2 Microstructuring by Laser Etching

Laser etching is carried out with a workpiece placed in a liquid etchant or surrounded by an atmosphere of a reactive gas (dry etching ablation). Both laser writing and laser projection lithography approaches have been applied for laser etching. Laser etching is especially suitable for applications where high-precision, low-damage structuring is required. This is possible because of the fact that laser stimulated chemical reactions occur at laser fluences/powers that are substantially below those required for structuring by direct ablation. Laser etching is of particular importance for compound materials that decompose non-congruently at elevated temperatures and, consequently, cannot be successfully processed by direct ablation. For instance, the vacuum ablation rate of InP achieved with a XeCl excimer laser operating at fluences approaching 120 mJ/cm^2 is very low, i.e., < 0.03 nm/pulse. A significant surface decomposition of InP (and other A^{III}B^V compounds) takes place under such conditions with the preferential removal of the group V element. However, if the process is carried out in a Cl$_2$ gas environment (16), a XeCl excimer-induced etch rate of InP is about 0.2 nm/pulse for laser fluence about 65 mJ/cm^2. It has been argued that laser etching leads to less damaged microstructures than reactive ion etching (17). The anisotropic nature of laser dry etching ablation, the smooth surface morphology of materials etched at low laser fluences, and the potential for high lateral resolution processing with deep-ultraviolet laser beams make this approach attractive for the fabrication of free-standing microstructures with feature sizes in submicrometer range. Laser etching ablation has been applied to small-scale fabrication of some semiconductor device structures and micro-electromechanical systems (MEMS). In the case of Si-based MEMS, this has been realized with an Ar$^+$ laser irradiating a sample surrounded by a Cl$_2$ ambient (18, 19). A schematic diagram of such a system is shown in Figure 2.

The system permits laser scanning of a 256 x 256 pixel field at up to 5 x 10^4 pixels per second in a random access mode or 10^6 pixels per second in a raster mode. The reaction profiles in the material are tightly confined to a zone of several micrometers in three dimensions. The 3D resolution of the laser writing process is 1 µm^3. An example of a laser microchemically etched microstructure is shown in Figure 3. In this case, several micrometer-thick planes of Si have been removed by scanning the laser beam at 20 mm per second. After a plane is etched, the focusing objective is lowered by an incremental amount, and a new pattern is etched.

Table 1. Examples of Microstructures Obtained by Laser Direct Ablation

Laser	Wavelength (nm)	Laser fluence (mJ/cm^2)	Material	Method of fabrication	Structure	Feature size	Ref.
Excimer	308	150–300	Polyimide	Dielectric mask	Vias for MCM	6 µm	8, 9
Excimer	248	150	Polyimide	Contour mask	Microlens array	15 µm	10
Excimer	248	500	Polyimide	Dielectric mask	Vias for printer heads	28 µm	11
Excimer	248	1000	Polyimide	Laser writing	Diffractive optical elements	1 µm	7
Excimer	193	12000 (air)	Diamond films	Quartz mask	Free-standing micro-gear	930 µm	12
Excimer	193	3500	Diamond films	Laser writing	Free-standing micro-gear	400 µm	13
Nd:YAG	1060	–	Poly-Si	Laser writing	Grooves for solar cells	20 µm	14
Nd:YAG	355	4000	Ag:Glass	Phase mask	Grating	1.06 µm (period)	15

Chapter 24: Laser-Produced Microstructures

The excimer laser is especially suited to ultraviolet or deep-ultraviolet-based projection lithography. Because of its large-size beam, the excimer laser has proved economical for high-resolution photolithography (0.2 μm feature size, or less) in semiconductor chip manufacturing.

Examples of excimer laser-based etching processes applied to various materials are listed in Table 2.

Table 2. Examples of Excimer Laser Etched Materials

Material	Wavelength (nm)	Etchant	Etch rate (nm/pulse)	Fluence (mJ/cm^2)	Ref.
Aluminum	308	Cl_2	100	500	20
Copper	308	Br_2 (liq.)	50 (nm/min)	–	20
	248	Cl_2	10	200	
Molybdenum	193	NF_3	0.02	60	20
Tungsten	193	COF_2	0.05	80	20
Poly-Si	193	NF_3	0.05	250	20
Si	308	Cl_2	0.05	500	21
	248	Cl_2	0.06	500	22
	248	Cl_2	0.06	700	23
	193	Cl_2	10^{-8} at./phot.	39–359	24
GaAs	193	Cl_2/Ar	0.5	25	25
	193–300	Cl_2	0.2 (digital)	20	26
	193	Cl_2 (cryo)	0.025	21	27
InGaAs/InAlAs	193	HBr/F_2	0.06	23	28
InP	193	HBr, HCl	0.23	120	29
	193	Cl_2	0.2	80	30
	248	Cl_2	0.2	150	31
	308	Cl_2/He	0.04	50	16
Bi-Sr-Ca-Cu-O	248	NF_3 (Cl_2)	15	250	32
Al_2O_3 (thin film)	193	H_3PO_4	0.1	10–20	33
	248	H_3PO_4	0.1	30–45	33
	308	H_2O	2700	25,000	34
SiO_2	193	NF_3/O_2	0.02	100	35
Glass	248	CF_2Br_2	0.1	1000	20
Pyrex	193	H_2	150	500	20
Diamond	193	Air	22	12,000	36
		Vacuum	0.6	12,000	36

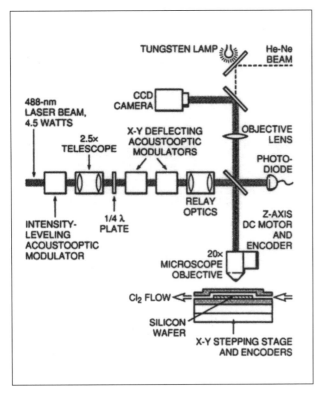

Figure 2. Schematic diagram of the laser etching system for the fabrication of micro-electromechanical systems (19).

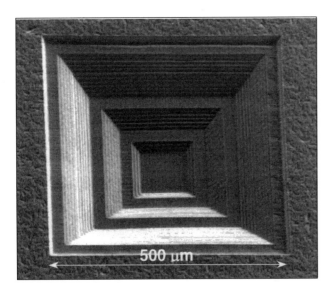

Figure 3. Terraced etch in Si with an Ar+ laser. Each small terrace is 10 μm deep, large terraces are 30 μm deep, and the total structure is 180 μm deep. Etch parameters: 4 W laser power, 20 mm/s galvo scanning, 1 μm line/space, 400 Torr chlorine pressure, 8 min. total etch time. The typical roughness of the etched surface is about several tens of nanometers with no clean-up (photograph courtesy of D. J. Ehrlich, Revise, Inc.).

References

1. W. Parker, *Solid State Technol.*, p. 124 (September 1996).
2. E. C. Harvey, P. T. Rumsby, M. C. Gower, S. Mihailov and D. Thomas, The Institute of Electrical Engineers, Savoy Place, London WC2R OBL, UK, p. 1 (1994).
3. J. F. Ready (Ed.), *Industrial Applications of Lasers,* Academic Press, San Diego, CA, p. 434 (1997).
4. S. M. Metev and V. P. Veiko, *Laser-Assisted Microtechnology,* Springer-Verlag, Berlin, Heidelberg, p. 81 (1994).
5. C. Schomburg et al., *Microelectronic Engineering* **35** (1), p. 509 (1997).
6. D. J. Ehrlich and J. Y. Tsao (Eds.), *Laser Microfabrication,* Academic Press, San Diego, CA, p. 51 (1989).
7. M. T. Duignan and G. P. Behrmann, SPIE Vol. 2991, p. 161 (1997).
8. R. S. Patel et al., *Laser Focus World,* 71–5 (January 1996).
9. T. Lizotte et al., *Solid State Technology,* 120–8 (September 1996).
10. K. Zimmer, D. Hirsch and F. Bigl, *Appl. Surf. Sci.* **96–98,** 425–9 (1996).
11. C. Rowan, *Laser Focus World,* 81–3 (August 1995).
12. S. S. M. Chan et al., *Diamond and Related Mater.* **5,** p. 317 (1996).
13. J. D. Hunn and C. P. Christensen, *Solid State Technology,* 57–60 (December 1994).
14. Ch. B. Honsberg and M. A. Green, *Mater. Sci. Forum* **173–174,** 311–18 (1995).
15. T. Koyama and Keiji Tsunetomo, *Jpn. J. Appl. Phys.* **36,** L244-L247 (1997).
16. J. J. Dubowski, M. Julier, G. I. Sproule and B. Mason, *MRS Symp. Proc.* **397,** 509–18 (1996).
17. J. J. Dubowski, B. E. Rosenquist, D. J. Lockwood, H. J. Labbé, A. P. Roth, C. Lacelle, M. Davies, R. Barber, B. Mason and G. I. Sproule, *J. Appl. Phys.* **78,** 1488–91 (1995).
18. T. M. Bloomstein, S. T. Palmacci, R. H. Mathews, N. Nassuphis and D. J. Ehrlich, *Proc. Laser Processing: Surface Treatment and Films Deposition,* Kluwer Academic Publishers, Dordrecht, Netherlands, 895–906 (1996).
19. T. M. Bloomstein and D. J. Ehrlich, *J. Vac. Sci. Technol.* **B10** (6), 2671–4 (1992).
20. J. Brannon, *IEEE Circuits and Device Magazine* **13,** N2, 11–18 (1997).
21. W. Sesselmann, E. Hudeczek and F. Bachmann, *J. Vac. Sci. Technol.* **B7** (5), 1284–94 (1989).
22. F. Foulon and M. Green, *Appl. Phys.* **A61,** 655–61 (1995).
23. H. Baumgärtner, W. Jiang and I. Eisele, *Appl. Surf. Sci.* **106,** 301–5 (1996).
24. X. H. Chen, J. C. Polanyi and D. Rogers, *Surf. Sci.* **376,** 77–86 (1997).
25. P. Tejedor and F. Briones, *J. Chem. Phys.* **101** (3), 2600–5 (1994).
26. M. Ishii, T. Meguro, K. Gamo, T. Sugano, and Y. Aoyagi, *Jpn. J. Appl. Phys.* **32** (12B), p. 6178 (1993).
27. M. C. Shih, M. B. Freiler, G. Haase, R. Scarmozzino and R. M. Osgood, Jr., *Appl. Phys. Lett.* **61** (7), p. 828 (1992).
28. H. Takazawa, S. Takatani and S. Yamamoto, *Jpn. J. Appl. Phys.* **35** (6B), L754 (1996).

29. R. Matz, J. Meiler and D. Haarer, *MRS Symp. Proc.* **158**, p. 307 (1990).
30. V. M. Donnelly and T. R. Hayes, *Appl. Phys. Lett.* **57** (7), p. 701 (1990).
31. R. Heydel, R. Matz and W. Göpel, *Appl. Surf. Sci.* **69**, p. 38 (1993).
32. T. Oohira, S. Sakai, Y. Kasai, T Shimizu, H. Tokumoto and K. Shimizu, *Jpn. J. Appl. Phys.* **35** (1B), L94 (1996).
33. K. Sugioka, J. F. Fan, K. Kita, S. Tanaka and K. Toyoda, *Jpn. J. Appl. Phys.* **30** (11B), p. 3182 (1991).
34. M. Geiger, W. Becker, T. Rebhan, J. Hutfless and N. Lutz, *Appl. Surf. Sci.* **96–98**, p. 309 (1996).
35. K. Kitamura and M. Murahara, *MRS Symp. Proc.* **334**, p. 439 (1994).
36. S. S. M. Chan, F. Raybould, G. Arthur, F. Goodall and R. B. Jackman, *Diamond and Related Mater.* **5** (3), p. 317 (1996).

J.J. DUBOWSKI

24.2 Other Methods of Laser Microstructuring

24.2.1 Laser-LIGA Processing

Laser-LIGA (the German acronym for "Lithographie, Galvanoformung und Abformung") technology is based on the combination of laser ablation of materials with replication processes (1). The steps involved in Laser-LIGA are described in Figure 1. A photoresist or a polymer film, deposited on a titanium wafer, is shaped directly by excimer laser ablation. Complicated 3D microstructures can be obtained with the use of a motor-driven aperture and computer-controlled laser fluence. In the next step, the laser ablated microstructure is covered with a thin metallic layer of nickel or gold (a few hundreds of nm) deposited by thermal evaporation. A thick metallic layer is deposited on top of this layer by electro-plating. A mould insert is obtained following separation of metal and polymer parts. Replicas of the original microstructure can be obtained either by injection moulding or by hot embossing.

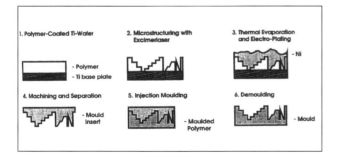

Figure 1. Schematic diagram of the steps involved in the Laser-LIGA process (1).

The Laser-LIGA approach has found application in rapid prototyping and large-scale production of micro-scale devices. Compared to deep X-ray lithography, the surface quality of microstructures made by Laser-LIGA is slightly poorer, and the maximum aspect ratios (up to 10) are considerably lower. However, because this technology is based on the application of direct laser ablation, it offers more flexibility in fabricating structures of almost any geometry, without the need of masks.

24.2.2 Laser Microstructuring of Glass

Texturing of Glass Surfaces

Texturing of glass, glass ceramic and fused silica surfaces is of great importance in the manufacture of optoelectronic devices. For instance, fabrication of small domes is required for the construction of stiction zones in magnetic hard disk drives (2). This can be achieved with a modulated high-power CO_2 laser. Using just the tip of the Gaussian laser beam makes possible the formation of extremely smooth micro-domes adjustable from 10 to 200 nm in height. This is truly a "tip-writing" process, since dome diameters of 10–30 μm can be formed with focused optical spot diameters 2–3 times greater. Figure 2 shows an atomic force microscopy (AFM) image of a series of micro-domes fabricated with a CO_2 laser in a glass substrate.

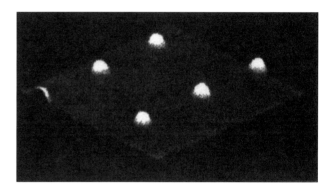

Figure 2. AFM (atomic force microscopy) image of dome microstructures fabricated in a glass substrate with a CO_2 laser. Each dome is approximately 25 nm in height and the base width is about 10 μm (2).

A waveguide CW CO_2 laser operating near the peak of the Si-O absorption band in glass, and an acousto-optic modulator were used for this purpose. Texturing was obtained with a train of pulses with adjustable widths from 0.5 to 50 ms, and repetition rates from 10 to 100 kHz. Various glass substrates can be textured by this method, including aluminosilicate, soda-lime, and borosilicate glasses.

Fiber Bragg Gratings

A fiber Bragg grating (FGB) is a periodic perturbation of the refractive index (n) along the fiber length which is formed by exposure of the core to an intense optical interference pattern (3). The main reasons for the photon-induced increase in the refractive index of the fiber are the formation of color centers and densification of the glass. Photosensitivity has been observed in a wide variety of different fibers; however, optical fiber having a Ge-doped SiO_2 core remains the most important material for the fabrication of FGBs. The Bragg gratings can be fabricated by a holographic technique, but the simplest and probably the most reliable approach is the phase mask technique. This method is illustrated in Figure 3.

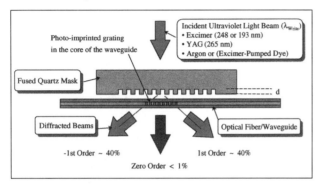

Figure 3. Zero-order nulled phase shift mask photolithography for the fabrication of Bragg gratings in optical fibers. For a square-wave mask, the zero order is nulled by setting $d = \lambda_{Write}/2(n-1)$, and by having a corrugation duty cycle of 50% (3).

Ultraviolet light incident normal to the phase mask passes through and is diffracted by the periodic corrugations of the phase mask. The two ±1 diffracted order beams interfere to produce a periodic pattern that photo-imprints a corresponding grating in the optical fiber. The most commonly used light sources are KrF and ArF excimer lasers. The typical irradiation conditions are exposure to the laser light (10 ns pulses at 50–75 Hz) at intensities ranging from 100 to 1000 mJ/cm². In addition, higher-harmonic Nd:YAG, Ar-ion, and excimer–pumped dye lasers have been used for this purpose. Typical changes in the refractive index are 10^{-5}–10^{-3}, but Δn as high as 10^{-2} can be obtained in specially processed glasses. Gratings with periods less than 1 μm have been routinely fabricated with this method. In comparison with the holographic technique, the phase mask technique offers easier alignment of the fiber for photo-imprinting, reduced stability requirements on the manufacturing station and lower coherence requirements on the ultraviolet laser beam, and thereby permits the use of a cheaper ultraviolet excimer laser source. FBGs have been used in fiber optic communications (e.g., reflectors for semiconductor lasers, fiber lasers, amplifiers, band rejection filters, wavelength selective devices), as well as in fiber optic sensor systems.

Photo-etching of 3D Microstructures

High aspect ratio 3D microstructures can be formed in a photosensitive glass by exposing it to ultraviolet laser radiation (photopatterning) followed by baking it at elevated temperatures. Partial crystallization of the glass results. Typical glasses used for this process are from the basic Li_2O/SiO_2 family containing traces of Ag_2O and CeO_2 (4). The crystalline phase of lithium silicate is much more soluble in hydrofluoric acid than the surrounding unexposed amorphous glass. This makes possible the fabrication of freestanding three-dimensional microstructures. Typical etch rates in 5–10% HF water solution are about 1–20 μm/min. A minimum feature size that can be achieved with this technique is about 25 μm. This is determined by the size of micro-crystals formed during heat treatment and that have to be etched away. Structures with an aspect ratio of 1:100 can easily be fabricated with this approach. Examples of machined parts include channels and nozzles for inkjet print heads (4) and satellite micro propulsion systems (5). Figure 4 shows a series of rings about a single tip that were etched in a photosensitive glass using 248 and 355 nm radiation from excimer and Q-switched Nd:YAG (3rd harmonic) lasers, respectively.

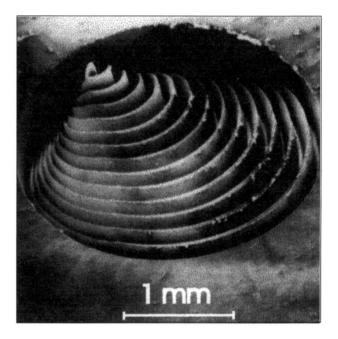

Figure 4. Off-axis tip in a circular hole fabricated with excimer (248 nm) and third-harmonic Nd:YAG (355 nm) lasers in photosensitive glass (Foturan). The tip is surrounded by a series of walls of variable height. Both the tip and rings share a common tangent (5).

Each laser beam is brought through a different ultraviolet-transparent achromatic microscope objective to irradiate the sample with spots of 5 to 10 μm diameter. Direct laser patterning is accomplished using a motorized XYZ microstep positioner under computer control. The varying structure heights observed in Figure 4 are due to various levels of overlap by the conical laser beam, while trenches of uniform depth are obtained because of a fixed laser focus depth and the nonlinear absorption characteristics of the photo-sensitive glass.

Femtosecond Laser Processing of Glass

Three-dimensional laser microstructuring of silica glass can be achieved directly using femtosecond lasers. Although the glass is transparent in the wavelengths ranging from 250 to 1000 nm, its refractive index can be increased by 0.01–0.035, without developing cracks or other damage, by irradiation with 120 fs pulses at 800 nm (6). The use of a tightly focused beam makes it possible to write three-dimensional dots (bits) inside the glass. Because of the self-focusing mechanism and/or non-linear response of the glass, individual bits can be fabricated with size smaller

Chapter 24: Laser-Produced Microstructures

than the wavelength of the laser. This method could be used to fabricate an optical memory with both an ultra-high density and a high recording speed.

24.2.3 Laser Microstructuring of Semiconductors

Lasers have been used in a variety of ways to produce microstructures in semiconductor materials. One important approach is photolithography, used to produce semiconductor chips with feature sizes less than 0.25 micrometers. This application is described extensively in Chapter 21.

Debris-free Texturing (Wafer Marking)

The technology of semiconductor wafer processing requires marking to record batch numbers and numerous process parameters. This application is covered in Section 18.2.1. The marking, which is carried out at various stages of the wafer processing, should be non-invasive, i.e., leave no debris that could become a source of defects in the final structure. The high-intensity laser light that is absorbed very close to the surface heats up the material until it melts. Consequently, a crater forms with a circular ridge or bulge around its heat-affected zone. This approach has been used since 1979 for the marking of semiconductor wafers. Debris is typically formed when the liquefied material is ejected as droplets and propelled by the expansion of the vapor formed. However, the proper choice of the laser parameters (wavelength, pulse energy, pulse duration) and processing environment (e.g., a reactive atmosphere of Cl_2) can reduce, or essentially eliminate debris in the area immediately surrounding the crater.

Nd:YAG laser-based technology can be used for debris-free marking of Si wafers in an ambient atmosphere (7). The principle of this process relies on depositing a high-energy laser pulse of duration sufficient to reach melting temperature only within a shallow absorption depth of about 2 µm. This allows the melt/flow cycle and subsequent cooling cycle to occur before any debris is ejected from the interaction region. An example of the dot obtained on a silicon wafer with the use of this technology is shown in Figure 5. Laser-made dots can be used in alphanumerics, bar codes, and two-dimensional symbols.

Laser Induced Selective Deposition/Epitaxy of Microstructures

Laser irradiation of a wafer during the epitaxial growth of semiconductor quantum well (QW) laser structures can be used for in-situ fabrication of QW lasers emitting at different wavelengths. The idea is schematically illustrated in Figure 6.

The role of a laser in this process is to modify the sticking coefficient of atoms/molecules in selective areas of a substrate, which is heated with a resistive heater in a growth chamber. The irradiation of a large wafer (typically of 2 in. diameter or more) with a small (millimeter size) laser beam results in selectively grown areas of material with a chemical composition different from that of the nonirradiated area of the wafer. Figure 7 shows that this approach can be used for the fabrication of a two-wavelength array of semiconductor QW lasers. The Ar-ion laser beam of 5 W was scanned at 10 Hz over a distance of 10 mm. This resulted in a 300-µm-wide stripe of material that was used for the fabrication of lasers diodes operating at 1.40 µm.

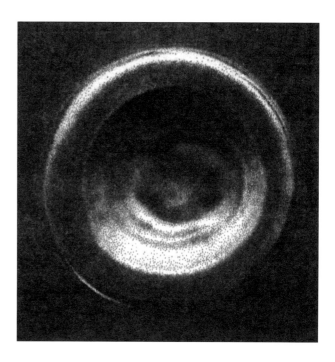

Figure 5. Scanning electron microscope picture of a dot made on a Si wafer with a *Q*-switched Nd:YAG laser. The dot is 2.6 µm deep and its diameter is 70 µm (7).

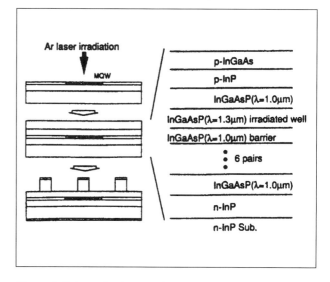

Figure 6. Schematic diagram of the fabrication method of multi-wavelength semiconductor lasers by Ar-ion laser irradiation during the growth of multiple quantum well (MQW) material. The shadowed area is the Ar-ion laser irradiated MQW active layer (8).

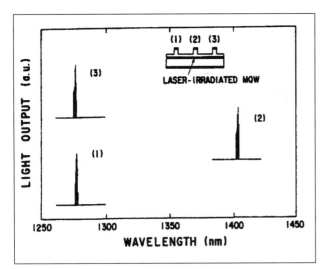

Figure 7. Operational spectra of the semiconductor laser array fabricated by laser-assisted epitaxy. The wavelength of the Ar-ion laser irradiated and nonirradiated laser diodes are 1.40 and 1.28 μm, respectively. The pitch of the laser array is 300 μm and the width of an individual ridge laser diode is 6 μm (8).

Selective Area Band-gap Tuning (Quantum Well Intermixing)

Localized annealing with powerful infrared laser radiation can be used to induce intermixing of the quantum well (QW) and barrier material of semiconductor microstructures. This results in the fabrication of material with an effectively different energy gap than that of the material surrounding it. A schematic illustration of the concept of selective area band-gap tuning by laser-induced QW intermixing (laser-QWI) is shown in Figure 8.

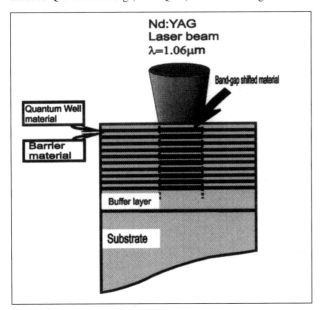

Figure 8. Selective area band-gap tuning in quantum well semiconductor microstructures realized by Nd:YAG laser post-growth processing. Band-gap shifting is caused by laser-induced intermixing of the well and barrier material (9).

Laser-QWI is carried out on a homogeneously grown wafer, thus offering some flexibility in design of optoelectronic devices and systems. It can be used for fine tuning the optical properties of individual devices (e.g., semiconductor lasers) analogously to the laser-based resistor trimming approach applied in microelectronics. Laser-QWI in $Si/Si_{1-x}Ge_x$ ($x = 0.30$) QW structures can be used to blueshift the band-gap of this material by about 142 meV (9). In GaInAs/InP QW microstructures, this process leads to the shifting of the material energy gap in excess of 90 meV (10). This technology has been applied to the fabrication of multi-wavelength semiconductor lasers from a single chip (10, 11). An example of emission spectra of a multi-wavelength laser array fabricated by laser-QWI is shown in Figure 9.

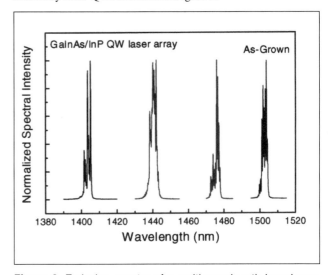

Figure 9. Emission spectra of a multi-wavelength broad-area (~ 40 μm) laser array fabricated by the laser-QWI technique. The cavity length is 500 μm and the spacing between the 1402 and 1502 nm lasers is 3 mm (11).

The spatial resolution of the laser-QWI process applied to the GaInAs/InP QW material is better than 25 μm (10), thus the process has potential for fabricating monolithically integrated photonic circuits comprising multifunction devices (modulators, waveguides, switches, etc.).

Selective area band-gap modulation in GaAs/AlGaAs QW microstructures can be realized by Ar-ion laser-induced Al/Ga interdiffusion (12). Because of strong nonlinear thermal effects, the lateral size of the interdiffused region can be substantially reduced when compared to the exciting laser spot size. This approach can be used for laser writing of less than 0.2-μm-wide nanostructures (quantum wires), with a Gaussian laser spot of 0.6-μm width (12).

References

1. M. Abraham, J. Arnold, W. Ehrfeld, K. Hesch, H. Möbius, T. Paatzsch, and C. Schulz, Proc. SPIE **2639**, 164–73 (1995).
2. A. C. Tam, J. Brannon, P. Baumgart, and I. K. Pour, *IEEE Trans. on Magnetics* **33** (5), 3181–3 (1997).

3. K. O. Hill and G. Meltz, *J. Lightwave Technol.* **15** (8), 1263–76 (1997).
4. T. R. Dietrich, W. Ehrfeld, M. Lacher, M. Krämer and B. Speit, *Microelectr. Eng.* **30,** 487–504 (1996).
5. W. W. Hansen, S. W. Janson and H. Helvajian, *Proc. SPIE* **2991**, 104–12 (1997).
6. J. Qiu, K. Miura, H. Inouye, J. Nishii and K. Hirao, *Nuclear Instr. Methods Phys. Res.* **B141,** 699–703 (1998).
7. J. Scaroni and T. McKee, *Solid State Technology,* July 1997, 245–51.
8. T. Yamada, R. Iga and H. Sugiura, *Appl. Phys. Lett.* **61,** 2449–51 (1992).
9. J. J. Dubowski, N. Rowell, G. C. Aers, H. Lafontaine and D. C. Houghton, *Appl. Phys. Lett.* April 5 (1999).
10. A. McKee, C. J. McLean, A. C. Bryce, R. M. De La Rue, J. H. Marsh and C. Button, *Appl. Phys. Lett.* **65,** 2263–5 (1994).
11. J. J. Dubowski, G. Marshall, Y. Feng, P. Poole, C. Lacelle, J. Haysom, S. Charbonneau and M. Buchanan, *Proc. SPIE* **3618,** (1999).
12. K. Brunner, G. Abstreiter, M. Walther, G. Böhm and G. Tränkle, *Surface Sci.* **267,** 218–22 (1992).

J.J. DUBOWSKI

Notes

Chapter 25

Electronic Packaging: Electrical Interconnects

25.0 Introduction

Packaging in microelectronics involves the integration of chips into a complete assembly to perform a specific function. A good example is the assembly of multichip modules that are collections of integrated circuits mounted onto a high-density interconnect substrate. The multichip module can require thousands of electrical connections, which have to be produced reliably and inexpensively within a very small space. As chip geometries continue to shrink, the performance of a system becomes limited by the packaging and interconnect technology. Lasers are being used increasingly to solve the problems of interconnecting multiple chips in high-density packages.

This chapter covers laser-based approaches to microelectronic interconnection and packaging—including via drilling to produce holes that allow interconnection between different circuit layers—bonding and soldering to form the electrical contacts, and stripping of insulation from wires to be used for connections.

25.1 Via Drilling

Laser via drilling is used for forming blind holes or through holes in printed circuit boards (PCBs) to allow electrical interconnections between circuit layers.

25.1.1 Lasers for Via Drilling

There are four laser types in common usage for via drilling: excimer, transverse excited CO_2 (TEA CO_2), RF excited sealed slab CO_2 (RF CO_2), and Nd:YAG using its ultraviolet harmonics (UV YAG). The pulse shapes of the lasers in use for this application are shown in Figure 1, and other operational characteristics are presented in Table 1.

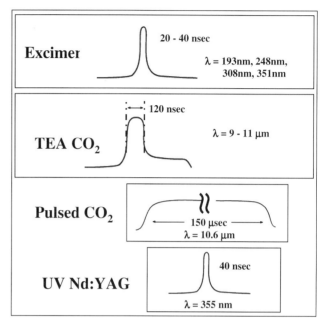

Figure 1. Relative pulse shapes of commercial lasers for via drilling.

Each of these lasers can drill blind holes in unreinforced polymers, such as epoxy or polyimide. The UV YAG can also drill through copper because of the available peak irradiance and material absorption at that wavelength. The tradeoff between laser technologies and other microvia formation methods is dependent on the hole size, the laminate construction, and the drilling depth. The choice of technology and the choice of laser for current applications are presented in Figure 2.

Table 1. Operational Characteristics of Lasers Used for Via Drilling

Type of laser	Wavelength	Practical beam size	Pulse repetition rate	Relative operating costs**
Excimer	193, *248, 308, 351 nm	15 x 10 mm	1–200 Hz	$15/hr
TEA CO_2	9–11, 9.4 µm	0.5 x 0.5 mm	1–300 Hz	$8/hr
Pulsed CO_2	9–11, *9.4, *10.6 µm	0.1 mm diameter	1–20,000 Hz	$1.50/hr
UV YAG	266, *355 nm	0.025 mm	1–24,000 Hz	$1.50/hr

*Most typical for laser via drilling
**Using typical figures applicable at the time of writing

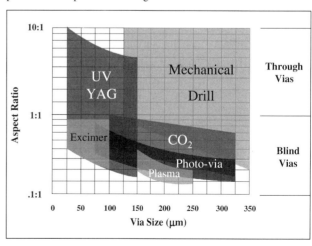

Figure 2. Optimal technology choice and laser choice as functions of via size and aspect ratio (the ratio of diameter to depth).

ISBN 0-912035-15-3

25.1.2 Optical Configurations

Because of the wide variation in power, repetition rate, operating costs, and beam size, different optics combinations are used to optimize each laser for via drilling. Some of these configurations are shown in Figure 3.

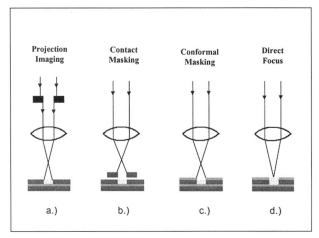

Figure 3. Mask and optics configurations used for laser via drilling.

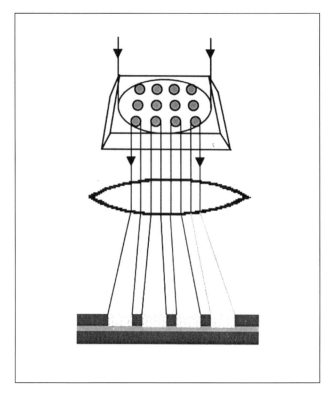

Figure 4. Projection mask imaging.

Mask Projection/Scanning

Mask imaging is typically used with excimer and TEA CO_2 lasers to make use of their large beam sizes and higher laser powers, and to overcome their high operating costs and low pulse repetition rates. Pattern-specific masks are used to "project" the laser onto the dielectric, creating multiple microvias at the same time. The size of the pattern is typically magnified by the imaging optics or objective lens. Typically, the masks are made of metals or metal films on appropriate transparent optical materials. Because of the damage thresholds of the masks, the laser fluence is kept < 1 J/cm^2.

The laser beam and projection mask are positioned over an area and pulsed several times until the dielectric is removed (typically 0.1 to 10 µm of material is removed per pulse), and then indexed to the next position as shown in Figure 4. This method has limited production applications, but is suited to repeating patterns where the mask can be made smaller than the beam size.

A special case of mask projection imaging is the use of an aperture in the beam path to improve the quality or modify the shape of the beam. In this case only a single via is drilled at a time, and the aperture is changed to adjust the diameter of the via. Because of the large size and poor shape of the beams from these lasers, it is necessary to use the aperture to image only a portion of the beam to form a via, rather than use all of the power available. An example of this is Figure 3a. Shapes other than circles can be imaged by changing the aperture. This technique significantly reduces the depth of field of the focused image, typically requiring additional optics to account for slight variations in the surface of the part being drilled.

Mask scanning can also be used with these lasers or with other lasers where the laser power is not the limiting factor. Here the mask is located between the objective lens and the work surface and the laser is scanned over the mask. Only the portion of the beam that passes through the mask aperature is used to form a via. While reusable masks are possible, the most typical configuration is to use the top copper layer of the circuit board as a conformal mask as shown in Figure 3c. In this case, the PCB has a resist applied, which is exposed and developed. The copper is chemically etched to form the conformal mask, and then the resist is removed. This process becomes expensive and has low yields for diameters below 125 µm, so UV YAG lasers are increasingly used to create the conformal masks. The conformal mask method is a common method for excimer and CO_2 lasers, and is also used with nonlaser technologies, such as plasma drilling and sand blasting.

UV YAG lasers can also be used with imaged aperatures or conformal masks, but are more typically used in a one- or two-step direct drilling described below.

Phase Mask Scanning

Phase mask scanning is a method used with excimer lasers to utilize the laser beam more efficiently than is possible with a projection mask. A phase mask is actually a quartz plate into which individual lenslets are machined at the location of each via, but the method is otherwise analogous to Figure 4. The masks are manufactured using focused ion beams, and can take several days and cost tens of thousands of dollars to produce each one, so this method is reserved for high-volume, high-density applications, in stable designs. While the efficiency of a projection mask is typically low (~1%) when drilling multiple vias simultaneously, a phase mask uses the beam more efficiently (> 50%), resulting in dramatically higher drilling rates.

Direct Laser Drilling

In direct laser drilling, the laser requires no masks in order to form vias. The laser beam is directly focused to drill vias one at a time, as shown in Figure 3d.

This method most commonly uses UV YAG lasers as well as CO_2 lasers with good beam mode quality. Since no mask is involved, fluence >> 1 J/cm^2 can be used. Holes can be made by pulsing, trepanning, or spiralling techniques. In pulsing, the via is the same as the size of the beam and the hole is formed by pulsing 1–100 pulses on a single location. For holes larger than the size of the beam, the laser is pulsed while the beam is moved in a spiral or trepanned in a circle of the desired diameter, as shown in Figure 5.

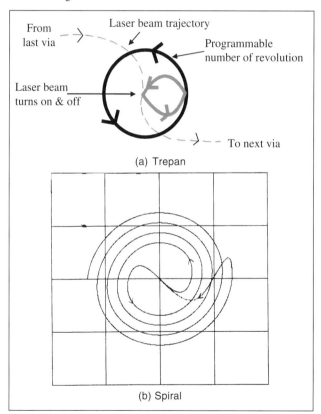

Figure 5. Vias can be formed with pulsed, trepan (a), or spiral (b) techniques.

The direct drilling approach has the most complex positioning system, but has the simplest optics, requires no custom tooling and allows the most flexibility in the applications possible. A special case of direct drilling uses the following two steps to form the vias (see Fig. 6):

1. A UV YAG (or sometimes an IR YAG laser operating at 1047 nm) is used to image the copper.
2. The imaged copper is used as a conformal mask for a UV YAG or CO_2 laser to remove the dielectric in a second step.

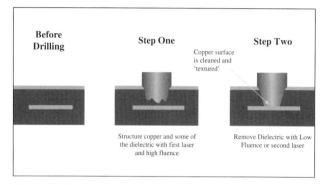

Figure 6. The two-step process for direct drilling.

25.1.3 Applications and Results

Laser via drilling is most commonly used for high-density applications, for portable products such as video cameras and cell phones, and with IC packaging, and computer controller boards. Despite the significantly different powers, wavelengths, repetition rates, pulse widths, and optics used in today's laser drilling systems, all produce via holes that have cost, speed, or quality advantages for some via drilling constructions. Figure 7 (next page) shows constructions, via sizes, materials, and laser choices qualified for production applications.

It is not possible to list all examples of laser via drilling. The following three examples will illustrate the range of these applications and show some typical parameters.

Example A: In a personal communication system (PCS) the use of laser vias allowed nearly 200 blind vias to be place into IC mounting pads directly, saving space on the board. A hybrid multilayer approach using epoxy resin was chosen for cost. (The UV YAG laser drills 150 µm blind vias at 1200 vias/min.) The result is shown in Figure 8.

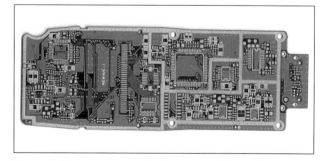

Figure 8. Personal communication system with 200 laser-drilled blind vias per board. Photograph courtesy of Samsung.

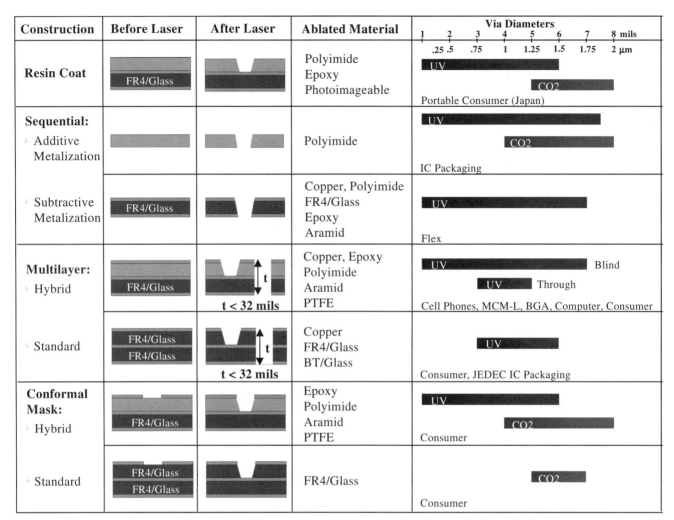

Figure 7. Construction chart (above).

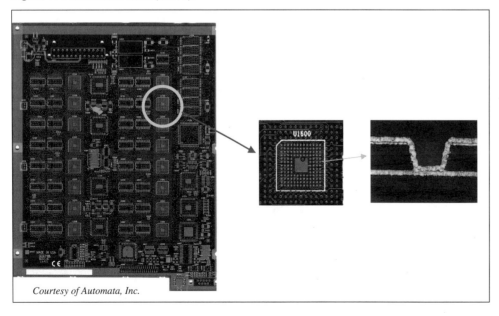

Example B: This network modem server uses 4600 blind holes to allow redistribution of the numerous contacts on the ball grid array device. FR4 is a low-cost, approved material. The UV YAG laser allows 4-mil (100-µm) holes to be drilled at 23 vias/sec. The holes are shown in Figure 9.

Figure 9. Via holes in a network modem server (left).

Chapter 25: Electronic Packaging: Electrical Interconnects

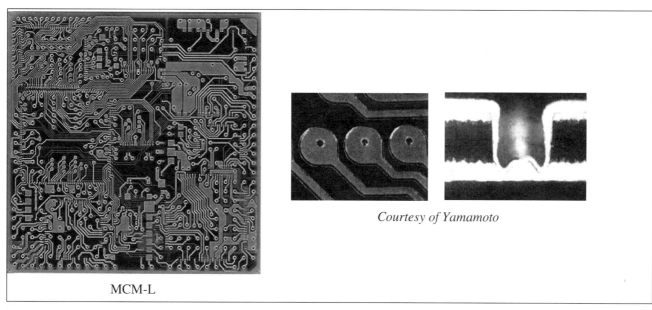

Courtesy of Yamamoto

MCM-L

Figure 10. Vias in an epoxy resin with glass fibers.

Example C: A very high-performance multichip module requires the use of an epoxy with glass fibers. Only the UV YAG laser could drill 80-μm blind vias in this material. The circuit and vias are shown in Figure 10 (above).

MARK D. OWEN

25.2 Bonding/Soldering

25.2.1 Laser Tape Automated Bonding (TAB)

This section describes laser-based processes used for making numerous interconnections required in the packaging of microelectronic assemblies.

Tape automated bonding (TAB) is a process first introduced about 1960 for interconnecting integrated circuit devices to a second-level assembly, such as a package or circuit board. The process is normally performed using a thermo-compression process wherein the connection between the TAB lead and the silicon die is accomplished by the application of heat and pressure forming a metallurgical bond between a gold- or tin-plated TAB lead and a gold bump on the die. This connection is known to as the inner lead bond (ILB). The inner lead on the tape is part of a continous conductor that terminates in an "outer lead" and makes the connection to the next-level assembly (1).

The problem with the thermocompression (TC) bonding process is that the silicon die is susceptible to damage from both the pressures and temperatures used. In a typical TC bonding operation, the bonding temperature may be ~500°C, and the applied pressure may be as high as 135 MPa. Both the device electrical characteristics and the mechanical integrity of the topside passivation layers may be degraded under these conditions. The process window for TC bonding is consequently narrow in order to avoid such damage. The use of tin-plated TAB tape has been tried in order to reduce the bonding temperature. Although the use of tin-plated tape is desirable because of the reduced cost compared to gold-plated tape, the gold-tin TC process has additional drawbacks.

The use of a laser-based bonding process for TAB relies on the fact that heat can be localized to the bonding site only and that little or no pressure is required to accomplish the bonding. This fact is most applicable to the gold-tin process, which is the more difficult process with TC bonding. The laser bonding process for the tin system was first described in 1990 (2) and a process for the gold/gold system was described in 1994 (3). The difference in the two processes reflects the variance in the material properties of tin and gold. Tin has a relatively low melting point (231°C) and a high absorptivity at 1.06 μm, whereas gold has a high melting point (1064°C) and a very low absorptivity at 1.06 μm. The tin-based laser process can utilize more conventional laser technology, such as Nd:YAG systems. The gold-based process requires a more complicated laser system to provide shorter wavelength light mixed with the fundamental 1.06 μm output. Thus, the majority of published data on laser TAB bonding has concentrated on the tin-based system.

The standard implementation of laser TAB bonding uses a two part workholder. A fixed mounting plate is used to support the TAB tape and a movable die pedestal is used to support and align the silicon die to the array of leads on the TAB tape (see Figs. 1 and 2). The rigid portion of the workholder should be designed so that the interior edge of the tape plate extends nearly to the inner edge of the TAB tape inner lead bond (ILB) window to provide sufficient mechanical support for the flexible TAB tape. The movable portion of the fixture must be large enough to support all of the die since silicon is a relatively brittle material and the die may be damaged if it is not fully supported. For purposes of alignment the die pedestal must have x, y, z and θ motion capability. Actual alignment of the die to tape can be performed manually or, preferably, through use of automated vision systems.

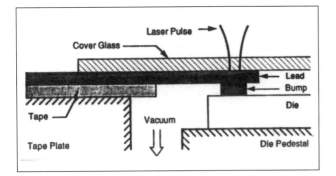

Figure 1. Cross-section view of laser bonder work fixture.

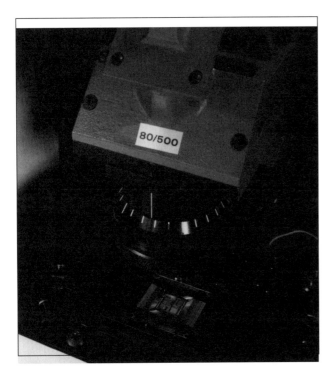

Figure 2. View of slide carrier containing TAB tape and die in position for bonding under laser beam optical head (cover glass removed for clarity).

As shown in Figure 1, a cover glass is placed over the tape and die during the bonding process. This is necessary to prevent the TAB leads from moving during the bonding operation. Without this cover glass, the instantaneous heat transfer from the laser pulse will cause the lead to jerk away from the contact bump on the die, because of differential thermal expansion. The amount of pressure needed to prevent the lead motion is relatively small and may be generated by application of a slight vacuum from within the work fixture. The vacuum is applied only after the tape and die have been aligned and is then released after the bonding operation. The cover glass forms the seal during bonding. This cover glass, which must be optically transparent at 1.06 μm, may have to be discarded after each use depending on the specific material and implementation. If reusability is not an issue, then an ordinary microscope cover slide is acceptable.

The bonding operation is a "single-point" process where each TAB to die connection is bonded in serial fashion. After placement of the TAB tape and die on the fixture, the die and tape are aligned, the cover glass is placed over the die and tape, and the die pedestal is raised to bring the die bumps into contact with the TAB leads. The laser beam optical head is then positioned over each bond site and the laser is pulsed to create the bond. In the tin/gold system, this joint is a metallurgical system created by melting the tin coating on the TAB tape which will then "solder" the gold bump on the die and the copper lead. Since tin forms stable alloys with both copper and gold, the resulting joint is very strong and reliable. Figures 3–6 illustrate the appearance of the laser bonded TAB bond.

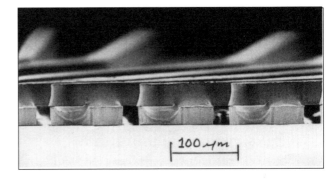

Figure 3. Frontal view of a series of laser-bonded TAB joints.

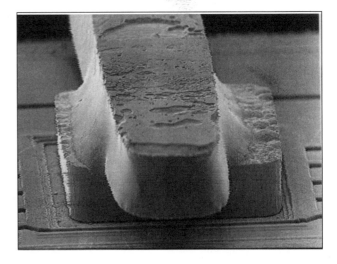

Figure 4. Overhead view of a single laser-bonded TAB joint

Chapter 25: Electronic Packaging: Electrical Interconnects

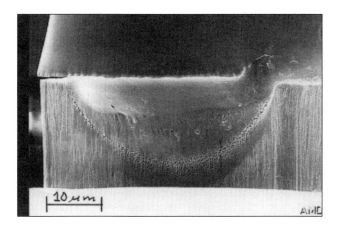

Figure 5. Underside view of laser-bonded TAB joint showing tin reflow on the inside edge of the lead and die bump.

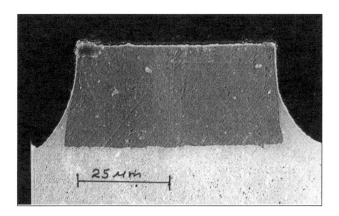

Figure 6. Cross-sectional view of laser-bonded TAB lead showing copper lead joined by tin/copper/gold relow to gold bump.

Formation of a continuous reflow zone at all the lead to bump interfaces as shown is a necesary condition for a reliable TAB bond.

The laser beam power required for each bond must be determined empirically or by use of thermal models for the bonding process. For most applications a laser power output of approximately 35 W (measured at the bond site) pulsed for 5 ms has been found to give acceptable results (4). But the exact power level for a specific application is a function of the lead and bump geometry and material characteristics. Power levels that are too low will result in incomplete tin reflow and voids in the joint; power levels that are too high will result in excessive melting of the copper lead. The selection of power level is especially sensitive if the die bump width is much larger than the TAB lead width. In such cases the gold bump acts as a heatsink and excess power is needed to heat the bump itself up to the bonding temperature.

For successful implementation of the tin/gold TAB system, specification of both the tape and die bump characteristics is required. Tin plating on the TAB tape should have minimum thickness of 0.5 μm on all surfaces and should be reflowed after plating to ensure uniformity. The critical parameter for the die bumps is the flatness of the top surface.

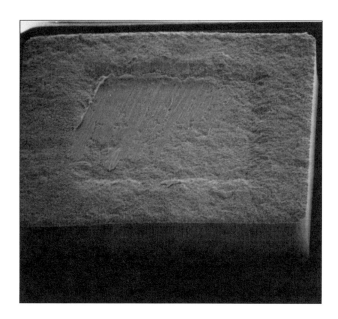

Figure 7. View of an unbonded die bump showing normal surface topography.

The variation in height across the surface of any bump should be in the range of 0–5 μm. With any greater variation in surface topography, the quantity of tin on the TAB lead will be insufficient to bridge gaps between the lead and bump surfaces during bonding.

References
1. John H. Lau (Ed), 1992: *Handbook of Tape Automated Bonding*, Van Nostrand Reinhold, New York, NY.
2. P. J. Spletter and R. T. Crowley, *Proceedings of Electronic Components and Technology Conference*, 757–61 (1990).
3. Phil Spletter, *IEEE Trans.* on CPMT-Part B, **17,** 554–58 (1994).
4. J. Hayward, *IEEE Trans.* on CPMT-Part B, **17,** 547–53 (1994).

JAMES HAYWARD

25.2.2 Laser Reflow Soldering

Introduction

Laser soldering is described in Chapter 9. This section discusses laser soldering with special emphasis on electronic applications. The most common method of interconnecting electronic packages to a printed wiring board (PWB) is via soldering. The majority of soldering operations are done by means of mass process techniques such as wave (flow) soldering or oven (reflow) soldering. But, technological advances now require microelectronic packaging and, thus, the need for interconnecting ever finer circuitry. The laser, with its unique characteristics and capabilities, is not only suited to the new demands for soldering, but offers some unequaled advantages and opportunities for electronics and the soldering process. Certainly mass flow and reflow soldering methods will continue to dominate the electronics industry, but it is clear that laser soldering has much to offer and will likely grow in importance as microelectronics continue to shrink in size. Methods and attributes of laser soldering will be discussed. A brief overview of the mechanics of soldering will provide the backdrop for better understanding the role of the laser and its benefits in this type of joining process.

The Soldering Process

Laser bonding can encompass a variety of techniques including welding and soldering with the latter the most prevalent and important for the joining of electronic circuitry. Soldering involves the use of a fusible filler metal between the items being joined such as IC components and circuit board contacts in the case of electronics soldering. The melting point of the fusible filler (the solder) is generally well below the melting point of the materials to be joined. The component contact is generally referred to as the lead and the substrate contact, the land or pad. When two pieces of metal are joined through soldering, the solder is heated to liquidus and wets to the metals to be joined. Upon resolidification of the molten solder, now in wetted contact with the lead and pad, the solder joint is formed. The ability of solder to wet a metal is dependent on the system's metallurgical characteristics. The base metal must be exposed to and compatible with the solder. The metal(s) to be joined must in some small part be soluble in the solder. Therefore, solder wettability will be highly dependent on the surface chemistry of the solder itself as well as the metal(s) to be joined.

Most materials bear a native oxide layer which is relatively inert and presents as an insoluble, nonwettable, barrier to soldering. Other surface contaminants (oils, sulfides, etc.) are typically present which interfere with bond formation. Therefore, the laser soldering process, as is the case for other soldering techniques, must encompass a method for oxide removal and exposure of the wettable base metal(s) during the bonding process. These barriers to soldering are removed with a fluxing agent (flux), that dissolves, reduces, or otherwise removes oxides and contaminants from the surfaces of the solder and metals to be joined. The most familiar forms of flux are liquid or paste. Gaseous phase fluxing agents (5, 6) and mechanical methods, such as ultrasonic oxide dispersal, are also effective in laser soldering. In some cases, more akin to welding than soldering, the violent convective forces established in the liquidus during high-energy short-duration laser bonding may be enough to disrupt the oxide layer allowing for a fluxless soldering method (7).

Once solder wets to the metals to be joined, crystalline intermetallic compounds (IMCs) begin to form and precipitate upon cooling. These are metallurgical alloys composed of the materials to be joined and solder constituents. Eutectic tin-lead (Sn-Pb) solder, the most commonly used alloy for electronic soldering applications, is composed of about 67 wt.% Sn and 37 wt.% Pb. In the case of a copper lead with eutectic tin-lead solder, Cu_6Sn_5 and Cu_3Sn are the intermetallic compounds formed. These IMCs are of highest concentration at the solder metal interface and become less prevalent through the bulk of the solder joint. They can distribute or grow in the solder itself in lesser concentration. The relationship of IMCs to laser soldering will be discussed shortly. The "glue" of the solder joint is the IMC layer(s) and joint properties are dominated by this brittle interface and its physical and chemical properties.

Advantages of Laser Soldering

There are several advantages provided by laser soldering. Since the laser is well suited for flexible manufacturing and close quarter soldering, it can precisely deliver high-density photonic energy rapidly and with an exceptionally small spot size. Therefore, heat sensitive components and substrates, which would not survive mass reflow processing, can be effectively soldered, if the beam is confined to the metal surfaces of the lead and/or pad.

Today's industrial lasers are stable and reliable enough for the demands of the modern manufacturing floor. The laser's monochromatic output is inherently reproducible and easily monitored, characteristics well suited for consistent high volume manufacturing. Other photonic heat sources are employed in industry for soldering, such as focused infrared radiation from a xenon lamp, but these noncoherent, polychromatic sources make tight spot focusing and beam monitoring more of a challenge. In addition, their spectral output can vary with time, further complicating process reproducibility.

1. Fine Grain Solder Joint and Thin Intermetallic Layer: With the short-duration, high-energy density laser irradiation used in the soldering process, the solder quench rate can be exceptionally rapid, sometimes as short as thousands of degrees/second. The energy density is several orders of magnitude higher than is achievable by the more conventional soldering processes used in the electronics industry. Since the grain size of the fusing metal alloy(s) (e.g., Sn-Pb) in the resolidifying solder mass is dependent upon the quench rate, the rapid solidification characteristic of laser soldering results in exceptionally fine grain crystallinity within the solder joint. Initially, smaller grain size translates to a stronger solder joint. As the joint ages, grain coarsening occurs as with any solder joint, and eventually the strength advantage is lost. But in today's disposable electronics consumer market, or in the case of high-reliability military or space electronics, any increase in joint strength may translate to an advantageous increase in product service life, so this advantage, characteristic of most forms of laser soldering, should be carefully considered.

Intermetallic compound formation rate is also time-temperature dependent and the rapid heat/quench cycle of laser soldering can have a profound effect on its minimization. Thinner intermetallic layers are advantageous as IMCs are notably brittle, the weakest interface within a solder joint. When soldering by more conventional methods, precise time-temperature profiles are used to avert thick intermetallic build up which is correlatable to weak solder joints and premature product field failures. The thermodynamics of metal/IMC/solder systems favor the growth intermetallics over time. Nonetheless, a thin intermetallic layer at the onset means greater initial solder joint strength and longer service life. This is an advantage for mechanical shock resistance and high reliability applications. The reproducible and easily monitored characteristics of laser output permits consistent laser soldering parameters and precludes undesirably thick IMC layer.

2. Some Independence from Thermal Mass: As with many laser-based techniques, short-duration, high-energy heating can be advantageous. In the case of laser soldering, heating is largely superficial and intense. This permits it to be somewhat less dependent on bulk thermal properties of the package and substrate as compared with conventional soldering methods. Therefore, substrate (printed wiring board) pre-heating, as required by hot bar soldering or hot gas soldering, is generally not required. Also, subtle changes in joint thermal mass or underlying circuit board thermal mass are of much less consequence than is the case in other soldering processes. The population density and spacing of packages on circuit boards is also of little consequence in the case of laser soldering. Typically, the presence or absence of a component heatsink has no effect on laser soldering since the heating is so localized and the duration of the soldering so short. Occasionally though, component heatsinks can be large enough to block line of sight access to component leads and board pads, in which case laser soldering will not be possible.

3. No Oxides or Lacquers to Impede Thermal Transfer: Conductive soldering methods (hand soldering iron or hot bar soldering) rely upon mechanical contact of the heating tool to the workpiece and thermal transfer from that heat source into the workpiece. If the bar or iron is not routinely cleaned, heated flux residues can polymerize into durable varnishes on the soldering iron tip or hot bar. Similarly, oxidation of the iron tip or bar cannot be avoided; this is the result of long-duration, high-temperature operation in an air environment.

Both lacquers and oxide coatings impede thermal transfer from the heating tool to the workpiece and interfere with and add variability to the soldering process. Since laser soldering is primarily a noncontact heating method, this is not a concern. Additionally, the laser also offers advantages over hot air soldering methods because thermal transfer through most gases is inefficient and achievable heat and quench rates are remarkably slow. Hot gas methods are far from localized and may result in unnecessary heating of adjacent components and overheating of the soldering substrate.

4. Permits Use of High Temperature Solders: Eutectic tin-lead solder (63% Sn/37%Pb, also symbolized by Sn63) has a melting point of 183°C and most circuit board materials are formulated to survive multiple reflow cycles well above this temperature. In some applications it is desirable to use noneutectic, higher lead alloy formulations such as 10Sn or even 5Sn with considerably higher melting ranges; 268°C–302°C and 301°C–314°C, respectively. This is well above the damage threshold of most common circuit board materials and if soldering by mass reflow were attempted at these higher temperatures, the circuit board would char and delaminate.

Since the thermal energy can be highly localized with laser soldering, this technique affords the opportunity to solder such high temperature alloys without adversely affecting the printed wiring board. This assumes, of course, that the laser exposure regime is of sufficiently short duration and high fluence to achieve solder fusion below the laser threshold damage limit of the circuit board material.

Hold-Down Strategies

As previously indicated, laser soldering can be an efficient, noncontact soldering method with unrivaled capability in terms of component lead pitch and application precision. However, the ideal of completely noncontact joining is rarely achieved in laser soldering. In most cases, some sort of hold-down fixturing is required to ensure intimate contact between the materials to be joined and the solder. The design and application of the fixture can have a significant impact on the laser soldering process. The use of wavelength appropriate windows (8–10) or optical fibers pushing leads into contact with pads has been demonstrated for laser soldering. This approach may be appropriate in laboratory scale soldering, but in high-volume manufacturing, the volatile by-products of the flux and oxides of the solder coat the underside of the window material or fiber tip and cause variations in soldering results. Also, the window hold-down approach is not flexible and will not conform well to the unevenness of component lead sets and undulating surfaces of laminated printed wiring boards in industrial electronic soldering.

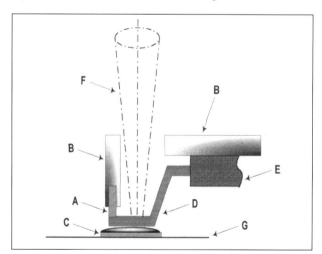

Figure 8. Hold-down tool (B) is used to ensure intimate contact of surface mount component lead (D) to printed wiring board solder coated land (C). The tool is made of a nonabsorptive metal, such as aluminum. A high-temperature, compressable polymeric foot (A) exerts pressure on the component lead tip while the hold-down tool gently compresses the IC body (E). This helps to compensate for lead and pan noncoplanarity and the uneven surface of the printed wiring board (G). The laser's beam (F) is directed through a windowless aperature in the hold-down tool to the component lead/pad combination for soldering.

The best solution for component lead hold-down is one which allows flexibility to account for uneven surfaces as in non-coplanar leads/pads and also provides a windowless approach for hold-down. An example of such a fixture is depicted in Figure 8 (previous page).

Flux for Laser Soldering

The high energy density of the laser beam makes for ideal fluxing conditions even with short irradiation times characteristic of laser soldering. It is best to test various fluxes for effectiveness. Some fluxes are more optically absorptive than others. An absorptive flux can be advantageous in helping to spread heat in the target area and minimize printed wiring board charring when a larger beam is used and lead/pad as well as interpad areas are irradiated during the soldering process. On the other hand, an overly absorptive flux may caramelize or even burn during laser irradiation. It is best to measure fluxes for optical absorption at the laser wavelength and test them for fluxing effectiveness with laser soldering. Often, even non-activated, "no-clean" fluxes are adequate for laser soldering applications.

Surface Finishes for Laser Soldering

Most of the standard metallurgical finishes for ICs and circuit substrates are appropriate for laser soldering. Matte tin plated surfaces, tin-lead alloys are common finishes for IC leads. Tin-lead solder, organic solderability protected copper and gold are the most frequently used circuit boards coatings. Even though copper and gold are highly reflective, if the laser energy is directed at a more absorptive surface finish, such as tin or tin-lead on the component lead, then enough thermal transfer may occur for solder joint formation. The converse is true also. If a gold leadframe is being soldered to a tin-lead circuit board pad, the laser's energy can be directed at the more absorptive tin-lead pad to effect soldering. With some forethought in board layout and material requirements, pad lengths can be extended to accommodate this method.

The solder for laser bonding can be supplied to the printed wiring board land, component lead, or both. Most solder deposition methods are adequate and requirements for laser soldering seem to be less stringent than for other soldering methods. A hot air solder leveled (HASL) surface is the most common finish available from circuit board vendors. In this process, the circuit board is dipped into molten solder and excess solder is blown off with an air knife. For fine pitch soldering (< 0.025-inch lead pitch) this may provide sufficient solder volume for laser bonded joint formation. The high heat and short duration of laser soldering tend to establish strong Marangoni flows. This draws much of the available solder up to the component lead. What results is a solder joint with rich fillet formation, formed with less solder than is typically required by other more common bonding methods. Ultimately, the amount of solder needed will be dictated by the product requirements for robustness in the field. If additional solder is needed beyond the HASL finish, it can be applied by plating or solder paste can be stenciled on to the lands and the board can be mass reflowed prior to laser soldering.

Raw solder paste should be avoided for laser soldering applications. Solder paste is composed of miniature spheres of solder held in a flux-based paste. When a high energy density laser beam is directed at a mass of solder paste, the paste volatiles boil rapidly. Some of the solder spheres fuse and splatter from the rapid volatilization of flux components. This results in loose, randomly dispersed solder balls which may lead to electrical shorting between leads of fine pitch componentry or between fine, unprotected traces on the circuit board. As for most soldering methods, one should strive for the best coplanarity of leads/pads to avoid solder opens. Solder bridging is never a problem with laser soldering even at the finest lead/pad pitches.

Reflectivity a Key Factor in Laser Soldering

The choice of laser should be tailored to the application. Materials reflectivities, power output, and required spot size are significant factors for laser soldering as in other laser processing applications. The laser output must be sufficient for material heating and its output must be kept below the laser damage threshold of the targeted materials. Most metals are good reflectors in the wavelength range of industrial lasers. In fact, some of the most common metals in soldering, such as gold and copper, are notably difficult to join by laser because of their high reflectivities. Even tin, another common element of soldering, can be quite reflective, so the choice of laser is important. Materials reflectivities at common laser wavelengths are presented in the Table 1. See Section 5.3 for more detailed information on surface reflectivity.

Table 1. Reflectivity of Solder Joint Materials at Common Laser Wavelengths

Laser type / λ (μm) Reflectivity	Nd:YAG 0.266	Nd:YAG 0.532	Nd:YAG 1.064	CO_2 10.6
~%R Sn	30	70	70	85
~%R Au	30	60	95	99
~%R Cu	25	50	90	98
~%R Ag	25	95	98	98
~%R solder 63/37 (Eut.) Sn/Pb	15	18	22	72
~%R laminate FR-4 (glass-epoxy)	5	15	25	2

The values in the table illustrate approximate magnitudes. Reflectivities will be greatly influenced by surface condition, oxidation, etc.

The wavelength-reflectivity data in Table 1 shows that the choice of laser will have a profound influence on the efficiency of thermal transfer into a given material. Therefore, the use of a particular metallurgical system necessitates careful consideration of the laser tool and the strategy for laser soldering.

Types of Lasers for Laser Soldering

Nd:YAG and CO_2 lasers are the ones most commonly used for soldering applications, with the former being preferable. Most metals increase in reflectivity with increasing wavelength. Conversely, the substrate materials, such as glass-epoxy laminate and polyimide, as commonly used in printed wiring boards, increase in absorptivity with increasing wavelength. CO_2 laser light is more likely to be absorbed by an organic circuit substrate and cause charring. Besides being cosmetically unappealing, this can cause electrical shorting from carbonaceous deposits, a product of the denatured circuit board surface.

The CO_2 laser may not be focusable to small enough spots for some electronic soldering applications. Also, because the CO_2 beam is more easily reflected by metals and absorbed by organics, stray reflectance off the soldering target is more prone to cause damage to adjacent IC packages or the circuit substrate, such as silicon die, printed wiring board, or ceramic substrate.

Strategies for Laser Soldering

The laser energy can be delivered in several ways:

1. Shuttered or Pulsed Laser Beam. This may use a gated CW laser or a pulsed laser. One can obtain a small spot size with beam energy density high enough that damage to substrate may occur. The beam must be restricted to irradiate the lead/pad combination only. This method offers a short dwell time. The user controls the pulse duration to yield a predetermined time, to effect heating and soldering. The pulses may cause damage (cutting, melting) to the lead if the delivered energy is excessive. The profile of laser energy delivered to the leads or pads as a function of distance is shown in Figure 9.

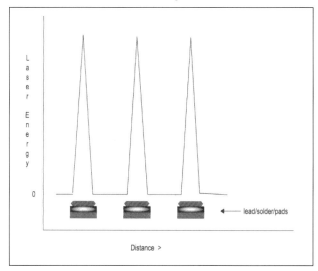

Figure 9. Laser energy versus distance with gated or pulsed beam delivery.

2. Scanned Laser Beam. This method uses a single sweep of a continuous wave beam directed at a lead/pad as well as interpad areas to effect soldering. The beam size is large as compared to the soldering target (lead/pad combination). The irradiation regime is below the laser damage threshold for the electronic substrate or circuit board. The heating is through direct absorption of laser energy into the lead/pad combination. Some degree of absorption into the substrate and/or flux augments the lead/pad heating. The profile of laser energy delivered to the leads or pads as a fuction of distance is shown in Figure 10.

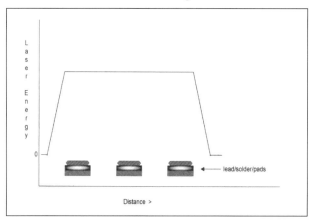

Figure 10. Laser energy versus distance with scanned continuous wave beam delivery.

3. Multiply Scanned (11) or Rastered Beam. In this method, the lead/pad as well as interpad areas are irradiated by a rapidly scanned, high energy laser beam. Each pass of the beam increases the temperature of the bonding area. The scan rate is adjusted such that each pass of the beam results in a net increase in the temperature of the lead/pad combinations. The number of scans (scanning time) and energy density are adjusted to coincide with the onset of solder joint formation without damage to the substrate. A galvanometer beam delivery system may be used. The profile of laser energy delivered to the leads or pads as a function of distance is shown in Figure 11.

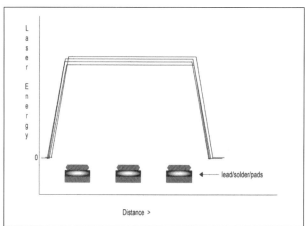

Figure 11. Laser energy versus distance with multiply scanned beam delivery.

ISBN 0-912035-15-3

Laser Soldering Applications

Lasers have been used for assembling multichip modules (MCMs), TAB tape and conventional gull-wing configured surface mount IC packages. No lead size or lead pitch is too small for laser soldering. Bonding of double-sided surface mount assemblies is possible. In doing so, components on one side of the printed wiring board can be reflowed without affecting previously soldered packages on the reverse side of the board; this is a product of rapid and highly localized heating attainable by laser soldering. As suggested previously, design rules required for conventional circuit assembly methods can be rewritten for laser soldering. The precision of beam delivery and the resulting localized heating allows much closer spacing of components to one another than is permitted for effective wave, reflow, hot bar, or hot gas soldering. Further, circuit board vias, vertical traces within circuit boards used for interconnecting one layer of the printed wiring board to another, can be placed directly in the surface mount pad. This is generally avoided when soldering by more conventional means because solder often wicks away through these layer-to-layer interconnects. Since laser soldering is so rapid and localized, there is neither enough liquidus time nor depth of heating for appreciable solder depletion through circuit board via capillarity.

Other laser soldering related applications include:

- Inner lead bonding of TAB tape (12) (connecting TAB leadframe to silicon die)
- Outer lead bonding of TAB tape (connecting TAB leads to circuit board)
- Attachment of punched or etched leadframes to silicon ICs
- Building multichip modules (MCMs)

As stated previously, the more conventional means of soldering will continue to dominate electronics soldering, but it is evident that lasers have some unique capabilities in this area. With development of a suitable infrastructure (production-ready systems suited to high-volume manufacturing), the electronics industry could more fully realize the benefits of laser soldering.

References

5. P. A. Moskawitz and A. Davidson, *J. Vac. Sci. Technol.* A, **3**, May/June 1985.
6. G. M. Freedman, U. S. Patent No. 5,227,604.
7. P. J. Spletter et al., U. S. Patent No. 5,164,566.
8. J. W. Benko and A. Coucoulas, U. S. Patent No. 4,785,156.
9. J. W. Benko and A. Coucoulas, U. S. Patent No. 5,021,630.
10. M. Jones, U. S. Patent No. 5,272,307.
11. S. Vickers and M. E. Connor, "Automated Laser Soldering of Electronic Components," presented at SME Lasers in Electronics Manufacturing, Wakefield, MA, October 13–15, 1987.
12. P. J. Spletter et al., *Hybrid Circuits* **22**, 12–15 (1990).

GARY M. FREEDMAN

25.3 Wirestripping

25.3.0 Introduction

Removal of the plastic insulation which typically covers electrically conducting wires has been performed by a variety of means in the aerospace, data storage, electronics, and electrical industries. Such wirestripping has been done by mechanical cutting, abrasive methods, electrical arching, chemical etching, and simple thermal methods such as burning. These thermo-mechanical techniques can be used when the wire is of sufficient durability, and when the processing speed, precision, or cleanliness of the stripped region are of no major concern. In contrast, laser stripping offers precision and speed without the necessity of contacting the insulated wire.

25.3.1 Important Parameters in Laser Wirestripping

Insulation Absorption of Laser Radiation

At the laser wavelength used in wirestripping operation, the absorption of the insulation is of considerable importance in determining the precision of the stripping, the laser power level employed, and the overall cleanliness of the stripped region. The absorption coefficient of the insulation (defined from Beer's Law: $T = (1-R)\exp(-ax)$, where T is the insulation transmission, R is the reflectivity, a is the absorption coefficient per cm, and x is the insulation thickness in cm), is a figure of merit for absorption strength. In general, the larger the absorption coefficient, the lower the required laser intensity for efficient stripping, and the higher the efficiency, precision, and cleanliness of the process. Insulation absorption coefficients of 10^4–10^5 cm^{-1} are typically found in the ultraviolet (where excimer lasers are utilized), whereas values of 10^2–10^3 cm^{-1} are found near the CO_2 laser wavelength of 10.6 micrometers. Usually, very low values of 10^0-10^2 cm^{-1} exist at the Nd:YAG wavelength near 1 micrometer.

Reflectivity of the laser radiation at the insulation surface is generally not a consideration because the reflectivity is 10% or less for organic insulators. However, if for some reason the reflectivity at the chosen laser stripping wavelength is significant, then the laser intensity must be increased accordingly.

Wire Reflectivity

The issue of wire reflectivity is important from the point of view of laser damage to the wire once the insulation is stripped away. During a wirestripping operation, the bare metal will be exposed to the laser radiation for some amount of time. This time depends on how precisely and quickly the laser exposure is terminated after the insulation has been removed. Usually, the time at which the last layer of insulation is removed is not precisely determined, and may vary from wire to wire. Consequently, a metal that possesses high reflectivity is able to shield itself against possible metal damage brought on by excessive laser exposure. Because metallic reflectivity can significantly decrease with decreasing wavelength, the choice of laser wavelength becomes important in this context. Laser stripping using ultraviolet wavelengths is a case in point. For common copper wire, the reflectivity at 0.248

micrometers wavelength is only about 36% for normally incident radiation. Consequently, some 60% of the incident radiation is absorbed. This large fraction of absorbed energy can lead to deleterious heating and even melting; aspects which may significantly impact the mechanical integrity of the wire. In contrast, the reflectivity of copper is near 97% at 1 micrometer, and greater than 98% near 10.6 micrometers.

Thermal Properties

The thermal properties of the plastic insulation, i.e., heat conduction, are rarely a consideration. Heat conduction within the insulation layer is at best poor, but does not lead to significant imprecision in the defined region to be stripped. The high thermal conductivity of most wire metals on the other hand, can, under certain circumstances, lead to imprecision in the stripped region. Exposure of the stripped wire to laser radiation may cause significant heat generation within the wire. Heat flow along the wire may thus cause non-irradiated insulation near the edge to char or burn away, leaving a ragged, poorly defined edge. Depending on the application, this thermal edge effect may or may not be of concern.

25.3.2 Lasers for Wirestripping

Engineering Issues

In laser wirestripping, a number of issues germane to laser choice must be considered. These issues include, but are not necessarily limited to, the following:

1. Precision, location, and sharpness of the required edge of the stripped region – how well defined must the edge region be?
2. Efficiency and degree of removal – can the process tolerate thin layers of remaining insulation, or splattered debris?
3. Amount of insulation to be removed – how fast must the stripping process be?
4. Cost – is the expense and maintenance of a particular laser system acceptable?
5. Cleanliness – will generated debris, or the production of noxious gases, be a problem?

Clear answers to these questions will greatly aid the engineer in proper design of a laser wirestripping system.

Common Laser Systems

Although many different types of lasers exist, just a few have been utilized for wirestripping. The common CO_2, Nd:YAG, and excimer lasers are discussed in the paragraphs below. Table 1 lists the conditions under which these lasers have been utilized, along with the type of insulation removed, and references to the original literature.

CO_2 Lasers

Because of its high power and relatively low cost, the CO_2 laser has been used in many wirestripping applications. The laser emits infrared radiation peaked at 10.6 µm wavelength – a spectral region where most plastic insulations absorb only moderately. Because of this limitation, CO_2 laser wirestripping requires focussing of the light in order to break down the insulation. Further, the moderate absorption can limit the efficiency with which the last insulation layers are removed, resulting in thin layers remaining on the wire. This may or may not be a problem for the process. The laser can operate either continuously, or as a pulsed TEA device. When running CW, the intense heat of the focused beam will cause rapid melting and vaporization of the insulation, leaving a charred residue near the edge. The gain-switched pulse from a TEA laser (~100 nsec pulse, followed by a several microsecond tail) can also remove insulation when it is focused near the plastic surface. Rather than a clear vaporization process, the focused pulse causes a dielectric breakdown of the material, resulting in a "bomb-like" micro-explosion and ejection of both molten and solid material. Stripping of the wire can be produced using just 2–3 pulses incident from a few circumferential directions. As a result, the edge definition for either CW or pulsed operation is not optimum, and debris generation can be problematic. Figure 1 (next page) displays a wire stripped by a pulsed TEA CO_2 laser. In particular, CW stripping can lead to dc wire heating accompanied by "edge rollback". Nevertheless, for many applications the edge definition is of acceptable quality. When exposed, the high reflectivity of the bare (stripped) wire to CO_2 radiation serves to protect the metal from unacceptable levels of heating and consequent mechanical fatigue.

Nd:YAG Lasers

Although there exist a few literature reports on wirestripping with a Nd:YAG laser, it has not been as commonly used as the CO_2

Table 1. Examples of Laser Wirestripping

Laser	λ	Irradiation conditions	Insulation	Wire	Ref
CO_2, CW	10.6 µm	Focused	Kapton	Cu	1
CO_2, pulsed	10.6 µm	Focused	Polyurethane	Au:Cu	2
Nd:YAG, CW	1.06 µm	Focused	Kapton	Cu	1
Nd:YAG, pulsed	0.53 µm	Imaged	Polyurethane, dye-doped	Au:Cu	3
KrF excimer, pulsed	0.248 µm	Imaged	Polyurethane	Au:Cu	2, 4

laser. Although the costs of the Nd:YAG and CO_2 lasers are not dissimilar, Nd:YAG performance may be diminished because of its wavelength. Compared to the CO_2 laser, insulation absorption near the 1 μm Nd:YAG wavelength is lower by 1–2 orders of magnitude. Thus, very high focused intensities would be required for stripping, with similar concerns about edge definition, debris generation, and the possibility of residual insulation remaining. The shorter wavelength of the Nd:YAG laser will permit smaller focused spot sizes and, in principle, better edge resolution. But because of the poor absorption, this perceived advantage may not be realized. Similar to the CO_2 laser, the Nd:YAG laser can operate with CW or pulsed (Q-switched, 10–100 nsec pulses). The recent generation of small footprint diode-pumped Nd:YAG lasers may appeal to engineers contemplating wirestripping systems. Again, while the quality of stripping may not be optimum, for many situation it may be "good enough" for Nd:YAG lasers to be seriously considered.

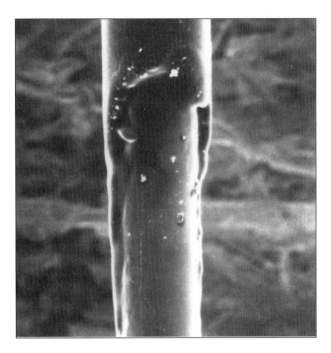

Figure 1. Electron microscope photogaph showing results of pulsed CO_2 laser wirestripping. Wire diameter: 40 μm. Polyurethane insulation thickness: 5 μm. Irradiation conditions: 2 pulses (focused) at approximately 20 J/cm² per pulse.

Excimer Lasers

Excimer lasers, which can operate at one of several ultraviolet wavelengths depending upon the gas mixture chosen, perhaps provide the highest-quality stripping action with regard to precision, edge definition, and cleanliness. The very large absorption coefficient of most plastic insulators in the ultraviolet, coupled with the pulsed (10–30 nsec) nature of the laser radiation, combine to produce high-quality stripping. As the pulsed excimer radiation interacts with the insulation, the light penetrates only a short distance (< 1 μm) because of the strong absorption. The shallow penetration depth causes only a thin layer to be ablated per pulse, with the result that many pulses are required to completely strip a wire. This promotes edge precision and definition as the material is "shaved off" pulse by pulse. The strong absorption also aids in the removal of residual insulation, helping to provide clean surfaces. Additionally, the ultraviolet light efficiently decomposes the organic material, significantly reducing the debris. Because of the high absorption, it is not necessary to focus the beam on the surface. Rather, the incident laser intensity must just be above some threshold value for insulation removal. Indeed, "blocks" of insulation can be removed by image projection rather than scanning a focused laser beam. This can lead to process efficiency and high throughput. Figure 2 shows a wire stripped by 0.248 μm excimer laser radiation. A major drawback to this desireable state of affairs is a costly laser system that is expensive to purchase and expensive to operate and maintain. This is further aggravated by the need to use toxic gases which must be replenished on a regular basis.

Once the metal surface is exposed, excessive irradiation may cause heating effects which prove deleterious to the mechanical strength of the wire. This is much more of an issue with ultraviolet lasers than with infrared lasers because the metal absorption is often significantly higher in the ultraviolet. For excimer laser stripping, the number of pulses, and their intensity (above the insulation removal threshold, but below the wire damage threshold) must be carefully chosen and maintained.

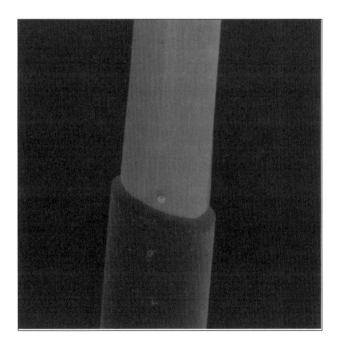

Figure 2. Electron microscope showing a KrF excimer laser stripped wire. Wire diameter: 40 μm. 5-μm polyurethane insulation thickness. Irradiation conditions: 15 nsec pulses at 350 mJ/cm² per pulse, 1 sec exposure at 100 pulses per sec. The stripped region was defined by mask image projection.

Alternative Lasers

While the above lasers represent the most common ones for wirestripping, it should be realized that many other lasers can potentially be utilized for a specific stripping application. Powerful Ar-ion, dye, Ti:Sapphire, and diode lasers are well known systems that may serve a particular wirestripping need. As an example, Figure 3 displays a wire stripped by use of the pulsed green radiation from a frequency-doubled Nd:YAG laser. In this case, the absorption of the insulator was dramatically increased by doping the insulator with an absorbing dye. The result is a stripped wire with an acceptable edge definition and cleanliness.

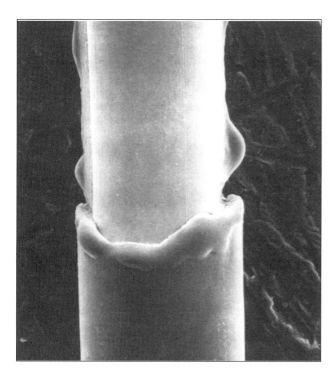

Figure 3. Electron microscope photograph showing pulsed Nd:YAG wirestripping using 0.532 μm radiation. Wire diameter: 35 μm. The 5-μm-thick polyurethane insulation has been doped with an absorbing dye. Only one side of this wire has been stripped. Irradiation conditions: 12 nsec pulses at 650 mJ/cm^2 per pulse, 5 sec exposure at 10 pulses per sec. The stripped region was defined by mask image projection.

References

1. W. F. Ireland, *SPIE Proc.* **86**, 68–72 (1976).
2. J. Brannon, A. Tam, and R. Kurth, *J. Appl. Phys.* **70** (7), 3881–6 (1991).
3. J. Brannon and C. Snyder, *Appl. Phys. A* **59**, 73–8 (1994).
4. J. Higgins, *Data Storage* **5**, 49–52 (May/June 1995).

JAMES F. BRANNON
ANDREW C. TAM

25.3.3 Wirestripping Procedures

Stripping can take place in one of three ways. The strip can be on cut lengths, at intervals on a roll-to-roll process or on a partial assembly or subassembly. Beam splitting techniques are desirable for maximum photon efficiency and for high throughput operation. The user also has three possibilities for integration of laser-based technology into the production line: contract the manufacturing to an outside vendor, purchase off-line equipment for the stripping process, or integrate the laser station into a production line controlled remotely through a single center responsible for overall control of the entire line. Integration is usually chosen for high-volume applications and especially when strips are made on partially assembled goods.

There are a variety of possibilities for the geometry of the stripped area. An end section of the wire may be stripped bare to prepare the wire for connection to a lead, or the wire may be stripped around its outer periphery ("cross cut") at a point away from the end of the wire. Or, the wire may be cross cut at two points and then stripped in a line along the length of the wire, leaving a section of insulation which may easily be removed mechanically. The choice of these procedures depends on the specific application.

The wires themselves are either solid copper or other metallic conductors or copper conductors with a thin gold coat sometimes used to enhance bonding efficiency. An acceptable strip will remove the insulation around the wire completely without burning, warping, or discoloring either the wire or remaining insulation, and without leaving debris behind. Many applications require a very well-defined and sharp "transition zone," while others are less demanding about this requirement if it impacts cost. As a matter of fact, it does impact cost, as the exact requirements will dictate the choice of laser and if the quality can only be met by using an excimer laser, hardware costs and operating costs will be higher than with a CO_2 laser.

A very active market for capital equipment used in the production of computer drive assemblies involves wire stripping with excimer lasers. One step of many in the process of assembly requires a precise amount of dielectric insulator to be removed from one or several locations on the wire. The material to be removed is usually polyurethane or polyimide, but it can also be composed of many other materials, some of which are Teflon based. The thickness of the wires is typically from 40 to 50 gauge, so more traditional means such as mechanical or chemical stripping are not practical.

Lasers are an obvious choice for a manufacturing tool. They are cost effective, and they process with unsurpassed quality; consequently they are currently involved in the manufacture of millions of wires daily.

Excimer lasers will produce the most pristine strip and a very sharp transition edge. Usually customers will accept the strip as good if the "transition" zone of the strip is less than half the diameter of the wire. Many customers can live with one diameter.

This requirement is fairly easily met by the excimer laser. In addition, the minimal thermal energy involved allows a fairly large process window in production. Because of the large, multi-mode beam, it is easy to split the excimer beam into several different beamlets for more efficiency.

Strip lengths from a few thousandths of an inch to one half inch long can be made with little change in the optical assemblies and one 75 W industrial laser can service three or more different beam delivery assemblies simultaneously. Light can be delivered to all points around the circumference of the wire by using either beam splitting and a dual delivery system or by using a retroreflector after the imaging lens to redirect the photons that passed the wire on the outward travel.

The aggressive nature of light interaction with organic materials at excimer wavelengths and the large difference in fluences required to machine organic materials with respect to that of metals contribute to the excellent quality results seen when using the excimer laser. Commercial excimer lasers made by manufacturers show a high degree of reliability and gas lifetimes of over 30 million shots per fill are routine.

Many applications are cost sensitive and may not need the quality of the excimer laser strip. In these cases, a good alternative is the transversely excited atmosphere (TEA) CO_2 laser. These lasers usually have large, multi-mode beams and are used in an imaging optical configuration much like an excimer. The choices range from high-energy, low-repetition-rate lasers to high-repetition-rate lasers with a smaller beam and output energy and with perhaps spectrally filtered output.

Although the potential quality of some strips using the CO_2-TEA laser is quite high with respect to a well defined edge, there is still one problem associated with the process. If the cut is observed under a high-power scanning electron microscope, it is apparent that there usually remains a thin, submicron layer of insulating material left after processing that it is very difficult to remove completely. In later processes, this might create a problem for subsequent bonding or plating steps.

Heavier-gauge wires can also be stripped with lasers, but when the wires are large enough so there is significant material to be removed, the laser is usually used to cut the insulation at some point and it is removed mechanically. Wires can be cut by rotating them individually in a chuck or by splitting the beam and then impacting the wire from two sides.

For larger wires where only a cut is required, the laser of choice is one with a focused beam and high reliability, such as a sealed CO_2 laser. These sealed units require very little maintenance, are highly reliable and frequently have fill lifetimes over 20,000 h. They are usually used in a near focal point machining mode where a high intensity of photons near the focal point causes a high local temperature and material removal. In many cases the heat-affected zone is actually desirable because the heat helps seal the cut insulation as for instance for braided insulators.

Laser wirestripping has made the transition from research to production and is being increasingly employed in the electronics industry.

References
R. D. Schaeffer, "Laser-based dielectric material removal," *Industrial Laser Review* (December 1996).

RONALD D. SCHAEFFER

Chapter 26

Electronic Packaging: Package Sealing and Ceramic Processing

26.0 Introduction

This chapter describes laser applications in packaging other than the technology of fabricating electrical interconnects. It emphasizes sealing of packages by laser welding, and the processing of ceramics, including cutting and scribing to separate chips and substrates and drilling of holes in ceramic substrates.

26.1 Package Welding

Laser welding is described extensively in Chapters 10 and 11. Laser welding of electronic packages is the subject of this section. Electronic packages often contain heat-sensitive components located near the area to be welded. That heating produced by lasers is localized makes them particularly useful for sealing electronic packages.

26.1.1 General Considerations

Applications

Laser welding is widely used in industry for both assembly and final case closure of high reliability electrical and electronic packages. Notable applications include television guns, sensors, relays, microwave modules, accelerometers, medical implants such as pacemakers, defibrillators, and insulin pumps, and power sources including batteries, capacitors, detonators, and neutron sources. Several packages that are laser welded are shown in Figure 1. Many of these long-standing applications date back to the first introduction of commercial laser welding equipment in the late 1960s. A laser is ideally suited for electrical and electronic packaging because it is a low heat input, noncontact, very small heat source. Conventional joining processes such as resistance welding, brazing, and soldering, are often not compatible with the sensitive internal features in these type devices. The presence of glass-to-metal seals, solid state devices, encapsulation materials, and reactive contents do not permit significant temperature excursions in these components. Owing to the small size of the weld and low heat input, packages are routinely laser welded without thermal damage. The noncontact nature of laser welding is also especially advantageous here since externally applied mechanical stresses are eliminated and there is no risk of electrodes passing electrical currents through sensitive internal devices.

CO_2 and Nd:YAG lasers in both the pulsed and continuous wave modes are used for package welding. The process is automated, but travel speeds (e.g., 10–30 mm/s) are not as fast as is typical of many laser seam welding applications. Continuous wave laser power greater than 1000 W is seldom required. The pulsed Nd:YAG laser is the laser typically selected for package welding; usually less than 400 W of average power is adequate in these applications. Continuous seam welds are made at pulse repetition rates of 10–50 Hz, creating a series of overlapping spot welds. Packaging welds are ordinarily autogeneous, the small size of the fusion zone is not compatible with the introduction of a filler wire.

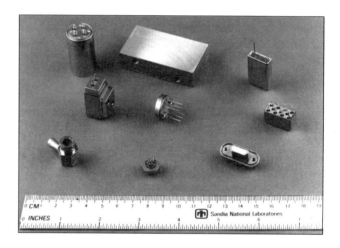

Figure 1. Typical high-reliability electronic and electrical packages that are laser welded.

Because of the critical service environment for many electrical and electronic packages, the metals selected are often corrosion resistant iron base or nickel base alloys which have good laser beam absorption characteristics. However, some common packaging metals are not good candidates for laser welding. Copper is extremely reflective to both Nd:YAG and CO_2 laser beams, and process control difficulties usually make welding of copper impractical. The presence of gold or copper platings also causes reflectivity problems and similarly should be avoided. Aluminum alloys are also very reflective and usually are not laser welded except with the pulsed Nd:YAG laser, which can achieve the high irradiance required. When a hot crack resistant aluminum alloy or combination is chosen, aluminum alloys are quite successfully joined with the pulsed Nd:YAG process (1).

Glass-to-Metal Seals

Glass-to-metals seals are often present in electrical and electronic packages. These hermetic seals facilitate electrical communication with the internal components of the device. Laser welding is successfully used for hermetic closure of many packages with either matched or compression type glass-to-metal seals that are integral with the housing or cover. In some applications, the glass and pin are grouped into headers, which are welded to the device individually. Despite the success of these assembly methods, cracking of the glass as a result of laser welding is still a widespread problem. Careful design of the device can minimize the chance of seal damage. Placement of the seals, as far as practical, away from the weld joint area can reduce thermally induced stresses at the glass seals. If possible, weld joints should be designed to create two-dimensional heat flow conditions around the weld. Edge welds as shown in Figure 2 are always preferable because they require less heat input to the part and the weld geometry minimizes shrinkage strains in the regions adjacent to the weld where the glass-to-metal seals are located (2). Welds labelled (c), (d), and (e) are preferred for package welding applications. Selection of reduced heat input weld schedule parameters has also proven effective in preventing glass-to-metal seal damage.

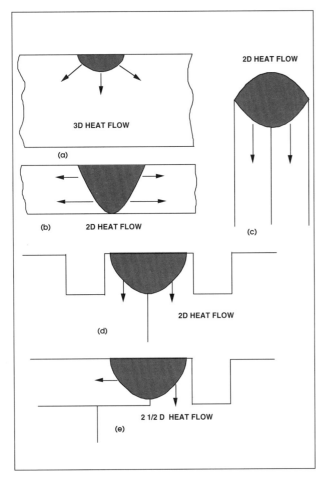

Figure 2. Weld joints that create two-dimensional heat flow are preferable for package welding.

Hot Cracking

An important requirement in welding of packages for high reliability is achieving maximum hermeticity. In addition to damaged glass-to-metal seals, defects in the fusion zone can result in significant leak rates that are often unacceptable in the intended service environment. Hot cracking is the most common defect, and occurs during weld metal solidification when mechanical strains induced by the restraining base metal pull the solidifying grains apart. The two requirements for hot cracking are a susceptible microstructure and sufficient mechanical stress. The high power density of laser welding creates thermal gradients that result in unusually high mechanical strains that can aggravate hot cracking tendencies in many engineering alloys (3). The microstructures are surprisingly susceptible to hot cracking because most of these alloys were developed for arc welding processes that do not create the high local strains seen with laser welding.

Table 1. Hot Crack Sensitivity of Packaging Alloys

Aluminum alloys	Austenic stainless steels	PH Martensitic stainless steels	Nickel alloys
Less susceptible			
A356	304	PH 13-8 Mo	Kovar*
4047	304L	17-4 PH	Alloy 52
4043	302	15-5 PH	Invar*
1100	321		Hast. B2
3003	316L		Hast. C4
5456	316		Hast. C276
5052	347		In. 625
5083	303		In. 718
5086			
2219			
6061			
7075			
More susceptible			

Compare materials within columns only. Materials in each row have less susceptibility to cracking than those in the rows below them. *Major constituent is iron.

Selection of process parameters to prevent hot cracking is extremely difficult and no clear guidance can be given. It is best to prevent hot cracking by proper material selection. Table 1 can be used as a guide in material selection, it indicates the hot cracking tendencies of some common packaging alloys. The table indicates alloys that are likely to have favorable hot crack microstructures. The rankings must be regarded as approximate, because the solidification microstructure and thus cracking susceptibility is strongly dependent on the actual levels of the alloy elements and impurities in each material. Free machining grades generally have a high propensity for hot cracking because of the addition of elements such as sulfur and selenium. Several other factors can readily make one material appear more weldable than another, including the grain size, type of weld joint, fusion zone dimensions, weld schedule, and whether the laser is pulsed or continuous. In general, pulsed lasers tend to cause hot cracking more than continuous wave lasers because of the rapid solidification event after each pulse.

Joint Preparation

The presence of platings and coatings on pins, headers, feedthroughs, and other subassemblies to be laser welded is often problematic. In some cases the plating melts into the fusion zone and becomes an impurity that can cause hot cracking, especially with gold, copper, and tin-lead platings. In other instances, the plating becomes a major cause of porosity in the weld pool because of a high concentration of hydrogen in the electroplated part. Vacuum heat treating before laser welding is sometimes helpful in reducing the porosity because of welding plated or anodized parts. Avoid electroless nickel platings, which contain phosphorous or boron, because these elements can aggravate hot cracking in some alloys. Sulfamate nickel plating is a good substitute that has proven to be weldable.

Surface finish roughness on parts to be laser welded is really not critical, provided it is consistent along the joint and from part to part. Most parts for packaging will be machined and therefore have a suitably uniform finish. The presence of contaminants on the surface is more of a concern. Surfaces should be free of any oils or lubricants that were used in fabrication. The best way to assure uncontaminated hardware is to solvent clean the parts before welding and only handle them subsequently with finger cots or gloves.

Traditional machine shop practice often involves deburring parts as a standard procedure. A file is usually used to break the sharp edges and create a small radius. In some instances, an edge radius is specified on the part drawing. These rounded corners can lead to poor weld joint fit-up and weld inconsistency. There is a direct correlation between the initial weld joint gap and the incidence of skips, pits, and other lack of fusion defects. These defects occur because a significant fraction of the small diameter laser beam passes right through the joint gap and no longer contributes to melting. To avoid this, the weld joint gap needs to be kept as small as is reasonably achievable. Sharp edges should be specified at the weld joint. The maximum gap that can be tolerated must be consistent with the width of the fusion zone. If the weld pool is disrupted significantly by gap variations, then energy absorption there will be reduced and the pool may collapse, causing a lack of fusion defect. Figure 3 shows two metallographic cross-sections taken at different locations along the same weld. The decreased fusion zone size in (b) is a direct result of the increased weld joint gap. In this case the gap is about 4% of the weld pool width; no defect was formed but weld penetration has been significantly reduced.

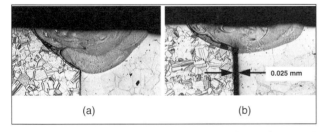

Figure 3. Pulsed Nd:YAG laser weld between Inconel 718 and Hastelloy B2 sectioned in two places along the joint. The laser parameters have not changed; the weld size variation is because of a change in joint gap.

It is important to perform a dimension tolerance analysis on parts to be laser welded before ordering hardware for production. The tolerance analysis should reveal the maximum joint gap that could occur after the parts are assembled for welding. The analysis assumes a worst case where the parts are machined to the dimensions that will produce the greatest weld joint gap. If the gap has the potential to become excessive, much difficulty in achieving consistent beam absorption can be expected. Rewelding of heat-sensitive parts to correct for an abnormally large weld joint gap is not recommended.

26.1.2 Weld Schedule Development

Methods

A weld schedule is a set of operation parameters for a particular laser welder that will yield the required weld performance characteristics. The list of required weld characteristics for packaging generally includes low heat input, hermeticity, and good weld appearance. Weld penetration is often secondary in importance because mechanical strength is not usually critical and only partial penetration welds may be required. Process feed rates are ordinarily of less significance as well. While high productivity is always a goal, obtaining a weld to meet the requirements is usually paramount. One must realize that package welding is often the final step of assembly for a very high value added product. Welds that do not pass inspection are costly to rework and in some cases the entire component must be scrapped. Early efforts invested to ensure high-quality welds during the weld schedule development period are often many times repaid later in a production run.

Typically, laser weld schedules result from the skill and experience of the laser operator or the welding engineer, rather than from any rigorous analytical approach. Previous empirically determined weld schedules are often used as a starting point and slightly modified as required for new applications. If the new performance characteristics are similar to the previous application, the weld will probably be acceptable. In other cases, more in depth weld schedule development must be undertaken. The task can be troublesome and time-consuming, and does not always lead to the best weld schedule for the application.

For applications where a better schedule is sought, weld schedule development is advanced by using statistically designed experiments such as fractional factorials, Taguchi methods, and response surface designs. In these experiments, the critical process parameters are identified and then carefully varied in a systematic way to reveal the best weld schedule. These experiments offer a rational approach, because the identification of a best schedule is based on an independent statistical method that narrows in on a desired response. Unfortunately, statistically designed experiments may require a large number of samples, and can be long and expensive to conduct and analyze. Another disadvantage with these experiments is that they seldom increase one's process understanding, because the results are usually specific to the application for which the experiment is designed, and are not directly extensible to a new material or configuration.

Few genuine alternatives to the designed experiment approach are available because multiple parameter interaction is complex. Finite element analysis models are difficult to apply because important physical inputs such as beam absorption, vaporization effects, and alloy properties are not known in general. Alternatively, computer programs that are based on empirically validated mathematical models of the laser welding process represent a recent encouraging trend and offer a more practical solution to the problem. By using the computational capabilities of a personal computer, the complex parameter interactions can be overcome and a weld schedule selected to achieve requirements, such as a narrow weld or low heat input can be obtained. Some software applications require the input of experimental results into the computer to actually build a neural net for the welding problem. Again, this approach is application-specific, and will require significant experimental effort, but welding-specific software does help expedite the process. More advanced software applications use more generic, physically based models to solve the optimization problem. With this approach, the number of test and evaluation welds can be reduced since the recommended weld schedule should already be close to optimized for the application (4).

Preferred Practices

Prior to the start of any weld schedule development effort, it is important to obtain at least a dozen weld development samples that can be used to optimize the weld schedule parameters. In too many cases, insufficient numbers of pre-production hardware are procured for this critical task. Weld development samples should be as similar as practical to the actual production hardware, including all prior processing steps such as glass sealing cycles, heat treatments, surface preparation, and cleaning. It is especially important to do development welding on material that is identical to what will be used in production. If more than one material is likely to be used during the production run, then all different materials should be obtained for weld development. Because shrinkage strains are also a significant cause of hot cracking, the development parts should have the same dimensions and overall size as the real component. The section size of the region adjacent to the fusion zone should be the same or very similar to the actual component. In special circumstances the strict rules given above may be relaxed, if through careful analysis of the application, someone quite familiar with the causes of hot cracking in laser welding recommends otherwise.

Focusing of the laser beam for small weld joints must be carefully implemented and controlled. Common lens focal lengths range between 50 and 200 mm, depending on the type of laser and the specific weld size requirements. For packaging applications, weld penetration depth is typically less than 1.0 mm. In many instances the laser has a power capacity many times greater than what is required to achieve the required penetration depth. With some laser power supplies it is a problem to achieve stable operation at these low powers. An intracavity or external aperture can be used to attenuate the laser beam and thereby allow operation at a higher and more stable average power. One should avoid running the laser at a higher power by sufficiently defocusing the laser beam so that only a small fraction of the laser power is absorbed. If for any reason the part is repositioned closer to focus, the consequences can be grave, with drilling and irreparable damage to the component resulting. If the goal of defocusing is to create a wider weld, then it is preferable to change to a lens which will produce a larger spot size; lenses to do this are available in many different focal lengths. Figure 4 indicates the effect of the lens focal length on the resulting weld pool width. One can see from the figure that for shallow penetration welds, choosing a lens that produces a larger spot size will also increase the weld pool width. The wider beam provides increased flexibility in lateral beam positioning along the weld joint and also can improve the weld appearance (5).

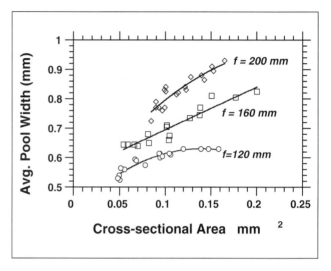

Figure 4. Effect of lens focal length on the weld pool width for pulsed Nd:YAG laser welding of 304L stainless steel (5).

Shielding of the fusion zone with an inert gas is a standard procedure in laser welding of packages. The gas shielding reduces formation of surface oxides and prevents reaction of the weld metal with the atmosphere, which may cause contamination and/or porosity. Argon shielding gas is most commonly used for package welding. Helium and nitrogen can also be used, but are not as effective as argon in preventing oxidation. Unlike high-power laser welding, plasma formation is inconsequential and does not need to be controlled in these applications. Achieving cosmetically appealing welds that are not discolored or oxidized can be a challenging problem. With some nozzle designs the shielding gas is also used to protect the focusing lens from the metal vapor plume. These nozzles may not provide sufficient gas coverage to prevent oxidation. If shielding is inadequate, it is best to provide a supplementary source of shielding gas directly behind the weld pool. A gas tungsten arc torch gas lens with the center hole plugged or similar device can be used for this purpose. For the welding of austenitic stainless steels, the addition of 5% hydrogen to the argon shielding gas can improve weld appearance by reducing oxidation. Postweld surface treatments to improve appearance of laser welded packages, such as wire brushing, are not recommended because they can hide significant flaws that need to be observed during inspection.

Reducing Heat Input

Minimizing heat input to the part is the primary goal of laser weld schedule development for packaging applications. Both shrinkage strains on glass seals and the thermal effects on heat-sensitive features can be decreased by reducing the heat input to the part. Despite the small spot size and high power density, laser welding does not always produce welds with the lowest heat input. The process parameters must be selected to produce low heat input. There are two fundamentally different ways that heat input can be reduced in welding. First, by decreasing the size of the fusion zone dimensions, the input energy required to melt the weld volume can be reduced. Because of the considerable enthalpy of melting, the overall size of the weld fusion zone is an important indicator of the magnitude of the heat input to the component. For many packaging applications, the small narrow weld that can only be attained with laser welding results in substantially lower heat input when compared to other welding processes. To reduce heat input in this way, one simply selects process parameters that decrease the cross-sectional area of the fusion zone, either increasing the travel speed, decreasing the power, or both. Conversely, if one increases the cross-sectional area by increasing the power or slowing the speed, then heat input to the part will also be increased.

Nd:YAG laser beam welding, the task of increasing melting efficiency is more convoluted, because one must deal with both average power and peak power. Figure 6 (below and next page) indicates the beneficial effect of increasing peak power in reducing glass-to-metal seal temperatures for three different focusing lenses (5). In the study, the average power was kept constant and the travel speed was varied to maintain a constant overlap. Despite the wide variations in several parameters, the temperatures were found to be primarily dependent on the travel speed as shown in Figure 7 (next page). One can see that the primary process parameter that reduces heat input to the part is the travel speed. Since these welds were approximately similar in size, it can be assumed that Figure 7 reflects an increase in melting efficiency.

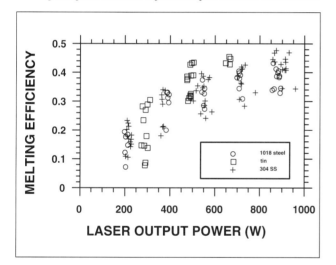

Figure 5. Dependence of measured melting efficiency on output power for continuous wave CO_2 laser beam welding. Five levels of travel speed account for the variation at each power (6).

The second way in which heat input can be reduced is to increase the melting efficiency. Melting efficiency is the ratio of the melted volume enthalpy to the energy absorbed by the workpiece. If one can increase the melted volume without increasing the energy absorbed, then the melting efficiency is increased. Melting efficiency indicates how effectively the energy absorbed by the workpiece is used to produce melting. Figure 5 shows the significant variation in melting efficiency versus output power for continuous wave laser beam welding. One can see that melting efficiency is clearly not always at a high level for laser beam welding (6). To increase melting efficiency, it is necessary to increase either the travel speed or the power independently, or increase them together. Since increasing the travel speed will often result in too small a weld, it is necessary to increase the power at the same time. For pulsed

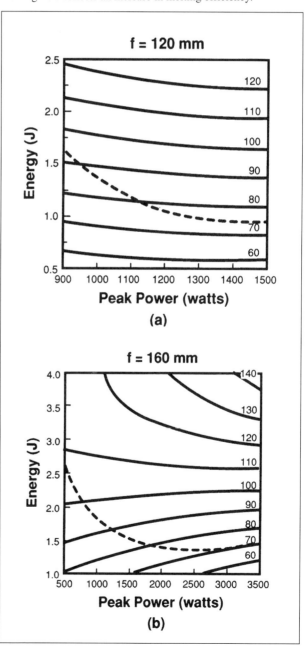

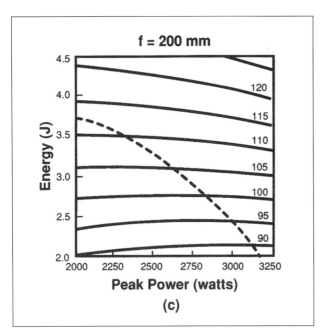

Figure 6. Response surface contour plots showing the effect of peak power and pulse energy on glass-to-metal seal temperatures (°C). The dashed line represents the contour line for constant penetration = 0.2 mm. Pulsed Nd:YAG at 200 W average power on 304L SS (5).

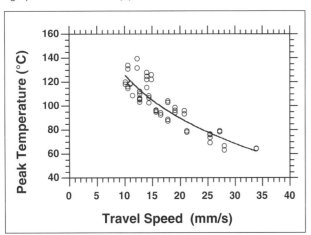

Figure 7. Dramatic effect of travel speed on measured glass-to-metal seal temperatures for welds with variable pulse energy, frequency, and duration. Pulsed Nd:YAG at 200 W average power on 304L SS (5).

26.1.3 Process Monitoring

Inspection

To truly distinguish process consistency, defect formation, and the effects of process parameters, metallographic cross-sections of package welds should be obtained. The sample specimens should be prepared periodically during weld schedule development, as a routine process control procedure, and as a part of a formal weld qualification. The considerable information that can be derived from a fusion zone micrograph includes the weld width, penetration depth, weld cross-sectional area, actual weld joint gap, base metal grain size, heat-affected zone size, and the presence of porosity, hot cracks, cold cracks, lack of fusion, and other similar defects. Furthermore, by sectioning the weld in several places along the joint, and examining the variation in sequential fusion zones, an important indicator of weld consistency can be obtained. Metallographic specimen preparation procedures vary and should be specifically developed for each material and weld application. Chemically etching the microstructure is not always necessary if there is sufficient contrast between the base metal and the fusion zone. In many cases etching can hide the presence of cracks and other defects in the fusion zone. The use of Nomarski interference contrast imaging can be advantageous in eliminating the need for etching. Scanning electron microscopy (SEM) is especially useful when one needs to clearly distinguish the presence of hot cracks on the weld surface.

To ensure hermeticity in laser-welded packages, a vacuum leak detector is typically employed to measure leak rates after welding. Both a mass spectrometer and vacuum pump are integral in the leak detector. The detector is used to sense for helium after the interior of the welded component has been attached to the vacuum pump and evacuated. Helium gas is flushed around the weld joint and a leak rate is assessed by the leak detector. Packages that are final-closure welded and cannot be evacuated after welding are tested in two ways. The package is closure welded in a helium-containing atmosphere such as a glovebox, and then placed in the leak detector to test for helium that escapes from the interior of the package. Alternatively, the closure-welded package is placed in the vacuum chamber, which is then evacuated and backfilled with helium. The leak detector then checks for helium that has entered the package interior during the evacuation and backfill. The influence of glass-to-metal seal cracking on helium leak rate and internal package atmosphere can be seen in Figure 8 (next page). In this application, electromechanical relays were welded in a 4% O_2, 10% He, Bal. N_2 atmosphere (7). Glass cracking from the laser welding process contributed to the increase in oxygen content shown in Figure 8.

Laser-welded packages are frequently examined under an optical microscope at 30X magnification or higher for cosmetic appearance. A 100% visual inspection of packages is typical, since leak testing will not always detect the presence of cracks, pores, or other defects. Fluorescent lighting of the weld surface is best for observing defects since it provides diffuse illumination. Pulse overlap is regularly measured, and is generally kept in the 70 to 80% range. Surface discoloration and oxidation may be allowed, depending on the application. In general, minor discoloration has little to do with weld hermeticity and reliability. The high value of the packages often requires that the part be free of any surface discontinuity, regardless of the effect on reliability. Porosity on the weld surface may be grounds for rejection if the pore diameter is greater than a minimum size, such as 5% of the penetration depth. The appearance of undercut in package welds is not of concern because weld mechanical performance is not critical. Similarly, mechanical testing of welds in laser-welded packages is not widely performed. The small size of the welds and the minimal weld strength requirements are factors that obviate the need for mechanical testing. Nondestructive pull testing of small leads is sometimes used for spot welding applications where weld consistency is difficult to determine.

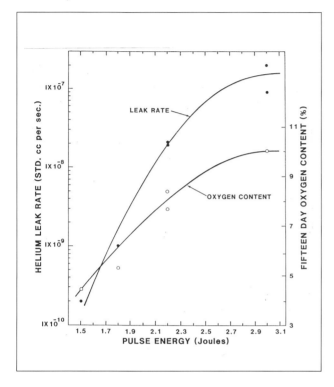

Figure 8. Effect of pulse energy on glass-to-metal seal cracking and relay package hermeticity. Pulsed Nd:YAG on 304L SS at 60 pps, 9.7 mm/s, 3.0 ms pulse duration, f = 100 mm (7).

For welds that are rejected by leak testing or visual examination, rewelding of the package may be necessary. Of course, rewelding cannot correct a leak if the glass seals are already damaged. Sometimes rewelding can correct hot cracking in certain alloys; in other instances rewelding can aggravate hot cracking. It is difficult to predict what will occur, given the uncertainties of alloy composition, the effects of dissolution, and alloy element vaporization. Rewelding can also increase the likelihood of thermal damage to glass-to-metal seals.

Calibration

Laser focal spot size is a key process parameter, so it is extremely important to ensure that the spot size remains constant from weld to weld. Calibrated measurements of the focal spot size are not typically recorded because of the obvious difficulties in measuring a focused high-power laser beam. The use of a video monitor or eyepiece to set the lens to workpiece distance, and thereby set spot size, is not recommended. The positioning uncertainty inherent in refocusing the lens in this manner can vary significantly from operator to operator. Even small variations (0.25 mm) in the lens-to-workpiece distance can affect the resulting weld size.

It is best to ensure repeatable lens positioning (i.e., spot size) by using either hard tooling or a micrometer to set and control the distance. Because laser beam quality can vary with power for most lasers, the lens-to-workpiece distance must be measured and set at the required laser power level.

Along with spot size, laser power is equally critical to process control for package welding. NIST traceable power meters of several designs are now widely available. The detector surface can be degraded so the detector and meter should be calibrated periodically (8). A power meter should be installed in the workstation and used on a schedule as defined in the welding procedure. The meter should measure the laser power that exits the focusing lens, since both laser performance decreases and degradation in the optical path will be observed in measurements there. Pulse energy can be determined by dividing the average power by the pulse repetition rate. Usually parameters such as pulse rate, pulse duration, shutter time, and travel speed are electronically controlled and should not need regular calibration.

Process Control Sample

To calibrate the weld performance directly, process control samples are widely used for package welding. High reliability manufacturers do daily functional checks of their lasers' output performance by welding a standardized test sample and measuring metallographically the depth of penetration. By optically examining the fusion zone geometry, one can determine that the laser is still producing the same power, the focal position is set properly, and the spot size is consistent. Ideally, actual production packages without internal subassemblies are welded as process control samples. By using production grade hardware, the metallography also serves to monitor uncontrolled changes in part tolerances and metallurgical characteristics. These samples are welded at both the beginning and end of a shift to bracket all welds made during that period (9). Depending on the production rate, a process control sample may need to be welded and sectioned periodically during the shift. For high reliability packages such as airbag actuators, process control samples are welded as often as after every 100 units. These control samples should also be processed after each time the laser system has been changed over to weld other products or has received major maintenance.

A lower-cost but less-informative alternative to the metallographically sectioned sample is also used to check process performance and consistency. In this approach, a very specific thickness specimen is welded with the standard welding conditions, so that the penetration depth is sufficient to melt just the backside of the sample. A second specimen of slightly larger thickness is also welded; it is selected so that the penetration depth cannot melt through the backside with the standard welding conditions. By carefully matching the thicknesses of the specimens to the weld requirements, one can quite successfully ensure that the process remains under control. These samples calibrate laser performance only and do not indicate uncontrolled changes in the packages that may affect welding. With either of the above process control samples, if the results of the test do not meet the inspection criteria the welding process will need to be adjusted.

References

1. T. Sakai, S. Okamoto, T. Iikawa, T. Sato, and Z. Henmi, "A New Laser Hermetic Sealing Technique for Aluminum Package," *IEEE Trans. on Components, Hybrids, and Manufacturing Technology* CHMT-**10** (3), 433–6 (1987).
2. P. W. Fuerschbach and M. J. Cieslak, "Restraint Effects in Laser Welding of an Aluminum MMC," *IEEE Transactions on Components, Hybrids, and Manufacturing Technology, Part B* **17** (1), 108–14 (1993).
3. J. C. Lippold, "Solidification Behavior and Cracking Susceptibility of Pulsed Laser Welds in Austenitic Stainless Steels," *Welding Journal* **73** (6), 129s–139s (1994).
4. G. R. Eisler and P. W. Fuerschbach, in: "SOAR: An Extensible Suite of Codes for Weld Analysis and Optimal Weld Schedules," *Seventh International Conference on Computer Technology in Welding*, TWI, San Francisco, CA (1997).
5. P. W. Fuerschbach and D. A. Hinkley, "Pulsed Nd:YAG Laser Welding of Heart Pacemaker Batteries with Reduced Heat Input," *Welding Journal* **76** (3), 103s–109s (1997).
6. P. W. Fuerschbach, "Measurement and Prediction of Energy Transfer Efficiency in Laser Beam Welding," *Welding Journal* **75** (1), 24s–34s (1996).
7. P. W. Fuerschbach, "Process Control Improvements in Pulsed Nd:YAG Laser Closure Welding of Electromechanical Relays," *International Power Beam Conference*, ASM, SanDiego, CA, 157–64.
8. P. D. Thacher, "Calibration of Beam Power Monitors for Laser Welding," *Laser Beam Radiometry*, SPIE: Los Angeles, CA (1988).
9. G. W. G. Janssen, "Laser Welding in the Manufacture of Heart Pacemakers," *Laser Weld, Cutting and Surface Treat*; 33–5, TWI: Cambridge, England (1984).

PHILLIP W. FUERSCHBACH

26.2 Cutting and Scribing of Substrates

26.2.0 Introduction

Ceramic processing applications include scribing and cutting of fired ceramic (alumina, AlN or BeO) or unfired ceramic (alumina, LTCC tape). The excellent pulse performance of lasers used is key in microelectronics applications because they minimize the heat-affected zone (HAZ). This is critical where thermally sensitive components are in close proximity to machined areas. Scribing, drilling, and dicing (cutting) of aluminum oxide (Al_2O_3) ceramic substrates or silicon (Si) wafers are among the most demanding laser processes. The optical quality of the laser beam and the pulsing characteristics of the laser directly affect the finished product. Optical beam delivery components must be of the finest quality and appropriate for their use. Motion tables and control systems must meet stringent requirements of tolerance and repeatability. System producers must use modern engineering tools to design a machine base around which components are integrated.

This section emphasizes the use of lasers for separating substrates into chips or other sections. Direct cutting by lasers has already been described in Chapter 12; here we emphasize the use of laser cutting of substrates in electronic packaging applications.

Laser scribing is a method for shaping and separating a workpiece into segments of desired shape without having to vaporize through the material. It provides separation of flat samples of material at a rate faster than cutting. Scribing is often used to dice wafers of material into smaller chips. Scribing is usually applied to shaping of brittle materials such as ceramics, silicon, and glass.

Scribing involves drilling a series of closely spaced blind holes. The substrate can then easily be separated by snapping it along the line defined by the holes. Direct cutting and scribing compete for substrate separation applications. Generally, for equal laser power, scribing produces faster separation rates. The use of lasers to drill holes through substrates will be described in the next section.

The main advantages of laser processing of alternative processes are:

1. High speed of processing
2. No physical contact of tool with part
3. No mechanical pressure on part
4. No tool wear
5. High automation capability
6. Ability to do prototyping of full-scale production
7. Laser systems are versatile; capable of performing multiple operation such as cutting, scribing, drilling, etc.

26.2.1 Laser Selection

For most ceramic processing applications the CO_2 laser (~300 W average power) is the most suitable because of its high absorptivity, pulse energy, excellent beam quality and speed of processing. The far-infrared wavelength is suitable for most ceramic materials including Al_2O_3, AlN, BeO and LTCC. The minimum spot size imaged on the ceramic with a CO_2 laser is typically 50 micrometers. For specific thin film applications, Nd:YAG lasers (~20 W) are preferred because of their short wavelength and their ability to produce a smaller spot size (20 micrometers). However, these lasers cannot penetrate more than 50 micrometers into the ceramic and hence, are limited to applications where lower penetration depths are required. Silicon wafer scribing is done with a *Q*-switched Nd:YAG laser. Silicon is extremely sensitive to thermal cracking and is susceptible to fracture when processed with the CO_2 laser. The near-infrared wavelength of the Nd:YAG minimizes thermal heat-affected zones and is preferred. Cutting of polycrystalline and single crystal Si wafers are being undertaken with both CO_2 and Nd:YAG lasers. CO_2 lasers offer the advantage of lower thermal damage. However, the advent of sealed CO_2 lasers, which can produce true square waveform pulses at higher frequencies, offer unique advantages of lower heat input and higher productivity.

26.2.2 Process Parameters

Scribing ceramic substrates requires very short, high-energy pulses. Lasers capable of producing pulses having very fast rise and fall times ($\cong$ 50 μseconds), yet with high pulse energy, can rapidly ablate ceramic, giving superior scribe holes. That is, there is very little resolidified ceramic in or around the holes, and no cracks. Conduction-cooled and diffusion-cooled CO_2 lasers are both capable of producing short, high energy pulses, with excellent optical brightness (low M^2). These lasers can produce pulses having an instantaneous power density in excess of 100 MW per cm^2. Figure 1 gives a schematic illustration of a scribing operation.

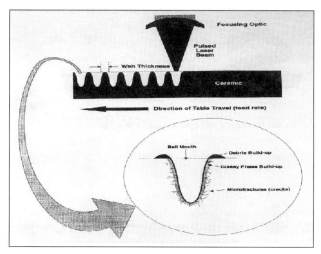

Figure 1. Laser scribing of fired ceramics – process and quality requirements.

The critical requirement of ceramic scribing is scribe depth and spacing between two adjacent scribe holes (pitch). Substrate thickness and processing methodology are considerations when establishing scribe depth. If the scribe depth is too shallow, partitioning of the substrate can be problematic. If the scribe depth is excessive, the substrate may spontaneously separate during subsequent processing. Typically, scribe depth is set to be from 30 to 40% of the substrate thickness. Scribe depth is controlled by pulse energy and rate of motion table travel. Additionally, the scribes must exhibit minimum microcracking, glassy phase build-up, bell mouthing, and show no variation in penetration depth. Figure 2 shows an example of CO_2 laser scribe on fired ceramic.

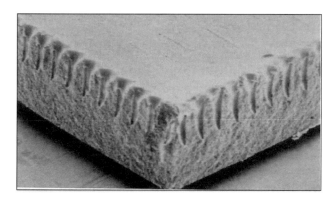

Figure 2. Example of a CO_2 laser scribe on fired ceramic.

Scribing silicon wafers is done using a Q-switched Nd:YAG laser, fitted with controls and apertures to produce an output approaching an M^2 value of 1. Average power at the workpiece is < 10 W, but pulse power is > 1 kW. The Q-switch produces pulse widths < 10 μseconds. Longer pulses would cause thermal damage to the wafer. In large, the process of scribing silicon wafers remains proprietary to those companies having empirically developed a satisfactory manufacturing process.

26.2.3 Pulse Parameters

The two main laser pulse parameters for sealed lasers are pulse length and pulse repetition rate (frequency). For ceramic scribing, the pulse length must be kept short to allow for high scribing speeds without elongating the holes. By using very short pulse lengths, holes smaller in diameter than the actual focused spot size can be created. Typically, pulse lengths for scribing range from 100 to 700 μseconds depending on type and thickness of ceramic. Pulse repetition rate in the case of scribing is determined by the scribing speed and scribe pitch. In the case of cutting, repetition rates are determined again by cutting speed and thickness of ceramic. The substrates are scribed at rates from 2 (50 mm) to 100 in. (250 mm) per second, with pulse repetition rates up to 2 kHz. The relationship between repetition rate, scribe speed and pitch can be calculated using the simple formula:

$$\text{Pulse repetition rate (Hz)} = \text{Speed/hole spacing}$$

For instance, a scribing speed of 8 in. per second with hole spacing of 0.005 in. would require 1600 pulses per second. As seen from Table 2, cutting speeds are significantly lower than scribing speeds (typically < 10 in. per min.). The reason why cutting and scribing speeds differ so dramatically is that in cutting more localized heat is generated than scribing. Fired ceramics are brittle and susceptible to thermal cracking. Therefore, to minimize thermal shock, cutting speeds must be reduced.

Table 1. Scribing Pulse Repetition Rate (Hz)

ips	Scribe pitch (in.)				
	0.005	0.006	0.007	0.008	0.009
1	200	167	143	125	111
2	400	333	286	250	222
3	600	500	429	375	333
4	800	667	571	500	444
5	1000	833	714	625	556
6	1200	1000	857	750	667
7	1400	1167	1000	875	778
8	1600	1333	1143	1000	889
9	1800	1500	1286	1125	1000
10	2000	1667	1429	1250	1111

To keep the scribe pitch constant, the system controller outputs to fire the laser by measurement of distance, not at a constant frequency. Motion table speed controls actual pulse repetition rate. When cutting, pulse repetition rate generally remains constant, although some controllers use vector velocity to modulate power.

Laser power required is relatively low, although the peak power of each pulse is quite high (> 500 W). Because the pulse length is short, the average, or integrated power of the pulses is low, typically between 50 to 150 watts. Peak power required increases with substrate thickness. When cutting ceramic substrates, power requirement is determined by the substrate thickness and consideration of thermal impact, especially when cutting complex shapes with acute angles. Typical power for cutting 0.025-in. (0.64 mm) thick substrates would be 50 W; for 0.060-in. (1.52 mm) substrates, 150 W.

26.2.4 Optical Considerations

Optical output from most CO_2 lasers used for processing ceramic substrates is linearly polarized. However, the rate of absorption of laser energy by the all materials varies with the orientation of plane of polarization with respect to the direction of travel. A quarter-wave phase shifting mirror is used to transform polarization of the light energy from linear to circular. Circularly polarized light energy is equally absorbed regardless of direction of travel. This device is commonly known as the circular polarizer of enhanced cut quality module (EQC), and is recommended for all microelectronics applications that involve more than one-dimensional processing.

Scribe hole diameter is dependent upon the focused spot size and pulse energy achieved from a given laser. For most cutting, scribing and drilling applications, short focal length lenses are used, typically a 2.5-in. (63.5 mm) focal length. There are different types of lenses available: aspheric, doublet, diffractive, meniscus, and plano-convex lenses. Aspheric and doublet lenses are aberration-free lenses and therefore can produce the smallest focused spots. The spot size for aberration-free lenses is given by the simple formula:

$$\text{Spot size} = \text{Focal length} \times \text{Beam divergence}$$

For example, a 2.5-in. f.l. aspheric lens used in conjunction with a 2 milliradian beam divergence will result in a 0.005-in.-diameter focused spot. However, the smaller the spot size, the narrower the depth-of-focus. Usually a 2.5-in. diffractive lens is used as a compromise between a smaller spot size and larger depth of focus. Typically a diffractive lens gives a 0.006-in. (0.15 mm) diameter spot with a depth of focus of ± 0.0075 in. (0.19 mm).

26.2.5 Assist Gas and Nozzle Configuration

Two types of gases are typically used as process assist gas – air and oxygen. Oxygen is necessary for aluminum nitride (AlN) machining but is optional for alumina. For reasons not entirely clear, oxygen appears to produce smoother cuts and cleaner scribes compared to air. However, air is cheaper and is preferred for less critical applications. Most CNC systems have provisions to be able to switch between oxygen and air automatically. Typical gas pressures vary between 30 psi (2 bar) for scribing to 75 psi (5 bar) for cutting and drilling. Gas jets used for cutting ceramic are similar to those used for cutting metals. The exit orifice of the cutting nozzle is nominally 0.050 in. (1.25 mm) diameter. The nozzles in gas jets used for ceramic scribing and drilling have large exit orifices, usually 0.125 in. (3.18 mm). Scribing gas jets

Table 2. Scribing and Cutting Parameters for Ceramics

Substrate material	Thickness (in.)	Process	Scribe depth (%)	Speed (ips)	Pitch (in.)	Pulse length (μsec)	Rep rate (Hz)	Average power (W)
Al_2O_3	0.010	Scribe	50	8	0.006	200	1333	88
Al_2O_3	0.025	Scribe	50	8	0.007	225	1143	84
Al_2O_3	0.040	Scribe	40	6	0.007	250	857	72
Al_2O_3	0.060	Scribe	40	4	0.007	300	571	65
AlN	0.025	Scribe	35	4	0.007	700	571	145
AlN	0.025	Cut	–	0.05	–	400	250	53
Al_2O_3	0.010	Cut	–	0.33	–	300	600	68
Al_2O_3	0.025	Cut	–	0.25	–	500	500	83
Al_2O_3	0.040	Cut	–	0.16	–	700	640	125
Al_2O_3	0.060	Cut	–	0.125	–	900	500	122
LTCC (unfired)	0.008	Cut	–	1.7	–	40	833	17
LTCC (unfired)	0.200	Cut	–	0.12	–	500	500	117

do not produce a columnar flow as do gas jets used for cutting ceramic. Nozzle stand-off is typically 0.250 (6.25 mm) to 0.500 in. (12.5 mm). Side jet (as opposed to coaxial jet) nozzles have also shown to benefit in very high precision scribing. In cases where scribing and cutting operations are performed on the same substrate, cutting nozzles may also be used for scribing. However, during the scribing operation the assist gas pressure must be decreased to 15 psi (1 bar).

26.2.6 Hardware Considerations

Depending on processing methodology, ceramic processing systems can have either a single focus head or multiple focus heads (typically 2 to 4 beams integrated to a common motion system). With multiple focus heads, output from the laser is optically split such that an equal amount of power is input to each focus head.

A well-designed system for scribing or cutting ceramic substrates should meet these minimum requirements:

Scribing
- Process rate of 8 in. per second, nominal for 0.025-in.-thick substrates
- Scribe pitch from 0.005 in. (0.125 mm)
- Scribe depth of 0.010 in. (0.25 mm) minimum
- X,Y axes repeatability and programmability within ± 0.0005 in. (12 micrometers)
- Capability of scribing at any angle relative to axes travel, and to scribe on arcs

Cutting
- 0.020 in. (0.5 mm) t at 20 in. (0.5 m) per min.
- 0.040in. (1 mm) t at 8in. (200 mm) per min.

Additional features worth investigating: vision systems for automatic theta correction or alignment of motion table travel, substrate auto load/off-load, programmable boring head, and multiple beam (2 or more focus heads) systems.

26.2.7 Comparison of Scribing and Cutting

Table 2 (previous page) presents typical results obtained with sealed CO_2 lasers for cutting and scribing of ceramic substrates. Note that for a given level of laser power, scribing yields a substantially higher separation rate than direct cutting.

WILLIAM SHINER
STEVE MAYNARD

26.2.8 Laser Scribing Results

Scribing is performed by drilling a series of closely spaced blind holes into the surface of the material. Typically the hole depth might be one-quarter of the thickness of the workpiece. Figure 3 shows how the relative force required for separation varies with the depth of the hole, expressed as a fraction of the thickness of the material. The relative force has a broad minimum near 30 per cent penetration.

The holes typically are spaced center-to-center by twice the diameter of the holes, which varies with laser wavelength and focusing conditions. The material will snap easily along the line described by the scribing. If a wafer is scribed with a series of lines in two perpendicular directions, it may easily be separated into a number of small chips. The quality of the edge defined by the scribing and snapping is of sufficient quality for applications such as dicing of silicon wafers and separation of ceramic chip carriers.

Most often, the holes are drilled along straight lines, but it is possible to separate employ gently curved contours. If the curves are too steep, the sample may fracture in an uncontrolled fashion.

Fixturing for laser scribing may be simple, similar to what is used for one-dimensional laser cutting. The workpiece may be held by a vacuum chuck and moved by a numerical controller, according to a pattern stored on a floppy disk. The scribing operation usually is carried out in ambient air.

The CO_2 laser is usually used for scribing ceramics, because of their high absorption at 10.6 μm. Both continuous and repetitively pulsed lasers have been used. Table 3 presents typical parameters for CO_2 laser scribing of alumina ceramic.

Table 3. Typical CO_2 Laser Parameters for Scribing of Alumina

Peak power	300 W
Pulse repetition rate	1 kHz
Pulse duration	100 μsec
Thickness	0.025 in.
Hole diameter	0.005 in.
Hole separation	0.01 in. (center to center)
Hole depth	0.007 in.
Scribe speed	6 in./s

For the scribing of silicon, Q-switched Nd:YAG lasers have been used because of the high absorption of silicon near 1 mm. The hole diameter and hole spacing will be smaller when an Nd:YAG laser is used.

Table 4 compares results of the laser scribing process for different types of lasers and different types of material.

Table 4. Characteristics of Laser Scribing

Laser	Wavelength (μm)	Power (W)	Material	Thickness (in.)	Speed (in./s)
CO_2	10.6	300 (peak)	alumina	0.025	6
CO_2	10.6	50 (avg.)	alumina	0.2	0.75–3
Nd:YAG	1.06	300 (peak)	silicon	–	0.25
CO_2	10.6	50–125	alumina	–	3–4
CO_2	10.6	340–560	silicon nitride	–	2–15
Nd:YAG	1.06	–	alumina	–	0.3
Nd:YAG	1.06	1000	tungsten carbide	–	0.04

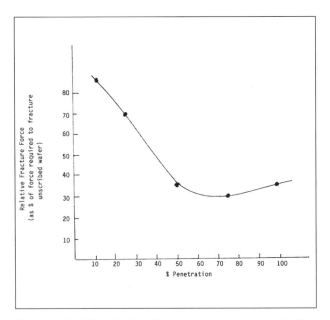

Figure 3. Relative fracture force versus percent penetration, for Nd:YAG laser scribing of silicon.

References
G. Chryssolouris, *Laser Machining, Theory and Practice,* Springer-Verlag, New York, 1991, Chapter 6.
R. M. Lumley, *Ceramic Bulletin* **48,** p. 650 (1969).

JOHN F. READY

26.3 Hole Drilling in Ceramics

26.3.0 Introduction

Drilling holes through ceramic substrates, such as alumina, has become a major application for lasers in the electronics industry. The general subject of laser-based hole drilling is described in Chapter 13. This section is specific to hole drilling in ceramic substrates for electronic packaging applications.

Section 25.1 describes via drilling, which is also a form of hole drilling for electronic applications. The thrust of the current section is somewhat different from that of Section 25.1. The properties of via drilling as described here and in Section 25.1 are compared in Table 1.

Table 1. Properties of Via Drilling and Hole Drilling

	Via drilling	Hole drilling
Typical materials	Printed circuit boards Polymide	Alumina ceramics
Lasers used	Excimer, TEA CO_2 Pulsed CO_2, UV Nd:YAG	Pulsed CO_2

Table 1. Properties of Via Drilling and Hole Drilling (cont.)

	Via drilling	Hole drilling
Hole diameter	25–350 µm	250–1000 µm
Typical applications	Interconnections of circuit layers	Electrical lead-throughs, mounting of components

26.3.1 Advantages and Laser Choice

The use of lasers to machine hard materials like ceramics and chemical vapor deposited diamond films can bring many benefits to the manufacturing process. Because of the hardness of these materials, there may be a limited number of options available for performing certain manufacturing tasks like drilling. Lasers become particularly attractive as a viable manufacturing technology when hole sizes become small. Hole diameters of 100 micrometers or less are extremely difficult to produce mechanically in high volume, but it is quite straightforward using lasers.

CO_2 lasers are employed in many commercial drilling operations. High drill speeds are possible, especially in thin material with most ceramics. With a 150 W laser one can easily drill through 0.10-in.-thick material; larger lasers can penetrate even deeper. Holes with as small as a 75-µm exit diameter with very little taper can be drilled by directly focusing the beam near the material surface. Larger holes can be drilled using a larger laser or by trepaning the beam or moving the part with respect to the beam.

The RF excited pulsed CO_2 laser is particularly well suited to ceramic hole drilling. The characteristics of this laser make it very suitable to micromachining because of the nearly square pulse shape and the adjustable pulse width. When conditions are properly optimized, high material removal rates with minimal surrounding damage can occur. The result is a smaller heat-affected zone (HAZ). Because thermal energy generated per pulse in the material is pulse-width dependent, it is often valuable to be able to vary this parameter.

Ceramic drilling is usually accompanied by an assist gas to remove molten material. This is often a high pressure flow of fairly pure, dry air through a nozzle concentric with the beam and positioned to within about 0.050 in. from the processing surface. The flow of air serves to blow molten material through the laser exit side and often results in droplets of recast material, or dross, on the backside. This is usually fairly easy to minimize and/or remove. Blind holes can also be drilled, but not with the same ease and consistency of through holes. One exception is the removal of thin ceramic film from highly reflective (Cu) substrates using a CO_2 TEA laser where, because of the high reflectivity, it is easy to stop at the materials interface.

Ceramics are also drilled with solid-state Nd:YAG lasers. Attainable feature quality tends to be as good as CO_2 or better in some cases, but the processing speeds are usually slower. Both pulsed and high-repetition-rate Q-switched lasers are used. One noticeable difference is the near lack of dross on the exit side. A typical production laser would have perhaps 10 mJ per pulse energy and 20 kHz repetition rate with a pulse length of 200 ns. Materials of thickness up to about 0.050 in. can be drilled and cut with this size laser. Larger lasers can cut thicker material. The primary material interaction is thermal, as with the CO_2 laser, but the solid-state laser pulse produces a more intense heat buildup, resulting in a more efficient process and better-quality features; that is less microcracking, cleaner walls and less debris. Focal point machining is normally used and the beam can be steered using galvanometers for trepaning larger holes.

The shorter wavelengths of the excimer laser makes it the laser of choice when neither other laser can give adequate quality or feature size. The excimer laser should be considered when hole diameters are less than 100 micrometers.

In terms of processing speed it is most practical to speak of the etch rate per pulse. In general for most ceramics the etch rate varies from about 0.08 μm per pulse at 10 J/cm^2 to about 0.16 μm at 30 J/cm^2. Fluences much below 10 J/cm^2 are quite close to the ablation threshold, below which material removal is non-existent. At fluences above 30 J/cm^2 the removal rate plateaus at its maximum value. All lasers will produce a tapered hole with the exit diameter being smaller than the entrance diameter, but the taper with the excimer laser will be greater than with red lasers, especially at low fluences. Tapers of 10° are common.

References
J. Angell and R. D. Schaeffer, *Laser Processing of Ceramics and CVD Diamond Film*, Proceedings from Advancements in the Application of Ceramics in Manufacturing, SME (1996).
J. Angell, W. Ho, and R. D. Schaeffer, *Effects of Taper on Drilling and Cutting with a Pulsed Laser*, SPIE, Photonics West (1997).
R. D. Schaeffer, L. Chen and W. Ho, *Laser Planarization of Chemical Vapor Deposited Film*; SPIE, Photonics West (1996).
H. K. Tonshoff and O. Gedrat, *Removal Process of Ceramic Materials with Excimer Laser Radiation*; SPIE Vol. 1132 (1988).

RONALD D. SCHAEFFER

26.3.2 Procedures and Results
Hole diameters less than 0.010 in. (0.25 mm) are most often drilled by focusing the laser beam to the desired hole diameter. Focus position and pulse energy both affect hole diameter. Rotating optical devices (boring heads) can be used to drill holes > 0.010 in. (0.25 mm). Holes 0.020 in. (0.5 mm) in diameter through 0.060 in. (1.5 mm) thick alumina can be drilled at a rate of up to 3 holes per second using a boring head; the same hole would take ≅ 1 second to drill by circular interpolation of linear axes.

Machining of fired ceramics is accomplished by use of a high-pressure gas jet. The intense focused beam melts the ceramic, while the compressed air or oxygen at 40 to 60 psi (2.6 to 4 bar) ejects molten ceramic from the cut slot (kerf). Nozzle stand-off is usually around 0.040 in. (1.0 mm) from the surface of the ceramic substrate.

Laser drilling of of fired ceramics offers substantial advantages compared to mechanical drilling, because of the hardness and brittleness of the material. With mechanical drilling, there is breakage and lower yield, plus high tool wear rates.

Green (unfired) ceramic is also drilled by CO_2 lasers, typically in the manufacture of multi chip modules (MCMs). Many of the laser parameters used to process green ceramic are similar to those used for fired ceramics. Unfired ceramics in general are easier to process than fired ceramics. For hole drilling applications, unfired ceramics (> 0.025 inch or 0.6 mm) drill at 30% higher rates than that for fired ceramics. For drilling holes < 0.010 in. (0.25 mm) in unfired ceramics less than 0.025 in. thick, drilling speeds in excess of 40 holes per second can be achieved by firing-on-the-fly technique. While green ceramic can be cut faster than fired ceramic, size of features and tolerances of dimension and position limit process speed.

Typical process parameters for ceramic drilling are listed below in Table 2.

Table 2. Ceramic Drilling Parameters for Sealed Lasers

Substrate	Thickness (in.)	Speed (holes per Sec)	Pulse length (μsec)	Rep rate (Hz)	Avg. power (W)
Al_2O_3	0.060	3	500	100	18
AlN	0.025	2	400	250	50

A well-designed system for drilling ceramic substrates should meet these minimum requirements:

- 1 hole/second by interpolation of linear motion tables
- 3 holes/second using boring head < 0.100-in. diameter
- 200 to 400 holes per second (green ceramic)

WILLIAM SHINER
STEVE MAYNARD

ISBN 0-912035-15-3

Notes

Chapter 27

Film Deposition and Doping

27.1 Thin Film Deposition

Thin film deposition by lasers can be broadly classified into two categories: laser chemical vapor deposition (LCVD) and pulsed laser deposition (PLD). In LCVD the laser is used to initiate a chemical reaction by heating (pyrolytic process) or photo-dissociating (photolytic process) a reactant gas as described in Sections 27.1.1–3. In general a laser with low power (~1 W) is required for the LCVD process. In PLD, laser pulses are used to vaporize a solid target as described in Section 27.1.4. Typically a laser with high peak power (> 1 MW) is required for the PLD process. A laser deposition system consists of a laser for initializing a reaction, a chamber that houses the substrate, and the reactant gas and/or source material for the coating. Laser deposition can be used to deposit a uniform film over a large area or can be used to deposit small features in a localized area defined by the laser beam.

27.1.1 Laser Chemical Vapor Deposition

Pyrolytic Process

As illustrated in Figure 1, in a pyrolytic LCVD process the laser light strikes the substrate surface, heating it locally to a few hundred degrees Celsius. Reactant gases impinge upon the heated region, undergo thermal decomposition, and one of the resultant species condenses onto the substrate surface. The wavelength of the laser is usually chosen so that it is absorbed by the substrate and is transmitted by the reactant gases. Typically a CW visible laser such as an Ar^+ laser is used in this process.

A pyrolytic process can operate in two different regimes, which offer different options for control of the deposition. The first regime is called a kinetic regime. In this regime, there is an adequate supply of reactant material at the surface, and the reaction rate increases exponentially with increasing temperature. The deposition rate is controlled by controlling the temperature.

The second regime, usually encountered at higher values of temperature, is called a mass-transport regime. The deposition is limited by the availability of reactant material at the surface. The deposition rate in this regime is controlled by controlling the pressure and flow rate of the reactant gas.

Pyrolytic processes are commonly used as a direct-writing process (Section 27.1.3). A typical set-up of a pyrolytic LCVD process is illustrated in Section 27.1.3.

Photolytic Process

In a photolytic LCVD process, the absorbed laser energy dissociates the reactant gas molecules nonthermally, and one of the resultant species condenses onto the nearby surface. In general, a photolytic process is insensitive to the kind of substrate as long as no specific surface reactions are involved. Normally a laser beam propagating parallel to the substrate surface is used to deposit a thin film onto the substrate surface as illustrated in Figure 2.

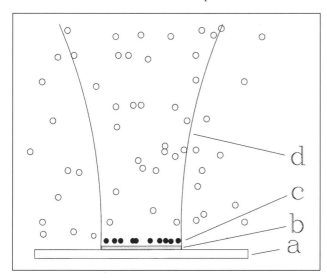

Figure 1. Pyrotolytic LCVD process: a - substrate; b - deposited film; c - reactant gas dissociated in the laser heated region; d - focused laser beam.

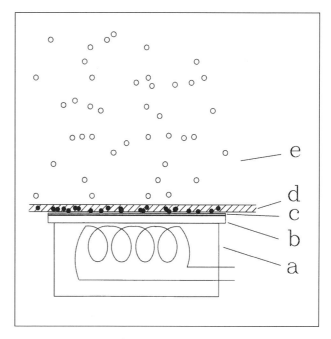

Figure 2. Photolytic LCVD process: a - heater; b- substrate; c - deposited film; d - laser beam initiates photo-dissociation of reactant gas; e - reactant gas.

Because the dissociation energy of a molecule is usually a few eV, an ultraviolet laser such as a frequency doubled Ar$^+$ laser or an excimer laser is usually used in this process. This process is generally used to deposit either small structures or uniform films over tens of square centimeters.

In many cases, to get a high-quality continuous film, one must heat the substrate to over two hundred degrees Celsius during deposition in order to provide adequate free energy for the nucleation process. A typical set-up for a photolytic LCVD process is illustrated in Figure 3.

Because the photolytic process usually has a relatively low deposition rate, it is less often used as a direct write process. However, it is difficult to direct-write a microstructure onto a transparent substrate using the pyrolytic process. In such a case the photolytic process is often used.

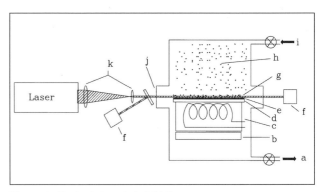

Figure 3. Typical photolytic LCVD set-up: a - to vacuum pump; b - translation stage for vertical motion; c - heater; d - substrate (proper cleaning required prior to deposition); e - deposited film; f - power meter; g - laser beam; h - reactant and buffer gases; i - incoming reactant and buffer gases; j - window; k - cylindrical lens telescope; translation stages.

Table 1. Some Electronic Materials Deposited by Pyrolytic LCVD

Film	Typical substrate	Reactant/ buffer gases	Typical pressures and flow rates (reactant / buffer)	Laser	Typical laser irradiance (MW/cm^2)	Typical focal spot diameter (µm)	Typical writing speed (µm/s)	Resistivity (µΩ-cm)	Ref.
Al	SiO$_2$	trimethyl amine alane, (Al H$_3$N C$_3$H$_9$)	2 torr	Ar$^+$	4	9	50	7.2	4
Ni	SiO$_2$	nickel tetracarbonyl, (Ni C$_4$O$_4$) / Helium, (He)	0.9 torr / 400 torr	Ar$^+$	0.1	17	24	7	5
Cu	SiO$_2$	copper (I) hexafluoro acetyl acetonate trimethyl vinylsilane^a, (Cu O$_2$C$_2$F$_6$ C$_3$H$_9$ SiH$_4$) / Helium, (He)	0.25 torr; 2 sccm^b /7.5 torr	Ar$^+$	0.3	17	24	3.7	5
Au	SiO$_2$	dimethyl gold hexafluoro acetyl acetonate, (Au C$_2$H$_6$ O$_2$C$_2$F$_6$)	0.35 torr	Ar$^+$	5	12	25	15	6
W	polyimide	tungsten hexafluoride, (WF$_6$) & Silane, (SiH$_4$)/ Argon, (Ar)	37 torr & 3 torr / 360 torr	Ar$^+$	2	2	50	25	7
Pt	pyrex	platinum-bis-hexafluoro acetyl acetonate, (Pt O$_4$C$_4$F$_{12}$)	0.5 torr	Ar$^+$	0.5	5	10	15	8
Si	Si	silane, (SiH$_4$)	100 torr	Ar$^+$	0.4	13	40	–	9

^{a}Cu(hfac)tmvs; CupraSelect™
^{b}standard cubic centimeter per minute

27.1.2 Coatings Made by LCVD

A variety of materials can be deposited by both pyrolytic and photolytic LCVD and several reviews (1–3) summarize materials that have been deposited by LCVD.

Pyrolytic Process

For metal deposition, the reactant gases used are usually organometallic compounds such as metal alkyls, metal carbonyls, and metal halides. A metal alkyl MR_n molecule consists of a metal (M) and a radical (R) of either methyl $(CH_3)_n$ or ethyl $(C_2H_5)_n$ where n is an integer. A metal carbonyl consists of a metal and a carbonyl $(CO)_n$ radical and a metal halide consists of a metal and a halide (F, Cl, Br, I)$_n$ radical. For the deposition of Ge and Si, the hydrides GeH_4 and SiH_4 are often used. In some cases a more complicated organometallic compound is utilized to give improved electrical conduction or higher vapor pressure. To deposit compounds, reactant gases that do not react spontaneously before deposition should be used. For pyrolytic LCVD the typical laser irradiance used is a few MW/cm^2 and the range of partial pressures for the reactant gases range from 0.1 to 100 Torr. Metals are the most common materials that are deposited by pyrolytic LCVD. Most of the deposited materials are amorphous or polycrystalline. Table 1 (previous page) lists some electronic materials that have been deposited with pyrolytic LCVD.

Photolytic Process

In this process reactant gases which have adequate absorption cross section should be used. For metal deposition, the reactant gases are similar to those used in the pyrolytic process. If an excimer laser is used, the typical peak laser irradiance is a few ten's of MW/cm^2. If a frequency doubled Argon ion laser is used the typical average laser irradiance is a few hundred W/cm^2. Table 2 lists the materials that are deposited by photolytic LCVD.

References

1. Y. Rytz-Froidevaux, R. P. Salathé, and H. H. Gilgen, *Appl. Phys. A* **37**, p. 121 (1985).
2. T. H. Baum and P. B. Comita, *Thin Solid Films* **218**, p. 80 (1992).
3. D. J. Ehrlich and J. Y. Tsao (Eds), 1989, *Laser Microfabrication*, Academic Press, CA, Chapters 7 and 8.
4. T. H. Baum, C. E. Larson, and R. L. Jackson, *Appl. Phys. Lett.* **55**, p. 1264 (1989).
5. S. Leppävuori, J. Remes and H. Moilanen, *SPIE* **2874**, p. 272 (1996).
6. T. T. Kodas, T. H. Baum, and P. B. Comita, *J. Appl. Phys.* **62**, p. 281 (1987).
7. J. G. Black, S. P. Doran, and M. J. Ehrlich, *Appl. Phys. Lett.* **56**, p. 1072 (1990).
8. D. Braichotto and H. van den Bergh, *Appl. Phys. A* **44**, p. 353 (1987).
9. D. Bäuerle, G. Leyendecker, D. Wagner, E. Bauser, and Y. C. Lu, *Appl. Phys. A* **30**, p. 147 (1983).
10. P. K. Boyer, C. A. Moore, R. Solanki, W. K. Ritchie, G. A. Roche and G. J. Collins, *Mat. Res. Soc. Symp. Proc.* **17**, p. 119 (1983).
11. T. H. Baum and E. E. Marinero, *Appl. Phys. Lett.* **49**, p. 1213 (1986).
12. R. W. Andreatta, D. Lubben, J. G. Eden, and J. E. Greene, *J. Vac. Sci. Technol.* **20**, p. 740 (1982).

YING TSUI

Table 2. Some Electronic Materials Deposited by Photolytic LCVD

Film	Reactant/buffer gases	Typical pressures and flow rates (reactant/buffer)	Laser	Typical (peak) laser irradiance (MW/cm^2)	Beam dimension	Typical substrate temperature (°C)	Ref.
Al	trimethyl aluminum, $(Al\ C_3H_9)$	vapor pressure at 50°C	ArF	40	1.2 cm x 0.15 cm	150	10
Cr	chromium hexacarbonyl, $(Cr\ C_6O_6)$	vapor pressure at 50°C	ArF	40	1.2 cm x 0.15 cm	150	10
Au	dimethyl gold acetylacetonate, $(Au\ C_2H_6\ C_5H_7O_2)$	9 mtorr	KrF	30	0.25 cm x 0.25 cm	150	11
Si	silane (SiH_4) / nitrogen, (N_2)	20 torr / 430 torr; 30 sccm	KrF	10	2 cmϕ	120	12
Ge	germane, (GeH_4) / helium, (He)	20 torr / 430 torr; 30 sccm	KrF	10	2 cmϕ	120	12
SiO_2	silane, SiH_4 / nitrous oxide (N_2O)	80 mtorr / 6 torr	ArF	40	1.2 cm x 0.15 cm	300	10
Si_3N_4	silane, SiH_4 / ammonia, (NH_3)	1 torr; 10 sccm / 1 torr; 10 sccm	ArF	40	1.2 cm x 0.15 cm	300	10
Al_2O_3	trimethyl aluminum, $(Al\ C_3H_9)$ / nitrous oxide (N_2O)	0.5 torr / 0.5 torr	ArF	40	1.2 cm x 0.15 cm	250	10

27.1.3 Direct Write Processing Using LCVD

In contrast to conventional lithographic techniques, the laser direct write process is a single-step technique that can save time and material. Laser direct writing technology has been developed for basic microelectronic fabrication steps that include deposition, etching, passivation, and doping. These steps are accomplished in a maskless fashion directly under software control. The direct-write process is useful in integrated circuit debugging, testing and repair, and it is particularly useful in processes that require creating complex three-dimensional (3D) microstructures. Thus the direct-write process is a useful tool for creating microstructures in a microelectromechanical system. It is also a useful tool for the multichip modules (MCMs) technology. Processes compatible with MCMs technology should permit the deposition of small microstructures on a irregular nonplanar surfaces. Those processes should also permit the deposition of small microstructures on a thermally fragile substrate such as polymide.

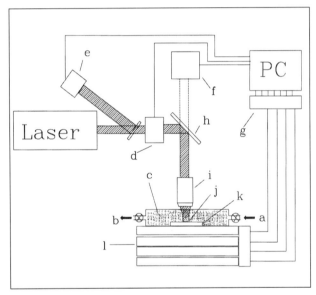

Figure 4. Typical direct-write deposition system: a - incoming reactant and buffer gases; b - to vacuum pump; c - reactant and buffer gases; d - laser shutter; e - power meter; f - CCD camera; g - controller for translation stages; h - dielectric mirror; i - microscope objective; j - deposited film; k - substrate (requires proper cleaning prior to deposition); l - translation stages.

Both photolytic and pyrolytic LCVD processes can be used to direct write small features. The pyrolytic process is more commonly used because of its higher deposition rate (vertical growth rate of 1–100 (m/s for pyrolytic processes versus 0.1–1 (m/s for photolytic processes). The photolytic process is often used when the substrate is either transparent to the laser light or thermally fragile. The photolytic process is sometimes used for pre-nucleation prior to the application of the pyrolytic process. As illustrated in Figure 4, a laser direct write instrument is essentially composed of five parts: a laser, a microscope objective, translation stages for substrate positioning, a gas cell containing the substrate, and a computer controller. The microscope objective is used to focus the laser beam to a spot of few micrometers to heat the substrate locally. It is also used to view the surface for accurate positioning and for process monitoring. The translation stages are driven by the computer to generate the desired patterns. The gas cell is normally evacuated to a low pressure ($< 10^{-5}$ torr) using an oil-free pump, such as a turbomolecular pump, and then filled with the reactant gas.

Laser writing of high-purity metals has been applied to a wide variety of microelectronics applications. Table 3 lists some of the metals and typical application areas.

Table 3. Typical Metals and their Application Areas in Microelectronic Industry

Metal	Properties	Applications
Al	low resistance; self passivation	integrated circuit (IC) metalization
Ni	good chemical and metallurgical inertness	diffusion barrier
Cu	low cost	IC packaging
Au	good chemical inertness; low resistance	contacts, bonding and wiring
W	good thermal and chemical stability	high current devices
Pt	low diffusion in Si at high temperature	ohmic contact

The most important criterion in laser writing of metals for microelectronics applications is the resistivity of the metal microstructure. The typical process parameters for laser direct-write process as well as the resistivity of the metals are summarized in Table 1. Laser parameters, reactant gas partial pressure, scanning speed of the laser beam are the common parameters that are varied in a direct-write process. Table 4 summarizes the effect of changing these parameters.

Table 4. Effect of Changing Parameters in a Direct-Write System Using Pyrolytic LCVD

Laser wavelength	Surface (substrate and deposited film) absorptivity
Laser intensity	Surface temperature; line width and line thickness
Reactant gas partial pressure and flow rate	Availabilty of reactant gas molecules; line width and line thickness
Scanning speed	Line width and line thickness

A direct-write process usually operates in the kinetic-limited regime when good spatial resolution is required. In such a regime, increases of pressure and mass flow of the reactant gas (beyond its threshold level) do not affect the deposition rate in a substantial manner. The deposition rate also increases exponentially with increasing temperature. The resolution of the line can be many times smaller than the focal spot of the laser, because the exponential dependence of the deposition rate limits the writing to the inner zone of the temperature profile, and thus helps to improve spatial resolution. For most applications, the scanning speed of the laser beam should be equal to the lateral growth speed of the film, so that a steady state growth of line is achieved. Instabilities can result in the direct-write process in certain ranges of laser power and scanning speed, because of changes in absorbed laser power caused by changes in surface absorptivity.

27.1.4 Pulsed Laser Deposition

The pulsed laser deposition (PLD) process consists of three stages: 1.) a laser beam strikes a solid target of certain composition and produces an outward plasma plume; 2.) the plume interacts with an ambient reactant gas if present; and 3.) the ablated material condenses on a substrate where a thin film nucleates and grows. As illustrated in Figure 5, a typical PLD system consists of five parts: a laser with beam delivery optics, a chamber, the target and its translation stage, a reactant gas and the substrate to be coated with its translation stages. The laser is usually a pulsed laser, such as an excimer laser. The peak power of the laser is typically in the MW range. The beam delivery optics are used to focus the beam onto the target. The target chamber is evacuated to a low pressure ($< 10^{-5}$ torr) using a vacuum pump and then filled with the reactant gas. The target is moved by translation stages so that the laser beam interacts with a fresh spot with each laser pulse and the substrate is rotated by a mechanical stage to give a uniform coating. In some cases the laser beam itself can be scanned in position using a tilt motion on one of the beam deflection mirrors.

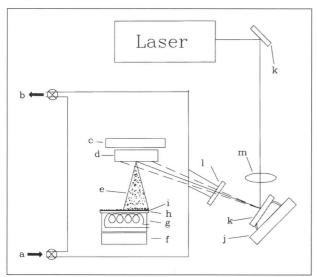

Figure 5. A typical PLD system: a - reactant and buffer gases; b - to vacuum pump; c - translation stage; d - target; e - plasma plume; f - rotational stage; g - heater; h - substrate (requires proper cleaning prior to deposition); i - deposited film; j - tilting motion stage; k - dielectric mirror; l - window; m - lens.

A wide variety of materials can be deposited by PLD with reasonable deposition rates. A recent review (1) summarizes simple and also complex materials that have been deposited by PLD. Table 5 lists some basic electronic materials that are deposited by PLD.

Table 5. Some Simple Electronic Materials Deposited by PLD

Material	Laser	Laser fluence (J/cm²)	Target to substrate distance (cm)	Deposition rate (Å/pulse)
Au	XeCl	5	1.7	0.05
Al	Nd:YAG (532 nm)	10	1.7	0.07
Cu	Nd:YAG (355 nm)	4	1.7	0.015
Co	XeCl	3	4	0.024
Fe	XeCl	3	4	0.032
Pt	KrF	4	4	0.1
Ti	XeCl	5	3.4	0.025
Ge (epitaxial)	KrF	1.5	3.7	1.5
Si (epitaxial)	KrF	1.5	3.7	1.5

While PLD can be used to deposit almost any material, it sometimes has advantages in depositing nonequilibrium materials such as diamond-like carbon (DLC). The deposition of DLC is made possible by the availability of the highly charged energetic ions which enhance the quality of the resulting coating. A DLC film can be produced by PLD using an Nd:YAG laser. Using a graphite target, a DLC thin film can be created when the PLD plume consists of energetic ions with kinetic energy greater than a hundred eV condensing onto a substrate surface. Table 6 presents typical parameters for Nd:YAG laser deposited DLC.

Table 6. Typical Parameters for Nd:YAG Laser Deposited DLC

Laser wavelength	1.064 μm
Pulse duration	10 ns
Laser fluence	500 J/cm² peak
Substrate temperature	20°C
Reactant gas	none

Multicomponent materials, such as $PbZr_xTi_{(1-x)}O_3$ (PZT), can also be deposited by PLD. The deposition of complex multicomponent materials by PLD is possible because of its ability to provide stoichiometric transfer of materials with complex composition. Multilayers of complex materials can be also deposited by

PLD because of its excellent control of the layer thickness by the number of laser pulses and laser energy. PLD can be used to fabricate novel devices made from compound semiconductor epitaxial layers with a predesigned compositional profile. This is used to produce a precise bandgap profile for the material to achieve specific electrical and optical properties. One such structure is the $Hg_{1-x}Cd_xTe$ superlattice, where x changes at different distance from the film surface. Table 7 summarizes some of the films that can be deposited using PLD. Also, Chapter 23 has a discussion of the use of PLD for depositing films of high-temperature superconductors.

Some of the nonmetallic materials that have been deposited by PLD are listed in Table 8.

Laser parameters, substrate temperature, reactant gas partial pressure, and target-to-substrate distance are the common parameters that are varied in a PLD process. Table 9 summarizes the effect of changing these parameters.

Table 7. Complex and Novel Structures that Can Be Deposited Using PLD

Structure	Process advantages	Example
Epitaxial (low temperature)	availability of large current density of 10–100 eV ions	epitaxial Ge on GaAs
Muticomponent	stoichemetric transfer of materials	$YBa_2Cu_3O_{7-\delta}$
Nonequilibrium	availability of large current density of 10–1000 eV ions	DLC
Mutilayer	excellent control in thickness of deposited material	PbO/TiO_2 layer
Epitaxial multicomponent multilayer	all of the above	$Hg_{1-x}Cd_xTe$ superlattice

Table 9. Effect of Changing PLD Parameters

Parameters	Effect on process	Possible effect on film properties
Laser wavelength	Charge states and kinetic energies of the ablated species; ablation rate	Target stoichiometry; formation of metastable structures; particulates; thickness per pulse
Laser intensity	Charge states and kinetic energies of the ablated species; ablation rate	Target stoichiometry; formation of metastable structures; particulates; thickness per pulse
Laser energy per pulse	Ablation rate	Thickness per pulse
Reactant gas partial pressure	Increase availabilty of reactant gas molecules	Film composition; establishment of epitaxy; control of crystal structure
Substrate temperature	Surface mobility of depositing material	Formation of metastable microstructures
Substrate to target distance	Deposition rate	Film thickness per pulse

Table 8. Some Complex and Novel PLD Deposited Electronic Materials

Film	Material type	Applications	Laser	Fluence (J/cm²)	Target to substrate distance (cm)	Substrate	Substrate temp. (°C)	Reactant gases and pressures	Ref.
SiC	High-temperature semiconductor	High-temperature electronics	XeF	1.5	7	Quartz	900	None	2
$Pb(Zr_xTi_{1-x})TiO_3$	Ferroelectric film	Nonvolatile random-access-memory (NVRAM)	KrF	1	4	MgO	550	O_2; 35 torr	1
$LiNbO_3$	Piezo-electric film	Surface acoustic wave devices	ArF	2	4	Sapphire	500	O_2; 10 mtorr	3
ITO	Semiconductor	Electronics	ArF	1	7	Glass	300	O_2; 15 mtorr	4
NiAl	Resistive element	Metallization of IC	KrF	10	5	Si	350	None	5
DLC	Thermal conductor	Electronic packaging	Nd:YAG (1064 nm)	500	8	Si	20	None	1
TiN	Diffusion barrier material	Circuit technology	XeCl	5	2.6	Si	400	None	6
HgTe/CdTe supperlattice	Bandgap engineering structure	IR detector	Nd:YAG (1064 nm)	2	4	CdTe	160	None	1

References

1. D. B. Chrisey and G. K. Hubler (Eds), *Pulsed Laser Deposition of Thin Films,* John Wiley & Sons, NY (1994).
2. L. Rimai, R. Ager, J. Hangas, and E. M. Logothetis, *J. Appl. Phys.* **73,** p. 8242 (1993).
3. Y. Shibata, K. Kaya, and K. Akashi, *J. Appl. Phys.* **77,** p. 1498 (1995).
4. J. P. Zheng and H. S. Kwok, *Appl. Phys. Lett.* **63,** p. 1 (1993).
5. R. K. Singh, D. Bhattacharya, S. Sharan, P. Tiwari and J. Narayan, *J. Mater. Res.* **7,** p. 2639 (1992).
6. J. C. S. Kools, C. J. C. M. Nilesen, S. H. Brongersma, E. van de Riet, and J. Dielman, *J. Vac. Sci. Technol. A* **10,** p. 1809 (1992).

YING TSUI

27.2 Deposition of Thick Films of Electronic Ceramics

Pulsed laser deposition (PLD), which has been described in Section 27.1, is a superior technique for growth of high-quality thin films (≤ 1 µm) of electronic ceramics. Some examples have been presented in Section 27.1.4. Deposition of such thin films has satisfied many important applications, but there is also a need for thick films (≥ 1 µm) of electronic ceramics (1). Two film qualities principally control the growth of thick films by PLD: the film surface morphology and film stress. This section gives several examples of PLD deposition parameters that affect these qualities including: film deposition rate, film-substrate lattice mismatch, film-substrate thermal coefficient of expansion mismatch, and film growth kinetics.

Introduction to PLD of Electronic Ceramics and Thick Films

Electronic ceramics are technologically important materials because they have a wide range of properties that lead to useful applications, ranging from solid-state electronics to optics and protective coatings. In many cases, it is required that the material be cast in thin-film form (~ 1 µm). Electronic ceramic materials are typically made up of several different elements, have a complex unit cell, and have anisotropic physical and chemical properties. This makes their processing by conventional coating techniques extremely difficult and novel approaches are required. PLD incorporates, typically, a high-powered excimer laser to deposit thin films of various types of electronic ceramics (1). It has many advantages over conventional physical vapor deposition techniques for ceramic thin films including: the ability to transfer the stoichiometry from the target to the growing film, the ability to add high pressures of reactive gases such as oxygen, simple vacuum requirements, high reproducibility, and the rapid production of smooth films. There are several electronic ceramic materials for which there is an application for thick films including ferroelectrics, ferrites, thermal barrier coatings, and biomaterials.

PLD has been applied to the problem of growing thick films (~ 50–100 µm) of ferroelectrics (e.g., $(Sr,Ba)TiO_3$) and all three classes of ferrites (e.g., YIG, $(Ni,Zn)Fe_2O_4$ and $BaFe_{12}O_{19}$). The problems associated with growing films of this thickness are different from the problems encountered with conventional PLD, e.g., stresses in the film can cause substrate warping and/or fracture or even film delamination, and the temperature, chemical, and morphological character of the substrate surface changes during the course of thick film depositions. In turn, the properties of the resulting film are often thickness-dependent. Films of this thickness also become prohibitively expensive for practical application, because of the long deposition times involved. These and other issues related to the deposition of thick films by PLD will be covered in this section.

Experimental Apparatus

The experimental apparatus used to grow thick films of electronic ceramics by PLD includes, typically, a KrF excimer laser operated at 248 nm, ~2 J/cm², ~150 mJ/laser shot, and 10–50 Hz. The films are deposited onto heated substrates. The targets rotate at ~0.5 Hz and are about 4–10 cm away from the substrate. The laser-target angle is nominally 45° and the laser spot should be rastered across the target to ensure film uniformity. Depositions are carried out in an oxygen ambient held constant in a dynamic equilibrium between 50 to 400 mTorr. The substrates are typically single-crystal ceramics, but polycrystalline or metal-coated substrates can be used. The film deposition rate is ~1–2 Å/laser shot with thick films taking several hours to deposit, depending on the laser repetition rate.

High Temperature Superconductors

Pulsed laser deposition has been applied to the important problem of depositing high-quality thin films of high T_c superconductors. This application has been described in more detail in Chapter 23. PLD achieved a great amount of success due to the rapid and reproducible deposition of $YBa_2Cu_3O_7$ (YBCO) films with state-of-the-art transport properties. For most applications, only thin HTS films (≤ 0.5 µm) were required, i.e., on the order of a couple magnetic penetration depths (~ 1200 Å). Several surface characterization techniques have shown that continued growth of YBCO beyond 0.5 µm thickness results in an extremely defective material (see Fig. 1). Thick film growth results in $YBa_2Cu_3O_7$ films which begin to contain different orientations, other phases, and grain boundaries. All of these features severely inhibit high-quality electrical transport.

Especially evident from Figure 1 (next page) is the importance of surface morphology and thermal expansion coefficient.

During the growth of a thick film, the importance of the substrate orientation and surface morphology becomes increasingly reduced. In time, the surface of the growing film acts as a substrate for further film growth. For materials like $YBa_2Cu_3O_7$ and most other electronic ceramics, the situation is even more complicated because these materials have highly anisotropic electrical transport properties requiring exclusively c-axis oriented growth. In addition, as the film gets thicker, it becomes comparable in volume to the substrate. At that point, bulk properties of the material being deposited, such as the coefficient of thermal expansion and film-substrate lattice mismatch, become very important. Catastrophic effects because of differences in these properties can occur, including film-substrate delamination or substrate fracture.

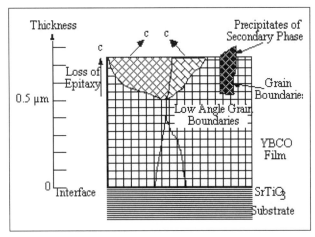

Figure 1. Schematic cross section through a $YBa_2Cu_3O_7$ film on a (100) $SrTiO_3$ substrate versus thickness.

Effect of Deposition Rate

Figure 2 shows $BaFe_{12}O_{19}$ ferrite film surface morphology as a function of deposition rate for two ~6-µm-thick films deposited under identical conditions except for the deposition rate.

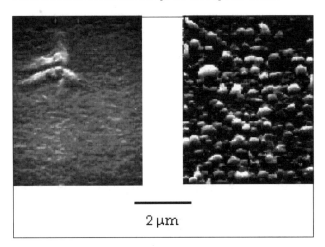

Figure 2. $BaFe_{12}O_{19}$ ferrite film surface morphology as a function of deposition rate. The film is ~6 µm for both films. The deposition rates for the left and right were 0.038 and 0.063 µm/minute, respectively.

Simple interpretation of these SEM micrographs suggest that thick film growth should be done at lower deposition rates to improve the surface morphology for subsequent layers. An important aspect of this conclusion is that for thick film growth, deposition time becomes an important factor. While depositing thick films at slow deposition rates will improve the surface morphology for this film-substrate system, and it may achieve the research goal of thick films with acceptable device properties, the onerous deposition time and thus cost may prohibit its ultimate application.

Effect of Nonuniform Strain

Ferroelectric films have many applications which typically require thin films (≤ 1 µm), but applications for thick films (~50 µm) of $(Sr,Ba)TiO_3$ exist in phased array antennas. Figure 3 illustrates the catastrophic effects that can occur when attempting to grow thick films.

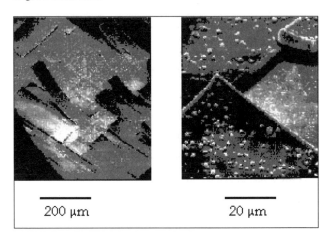

Figure 3. Surface morphology of a 7-µm-thick $(Sr,Ba)TiO_3$ film on a (100) $LaAlO_3$ substrate.

The SEM micrograph in Figure 3 shows that while the $(Sr,Ba)TiO_3$ film on a (100) $LaAlO_3$ substrate was relatively smooth, dense, and single crystalline in appearance, it obviously contained a great deal of nonuniform strain, causing the film to delaminate from the substrate at the deposition temperature of 750°C. Because this occurred at the deposition temperature, the nonuniform strain cannot be caused by a difference in the thermal expansion coefficient.

Evolution of Surface Morphology with Film Thickness

Figure 4 shows the surface morphology for $(Sr,Ba)TiO_3$ films grown on MgO substrates as a function of film thickness.

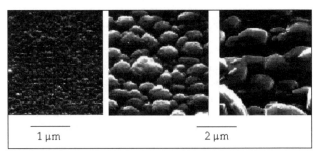

Figure 4. Surface morphology as a function of thickness for a $(Sr,Ba)TiO_3$ film on an (100) MgO substrate. The approximate film thicknesses from left to right are ≤ 1, 10, and 30 µm, respectively.

For 1-µm thickness, the films were smooth with a fine grain texture. At 10 µm, the small grains coalesce into larger grains and at 30 µm the films continue to coalesce into even larger grains. There is also the presence at 30 µm of some material nucleating which appears to be either another phase or another orientation. X-ray

Chapter 27: Film Deposition and Doping

diffraction characterization of films similar to that shown in Figure 4 indicates that the new material is another orientation and not another phase. Unlike the case for thick (Sr,Ba)TiO$_3$ films on a (100) LaAlO$_3$ substrates shown in Figure 3, these films showed no sign of delamination even for the largest thicknesses (~40 μm).

The difference between the surface morphology for the films of Figures 3 and 4 can be understood by examining their respective amounts of film-substrate lattice mismatch. The lattice constant for (Sr,Ba)TiO$_3$ films with a 50/50 stoichiometry is 3.947 Å, whereas the lattice constant for (100) LaAlO$_3$ and MgO is 3.787 and 4.210 Å, respectively. This represents a 4.1 and 6.7% lattice mismatch for LaAlO$_3$ and MgO, respectively. It is clear from the morphology of these two films that the (Sr,Ba)TiO$_3$ film grown on LaAlO$_3$ grew epitaxially and was nearly single crystalline. The better film-substrate lattice match for this substrate compared to MgO still left the film with a great deal of stress. On the other hand, for the MgO substrate the film-substrate lattice mismatch was large enough that it caused the film to be oriented, but polycrystalline with a large number of grain boundaries, i.e., not single crystalline. Therefore, these grain boundaries contained lattice mismatch accommodating defects which allowed the film to grow without any signs of delamination. For thin films, the crystalline quality of the (Sr,Ba)TiO$_3$ film material on LaAlO$_3$ would be typically better than for MgO because of the better film-substrate lattice match, but for thick film growth the good match results in catastrophic film delamination. It is important to note that the difference between Figures 3 and 4 had nothing to do with differences in thermal expansion coefficients because the delamination was observed to occur at the deposition temperature.

It is difficult to draw strong conclusions from the examples in Figures 3 and 4, except that the film-substrate lattice mismatch is a factor in the film growth kinetics. For the case of LaAlO$_3$ substrate, the closeness of the lattice match caused the (Sr,Ba)TiO$_3$ film to grow with near perfect registry. But this was not the equilibrium lattice distance for the (Sr,Ba)TiO$_3$ material, and it resulted a highly strained material. The cumulative effect of this strain increased with thickness until the energetics favored delamination over continued growth. For applications where polycrystalline material is acceptable, this problem can be overcome. But for applications in which a high degree of orientation is required (see below), the choice of substrate may be the most important for thick film growth.

Issues for the Growth of Highly Oriented Thick Films: Oxygen Pressure

Most of the applications for ferrite films require film thicknesses between 50 and 400 μm. Isolators and circulators make up a class of devices called nonreciprocal devices because they work differently in one direction as compared to another. This effect is caused by the alignment of magnetic moments on the various sublattices. Aligning the magnetic moments requires an external biasing magnet. Electromagnetic waves passing through polarized ferrites are exposed to a asymmetric vector potential as opposed to a scalar potential, which is seen in conventional dielectrics, and this results in the nonreciprocal effect. The large film thickness is required because the nonreciprocal effect is a volume effect. There are three crystallographic types of ferrites (spinels, garnets, and hexagonals).

Hexagonal ferrites possess a large uniaxial anisotropy, which means that there is an easy and a hard crystallographic direction with which to pole the material. For device applications this is useful because it may eliminate the need for external biasing magnets, but it adds the difficult requirement that the film is highly c-axis oriented, in addition to just obtaining a thick film which is single phase and adherent.

Figure 5 shows the surface morphology of a BaFe$_{12}$O$_{19}$ ferrite film growth as a function of thickness. These films were deposited at 900°C and 400 mTorr oxygen on a (0001) Al$_2$O$_3$ substrate. Under these conditions, BaFe$_{12}$O$_{19}$ grows as a smooth thin film. Then for increasing thicknesses hexagonal crystallites begin to nucleate and grow highly c-axis oriented. In time, though, for thicker films the presence of other material which is either of another orientation or another phase begins to nucleate. The surface structure for the thickest film in Figure 5 shows a hexagonal crystallite growing on edge. This feature, as well as the other surface features, will inhibit the subsequent growth of device quality highly c-axis oriented (self-biased) hexagonal ferrite material. Continued BaFe$_{12}$O$_{19}$ ferrite film growth on a surface like that shown in Figure 5 results in a layers that are weakly adherent and randomly oriented.

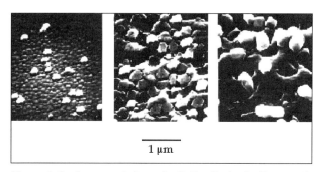

Figure 5. Surface morphology of a BaFe$_{12}$O$_{19}$ ferrite film growth as a function of thickness. The approximate film thicknesses from left to right are ≤ 1, 5, and 10 μm, respectively. The films were deposited at 900°C and 400 mTorr oxygen.

The resulting surface morphology shown in Figure 5 does not support thick film growth. One approach to resolving this problem is to adjust a PLD growth parameter similar to what was observed in Figure 2. The surface morphology of a growing BaFe$_{12}$O$_{19}$ film can be modified by adjusting the background oxygen pressure during deposition. Figure 6 shows the evolving surface morphology of a BaFe$_{12}$O$_{19}$ ferrite film grown at a lower oxygen deposition pressure.

Reducing the deposition pressure has a dramatic effect on surface morphology. During PLD film growth, the background gas has many functions: it provides stopping for some of the energetic ions and neutrals in the plasma plume which prevents surface damage, it provides oxidation of the target surface, the film, and the ablated ejecta, and it provides a high-pressure ambient to prevent re-evaporation of volatile species from the heated substrate. There are likely other effects of the background gas on film growth. The effect on film nucleation and growth kinetics is not well understood, but it is clear from Figure 6 that it has a positive effect on the morphology.

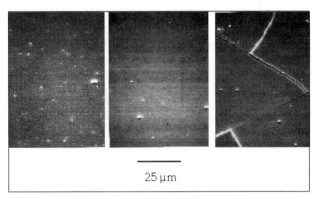

Figure 6. Surface morphology of a $BaFe_{12}O_{19}$ ferrite film as a function of oxygen deposition pressure. The approximate film thicknesses from left to right are 1, 10, and 20 µm, respectively.

An interesting feature of the 20-µm thick film of Figure 6 is the appearance of cracking during thick film growth. This effect is similar to the $(Sr,Ba)TiO_3$ film of Figure 3 and is caused by stress present in the growing film. Therefore, while lowering the oxygen deposition pressure does improve the surface morphology of the growing film, it is at the expense of added strain present in the film.

The goal of a self-biased $BaFe_{12}O_{19}$ ferrite thick film device is even more difficult to obtain when the film is characterized for its magnetic properties. Figure 7 plots the full-width-at-half-maximum for x-ray diffraction scans for the (008) peak of a c-axis oriented $BaFe_{12}O_{19}$ ferrite films as a function of thickness.

As expected, the quality of the growing film degrades with thickness. The magnetic characterization, also shown in Figure 7, indicates that long before the film shows visible signs of cracking, the quality of the orientation has degraded to the point that it appears magnetically isotropic. For the case of thick $BaFe_{12}O_{19}$ ferrite film growth, an extremely high degree of orientation must be obtained.

Conclusions and Future Work

PLD is a superior technique for the growth of high quality thin films (≤ 1 µm) of electronic ceramics. For thick films (≥ 1 µm), the results presented in this section suggest that two film qualities principally control the growth: film surface morphology and film stress. Several PLD deposition parameters affect these qualities including: film deposition rate, film-substrate lattice mismatch, film-substrate thermal coefficient of expansion mismatch, and film growth kinetics. The major conclusion of this section is that it will be difficult to fabricate thick ceramic films of suitable electronic quality by conventional physical vapor deposition techniques. Other modifications such as some form of particle-assist (laser, low-energy ion) during the deposition may be required to maintain good morphology and adequate crystalline quality during growth.

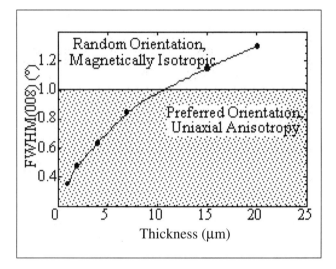

Figure 7. X-ray diffraction full-width-at-half-maximum scans of (008) peak for $BaFe_{12}O_{19}$ ferrite films as a function of thickness for depositions in low-oxygen pressure. Also shown are the regions of isotropic and oriented magnetic anisotropy.

References
1. D. B. Chrisey and G. K. Hubler (Eds), *Pulsed Laser Deposition of Thin Films,* Wiley-Interscience, New York (1994).

D. B. CHRISEY
J. S. HORWITZ
P. C. DORSEY
L. A. KNAUSS

27.3 Gas Immersion Laser Doping (GILD)

The doping of semiconductors with electrically active impurity elements may be performed in a manner similar to laser deposition.

27.3.1 Theory of Operation

The controlled incorporation of impurities into Si at the 10^{14}–10^{21} cm^{-3} concentration level is a critical process in the manufacturing of semiconductor devices. Gas immersion laser doping (GILD) provides a unique method of introducing dopants including phosphorus, boron, arsenic, and antimony into the near surface region (20–300 nm), while simultaneously electrically activating the dopants at concentrations which can exceed the solid solubility. An excellent review may be found in Reference 1.

The basic principle behind GILD is the adsorption of gas phase dopant precursors (hydrides, fluorides) on a semiconductor surface followed by irradiation with a pulsed laser at a fluence sufficient to melt the near surface region of the wafer. The precursor is decomposed upon heating, the dopant is incorporated at near uniform concentration throughout the molten zone, while the residual gas component is released into the ambient. This adsorption/melt cycle is typically repeated 10–100 times to achieve the required dopant concentration. The adsorption process and number of laser pulse cycles controls the doping concentration, while the junction depth is determined solely by the laser fluence.

27.3.2 GILD Equipment and Sample Preparation

A GILD system consists of:

- A gas cell containing the wafer and appropriate dopant gases (static or flowing)
- A laser, beam homogenizer, and fluence adjustment
- A translation system for rastering the beam (or wafer)

The laser and homogenizer are discussed below. Since the doping gases are typically hydrides or fluorides, toxic gas safety policies must be followed for the gas cell design and operation. The cell typically is evacuated to the 10^{-4} Torr level before filling with dopant gas at pressures below ambient (typically 300 Torr). An ultraviolet laser grade and vacuum-compatible window provides access for the irradiation beam.

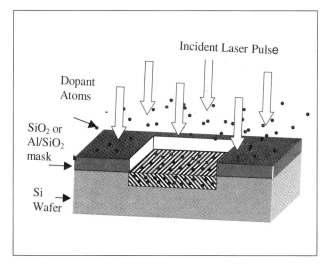

Figure 1. Selective doping using a masking layer (SiO_2 or Al/SiO_2).

Doping is accomplished on any area of the wafer directly exposed to the laser and dopant gases. For selective doping, areas that are to remain undoped must be masked using oxide or metal/oxide layers, as depicted in Figure 1. An oxide only mask should be designed with maximum reflectivity at the laser wavelength (i.e., multiples of 102-nm-thick SiO_2 for a 308-nm XeCl laser). To further reduce heating of the undoped regions, a metal reflective mask over an oxide (now acting as a thermal barrier) can be used. For large features where lateral thermal diffusion is insignificant, aluminum can be used. For small (micrometer-scale) features though, aluminum may melt and flow, and thus metals with higher melting temperatures (tungsten or tantalum) must be used.

Since surface contaminants are equally incorporated during the laser induced melting, sample preparation prior to loading the gas cell is also critical. A standard cleaning sequence, excluding the final oxide etch, should be used to prepare the surface. A final dip in a 50:1 DI:HF solution should immediately precede loading of the gas cell.

27.3.3 Laser Sources

Although numerous commercial laser sources can be used, pulsed excimer lasers operating either with XeCl (308 nm), KrF (248 nm), or ArF (193 nm) gas mixtures provide near optimum conditions. Lasers operating at wavelengths above the direct gap for Si (~365 nm) can be used, but it is more difficult to control the melt depth because of the absorption coefficient discontinuity between liquid and crystalline Si. Besides operating at appropriate wavelengths, commercially available excimer lasers also provide appropriate single pulse energy (600 mJ), repetition rates (300 Hz), total power (200 W), beam uniformity, and short temporal coherence lengths (required for beam homogenization).

The choice of excimer laser wavelength is dictated by three criteria; minimum junction depth, pyrolytic or photolytic decomposition of the dopant precursor, and gas fill lifetime. Because the optical absorption coefficient in Si is weakly wavelength dependent, slightly shallower junctions can be obtained using 193/248 nm compared to the 308 nm line. Operating at 193 nm shifts the precursor decomposition from primarily pyrolytic (at 248/308 nm) to primarily photolytic, permitting per-pulse doping levels to be increased by as much as an order of magnitude. The levels achieved are suitable for source-drain doping but generally too high for bipolar or diode junctions. Operation at shorter wavelengths is also penalized by the lower fluences and powers (especially at 193 nm), optical materials costs (at 193 nm), and the reduced gas fill lifetimes. Current GILD systems operate primarily at 308 nm.

Laser pulse widths (FWHM) of 30–50 ns yield solidification velocities in Si of 3–5 m/s for shallow melts. For shorter pulse lengths, the solidification velocity increases as the square root of the pulse duration. Above 10 m/s, twinning occurs during solidification even for (100) oriented Si wafers (other orientations twin at lower velocities and limits for other semiconductors are generally not known). Longer pulse widths reduce the solidification velocity at the expense of higher melt threshold fluences and hence lower total throughput. Multiple peaks in the laser temporal profile should be avoided, because they lead to re-melting of the solidified surface during a single cycle.

Although excimer lasers provide moderately uniform beam profiles, junction control during GILD requires a uniformity to ± 5% top-hat with steep side slopes. Excessive slope on the trailing side and edge of the beam profile leads to non-uniform doping profiles. Adequate beam homogenization can be achieved using either a fly's eye square beam spot homogenizer (2) or more recently developed line-scan homogenizers (3). Line scan widths approaching 200 mm (wafer scale) are currently being developed.

27.3.4 Gas Sources

Because the GILD process can potentially incorporate any gas component adsorbed on the Si surface, the gas delivery system and gas cell must be constructed for ultra-high vacuum operation. To avoid hydrocarbon contamination, turbomolecular pumps exhausting to an appropriate scrubber must be used. Prior to gas filling, the cell should be evacuated to high vacuum and tested for leaks.

Because of their availability in semiconductor grade purity, arsine (AsH_3), boron trifluoride (BF_3) and phosphine (PH_3) are preferred doping gases. $SbCl_5$ can be used at elevated temperatures, although the segregation of Sb during solidification prevents formation of uniform doping layers. Diborane (B_2H_6) may also be used for boron doping, but the wafer temperature must be actively maintained due to the thermal instability of the molecule. Minor fluctuations in temperature can lead to significant changes in doping levels, a behavior not observed with boron triflouride. Dopant gases are typically diluted with helium, hydrogen, or nitrogen when reduced doping concentrations are required. Total cell pressures are typically 100–500 Torr with dopant gas fractions ranging from 0.1 to 100%.

For photolytically catalyzed dissociation doping, using for example a 193-nm ArF laser, organometallics such as trimethylaluminum ($Al(CH_3)_3$), trimethylboron, ($B(CH_3)_3$), and triethylboron ($B(C_2H_5)_3$) have been used. Although enhanced doping efficiencies are possible, the organic radicals cannot be fully desorbed during the laser melt and significant carbon contamination is observed.

During GILD processing, dopant gases are both chemisorbed and physisorbed on the surface, although it is thought that physisorbed molecules desorb during the laser heating prior to melt formation. Experimental data indicate a maximum effective surface coverage of 5–10%, with typical doping efficiencies (absent pyrolytic processes) of 5×10^{13} ions/cm² per cycle. This doping level is nearly independent of junction depth because melt durations are insignificant compared to gas-surface collision times.

Because the time between laser irradiations is long compared to gas adsorption times, the surface approaches steady state conditions between cycles. Significant reductions in the per-cycle doping levels can thus only be achieved by dilution with inert gases. Dilutions of 0.1–1% are typically required to affect the surface coverage (and thus doping efficiency) since the inert gases are not strongly adsorbed on the clean surface. At very low dopant partial pressures, care must be taken to ensure that no significant depletion of the dopant gases occurs during full wafer processing.

The maximum dopant concentration is limited only by the number of melt cycles and the ultimate solubility of dopants in the molten phase. For electrically active dopants, the liquid phase is fully miscible. Thus only at very low partial pressures of dopant gases should saturation of the liquid phase become significant. However, above 50–100 laser pulses at fixed energy, the Si surface roughens and begins to damage, limiting the ultimate concentration. This damage can, to some degree, be reversed with a single higher fluence anneal.

27.3.5 Process Monitoring and Calibration

In-situ monitoring of the melt duration using either a transient reflection or transmission technique is essential for control of the junction depth. One-dimensional computer simulation codes are available to predict melt depths based on laser pulse profile, fluence, and wafer configuration (absorber and/or reflection layers) (4). Because of the difficulty of accurately determining the laser fluence at the sample plane (J/cm²), the melt duration is normally measured and a calibration curve relating melt duration to fluence and melt depth is used. For a 30-ns FWHM, 308-nm XeCl excimer laser, the melt threshold is approximately 650 mJ/cm² with a melt depth versus fluence slope of 350 nm/(J/cm²) and melt duration versus fluence slope of 100 ns/(J/cm²).

Simulations for the melt duration and melt depth versus fluence, and melt depth versus melt duration, are shown in Figure 2 (next page) for 308-nm irradiation of crystalline Si with the laser shape shown in the inset. As can be seen, the laser pulse shape has a very significant influence on the melt calibration. Exact calibrations are thus required for individual lasers, especially for shallow melts.

The melt duration may be measured either in a reflection or transmission mode. Liquid Si (like most semiconductors) is metallic and hence both the reflectivity and absorption coefficients (below the direct gap) increase. For Si wafers, reflection measurements using either a HeNe laser (633 nm) or semiconductor diode laser (790–650 nm) and a high-speed Si photodetector are adequate. The semiconductor diode lasers have an advantage because mode beating occurs on a time scale much shorter than the reflectance measurements.

For thin film work, interference effects arising from the temperature dependent optical properties complicate reflectance measurements. In these cases, a transmission measurement will provide a more accurate determination of the melt duration. For thin films on transparent substrates (i.e., silicon on glass), the same semiconductor diode or HeNe laser can be used for transmission and reflectance measurements. For nontransparent substrates (oxidized Si wafers), a 1.5–1.9 µm diode laser must be used, coupled with either backside polishing or collection optics to direct the transmitted beam into a detector. Transmission data is superior to reflectance data for melts of a few skin depths (10–30 nm) since the temperature dependence of the optical properties of the solid phase do not affect the results. In both cases, melt duration should be measured from the 10% rise to fall time, not FWHM.

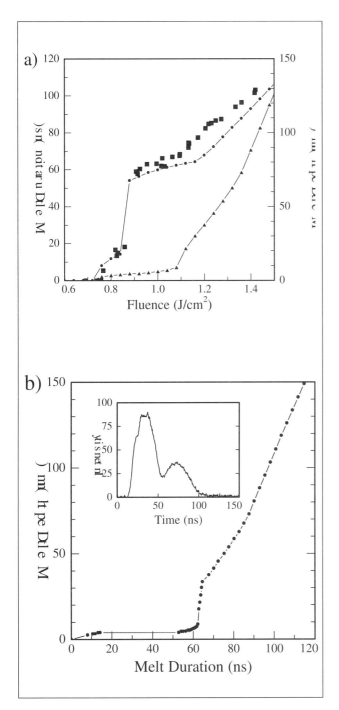

Figure 2. a) Comparison of simulated melt durations (circles) and experiment (squares) for XeCl irradiation of a single-crystal silicon wafer. Melt depths are indicated with triangles. b) Correlation of melt duration and melt depth from heat flow simulations, using the XeCl excimer laser pulse depicted in the inset.

For shallow junctions (on the order of 10–30 nm), it is critical to simultaneously measure the melt duration and temporal laser profile, and couple both to the simulation code for immediate determination of the melt depth. Near the melt threshold, small changes in the temporal laser profile strongly modify the calibration of melt duration to melt depth. Alternatively, the minimum transmission level (for melts up to 2–3 skin depths) can be related directly to melt thickness using independent melt measurements for calibration, such as secondary ion mass spectroscopy (SIMS).

At extremely high dopant concentrations ($> 10^{21}$ cm^{-3}), the solidification velocity is reduced in the alloy. In addition, the thermal conductivity of heavily doped Si is slightly reduced and the optical properties are slightly modified (though minimally for ultraviolet wavelengths). These effects result in substantially longer melt duration at constant fluence. The reduced solidification velocity is the dominant effect, and the melt depths are only slightly extended. Extensive twinning and defect incorporation in the layer will similarly modify the solidification velocity and thermal conductivity. No adequate models for this concentration dependence exist, and direct calibration of the melt thickness is required for extremely high dopant levels.

27.3.6 Doping Profiles

The GILD process ideally produces box-like impurity concentration profiles extending to the maximum melt depth. This situation is approached in practice, constrained only by two fundamental limitations. First, dopants are incorporated in the surface and must be diffused in the liquid phase to the full melt depth. For a typical liquid phase diffusivity (2.3×10^{-4} cm^2/s for As), impurities can redistribute over 50 nm during a typical single-pulse 30 ns melt cycle. While adequate for shallow junctions, multiple irradiation cycles must be used to provide adequate diffusion for deep junctions.

The second effect involves segregation of dopant impurities during solidification. For arsenic and phosphorus, there is general agreement that no significant segregation occurs during solidification at typical laser annealing velocities (1–6 m/s). Although boron should also show no segregation behavior, there is some evidence of boron trapping near the maximum melt depth, which cannot be adequately explained. Antimony segregates with an effective segregation constant near 0.7 for 3 m/s velocities. One-dimensional impurity diffusion computer codes incorporating velocity dependent segregation models are available from the same sources (4).

High-concentration doping may require in excess of one hundred dopant adsorption and melt cycles. Stress-induced trap states have been observed following such irradiation cycles and generally are unacceptable for junction formation. To eliminate these traps, doping is typically performed in a two-step sequence:

- Low fluence doping irradiations to incorporate the required total dopant dose
- Small number (2–3) higher fluence irradiations (either with or without the dopant gas) to "drive-in" dopants to the desired junction depth

The second step relieves the stress induced by the multiple lower fluence cycles. The number of drive-in cycles is determined only by the requirement of liquid phase diffusion of impurities to the maximum melt depth.

27.3.7 Wafer Throughput

With currently available lasers, the GILD process requires numerous laser-doping cycles to fully process a wafer at required dopant levels. If the single pulse fluence is adequate to irradiate a full die (or multiples), step and repeat at each die is the preferable operating mode since the nonuniform effects at the edge of the irradiation beam can be avoided. However, raster scanning in either area-scan or line-scan mode is more commonly required to process the required area and cycles. The wafer should be over scanned, or additional laser cycles should be used at the beginning and end of each to correct for the overlap.

The overall throughput is limited by the total laser power available. The time to process a wafer is nEA/P where n is the number of laser pulses required, E the fluence per pulse, A the total area, and P the total laser power. Shallow junction doping of a 100-mm single-crystal wafer with 20 pulses, using a 300 W laser, requires approximately 10 minutes. Since the total time is essentially inversely proportional to the melt threshold fluence, much less time is required for TFT (thin film transistor) fabrication.

References

1. Paul G. Carey, Ph.D. Thesis, Stanford University, 1988; Kurt H. Weiner, Ph.D. Thesis, Stanford University, 1989.
2. XMR, Inc., 47281 Bayside Parkway, Fremont, CA 94538.
3. Lambda Physik GmbH, Hans-Böckler Str. 12, D-37079 Göttingen, Germany.
4. Contact Michael O. Thompson, Cornell University (mot1@cornell.edu) or Patrick M. Smith, Lawrence Livermore National Laboratory (psmith@post.harvard.edu).

MICHAEL O. THOMPSON
T. W. SIGMON
PATRICK M. SMITH

Index

A

Ablation 190, 195, 651
Abrasive water jet cutting 466–469
ABS 457
Absorbance 168, 169
Absorption 173, 174, 182, 183, 184, 426, 431
Absorption coefficient 5, 182, 183, 348, 436, 460
Absorption coefficients for metals 6
Absorptive index 176, 181, 182, 183
Absorptivity 95, 167, 175, 176, 180, 181, 182, 183, 186, 193, 194, 200, 223, 224, 225, 232, 234, 237, 238, 280, 375, 376, 387, 389, 392, 396, 413, 429, 430, 417, 472, 606
Accurate clear epoxy solid 546, 548
Acetal 474
Acetate 490
ACGIH 205, 206, 209, 210, 212, 214, 218, 220
Acoustic emission 161
Acousto-optic devices 12, 39
Acousto-optic (AO) Q switch 12, 39, 40, 327, 527, 637
Acousto-optic Q switched laser 41
Acousto-optic modulator 655
Acrylate 549
Acrylate photopolymer 543
Acrylic 293, 294, 366, 426, 458, 533
Acrylic resin 484
Acrylonitrile butadiene 522
ADA 72
Adaptive mirror 113, 114, 230
Airborne contaminants 209, 214
Alexandrite 45, 46
Alexandrite laser 14, 16, 17, 44, 45, 73
Alignment 427
Alloying 185, 190, 197, 232, 233, 263, 267, 279, 280, 281, 282, 283, 284
Alumina 172, 181, 182, 486, 493, 495, 556, 566, 569, 578, 587, 619, 684, 686, 687, 688, 689
Aluminum 68, 147, 151, 171, 172, 173, 177, 181, 182, 183, 196, 198, 200, 201, 202, 213, 253, 299, 301, 302, 303, 554, 560, 565, 575, 618, 636, 653, 678, 692, 693, 694, 695, 696, 701

Aluminum, cutting of 425, 426, 429, 430, 438, 440, 445, 448, 467, 468,
Aluminum, drilling of 472, 479, 480, 481, 482, 505, 506,
Aluminum, link cutting 595, 596, 597, 599, 600, 601, 603, 605, 608, 609, 612, 613, 614
Aluminum, marking of 524, 527, 536
Aluminum, surface treatment of 263, 264, 271, 272, 283, 288, 290, 291, 294, 296, 297
Aluminum, welding of 309, 315, 316, 318, 321, 324, 326, 327, 328, 335, 338, 339, 342, 345, 351, 352, 353, 354, 355, 365, 367, 368, 370, 371, 372, 373, 374, 375, 376, 377, 378, 379, 382, 383, 384, 385, 386, 387, 389, 392, 398, 401, 403, 404, 405, 409, 410, 411, 413, 414, 420, 421
Aluminum alloys 174, 210, 252, 257, 258, 284, 472, 499
Aluminum gallium arsenide 61, 62, 63, 64, 658
Aluminum gallium arsenide laser 15, 143
Aluminum gallium indium arsenide 61
Aluminum gallium indium nitride 61
Aluminum gallium indium phosphide 61
Aluminum honeycomb 570
Aluminum nitride 485, 486, 495, 684, 686
Aluminum oxide 46, 118, 282, 284, 290, 291, 368, 398, 445, 461, 523, 653, 693
American Conference of Governmental Industrial Hygienists (see ACGIH)
Ammonia 282
Ammonium dideuterium arsenate (AD*A) 72
Ammonium dideuterium phosphate (AD*P) 72
Ammonium dihydrogen arsenate (ADR) 72
Ammonium dihydrogen phosphate (ADP) 71, 72, 74
Amplitude modulation 11
(ANSI) American National Standards Institute 206, 207, 208, 210, 211, 212, 214, 218, 219, 220
Antimony 703
Antimony-bismuth 145
Antimony chloride 702
Anti-reflection (AR) coating 117, 183, 227
Application specific integrated circuit 629

Arc welding 377, 422
ArF laser 3, 16, 17, 48, 290, 492, 493, 494, 524, 528, 623, 624, 625, 626, 628, 631, 656, 693, 701, 702
Argon 425, 625
Argon fluoride laser (see ArF laser)
Argon gas shielding 302
Argon laser 3, 7, 14, 16, 45, 55, 56, 58, 76, 98, 99, 143, 175, 595, 614, 619, 621, 625, 636, 647, 648, 651, 652, 654, 656, 657, 658, 691, 692, 693
Argon laser, and RP 545, 548, 551–552, 576
Arrhenius equation 196, 198
Arsenic 703
Arsine 702
Asbestos 459
Aspect ratio 329, 330, 331, 333
Asphalt 5
Assist gas 409
Atmospheric breakdown 202
Austenite 223, 224, 232, 234, 235, 237, 246, 247, 248, 254, 257, 277, 281
Austenization 232, 244, 276, 277
Autogenous welding 318, 320
Avalanche ionization 7, 264, 501
Axial modes 9, 10
Axial-flow laser 29, 30
Axicon 123, 130, 229

B

Back-spatter 409
$BaFe_{12}O_{19}$ 697, 698, 699, 700
Bainite 224, 378
Balancing 513, 514, 515, 516, 517, 518, 519, 520
Bar codes 522
Barium fluoride 134
Barium oxide 649
Barium sodium niobate 41, 73
Barium titanate 486
BBO 41, 59, 69, 71, 72, 73, 74, 76, 77, 79, 484
Beam bending unit 112, 113
Beam delivery 96–98, 101, 337
Beam delivery system 109, 110, 113, 114, 115, 125, 153
Beam delivery, CO_2 laser 23
Beam delivery, fiber optic 18, 23, 98–102, 127, 233, 238, 288, 293, 330, 342, 383, 392, 404, 465

Beam divergence (see also divergence) 91, 92, 93, 94, 100, 104, 106, 111, 149, 173, 326
Beam guiding system 428
Beam profiler 149, 150
Beam quality (see also M²) 28, 32, 43, 106, 107, 112, 121, 149, 225, 299, 300, 427, 431, 474, 475, 478
Beam sampler 144, 146
Beam sampling methods 146
Beam shaping optics 128
Beam splitter 132, 133
Beer's law 170, 542, 672
Beryllium 182, 271, 355
Beryllium copper 435
Beryllium oxide 56, 684
Beta-barium borate (see also BBO) 41, 74, 79, 484
Biological effects 205
Birefringence 70
BiSrCaCuO 653
Black velvet 5
Blech effect 612
Boiling point 309
Bolometer 144, 145
Boltzmann's constant 201
Bonding 661
Bone 499
Borax 282
Boron 251, 279, 282, 283, 284, 703
Boron anhydride 282
Boron carbide 282, 283, 284
Boron trifluoride 702
Boronizing 281
Borosilicate crown glass 134, 271
Borosilicate glass 493
Bragg grating 100, 655, 656
Branding 589
Brass 172, 173, 310, 356, 446, 472, 479, 481, 482, 536
Brazing 299, 300, 301, 302
Breakdown threshold 7, 202
Bremsstrahlung 202
Brewster absorption 225, 229
Brewster plate 11
Brewster window 56, 60, 119
Brewster's angle 38, 39, 56, 180, 226, 228, 436
Brightness (see also radiance) 91, 94, 106, 107
Bronze 356, 563

C

Cadmium 444, 481
Cadmium dideuterium arsenate (CD*A) 71, 72, 73, 74, 76, 77

Cadmium dihydrogen arsenate (CDA) 71, 72
Cadmium sulfide 118
Cadmium sulfide selenide 61
Cadmium telluride 118, 134, 144
Cadmium zinc selenide 61
Calcium fluoride 134, 135, 137, 624, 628, 633
Calorimeters 148
CAM-LEM processing 567
Capacitive discharge welding 422
Carbamide 282
Carbides 273, 274, 275, 276, 280, 282
Carbon (see also C) 172, 182, 223, 235, 236, 237, 243, 245, 246, 249, 251, 253, 254, 255, 256, 257, 258, 273, 276, 278, 279, 281, 282, 284, 348, 371, 378, 382, 403, 404, 413, 442, 457, 461, 495, 496, 528, 618
Carbon black 523
Carbon dioxide lasers (see also CO_2 lasers)
Carbon fiber 493
Carbon monoxide lasers (see also CO lasers) 52, 431
Carbon steel (see also steel) 192, 472
Carbon steel, surface treatment 223, 224, 232, 233, 234, 236, 237, 239, 245, 252, 253, 254, 255, 256, 257, 258, 279, 281, 282, 284
Carbon steel, welding of 328, 347, 348, 349, 353, 372, 376, 378, 381, 382, 383, 384, 385, 386, 387, 391, 398, 404, 408, 409, 412, 418, 419, 420, 421, 439, 441–443, 464, 467
Carbonizing 283
Cardboard 457
Carpet 459
Cavity dumping 11, 12
Cavity modes 2
(CDRH) Center for Devices and Radiological Health 211, 219–220
Cellulose 493
Cellulose acetate 493
Cementite 257, 277, 278
Ceramics 272, 284, 347, 354, 425, 426, 431, 457, 458, 460, 461, 466, 467, 469, 478, 483, 484, 494, 495, 496, 499, 509, 511, 524, 535, 556, 566–567, 578, 677, 684, 685, 686, 687, 688, 689
Ceramic green parts 574
Ceramic tile 459
Cerium oxide 645
Cermets 280, 556, 574
Cesium 289
Cesium-lithium borate (CLBO) 69, 627

Charpy impact test 413
Charpy V-notch 382, 383
Chemical laser 66
Chemical oxygen iodine laser (see also COIL) 66, 68, 404, 431, 454
Chemical stability of HTSC 648
Chiller 83, 84, 85, 88, 89, 408, 428, 464, 465
Chip resistors 587
Chrome-on-glass 631
Chromium 4, 182, 201, 214, 223, 236, 237, 251, 252, 253, 254, 255, 256, 273, 279, 280, 282, 284, 291, 324, 348, 355, 356, 362, 370, 403, 439, 445, 481, 618, 621, 636, 693
Chromium boride 282, 283
Chromium oxide 290
Chromium steel (see also steel) 235, 253, 257, 258, 282
Cladding 185, 197, 199, 232, 233, 263, 279, 281, 284, 285, 286, 287
Classes of lasers 206
Cleaning 263, 287, 288, 289
Cloth 459
CNC control 19, 20, 24, 155, 300, 428
CO laser (see also carbon monoxide laser) 16, 52, 53, 404, 405, 406, 407, 453, 454, 558
CO_2 laser, balancing 515, 516, 519
CO_2 laser, brazing 299, 300
CO_2 laser, cutting 428, 431, 434, 435, 436, 439, 444, 446, 447, 453, 454, 456, 457, 458, 459, 460, 462, 464, 466, 467, 468, 470
CO_2 laser, displays 637, 638
CO_2 laser, drilling 471, 473, 475, 478, 479, 490, 499
CO_2 laser, hardening 223, 224, 225, 226, 227, 228, 229, 230, 232, 233, 234, 235, 236, 238, 239, 240, 242, 244, 249, 252, 254, 257, 258, 259, 260
CO_2 laser, HTSC 647, 648, 649, 650
CO_2 laser, interactions of 173, 174, 175, 177, 181, 183, 184, 201, 202
CO_2 laser, marking 522, 523, 524, 525, 526, 529, 531, 532, 535, 537, 538, 539, 589, 590, 592
CO_2 laser, microstructures 655
CO_2 laser, packaging 661, 663, 670, 671, 672, 673, 674, 675, 676, 677, 681, 684, 685, 686, 687, 688, 689
CO_2 laser, properties 3, 5, 13, 16, 17, 18, 19, 20, 21, 22, 27, 28, 30, 31, 32, 33, 34, 35, 36, 44, 51, 52, 53, 54,

55, 61, 66, 67, 68, 76, 77, 96, 98, 99, 101, 102, 109, 112, 117, 118, 119, 122, 124, 127, 134, 144, 165, 166
CO_2 laser, RP 542, 557–559, 560, 562, 566, 576, 578–579
CO_2 laser, safety 205, 212, 213, 215
CO_2 laser, surface treating 271, 273, 276, 279, 281, 282, 283, 284, 286, 288, 290, 291, 292, 293, 294, 295, 296
CO_2 laser, trimming 585
CO_2 laser, welding 307, 312, 314, 315, 316, 317, 320, 322, 324, 325, 338, 347, 348, 349, 351, 353, 354, 358, 361, 362, 363, 364, 365, 366, 368, 370, 371, 375, 376, 377, 378, 379, 380, 381, 382, 383, 384, 386, 399, 404, 406, 408, 410, 411, 412, 413, 414, 416, 417, 422
Coating, absorption 224, 225, 227, 237, 240, 259
Coating, antireflective 117, 133, 227
Coating, multilayer 366, 511
Coatings (see also absorption, antireflective, reflective, dielectric) 122, 123, 124, 148, 234, 235
Coatings, dielectric 97
Coatings, by PLD 572
Coatings, reflective 97, 271
Cobalt 282, 283, 284, 286, 342, 353, 481, 509, 618, 695
Coherence 28, 91, 92, 93, 94, 173
Coherence length 70, 91, 93, 94, 106
Coherence time 93
Coherence width 93, 94, 106
COIL (see also chemical oxygen iodine laser) 66, 67, 404, 405, 406, 407, 454, 455
Collimators 110, 111, 316
Complex dielectric constant 168, 170
Complex index of refraction 176, 177
Composite tooling 574
Composites 496, 578
Concrete 172, 292, 459, 468
Conduction of heat 190
Conduction welding 307, 311, 312, 314, 317, 322, 330, 331, 333, 335, 339, 347, 348, 350, 361, 364, 379, 380, 389, 390, 392, 397
Contour cut 432
Controllers 153
Convection 190, 194, 195, 197
Coolers 511
Copper 4, 5, 33, 37, 112, 113, 117, 122, 123, 143, 158, 162, 169, 171,

172, 173, 177, 182, 183, 184, 200, 201, 213, 305, 595, 609, 612, 613, 617, 618, 620, 653
Copper, cutting 429, 431, 440, 446, 447, 448, 450, 467, 470, 479
Copper, deposition 692, 694, 695
Copper, drilling 481, 482, 483
Copper, marking 527, 536
Copper, packaging 661–664, 666–668, 670, 673, 675, 677, 678, 688
Copper, rapid prototyping 556, 563
Copper, surface treatment 227, 236, 237, 244, 253, 263, 264, 271, 272, 283, 290
Copper, welding 309, 310, 313, 315, 327, 328, 335, 338, 339, 342–345, 366, 376, 379, 389, 392, 398, 403, 404, 414, 420, 421
Copper alloy 472, 481
Copper oxide 649
Copper, in packaging 661, 662, 663, 664, 666, 667, 668, 670, 673, 675
Copper , welding of 309, 310, 313, 315, 327, 328, 335, 338, 339, 342, 343, 345, 352, 355
Copper vapor laser (see also CVL) 16, 17, 53, 175, 364, 431, 619
Copper vapor laser, and drilling 475, 479, 481, 483, 484, 494, 495, 496, 499
Copper-zinc alloy 272
Cork 172
Corrosion 404
Corrosion resistance 356, 433
Cost 358, 359, 366, 371, 372, 407, 408, 415, 417, 464, 466, 467, 468, 470, 510, 511, 512, 538
Coupling of laser energy 308, 311, 318, 370, 375, 386
Critical exposure 548
Critical temperature 644, 649
Cr:LiSAF laser 44, 45
Cr,Tm,Ho:YAG laser (CTH:YAG) 44, 46
Cupronickel 349
Cut quality 457, 460, 466, 467
Cutting 158, 159, 160, 161, 185, 190, 195, 204, 210, 233, 242, 417, 425, 427, 428, 432, 433, 436, 438
  head 428
  process 425, 429
  quality 442
  speed 425, 427, 428, 429, 430, 444, 445, 447, 448, 453, 460, 466, 467, 468, 470
  system 428
  abrasive water jet 466, 468
  water jet 465

fusion 425, 427, 429–430, 440
melt shear 440, 457
Cutting nozzle (see also nozzle) 158, 571
CVL (see also copper vapor laser) 53, 54, 55, 479, 480, 481, 482, 484, 494, 495, 496
Cyaniding 281, 282
Czochralski method 37

D

Damage, lens 633
Damage threshold 7, 8, 70, 71, 73, 118, 119, 150, 500, 501, 502, 503, 504, 505
Damage thresholds for thin film optical coatings 8
Damkohler number 198
Damping constant 167, 168, 169
Debye temperature 170, 172
Deep penetration welding 66, 96, 327, 329
Depth of focus 104, 105, 173, 174
Depth of penetration 186
Detectivity 140, 141, 142, 143, 144
DF laser 3, 14
Diamond 82, 118, 172, 318, 461, 483, 484, 486, 495, 496, 499, 651, 652, 653, 688
Diamond-like carbon 695, 696
Diborane 702
Diborides 282
Dicing 684, 687
Dielectric mirror 227
Die cast parts 554
Die casting inserts 575
Die casting tools 573
Difference-frequency generation 16
Difference frequency mixing 70
Diffraction-limited spot size 121, 174
Diffractive optical element 485, 492
Diffractive optics 125
Dimethyl-Au-acetylacetonate 619
Diode lasers (see also laser diode and semiconductor laser) 34, 38, 39, 42, 45, 46, 60, 61, 62, 63, 64, 65, 66, 76, 77, 98, 99, 100, 101, 118, 175, 300, 303, 304, 305, 348, 350, 675, 702
Diode lasers (and hardening) 225, 226, 227, 229, 241, 242, 243, 249
Diode-pumped laser 586
Diode-pumped Nd:YAG laser 225, 638
Diode pumped solid-state laser 39, 64, 551
Direct AIM 553
Directed light fabrication (DLF) 541, 559, 560

Direct-write process 614, 694
Directionality 91
Dispersion 167
Displays 635
    liquid crystal 635
    repair 636
Disulfides 282
Divergence (see also beam divergence) 92, 95
Divergence angle 151
Doping 701, 702, 703
Dot matrix 524, 529, 530, 535, 536
Doubled Nd:YAG laser 44, 45, 47
Drilling 185, 204, 232, 307, 432, 471, 473, 474, 476, 479, 480, 481, 484, 485, 491, 494, 495, 496, 684, 686, 687, 688, 689
Drilling nonmetals by excimer laser 492, 493, 494
Drilling, shaped hole 490
Drilling speed 494, 495
Drude theory 177, 181
Dye laser 2, 15, 72, 76, 173, 364, 656, 675

E

Edge emitter 64
Edge emitters 65
Edge-emitting laser 100
EDM (see also electron discharge machining) 465, 512
Efficiency 431
Electrical discharge milling 449
Electrical resistance welding 421, 422
Electro-optic shutter 12
Electro-optical Q-switch 39, 40
Electron beam 509, 510, 512
Electron beam welding (EBW) 357, 359, 362, 367, 368, 374, 413, 421, 422, 423
Electron discharge machining (see also EDM) 483, 499, 509, 511
Emissivity 176, 178, 179, 181
Enamel 484
Energy balance 473
Energy meters 146, 148
Energy transport 184
Engraving 530, 531, 532, 533, 537
Epoxy 543, 546, 548, 549, 661, 664
Epoxy material 485
Epoxy resin 459
Er laser 46
Er:YAG laser 14, 44, 46, 291
Er^{3+} fiber laser 14
Excimer laser 5, 15, 16, 18, 20, 47, 48, 49, 50, 51, 52, 54, 77, 98, 99, 174, 175, 181, 288, 291, 431, 473, 491, 492, 495, 499, 558, 572
Excimer laser, deposition and doping 692, 693, 695, 697, 701
Excimer laser, displays 636, 637, 638, 639
Excimer laser, HTSC 650
Excimer laser, link cutting 595
Excimer laser, marking 522, 523, 524, 528, 529, 534, 535, 536, 538, 591, 593
Excimer laser, microstructures 651, 652, 655
Excimer laser, packaging 661, 662, 673, 674, 675, 676, 688, 689
Excimer laser, photolithography 623, 625, 626, 628, 629, 633
Excimer laser, repair 617, 618, 620
Excimer laser etched materials 653
Exothermal reaction 425, 429, 430
Explosives 502, 503
Extinction coefficient 168
Eye protection (see also protective and safety eyewear) 207–208, 211–212, 217

F

F_2 excimer laser 17, 492, 528, 623, 624, 631, 651
Fabrics 469, 495
Fabry-Perot 91, 100
Fabry-Perot etalon 10
Faraday effect 133
Faraday rotator 133
Fast Fourier transform 160
FEL (see free-electron laser)
Felt 459
Ferrite 223, 232, 234, 235, 237, 247, 257, 276, 290, 378, 461
Ferrite-cementite 232, 234
Ferroboron 280, 282
Ferrochrome 280
Ferrosilicium 280
Ferrous alloys 309, 311, 318, 321
Fiberglass 296, 458
Fiber laser 9, 46
Fiber-optic cable 387, 388, 389
Fiber optic laser system 26
Fick's second law 173
Filler 318, 345, 346, 352, 354, 355, 357, 368, 373, 374, 375, 382, 400, 401, 403, 406, 409, 412, 413, 417, 418, 420
Film deposition 691
Flame cutting 369
Flat panel displays 635

Flow visualization 549
Fluorine 625
Fluoropolymer 523
Flushing 473
Flux cored arc welding (FCAW) 419, 422
Focusing 104, 116, 409
Focusing head 125, 126, 127
Fokker-Planck equation 504
Fourier number 395, 396
Fourier Transform Infrared Spectroscopy 503
Free-electron laser (FEL) 16, 78
Frequency-doubled laser 587
Frequency doubling 40, 69, 70, 76, 484
Frequency modulation 11
Fresnel lens 125
Fresnel losses 72
Fresnel number 30, 32, 498
Fresnel reflection 63
Fresnel's equations 176–180, 348, 434
Friction stir welding 420, 421, 422
Froude number 368
Full-penetration welding 329
Fused deposition modeling 541
    comparison with other methods 578
Fused silica 39, 98, 99, 135, 146, 227, 493, 494, 499, 500, 501, 502, 511, 624, 633, 655
Fusion welding 327

G

GaAlAs laser 16, 17
Gadolium gallium garnet 643
Gain switching 12
Gain-switched laser 12
Galilian telescope 111
Gallium 200, 201
Gallium aluminum arsenide 100
Gallium arsenide 28, 62, 63, 116, 118, 135, 136, 138, 172, 227, 271, 316, 486, 494, 499, 524, 591, 646, 653, 658, 696
Gallium arsenide antimonide 61, 100
Gallium arsenide phosphide 61
Gallium indium arsenide 658
Gas immersion laser doping (GILD) 700, 701, 702, 703
Gas laser 13, 16, 17
Gas shield 410
Gas shielding 302, 398, 406, 413, 680
Gas tungsten arc welding (GTAW) 357, 359, 420, 422
Gas-metal-arc welding (GMAW) 357, 371, 419, 420
Gaussian beam 28, 30, 31, 32, 61, 63, 71, 92, 93, 94, 95, 99, 105–107, 120,

121, 128, 193, 228, 234, 236, 263, 300, 388, 389, 395, 501, 507, 526, 527, 598, 607, 641
Gaussian source 191, 192
Germanium 32, 35, 62, 116, 117, 118, 119, 135, 136, 142, 143, 145, 150, 182, 201, 271, 299, 693, 695, 696
Gibbs potential 648
Glass 28, 34, 97, 99, 101, 173, 179, 180, 290, 347, 366, 458, 461, 466, 468, 490, 494, 499, 524, 533, 535, 655, 684, 702
Glass, borosilicate 524
Glass cloth 458, 459
Glass epoxy 671
Glass fabric 486
Glass fibers 66, 493
Glass, soda-lime 524
Glass-to-metal seal 677, 678, 681, 682, 683
Glass wool 172
Glassy carbon 496
Glazing 185, 190, 263, 272, 273
Gleeble 244, 245, 247
Gold 33, 37, 143, 169, 172, 182, 183, 291, 304, 309, 318, 345, 355, 362, 366, 389, 392, 447, 464, 470, 472, 481, 504, 505, 524, 595, 600, 618, 619, 620, 636, 655, 665, 666, 667, 670, 673, 675, 677, 678, 692, 693, 694, 695
Gold vapor laser 16, 17, 53
Graphite 171, 223, 235, 237, 249, 258, 276, 277, 278, 439, 495, 496
Green parts 542, 566, 574
Green sheet feedstock 569
Green sintered densities 566
Green stainless steel 568
Green strength 541, 547, 556
Green tape 567, 568

H

Hagen-Rubens relation 171, 177, 178
Hardening 185, 190, 224, 225, 229, 232, 236, 239, 240, 242, 243, 244, 245, 248, 249, 251, 252, 254, 256, 259, 260, 261
Harmonic generation 40
Hastalloy 286, 290, 345, 346, 347, 355, 446, 477, 679
Haynes alloy 290, 346, 384, 414, 563
Hazards, health 205, 209, 211
   to skin 207
   to eyes 206
   from beam delivery 213
   from plasma radiation 216

   from nonbeam sources 214
   from plastics 210
   from welding 210
   laser classes 206
Heat balance 189, 190
Heat capacity 170, 171, 172, 173, 309, 310, 331, 362, 364, 403, 429, 472
Heat conduction 172, 429, 432
Heat conduction losses 429, 430
Heat of fusion 362, 364
Heat treating 223, 224, 260
Heat treatment 232, 233, 238, 239, 242, 243, 307
He-Cd laser 14, 16
He-Cd laser, RP 542, 550, 551, 552, 576
He-Ne laser 7, 13, 33, 34, 114, 115, 122, 288, 628, 702
Hermeticity 322, 341
Hermite mode 228
Heterojunction 62, 63
Heterostructure 62
Heterostructure diode laser 63
HF laser 3, 14, 481
HF-DF laser 118
High-absorptivity coating 223
High-frequency resistance welding 422
High-temperature superconductors (HTSC) 641
   monitoring of 649
   optical properties 649
   polishing of 650
Ho laser 46
Ho:YAG laser 14, 44, 76
Holographic beam sampler 148, 149
Holographic sampler 145, 146
Homojunction 62, 63
Hydrogen discharge laser 15

I

(IEC) International Electrotechnical Commission 206, 210, 211, 218–220
Image micromachining 534
Inconel 290, 346, 349, 355, 373, 384, 395, 398, 414, 446, 450, 472, 477, 556, 560, 563, 578, 679
Index of refraction (see also refractive index) 167, 168, 169, 170, 434
Indium 200, 299
Indium aluminum arsenide 653
Indium antimonide 142, 143, 145
Indium arsenide 142, 143, 145
Indium arsenide phosphide 61
Indium gallium arsenide 61, 64, 143, 150, 653
Indium gallium arsenide phosphide 15, 61, 64, 100

Indium phosphide 62, 172, 652, 653, 658
Indium tin oxide (ITO) 635, 637
Inert gas 425, 426
Inert gas cutting 425
Inert gas shielding 309
Infrared materials 134
InGaAs 61, 64
InGaAs diode laser 15
InGaAsP 15, 61, 64, 100
Injection-mold 553
Inox 342, 450
Integrated circuit 592
Integrator 128, 129, 231
Invar 173, 678
Inverse Bremsstrahlung 370, 375, 501, 504
Iodine laser 14, 66
Ion laser 14, 55, 56, 57, 58, 59, 60
Ion milling 510, 511
Ionization potential 370, 380
Irradiance (see also power density) 94, 95, 107, 108
Iron 171, 172, 173, 182, 183, 200, 201, 225, 233, 235, 258, 263, 264, 281, 282, 283, 284, 310, 324, 342, 355, 356, 370, 376, 379, 403, 436, 443, 472, 481, 562, 625, 695
Iron alloy 272, 472, 481
Iron carbide 223
Iron, cast 223, 232, 233, 235, 236, 237, 239, 252, 253, 254, 255, 256, 257, 258, 259, 260, 272, 273, 276, 277, 278, 414, 420, 482
Iron, gray 372
Iron nitride 249
Iron-graphite 258
Iron sulfide 378
Irtran 118, 136
(ISO) International Standards Organization 219, 220
Isolation reflector 124
Isolator 133, 134

J

Jade 462
Jewelry 462
Joint design 318, 319, 320, 333, 345, 357, 368
Joint preparation 357
Jominy test 244, 245, 248
Josephson junction 649
Joulemeter 146, 147

K

Kaleidoscope 228
Kaolin 523

Kapton 394, 409, 673
KDP (see also potassium dihydrogen phosphate) 41, 70, 71, 72, 73
Keplerian telescope 111
Kerf cross section 468
Kerf volume 429
Kerf width 429, 431, 453, 467, 470, 568, 571
Kerr effect 13
Kevlar 456
Keyhole 159, 160, 161, 165, 237, 310, 311, 312, 313, 314, 315, 317, 321, 325, 329, 335, 348, 361, 362, 363, 366, 368, 369, 370, 371, 372, 374, 375, 376, 377, 378, 379, 380, 382, 386, 390, 392, 393, 397, 402, 405, 410, 413, 420, 434
Keyhole welding 174, 185, 196, 197, 201, 203
Kinoform 125
Kirchoff's law 176
Kovar 355, 387, 524, 678
Kr lamp 38, 41
Kr laser 15, 16, 48, 50, 51, 55–58, 59
KrF laser 3, 16, 17, 290, 291, 492, 493, 494, 499, 524, 528, 623, 624, 625, 626, 631, 642, 647, 648, 649, 656, 673, 674, 695, 696, 697, 701
Krypton 625

L

Laminated object manufacturing (LOM) 541, 564, 565
Langmuir 196
Lanthanum aluminate 642, 643, 644, 646, 698, 699
Lanthanum scandium borate 484
Laser absorption wave 203
Laser annealing 638, 639, 640, 649
Laser chemical vapor deposition (see also LCVD) 185, 197, 198, 618, 619, 691
Laser damage 7–9, 116–117
Laser deposition, liquid phase 620
Laser diode (see also diode laser) 38, 39, 42, 45, 46, 64–66, 100, 484
Laser engineered net shaping (LENS) 541, 561, 573
    comparison with other methods 578
Laser microstructuring 655
Laser safety officer (LSO) 207, 211, 214, 215, 216, 219

Lasers(s)
    see specific types, i.e.,CO_2, Nd:YAG, etc.
Laser-supported absorption wave 203, 204, 479
Laser-supported combustion (LSC) 203
Laser-supported detonation (LSD) 203, 204
Laser-supported radiation (LSR) 203, 204
Laser-sustained plasma 202
Laser sonic bonding 620
$LaSrGaO_4$ 643, 644
Latent heat 186, 189, 193, 200, 201, 309, 472
Latent heat of fusion 429
Latex 478
Laval nozzle 155, 156, 158, 431, 432
Lavsan 459
Layered object manufacturing 578
LBO 69, 70, 71, 72, 73, 76, 77, 627, 628
LCVD (see also laser chemical vapor deposition) 618, 619, 691, 692, 693, 694
Lead 171, 172, 173, 201, 304, 342, 352, 353, 354, 355, 356, 447, 481, 618, 669
Lead brick 290
Lead glass 494
Lead oxide 696
Lead selenide 145
Lead sulfide 145
Lead-salt laser 15
Lead zirconate titanate (PZT) 493, 695, 696
Leather 426, 458, 459, 460, 532
Ledeburite 281
Lenses 116, 117, 120, 121, 122, 134
LiB_3O_5 75
LIGA processing 655
Limestone 5
Linear expansion coefficient 170, 173
Link cutting 595, 597, 598, 599, 600, 602, 605, 606, 607, 608, 614
    processing speed 602
    repairs 604
Link making 608, 609, 610, 611, 612, 613, 614
Liquid crystal displays 635
Lithium 401
Lithium borate (see also LBO) 69–73, 76, 77, 627, 628
Lithium fluoride 136, 137
Lithium iodate 41, 72, 74, 76, 77
Lithium niobate 41, 73, 74, 76, 627, 643, 696
Lithium silicate 656

Lithium tantalate 144, 145, 493
Lithium triborate (see Lithium borate)
Longitudinal coherence 93
Longitudinal modes 2, 10, 59, 91
Lorentzian 93
Lucite 533

M

M^2 (see also beam quality) 24, 25, 28, 30, 32, 42, 44, 54, 58, 95, 102, 106, 107, 121, 146, 151, 388, 431, 474, 478, 497, 498, 550, 551, 685
Magnesium 200, 201, 253, 299, 355, 401, 403, 404, 405, 430, 481, 554, 575
Magnesium aluminate 643
Magnesium carbonate 439
Magnesium fluoride 137, 146, 624
Magnesium oxide 5, 182, 486, 643, 644, 646, 698, 699
Manganese 200, 201, 236, 237, 251, 252, 253, 254, 255, 258, 272, 273, 276, 277, 278, 348, 353, 401, 403, 404, 481
Manganese phosphate 234, 235, 237, 259
Marangoni flows 670
Marangoni number 267, 268
Marble 462, 468
Marking 521, 522, 523, 524, 525, 527, 535, 538, 589, 590, 592, 636
Martensite 223, 224, 232, 234, 235, 252, 257, 273, 277, 281, 282, 378
Martensitic steel 275
Martensitic transformation 232, 277
Mask
    image 662, 674, 675
    imaging 534, 535, 592
    projection 589
Mass diffusion 197
Master oscillator-power amplifier (MOPA) 39
Maximum permissible exposure 206
Maxwell's equations 69
Melt ejection 425, 432
Melt-quenching 232
Melting efficiency 329
Melting point 309
Melting temperature 201, 429
Memory 629
Memory arrays 617
Memory repair 595
Memory yield enhancement 604, 606
Mercury cadmium telluride (HgCdTe) 142, 143, 145, 696
Mercury cadmium zinc telluride 145
Mercury lamp 623, 624, 632

Mercury xenon lamp 628
Metal, marking of 532, 533
Metal mold insert 563
Metal optics 409
Metal-vapor laser 14, 53
Mica 523
Microcutting 450
Microelectronics 617
Micro-joining 332, 344
Microlithography 623, 624, 625, 626, 628
Micromachining 431
Micropositioning equipment 151, 152
Microprocessing 431
Microprocessors 629
Microstructure 561
Microstructuring 651
Mirror 122, 123, 426
Mixed-gas ion laser 55
Mode locking 11, 12, 13
Mode-locked dye laser 15
Mode-locked laser 12
Molybdenum 182, 201, 223, 237, 251, 253, 255, 260, 271, 273, 280, 282, 284, 328, 355, 365, 366, 394, 447, 450, 481, 621, 653
Molybdenum disulfide 223
Molybdenum sulfide 282, 284
Monel 349, 446, 472
Monochromaticity 91, 173
Moore's law 631
Mother-of-pearl 463
Motion system 151
Multijet modeling 580
Multilayer dielectrics 32
Multimaterial feed stream 567
Multimetal materials 574
Multiphoton absorption 7, 183, 264
Multiphoton ionization 500, 501, 502, 503

N

N_2 laser 307
Navier-Stokes equation 194
Nd:glass laser 14, 17, 44, 45, 81, 174, 175, 183, 281, 282, 314, 315, 317, 473, 515
Nd:YAG 38, 46
Nd:YAG laser (see also YAG laser) 14, 16, 17, 18, 20, 22, 23, 25, 37, 38, 40, 41, 42, 43, 44, 45, 46, 47, 54, 55, 61, 63, 66, 67, 68, 69, 73, 76, 77, 98, 99, 101, 102, 109, 118, 119, 126, 127, 143, 149, 165, 166, 173, 174, 175, 177, 181, 198
Nd:YAG laser, balancing 515, 519
Nd:YAG laser, brazing 299, 300, 301, 302, 303, 304
Nd:YAG laser, cutting 431, 435, 436, 439, 447, 448, 449, 454, 456, 457, 460, 461, 465, 466, 467, 470
Nd:YAG laser, deposition and doping 695, 696
Nd:YAG laser, displays 636, 637, 638
Nd:YAG laser, drilling 471, 472, 473, 474, 475, 476, 477, 479, 484, 486, 488, 496, 498, 499, 509
Nd:YAG laser, hardening 224, 225, 226, 227, 228, 229, 230, 233, 238, 239, 242, 244, 249
Nd:YAG laser, HTSC 647, 648, 649
Nd:YAG laser, link cutting 595, 597, 604, 605, 614
Nd:YAG laser, marking 522, 523, 524, 525, 527, 529, 531, 532, 534, 535, 536, 589, 590, 591, 592
Nd:YAG laser, microstructures 651, 652, 656, 657
Nd:YAG laser, packaging 661, 665, 670, 671, 672, 673, 674, 677, 679, 680, 681, 682, 683, 684, 685, 687, 688
Nd:YAG laser, photolithography 624, 626, 627
Nd:YAG laser, repair 617, 618, 619, 620, 621
Nd:YAG laser/robot 23
Nd:YAG laser, RP 542, 557–559, 561, 563–564, 572, 579
Nd:YAG laser, safety 205, 211, 213
Nd:YAG laser, surface treating 271, 273, 276, 281, 282, 284, 286, 288, 289, 290, 292, 293, 294, 296
Nd:YAG laser, trimming 585, 586, 587
Nd:YAG laser, welding 307, 309, 311, 314, 315, 316, 317, 322, 324, 325, 326, 327, 329, 330, 332, 333, 334, 338, 339, 340, 341, 342, 344, 345, 348, 351, 353, 354, 358, 362, 364, 365, 370, 375, 376, 377, 383, 386, 387, 388, 389, 390, 392, 394, 396, 399, 404, 405, 406, 408, 409, 410, 411, 412, 413, 416, 417, 418, 422
Nd:YAG laser writer 592
Nd:YAG robot 23
Nd:YLF laser 16, 17, 44, 76, 297, 486, 586, 587, 597, 598, 605, 606, 610, 613
Nd:YVO$_4$ laser 44, 76, 597, 598, 605, 606

Nd:YVO$_4$ laser, RP 551, 576
NdGaO$_3$ 646
Neodymium 37, 44, 365
Neural network 161
Nichrome 587
Nickel 4, 169, 171, 172, 182, 198, 201, 214, 223, 236, 237, 251, 253, 258, 263, 264, 272, 279, 282, 283, 284, 286, 304, 305, 309, 313, 318, 330, 342, 345, 347, 348, 349, 353, 355, 356, 446, 471, 473, 481, 497, 498, 509, 524, 536, 562–563, 572, 578, 590, 595, 618, 636, 655, 678, 679, 692, 694, 696
Nickel alloys 172, 198, 272, 273, 282, 284, 291, 446, 472, 477
Nickel-chromium 583
Nickel-iron 353
Nickel phosphide 297
Nickel, welding of 362, 366, 383, 384, 387, 388, 403, 414, 418
Nimonic 446
Niobium 282, 481
Nitralloy 282
Nitrides 280, 282
Nitriding 281, 282
Nitrocellulose 492
Nitrogen discharge laser 15
Nitronic 384
(Ni,Zn)Fe$_2$O$_4$ 697
Noise equivalent power 140
Nomarski interference contrast 682
Nominal hazard zone 207, 211, 212, 214
Nonbeam hazards 214
Nonlinear optical effects 40, 69
Nonlinear optics 69, 627
Nonlinear susceptibility 71, 74, 75
Nonmetal cutting 431
Nozzle (see also laval nozzle) 153, 155, 156, 157, 158, 159, 285, 286, 322, 323, 337, 400, 402, 406, 410, 420, 425, 427, 428, 431, 432, 438, 441, 442, 444, 454, 462, 464, 474, 475, 571, 686, 687, 688
Nylon 459, 522, 549, 576

O

Ocular injury 205
Optical parametric oscillator (OPO) 16, 70, 72, 76, 77, 627
(OSHA) Occupational Safety and Health Administration 214, 216, 218, 219, 220
Oxidation 427, 431, 433

Oxidation cutting 425, 426, 427, 429, 430, 431, 439, 440
Oxyacetylene welding 357
Oxyfuel cutting 465–466
Oxygen 425, 426, 427, 430, 431
Oxygen cutting 425
Oxygen-flame cutting 465–466
Oxygen-iodine laser 3

P

P-hydroxystyrene 633, 634
Packaging 661, 677, 679, 681
    alloys 678
        cutting 684, 687
        cutting speeds 685
        hot crack sensitivity 678
        scribing speeds 685
Paint 234, 237, 260, 261, 441, 444
Paint removal 293
Palladium 272, 355, 618, 620
Palladium acetate 620
Paper 426, 457, 484, 490, 495, 525, 532, 535
Peak power 326, 330
Pearlite 224, 237, 248, 276
Peclet number 186, 192, 193, 429
Penetration depth 168, 169, 326, 327, 328, 329, 333
Penetration welding 307, 311, 312, 313, 314, 322, 329, 330, 331, 338, 339, 340, 361, 362, 363, 364, 379, 380, 399, 407, 423
Percussion drilling 473, 474, 475, 476, 480, 481, 485, 490, 495, 497, 498
Personalization 595, 614
Perspex 409, 457
Phase changes 200
Phase-matching 70, 72, 73, 74
Phenolic 523
Phosphate glass 44
Phosphine 702
Phosphor bronze 349, 472
Phosphorous 236, 237, 253, 318, 353, 403, 703
Photoablation 491
Photoconductive detector 142, 143
Photoconductive effect 139, 145
Photoconductivity 142
Photodetector 139, 148, 149
Photodiode 142, 143, 149, 159
Photoelastic stress analysis 549
Photoemissive cathode 141, 142
Photoemissive detector 142
Photoemissive effect 140, 141

Photolithography 623, 629
Photolytic iodine laser (see also PIL) 66, 67, 351, 455
Photolytic process 692, 693, 694
Photomask imaging 491
Photomask repair 621, 636
Photomultiplier tube 141, 142
Photon detector 139, 141, 142, 143, 144
Photoresist processing 620
Photovoltaic detector 141, 142, 143
Photovoltaic effect 140, 141, 142, 145
Piercing 427, 432, 441, 447, 462, 463
PIL (see also photolytic iodine laser) 66, 67, 68, 455, 456
Plasma 205, 210, 368, 375, 376, 405
Plasma arc welding (PAW) 357, 420
Plasma arc cutting 465–467
Plasma cutting 369
Plasma formation 362, 370
Plasma shielding 202, 203, 472, 481
Plasma suppression 28, 337, 371, 372
Plastics 210, 354, 409, 413, 414, 426, 460, 469, 499, 511, 531, 532
Platinum 177, 180, 182, 310, 355, 600, 618, 620, 692, 694, 695
Plexiglass 457
Plywood 457
Pockel's cell 12, 40
Polarization 3, 11, 95, 96, 97, 98, 110, 123, 124, 128, 133, 168, 177, 180, 238, 348, 427, 433, 434, 435, 436, 437, 471, 686
Polarizer 133
Polarizing angle 180
Polyacetylene 492
Polyamide 457, 492, 522
Polybutylene terephthalate 522
Polycarbonate 492, 522, 549
Polyester 532
Polyethylene 522, 523
Polyetheretherketone 492
Polyetherimide 492
Polyethersulfone 492
Polyethylene 37, 172, 457, 458, 474, 490, 492
Polyethylene terephthalate 492, 522, 523
Polyimide 484, 485, 486, 595, 596, 617, 619, 651, 652, 661, 664, 671, 675, 692
Polymer 466, 468, 473, 495, 496, 549, 556, 576, 578
Polymer repair 619
Polymethyl methacrylate 492
Polymide 688
Polyolefin 522

Polyparaxylylene 492
Polypropylene 414, 457, 458, 484, 486, 522, 523, 549
Polysilicides 600
Polysilicon 595, 596, 599, 600, 605, 608, 609, 635, 638
Polystyrene 492
Polytetrafluoroethylene 492
Polyurethane 492, 553, 673, 675
Polyvinyl chloride 459, 492, 522
Polyvinylidene fluoride 492
Post-cured materials 549
Post treatment 427, 433
Potassium chloride 28, 137, 317
Potassium dideuterium arsenate (CD*M) 77
Potassium dideuterium phosphate (KD*P) 70
Potassium dihydrogen arsenate (KD*A) 72
Potassium dihydrogen phosphate (see also KDP) 40, 70
Potassium ferrocyanide 282, 284
Potassium niobate 70, 73, 75–77
Potassium silicate 237
Potassium titanyl phosphate (KTP) 41, 47, 69, 70–73, 75, 77, 628
Powder metallurgy 567
Power density (see also irradiance) 94
Power meters 148, 149
Prandtl number 267
Pressure die casting 564, 573
Printed circuit board 484
Problem of Stefan 200, 201
Process temperature 429
Protective eyewear (see also eye protection) 207, 208, 211–212, 217
Proustite 76
Pulse-compression 13
Pulsed laser deposition (PLD) 572, 573, 641, 644, 646, 691, 693, 694
    as PLD 643, 644, 691, 695, 696, 697, 699, 700
Pulsed mode 307
Pyrex 28, 653, 692
Pyroelectric detector 144, 145
Pyroelectric effect 144, 145, 150
Pyroelectric material 147
Pyrolytic deposition 618, 621
Pyrolytic process 691, 693, 694
PZT 695

Q

Q-switched laser 39
Q-switched operation 2
Q-switching 3, 11, 12, 527
Quantum-well 63

Handbook of Laser Materials Processing

Quartz 5, 28, 137, 138, 173, 271, 290, 366, 405, 458, 461, 639, 662
Quartz glass 485, 494
QuickCast 546

R

Radiance (see also brightness) 91, 94, 173
Rapid prototyping (RP) 541
    and, Ar lasers 542, 551
    brown part 574
    CAM-LEM processing 567
    comparison of systems 557–581
    CO_2 lasers 542
    cost 552
    green parts (see also under green) 542, 566, 574
    He-Cd lasers 542, 551
    injection molding 550, 553, 563
    investment casting 541, 546, 553, 564–565
    manufacturing 541
    laser cutting based 566
    lasers for 542
    metal parts 564
    Nd:YAG lasers 542
    part building 546
    part density 566
    photopolymerization 542
    powder feeds 560
    processes for ceramics 566
    solid-state lasers 551
    system parameters 544
    tooling 545, 553
    working distance 544
Rayleigh range 2, 106, 544
Rayleigh scaling equations 630
Redundancy 604, 605
Reflective optics 431, 432
Reflectivity 5, 167, 168, 169, 170, 171, 174, 175, 176, 177, 178, 179, 180, 181, 183, 184, 201, 227, 308, 309, 316, 331, 345, 348, 353, 355, 362, 363, 365, 376, 379, 386, 434, 435, 440, 441, 445, 446, 447, 471, 472, 473, 475, 600, 670, 672, 673
Reflectivity, metals 4, 176
Reflectivity of nonconductors 178
Reflectivity of some nonmetals 5
Refraction 167, 168
Refractive index (see also index of refraction) 70, 71, 74, 75, 176, 178, 179
Relaxation oscillation 11
Remelting 263, 273, 275, 276
Rene 446
Repair 617
Repetition rates 431
Resistance welding 365, 422
Resistor 583, 585, 586, 588
Resistor paste 584
Response time 140
Responsivity 140, 141, 143, 145
Reststrahlen 178, 179
Retina 205
Reynolds number 267
Rhodium 182
Robot 22, 102, 103, 303, 448, 449
Rosenthal solution 192
Rubidium dideuterium arsenate (RD*A) 72
Rubidium dideuterium phosphate (RD*P) 72
Rubidium dihydrogen arsenate (RDA) 71–73
Rubidium dihydrogen phosphate (RPP) 71, 72
Rubber 173, 426, 458, 459, 460, 469, 511, 532
Rubber plaster casting 544
Ruby 461, 494
Ruby laser 14, 16, 17, 47, 69, 73, 174, 175, 291, 292, 473, 618

S

Safety eyewear (see also eye protection) 207, 208, 211–212
Safety standards 205, 206, 207, 218, 220
Sand casting 563, 564, 565
Sapphire 82, 102, 118, 461, 463, 494, 499, 643, 646
Scanner 130, 131, 132
Scribing 467, 521, 531, 637, 684, 685, 686, 687
Seam tracking 162, 163, 164, 165
Seam welding 331, 332
Second-harmonic generation (SHG) 69, 70, 71
    as SHG 69, 70, 71, 72, 73, 74, 75, 76
Seebeck effect 147
Selective laser sintering (SLS) 541, 542, 554, 555, 557, 573
    comparison with other methods 576
    lasers for 557
    machine layout 555
    materials used 556
Semiconductor laser (see also diode laser and laser diode) 3, 9, 15, 16, 17, 702
Shear cutting 440
Shield gas delivery 341
Shield gas nozzle 337
Shielded-metal-arc welding 357
Shielding 337, 354, 371, 375, 378, 381, 406, 425
Shielding gas 210, 273, 285, 329, 338, 350, 354, 362, 371, 380, 384, 387, 402, 406, 408, 410, 412, 413, 416, 419, 420, 680
Shielding of the molten pool 322
Shielding plasma 427
Shock hardening 204, 232
Shock processing 204
Silica 101, 102, 181, 182, 284, 291, 330, 387
Silicon 32, 33, 62, 97, 118, 122, 123, 138, 143, 145, 149, 150, 151, 169, 172, 178, 182, 200, 201, 236, 237, 253, 258, 272, 276, 278, 279, 283, 284, 287, 290, 291, 348, 353, 355, 403, 404, 405, 444, 447, 488, 490, 494, 499, 524, 528, 586, 587, 588, 590, 591, 592, 595, 596, 599, 606, 609, 612, 613, 614, 623, 638, 639, 640, 643, 646, 653, 654, 657, 658, 665, 684, 685, 687, 692, 693, 695, 701–703
Silicon aluminate oxynitride 493
Silicon carbide 82, 172, 181, 182, 271, 461, 493, 572
    as SiC 486, 488, 495, 499, 696
Silicon dioxide 596
Silicon/gold 145
Silicon nitride 182, 462, 486, 493, 495, 499, 569, 578, 596, 609, 610, 687, 693
Silicon nitride tape 569
Silicon oxide 172, 181, 488, 608, 609, 613, 653, 655, 692, 693, 701
Silicon photodiode 143
Silicon resistor trimming 587
Silicone 532
Silicone rubber 492
Silicone rubber molding 566
Siliconizing 283
Silver 4, 5, 33, 102, 169, 171, 172, 177, 182, 183, 184, 271, 301, 304, 309, 342, 345, 355, 362, 447, 464, 470, 472, 481, 620, 636, 652
Silver arsenide sulfide 76
Silver bromide 118
Silver chloride 118
Silver-copper 269
Silver gallium selenide 75, 76, 77
Silver gallium sulfide 75, 76
Silver-lead solder 305
Sintering 66, 563

Skin injury 206
Slab lasers 31
Slate 5
Slate tile 488
Slitting 426
Snell theorem 434
Snow 172
Soda-lime glass 172, 494
Sodium chloride 28, 138, 173, 317
Sodium silicate 237
Soldering 66, 299, 300, 303, 304, 661, 667, 668, 669, 670, 671, 672
Solid-state laser 3, 14, 16, 17, 24, 25, 37, 39, 40, 42, 44, 45, 47, 52, 63, 64, 65, 69, 82, 156, 315, 326, 473, 474, 484, 485, 617, 627
Sonic speed 431
Sonic nozzle 155, 156
Sormite 280
Spatial coherence 93, 94
Specific heat 472
Spin-on deposition 620
Spot diameter 92, 94
Spot welding 329, 330
Spray metal tooling 566
SQUID 644
Stainless steel (see also steel) 37, 82, 151, 158, 162, 184, 196, 210, 237, 678, 680, 682, 683
Stainless steel, cutting of 425, 428, 430, 439, 441, 444, 446, 448, 449, 450, 454, 455, 465, 467, 468
Stainless steel, drilling of 472, 475, 476, 477, 478, 479, 483, 503, 504, 507, 508
Stainless steel, marking of 534, 536
Stainless steel, surface treating 281, 282, 284, 290, 559, 560, 562, 563, 564, 566, 569, 572, 578
Stainless steel, welding of 310, 321, 323, 324, 327, 330, 335, 338, 339, 341, 346, 347, 348, 349, 350, 351, 352, 353, 355, 356, 364, 365, 376, 377, 380, 381, 382, 383, 384, 386, 387, 388, 389, 390, 409, 410, 411, 414, 419, 420, 423
Steel (see also stainless, carbon, tool steel) 4, 5, 66, 126, 157, 162, 165, 166, 183, 184, 194, 195, 210, 223, 224, 226, 232, 233, 234, 235, 236, 237, 238, 239, 240, 242, 244, 245, 246, 247, 248, 249, 251, 252, 253, 254, 257, 258, 273, 274, 275, 276, 281, 282, 284, 287, 293, 294, 296, 299, 300, 301, 302, 303, 324, 327, 328, 330, 331, 332, 335, 342, 345, 351, 352, 353, 356, 425, 426, 427, 429, 430, 432, 439, 442, 443, 444, 448, 450, 467, 468, 520, 563
Steel, drilling of 471, 476, 477, 478
Steel, welding of 364, 366, 368, 371, 372, 374, 376, 377, 378, 379, 382, 385, 386, 388, 389, 399, 401, 403, 406, 409, 410, 411, 412, 413, 414, 415, 416, 420, 421
Stellite 286
Step-and-repeat machines 623
Step-and-scan machines 623
Stereolithography (SL) 545
    build platform 546
    CAD to .stl translators 545
    Critical exposure 548
    lasers for 551
    material properties 549
    part building 546
    rapid tools 545, 553, 572
    SL process 545
    thermoplastic materials 549
Strehl ratio 106, 107, 108
Strontium barium titanate 697, 698, 699, 700
Strontium titanate 643, 644, 646, 698
Submerged-arc welding (SAW) 357, 378, 403, 419, 420
Sulfur 172, 236, 237, 253, 259, 353, 356, 378, 403
Sum frequency mixing 70, 76
Superconductors 641, 644, 697
Superpulsed laser 31, 431
Surface alloying 185, 197
Surface emitters 65
Surface hardening 185
Synthetic cloth 459
Synthetic crystals 326

T

Tailored blank welding 110
Tailored blanks 332, 414, 415, 416, 417
Tantalum 282, 352, 354, 355, 450, 481
Tantalum nitride 587
Tape automated bonding (TAB) 665–667, 672
Tape-cast ceramic sheets 566
Tape-cast metal sheets 566
TEA (transversely excited atmospheric-pressure) laser 14, 31, 119, 175, 184, 307, 478, 479, 495, 525, 534, 649, 662
Teflon 172, 402
Telescope 110, 111, 112
TEM_{00} mode 9, 58, 63, 77, 92, 93, 95, 105, 106, 109, 121, 234, 235, 236, 526, 527, 542, 544, 551
Temporal coherence 94
Texturing 297
Thallium arsenic selenide (TAS) 76
Thallium bromide 118
Thermal conductivity 74, 75, 170, 172, 173, 186, 193, 200, 201, 309, 310, 313, 326, 329, 348, 355, 363, 365, 375, 376, 378, 379, 380, 387, 392, 445, 446, 447, 472, 600
Thermal detector 139, 143, 144
Thermal diffusivity 170, 173, 186, 310, 313, 316, 329, 364, 371, 375, 376, 387, 429, 472, 504
Thermal expansion stress 546
Thermal injury 205, 206
Thermal penetration depth 504
Thermal runaway 136, 183
Thermistor 144
Thermocapillary forces 195
Thermocouple 144, 145
Thermopile 144, 145, 147, 148
Thermoplastic materials 549, 578
Thermoplastics 413, 425, 426, 522
Thermoset epoxy 523
Thermoset polymer 426, 459
Thermoset resin 457
Thick-film resistor trimming 586, 587
Thick-film resistors 583
Thin-film deposition 185
Thin-film resistors 583, 587
Thin-film transistors 638
Third harmonic generation (THG) 69, 76, 77, 551
Thorium 356
Thorium fluoride 35
Three-dimensional printing 580
Time-temperature-transformation (TTT) 223, 224
Tin 200, 282, 342, 343, 355, 404, 481, 618, 665, 666, 667
Tin-lead 668, 669, 670, 678
Ti:Sapphire 45, 82
Ti:Sapphire laser 2, 16, 17, 44, 45, 73, 76, 82, 486, 503, 675
Titanium 198, 201, 263, 264, 272, 280, 281, 282, 284, 299, 302, 425, 429, 438, 440, 441, 445, 448, 467, 468,

472, 477, 481, 556, 560, 562, 563, 566, 578, 598, 618, 620, 655, 695
Titanium alloy 252, 253
Titanium boride 283
Titanium bromides 198
Titanium carbide 82, 282, 284, 291, 563
Titanium dioxide 181, 523
Titanium nitride 282, 284, 612, 696
Titanium oxide 696
Titanium, welding of 309, 321, 323, 324, 325, 328, 342, 349, 352, 354, 355, 368, 373, 382, 383, 386, 403, 410, 414, 420, 421
Tm laser 46
Tm:YAG 46
Tm:YAG laser 44
Tm,Ho:YAG 46
Tool steel (see also steel) 232, 233, 234, 237, 239, 245, 246, 253
Transformation hardening 66, 190, 223, 224, 232, 236, 258, 259, 273
Transmissivity 168, 169, 176, 182, 183
Transverse-flow laser 30
Transverse mode 2, 9, 10
Trepanning 473, 474, 475, 477, 479, 481, 482, 484, 485, 498
Triethylboron 702
Trimethyl aluminum 702
Trimethylboron 702
Trimming 583, 584, 585, 586, 587
Tungsten 4, 172, 178, 182, 201, 251, 252, 253, 254, 255, 263, 264, 273, 280, 282, 283, 284, 327, 328, 352, 354, 355, 402, 477, 481, 563, 578, 598, 600, 601, 653, 692, 694
Tungsten carbide 282, 284, 495, 687
Turquoise 464

U

Ultrafast laser 82
Ultrashort-pulse laser 82, 499
Ultraviolet emission 209, 210
Ultraviolet materials 134
Unstable resonator 32, 366
Urethane 549

V

Vanadate laser 597
Vanadium 253, 259, 272, 273, 282, 326, 481
Van Cittert-Zernike theorem 93
Vaporization 195, 204, 426
Vaporization cutting 425, 426, 429

Vaporization temperature 201
Verdet constant 133, 134
Via drilling 661, 688
Vickers hardness 242, 243

W

Wafer serialization 590, 591
Waspalloy 414, 498
Water 171, 172
Water chiller 83
Water jet cutting (see also abrasive water jet cutting) 465, 466–469, 470
Water jet drilling 465, 510, 512
Waveguide laser 31
Waxicon 130
Weld spatter 409
Weld trouble-shooting 337
Welding 157, 160, 161, 162, 165, 166, 185, 190, 195, 197, 200, 203, 204, 233, 242, 263, 302, 307, 310, 313, 315, 317, 318, 319, 320, 321, 323, 325, 326, 327, 328–330, 331, 332, 333, 334, 335, 339, 340, 341, 342, 344, 345, 347, 348, 349, 350, 353, 354, 356, 357, 358, 359, 361, 362, 363, 365, 367, 368, 369, 370, 371, 372, 373, 374, 375, 376, 377, 379, 380, 381, 382, 383, 384, 385, 386, 387, 388, 389, 396, 398, 399, 400, 401, 406, 408, 409, 410, 411, 412, 413, 415, 416, 417, 418, 419, 420, 421, 433, 434
Welding, butt joint 351
    coatings 318
    resistance 357, 359
    plume 409
Welding, in packaging 677, 678, 680, 681, 682, 683
White marble 5
Wirestripping 672, 673, 675, 676
Wood 172, 426, 457, 460, 469, 495, 531, 532, 533
Wool cloth 459
Working range 544

X

X-ray laser 16, 78, 79, 80, 81
Xe lamp 38, 41
Xe laser 15, 17, 636
XeCl laser 16, 17, 48, 50, 291, 492, 493, 494, 499, 617, 647, 652, 695, 696, 701, 702, 703
XeF laser 16, 17, 48, 50, 696

Y

YAG laser (see also Nd:YAG laser) 177, 661, 662, 663, 664
YAG (see also yttrium aluminum garnet) 37, 38, 42, 46, 365, 542
$YBa_2Cu_3O_{8-\delta}$, (YBCO) chemical reactions of 648
$YBa_2Cu_3O_{7-\delta}$ (YBCO) 641, 644, 648, 696, 697, 698
YBCO 641, 642, 643, 644
    deposition of 642
    films on $LaAlO_3$ 645
$Yb:SiO_2$ laser 44
Yb:YAG laser 44, 46
Yttria-stabilized zirconia (YSZ) 643, 645, 646
Yttrium 37
Yttrium aluminum garnet ($Y_3Al_5O_{12}$) (see also YAG) 37, 494
Yttrium iron garnet 697
Yttrium lithium flouride (YLF) 484, 542
Yttrium vanadate (YVO_4) 484, 542

Z

Zinc 117, 200, 201, 300, 302, 310, 318, 324, 342, 355, 356, 385, 386, 398, 399, 403, 444, 447, 481, 554
Zinc germanium phosphide 75, 76
Zinc oxide 240
Zinc phosphate 237
Zinc selenide 28, 33, 116, 118, 119, 120, 121, 134, 135, 138, 139, 146, 227, 271, 273, 316, 366, 409
Zinc selenide lenses 466
Zinc sulfide 35, 118, 136, 139
Zircalloy 368, 371
Zirconia 182, 493
Zirconium 283, 309, 352, 354, 404, 450, 481, 578
Zirconium alloy 193
Zirconium carbide 179
Zirconium dioxide 495, 499
Zirconium oxide 272, 290